D1064374

THE HEART AND
THE VASCULAR SYSTEM
IN ANCIENT GREEK
MEDICINE

FROM ALCMAEON TO GALEN

THE HEART AND
THE VASCULAR SYSTEM
IN ANCIENT GREEK
MEDICINE

FROM ALCMAEON TO GALEN

C. R. S. HARRIS

OXFORD
AT THE CLARENDON PRESS
1973

Oxford University Press, Ely House, London W. 1

GLASGOW NEW YORK TORONTO MELBOURNE WELLINGTON
CAPE TOWN IBADAN NAIROBI DAR ES SALAAM LUSAKA ADDIS ABABA
DELHI BOMBAY CALCUTTA MADRAS KARACHI LAHORE DACCA
KUALA LUMPUR SINGAPORE HONG KONG TOKYO

*Printed in Great Britain
at the University Press, Oxford
by Vivian Ridler
Printer to the University*

TO

ARTHUR SALTER

but for whose encouragement this book
would never have been written

PREFACE

IT may perhaps seem a little presumptuous for a man who is professionally neither a classical scholar nor a physician to have embarked upon a work of this kind. I must therefore explain how and why I was induced to attempt it. From 1958 to 1965 I had the good fortune to teach in the University of Adelaide, where I held the interesting post of Reader in Studies in Humanities for medical students, a substantial part of my course being devoted to the outlines of the history of medicine. In preparing my lectures on medicine in Greco-Roman times, I found that comparatively little even of the principal authorities had been translated into English, and what was even worse, very little had been written about them in our native tongue, so that for the student of medical history there was an important gap which needed filling. It is, of course, true that a substantial amount of the Hippocratic corpus does exist in readily available English versions, notably those published in the Loeb series, but a large number of important treatises are still untranslated. Of the medical writers between Hippocrates and Galen—a period of some six centuries—practically nothing exists in the English tongue except the remaining works of Aretaeus; and of Galen himself, when I was beginning to lecture, only a very few of his hundred-odd treatises had been translated, a deficiency which is now fortunately being remedied by American scholars. But there are still practically no books in English on either Hippocrates or Galen which give a reliably detailed account of the contents of the Hippocratic corpus or of the vast system of medical theory and practice evolved by Galen. I therefore proposed to myself as a task for my retirement the writing of a book on the Prince of Physicians. But the world-wide interest aroused by the tercentenary of Harvey's death in the discovery of the circulation of the blood led me to design this work, on the advice of my old friend and one-time colleague at All Souls Lord Salter, as a preliminary study for a later book on Galen.

The guiding thread of my argument in this volume is the endeavour to explain how it was that the ancient Greeks, in spite of their accurate knowledge of anatomy, failed to discover the circulation of the blood. I therefore trace in detail the development of their ideas on the functions of the heart and the vascular system from the days of Alcmaeon to the time of Galen, confining my attention chiefly to the physiological aspects. To have included the clinical would have involved enlarging an already bulky volume to an impracticable size, besides reproducing a confusing mass of detail which could have no interest for the general reader, and probably very little even for the specialist student of medical history. This has meant, for example, abbreviating very considerably the account given of Galen's sphygmology, particularly in respect of his very detailed descriptions of the behaviour of the pulse—not, be it noted, the heart— in various kinds and stages of disease. The justification of these omissions can be summed up in a single sentence. The ancient Greeks never arrived at any clear conception of what we today would call heart disease, in spite of their accurate anatomical knowledge of that organ's structure, largely because of the limits imposed on their pathological discoveries by the convention forbidding human dissection.

In planning this study it has been my chief concern to provide as complete an account as possible of the development of Greek ideas on the heart and the vascular system almost in the form of a source-book. This has entailed the inclusion in the text of a very large number of quotations and a still greater number of abstracts and précis of passages from the ancient authors. In spite of the fact that today the number of students of medical history who are acquainted with a working knowledge of Greek is very small, I nevertheless decided to give the full source-texts in my footnotes, so that the whole of the evidence could be assembled for the classical scholar, since mere references would not in my opinion be enough, because many of the texts in question are not readily accessible without reference to a library like the Bodleian. In my translations, where these have not been borrowed from existing modern versions, I have preferred, a little naïvely perhaps, the blemishes of literal accuracy to the seductions of elegance, for which I must in advance beg my reader's pardon.

The purpose of these arrangements has been to provide a text which can be read quite independently of footnotes, most of these being of interest only to the classical scholar, whose special and critical interests have in other respects been but poorly provided for. Thus, for example, the enormously complicated and fascinating question of the dates and authorships of the various treatises of the Hippocratic corpus has been barely touched on. I have been forced to neglect the growing volume of work on this subject. What I hope I have succeeded in producing is an account, as complete as possible, of the development of Greek medical ideas in this restricted field, which can be followed without difficulty by the general reader, who will I hope not be deterred by the formidable appearance of my footnotes.

It remains for me to thank all those persons and institutions who so generously lent me their time and aid. First and foremost I am grateful to my old friend the late Sir Maurice Bowra, who read through my far from tidy draft, suggested many improvements, and smoothed my way to the Clarendon Press. Secondly, to Dr. Walter Pagel whose advice and criticisms have proved invaluable, from the depths of whose bottomless well of learning I have been privileged to draw so many refreshing potions. And thirdly, to Dr. Richard Lebowich of New York, whose interest in Greek medical and philosophical achievements has furnished me with much matter for useful discussions on my work. My thanks are also due to Professor Ackerknecht, the head of the Institute of Medical History of the University of Zürich and his staff, for the warm welcome they offered me and the hospitality of its great library, to the directors of the libraries of the faculty of medicine in the universities of Montpellier and Madrid and to their staffs, whose help in the collection of material was so useful, and to Mr. Gaskell, the librarian of the Wellcome Institute of Medical History and his colleague Mr. R. M. Price, without whose aid I should have missed many important sources of material. Last, but not least, I have to thank the staff of the Clarendon Press for their patience and scholarly revision.

CONTENTS

ABBREVIATIONS   xii

1. BEFORE HIPPOCRATES   I

2. 'HIPPOCRATES'   29

3. AFTER HIPPOCRATES   97

4. THE ALEXANDRIANS   177

5. THE ROMAN PERIOD BEFORE GALEN   234

6. GALEN   267

7. GALEN'S PULSE-LORE   397

8. HEART AND VASCULAR DISEASE   432

FIGURES 1-5   456

INDEX   461

LIST OF WORKS CITED   473

ABBREVIATIONS

AMG   R. Fuchs, 'Anecdota Medica Graeca', *Rheinisches Museum* 49 (1894), 50 (1895).

CMG
(Corp. Med.
Graec.)   *Corpus Medicorum Graecorum* (Leipzig and Berlin, 1927–).

D–K   Diels–Kranz, *Die Fragmente der Vorsokratiker*, 11th edn., Berlin, 1964.

D–R   *Œuvres de Rufus d'Ephèse*, ed. Ch. Daremberg and E. Ruelle, Paris, 1879.

J.   W. H. S. Jones, *The Medical Writings of Anonymus Londinensis*, Cambridge, 1947.

K.   *Galeni Omnia Opera*, ed. C. G. Kühn, 20 vols., Leipzig, 1821–33.

Littré (L.)   *Œuvres complètes d'Hippocrate*, ed. É. Littré, 10 vols., Paris, 1839–61.

RE   Pauly–Wissowa, *Real-Encyclopädie*.

1 · BEFORE HIPPOCRATES

It is surely one of the greater paradoxes of the history of medicine that the ancient Greek physicians, who laid the foundations of our Western knowledge of anatomy and physiology with a degree of accuracy and understanding which contrasts most favourably with the methods and speculations of the other civilizations of the ancient world, should have failed entirely to arrive at any conception of the circulation of the blood, whereas the Chinese, whose anatomy has been described by most of the more recent historians of medicine as 'almost entirely fanciful', nevertheless succeeded in divining, if not in establishing, some notion of a perpetual circulatory movement. Yet so in fact it was. The great Chinese canon of medicine, *Nei Ching*, the author of which was supposed to be the legendary Emperor Hwang-Ti whose traditional date was 2689–2599 B.C.—a compendium which does not, in the form in which we now possess it, go back further than the third century A.D.—contains a number of sayings which can only be interpreted to indicate some such intuition. Thus we are told that 'All blood is under control of the heart', that 'The heart regulates all the blood of the body', that 'The blood flows continuously and never stops', and that 'The blood cannot but flow continuously like the current of a river, or the sun and the moon in their orbits'. The exact significance of these statements cannot of course be grasped outside their context and without a general survey of Chinese physiological and anatomical doctrines, which I am quite incompetent to make. But a modern Chinese authority remarks that the claim that Harvey's discovery had been anticipated about two thousand years ago in China rests on rather scanty evidence, even if the ancients made a very near guess at the facts. Beyond this guess no further investigations were made. 'The systemic and pulmonary circulations were not understood. According to one passage, the blood stream is said to start from the foot and to circulate to the kidneys, the heart, the lungs, the liver, and the spleen, in the order named, and from the spleen back to the kidneys, thus making a complete circuit.'[1] It is true that the Chinese elaborated a most

---

[1] Wong and Wu, *A History of Chinese Medicine* (Tientsin, 1932), p. 20.

B

complicated pulse-lore, even more complicated than that of Galen, but its very complications indicate that they could not have understood the way in which the pulse is produced, nor is there, as far as I am aware, any indication that they had the slightest acquaintance with the way in which the heart really works.

Before embarking on the task of explaining this apparent paradox, it may perhaps be convenient to dispose of what parliamentarians might call the previous question. For there are several eminent students of Greek medicine who have maintained that the ancient Greeks were in fact, no less than the Chinese, acquainted with the circulation of the blood. This claim has been put forward on behalf both of Hippocrates and of Galen. Of the recent protagonists of the view that Hippocrates was so acquainted, the most pertinacious was the late Dr. Richard Kapferer,[1] who made himself responsible for the most recent German translation of the entire *Corpus Hippocraticum*. He was by no means the only medical historian who held this view, since his main thesis was supported among others by Sticker[2] and J. Wiberg,[3] as well as by Fredrich,[4] and by Gossen[5] in his article on Hippocrates in the eighth volume of Pauly–Wissowa's *Real-Encyclopädie*. Both these last appear to uphold opinions rather similar to those of Kapferer, which can be traced back as far as Littré.[6] They have received some reinforcements more recently from Athens in the shape of a pamphlet by Pezopoulos and Lamera[7] which betrays no doubt on the opinion, temerarious to say the least of it, that both Hippocrates and Galen had anticipated Harvey. Kapferer's opinions have been refuted, in my view quite conclusively, by Diepgen,[8] Diller,[9] and Abel.[10] The details of this controversy need not detain us at this stage of our exposition, though as we proceed they will, of course, be referred to from time to time during the course of our argument.

The best example of similar claims on behalf of Galen which I have been able to discover comes from Spain in the writings of Bañuelos,[11] who

[1] Kapferer, 'Der Blutkreislauf, seine Darstellung in den hippokratischen Schriften', *Hippokrates* 8 (1937); and also his introduction to the Hippocratic *De corde* in vol. 16 of his translation of the *Corpus* (Stuttgart–Zürich, 1937).

[2] In an article in *Münchener medizinische Wochenschrift* 85 (1938). See also his essay on the *Blutkreislauf* attached to vol. 15 of Kapferer's translation of the *Corpus*.

[3] Wiberg, 'The medical science of Ancient Greece, the doctrine of the heart', *Janus* 41 (1937).

[4] Fredrich, *Hippokratische Untersuchungen*, Heft 15 (Berlin, 1899), p. 65.

[5] Pauly–Wissowa, *RE* 8 (2), cols. 180 ff.　　　　　　　　　　[6] Vol. 1, 222 ff.

[7] *The Knowledge of the Circulation of the Blood of the Old Physicians* (trs.) (Athens, 1947).

[8] Diepgen, 'Haben die Hippokratiker den Blutkreislauf gekannt?', *Klinische Wochenschrift* Dec. 1937, 1820–3.

[9] Diller, 'Die Lehre vom Blutkreislauf, eine verschollene Entdeckung des Hippokrates?', *Arch. f. Gesch. d. Med.* xxxi (1938).

[10] 'Die Lehre vom Blutkreislauf im Corpus Hippocraticum — H. Schumacher zum Gedächtnis', *Hermes* 86 (1958), 192–219; also *Gesnerus* 15 (1958).

[11] See *El problema de la circulación de la sangre—nuevos hechos y nuevas ideas* (Barcelona, 1946); as well as three articles, 'De nuevo sobre Galeno y la circulación', *Gac. Méd. Esp.* 21 (Sept.

tries to prove that Galen was acquainted with the pulmonary circulation and, by implication, with the systemic as well. This idea, so far as the pulmonary circulation is concerned, has also been maintained in the United States by Peller,[1] and in England by Prendergast.[2] Bañuelos's views have been very competently contested by De la Granda and by Granjel and Lain Entralgo in Spain,[3] while those of Peller and Prendergast have been criticized in the United States by Fleming.[4] A balanced account of Galen's teaching in this field has been sketched out by Hall,[5] to which reference will be made below.

Having disposed for the moment of the previous question, we will now try to trace in some detail the history of the ideas of the early Greek physicians on the anatomy and physiology of the cardio-vascular system. The beginnings of Greek medicine, like those of Greek science, are not easy to investigate because no more than a few fragments in disconnected quotations, supplemented by reports of doxographers, have come down to us. No complete treatises of Greek medicine earlier than those contained in the *Hippocratic corpus* have survived, and the earliest of these probably dates from the second half of the fifth century B.C. The Hippocratic collection itself is an amalgam of very different dates and authorships, while the pre-Hippocratics, like the pre-Socratics, are largely if not entirely subjects for imaginative reconstruction, or, to speak plainly, guess-work. The surviving fragments have been subject to a variety of often contradictory interpretations, most of which require to be treated, if not with scepticism, with considerable reservation.

The earliest references to matters anatomical and physiological occur, as we might expect, in Homer. The descriptions of the various wounds caused in battle have been analysed by Daremberg.[6] Interesting as they are for the light they throw on the conceptions current, shall we say, in the eighth century B.C., they do not call for any elaborate analysis here, and it is hard to understand how Körner could have come to the

1947); 'Conoció Galeno la circulación?', ibid. 22 (Feb. 1948); and 'Opiniones de Galeno sobre la respiración y sobre el uso de los pulmones', ibid. (April, 1948).

[1] Peller, 'Harvey's and Cesalpino's role in the history of medicine', *Bull. Hist. Med.* 23 (1949).

[2] Prendergast, 'Galen's view of the vascular system', *Proc. R. Soc. Med.* 21 (1928), 1839–48.

[3] See De la Granda's article, 'Galeno y Servet', in the *Gac. Méd. Esp.* 21 and 22 (Dec. 1947, Apr. 1948). De la Granda, while denying Galen's discovery of the circulation, appears to believe that it was known to many Spanish physicians before Harvey. For the views of Granjel and Entralgo see below, p. 311.

[4] Fleming, 'Galen on the motion of the blood in the heart and the lungs', *Isis* 46 (1955), 14–21.

[5] R. Hall, 'Studies in the history of the cardio-vascular system—Galen', *Bull. Hist. Med.* 34 (1960), 391–413.

[6] Daremberg, 'La médecine dans Homère', *Revue archéol.* (1865); 'État de la médecine entre Homère et Hippocrate', ibid. (1869). Sigerist notes (*A History of Medicine* (Oxford, 1961), 2. 26) that he analyses no less than 141 wounds affecting different parts of the body.

conclusion that they could only have been derived in certain cases from evidence obtained from the dissecting table.[1]

The first Greek writer on medicine of whom tradition affords any coherent outline is Alcmaeon of Croton, who was supposed to have been a pupil of Pythagoras, himself a figure shrouded in mystery. Concerning the date of his birth modern research has raised, since Edelstein, quite a number of uncertainties. Earlier historians had assumed that he was probably born some time at the end of the sixth century B.C., but Sigerist[2] believed that he flourished about the middle of the fifth century, and Edelstein[3] would place him even later. Wellmann[4] places his *floruit* early in the fifth century. Edelstein's late dating is not accepted by Erhard,[5] Michler,[6] or Guthrie.[7] Alcmaeon's traditional date rests on two references: a statement of Diogenes Laertius in his *Vitae philosophorum* to the effect that he was a pupil of Pythagoras,[8] and another from Aristotle himself[9] that he was a young man in Pythagoras' old age. This latter statement is not contained in what have been regarded as the most reliable of Aristotelian manuscripts, and is not included in Ross's text of the *Metaphysics* (Oxford edition). Heidel[10] pointed out that Diogenes Laertius' statement may be a later interpolation from Porphyrius' life of Pythagoras, and Deichgräber[11] also refused to accept it and expressed the view that he flourished about 450 B.C. This would make him an almost exact contemporary of Empedocles. But as Guthrie points out there is no solid reason for refusing to accept the statement that he was a pupil of Pythagoras, which would not force us to place his birth earlier than about 510 B.C., assuming that Pythagoras died about 490 B.C.

The juxtaposition of Alcmaeon and Empedocles, even if the latter was considerably the younger,[12] forms a convenient starting-point for our

[1] O. Körner, 'Wie entstanden die anatomischen Kenntnisse in Ilias und Odyssee?', *Münch. med. Wschr.* 42 (1922). For a recent account of the traditional origins of ancient Greek medical thought, see F. Kudlien, *Der Beginn des medizinishen Denkens bei den Griechen, von Homer bis Hippokrates* (Artemis Verlag, Zürich–Stuttgart, 1967). [2] Sigerist, op. cit. 2. 101.

[3] See his review in the *Am. J. Philol.* (1948) of L. A. Stella's monograph, *L'importanza di Alcmeone nella storia del pensiero greco*, Ac. Naz. Lincei, ser. vi, vol. 8, fasc. 4 (Rome, 1939).

[4] See his article on the Hippocratic work *On the sacred disease*, *Arch. f. Gesch. d. Med.* xxii (1929), 302; also his article on Alcmeon in *Archeon* 11 (1929), 156.

[5] Erhard, 'Alkmaeon der erste Experimentalbiologe', *Arch. f. Gesch. d. Med.* xxxiv (1941), 77–89.

[6] Michler, 'Das Problem der westgriechischen Heilkunde', *Arch. f. Gesch. d. Med.* xlvi (1962), 137–52.

[7] Guthrie, *History of Greek Philosophy*, vol. 1 (Cambridge, 1962). See especially the footnote to p. 342.

[8] Diogenes Laertius, viii. 83: Ἀλκμαίων ὁ Κρωτωνιάτης, καὶ οὗτος Πυθαγόρου διήκουσε.

[9] Aristotle, *Metaph.* 1. 5, 986ª29–30: καὶ γὰρ ἐγένετο τὴν ἡλικίαν ὁ Ἀλκμαίων ⟨νέος⟩ ἐπὶ γέροντι Πυθαγόρᾳ. [10] Heidel, *Hippocratic Medicine* (New York, 1941), pp. 43 ff.

[11] Deichgräber, *Hippokrates über Entstehung und Aufbau des menschlichen Körpers* (Leipzig, 1935) (Text and translation of the Περὶ σαρκῶν), p. 37.

[12] I can, however, find no evidence for the statement made in G. A. G. Mitchell and E. L. Patterson's *Basic Anatomy* (2nd edn., Edinburgh, 1967), p. 1, that Empedocles was one of

inquiry, since it introduces us to one of the earlier controversies of pre-Hippocratic medicine, that of the primacy of the organs of the body, the issue of the heart versus the brain as the seat of the intelligence, a question of much more than merely logical importance, since upon the answer given to it depended to a large extent the interpretation given to the physiological functions of the various organs. Of these two thinkers, Alcmaeon, of whose works only a few fragments have survived—much less than the fragments of Empedocles—will certainly strike the modern ear as much the more scientific,[1] though in fact the influence of Empedocles was in some ways even greater. His importance rests on two fundamental contributions to medical thinking, first, the conception of the brain as the seat of consciousness, and secondly, his theory of disease as the 'unbalance' of opposite qualities, which constitutes the first purely rational explanation of disease which has come down to us. These contributions, quite apart from some scarcely less important, have led some historians to question whether the title of the Father of Medicine should not more appropriately be bestowed on Alcmaeon than on Hippocrates,[2] a question which recent criticism of the Hippocratic tradition by Edelstein and others renders all the more relevant. Whether the notion that the brain was the seat of consciousness was in fact derived from Pythagoras' teaching cannot be decided with any degree of certainty, for we know all too little about what Pythagoras himself really taught. However, he was teaching at Croton where Alcmaeon lived, at the most a generation before, and it is interesting to record that this doctrine was attributed to Pythagoras by Diogenes Laertius and by the late doxographer, Aetius.[3] Some confirmation is perhaps supplied by the passage from

Alcmaeon's pupils, though there is a tradition that according to Timaeus (*F.H.G.*, fr. 81, vol. 1), quoted in D–K, that Empedocles was also a pupil of Pythagoras. This can hardly be correct, since he cannot have been born much before 490 B.C., since he was, as Burnet has put it, 'contemporary with the meridian splendour of Periclean Athens', and must have met at Thurii, to which he went shortly after its foundation in 444/3, both Herodotus and Protagoras. See J. Burnet, *Greek Philosophy from Thales to Plato* (London, 1943), p. 71.

[1] In spite of the theory imputed to him by Aristotle, that goats breathe through their ears, in *Hist. an.* 1. 11, 492ᵃ13, Ἀλκμαίων γὰρ οὐκ ἀληθῆ λέγει φάμενος ἀναπνεῖν τὰς αἶγας κατὰ τὰ ὦτα, and the no more scientific view attributed to him by Clement of Alexandria, that the stars are gods, which was to exercise so curious an influence on European thought, largely through Aristotle. See Clement, *Protrept.* 66: ὁ γάρ τοι Κροτωνιάτης Ἀλκμαίων θεοὺς ᾤετο τοὺς ἀστέρας εἶναι ἐμψύχους ὄντας. (Both quotations in D–K, vol. 1, 212–13.)

[2] e.g. J. R. Beltrani's article, 'Alcmeon de Crotona y la psicología', *Revta Assoc. Méd. Argent.* 54 (Oct. 1940), in which he remarks: 'Con justicia Alcmeon es considerado el verdadero padre de nuestra medicina.' Wellmann considers him to have been the father of psychology, the creator of psychiatry, and the founder of gynaecology: see his article on the Περὶ ἱερῆς νούσου in *Arch. f. Gesch. d. Med.* (1929), 303 ff.; also Arcieri's essay '*Alcmeone*' (Catanzaro, 1950), which takes the same view as Beltrani—a view contested by Piccinini in *Castalia* (1960), pp. 51–8, 176–81.

[3] See the passage from *De plac. phil.* (i. 3. 8), quoted in D–K, vol. 1, 455, where this doctrine is implicitly attributed to the master. Aetius has just explained Pythagoras' doctrine of the

Philolaus of Tarentum, quoted by Sigerist.[1] Philolaus was almost certainly a contemporary of Alcmaeon and himself a follower of Pythagoras. In a fragment of his included in D–K, we are told that 'There are four vital organs in the rational living being, the brain, the heart, the navel, and the genital organs. The brain is the seat of the mind, the heart of the "soul" or "vital principle" and of sensation. . . . The brain signifies the ruling principle of man, the heart that of the animal, the navel that of the plant, and the genital organ that of all of them, for they all sprout and grow from the sperm.'[2] The similarity of this doctrine to the teaching both of Plato and of Aristotle, not to mention even Galen himself, certainly becomes obvious to all who read the story told in these pages.

It would appear that Alcmaeon did not found his doctrine of the primacy of the brain merely on speculative reasoning. He is known to have performed anatomical experiments; indeed, he is generally regarded as the first of the Greek physicians to have done so. Our authority for this statement is indeed late, but not therefore necessarily unreliable. Chalcidius, in his commentary on Plato's *Timaeus*, says that Alcmaeon was the first who dared to attack, that is, cut out or open, the eye.[3] The natural interpretation of this statement would certainly suggest that the eye referred to was a human eye, otherwise the use of the word 'dare' would be meaningless. But it would be going much too far to suppose that Alcmaeon practised the dissection of the human body.[4] He might very well have been operating on a severely wounded or injured person. Tradition is agreed that he dissected animals, and it is certainly tempting to believe that the distinction he made between reason and perception,

decade and the number four, finishing up with the words, ὥστε ὁ ἀριθμὸς κατὰ μὲν μονάδα ἐν τοῖς δέκα κατὰ δὲ δύναμιν ἐν τοῖς τέσσαρσι. He then refers to the 'greatest oath of the Pythagoreans',

οὐ μὰ τὸν ἁμετέραι κεφαλᾶι παραδόντα τετρακτὺν
παγὰν ἀενάου φύσεως ῥίζωμά τ' ἔχουσαν,

which seems to imply that Pythagoras believed the brain to be the seat of reason. It would however be distinctly temerarious to build too heavy a reconstruction of Pythagoras' physiology on this slender foundation. But for Diogenes Laertius' account of Pythagoras' teaching see below, p. 9.

[1] Sigerist, op. cit., 2. 99.

[2] Fr. 13 *Theol. Arithm.* p. 25. 17 de falco (D–K, vol. 1, 413): καὶ τέσσαρες ἀρχαὶ τοῦ ζῴου τοῦ λογικοῦ, ὥσπερ καὶ Φιλόλαος ἐν τῷ περὶ φύσεως λέγει, ἐγκέφαλος, καρδία, ὀμφαλός, αἰδοῖον· κεφαλὰ μὲν νόου, καρδία δὲ ψυχᾶς καὶ αἰσθήσιος . . ἐγκέφαλος δὲ (σαμαίνει) τὰν ἀνθρώπω ἀρχάν, καρδία δὲ τὰν ζῴου, ὀμφαλὸς δὲ τὰν φυτοῦ, αἰδοῖον δὲ τὰν συμπάντων· πάντα γὰρ ἀπὸ σπέρματος καὶ θάλλοντι καὶ βλαστάνοντι.

[3] Chalcidius, *In Timaeum* (Wrob.), p. 279 D–K, vol. 1, 212: 'Demonstranda igitur oculi natura est, de qua cum plerique alii, tum Alcmaeon Crotoniensis in physicis exercitatus quique primus exsectionem aggredi est ausus.' Might not this operation have been undertaken in the case of severe cranial injury involving an eye 'hanging out' and crushed or mangled? In such a situation Alcmaeon may very well have 'dared' to sever the optic nerve.

[4] There seems to be no agreement among the historians of Greek medicine on this subject. Stella, in the paper cited in p. 4, n. 3 above, refers to some of the historians' comments on this case.

the former of which belongs to man alone, was founded on a comparison of the human and the animal brain—at least it would be were there any evidence. Alcmaeon is also credited, this time with some degree of probability, with the discovery of the optic nerve.[1] Sigerist points out that, though there is no evidence that he dissected human cadavers,[2] the testimonies show unmistakably that he did dissect eyes, and that he found the eye to be connected with the brain by certain light-giving 'paths'.[3] Theophrastus in his treatise *De sensu* tells us that Alcmaeon taught that all the senses were somehow connected with the brain, or somehow joined on to it; hence when the brain was shaken, and made to change its position, the paths through which perception would come were blocked.[4] This doctrine of the brain as the seat of the intelligence was to be confirmed two centuries later by the anatomical and physiological discoveries of the Alexandrians, and adopted by most, but by no means all, of their successors. The important 'Pneumatic' school, influenced in this matter by the teaching of the Stoic philosophers, still insisted in placing the intelligence, for the most part, in the heart. Alcmaeon's other important contribution to medical thought, the theory of 'disequilibrium' as the cause of disease, which must be regarded as the original formulation of the Hippocratic theory of 'dyscrasia', cannot be discussed except very briefly in this essay; but to Alcmaeon have also been traced by several historians the roots of some conceptions which were to play an important part in the development of some of the ideas about the vascular system and its functions.

Wellmann believed that the main ideas expressed in the Hippocratic treatise *On the sacred disease*, which we shall examine in due course,[5] were derived from Alcmaeon, whom he looked upon as the originator of the notion that *pneuma* was breathed in directly into the brain, and that it was the instrument if not the actual principle of thought and sensation and all

[1] This is denied by some authorities, e.g. Tannery and Souques.

[2] Sigerist, op. cit., pp. 101 ff., and notes 51, 52, and 53 on p. 114.

[3] Stella disagrees with Sigerist here and maintains (op. cit.): 'Alcmeone non solo non esita ad estrarre il globo oculare, ma con audacia del tutto nuova apre il cranio per studiare la connessione dell'occhio col cervello.' In this connection it may perhaps be relevant to remember that Alcmaeon was one of the first Greek thinkers to maintain an absolute distinction between thought and sensation and to insist on the immortality of the soul. Might not this separation have rendered a little less repugnant the notion of cutting up a corpse? There was of course no question of any resurrection of the body.

[4] Theophrastus, *De sensu*, 26 (D–K, vol. 1, 212): διὸ καὶ πηροῦσθαι κινουμένου καὶ μεταλλάττοντος τὴν χώραν· ἐπιλαμβάνειν γὰρ τοὺς πόρους δι᾽ ὧν αἱ αἰσθήσεις. J. Hirschberg, 'Alcmäions Verdienst um die Augenheilkunde', *Albrecht v. Gräfes Archiv Ophthal.* 105 (1921), 129 ff., says that Alcmaeon cut through the connections between the eye and the brain in an animal and showed that the result was blindness. He explains the use of the word 'dared' quite unconvincingly: 'das Wort „wagen" bezieht sich auf das neue Verfahren der Forschung.' Erhard, op. cit., attributes to him a correct description of the optic nerve and the optic chiasma.

[5] See below, pp. 39–43.

mental activity,[1] a fundamental theory underlying all subsequent thinking on this subject by later Greek physicians. The quotations upon which he bases this notion are perhaps a little tenuous. Two of them are perhaps worth examining. He tells us that the sense of smell is dependent upon the drawing of *pneuma* through the nostrils into the brain;[2] indeed he discovered the connections not only of the optic nerve, but also of the olfactory nerve with the brain. But it is a little difficult to justify on these fragments the notion that he anticipated Diogenes of Apollonia in borrowing Anaximenes' theory of the monistic air-substance, though this is not, of course, impossible. It should be noted that Stella does not consider there is sufficient evidence to regard Alcmaeon as the founder of the theory of the 'psychic' spirit which was to play such an important part in the doctrines of Erasistratus and Galen.

Two other important conceptions have also been attributed to Alcmaeon by Fredrich, who believed that he foreshadowed the distinction between arteries and veins in his distinction between αἱμόρροι φλέβες and φλέβες without qualification, which is implied in his theory of sleep. For we are told in Aetius that 'Alcmaeon says that sleep occurs through the retreat of the blood into the blood-running veins, that awakening occurs through its dispersal, and that complete retreat is death'.[3] Fredrich draws the conclusion from this passage that Alcmaeon, who was the first Greek physician we know of to practise the dissection of animals, had noted that on dissecting the body of a dead animal certain of the important blood vessels, to wit the principal arteries, were either bloodless or else contained very little blood, and that Alcmaeon wrongly concluded that this was also the case in the living body. Hence (*a*) the distinction between the two kinds of blood vessel, and (*b*) the theory that arteries contained not blood but *pneuma*. If he is correct—a matter which in view of the very slender textual foundation must be open to some doubt— Alcmaeon, besides being the Father of Greek medicine, was also, more like a wicked uncle, the originator of a *damnosa haereditas*, developed with disastrous consequences by Praxagoras and Erasistratus, which proved in the last resort one of the chief factors which prevented the Greeks from anticipating Harvey. Fredrich also concludes that Alcmaeon, in view of the importance which he attached to the brain, was also the inventor of

---

[1] Wellmann, op. cit., p. 291 : 'Der Träger aller seelischen Vorgänge ist nach Alkmaion das Pneuma daß durch die Atmung durch Mund und Nase dem Gehirn zugeführht wird.' He adds a footnote to the effect that 'Alkmaion ist also der Begründer der Pneumalehre in der Medizin, soweit unsere Kenntnis reicht. Entnommen hat er sie dem Milesier Anaximenes, der alle Dinge aus der Luft durch Verdichtung und Verdünnung entstehen ließ.'

[2] In a passage from Theophrastus, *De sensu*, 25, which runs as follows : ὀσφραίνεσθαι δὲ ῥισὶν ἅμα τῷ ἀναπνεῖν ἀνάγοντα τὸ πνεῦμα πρὸς τὸν ἐγκέφαλον (D–K, vol. 1, 212).

[3] Aetius, *De plac. phil.* v. 24 (D–K, vol. 1, 214): Ἀλκμαίων ἀναχωρήσει τοῦ αἵματος εἰς τὰς αἱμόρρους φλέβας ὕπνον γίνεσθαί φησι, τὴν δὲ ἐξέγερσιν διάχυσιν, τὴν δὲ παντελῆ ἀναχώρησιν θάνατον.

the theory that all blood vessels originate in the head, which may be correct but is again not proven.[1] These elementary mistakes in anatomy should not, however, blind us to the fact that Alcmaeon was certainly one of the great pioneers of rational if not of scientific medicine. Indeed it was precisely this quality which induced Edelstein to place his *floruit* at the end rather than the beginning of the fifth century B.C.

We cannot leave Alcmaeon without a paragraph on his relation to the shadowy Pythagoras, of whom we may believe that in his youth he was a pupil. If we can trust the account of his medical doctrines given by Diogenes Laertius, many of the features bear a considerable resemblance to those of Alcmaeon. Thus, on the question of the brain as the seat of the intelligence, we are told that Pythagoras taught that the soul was divided into three parts: into νοῦς, which we may translate as consciousness, φρένες, which we might call mind, and θυμός or emotion. The first and the last of these are common to man and the animals, but the second exists only in man. And the principle of the soul or life was located in and moved from the heart to the brain, the emotional part existed in the heart, but both consciousness and mind were seated in the brain.[2] And the senses were as it were 'drops' of these, and reason or the mind was eternal and the rest mortal,[3] implying a distinction between animals and men very similar to that we have just noticed in Alcmaeon. But, as Vlastos[4] has pointed out, it would be a mistake to derive from Pythagorean sources Alcmaeon's doctrine of health as the balance or equality between the opposite tendencies or powers. His notion of ἰσονομία must not be confused with the Pythagorean doctrine of 'harmony', which referred rather to 'proportion', being in most cases unequal, not equal. For the rest, Pythagoras' specifically medical doctrines appear to be those of a philosopher rather than a physician. He seems to have been attracted by the Ionian doctrine of Anaximenes equating air with the soul. The 'soul'

[1] Fredrich, op. cit., p. 67: 'Alkmaion von Kroton, dieser Heros der Aertzte, der zuerst Tiersektionen vorgenommen haben soll, ist für uns der erste, der blutführende (αἱμόρρους) und Adern ohne Zusatz unterschieden hat. Da er nämlich den Schlaf durch Zurückweichen des Blutes in die blutführenden Adern erklärt, so hat man volkommen korrekt daraus geschlossen, daß er beim Sezieren die jetzt Arterien genannten Gefaße bemerkt, ziemlich oder ganz blutleer gefunden, und aus dem toten auf das lebende Wesen geschlossen habe. Nach ihm gab es also φλέβες, die wenig und zuweilen fast gar kein Blut führen, und αἱμόρροι φλέβες. Und ich möchte vermuten, daß Alkmaion der dem Gehirn eine so große Bedeutung beigemessen hat . . . alle Adern aus dem Kopfe oder Gehirn hergeleitet hat und für den Stammvater der ersten Gruppe [i.e. the cephalo- as opposed to the cardio-centrics] zu halten ist.'

[2] Diogenes Laertius, viii. 30: τὴν δ' ἀνθρώπου ψυχὴν διηρῆσθαι τριχῇ, εἴς τε νοῦν καὶ φρένας καὶ θυμόν. νοῦν μὲν οὖν καὶ θυμὸν εἶναι καὶ ἐν τοῖς ἄλλοις ζῴοις, φρένας δὲ μόνον ἐν ἀνθρώπῳ· εἶναι δὲ τὴν ἀρχὴν τῆς ψυχῆς ἀπὸ καρδίας μέχρις ἐγκεφάλου· καὶ τὸ μὲν ἐν τῇ καρδίᾳ μέρος αὐτῆς ὑπάρχειν θυμόν, φρένας δὲ καὶ νοῦν τὰ ἐν τῷ ἐγκεφάλῳ.

[3] Ibid.: σταγόνας δ' εἶναι ἀπὸ τούτων τὰς αἰσθήσεις. καὶ τὸ μὲν φρόνιμον ἀθάνατον, τὰ δὲ λοιπὰ θνητά.

[4] See his article on Isonomia, *Am. J. Philol.* 74 (1953), 337 ff.

is nourished by the blood, and its reasonings are 'winds'. For the soul is invisible, and so is the aether.[1] The bonds of the body are the veins, the arteries, and the nerves, a statement than can hardly be taken *au pied de la lettre*, since Pythagoras could certainly not have known the distinction between arteries and veins; but he may very well have had some notion that the air-soul was distributed and worked through the blood vessels and that sinews were instruments for moving the limbs. He may also have used the word 'artery' in its original sense for windpipe. And just as the blood vessels were the bonds of the body which held it together, so arguments or acts of reason held together the soul.[2] But his notion of the causes of disease was far from progressive. The air, he thought, was full of spirits, heroes, and 'demons', who sent men (and animals as well) not only their dreams, but also their diseases.[3] It would appear that Alcmaeon, if he studied philosophy under Pythagoras, went to his medical school elsewhere, since, as Heidel[4] has observed, the school of medicine at Croton was in existence before Pythagoras' arrival.

With Empedocles we seem to breathe a very different atmosphere from that contained in the surviving fragments of Alcmaeon. His ideas seem to match much more closely those of Pythagoras. In the first place his works were written in hexameters, not exactly an ideal medium for scientific accuracy or conciseness; and in the second place, the fragments of his poems which have survived contain a great deal of what today cannot fail to look like charlatanism to the unsophisticated 'modern'. He can, and does 'call spirits from the vasty deep', and his reported behaviour cannot fail to appear, even to those scholars unacquainted with the work of Professor Dodds, very different from the Victorian ideal of the 'scientific' Greek thinker. Dodds makes no bones about calling Empedocles a Shaman, and suggests 'a tentative line of spiritual descent which starts in Scythia, crosses the Hellespont into Asiatic Greece, is perhaps combined with some remnants of Minoan tradition surviving in Crete, emigrates to the far West with Pythagoras, and has its last outstanding representative in the Sicilian Empedocles. These men diffused the belief in a detachable self, which by suitable techniques can be withdrawn from the body even during life, a self which is older than the body and will outlast it.'[5] He also is inclined to connect Empedocles with Pythagoreanism rather than with Orphism, but thinks that it is probably a mistake to

---

[1] Diogenes Laertius, loc. cit.: τρέφεσθαί τε τὴν ψυχὴν ἀπὸ τοῦ αἵματος· τοὺς δὲ λόγους ψυχῆς ἀνέμους εἶναι. ἀόρατόν τ᾽ εἶναι αὐτὴν καὶ τοὺς λόγους, ἐπεὶ καὶ ὁ αἰθὴρ ἀόρατος.

[2] Ibid., viii. 31: δεσμά τ᾽ εἶναι τῆς ψυχῆς τὰς φλέβας καὶ τὰς ἀρτηρίας καὶ τὰ νεῦρα ... ὅταν δ᾽ ἰσχύῃ καὶ καθ᾽ αὑτὴν γενομένη ἠρεμῇ, δεσμὰ γίνεσθαι αὐτῆς τοὺς λόγους καὶ τὰ ἔργα.

[3] Ibid., 32: εἶναί τε πάντα τὸν ἀέρα ψυχῶν ἐμπλέων· καὶ ταύτας δαίμονάς τε καὶ ἥρωας ὀνομάζεσθαι· καὶ ὑπὸ τούτων πέμπεσθαι ἀνθρώποις τούς τ᾽ ὀνείρους καὶ τὰ σημεῖα νόσους τε, καὶ οὐ μόνον ἀνθρώποις ἀλλὰ καὶ προβάτοις καὶ ἄλλοις κτήνεσιν.

[4] See his article, 'The Pythagoreans and Greek mathematics', *Am. J. Philol.* (1940).

[5] E. R. Dodds, *The Greeks and the Irrational* (University of California Press, 1951), pp. 146 f.

regard him as a member of any school;[1] he was an independent Shaman who had his own way of putting things, and was a true poet, not a philosopher who happened to write in verse.[2] But it would appear that in this respect his Pythagoreanism was less orthodox than that of Alcmaeon, since (as Theophrastus informs us) Alcmaeon was the first to separate sense perception from intelligence and confine the latter to the human species, refusing to identify them in the way that Empedocles did.[3] But both would appear to have accepted the doctrine of the immortality of the soul, an immortality shared, according to Alcmaeon, with the heavenly bodies and the whole sky, so Aristotle informs us in the *De anima*.[4]

Renan has described Empedocles as a mixture of Newton and Cagliostro, but Sigerist sees more of Newton in him and insists that he was not a quack, but 'an outstanding representative of a period in which scholars and scientists were not specialized, when one individual could embrace all science and learning, and be active in many fields'.[5] But whether sage, Shaman, scientist, or magician, Empedocles accomplished much more than miraculous cures. He provided a basis for ancient Greek science, upon which the fabric of many centuries of discovery was able to be erected—even if in the last resort his hypothesis proved less fruitful than the unverifiable alternative proposed by his contemporaries, Leucippus and Democritus. Empedocles' theory of the four elements remained the most generally accepted physical hypothesis during the whole of the classical age. On it Aristotle built the vast fabric of his system, in the form of the doctrine that all sublunary bodies are composed of earth, water, fire, or air, or their mixtures, with their combination of the four opposite qualities, heat, cold, wetness, and dryness. These four elements and their qualities, which have been related by many historians to the Pythagorean tetrad and the Pythagorean 'opposites', may perhaps be derived only from the first common-sense rationalization of sense experience. Anything you touch is either hot or cold and wet or dry, and touch is the most fundamental of the senses, not confined to the operation of any special organ like the eye or the ear. Early medical theory seems

---

[1] Ibid., footnote to chapter 5, no. 81.

[2] Ibid., footnote no. 115.

[3] Theophrastus, *De sensu*, 25: τῶν δὲ μὴ τῷ ὁμοίῳ ποιούντων τὴν αἴσθησιν Ἀλκμαίων μὲν πρῶτον ἀφορίζει τὴν πρὸς τὰ ζῷα διαφοράν· ἄνθρωπον γάρ φησι τῶν ἄλλων διαφέρειν ὅτι μόνος συνίησι, τὰ δ' ἄλλα αἰσθάνεται μέν, οὐ συνίησι δέ, ὡς ἕτερον ὂν τὸ φρονεῖν καὶ αἰσθάνεσθαι, καὶ οὐ καθάπερ Ἐμπεδοκλῆς ταὐτόν. (D–K, vol. I, 211.)

Aristotle, *De anima*, I. 2, 405[a]29–[b]1: παραπλησίως δὲ τούτοις καὶ Ἀλκμαίων ἔοικεν ὑπολαβεῖν περὶ ψυχῆς· φησὶ γὰρ αὐτὴν ἀθάνατον εἶναι διὰ τὸ ἐοικέναι τοῖς ἀθανάτοις· τοῦτο δ' ὑπάρχειν αὐτῇ ὡς ἀεὶ κινουμένῃ. κινεῖσθαι γὰρ καὶ τὰ θεῖα πάντα συνεχῶς ἀεί, σελήνην, ἥλιον, καὶ τοὺς ἀστέρας καὶ τὸν οὐρανὸν ὅλον.

[5] Sigerist, op. cit. 2. 105. But the quotations which he makes from the translation of W. E. Leonard's *The Fragments of Empedocles* (Chicago, 1905) make it a little difficult to look upon him as a scientist. Dodds's Shaman seems more to the point.

to have distinguished quite a number of opposites, adding to the traditional Pythagorean ten an indefinite number of pairs, e.g. sour and sweet, etc. Aristotle indeed informs us that Alcmaeon did so, and even suggests that he may have invented the Pythagorean decad of opposite qualities.[1] But the four elements of Empedocles, with their corresponding qualities, were eventually embodied in the physiological tradition of the Hippocratic school and its descendants up to Galen and beyond. They did not, however, hold undisputed sway in the realm of Greek physical or medical thinking. Atomists and their like crop up continually in the history of ancient Greek medicine, for example Erasistratus and Asclepiades, though, as we shall see, the first of these was not strictly speaking an atomist in the modern sense.[2] And even Empedocles himself did not altogether escape the imputation of atomism. As Schumacher has pointed out,[3] Galen criticizes his conception of the mixture of the four elements as being, unlike that of Hippocrates, what we should today call 'mechanical', and therefore open to the same criticism as that which he has applied to the atomists. Indeed Galen claims that Hippocrates was the first to formulate the doctrine of the true mixture of the elements.[4]

It would appear that the doctrine of the four elements did appeal to the earliest writers of the *Hippocratic corpus*; the doctrine of the four humours seems to be unquestionably older. It was probably only after Aristotle that the four sublunary elements were adopted as the constituents of the four fluids which were, at any rate after Polybus, regarded as composing the human body. And it would appear to be possible to trace the migration of the Empedoclean theory to eastern Greece. It should be noted that the first generalizations of Ionian scientists received little support from some professional physicians. The author of the first section of the 'Hippocratic' treatise *On the nature of man* has no patience for those who say

---

[1] Aristotle, *Metaph.* i. 5, 986ᵃ22–ᵇ1 : ἕτεροι δὲ τῶν αὐτῶν τούτων τὰς ἀρχὰς δέκα λέγουσιν εἶναι, τὰς κατὰ συστοιχίαν λεγομένας, πέρας ἄπειρον· περιττόν, ἄρτιον· ἕν, πλῆθος· δεξιόν, ἀριστερόν· ἄρρεν, θῆλυ· ἠρεμοῦν, κινούμενον· εὐθύ, καμπύλον· φῶς, σκότος· ἀγαθόν, κακόν· τετράγωνον, ἑτερόμηκες· ὅνπερ τρόπον ἔοικε καὶ Ἀλκμαίων ὁ Κροτωνιάτης ὑπολαβεῖν. καὶ ἤτοι οὗτος παρ' ἐκείνων, ἢ ἐκεῖνοι παρὰ τούτου παρέλαβον τὸν λόγον τοῦτον. καὶ γὰρ . . . Ἀλκμαίων . . . ἀπεφήνατο δὲ παραπλησίως τούτοις. φησὶ γὰρ εἶναι δύο τὰ πολλὰ τῶν ἀνθρωπίνων, λέγων τὰς ἐναντιότητας, οὐχ ὥσπερ οὗτοι διωρισμένας, ἀλλὰ τὰς τυχούσας· οἷον λευκόν, μέλαν· γλυκύ, πικρόν· ἀγαθόν, κακόν· μικρόν, μέγα. οὗτος μὲν οὖν ἀδιορίστως ἐπέρριψε περὶ τῶν λοιπῶν.

[2] See below, pp. 216 ff.

[3] Schumacher, 'Der Physis-Begriff bei Empedokles', *Arch. f. Gesch. d. Med.* xxxiv (1941), 179–96.

[4] Galen, *Comment. I in Hipp. de nat. hom.*, par. 12, K. xv. 49 f. : μεμνῆσθαι δὲ χρὴ τοῦ κατ' αὐτὴν ὀνόματος εἰρημένου τοῦ τῆς κράσεως, ὅπερ διὰ τοῦ κρήσιος εἶπεν. ὅτι πρῶτος ὧν ἴσμεν Ἱπποκράτης ἀπεφήνατο κεράννυσθαι τὰ στοιχεῖα, καθάπερ καὶ μικρὸν ἔμπροσθεν ἐδείχθη. καὶ ταύτῃ διήνεγκεν Ἐμπεδοκλέους. κἀκεῖνος γὰρ ἐκ μὲν τῶν αὐτῶν στοιχείων, ὧν καὶ Ἱπποκράτης γεγονέναι φησὶν ἡμᾶς γε καὶ τὰ ἄλλα σώματα πάντα τὰ περὶ τὴν γῆν, οὐ μὴν κεκραμένων γε δι' ἀλλήλων, ἀλλὰ κατὰ μικρὰ μόρια παρακειμένων τε καὶ ψαυόντων. ὅτι δὲ καὶ ἥδε ἡ δόξα τοὺς αὐτοὺς ἐλέγχους ἔχει ταῖς ἐξ ἀναισθήτων καὶ ἀπαθῶν τῶν πρώτων σωμάτων τὸ αἰσθητικὸν σῶμα γεννώσαις δόξαις, ἐπιδέδεικται διὰ τοῦ περὶ τῶν καθ' Ἱπποκράτην στοιχείων ὑπομνήματος.

'all is air or fire or water or earth',[1] nor even for the monistically inclined physician, who says 'man is all blood, all phlegm, or all bile'.[2] The unity of his nature is something much more complex. Man's body is made up of four elemental fluids, blood, phlegm, and yellow and black bile,[3] but the inference is drawn that these in their turn are made up of the four Empedoclean elements, even if this is not expressly stated; though to my mind that inference is by no means certain, however plain it was to Galen. Be that as it may, what the author is interested in is not the chemistry so much as the visible changes in the various and diverse parts of the body. A similar distrust of medical metaphysics is also displayed by the author of *Ancient medicine*, who especially singles out Empedocles as the target of his criticism.

Certain physicians and philosophers assert that nobody can know medicine who is ignorant of what a man is; he who would treat patients properly must, they say, learn this. But the question they raise is one for philosophy: it is the province of those who like Empedocles have written about natural science (φύσιος), what man is from the beginning, how he came into being at the first, and from what elements he was originally constructed. But my view is, first, that all that philosophers or physicians have said or written on natural science no more pertains to medicine than to painting.[4]   (trs. Jones.)

But the doctrine of the four elements did come from certain medical circles from Sicily to the mainland and to Asia Minor in the teaching, as we shall see in due course, of Plato's Sicilian doctor-friend Philistion, who, as the Anonymous Londoner informs us, taught that man's body was composed of four 'forms' or elements.[5] But, as Schöner has pointed out,[6]

---

[1] Hippocrates, *De nat. hom.* 1: οὔτε γὰρ τὸ πάμπαν ἠέρα λέγω τὸν ἄνθρωπον εἶναι, οὔτε πῦρ οὔτε ὕδωρ, οὔτε γῆν. οὔτ' ἄλλο οὐδὲν ὅ τι μὴ φανερόν ἐστιν ἐνεὸν ἐν τῷ ἀνθρώπῳ . . . λέγει δ' αὐτῶν ὁ μέν τις φάσκων ἠέρα τοῦτο εἶναι τὸ ἕν τε καὶ τὸ πᾶν, ὁ δὲ πῦρ, ὁ δ' ὕδωρ, ὁ δὲ γῆν, καὶ ἐπιλέγει ἕκαστος τῷ ἑωυτοῦ λόγῳ μαρτύριά τε καὶ τεκμήρια, ἅ ἐστιν οὐδέν. ὁπότε δὲ γνώμῃ τῇ αὐτῇ προσχρέονται, λέγουσι δ' οὐ τὰ αὐτά, δῆλον ὅτι οὐδὲ γινώσκουσιν αὐτά.

[2] Ibid., 2: τῶν δὲ ἰητρῶν οἱ μέν τινες λέγουσιν ὡς ἄνθρωπος αἷμά ἐστιν, οἱ δ' αὐτῶν χολήν φασιν εἶναι τὸν ἄνθρωπον, ἔνιοι δέ τινες φλέγμα· ἐπίλογον δὲ ποιέονται καὶ οὗτοι πάντες τὸν αὐτόν· ἐν γὰρ εἶναί φασιν, ὅ τι ἕκαστος αὐτῶν βούλεται ὀνομάσας, καὶ τοῦτο μεταλλάσσειν τὴν ἰδέην καὶ τὴν δύναμιν.

[3] Ibid., 5: εἶπον δὴ ἃ ἂν φήσω τὸν ἄνθρωπον εἶναι, ἀποφανεῖν αἰεὶ ταῦτα ἐόντα καὶ κατὰ νόμον καὶ κατὰ φύσιν· φημὶ δὴ εἶναι αἷμα καὶ φλέγμα καὶ χολὴν ξανθὴν καὶ μέλαιναν. καὶ τούτων πρῶτον μὲν κατὰ νόμον τὰ ὀνόματα διωρίσθαι φημὶ καὶ οὐδενὶ αὐτῶν τὸ αὐτὸ ὄνομα εἶναι, ἔπειτα κατὰ φύσιν τὰς ἰδέας κεχωρίσθαι, καὶ οὔτε τὸ φλέγμα οὐδὲν ἐοικέναι τῷ αἵματι, οὔτε τὸ αἷμα τῇ χολῇ, οὔτε τὴν χολὴν τῷ φλέγματι.

[4] Hippocrates, *De vet. med.* 20: λέγουσι δέ τινες ἰητροὶ καὶ σοφισταὶ ὡς οὐκ εἴη δυνατὸν ἰητρικὴν εἰδέναι ὅστις μὴ οἶδεν ὅ τί ἐστιν ἄνθρωπος. ἀλλὰ τοῦτο δεῖ καταμαθεῖν τὸν μέλλοντα ὀρθῶς θεραπεύσειν τοὺς ἀνθρώπους. τείνει δὲ αὐτοῖς ὁ λόγος ἐς φιλοσοφίην, καθάπερ Ἐμπεδοκλῆς ἢ ἄλλοι οἱ περὶ φύσιος γεγράφασιν ἐξ ἀρχῆς ὅ τί ἐστιν ἄνθρωπος, καὶ ὅπως ἐγένετο πρῶτον καὶ ὁπόθεν συνέπαγη. ἐγὼ δὲ τοῦτο μέν, ὅσα τινὶ εἴρηται ἢ σοφιστῇ ἢ ἰητρῷ ἢ γέγραπται περὶ φύσιος, ἧσσον νομίζω τῇ ἰητρικῇ τέχνῃ προσήκειν ἢ τῇ γραφικῇ.

[5] See below, pp. 37 ff.

[6] Schöner, 'Das Viererschema in der antiken Humoralpathologie', Beiheft 4 to vol. xlviii of *Arch. f. Gesch. d. Med.* (1964): 'Von einer Behauptung der Körper bestehe aus Feuer,

the doctrine that the body is composed of the four elements appears neither in the treatise *On the nature of man* nor in any of the principal works of the *Hippocratic corpus*. It was only, it would appear, after Aristotle that the theory of the four elements with their two qualities became the physical basis of medical theory. And even so, there were evolved, by the Stoics in particular, certain variations of this basis of what we might call 'orthodox' physics.

In Empedocles' physiological thinking, as Rüsche has explained,[1] these four elements play an important part as the instruments of sensation and thought, but in the constitution of living things particularly, fire fills the predominant role. So much so that Aristotle observes that he reduced the four to a sort of dualism: fire, and the rest.[2] Warmth is the essence of life and, in the form of the innate heat, also the principle of growth.[3] The vehicle of the innate heat is the blood, which is also the principal instrument of thought, because it constitutes the most intimate mixture of the elements which form the body,[4] according to Theophrastus' account of Empedocles' teaching. We have here one source of one of the fundamental notions of Hippocratic medicine, that of eucrasia, the earliest ancestor of which would appear to be Alcmaeon's theory of ἰσονομία, the disturbance of which was the fundamental cause of disease. For, as Theophrastus goes on to explain, the psychological qualities of intelligence and prudence depend upon the nature of the elemental mixture, presumably of the blood. Where the elements are equally mixed or in not too large

Wasser, Luft und Erde, oder einer direkten Koncordanz dieser vier Elemente mit den vier Säften, kann ich allerdings nicht finden, weder in De nat. hom. noch im übingem C. H. Ebensowenig kann von einer volkommenen Zuordnung der Elemente zu Qualitäten die Rede sein, Daß die Verknüpfung der Elemente mit den Qualitäten systematisch erst durch Aristoteles geschah, hat bereits Link mit Recht betont, wenn er auch den falschen Schluß zog alle Schriften, die irgend ein Vierschema mit Parallelisierung zu den vier Säften enthielten seien nacharistotelisch.' (Link, 'Über die Theorien in den hippokratischen Schriften, nebst Bemerkungen über die Echtheit dieser Schriften', *Abh. Kgl. Akad. Wiss. Berlin*, 1814/15, 224–40.)

[1] Rüsche, *Blut, Leben und Seele, ihr Verhältnis nach Auffassung der griechischen und hellenistischen Antike*, etc., Ergänzungsband Studien zur Geschichte des Altertums (Paderborn, 1930), pp. 127 ff., to which I am indebted for the quotations given in this paragraph.

[2] Aristotle, *Metaph.* 1. 4, 985ᵃ31–ᵇ2: ἔτι δὲ τὰ ὡς ἐν ὕλης εἴδει λεγόμενα στοιχεῖα τέτταρα πρῶτος εἶπεν· οὐ μὴν χρῆταί γε τέτταρσιν, ἀλλ' ὡς δυσὶν οὖσι μόνοις, πυρὶ μὲν καθ' αὑτό, τοῖς δ' ἀντικειμένοις ὡς μιᾷ φύσει, γῇ τε καὶ ἀέρι καὶ ὕδατι. Cf. *De gen. et corr.* 2. 3, 330ᵇ19–21: ἔνιοι δ' εὐθὺς τέτταρα λέγουσιν, οἷον Ἐμπεδοκλῆς. συνάγει δὲ καὶ οὗτος εἰς τὰ δύο· τῷ γὰρ πυρὶ τἆλλα πάντα ἀντιτίθησιν.

[3] Aetius, *De plac. phil.* v. 27: Ἐμπεδοκλῆς (φησί) τρέφεσθαι μὲν τὰ ζῷα διὰ τὴν ὑπόστασιν τοῦ οἰκείου, αὔξεσθαι δὲ διὰ τὴν παρουσίαν τοῦ θερμοῦ, μειοῦσθαι δὲ καὶ φθίνειν διὰ τὴν ἔκλειψιν ἑκατέρου.

[4] Theophrastus, *De sensu*, 9: διαριθμησάμενος γάρ, ὡς ἕκαστον ἑκάστῳ γνωρίζομεν, ἐπὶ τέλει προσέθηκεν ὡς

ἐκ τούτων γὰρ πάντα πεπήγασιν ἁρμοσθέντα
καὶ τούτοις φρονέουσι καὶ ἥδοντ' ἠδ' ἀνιῶνται.

διὸ καὶ τῷ αἵματι μάλιστα φρονεῖν· ἐν τούτῳ γὰρ μάλιστα κεκρᾶσθαι τὰ στοιχεῖα τῶν μερῶν.

or too small pieces not too far separated from each other, prudence and accurate senses are the result.[1] The kinship of these ideas with those of Alcmaeon is certainly striking, and Empedocles' theory of sleep, though not identical, shows also a distinct resemblance. Sleep is due to the moderate cooling of the blood's heat, the complete extinction of which means death.[2]

Another widely spread doctrine was contributed by Empedocles to ancient Greek medicine, the notion of poral respiration. This theory, contained in the famous fragment describing the experiment with the water-clock—an experiment designed to prove the material character of air—is the first Greek physiological theory which has come down to us connecting the act of respiration with the movement of the blood. It has been thought that the influence of Alcmaeon's theory of sleep can be detected in it, but the chronological relation between Alcmaeon and Empedocles is uncertain, and Empedocles' own theory of sleep was rather different. Moreover, the exact meaning of the theory has been disputed. The fragment in which it is contained has come down to us only in a quotation from Aristotle's treatise *On respiration*, the text of which forms fragment no. 100 in Diels–Kranz.[3] A translation into English

---

[1] Ibid., 11: ὅσοις μὲν οὖν ἴσα καὶ παραπλήσια μέμεικται καὶ μὴ διὰ πολλοῦ μηδ' αὖ μικρὰ μηδ' ὑπερβάλλοντα τῷ μεγέθει, τούτους φρονιμωτάτους εἶναι καὶ κατὰ τὰς αἰσθήσεις ἀκριβεστάτους, κατὰ λόγον δὲ καὶ τοὺς ἐγγυτάτω τούτων, ὅσοις δ' ἐναντίως, ἀφρονεστάτους. καὶ ὧν μὲν μανὰ καὶ ἀραιὰ κεῖται τὰ στοιχεῖα, νωθροὺς καὶ ἐπιπόνους. ὧν δὲ πυκνὰ καὶ κατὰ μικρὰ τεθραυσμένα, τοὺς δὲ τοιούτους ὀξεῖς φερομένους καὶ πολλοῖς ἐπιβαλλομένους ὀλίγα ἐπιτελεῖν διὰ τὴν ὀξύτητα τῆς τοῦ αἵματος φορᾶς. οἷς δὲ καθ' ἕν τι μόριον ἡ μέση κρᾶσίς ἐστι, ταύτῃ σοφοὺς ἑκάστους εἶναι.

[2] Aetius, *De plac. phil.* v. 24: Ἐμπεδοκλῆς τὸν μὲν ὕπνον καταψύξει τοῦ ἐν τῷ αἵματι θερμοῦ συμμέτρῳ γίνεσθαι, τῇ δὲ παντελεῖ θάνατον.

[3] The text of this runs as follows:

"Ὧδε δ' ἀναπνεῖ πάντα καὶ ἐκπνεῖ· πᾶσι λίφαιμοι
σαρκῶν σύριγγες πύματον κατὰ σῶμα τέτανται
καί σφιν ἐπὶ στομίοις πυκναῖς τέτρηνται ἄλοξιν
ῥινῶν ἔσχατα τέρθρα διαμπερές, ὥστε φόνον μὲν
κεύθειν αἰθέρι δ' εὐπορίην διόδοισι τετμῆσθαι,
ἔνθεν ἔπειθ' ὁπόταν μὲν ἐπαΐξῃ τέρεν αἷμα
αἰθὴρ παφλάζων καταΐσσεται οἴδματι μάργῳ
εὖτε δ' ἀναθρώσκῃ πάλιν ἐκπνέει ὥσπερ ὅταν παῖς
κλεψύδρῃ παίζῃσι διειπετέος χαλκοῖο—
εὖτε μὲν αὐλοῦ πορθμὸν ἐπ' εὐειδεῖ χερὶ θεῖσα
εἰς ὕδατος βάπτῃσι τέρεν δέμας ἀργυφέοιο
οὐδεὶς ἄγγος ὄμβρος ἐσέρχεται, ἀλλά μιν εἴργει
ἀέρος ὄγκος ἔσωθε πεσὼν ἐπὶ τρήματα πυκνά,
εἰσόκ' ἀποστεγάσῃ πυκινὸν ῥόον· αὐτὰρ ἔπειτα
πνεύματος ἐλλείποντος ἐσέρχεται αἴσιμον ὕδωρ
ὡς δ' αὔτως, ὅθ' ὕδωρ μὲν ἔχῃ κάτα βένθεα χαλκοῦ
πορθμοῦ χωσθέντος βροτέῳ χροῒ ἠδὲ πόροιο,
αἰθὴρ δ' ἐκτὸς ἔσω λελιημένος ὄμβρον ἐρύκει
ἀμφὶ πύλας ἰσθμοῖο δυσηχέος. ἄκρα κρατύνων,
εἰσόκε χειρὶ μεθῇ· τότε δ' αὖ πάλιν, ἔμπαλιν ἢ πρὶν
πνεύματος ἐμπίπτοντος ὑπεκθέει αἴσιμον ὕδωρ·
ὡς δ' αὔτως τέρεν αἷμα κλαδασσόμενον διὰ γυίων

verse was included by W. Ogle in his translation of the Aristotelian
treatise. It runs as follows.

> Thus all breathe in and all breathe out, in all
> Are tubes unfilled by blood, that through the flesh
> Stretch surface-wards, to where the projecting nose
> Is tunnelled through with close-set passages.
> In these have they such openings as give
> Free pass to air, to keep the gore confined.
> When inwards from the surface ebbs the Blood,
> Tempestuous air with eager wave flows in,
> Again to be expelled, with course reversed,
> When turns the tide. So, when some girl at play,
> Taking a bronze clepsydra for her toy,
> Blocks up with shapely hand its open tube,
> And dips the vessel 'neath the silvery sheen
> Of limpid water, not a drop of this
> As yet makes entrance; for the air within,
> Pressing with force upon each orifice,
> Forbids all ingress, till the girl withdraws
> Her hand, when straight the yielding air gives way,
> And in its stead flows in an equal stream.
> Now is the vessel full; the girl, again,
> Blocks with her palm the bronze-wrought pipe, and now
> The outer air, besieging all the pores,
> Forbids the imprisoned flood to percolate
> With pattering drops the strainer's openings,
> Till the child lifts her hands. Then the strong air,
> Conquered before, but now the conqueror,
> In-rushing through the tube, drives out the stream
> In headlong rout before it through the pores.
> So when the thin blood coursing through the limbs,
> Retires with ebbing stream to inner depths,
> Straightway the air flows in with surging wave,
> Again to harry forth, with equal force
> Of expiration, when the blood rebounds.[1]

This fragment has given rise to a certain amount of controversy depending upon the meaning given to the words ῥινῶν ἔσχατα τέρθρα διαμπερές.
Did Empedocles mean breathing through the nose or through the skin,
and how does the simile fit either case? Aristotle's comments on this
fragment are far from clear. He criticizes Empedocles on the ground

> ὁππότε μὲν παλίνορσον ἀπαΐξειε μυχόνδε,
> αἰθέρος εὐθὺς ῥεῦμα κατέρχεται οἴδματι θῦον,
> εὖτε δ' ἀναθρώσκῃ, πάλιν ἐκπνέει ἴσον ὀπίσσω.
> (De resp. 7, 473ᵇ9–474ᵃ6.)

[1] *Aristotle on Youth and Age, Life and Death and Respiration*, trans. W. Ogle (London, 1897),
p. 81.

that breathing is not merely through the nostrils but takes place also through the mouth with its direct passage into the throat,[1] having previously described his theory of breathing as follows:

And he says that inspiration and expiration take place because there are certain blood vessels in which there is some blood, though they are not filled with blood. They have passages into the outside air, smaller than the particles of the body, but greater than those of air. Wherefore, since blood has a natural motion up and down, when it moves down (i.e. from the exterior to the interior) the air flows in, and inspiration takes place. When it (the blood) goes up, the air is expelled outwards and expiration takes place. He compares the process to the working of the water-clock.[2]

The various aspects of this clepsydra puzzle have been set out in three articles in the *Journal of Hellenic Studies*.[3] In the first, Professor Furley puts the case for cutaneous breathing, attributing to Empedocles a theory on the lines of that laid down by Plato in the *Timaeus*, which we shall consider in due course. In the second, Mr. Booth maintains that there is no question of cutaneous, but only of oral breathing. In the third, Mr. O'Brien also rejects cutaneous breathing and puts forward the interesting suggestion that the 'pores' referred to by Aristotle are in the lungs, not on the surface of the skin. Be that as it may, it seems fairly certain that a theory of double respiration had been put forward, if not by Empedocles himself, before the end of the fifth century, one of its principal propounders being Plato's friend Philistion, of whom more below. It also looks as if the author of the 'Hippocratic' treatise *On the sacred disease*, held a similar theory.

This theory of cutaneous respiration was widely accepted by most later physicians as an auxiliary method of breathing, and we have no evidence that Empedocles regarded it as the sole method of breathing. If we can accept Wellmann's notion of a Sicilian school with Empedocles as one of its founders and Philistion as one of his successors, it would be reasonable to regard the theory of respiration by περίωσις which is described in the *Timaeus*[4] as being ultimately derived from the Master of Akragas.

---

[1] Aristotle, *De resp.* 7, 474ª17–20: εἰ δὲ περὶ τῆς κατὰ τοὺς μυκτῆρας λέγει μόνης, πολὺ διημάρτηκεν· οὐ γάρ ἐστιν ἀναπνοὴ μυκτήρων ἴδιος, ἀλλὰ παρὰ τὸν αὐλῶνα τὸν περὶ τὸν γαργαρεῶνα.

[2] Ibid., 473ᵇ1–8: γίνεσθαι δέ φησι τὴν ἀναπνοὴν καὶ ἐκπνοὴν διὰ τὸ φλέβας εἶναί τινας, ἐν αἷς ἔνεστι μὲν αἷμα, οὐ μέντοι πλήρεις εἰσὶν αἵματος· ἔχουσι δὲ πόρους εἰς τὸν ἔξω ἀέρα, τῶν μὲν τοῦ σώματος μορίων ἐλάττους, τῶν δὲ τοῦ ἀέρος μείζους. διὸ τοῦ αἵματος πεφυκότος κινεῖσθαι ἄνω καὶ κάτω, κάτω μὲν φερομένου, εἰσρεῖν τὸν ἀέρα, καὶ γίνεσθαι ἀναπνοήν· ἄνω δ' ἰόντος, ἐκπίπτειν θύραζε, καὶ γίνεσθαι τὴν ἐκπνοήν, παρεικάζων τὸ συμβαῖνον ταῖς κλεψύδραις.

[3] P. J. Furley, 'Empedocles and the clepsydra', *JHS*, lxxvii (1957); N. B. Booth, 'Empedocles' account of breathing', ibid., lxxx (1960); and D. O'Brien, 'The effect of a simile: Empedocles' theories of seeing and breathing', ibid., xc (1970). See also Guthrie, op. cit., ii. 220–6 and G. E. Lloyd, *Polarity and Analogy* (Cambridge, 1966).

[4] See below, p. 120.

It seems clear enough that Empedocles thought of the blood as being in perpetual motion through the alternative in- and out-breathing of air, through both the nostrils and the skin. But there is little evidence that he connected the movements of the heart with the propulsion of the blood. Indeed his mention of the heart that has come down to us is very brief. The only place in which he refers to it in his existing fragments consists of three lines in which he speaks of it as nourished in the seas of blood which leap against it. For the blood that is round the heart is man's mind.[1]

Empedocles is not interested in the heart but in the blood. For in the last resort it is the blood which is identified with man's 'soul'. Cicero, Macrobius, and Tertullian all tell us that he identified the soul with the blood, or at any rate with a certain portion of the blood.[2] But the heart, if we may credit Censorinus, had its importance for him, for we are told that he anticipated Aristotle in discovering that the heart was the first-formed of all the organs 'because it in greatest measure contains man's life'.[3] From this point it would not seem to be a long or difficult transition to the theory that the heart is the seat of the intelligence.[4] Indeed, later doxographers attributed precisely this doctrine to him, almost certainly incorrectly. Before leaving Empedocles it may be as well to add a footnote. For him, it is true, the blood is in perpetual motion, but it is a motion to and fro, not a circulation in any but an Italian sense.[5] This idea of the blood moving up and down the same blood vessels was to haunt Greek medical theory down to Galen and beyond. One of Galen's most perplexing problems was how to connect these movements of blood with those of the heart, the structure of which, owing to the

---

[1] D–K, fr. 105:

αἵματος ἐν πελάγεσσι τεθραμμένη ἀντιθορόντος,
τῇ τε νόημα μάλιστα κικλήσκεται ἀνθρώποισιν·
αἷμα γὰρ ἀνθρώποις περικάρδιόν ἐστι νόημα.

[2] The passages cited in this connection by Rüsche, op. cit, p. 128, are the following: Macrobius, *In somnium Scipionis*, i. 14, 'Empedocles et Critias a sanguine (sc. dixerunt animam)'; Tertullian, *De anima*, 5, 'Empedocles et Critias ex sanguine (sc. animam effingunt); Cicero, *Tusculan*. i. 9, 'Empedocles animum esse censet cordi suffusum sanguinem.' Rüsche also quotes Galen, *De plac. Hipp. et Plat*. 2. 8, K. v. 283: αἷμά φησιν εἶναι τὴν ψυχήν, ὡς Ἐμπεδοκλῆς καὶ Κριτίας ὑπέλαβον. The Critias mentioned is identified by Philoponus with the celebrated member of the thirty tyrants in *De an. prooem*. 9, but in another passage (ibid., 89) he expresses some doubt as to this identification: it may have been another Critias. Rüsche, op. cit., p. 134, n. 1.

[3] Censorinus, *De die natali*, 6: 'Empedocles, quem in hoc Aristoteles secutus est, ante omnia cor iudicavit increscere, quod hominis vitam maxime contineat.' (D–K, fr. 84, vol. 2, 301.)

[4] Cf. the passage from Theodoret, v. 22, quoted by Wellmann, *Die Fragmente der sikelischen Ärtzte Akron, Philistion und des Diokles von Karystos* (Berlin, 1901), p. 14: Ἐμπεδοκλῆς δὲ καὶ Ἀριστοτέλης, Διοκλῆς καὶ τῶν Στωικῶν ἡ ξυμμορία τὴν καρδίαν ἀπεκλήρωσαν τούτῳ (τῷ ἡγεμονικῷ) καὶ τούτων δ' αὖ πάλιν οἱ μὲν ἐν τῇ κοιλίᾳ τῆς καρδίας, οἱ δ' ἐν τῷ αἵματι (D–K, vol. 1, 307).

[5] 'Circolare' can mean 'walk up and down'.

great discoveries of the Alexandrians, had been more or less correctly worked out.[1]

The origins of the theory that the heart was the seat of the intelligence have been explored by Wellmann in his important work on the fragments of the Sicilian physicians, where they are traced back to the teaching of the school of Cnidos. Wellmann postulates the existence of a Sicilian school with Empedocles as one of its founders, though as we have seen he did not regard the heart but the blood around the heart as the seat of the intelligence. The other 'founding father' of the school was Philistion of Locri, who practised in Syracuse at the court of Dionysius the elder and was the friend of Plato. He also adopted the theory of Empedocles of respiration through pores of the skin as well as through the throat and lungs, in contrast to the teaching of his contemporary, Diogenes of Apollonia, who confined it to the latter.[2] Wellmann implies that he was the chief influence responsible for the doctrine expressed in the fragment in the Hippocratic collection known as the *De corde*,[3] an opinion which has not been accepted by all modern critics,[4] though the latest translator of the fragment, the American Hurlbutt, whose version was published in 1939, still did so.[5] Wellmann implies that like other members of the Sicilian as well as of the Cnidian school, Philistion believed that the heart was the seat of the intelligence as opposed to the head, and that this was one of the characteristic differences which divided the two schools of Asia Minor.[6] Too little is known about either the Sicilian or the Cnidian schools to trace their influence upon each other. In the past it has generally been assumed that the predominating influence on Sicilian thought must have come to the West from Asia, but Michler has hinted that the current may have flowed the other way.[7] It is therefore impossible to assert with any degree of certainty where Philistion found the source of his doctrine of *pneuma*. For he is reported by the Anonymous Londoner to have maintained that one, at any rate, of the causes of disease was the obstruction of the passage of the *pneuma*, presumably

---

[1] See below, Chapter 4.

[2] Wellmann, *Fragmente*, p. 71.

[3] Ibid., p. 107: 'So wird es niemanden zu kühn denken, wenn ich behaupte daß die Schrift περὶ καρδίας unter dem Einfluß der sikelischen Lehren, speziell des Philistion entstanden ist.'

[4] See below, pp. 83 f.

[5] See his translation with introduction, published in *Bull. Hist. Med.* 7 (1939), 104 ff.

[6] Wellmann, *Fragmente*, p. 77: 'Der fundamentale Unterschied der Lehre der koischen und sikelischen Schule vom Sitz der Seele'; and p. 17: 'so ergiebt sich für uns als eine zweifellose Thatsache, daß die fundamentale Lehre vom Sitz der Seele ein wichtiges Unterschiedungsmerkmal der koischen und sikelischen resp. knidischen Schule gewesen ist.'

[7] Michler, op. cit.: 'Auf solchen Ergebnissen liesse sich am Ende vielleicht eine Hypothese aufbauen, die noch zu zeigen vermag daß die westgriechische Medizin in ihren Anfangsstadien möglicherweise sogar die Voraussetzung für Kos und Knidos bildete, und auch später noch für geraume Zeit ihren eigenen Weg ging.'

through the blood vessels over the whole body.[1] This notion may be compared with the theory of Diogenes of Apollonia, who was probably an older contemporary of Hippocrates. Diogenes borrowed the main idea which underlay his physiological thinking from Anaximenes. He was a thorough-going monist. The universe was composed of a single substance, air, which he seems to have looked upon as the substance of body as well as soul.[2] He was also the first physician that we know of to make a systematic description of the vascular system, to which we must turn before discussing his psycho-physical notions.

But before dealing with this there is one predecessor, it would appear, of the Apollonian,[3] whose account is worth considering.

Diogenes' description, pace Erhard, is not absolutely the first which has survived, since Aristotle, in his account of the opinions on the blood vessels given by earlier authorities which he places before his own account in the History of animals, mentions before Diogenes a short account of the theory of an otherwise obscure physician, Syennesis of Cyprus, about whom nothing more is known. Syennesis in his description of the main blood vessels makes them start from the head, and execute in the thorax a kind of chiasma, passing from left to right and right to left. No mention is made of the heart, any more than in the description by Diogenes. Syennesis taught, we are told, that (see Fig. 1)

The thick veins grow as follows. From the eye along the eyebrow, passing down the back, past the lung, under the breast, one from the right to the left, the other from the left to the right. The one from the left goes through the liver to the kidney and the testicle, and the one from the right goes to the spleen and the kidney and the testicle, and from there to the penis.[4]

Though the heart is not mentioned at all, the impression which this description leaves is that the crossing place of these diagonals must have

---

[1] Anonymus Londinensis, xx, J. 80: ὅταν γάρ, φησίν, εὐπνοῇ ὅλον τὸ σῶμα καὶ διεξίῃ ἀκωλύτως τὸ πνεῦμα, ὑγίεια γίνεται· οὐ γὰρ μόνον κατὰ τὸ στόμα καὶ τοὺς μυκτῆρας ἡ ἀναπνοὴ γίνεται, ἀλλὰ καὶ καθ' ὅλον τὸ σῶμα. ὅταν δὲ μὴ εὐπνοῇ τὸ σῶμα, νόσοι γίνονται, καὶ διαφόρως· καθ' ὅλον μὲν γὰρ τὸ σῶμα τῆς ἀναπνοῆς ἐπεχομένης, νόσος . . .

[2] Diogenes, frg. 5 (D–K, vol. 2, 61): καὶ ἔστιν οὐδὲ ἕν ὅ τι μὴ μετέχει τούτου· μετέχει δὲ οὐδὲ ἓν ὁμοίως τὸ ἕτερον τῷ ἑτέρῳ, ἀλλὰ πολλοὶ τρόποι καὶ αὐτοῦ τοῦ ἀέρος καὶ τῆς νοήσιός εἰσιν. ἔστι γὰρ πολύτροπος καὶ θερμότερος καὶ ψυχρότερος καὶ ξηρότερος καὶ ὑγρότερος . . . καὶ ἄλλαι πολλαὶ ἑτεροιώσιες ἔνεισι καὶ ἡδονῆς καὶ χροιῆς ἄπειροι.

[3] Simplicius, Phys. 25, 1 (D–K, loc. cit. 52): τὴν δὲ τοῦ παντὸς φύσιν ἀέρα καὶ οὗτός φησιν ἄπειρον εἶναι καὶ ἀίδιον, ἐξ οὗπυκνουμένου καὶ μανουμένου καὶ μεταβάλλοντος τοῖς πάθεσι τὴν τῶν ἄλλων γίνεσθαι μορφήν. καὶ ταῦτα μὲν Θεόφραστος ἱστορεῖ περὶ τοῦ Διογένους, καὶ τὸ εἰς ἐμὲ ἐλθὸν αὐτοῦ σύγγραμμα Περὶ φύσεως ἐπιγεγραμμένον ἀέρα σαφῶς λέγει τὸ ἐξ οὗ πάντα γίνεται τὰ ἄλλα.

[4] Aristotle, Hist. an. 3. 2, 511ᵇ24–30: Συέννεσις μὲν (γὰρ) ὁ Κύπριος ἰατρὸς τόνδε τὸν τρόπον λέγει. Αἱ φλέβες αἱ παχεῖαι ὧδε πεφύκασιν· ἐκ τοῦ ὀφθαλμοῦ παρὰ τὴν ὀφρὺν διὰ τοῦ νώτου παρὰ τὸν πνεύμονα ὑπὸ τοὺς μαστούς, ἡ μὲν ἐκ τοῦ δεξιοῦ εἰς τὰ ἀριστερὰ ἡ δ' ἐκ τοῦ ἀριστεροῦ εἰς τὸ δεξιόν. ἡ μὲν οὖν ἐκ τοῦ ἀριστεροῦ διὰ τοῦ ἥπατος εἰς τὸν νέφρον καὶ εἰς τὸν ὄρχιν, ἡ δ' ἐκ τοῦ δεξιοῦ εἰς τὸν σπλῆνα καὶ νεφρὸν καὶ ὄρχιν, ἐντεῦθεν δ' εἰς τὸ αἰδοῖον.

been the heart, which is described by Plato in the famous passage in the *Timaeus* as the 'knot of the veins'.[1] One cannot help asking oneself, too, how this picture of the main blood vessels crossing one another can have arisen. Was it based on some dissection of an animal body, or even of human body subjected to some fearful mishap, or perhaps more probably cut open in battle by a gaping wound, which exposed the crossing of the innominate artery and the left innominate vein?

After quoting Syennesis' description of the main vessels, Aristotle goes on to quote that of Diogenes (see Fig. 2). This passage Erhard[2] regards as the first systematic description of the vascular system which has survived. The passage reads as follows:

And the veins in man are like this. There are two very large (or the greatest) ones. These stretch through the belly along the spine, one on the right and the other on the left. Each of them extends to the corresponding leg, and up to the head, past the collar-bones and through the throat. And from these two, veins branch off and extend to the whole body, from the large vein on the right to the parts on the right side, and from the large vein on the left to the parts on the left side: two very big ones to the heart, on each side of (or near) the spine, and others a little higher up, through the chest under the armpit to the hand on each side. [And one is called the spleen vein and the other the liver vein.[3]] And each of these is divided at the top end, one branch extending to the thumb, and the other to the palm. [*Handwurzel*, Erhard.] And from these there are thin veins with many branches to the rest of the hand and to the fingers. And other thinner veins branch out from the first veins, from the one on the right to the liver, and from the one on the left to the spleen and to the kidneys. And those which extend to the legs are divided at the point where the leg grows on to the trunk, and extend through the whole of the thigh. The biggest of them extends along the back of the thigh and is visibly a thick vein, and the other, which runs inside the thigh, is a little less thick than the former. Further on, past the knee, they extend to the calf and the foot, just as [the ones mentioned above] go to the hand. And they stretch down to the flat of the foot, and from thence to the toes. And many thin veins branch off from the great vessels, to the belly and the ribs. And those which extend to the head through the throat are plainly visible in the neck as large veins. From each of them, where they end, there are many branches that divide into the head, some going from the right to the left, and some from the left to the right. And on each side they end by the ear. And there is another vein in the neck, running along the big one on each side, a little smaller than it, with which most of the veins coming

---

[1] Plato, *Timaeus*, 70 b, c: τὴν δὲ δὴ καρδίαν ἅμμα τῶν φλεβῶν καὶ πηγὴν τοῦ κατὰ πάντα τὰ μέλη σφοδρῶς αἵματος εἰς τὴν δορυφορικὴν οἴκησιν κατέστησαν.

[2] See his article, 'Diogenes von Apollonia als Biologe', *Arch. f. Gesch. d. Med.* xxxiv (1941), 335–56.

[3] This sentence is regarded by Erhard as an interpolation, since it obviously interrupts the description of the blood vessels in the arms and the hands, and does not appear to be consistent with the account given later of the thinner branches from the first veins to the liver and the spleen.

from the head unite. And these stretch along the throat inwards [i.e. down into the chest]. And from each of them [the smaller veins in the neck] other branches extend under the shoulder-blade into the hands. They can be seen running alongside of the splenetic and hepatic, a little smaller than these. They are the ones which they cut when there is a pain under the skin; but when the pain is in the belly, it is the hepatic and the splenetic which they cut. And from these other branches extend under the breasts. And there are others, thin ones, which extend from each of the big veins through the marrow of the spine to the testicles. And others, too, extend under the skin through the flesh to the kidneys, and they extend in man to the testicles, and in women to the womb.

In the Aristotelian text there follows a sentence which seems to be an interpolation, and has been bracketed in D–K. It reads:

Now the first veins, those that come from the belly, are rather broad and then become thinner up to the point where they change from right to left and left to right.

The passage then continues in words which follow quite appropriately on those occurring before the interpolated sentence:

These are called the spermatic veins, and the thickest blood is absorbed by the flesh-like parts, but the blood which gets up into these parts becomes thin and hot and foamlike.[1]

---

[1] Aristotle, *Hist. an.* 3. 2, 511^{b}31–512^{b}11, quoted in D–K, vol. 2, 63–5: αἱ δὲ φλέβες ἐν τῷ ἀνθρώπῳ ὧδ' ἔχουσιν. εἰσι δύο μέγισται. αὗται τείνουσι διὰ τῆς κοιλίας παρὰ τὴν νωτιαίαν ἄκανθαν, ἡ μὲν ἐπὶ δεξιὰ ἡ δ' ἐπὶ ἀριστερά, εἰς τὰ σκέλη, ἑκατέρα (εἰς τὸ) παρ' ἑαυτῇ, καὶ ἄνω εἰς τὴν κεφαλὴν παρὰ τὰς κλεῖδας διὰ τῶν σφαγῶν. ἀπὸ δὲ τούτων καθάπαν τὸ σῶμα φλέβες διατείνουσιν, ἀπὸ μὲν τῆς δεξιᾶς εἰς τὰ δεξιά, ἀπὸ δὲ τῆς ἀριστερᾶς εἰς τὰ ἀριστερά, μέγισται μὲν δύο εἰς τὴν καρδίαν περὶ αὐτὴν τὴν νωτιαίαν ἄκανθαν, ἕτεραι δ' ὀλίγον ἀνωτέρω διὰ τῶν στηθῶν ὑπὸ τὴν μασχάλην εἰς ἑκατέραν τὴν χεῖρα τὴν παρ' ἑαυτῇ. [καὶ καλεῖται ἡ μὲν σπληνῖτις, ἡ δ' ἡπατῖτις.] σχίζεται δ' αὐτῶν ἄκρα ἑκατέρα, ἡ μὲν ἐπὶ τὸν μέγαν δάκτυλον, ἡ δ' ἐπὶ τὸν ταρσόν· ἀπὸ δὲ τούτων λεπταὶ καὶ πολύοζοι ἐπὶ τὴν ἄλλην χεῖρα καὶ δακτύλους. ἕτεραι δὲ λεπτότεραι ἀπὸ τῶν πρώτων φλεβῶν τείνουσιν, ἀπὸ μὲν τῆς δεξιᾶς εἰς τὸ ἧπαρ, ἀπὸ δὲ τῆς ἀριστερᾶς εἰς τὸν σπλῆνα καὶ τοὺς νεφρούς. αἱ δ' εἰς τὰ σκέλη τείνουσαι σχίζονται κατὰ τὴν πρόσφυσιν, καὶ διὰ παντὸς τοῦ μηροῦ τείνουσαι. ἡ δὲ μεγίστη αὐτῶν ὄπισθεν τείνει τοῦ μηροῦ, καὶ ἐκφαίνεται παχεῖα· ἑτέρα δ' εἴσω τοῦ μηροῦ, μικρὸν ἧττον παχεῖα ἐκείνης. ἔπειτα παρὰ τὸ γόνυ τείνουσιν εἰς τὴν κνήμην τε καὶ τὸν πόδα, καθάπερ αἱ εἰς τὰς χεῖρας· καὶ ἐπὶ τὸν ταρσὸν τοῦ ποδὸς καθήκουσι, καὶ ἐντεῦθεν ἐπὶ τοὺς δακτύλους διατείνουσιν. σχίζονται δὲ καὶ ἐπὶ τὴν κοιλίαν καὶ τὸ πλευρὸν πολλαὶ ἀπ' αὐτῶν καὶ λεπταὶ φλέβες.

Αἱ δ' εἰς τὴν κεφαλὴν τείνουσαι διὰ τῶν σφαγῶν φαίνονται ἐν τῷ αὐχένι μεγάλαι· ἀφ' ἑκατέρας δ' αὐτῶν, ᾗ τελευτᾷ, σχίζονται εἰς τὴν κεφαλὴν πολλαί, αἱ μὲν ἐκ τῶν δεξιῶν εἰς τὰ ἀριστερά, αἱ δ' ἐκ τῶν ἀριστερῶν εἰς τὰ δεξιά· τελευτῶσι δὲ παρὰ τὸ οὖς ἑκάτεραι. ἔστι δ' ἑτέρα φλὲψ ἐν τῷ τραχήλῳ παρὰ τὴν μεγάλην ἑκατέρωθεν, ἐλάττων ἐκείνης ὀλίγον, εἰς ἣν αἱ πλεῖσται ἐκ τῆς κεφαλῆς συνέχουσιν αὐταί· καὶ αὗται τείνουσιν διὰ τῶν σφαγῶν εἴσω. καὶ ἀπ' αὐτῶν ἑκατέρας ὑπὸ τὴν ὠμοπλάτην τείνουσι καὶ εἰς τὰς χεῖρας, καὶ φαίνονται παρά τε τὴν σπληνῖτιν καὶ τὴν ἡπατῖτιν ἕτεραι ὀλίγον ἐλάττους, ἃς ἀποσχάζουσιν, ὅταν τι ὑπὸ τὸ δέρμα λυπῇ· ἐὰν δέ τι περὶ τὴν κοιλίαν, τὴν ἡπατῖτιν καὶ τὴν σπληνῖτιν. τείνουσι δὲ καὶ ὑπὸ τοὺς μαστοὺς ἀπὸ τούτων ἕτεραι.

Ἕτεραι δ' εἰσὶν αἱ ἀπὸ ἑκατέρας τείνουσαι διὰ τοῦ νωτιαίου μυελοῦ εἰς τοὺς ὄρχεις, λεπταί. ἕτεραι δ' ὑπὸ τὸ δέρμα καὶ διὰ τῆς σαρκὸς τείνουσιν εἰς τοὺς νεφρούς, καὶ τελευτῶσιν εἰς τοὺς ὄρχεις τοῖς ἀνδράσι, ταῖς δὲ γυναιξὶν εἰς τὰς ὑστέρας. [αἱ δὲ φλέβες αἱ μὲν πρῶται ἐκ τῆς κοιλίας εὐρύτεραί εἰσιν, ἔπειτα λεπτότεραι γίγνονται, ἕως ἂν μεταβάλωσιν ἐκ τῶν δεξιῶν εἰς τὰ ἀριστερὰ καὶ ἐκ τούτων εἰς τὰ δεξιά.] αὗται δὲ σπερματίτιδες καλοῦνται. τὸ δ' αἷμα τὸ μὲν παχύτατον ὑπὸ τῶν σαρκῶν ἐκπίνεται· ὑπερβάλλον δ' εἰς τοὺς τόπους τούτους λεπτὸν καὶ θερμὸν καὶ ἀφρῶδες γίγνεται.

From the facts stated in the last two sentences, Diogenes, so Clement of Alexandria informs us, derived the term 'aphrodisia' applied to the sexual act.[1]

The text as it stands raises a number of difficulties which have puzzled scholars. Neither Aubert and Wimmer, nor Dittinger, nor Pierre Louis, the producer of the Budé text, nor Peck in the Loeb translation have secluded or transposed the two passages rejected by Erhard. It seems clear, as both Weygoldt[2] and Krause[3] pointed out, that Aristotle cannot be quoting Diogenes verbatim, since Diogenes would have written in the Ionian dialect. The passage must therefore be regarded as a précis. Moreover the *History*, like all the Aristotelian main treatises, was almost certainly made up of lecture-notes, either by a pupil or by the Master himself. This would appear sufficient to account for a certain incoherence, which obviously exists. The main problem concerns the veins in the arms which Diogenes here appears to name the 'hepatic' and the 'splenetic' in the right and left arms respectively. What is their connection with the two main blood vessels? Weygoldt[4] would appear to identify them. Krause, on the other hand, keeps much more closely to the text, and makes the hepatic and splenetic veins branch off from the two main blood vessels, which he identifies rather more plausibly as the vena cava and the aorta, above the heart. If this is correct, why are they named 'hepatic' and 'splenetic'? The problem is made all the more puzzling by the fact that in the citation from 'Polybus' (see Fig. 3)—made verbatim this time—we do find veins connecting the liver and the spleen with the right and left arms respectively, as well as in the 'Hippocratic' treatise *On the sacred disease*, which has rightly been interpreted as showing strongly the influence of Diogenes. The second sentence, regarded by Erhard as an interpolation, would seem to make quite good sense if we transpose it to follow the description of the various veins lanced, which forms the concluding sentence of p. 512[a] of the Berlin text. Below the neck the two main blood vessels send off branches in only one direction, the one on the right to the right,

Cf. the passage from Vindicianus quoted by Wellmann, op. cit., p. 210: 'Diogenes autem Apolloniates essentiam (seminis) similiter (sc. Diocli) spumam sanguinis dixit libro physico. Etenim spiratione adductus spiritus sanguinem suspendit, cuius alia pars carne bibitur, alia superans in seminales cadit vias et semen facit, quod (non) est aliud quam spuma sanguinis spiritu collisi.'

[1] Clemens Alexandrinus, *Paedag.* i. 6, D–K 2. 57. 24: τινὲς δὲ καὶ τὸ σπέρμα τοῦ ζῴου ἀφρὸν εἶναι τοῦ αἵματος κατ' οὐσίαν ὑποτίθενται· ὃ δὴ τῇ ἐμφύτῳ ἄρρενος θέρμη παρὰ τὰς συμπλοκὰς ἐκταραχθὲν ἐκριπιζόμενον ἐξαφροῦται κἂν ταῖς σπερματικαῖς παρατίθεται φλεψίν. ἐντεῦθεν γὰρ ὁ Ἀπολλωνιάτης Διογένης τὰ ἀφροδίσια κεκλῆσθαι βούλεται.

[2] G. P. Weygoldt, 'Zu Diogenes von Apollonia', *Arch. Gesch. Philos.* 1. 2, 166; also a note in *Jahrbücher f. Klassische Philologie* (Leipzig, 1881), 508–11.

[3] E. Krause, 'Diogenes von Apollonia' (*Beilage zu dem Jahresberichte des Königlichen Gymnasiums zu Gnesen*, Ostern, 1909. Posen, 1909).

[4] Weygoldt, note, *Jahrb. f. Klass. Philol.* (op. cit.), 509.

and the one on the left to the left, but above the neck these directions are reversed. This would appear to involve a sort of chiasma, the veins branching off from the right jugular ending by the left ear, and those from the left jugular by the right ear. This arrangement is then amplified by the statement that the two main blood vessels are at their thickest in the belly, the jugular portions being narrower.

This description by Diogenes is interesting, not only because it represents such a great advance over Syennesis and in some ways, too, over some of the descriptions in the *Hippocratic corpus* (e.g. those in the treatises *On places* and *On the nature of man*), but also because of the way in which it foreshadows some of the later discoveries. Before passing on to these, two points are perhaps worth considering. First, there is no distinction made between arteries and veins, both are called φλέβες. The word *arteria* is not used, for the simple reason that *arteria* in common parlance meant the windpipe. It was only later that the same word was applied to the arteries. The first person who made any clear distinction between the two types of blood vessel would appear to be Praxagoras, a physician of the school of Cos who lived towards the end of the fourth century B.C. and was probably the grandson of the Praxagoras who is reputed to have been a disciple of Hippocrates himself, though the distinction has been traced back as far as Euryphon of Cnidos by Wellmann[1] and Fredrich.[2] It would appear, however, that the anatomical difference between the two kinds of blood vessels was first described by Herophilus. Secondly, the description expressly purports to be that of the blood vessels in man. This once more raises the question touched on in connection with Alcmaeon. Was Diogenes' description based on the dissection of human corpses? That the Greeks knew a good deal about the insides of the human, as opposed to the animal body, would be impossible to deny. They were acquainted with the cavities in the lung resulting from tuberculosis and also, it would appear, with the tubercles themselves, probably as Dr. Walter Pagel has pointed out from postmortem observation,[3] since it is difficult to see how otherwise they could have known them. Yet the general opinion of medical historians, though it is divided upon this subject, would seem to reduce the direct acquaintance of Greek physicians, with the exception of the Alexandrians, to a minimum. Before the days of Herophilus and Erasistratus the ban on human dissection is generally considered to have been exceedingly strict, but it is difficult not to suspect that Hellenic curiosity did lead

---

[1] Wellmann, *Fragmente*, p. 91, who refers to Caelius Aurelianus, *Morb. chron.* ii. 10: 'Differentias etiam fluoris sanguinis veteres quaesierunt. Et quidam aiunt unum solum esse vel intelligi, hoc est, vulnerationis, ut Themison libro tardarum passionum. Alii vero eruptiones, ut Hippocrates, Eurypho. Sed Hippocrates solarum venarum, Eurypho vero etiam arteriarum.'

[2] Fredrich, op. cit., p. 68.

[3] See below, p. 100.

to the occasional, if surreptitious, contravention of traditional taboos. Be that as it may, Diogenes' description would certainly appear to indicate only the briefest inspection of the human corpse, if any at all, and little, if anything, which could not have been observed in a domestic animal. The course of a large number of superficial veins in the limbs can be traced by the naked eye, while the existence of a double set of vessels going along each side of the neck can be inferred from the sacrificial altar, and the two main internal 'veins' from the operations of any butcher.

It is to be noticed that the heart has not yet become the centre of the vascular system, though Diogenes was credited by Littré[1] with a knowledge of the two ventricles, since, in a passage from 'Plutarch', we are told that he placed the 'commanding element' in the left ventricle of the heart —an attribution which is not accepted by Wellmann, Zeller, Weygoldt, or Krause. Indeed the attribution may be dismissed as a gross anachronism, implying a conception of the heart and vascular system which can only have been formed in the Hellenistic epoch.[2] The discovery of the heart as the focus from which all the blood vessels emerge has generally been attributed to Aristotle. But even after Aristotle's time it was not universally accepted. It was, for instance, denied by Galen, who, following what may have been an older tradition, placed the origin of the veins in the liver.[3] But Diogenes has pointed the way to Aristotle. His 'two biggest veins' each have two large branches leading to the heart, and were soon to be interpreted to represent the vena cava and the aorta. In this connection it is perhaps worth while noting that for most later authorities, including Erasistratus and Galen, the auricles were not considered to be part of the heart, but were regarded as terminal processes of the blood vessels, the vena cava and the pulmonary vein, which brought matter into it. Diogenes seems also to foreshadow, however faintly, the distinction between arteries and veins. He postulates a double system of vessels in the neck, which seems to indicate that he had observed the jugular veins and the carotid arteries, without, of course, noting any difference of character between the two sets of vessels. He also has a double set of vessels leading to the liver and the spleen and to the kidneys and the genitals, which would again suggest that he had observed, without knowing it, the double system of veins and arteries.

---

[1] Vol. 1, 204 ff., where he cites the following from Aetius iv. 5. 7: Διογένης (τὸ τῆς ψυχῆς ἡγεμονικὸν τίθησι) ἐν τῇ ἀρτηριακῇ κοιλίᾳ τῆς καρδίας, ἥτις ἐστὶ πνευματικὴ (D-K, vol. 2, 57).

[2] Wellmann, *Fragmente*, p. 15, n. 4, does not accept this statement as representing Diogenes' doctrine, and believes that for Diogenes should probably be substituted Diocles. Krause, following Zeller, thinks that the mistake has arisen through the confusion of Diogenes of Apollonia with Diogenes of Babylon, a Stoic pupil of Chrysippus. This suggestion seems the more probable, since he wrote a work—now lost—Περὶ τῆς ψυχῆς ἡγεμονικοῦ.

[3] See below, pp. 324 ff.

But it is as the founder or one of the founders of the doctrine of *pneuma*
that Diogenes is particularly important, seeing that he developed the
theory of *pneuma* co-existing with, and indeed moving, the blood in the
blood vessels not yet differentiated into arteries and veins. For air, as we
have seen, exists in many forms. In its more condensed forms it exists as
solids or liquids, but in its rarest as soul or in its supremely spirituous
form as God. We have here in a more primitive form the doctrine which
will identify *pneuma* in the Stoic teaching with the spark of the world-soul.[1]

And it seems to me that that which possesses thought is air. By that all things
and people are governed and govern everything. For this seems to be God and
to reach everything, to dispose or arrange everything and to be in everything
. . . And the soul of all animals is the same thing, air, hotter than the air outside
us, in which we live, but much colder than the air which is in the sun.[2]

According to Erhard,[3] Diogenes assumed that normally only *pneuma* not
blood was contained in the arteries, but there does not seem to be any
real evidence for this statement beyond a rather insecure conjecture made
from his theory of sleep, which seems to be derived from that of Alcmaeon, if Aetius' attribution is correct. According to this theory, when all
the blood dispersed fills the veins and pushes the air contained in them
into the breast and the belly, which lies underneath them, sleep comes
about and the chest becomes hotter. But if all the air-like substance
disappears from the veins, death takes place.[4] This seems to me to imply
that Diogenes thought all the blood vessels contained both blood and air.
According to Theophrastus, Diogenes taught that the brain is surrounded
by an inner *pneuma* which receives the sensory impressions. This *pneuma*
is a little bit of God, a conception which is proved by the fact that, when
we are thinking hard, we sometimes neither hear nor see. This is because
when we think vigorously we hold our breath and so no air can get to the
brain.[5] Diogenes thought, like Alcmaeon, that in respiration air is directly

---

[1] See below, p. 236.

[2] D–K, fr. 5 (vol. 2, 61): καί μοι δοκεῖ τὸ τὴν νόησιν ἔχον εἶναι ὁ ἀὴρ καλούμενος ὑπὸ τῶν
ἀνθρώπων, καὶ ὑπὸ τούτου πάντας καὶ κυβερνᾶσθαι καὶ πάντων κρατεῖν. αὐτὸ γάρ μοι τοῦτο θεὸς
δοκεῖ εἶναι καὶ ἐπὶ πᾶν ἀφῖχθαι καὶ πάντα διατιθέναι καὶ ἐν παντὶ ἐνεῖναι . . . καὶ πάντων τῶν
ζῴων δὲ ἡ ψυχὴ τὸ αὐτό ἐστι, ἀὴρ θερμότερος μὲν τοῦ ἔξω ἐν ᾧ ἐσμεν τοῦ μέντοι παρὰ τῷ ἡλίῳ
πολλὸν ψυχρότερος. Cf. Aristotle, De an. 1. 3, 405ᵃ21–5: Διογένης δ' ὥσπερ καὶ ἕτεροί τινες, ἀέρα
(τὴν ψυχὴν εἶναι ὑπέλαβε) τοῦτον οἰηθεὶς πάντων λεπτομερέστατον εἶναι καὶ ἀρχήν· καὶ διὰ τοῦτο
γινώσκειν τε καὶ κινεῖν τὴν ψυχήν, ᾗ μὲν πρῶτόν ἐστι, καὶ ἐκ τούτου τὰ λοιπὰ γινώσκειν, ᾗ δὲ
λεπτότατον κινητικὸν εἶναι.

[3] Erhard, op. cit., p. 339: 'Im Sinne der übrigen Vorsokratiker nimmt auch Diogenes an,
daß im normalen Leben in den Arterien Luft enthalten sei, und nur in den Venen Blut.'

[4] Aetius, v. 24. 3 (D–K, vol. 2, 57): ἐὰν ἐπὶ τὸ πᾶν τὸ αἷμα διαχεόμενον πληρώσῃ μὲν τὰς
φλέβας τὸν δ' ἐν αὐταῖς περιεχόμενον ἀέρα ὤσῃ εἰς τὰ στέρνα καὶ τὴν ὑποκειμένην γαστέρα,
ὕπνον γεγενῆσθαι καὶ θερμότερον ὑπάρχειν τὸν θώρακα. ἐὰν δὲ ἅπαν τὸ ἀερῶδες ἐκ τῶν φλεβῶν
ἐκλίπῃ, θάνατον συντυγχάνειν.

[5] Theophrastus, De sensu, 42, explains his theory as follows: ὅτι δὲ ὁ ἐντὸς ἀὴρ αἰσθάνεται,
μικρὸν ὢν μόριον τοῦ θεοῦ, σημεῖον εἶναι διότι πολλάκις πρὸς ἄλλα τὸν νοῦν ἔχοντες, οὔθ' ὁρῶμεν
οὔτ' ἀκούομεν (D–K, vol. 2, 56).

drawn into the brain, a doctrine we shall meet again in the Hippocratic writings. Clean dry air in the body stimulates thought, thick damp air impedes it. Hence we think less well when we are drunk, or on a full stomach, or in sleep.[1] Because of this theory of *pneuma* as the principle of intelligence, and its direct inspiration into the brain, Diogenes does not appear to have located 'the governing element', τὸ ἡγεμονικόν, in any particular organ. There seems to be little doubt that he conceived the *pneuma*, which is specifically identified with air, apparently unchanged, as going up and down in the blood vessels.[2] The amount of air in the mixture with the blood varied from time to time. If a lot of air mixed with the blood and lightening it in a natural condition goes all over the entire body, pleasure takes place, but if the blood in an unnatural manner does not mix with the air, but coagulates and becomes weaker and thinner, pain is the result. And in the same way courage and health and their opposites are produced.[3] Unfortunately the fragments of Diogenes' work *On nature* which have survived and the doxographical accounts of Theophrastus, Simplicius, etc., do not enable us to form any precise picture of his teaching. He was not, as far as we know, a physician, and does not seem to have shown much, or indeed any, interest in the controversy concerning the primacy of the organs. Zeller was convinced that he refused to confine the seat of the soul to a single organ,[4] though at the same time he emphasizes the importance of the brain as the locus of sensation.[5] But Nestle the editor of his sixth edition adds to his footnote the suggestion that he may, like Alcmaeon, have located intelligence in the brain, and that his doctrine attributing sensation to the air passing through the brain, was adopted by 'Hippocrates' in the sixteenth chapter of the treatise *On the sacred disease.*[6]

Erhard, following Krause, comes to the conclusion that Diogenes regarded all parts of the body which contained air, including empty arteries and the (empty?) left ventricle of the heart, as parts of the

---

[1] Ibid., 44: φρονεῖν δ' ὅπερ ἐλέχθη τῷ ἀέρι καθαρῷ καὶ ξηρῷ, κωλύειν γὰρ τὴν ἰκμάδα τὸν νοῦν· διὸ καὶ ἐν ταῖς μέθαις καὶ ἐν ταῖς πλησμοναῖς ἧττον φρονεῖν (ibid.).

[2] Simplicius, *In phys.*, p. 153: δείκνυσιν ὅτι καὶ τὸ σπέρμα τῶν ζῴων πνευματῶδές ἐστι καὶ νοήσεις γίνονται τοῦ ἀέρος σὺν τῷ σώματι τὸ ὅλον σῶμα καταλαμβάνοντος διὰ τῶν φλεβῶν (D-K, vol. 2, 62).

[3] Theophrastus, *De sensu*, 43: ἡδονὴν δὲ καὶ λύπην γίνεσθαι τόνδε τὸν τρόπον· ὅταν μὲν πολὺς ὁ ἀὴρ μίσγηται τῷ αἵματι καὶ κουφίζῃ κατὰ φύσιν ὢν καὶ κατὰ πᾶν τὸ σῶμα διεξιών, ἡδονήν. ὅταν δὲ παρὰ φύσιν καὶ μὴ μίσγηται συνιζάνοντος τοῦ αἵματος καὶ ἀσθενεστέρου καὶ πυκνοτέρου γινομένου, λύπην. ὁμοίως καὶ θάρσος καὶ ὑγίειαν καὶ τἀναντία (D-K, vol. 2, 56).

[4] E. Zeller, *Die Philosophie der Griechen* (6th edn., Leipzig, 1919), i. 350 n. 4: 'Aus diesen Stellen ergiebt sich, daß Diogenes den Sitz der Seele auf kein einzelnes Organ beschränkte.'

[5] Loc. cit. p. 351: 'Den Sitz der Empfindung suchte Diogenes in der das Gehirn durchziehenden Luft.'

[6] Loc. cit., note 4: 'Diese Ansicht Zeller's übernimmt Krause. Immerhin könnte Diogenes das Denken nach dem Vorgang Alkmaion von Kroton in das Gehirn verlegt haben: wenigstens schrieb er der das Gehirn durchziehenden Luft für die Sinnesempfindung große Bedeutung. Hippokrates, *de morbo sacro*, 16, hat dann hier angeknüpft.'

commanding organ, though he was quite clear that the seat of sensation and intelligence is the brain.[1] One other interesting theory is credited to Diogenes by Aristotle, namely the idea that fishes breathe through their gills by absorbing air dissolved in the water, a notion which, as we shall see later, is repudiated by the Master of those that know.[2]

Thus by the end of the fifth century B.C. two notions had been evolved which were to divide Greek medicine well into Roman times: the idea that the heart was the seat of consciousness, and the idea that intelligence was centred in the brain. Another difference, which was eventually to be reconciled in a higher synthesis by Galen, had also begun to make its appearance, a difference derived, as Rüsche has shown, from a difference in the conceptions of the pre-Socratic 'philosophers' Anaximenes and Empedocles as to the nature and location of the soul. Anaximenes identified it with air, and his disciple or follower Diogenes with the air, moving up and down the blood vessels. And both associated it with heat, Empedocles with hot blood, and Anaxagoras with hot air. For Empedocles the hot blood near the heart was the vehicle of the intelligence or soul, for Anaximenes the hot air was the soul itself.[3] We shall have the opportunity in the chapter which follows to examine the variations of these doctrines in the *Hippocratic corpus*.

[1] Erhard, op. cit., p. 353: 'Über seine Vorstellung vom Zentralorgan schreibt E. Krause, "Das Denken verlegte er weder in das Herz, noch in das Hirn, überhaupt in kein bestimmtes Organ, sondern in dem ganzen Leib." . . . Außerhalb des Kopfes hat Diogenes, wie mir scheint, all die Räume die er im Korper für lufthaltig hielt, für ein Zentralorgan gehalten. Bei der Anatomie am Toten mußte er alle Arterien und linke Vorkammer und linke Kammer des Herzens blutleer luftgefüllt gefunden haben. Im Kopfe dagegen scheint mir, hat er als Vermittlungsorgan für die Sinnesempfindungen die von ihm in das Gehirn angenommene Luft betrachtet. Dagegen war für Diogenes für das Zustandekommen der Sinnesempfindung und des Denkens das Gehirn, das er sich locker vorgestellt hat Zentralorgan. Vielleicht ist er dieser Auffassung von Alkmaion beeinflußt worden.'

[2] Aristotle, *De resp.* 1, 470ᵇ30–471ᵃ5: Ἀναξαγόρας δὲ καὶ Διογένης, πάντα φάσκοντες ἀναπνεῖν, περὶ τῶν ἰχθύων καὶ τῶν ὀστρείων λέγουσι τίνα τρόπον ἀναπνέουσι· καί φησιν Ἀναξαγόρας μέν, ὅταν ἀφῶσι τὸ ὕδωρ διὰ τῶν βραγχίων, τὸν ἐν τῷ στόματι γινόμενον ἀέρα ἕλκοντας ἀναπνεῖν τοὺς ἰχθῦς· οὐ γὰρ εἶναι κενὸν οὐδέν. Διογένης δέ, ὅταν ἀφῶσι τὸ ὕδωρ διὰ τῶν βραγχίων, ἐκ τοῦ περὶ τὸ στόμα περιεστῶτος ὕδατος, ἕλκειν τῷ κενῷ τῷ ἐν τῷ στόματι τὸν ἀέρα· ὡς ἐνόντος ἐν τῷ ὕδατι ἀέρος. ταῦτα δ' ἐστὶν ἀδύνατα.

[3] Rüsche, op. cit., p. 117, where he says of Diogenes: 'So ist das Blut Lebens- und Seelenträger, insofern es die Lebens- und Seelenluft in sich aufnimmt und mit ihr durch die Adern wallt. Von der Mischung der beiden und ihrere Verteilung im Körper hängen Leben und Gesundheit, Gemütszustande, Bewußtsein und Denkkraft ab.'
And p. 132, where speaking of Enpedocles, he says: 'Das Blut ist die Seele, das wird als Meinung des Empedocles überliefert. Nach vorstehenden Auseinandersetzungen ist das Wort zu nächst nach der psychologischen Seite hin so zu verstehen, daß das Blut infolge der vorzüglichen Mischung der Elemente in ihm der vorzügliche Träger der Geistestätigkeit ist.'

2 · 'HIPPOCRATES'

So far we have been dealing with authors whose doctrines can only be reconstructed piecemeal from a few fragments of quotation or doxographical *reportata*, some of them many centuries later. When we come to the *Hippocratic corpus* we are on quite different ground. The Hippocratic collection consists of a number of complete treatises or essays (though one at least would appear to be only a fragment) of varying dates and authorships, some, at any rate, of which go back to the later years of the fifth century B.C. But when we come to Hippocrates himself, difficulties at once occur. Some modern criticism has gone so far as to maintain that there is no evidence that even one single treatise of the works attributed to him was actually written by the Father of Medicine. Such, indeed, was the view of Edelstein,[1] who pursued much more radically the work of criticism inaugurated at the beginning of the century by Wilamowitz-Moellendorff. But as Pohlenz[2] has pointed out, Edelstein's view remains something of a paradox. It would certainly be something of a prank on the part of providence if really nothing of his genuine writings had survived. For the purposes of this work, it does not matter at all whether these treatises were written by 'Hippocrates', or by someone of the same or of a different name.[3] What is important is that we have here a unique collection of medical treatises written at various dates between 450 and 350 B.C. by persons who were for the most part experienced physicians, who held differing theories about the constitution of the human body and

[1] Edelstein, 'Περὶ ἀέρων und die Sammlung der Hippokratischen Schriften', *Problemata* 4 (Berlin, 1931); and 'The genuine works of Hippocrates', *Bull. Hist. Med.* 7 (1) 1939, 236–48.
[2] Pohlenz, *Hippokrates und die Begründung der wissenschaftlichen Medizin* (Berlin, 1938), pp. 3 f.: 'Es wäre eine schier unbegreifliche Tücke des Schicksals, wenn gerade die Werke des anerkannten Meisters spurlos verschwunden sein sollten. Es ist also einfach ein methodisches Postulat, daß unter den uns erhaltenen Schriften auch solche von Hippokrates selber sein müßen. Und damit ist der Forschung eine Aufgabe gewiesen, der sie sich nicht entziehen darf, mach sie auch diese Lösung noch so schwierig erscheinen.'
[3] For the controversy on the genuineness of the works of the Hippocratic collection, see, besides the works mentioned above: Edelstein's article 'Hippocrates', Pauly–Wissowa, *RE* Suppl. 6, 1290–1345; W. H. S. Jones, 'Hippocrates and the corpus Hippocraticum', *Proc. Br. Acad.* 31 (1945); Sigerist, 'On Hippocrates', *Bull. Hist. Med.* 2 (1934).

the treatment of disease, which, however inadequate by modern standards, were based on actual observations and on deductions from them, not merely on traditional folk-theories or superstitions. It is precisely this fact which has earned for the ancient Greeks the title of founders of scientific medicine, though this title has recently been disputed by Joly, who in his book on the scientific level of the Hippocratic works, points out the ambiguous use of the term 'scientific', which is properly applicable only to modern medicine from the nineteenth century onwards, and remarks that it would be preferable to call Hippocratic medicine rational rather than scientific.[1]

We are not, I believe, compelled to accept in all their rigour the nihilistic conclusions so alluringly displayed by Edelstein in the following words:

I feel however that the failure of the recent interpreters, as of all the previous ones, is fundamentally due to the peculiar difficulties of the problem with which they are faced. For the task set them is not to show the genuineness or spuriousness of some writings, which can be compared with those whose genuineness is unquestioned. Rather, it is demanded that without any possible comparison, one of the books of Hippocrates be identified, one book which then in turn can be used as a standard for other identifications . . . Yet neither Plato nor Meno quotes verbally from Hippocrates' works. They seem not even to use the specific terminology of Hippocrates, but to write them in their own terminology.[2]

Edelstein propounded the hypothesis that the works composing the *Corpus* all arrived in the library at Alexandria anonymously, and that they remained there until, in the third century B.C., the schools of Herophilus and Erasistratus developed the techniques of historical interpretation and set up the figure of the Father of Medicine, the completer of the traditional system of Greek dietetics, Hippocrates,[3] attributing to him an increasing

---

[1] R. Joly, *Le Niveau de la science hippocratique* (Paris, 1966), pp. 14 f.: 'Les rapports néo-hippocratiques cités plus haut affirment plusieurs fois que la médecine grecque classique n'étant plus magique ni religieuse, est scientifique. Voilà précisément le point où doit porter une analyse plus exigeante. Il est clair selon nous qu'une médecine qui a rompu avec la magie et l'explication religieuse n'est pas encore nécessairement et par le fait même scientifique. Elle est certainement rationnelle, mais il peut y avoir encore un abîme entre «rationnel» et «scientifique». C'est cet abîme que nous proposons de sonder.'

[2] Edelstein, 'The genuine works of Hippocrates', *Bull. Hist. Med.* 7 (1939).

[3] The passages from Plato and Aristotle in which Hippocrates is mentioned are reproduced in Jones, op. cit., in English translation. The Greek texts are as follows:

A. Plato, *Protagoras*, 311 b: Εἰπέ μοι, ἔφην ἐγώ, ὦ Ἱππόκρατες, παρὰ Πρωταγόραν νῦν ἐπιχειρεῖς ἰέναι ἀργύριον τελῶν ἐκείνῳ μισθὸν ὑπὲρ σεαυτοῦ, ὡς παρὰ τίνα ἀφιξόμενος καὶ τίς γενησόμενος; ὥσπερ ἂν εἰ ἐπενόεις παρὰ τὸν σαυτοῦ ὁμώνυμον ἐλθὼν Ἱπποκράτη τὸν Κῷον, τὸν τῶν Ἀσκληπιαδῶν, ἀργύριον τελεῖν ὑπὲρ σαυτοῦ μισθὸν ἐκείνῳ, εἰ τίς σε ἤρετο· εἰπέ μοι, μέλλεις τελεῖν, ὦ Ἱππόκρατες, Ἱπποκράτει μισθὸν ὡς τίνι ὄντι; τί ἂν ἀπεκρίνω; Εἶπον ἄν, ἔφη, ὅτι ὡς ἰατρῷ. ὡς τίς γενησόμενος; ὡς ἰατρός, ἔφη.

B. Plato, *Phaedrus*, 270 c, d: Ψυχῆς οὖν φύσιν ἀξίως λόγου κατανοῆσαι οἴει δυνατὸν εἶναι ἄνευ τῆς τοῦ ὅλου φύσεως; Εἰ μὲν Ἱπποκράτει γε τῷ τῶν Ἀσκληπιαδῶν δεῖ τι πείθεσθαι, οὐδὲ περὶ

number of these anonymous manuscripts. Though why Hippocrates should have been chosen as the peg to hang them on is not very convincingly demonstrated, nor is it explained why these manuscripts should have all arrived anonymously. Moreover, the one work that Hippocrates is reported to have written, according to Aristotle's pupil Meno, dealt not with dietetics, but with the causes of disease, which he attributed to 'blasts' or 'airs' (φῦσαι).[1] As an explanation of the origin of the *Corpus*, it seems to me that Jones's notion that it represents an actual collection of books belonging to the school of Cos or even to Hippocrates himself, though not very satisfying, is a good deal more probable.

It is, of course, true that, as Poschenrieder was the first to work out, passages in Plato, chiefly the *Timaeus*, and in Aristotle's biological works reproduce almost verbatim a number of sentences which are to be found in various treatises of the *Corpus*, without acknowledgement or the faintest indication that they are quotations. But the ethics of plagiarism were late to develop and scientific copyright is a comparatively modern notion. Moreover it might well have been considered that in a treatise which would be read by a small body of 'experts' quotation marks were obviously unnecessary, more particularly in the case of the works of a great master whose views were widely known. It is a little difficult to believe that absolutely no genuine work of Hippocrates was known to the generation which followed his death at an advanced age at the traditional date of 357 B.C. For it would appear from the way in which both Plato and Aristotle mention him that his fame must have been very considerable and very widespread in the Hellenic world. Had he really been, as Wilamowitz put it, a name without works,[2] this fact would scarcely have escaped later commentators or the writers of immediately succeeding

σώματος ἄνευ τῆς μεθόδου ταύτης. Καλῶς γάρ, ὦ ἑταῖρε, λέγει. χρὴ μέντοι πρὸς τῷ Ἱπποκράτει τὸν λόγον ἐξετάζοντα σκοπεῖν, εἰ συμφωνεῖ. Φημί. Τὸ τοίνυν περὶ φύσεως σκόπει, τί ποτε λέγει Ἱπποκράτης τε καὶ ὁ ἀληθὴς λόγος. ἆρ' οὐχ ὧδε δεῖ διανοεῖσθαι περὶ ὁτουοῦν φύσεως; πρῶτον μέν, ἁπλοῦν ἢ πολυειδές ἐστιν οὗ πέρι βουλησόμεθα εἶναι αὐτοὶ τεχνικοὶ καὶ ἄλλον δυνατοὶ ποιεῖν, ἔπειτα δέ, ἐὰν μὲν ἁπλοῦν ᾖ, σκοπεῖν τὴν δύναμιν αὐτοῦ, τίνα πρὸς τί πέφυκεν εἰς τὸ δρᾶν ἔχον ἢ τίνα εἰς τὸ παθεῖν ὑπὸ τοῦ; ἐὰν δὲ πλείω εἴδη ἔχῃ, ταῦτα ἀριθμησάμενος, ὅπερ ἐφ' ἑνός, τοῦτ' ἰδεῖν ἐφ' ἑκάστου, τῷ τί ποιεῖν αὐτὸ πέφυκεν ἢ τῷ τί παθεῖν ὑπὸ τοῦ; Κινδυνεύει, ὦ Σώκρατες. Ἡ γοῦν ἄνευ τούτων μέθοδος ἐοίκει ἂν ὥσπερ τυφλοῦ πορείᾳ.

C. Aristotle, *Politics* 7. 4, 1326ᵃ13–16: ἔστι γάρ τι καὶ πόλεως ἔργον· ὥστε τὴν δυναμένην τοῦτο μάλιστ' ἀποτελεῖν, ταύτην οἰητέον εἶναι μεγίστην· οἷον Ἱπποκράτην οὐκ ἄνθρωπον ἀλλ' ἰατρὸν εἶναι μείζω φήσειεν ἄν τις τοῦ διαφέροντος κατὰ τὸ μέγεθος τοῦ σώματος.

Edelstein, loc. cit., quotes in this connection an Alexandrian scholion to Homer, which reads: τοῦ (γὰρ) διαιτητικοῦ Ἡρόδικος μὲν ἦρξατο, συνετέλεσε δὲ καὶ Ἱπποκράτης, Πραξαγόρας, Χρύσιππος.

[1] That is, assuming that the doctrine attributed to Hippocrates is that contained in the work Περὶ φυσῶν of the Hippocratic collection, which is however doubtful, as this has been usually considered as the work of a 'sophist', and the doctrine contained in it does not correspond at all accurately with the account given in the fragment of Meno.

[2] As Jones remarked, op. cit.: 'The quotation from Wilamowitz reads: "Hippokrates ist zur Zeit ein berühmter Name, ohne Hintergrund irgend einer Schrift."'

generations. Nor, in my opinion, should too much stress be laid on the presumed fragment from the *Menoneia* contained in the papyrus known as the *Anonymus Londinensis*. Jones agreed with Edelstein that there was no absolute proof that any of the works in the *Corpus* were genuine, but both he and most other critics have been content to consider some of the works in the collection as really Hippocrates' work; in the last resort because they form a fairly coherent body of doctrine, and because they were written by a man who was without question an outstanding physician. In the list given in the footnote below,[1] it will appear that various critics have made various choices, and show a considerable coefficient of agreement. Moreover there can have been little doubt even in the mind of Edelstein, that most of the works included in the *Corpus* were written in the fifth or in the fourth centuries B.C. Among the most recent critics must be numbered Kudlien, who seems to be inclined to treat *Prognostic* and *Epidemics* i and iii as genuine. He believes them to have been written about 410 B.C., and remarks that if they are not by Hippocrates, then Hippocrates becomes a legend, although he admits that even in these three treatises there are inconsistencies. *Ancient medicine*, *Airs, waters, and places*, *Nature of man*, *Regimen*, *Regimen in acute diseases*, and *The art* all belong to the later half of the fourth century B.C., as well as the other books of the *Epidemics*. Sigerist, though he regarded Edelstein's thesis as 'the most illuminating hypothesis on the subject ever posed', and his monograph 'the most important contribution to the Hippocratic problem since the time of Littré', did not himself accept Edelstein's conclusions. He adopted an attitude to be justified perhaps by the Jamesian 'will to believe' which in the circumstances would appear to be reasonable: 'Personally I incline to the belief that the *corpus Hippocraticum* does contain books written by the master, though I cannot prove it, and cannot tell which books must be his work.'[2]

The higher criticism of the Hippocratic canon is scarcely less complicated than its Biblical homonym, and its conclusions far from certain.

---

[1] As Edelstein noted, op. cit.: Littré regarded as genuine *Ancient medicine*, *Prognostic*, *Aphorisms*, *Epidemics* i and iii, *Regimen in acute diseases*, *Airs, waters, and places*, *Fractures*, *Joints*, *Instruments of reduction*, *Wounds in the head*, the *Oath*, and *Law*.

Deichgräber considered genuine *Epidemics* i and ii, iii, iv, and vi, the *Surgery*, *Instruments of reduction*, and *Humours*, and found a close relation between these and *Prognostic*, *Fractures*, *Joints*, and *Nature of man* as well as *Airs, waters, and places*, *Sacred disease*, and even *Epidemics* v and vii.

Pohlenz holds to be authentic *Sacred disease*, *Airs, waters, and places*, *Prognostic*, *Epidemics* i and iii, but he is undecided about *Fractures*, and *Joints*.

Nestle, *Hermes* 73 (1938) asserts the authenticity of *Prognostic*, *Epidemics* i and iii, *Airs, waters, and places*, *Fractures*, *Joints*, *Instruments of reduction*, *Sacred disease*, parts of the *Aphorisms*, *Regimen in health*, and *Epidemics* ii, iv, and vi.

Sticker, the collaborator of Kapferer, assumed that the whole *Corpus* was written by the same author, who was of course Hippocrates, a belief which Sigerist calls a kind of fairy tale; 'On Hippocrates', *Bull. Hist. Med.* 2 (1934).

[2] Sigerist, *History of Medicine*, 2. 266.

The word 'Hippocratic' could thus be very misleading. In view of all these doubts I prefer henceforward to print 'Hippocrates' in inverted commas.

The bulk of the *Corpus* consists of about sixty treatises, a large part of which we may for convenience label as pre-Aristotelian.[1] Only comparatively few of them are devoted exclusively to anatomical or physiological topics, and those that deal with these questions are certainly not the works of a single author, a fact that was already recognized in the school of Alexandria in which the *Corpus* was assembled. Among them are works belonging to at least three different schools of early Greek medical thought, which has generally been divided by historians into three main groups, the Coan, the Cnidian, and the Italo-Sicilian. Many of the treatises as they have come down to us contain discrete passages from various sources, and much of their anatomical and physiological content is in the form of notes to therapeutic or surgical essays or handbooks. For our present purposes we may divide the physiological works into two classes, those which regard the head as the seat of the intelligence, and those which assign this function to the heart. Of these two doctrines, the former has been regarded as 'Hippocratic' and identified with the school of Cos. It is the doctrine expressed most fully in the treatise *On the sacred disease*, a work which, though its authenticity is not now generally accepted, has by tradition been reckoned as typically 'Hippocratic'. And it was, perhaps, this treatise, or at any rate the doctrine expressed in it, which inspired the Anonymous Parisian of Fuchs's *Anecdota medica* in his picturesque description of 'Hippocrates' ' teaching, that the mind was installed in the brain like the sacred image in the Acropolis of the body.[2] The same doctrine seems also to be implied in the treatise *On the nature of man*, which has generally been attributed to Polybus, Hippocrates' son-in-law, since Aristotle, in the *History of Animals* Bk. III cap. iii quotes verbatim the chapter (xi) giving the description of the principal blood vessels. These all start from the head.[3] Several of the treatises of the *Corpus* on

---

[1] Sigerist, op. cit., regards as definitely post-Aristotelian among others the treatise *On nourishment* and Book vii of the *Epidemics*, to which we must almost certainly add the fragment *On the heart*.

[2] AMG (1894), fr. 1 contains the following sentence: ὁ δὲ ῾Ιπποκράτης τὸν μὲν νοῦν φησὶν ἐν τῷ ἐγκεφάλῳ τετάχθαι καθάπερ τι ἱερὸν ἄγαλμα ἐν ἀκροπόλει τοῦ σώματος. χρῆσθαι δὲ τροφῇ τῷ περὶ τὴν χοριοειδῆ μήνιγγα αἵματι. The same figure of the sacred image is also found in Galen's treatise *De remediis potabilibus*, K. xiv. 313: ἀπὸ κεφαλῆς ἀρξάμενος· αὕτη γὰρ καθάπερ τις ἀκρόπολίς ἐστι τοῦ σώματος κατὰ τῶν τιμιωτάτων καὶ ἀναγκαιοτάτων ἀνθρώποις αἰσθήσεων οἰκητήριον. But it is not found, as far as I am aware, in the *Corpus* itself. Is it perhaps an invention of the Anonymous Parisian himself, who has been taken by some critics to be Soranus? Or is it, as Wellmann has suggested, contained in a lost work of Hippocrates himself? See Wellmann, *Fragmente*, p. 19.

[3] It is, however, probable that this chapter is an insertion taken from some other work. It seems to have little or no connection with the preceding or succeeding chapters. Galen, as we shall see, refused to attribute it either to Polybus or to Hippocrates.

C

the other hand, like that *On places in man* and *On diseases*, not to mention the fragment *On the heart*, follow the Cnidian tradition which make the heart the centre of consciousness.[1]

Before proceeding to the task of analysing the various treatises of the *Corpus* with respect to their doctrines on the heart and the vascular system, it may perhaps be well to consider, very briefly, the general ideas on human physiology which had been developed by the second half of the fifth century B.C. It needs a considerable effort of the imagination to form any picture in one's mind of the state of knowledge in the age of Pericles, before any but the simplest forms of measurement had been thought of, and before even the most elementary notions of physics and chemistry were understood. The behaviour of 'things', including, of course, animal and human bodies, while they could no longer be attributed to any personal agency, had to be interpreted in terms of sensible qualities and the still comparatively simple techniques of agriculture, ceramics, and metallurgy. Hence the enormous importance attributed to form or shape, which under Plato was to become a metaphysic, and to the qualities perceived by touch—heat and cold, and wetness and dryness, which with the addition of the elements of geometry, provided the only principles by which observed changes could be interpreted. The genius of the Greek mind, something altogether new in the history of human thought, was really the passion for explanation—the itch to generalize, often, too often alas, on insufficient grounds and wholly unsatisfactory evidence. But it was this passion which succeeded in laying the foundations of what we today call science.

The attempts to interpret physical changes in terms, not of a God, but of a single substance was the great problem of the early Milesians. The hypotheses advanced by the earlier thinkers, 'all is water' (Thales); 'all is air' (Anaximenes); 'all is fire' (Heracleitus), had all broken down under criticism. A brilliant hypothesis, that of atoms existing in a void, had been formulated by Leucippus and Democritus, but this, too, presented metaphysical difficulties, and all evidence for it was lacking *ex hypothesi*, since atoms were far too small to be seen, and the void was of course invisible. The way out of the paradoxes presented by Parmenides and the Eleatics was therefore sought in another direction—a 'common-sense' explanation of change in terms of four elementary substances with which everybody in his practical life was necessarily acquainted, earth, air,

---

[1] For a discussion of the so-called Cnidian treatises in the *Hippocratic corpus*, see the article by I. M. Lonie, *Classical Quarterly* N.S. 15 (1965). According to Lonie the only works which are certainly Cnidian are the following: Περὶ παθῶν, Περὶ νούσων i and ii (1–40), and iii, and Περὶ τῶν ἐντὸς παθῶν. Lonie gives good reasons for supposing that none of the others is, whereas Ilberg looked upon no less than twelve works of the *Corpus* as Cnidian. The treatise *On regimen in acute diseases* has also been regarded as showing Cnidian influence or even provenance by some critics, e.g. Edelstein, article in *Problemata*, op. cit.

fire, and water; a solution to the problem of change put forward by the
least common-sensible of the earlier sages, namely Empedocles. It was in
terms of these four elementary substances with their four primary
qualities that most of the physicians of the later fifth and even more of the
fourth century B.C. tried to explain the workings of the human body.

Now what did the most elementary acquaintance with the facts of life
suggest? What must all living creatures do to keep alive, and how does
the touch and feel and behaviour of a corpse differ from that of a living
body?[1] In order to keep alive, all animals and all men have to breathe
and to take nourishment. We know by direct experience that as soon as
a man altogether stops breathing, even for a very short time, he dies, and
we know, too, that if he is deprived of food, and more particularly of
drink, for more than quite a limited number of days, he also dies. We
know, too, that when he stops breathing he loses consciousness, that is, he
ceases to be aware of any sense perceptions. Indeed, we have often observed that before death takes place, hearing, sight, touch, and taste have,
sometimes for a considerable period, ceased to function. And when a man
is dead, his body looks and feels and behaves quite differently from the
way in which it did when he was still alive, several hours before the
repellent but striking phenomena of putrefaction have set in. Moreover a
corpse is cold, whereas a living body is warm; moreover it does not move,
and becomes stiff, nor does it bleed when cut or pricked in the same way
as a living body—one of the prime discoveries of forensic medicine which
must have revealed itself at a very early date.

From these elementary observations common to all mankind, the Greek
physicians of the fifth century B.C. and their immediate successors
attempted to build up a physiological system connecting the phenomena
of respiration, blood-flow, alimentation, sensation, and thought in a
coherent scheme. On the purely anatomical side they had a pretty
thorough knowledge of external features of the human body. The training of athletes must have given them considerable insight into the way the
body works, fairly intimate acquaintance with the articulation of the
limbs, and some knowledge of the skeleton and the externally traceable
blood vessels, almost entirely veins. The trainer in the palaestra may have
acquired something of the technique of the bone-setter which we know
that he passed on to the physician, who in certain cases studied under him.
But, as some of the earlier works of the *Hippocratic corpus* show quite
plainly, his knowledge of the internal organs was incredibly primitive.
With the outward shape and situation of the major internal organs, he
was, of course, familiar. So much he must have gathered from the
butcher, but not, it would appear, very much more before the end of the
fifth century B.C. But the practice of animal dissection was probably not

[1] Cf. Hippocrates, *Regimen*, i. 12: οὐχ ὅμοιον ἀποθανὼν ζώοντι.

uncommon at the beginning of the fourth century B.C., and Galen informs us that Diocles was the first to write a book on anatomy, i.e. dissection. A more detailed knowledge of the animal organism must have started to accumulate early in the fourth century B.C., but it was not until the third that the great anatomical discoveries were made. Before the end of the fifth century the kitchen and the butcher's yard had given them a fair acquaintance with the stomach and intestines, the liver and the gall-bladder, the spleen, the kidneys, the bladder, as well as the lungs and the heart, the bronchi, and the oesophagus. They were also acquainted with the diaphragm and the peritoneum, and the division of the trunk into the thoracic and abdominal cavities. As Sigerist has remarked:

The keen sense of observation that these doctors showed at the bedside of patients did not fail them when they looked at organs. Anatomical data are scattered all through the Hippocratic collection, and the surgical treatises obviously presuppose anatomical knowledge. Surgery, however, requires familiarity with topographical anatomy, and an ancient surgeon might have known the shoulder in every detail without having the faintest idea of the pancreas in its relation to the intestinal tract. Still, the ancients knew more anatomy than we commonly assume. In a seminar course we once made a study of the ancient physicians' knowledge of the liver and were astonished to find that the Alexandrian anatomists and Galen added very little to what the Hippocratic doctors knew about this organ.[1]

This means that they had already discovered not only the gall-bladder and its connections with the liver and the intestinal tract (yellow bile was to play an important part in their physiological and nosological inter-pretations), but also the portal system of veins, the veins leading from the intestinal tract to the liver. They also had some acquaintance with the main blood vessels of the belly and the thorax, the superior and inferior venae cavae, as well as the thoracic and descending aortae. But of the heart itself their knowledge seems to have been surprisingly limited, if we except the treatise *On the heart* which, as we shall see, is certainly much later than Hippocrates, whose dates are quite firmly established beyond the assault of any sceptical criticism.[2] Of the distinction between arteries and veins there is as yet little trace. The word φλέψ is applied to both quite indiscriminately, though there is some evidence that the distinction between the 'hollow or big vein' and the aorta was made at any rate early in the fourth century B.C. The distinction between the two is to be found in the treatise *On fleshes*,[3] though this is almost certainly one of the late works of the Hippocratic collection. Even as late as Aristotle the

---

[1] Sigerist, op. cit., p. 277.
[2] For a discussion of the date of the *De corde*, see below, pp. 83 ff.
[3] *De carnibus*, 5: δύο γάρ εἰσι κοῖλαι φλέβες ἀπὸ τῆς καρδίης, τῇ μὲν ὄνομα ἀρτηρίη, τῇ δὲ κοίλη φλέψ.

anatomy of the heart was only imperfectly understood, since this physician's son, though acquainted with the aorta,[1] believes that the hearts of the larger animals, including man, have three ventricles,[2] and of the valves he does not appear to have had the faintest conception. Of the nervous system their knowledge was practically nil. The word νεῦρον, which originally means a tendon or a sinew, is used indifferently for these anatomical features, as well as for what we now call nerves (compare the French words *nerf* and *nerveux*) and is used sometimes in earlier works to denote muscles as well as ligaments. Even Galen believed that nerves usually ended in tendons, while before the discovery by the Alexandrians of the nervous system, the functions which were later attributed to it were supposed to be performed by blood vessels. Thus in the 'Hippocratic' treatise *On the nature of bones* we are told that it is the veins which distribute the power of action. It was left to the Alexandrians Herophilus and Erasistratus to discover this important system of the animal anatomy. Yet, in spite of these deficiencies, an intelligible physiological picture was beginning to emerge.

The connection of breathing with life was conceived somewhat differently by the various schools: those who like the 'Hippocratic' school of Cos followed Alcmaeon in giving the primacy to the brain, and those who like the Cnidians and the Sicilians regarded the heart as the principle organ. The latter followed in the path of Empedocles and adopted his theory of respiration in believing that inspiration took place not only through the nostrils but also throughout the whole body, through the 'pores'.[3] They regarded the *pneuma* as the 'vehicle' of reason. It was Philistion of Locri who, according to Wellmann,[4] was the first propounder of this theory. But what exactly the mechanics of the process were we are not informed. Empedocles wrote of 'pipes' (σύριγγες) through which air was sucked in, too narrow for the blood to pass, at any rate through their terminations; but they would appear to be continuous with the blood vessels, of which we have no description, nor have we of their connections with the heart. He seems to have conceived the blood vessels as ending in capillaries opening into the pores of the skin; the word *poros* means channel. Nor does our only account of the teaching of Philistion throw any light on the conception that he had of the vascular system. But there can be no doubt that we have here the origin of the doctrine of arterial respiration, which was to play so important a part in the physiology of Galen. Philistion is also important because he was the first we know of to adopt the theory that the body was made up of the

---

[1] The use of the word ἀόρτη would appear to have been originally as ambiguous as that of ἀρτηρίη, so Rufus of Ephesus tells us, *De nominibus partium hominis* (Daremberg–Ruelle), p. 155: αἱ δὲ εἰς τὸν πλεύμονα ἀποφύσεις βρόγχαι καὶ σήραγγες καὶ ἄορται.

[2] For Aristotle's teaching on the heart, see below, pp. 160 ff.

[3] See *Anon. Lond.* xx, J. 80.   [4] *Fragmente*, pp. 69 f.

four Empedoclean elements. We know, too, that he was the master of the two Cnidian physicians Eudoxus and Chrysippus of the fourth century B.C., who likewise made the heart the seat of the intelligence.

If Wellmann's suggestion is correct, Philistion's physiology, which exercised so great an influence on Diocles, appears to have borrowed elements both from Empedocles and from Diogenes of Apollonia; the theory of the four elements from the former and the theory of the air-soul from the latter, only in his case *pneuma* is no longer the soul itself, but only the instrument or vehicle of life and thought. We shall see later how this combination of the doctrine of the supremacy of the heart, together with the notion of *pneuma* as the life-spirit, was to be refurbished in the pneumatism of the Stoic philosophy and the Pneumatic school of medicine.

The role assigned to the *pneuma* by the school of Cos, since we are no longer entitled to attribute the treatises to be discussed to Hippocrates himself, was scarcely less important, though its physiological mechanism was conceived rather differently. Thus in the famous work *On the sacred disease*, the author describes the course of the *pneuma* in the process of respiration as going first to the brain, then, most of it, to the belly, and then some of it to the lungs and the veins. It appears to have a double transit to that organ, since all of it goes there in the first place, while some of it returns via the veins. The heart is not mentioned except incidentally, because the head, not the heart, is regarded as the source or focus of the blood vessels, which come up to the brain from every part of the body. And it is through the blood vessels in the head that respiration principally takes place. The idea that some of the *pneuma* returns to the brain via the veins is interesting, since it would appear to be one of the origins of the theory of psychic *pneuma* which was to be developed first by Erasistratus and later by Galen.

Other treatises of the *Corpus*, notably the one miscalled *On the nature of bones*, devote some passages to the description of the blood vessels connecting the lungs and the heart. Kapferer would have us believe that the author of this treatise was acquainted with both the pulmonary arteries and the pulmonary veins and their mutual connections.[1] But the ambiguity of the word ἀρτηρία, especially in connection with the lungs, makes the interpretation of this text, which as we shall see is a collection of paragraphs taken from very different sources, more than usually difficult.[2] In another treatise of the *Corpus*, *On diseases*, we find, if not expounded, at any rate foreshadowed the discovery, generally attributed to Aristotle,[3]

---

[1] Kapferer (with A. Fingerle and F. Lommer), *Die anatomischen Schriften, die Anatomie, das Herz, die Adern, in der Hippokratischen Sammlung* (Stuttgart, 1951), pp. 19, 21, 32, 40 f., 47, etc. See also his article 'Die Lungenadern in der antiken Literatur', *Münch. med. Wschr.* (1955), 672–4.

[2] See below, pp. 63 f.

[3] Littré, i. 222; ix. 163.

that the heart is the centre of the vascular system.[1] The connections between the heart and the lungs having been established correctly (if, as Kapferer asserts, this was really done, for Aristotle, as we shall see, had no very clear notions on this subject), the next step might be expected to have been the discovery of the circulation, but that was not to be. We really have no evidence when, if indeed at all, the gross anatomy of the heart and the main blood vessels was established before Herophilus. But this is to anticipate.

Our present task is to examine in some detail the principal treatises in the *Corpus* which deal with the heart and the vascular system, without going into the question of their exact dates and reputed authenticity, except in so far as concerns the fragment *On the heart*. Apart from this document there are a large number of treatises in the collection, which contain long passages devoted to our subject, one of them dealing almost exclusively with the description of the vascular system. This is the treatise misnamed *On the nature of bones*, of which only two short paragraphs are devoted to the subject of the title. It is obviously a collection of material from various sources; two chapters are taken from other works in the *Corpus*, another from Aristotle, but a succession of consecutive chapters constitutes the longest treatise in the *Corpus* dealing with our subject. The essay *On the nature of man*, that *On the sacred disease*, the treatises *On the fleshes* and *On nourishment*, the fragment *On anatomy*, the book *On diet*, the treatise *On diseases*, two of the books *On epidemics*, as well as the treatises *On interior ailments* and *On joints*, and the essay *On places in man* all contain passages dealing with the vascular system, the more important of which will be quoted. The theories put forward in these different passages are by no means consistent. Thus, as we shall see, the author of the *Sacred disease* has quite a different conception of the blood vessels from that of the author of the fragment *On the heart*, while the description given in the work *On the nature of the bones* contains a passage taken from the work *On the nature of man* which is quite inconsistent with that given in the rest of the treatise.

In analysing the various passages, it would appear to be convenient to begin by classifying them in accordance with their apposite views concerning the primacy of the organs, the head or the heart. The description given in two of the more important treatises, that *On the sacred disease* and that *On the nature of man*, is in both cases based on the primacy of the head, this primacy being explicitly asserted in the former, though only implied in the latter. Both regard the head as the starting-point or focus of the

---

[1] See Hippocrates, *De morbis*, 33, 34; also *De alimento*, 31. Compare also the remark in the treatise *On joints*, 45: αἱ δὲ φλεβῶν καὶ ἀρτηριῶν κοινωνίαι ἐν ἑτέρῳ λόγῳ δεδηλώσονται, ὅσαι τε καὶ οἷαι καὶ ὅθεν ὡρμημέναι καὶ ἐν οἷοισι οἷα δύνανται. *Pace* Kapferer, no 'Hippocratic' text answering this description has come down to us.

'veins', i.e. the blood vessels. This notion, quite apart from any hierarchical consideration of precedence, would appear to have suggested itself very naturally to people habituated, through the course of many centuries, to sacrificial throat-cutting,[1] who had observed, as the Greeks already had, the double jugular veins and carotid arteries going up each side of the neck.

The description of the process of respiration, given in the first of these works to which we have already alluded, runs as follows:

For when a man draws in breath through the mouth and nostrils, the *pneuma* passes first to the brain, and then the greater part goes to the belly, but some to the lungs and to the veins. From these places it is distributed throughout the whole body by means of the veins. The *pneuma* which flows to the stomach cools it, but makes no other contribution. But that which goes to the lungs and the veins enters from these into the cavities of the body and the brain, and has a further purpose. It induces intelligence, and is necessary for the movement of the limbs. For when the veins are shut off from the air by phlegm and do not receive any, it makes a man speechless and mindless.[2]

The main blood vessels leading to the brain are also described:

And veins reach it [sc. the brain] from all parts of the body, many of them thin veins, but two thick ones, one from the liver and the other from the spleen. And the one that comes from the liver runs like this. Part of the vessel reaches down through the parts on the right side past the kidney itself, and the loin into the interior of the thigh, and it reaches the foot. It is called the 'hollow' vein. And the other part goes upwards through the right side of the diaphragm and the lung, and it has a branch going to the heart and to the right arm. And the rest of it goes upwards, passing beyond the collar-bone to the right side of the neck, quite close to the skin, so as to be plainly visible. And by the ear it disappears from sight, and there it branches into two, and the thickest and biggest and most hollow branch ends up in the brain, but the smaller branch puts forth a thin little vein into the right ear, and another into the right eye, and another into the nostril. These are the veins that come from the liver. And from the spleen there is also a vein which extends both upwards and downwards on the left side, like that from the liver, but it is thinner and weaker.[3]

[1] Cf., e.g., Homer, *Iliad*, iii. 292 ff.:

Ἦ καὶ ἀπὸ στομάχους ἀρνῶν τάμε νηλέϊ χαλκῷ
καὶ τοὺς μὲν κατέθηκεν ἐπὶ χθονὸς ἀσπαίροντας
θυμοῦ δευομένους· ἀπὸ γὰρ μένος εἵλετο χαλκός.

[2] *De morbo sacro*, 10: ὅταν γὰρ λάβῃ ἄνθρωπος κατὰ τὸ στόμα καὶ τοὺς μυκτῆρας τὸ πνεῦμα, πρῶτον μὲν ἐς τὸν ἐγκέφαλον ἔρχεται. ἔπειτα δὲ ἐς τὴν κοιλίην τὸ πλεῖστον μέρος τὸ δὲ ἐπὶ τὸν πλεύμονα, τὸ δὲ ἐπὶ τὰς φλέβας. ἐκ τούτων δὲ σκίδναται ἐς τὰ λοιπὰ μέρεα κατὰ τὰς φλέβας· καὶ ὅσον μὲν ἐς τὴν κοιλίην ἔρχεται, τοῦτο μὲν τὴν κοιλίην διαψύχει, καὶ ἄλλο οὐδὲν συμβάλλεται· ὁ δ' ἐς τὸν πλευμονά τε καὶ τὰς φλέβας ἀὴρ συμβάλλεται ἐς τὰς κοιλίας ἐσιὼν καὶ ἐς τὸν ἐγκέφαλον, καὶ οὕτω τὴν φρόνησιν καὶ τὴν κίνησιν τοῖς μέλεσι παρέχει, ὥστε ἐπειδὰν ἀποκλεισθῶσιν αἱ φλέβες τοῦ ἠέρος ὑπὸ τοῦ φλέγματος, καὶ μὴ παραδέχωνται ἄφωνον καθιστᾶσι καὶ ἄφρονα τὸν ἄνθρωπον.

[3] Ibid., 6: καὶ φλέβες δ' ἐς αὐτὸν τείνουσιν ἐξ ἅπαντος τοῦ σώματος, πολλαὶ καὶ λεπταί, δύο δὲ παχεῖαι, ἡ μὲν ἀπὸ τοῦ ἥπατος, ἡ δὲ ἀπὸ τοῦ σπληνός. καὶ ἡ μὲν ἀπὸ τοῦ ἥπατος ὧδ' ἔχει· τὸ μέν τι

And along these veins we also bring in most of the *pneuma*. For these are our channels of inspiration which draw air into themselves, and channel it into the rest of the body along the veins, and cool it and again send it out. For *pneuma* is unable to stay still, but goes up and down. For if it stands still anywhere and is blocked, that part wherever it stays still becomes powerless, i.e. incapable of motion. And the proof of this is the fact that whenever the veins of a man are compressed, through sitting or lying down, so that the *pneuma* can no longer pass through the veins, numbness immediately supervenes.[1]

This topographical description of the 'veins' would seem to be a simplified version of that given by Diogenes of Apollonia, which fails altogether to distinguish the vascular from the tracheal system. The author of the treatise we have for a long time ceased to call Hippocrates, since Littré did not consider it as genuine,[2] even though on account of its insistence on the natural, as opposed to the supernatural, origin of disease, it is one of the writings which, almost more than any other, earned for Hippocrates the title of the Father of Medicine. Like Diogenes, the author of this treatise regards air as the vital principle. In the passage we have just quoted he insists that it 'provides thought', and in another place he tries to give a physical explanation of this fact in terms of respiration.

It ought to be generally known that the source of our pleasure, merriment, laughter, and amusement, as of our grief, pain, anxiety, and tears is none other than the brain.[3]

τῆς φλεβὸς κάτω τείνει, διὰ τῶν ἐπὶ δεξιὰ παρ' αὐτὸν τὸν νεφρὸν καὶ τὴν φυὴν ἐς τὸ ἐντὸς τοῦ μηροῦ, καὶ καθήκει ἐς τὸν πόδα καὶ καλέεται κοίλη φλέψ. ἡ δ' ἑτέρη ἄνω τείνει διὰ φρενῶν τῶν δεξιῶν καὶ τοῦ πλεύμονος· ἀπέσχισται δὲ καὶ ἐς τὴν καρδίην καὶ ἐς τὸν βραχίονα τὸν δεξιόν. τὸ δὲ λοιπὸν ἄνω φέρει διὰ τῆς κληῖδος ἐς τὰ δεξιὰ τοῦ αὐχένος, ἐς αὐτὸ τὸ δέρμα ὥστε κατάδηλος εἶναι. παρὰ δὲ τὸ οὖς κρύπτεται καὶ ἐνταῦθα σχίζεται, καὶ τὸ μὲν παχύτατον καὶ μέγιστον καὶ κοιλότατον ἐς τὸν ἐγκέφαλον τελευτᾷ, τὸ δὲ ἐς τὸ οὖς τὸ δεξιὸν φλέβιον λεπτόν, τὸ δὲ ἐς τὸν ὀφθαλμὸν τὸν δεξιόν, τὸ δὲ ἐς τὸν μυκτῆρα. ἀπὸ μὲν τοῦ ἥπατος οὕτως ἔχει τὰ τῶν φλεβῶν. διατέταται δὲ καὶ ἀπὸ τοῦ σπληνὸς φλέψ ἐς τὰ ἀριστερὰ καὶ κάτω καὶ ἄνω, ὥσπερ καὶ ἀπὸ τοῦ ἥπατος, λεπτοτέρη δὲ καὶ ἀσθενεστέρη.

[1] Ibid., 7: κατὰ ταύτας δὲ τὰς φλέβας καὶ εἰσαγόμεθα τὸ πουλὺ τοῦ πνεύματος· αὐταὶ γὰρ ἡμέων εἰσὶν ἀναπνοαὶ τοῦ σώματος τὸν ἠέρα ἐς σφᾶς ἕλκουσαι. καὶ ἐς τὸ σῶμα τὸ λοιπὸν ὀχετεύουσι κατὰ τὰ φλέβια, καὶ ἀναψύχουσι καὶ πάλιν ἀφιᾶσιν. οὐ γὰρ οἷόν τε τὸ πνεῦμα στῆναι, ἀλλὰ χωρέει, ἄνω τε καὶ κάτω· ἢν γὰρ στῇ που καὶ ἀποληφθῇ, ἀκρατὲς γίνεται ἐκεῖνο τὸ μέρος, ὅπου ἂν στῇ. τεκμήριον δέ· ὁκόταν καθημένῳ ἢ κατακειμένῳ φλέβια πιεσθῇ, ὥστε τὸ πνεῦμα μὴ διεξιέναι διὰ τῆς φλεβός, εὐθὺς νάρκη ἕλκει.

[2] Littré does not regard it as genuine and most critics have agreed with him. He informs us of a gloss attached marginally to some manuscripts to the effect that Galen too regarded it as spurious. Its reproduction of Diogenes of Apollonia's scheme of blood vessels suggests that it is at any rate one of the earlier treatises in the *Corpus*. The gloss reads as follows: οὐ γνήσιον Ἱπποκράτους ἀξιόλογον δὲ ἀνδρός φησιν ὁ Γάληνος, καὶ κατὰ ἑρμηνείαν καὶ κατὰ τὴν διάνοιαν. Ἱπποκράτους δὲ οὐδὲν ἐν αὐτῷ, οὔτε κατὰ τὸν τρόπον τῆς ἑρμηνείας, οὔτε κατὰ τὸ τῆς διανοίας ἀκριβές (Littré i. 353 ff.).

[3] *De morbo sacro*, 17: εἰδέναι δὲ χρὴ τοὺς ἀνθρώπους, ὅτι ἐξ οὐδενὸς ἡμῖν αἱ ἡδοναὶ γίνονται καὶ εὐφροσύναι καὶ γέλωτες καὶ παιδιαὶ ἢ ἐντεῦθεν, καὶ λῦπαι καὶ κλαυθμοί. καὶ τούτῳ φρονέομεν μάλιστα καὶ βλέπομεν καὶ ἀκούομεν καὶ διαγινώσκομεν τά τε αἰσχρὰ καὶ καλὰ καὶ ἀγαθὰ καὶ ἡδέα καὶ ἀηδέα.

For these reasons I believe the brain to be the most powerful organ in the body. For it is the interpreter of the things that affect us from the air. Consciousness is caused by air. The eyes, ears, tongue, hands, and feet perform actions which are planned by the brain, for there is a measure of conscious thought throughout the body in proportion to the amount of air it receives. The brain is also the organ of understanding, for when a man draws in a breath it reaches the brain first, and thence is distributed to the rest of the body having left behind in the brain its vigour and whatever pertains to understanding and intelligence. For if the air went first to the body and then to the brain, it would only come there after leaving behind its power of judgement in the tissues and in the veins, and would come to the brain in a heated condition and not pure but mixed with the fluid from the tissues and the blood, which would blunt its precision.[1]

This theory of the evil effects of moisture on the mind-*pneuma* we have just met in Diogenes, but the notion of the brain as the controlling organ would appear, as Wellmann suggests, to be derived from Alcmaeon.[2]

The cause of the sacred disease is described as the blocking of the passage of respired air into the blood vessels of the brain by phlegm, which has just been described, and the symptoms resulting from it are those usually associated with an epileptic fit.

The hands are paralysed and twisted when the blood is still and is not distributed as usual. The eyes roll when the minor veins are shut off from the air and pulsate. The foaming at the mouth comes from the lungs: for when the breath fails to enter them they foam and boil as though they were dying, and excrement is discharged as they are forcibly compressed, etc.[3]

A similar theory of the causation of various mental diseases is also to be found in the *Timaeus*,[4] presumably derived from the teaching of Philistion. Our 'Hippocratic' treatise also contains a rather curious theory of cardiac palpitations caused by cold phlegm.

[1] De morbo sacro, 19: κατὰ ταῦτα νομίζω τὸν ἐγκέφαλον δύναμιν ἔχειν πλείστην ἐν τῷ ἀνθρώπῳ· οὗτος γὰρ ἡμῖν ἐστι τῶν ἀπὸ τοῦ ἠέρος γενομένων ἑρμηνεύς, ἢν ὑγιαίνων τυγχάνῃ· τὴν δὲ φρόνησιν ὁ ἀὴρ παρέχεται. οἱ δὲ ὀφθαλμοὶ καὶ τὰ ὦτα καὶ ἡ γλῶσσα καὶ αἱ χεῖρες καὶ οἱ πόδες οἷα ἂν ὁ ἐγκέφαλος γινώσκῃ, τοιαῦτα πρήσσουσι· γίνεται γὰρ ἐν ἅπαντι τῷ σώματι τῆς φρονήσιος, ὡς ἂν μετέχῃ τοῦ ἠέρος. ἐς δὲ τὴν σύνεσιν ὁ ἐγκέφαλός ἐστιν ὁ διαγγέλλων· ὅταν γὰρ σπάσῃ τὸ πνεῦμα ὥνθρωπος ἐς ἑωυτόν, ἐς τὸν ἐγκέφαλον πρῶτον ἀφικνεῖται, καὶ οὕτως ἐς τὸ λοιπὸν σῶμα σκίδναται ὁ ἀήρ, καταλελοιπὼς ἐν τῷ ἐγκεφάλῳ ἑωυτοῦ τὴν ἀκμὴν καὶ ὅ τι ἂν ᾖ φρόνιμόν τε καὶ γνώμην ἔχον· εἰ γὰρ ἐς τὸ σῶμα πρῶτον ἀφικνεῖτο καὶ ὕστερον ἐς τὸν ἐγκέφαλον, ἐν τῇσι σαρξὶ καὶ ἐν τῇσι φλεψὶ καταλελοιπὼς τὴν διάγνωσιν ἐς τὸν ἐγκέφαλον ἂν ἴοι θερμὸς ἐὼν καὶ οὐκ ἀκραιφνής, ἀλλ' ἐπιμεμιγμένος τῇ ἰκμάδι τῇ ἀπό τε τῶν σαρκῶν καὶ τοῦ αἵματος, ὥστε μηκέτι εἶναι ἀκριβής.

[2] See his essay on the Περὶ ἱερῆς νούσου, op. cit.

[3] De morbo sacro, 10: αἱ δὲ χεῖρες ἀκρατεῖς γίνονται καὶ σπῶνται, τοῦ αἵματος ἀτρεμίσαντος καὶ οὐ διαχεομένου ὥσπερ εἰώθει. καὶ οἱ ὀφθαλμοὶ διαστρέφονται, τῶν φλεβίων ἀποκλειομένων τοῦ ἠέρος καὶ σφυζόντων. ἀφρὸς δὲ ἐκ τοῦ στόματος προέρχεται ἐκ τοῦ πλεύμονος· . . . ἡ δὲ κόπρος ὑπέρχεται ὑπὸ βίης πνιγομένου, κτλ.

[4] See Wellmann, op. cit., p. 78; Timaeus, 86 e: ὅπου γὰρ ἂν οἱ τῶν ὀξέων καὶ ἁλυκῶν φλεγμάτων καὶ ὅσοι πικροὶ καὶ χολώδεις χυμοὶ κατὰ τὸ σῶμα πλανηθέντες ἔξω μὲν μὴ λάβωσιν ἀναπνοήν, ἐντὸς δὲ εἱλλόμενοι τὴν ἀφ' αὑτῶν ἀτμίδα τῇ τῆς ψυχῆς φορᾷ ξυμμίξαντες ἀνακερασθῶσι, παντοδαπὰ νοσήματα ψυχῆς ἐμποιοῦσι, μᾶλλον καὶ ἧττον καὶ ἐλάττω καὶ πλείω.

When cold phlegm gets down into the lungs and the heart, the blood is made cold, and the veins, being forcibly cooled, leap up against the lungs and the heart. The heart palpitates, so that as a result of this forced condition, asthma and orthopnoea supervene. For the heart cannot get as much *pneuma* as it wants, until the phlegm that has flowed in has been overpowered and dissolved. Then the palpitations and asthma cease.[1]

This passage is interesting as it mentions the beating of the heart, a phenomenon which is not regarded as normal but only the result of pathological conditions.

Like Diogenes, our 'Hippocratic' author believes that air (or *pneuma*) and blood are contained in the same blood vessels. He seems to look upon the blood as the vehicle of the vital or innate heat, for it is the influx of the cold phlegm which fixes the blood coagulating it, as it were, and causing a blockage of the *pneuma*, and in the severest cases causing instant death.[2]

The influence of Anaximenes and Diogenes of Apollonia is also found in another treatise in the *Hippocratic corpus*, the essay *On breaths*, which is regarded by Rüsche as the work of a 'medical sophist' who wrote about the turn of the fifth century B.C.[3] He too looks upon air as the most powerful of all things, lord of all.[4] And as such, it is the cause not only of life but also of disease.[5] Thus all diseases, though their seats and symptoms may vary, all have one fundamental cause.[6] Some, like the plague or epidemic fevers, are caused by the inhalation of a particular kind of polluted external air, others by airs produced within the body itself by faulty regime.[7] Airs produce disease because by causing accumulation

---

[1] De morbo sacro, 9: ὅταν γὰρ ἐπικατελθῇ τὸ φλέγμα ψυχρὸν ἐπὶ τὸν πλεύμονα καὶ τὴν καρδίην ἀποψύχεται τὸ αἷμα· αἱ δὲ φλέβες πρὸς βίην ψυχόμεναι πρὸς τῷ πλεύμονι καὶ τῇ καρδίῃ πηδῶσι, καὶ ἡ καρδίη πάλλεται, ὥστε ὑπὸ τῆς ἀνάγκης ταύτης τὸ ἄσθμα ἐπιπίπτειν καὶ τὴν ὀρθοπνοίην. οὐ γὰρ δέχεται τὸ πνεῦμα ὅσον ἐθέλει, ἄχρι κρατηθῇ τοῦ φλέγματος τὸ ἐπιρρυὲν καὶ διαθερμανθὲν διαχυθῇ ἐς τὰς φλέβας· ἔπειτα παύεται τοῦ παλμοῦ καὶ τοῦ ἄσθματος.

[2] De morbo sacro, 9: ταῦτα δὲ πάσχει πάντα, ὁπόταν τὸ φλέγμα παραρρυῇ ψυχρὸν ἐς τὸ αἷμα θερμὸν ἐόν· ἀποψύχει γὰρ καὶ ἵστησι τὸ αἷμα· καὶ ἢν μὲν πολὺ ᾖ τὸ ῥεῦμα καὶ παχύ, αὐτίκα ἀποκτείνει· κρατεῖ γὰρ τοῦ αἵματος καὶ πήγνυσιν· ἢν δὲ ἔλασσον ᾖ, τὸ μὲν παραυτίκα κρατεῖ ἀποφράξαν τὴν ἀναπνοήν.

[3] Rüsche, *Blut, Leben und Seele, ihr Verhältnis nach Auffassung der griechischen und hellenistischen Antike* . . . , p. 124.

[4] Hippocrates, *De flatibus*, 3: πνεῦμα δὲ τὸ μὲν ἐν τοῖσι σώμασι φῦσα καλεῖται, τὸ δὲ ἔξω τῶν σωμάτων ὁ ἀήρ. οὗτος δὲ μέγιστος ἐν τοῖσι πᾶσι τῶν πάντων δυνάστης ἐστίν.

[5] Ibid., 4: τοῖς δ' αὖ θνητοῖσιν οὗτος τοῦ τε βίου, καὶ τῶν νούσων τοῖσι νοσέουσι.

[6] Ibid., 2: τῶν δὲ δὴ νούσων ἁπασέων ὁ μὲν τρόπος ωὑτός, ὁ δὲ τόπος διαφέρει· δοκεῖ μὲν οὖν οὐδὲν ἐοικέναι τὰ νοσήματα ἀλλήλοισι διὰ τὴν ἀλλοιότητα τῶν τόπων, ἔστι δὲ μία πασέων νούσων καὶ ἰδέη καὶ αἰτίη.

[7] Ibid., 6: ἔστι δὲ δισσὰ ἔθνεα πυρετῶν, ὡς ταύτῃ διελθεῖν· ὁ μὲν κοινὸς ἅπασι καλεόμενος λοιμός· ὁ δὲ διὰ πονηρὴν δίαιταν ἰδίῃ τοῖσι πονηρῶς διαιτεομένοισι γινόμενος· ἀμφοτέρων δὲ τούτων ὁ ἀὴρ αἴτιος. ὁ μὲν οὖν κοινὸς πυρετὸς διὰ τοῦτο τοιοῦτός ἐστιν, ὅτι τὸ πνεῦμα τωὐτὸ πάντες ἕλκουσιν . . . ὅταν μὲν οὖν ὁ ἀὴρ τοιούτοισι χρωσθῇ μιάσμασιν, ἃ τῇ ἀνθρωπείῃ φύσει πολέμιά ἐστιν, ἄνθρωποι τότε νοσέουσιν.

of air in the blood vessels they do not leave room for the blood to pass. Our author regards blood rather than air as the instrument of consciousness, even if air is the fundamental cosmic substance.

No constituent in the body contributes more to intelligence than does blood. So long as blood remains in its normal state, consciousness or intelligence also remains. But when the condition of the blood changes, consciousness or intelligence also change. There are many testimonies to this fact. First sleep . . . For when sleep comes to the body the blood is chilled, for sleep is by nature a cooling agent. And when the blood is chilled the outlets of the blood become more torpid.[1]

The sacred disease is caused when much air is mixed with the blood throughout the body, with the result that the veins do not have enough room to let both pass. The result is that many barriers are created in many places. Accumulations of air weigh or press heavily upon the blood so that its movement becomes irregular, giving rise to the well-known symptoms.[2] So greatly does a disturbance of the air disturb and pollute the blood.[3]

The most interesting feature of this theory is the explanation of epidemics as air-borne diseases. It resembles in some respects the doctrine attributed to Hippocrates in the *Menoneia*, but differs very considerably from it in others. For while Hippocrates seems to regard the unimpeded passage of the *pneuma* as the fundamental condition of health,[4] the author of *Breaths* lays much more stress on the unimpeded passage and condition of the blood. It is therefore very doubtful whether our medical sophist derived his teaching from any actual writing of Hippocrates.

To return now to the vascular system. A rather similar description of the blood vessels to that which we have been examining occurs in the

---

[1] Hippocrates, *De flatibus*, 14: ἡγεῦμαι δὲ οὐδὲν ἔμπροσθεν οὐδενὶ εἶναι μᾶλλον τῶν ἐν τῷ σώματι συμβαλλομένων ἐς φρόνησιν ἢ τὸ αἷμα· τοῦτο δὲ ὅταν ἐν τῷ καθεστεῶτι μένῃ, μένει καὶ ἡ φρόνησις· ἑτεροιουμένου δὲ τοῦ αἵματος μεταπίπτει καὶ ἡ φρόνησις. ὅτι δὲ ταῦτα οὕτως ἔχει, πολλὰ τὰ μαρτυρέοντα· πρῶτον μὲν ὅπερ ἅπασι ζῴοις κοινόν ἐστιν, ὁ ὕπνος, οὗτος μαρτυρεῖ τοῖς εἰρημένοισιν· ὅταν γὰρ ἐπέλθῃ τῷ σώματι, τὸ αἷμα ψύχεται, φύσει γὰρ ὁ ὕπνος πέφυκεν ψύχειν· ψυχθέντι δὲ τῷ αἵματι νωθρότεραι γίνονται αἱ διέξοδοι.

[2] Ibid.: φημὶ δὲ τὴν ἱερὴν νοῦσον ὧδε γίνεσθαι· ὅταν πνεῦμα πολὺ κατὰ πᾶν τὸ σῶμα παντὶ τῷ αἵματι μιχθῇ, πολλὰ ἐμφράγματα γίνεται πολλαχῇ κατὰ τὰς φλέβας· ἐπειδὰν οὖν ἐς τὰς παχείας καὶ πολυαίμους φλέβας πολὺς ἀὴρ βρίσῃ, βρίσας δὲ μείνῃ, κωλύεται τὸ αἷμα διεξιέναι· τῇ μὲν οὖν ἐνέστηκε, τῇ δὲ νωθρῶς διεξέρχεται, τῇ δὲ θᾶσσον· ἀνομοίῃς δὲ τῆς πορείης τῷ αἵματι διὰ τοῦ σώματος γενομένης, παντοῖαι αἱ ἀνομοιότητες· πᾶν γὰρ τὸ σῶμα πανταχόθεν ἕλκεταί καὶ τετίνακται τὰ μέρεα τοῦ σώματος ὑπηρετέοντα τῷ ταράχῳ καὶ θορύβῳ τοῦ αἵματος, διαστροφαί τε παντοῖαι παντοίως γίνονται.

[3] Ibid.: οὕτως ὁ ἀὴρ ταραχθεὶς ἀνετάραξε τὸ αἷμα καὶ ἐμίηνεν.

[4] *Anonymus Londinensis*, v and vi, J. 34–6: Ἱπποκράτης δέ φησιν αἰτίας εἶναι τῆς νόσου τὰς φύσας, καθὼς διείληφεν περὶ αὐτοῦ Ἀριστοτέλης. ὁ γὰρ Ἱπποκράτης λέγει τὰς νόσους ἀποτελεῖσθαι κατὰ λόγον τοιοῦτον· ἢ παρὰ τὸ πλῆθος τῶν προσφερομένων ἢ παρὰ τὴν ποικιλίαν ἢ παρὰ τὸ ἰσχυρὰ καὶ δυσκατέργαστα εἶναι... τὸ γὰρ πνεῦμα ἀναγκαιότατον καὶ κυριώτατον ἀπολείπει τῶν ἐν ἡμῖν, ἐπειδή γε παρὰ τὴν τούτου εὔροιαν ὑγίεια γίνεται, παρὰ δὲ τὴν δύσροιαν νόσοι.

treatise *On the nature of man*. This description was attributed by Aristotle to Polybus, though Galen vigorously denied that the description could possibly have been written by him, let alone by Hippocrates, as we have already noted. Here too the blood vessels are described as issuing from the head:

The thickest of the veins grow as follows. There are four pairs in the body. One pair starts from the head at the back, and runs through the neck, and passing on each side just on the outside of the spine, and parallel to it, one on each side of it, passes the hips and goes into the legs, thence through the calves to the outside of the ankles and reaches the feet. Now in venesections performed to ease pains in the back and the hips, blood should be drawn from the parts behind the thigh and from the outer parts of the ankles. The second pair of veins runs from the head near the ears through the neck, they are called the jugular, and they run on the outside of the spine parallel to it, and on each side they pass close to the muscles of the loins to the testicles and the thighs, and through the back part of the thighs on the inward side, and then through the calves past the outer side of the ankles into the feet. Now in venesections made to relieve pain in the loins and the testicles, blood must be taken from the back of the thigh and the outer side of the ankles. The third pair goes from the temples through the neck, and under the shoulder-blades. They then come together into the lungs, and the one from the right side crosses over to the left, and the one from the left side over to the right. The right hand one passes out of the lung under the breast and into the spleen and kidney. The left hand one passes to the right from the lungs, under the breast and into the liver and the kidney, and on each side they terminate in the anus. The fourth pair goes from the front of the head and the eyes down the neck and under the collar-bones. They then run on the upper surface of the arms down to the elbows, then through the forearms to the wrists and to the fingers, then from the fingers backwards through the 'chests' [palms?] of the hands and the forearms on the upper side to the elbows, and through the underside of the arms into the armpits and from the upper side of the ribs, one goes to the spleen and the other to the liver. Then they run on above the stomach and end in the penis, both of them. That is how the thick veins run. And there are many veins running from the belly of all kinds and sizes, through which the nourishment to the body passes. And they carry it from the inward parts and communicate with one another, those going from the inside outwards and those going from the outside inwards. Now venesections must be performed on these principles. Care must be taken that the cuts should be made as closely as possible to the places where the pain has been ascertained to be and the blood has collected. For in this way the sudden change induced by bleeding becomes as small as possible, and you will be able to change the habitual condition, so that blood no longer collects in the same place.[1]

[1] Hippocrates, *De natura hominis*, 11 : αἱ παχύταται δὲ τῶν φλεβῶν ὧδε πεφύκασιν. τέσσαρα ζεύγεά ἐστιν ἐν τῷ σώματι, καὶ ἕν μὲν αὐτέων ἀπὸ τῆς κεφαλῆς ὄπισθεν διὰ τοῦ αὐχένος, ἔξωθεν ἐπὶ τὴν ῥάχιν ἔνθεν τε καὶ ἔνθεν παρὰ τὰ ἰσχία ἀφικνέεται καὶ ἐς τὰ σκέλεα, ἔπειτα διὰ τῶν κνημέων ἐπὶ τῶν σφυρῶν τὰ ἔξω καὶ ἐς τοὺς πόδας διήκει. δεῖ οὖν τὰς φλεβοτομίας τὰς ἐπὶ τῶν ἀλγημάτων

There does not seem to be much point in attempting to relate the details of this description to the observed facts of anatomy. As Littré pointed out, Galen, and he was not the first, condemns this description of the blood vessels as spurious, as being that of neither Polybus nor Hippocrates.[1] Having just told us that his master Pelops used to teach a somewhat similar doctrine, which he falsely attributed to Hippocrates, he points out that none of the anatomists supported it.[2] There are, however, one or two features of this description which are perhaps worth noting. There is no mention of the heart at all. The crossing-place of the great vessels is in the chest, where the chiasmus first described by Syennesis is located. To attempt to identify these as the pulmonary arteries or pulmonary veins is obviously futile, but the two big crossing vessels seem to fit fairly well as a first approximation to the vena cava and the aorta. The other point of interest is the conception of intercommunicating blood vessels, which has evidently helped to give some historians the impression that Hippocrates was acquainted with the circulation of

τῶν ἐν τῷ νώτῳ καὶ τοῖσιν ἰσχίοισιν ἀπὸ τῶν ἰγνύων ποιέεσθαι καὶ ἀπὸ τῶν σφυρῶν ἔξωθεν. αἱ δ' ἕτεραι φλέβες ἐκ τῆς κεφαλῆς παρὰ τὰ οὔατα διὰ τοῦ αὐχένος, αἱ σφαγίτιδες καλεόμεναι, ἔσωθεν παρὰ τὴν ῥάχιν ἑκατέρωθεν φέρουσι παρὰ τὰς ψόας ἐς τοὺς ὄρχιας καὶ ἐς τοὺς μηροὺς καὶ διὰ τῶν ἰγνύων ἐκ τοῦ ἔσωθεν μέρεος, ἔπειτα διὰ τῶν κνημέων παρὰ τὰ σφυρὰ τὰ ἔσωθεν καὶ ἐς τοὺς πόδας. δεῖ οὖν τὰς φλεβοτομίας πρὸς τὰς ὀδύνας ποιέεσθαι τὰς ἀπὸ τῶν ψόων καὶ τῶν ὀρχίων, ἀπὸ τῶν ἰγνύων καὶ ἀπὸ τῶν σφυρῶν ἔσωθεν. αἱ δὲ τρίται φλέβες ἐκ τῶν κροτάφων διὰ τοῦ αὐχένος ὑπὸ τὰς ὠμοπλάτας. ἔπειτα συμφέρονται ἐς τὸν πλεύμονα, καὶ ἀφικνέονται, ἡ μὲν ἀπὸ τῶν δεξιῶν ἐς τὰ ἀριστερά, ἡ δὲ ἀπὸ τῶν ἀριστερῶν ἐς τὰ δεξιὰ ἐκ τοῦ πλεύμονος ὑπὸ τὸν μαζὸν καὶ ἐς τὸν σπλῆνα καὶ ἐς τὸν νεφρόν, ἡ δὲ τῶν ἀριστερῶν ἐς τὰ δεξιὰ ἐκ τοῦ πλεύμονος ὑπὸ τὸν μαζὸν καὶ ἐς τὸ ἧπαρ καὶ ἐς τὸν νεφρόν, τελευτῶσι δὲ ἐς τὸν ἀρχὸν ἑκάτεραι. αἱ δὲ τέταρται ἀπὸ τοῦ ἔμπροσθεν τῆς κεφαλῆς καὶ τῶν ὀφθαλμῶν ὑπὸ τὸν αὐχένα καὶ τὰς κληῖδας, ἔπειτα δὲ ὑπὲρ τῶν βραχιόνων ἄνωθεν ἐς τὰς συγκαμπάς, ἔπειτα δὲ διὰ τῶν πήχεων ἐπὶ τοὺς καρποὺς καὶ τοὺς δακτύλους, ἔπειτα ἀπὸ τῶν δακτύλων πάλιν διὰ τῶν στηθέων τῶν χειρῶν καὶ τῶν πήχεων ἄνω ἐς τὰς συγκαμπάς, καὶ διὰ τῶν βραχιόνων τοῦ κάτωθεν μέρεος ἐς τὰς μασχάλας, καὶ ἀπὸ τῶν πλευρέων ἄνωθεν, ἡ μὲν ἐς τὸν σπλῆνα ἀφικνέεται, ἡ δ' ἐς τὸ ἧπαρ, ἔπειτα ὑπὲρ τῆς γαστρὸς ἐς τὸ αἰδοῖον τελευτῶσιν ἀμφότεραι. καὶ αἱ μὲν παχεῖαι τῶν φλεβῶν ὧδε ἔχουσιν. εἰσὶ δὲ καὶ ἀπὸ τῆς κοιλίης φλέβες ἀνὰ τὸ σῶμα πάμπολλαί τε καὶ παντοῖαι καὶ δι' ὧν ἡ τροφὴ τῷ σώματι ἔρχεται· φέρουσι δὲ καὶ ἀπὸ τῶν παχειῶν φλεβῶν ἐς τὴν κοιλίην καὶ τὸ ἄλλο σῶμα καὶ ἀπὸ τῶν ἔξω καὶ ἀπὸ τῶν εἴσω καὶ ἐς ἀλλήλας διαδιδόασιν, αἵ τε εἴσωθεν ἔξω καὶ αἱ ἔξωθεν εἴσω. τὰς οὖν φλεβοτομίας δεῖ ποιέεσθαι κατὰ τούτους τοὺς λόγους· ἐπιτηδεύειν δὲ χρὴ τὰς τομὰς ὡς προσωτάτω τάμνειν ἀπὸ τῶν χωρίων, ἔνθ' ἂν αἱ ὀδύναι μεμαθήκωσι γίνεσθαι καὶ τὸ αἷμα συλλέγεσθαι· οὕτω γὰρ ἂν ἥ τε μεταβολὴ ἥκιστα γίνοιτο μεγάλη ἐξαπίνης, καὶ τὸ ἔθος μεταστήσαις ἂν ὥστε μηκέτι ἐς τὸ αὐτὸ χωρίον συλλέγεσθαι.

[1] See Littré i. 12. Cf. Galen's *Commentaries on the De natura hominis*, K. xv. 1–173; he divides the treatise into two books, the first of which he regards as genuine, but he rejects altogether much of the second book, including the chapter just quoted. See also the following passage, *De plac. Hipp. et Plat.* vi. 3, K. v. 529: ἀλλ' ὅτι μὲν οὔκ ἐστι γνήσιος οὔθ' Ἱπποκράτους οὐδὲ Πολύβου τῶν εἰρημένων φλεβῶν ἡ ἀνατομή, καὶ πρὸ ἡμῶν ἑτέροις ἀποδέδεικται· καὶ ἡμεῖς δέ, εἰ θεὸς δοίη ποτὲ περὶ τῶν γνησίων Ἱπποκράτους γραμμάτων πραγματεύσασθαι, διὰ πλεόνων ὑποδείξομεν ἥτις ἐστὶν Ἱπποκράτους γνώμη περὶ φλεβῶν ἀρχῆς.

[2] Ibid., 527 f.: ἐγὼ τοῦτον τὸν λόγον οὐδ' ὅτε μειράκιον ὂν ἤκουσα παρὰ τοῦ διδασκάλου Πέλοπος ἐπιδεικνύναι πειρωμένου τὸν ἐγκέφαλον ἁπάντων τῶν ἀγγείων ἀρχήν ... τὰ δ' ἀπὸ τῆς κεφαλῆς καταφέρεσθαι λεγόμενα τέτταρα ζεύγη φλεβῶν, ἐμβεβλῆσθαί τέ μοι δοκεῖ τοῖς ἐπιγραφομένοις Ἱπποκράτους συγγράμμασι ... τὰ δὲ τέτταρα ἐκεῖνα ζεύγη πρὸς τὸ μηδ' ὑφ' ἑνὸς ἄλλου λέγεσθαι τῶν ἀνατομικῶν, οὐδὲ δείκνυται πρός τινος.

the blood.[1] A similar intercommunication of 'veins' is also postulated in the treatise *On places in man*. Here we have again pairs of 'veins' running from the head through the neck to the chest, and a rather peculiar pair in the head which are responsible for the pulse, obviously the temporal arteries. The relevant passage reads as follows:

And those which turn to the lower portions of the body are two veins running alongside the tendons of the neck; they also run parallel to the vertebrae and end in the kidneys. They also reach the testicles. And when these become diseased, a man pisses blood. There are two other veins which go from the top of the head to the shoulders, and they are called the shoulder-veins. Two other veins run from the top of the head past the ears along the front of the neck one on each side into the so-called hollow vein. Now the hollow vein travels like the oesophagus, and grows between the windpipe and the oesophagus. And it travels through the diaphragm and the heart in the middle of the diaphragm, and splits into two, a branch going into each buttock and into the interior of each thigh. And it makes its division in the thigh and runs to the calves on the inside by the ankle. These are the veins which, if they are cut, make a man unfruitful. They also end in the big toes. And from the hollow vein there is a branch going to the left flank, and it runs underneath the spleen into the left flank, where the spleen grows out of the omentum, and it ends by going up into the chest. And it branches off by the diaphragm and joins up with the shoulder vein. This vein is divided, at a level lower down than the elbow joint and the spleen. And another branch grows out of the hollow vein in the same manner into the right flank. And all the veins communicate with and run into one another, some of them running into their own branches, and others through the little branch veins that fan out from them which give nourishment to the tissues. In this way do they flow into one another.[2]

Here we seem to be on rather firmer anatomical ground. The existence of a main system of blood vessels going through the heart, the so-called

[1] See for example L. Stroppiana's paper, 'Può risalire al periodo Ippocratico l'intuizione dei capillari?', *Proceedings of the Fifteenth Italian Congress of the History of Medicine*, which makes a not at all convincing attempt to date back the 'invention' of the capillaries to Hippocratic times.

[2] *De locis in homine*, 3: αἱ δὲ κάτω τοῦ σώματος τετραμμέναι δύο μὲν φλέβες παρὰ τοὺς τένοντας τοῦ τραχήλου, φέρονται δὲ καὶ παρὰ τοὺς σπονδύλους καὶ τελευτῶσιν ἐς τοὺς νεφρούς. αὗται δὲ καὶ ἐς τοὺς ὄρχιας περαίνουσι. ὅταν αὗται πονέωσιν, αἷμα οὐρέει ὤνθρωπος. ἄλλαι δύο φλέβες ἀπὸ τῆς κορυφῆς φέρονται ἐς τοὺς ὤμους, καὶ δὴ καὶ ὠμαῖαι καλέονται. ἄλλαι δύο φλέβες ἀπὸ τῆς κορυφῆς παρὰ τὰ ὦτα ἐν τοῖς ἔμπροσθεν τοῦ τραχήλου ἑκατέρωθεν ἐς τὴν κοίλην φλέβα καλεομένην φέρονται. ἡ δὲ κοίλη φλὲψ περαίνεται μὲν ὡς ὁ οἰσοφάγος, πέφυκε δὲ μεταξὺ τοῦ τε βρόγχου καὶ τοῦ οἰσοφάγου· φέρεται δὲ διὰ τῶν φρενῶν καὶ διὰ τῆς καρδίης καὶ μεταξὺ τῶν φρενῶν καὶ σχίζεται ἐς τοὺς βουβῶνας καὶ ἐς τοὺς μηροὺς ἐντός, καὶ τὰς διασφαγὰς ἐν τοῖσι μηροῖσι ποιέεται, καὶ ἐς τὰς κνημὰς φέρεται ἐντὸς παρὰ τὰ σφυρά. αὗται καὶ ἄκαρπον ποιέουσι τὸν ἄνθρωπον ὅταν ἀποτμηθῶσι, αἳ καὶ ἐς τοὺς μεγάλους δακτύλους τελευτῶσιν. ἐκ δὲ τῆς κοίλης φλεβὸς ἀποπέφυκεν ἐς τὴν λαπαρὴν τὴν ἀριστερήν, φέρεται δ' ὑποκάτω τοῦ σπληνὸς ἐς τὴν λαπαρὴν τὴν ἀριστεράν, ὅθεν ὁ σπλὴν ἀποπέφυκε διὰ τοῦ ἐπιπλόου, καὶ τὴν ἀποτελεύτησιν ἴσχει ἐς τὸν κιθαρόν, ἀποπέφυκε δὲ κατὰ τὰς φρένας καὶ συμβάλλει τῇ ὠμειῇ, κάτω τοῦ ἄρθρου τοῦ ἀγκῶνος καὶ τοῦ σπληνὸς τάμνεται αὕτη. καὶ ἄλλη ἐς τὴν δεξιὴν τὸν αὐτὸν τρόπον ἀποπέφυκεν ἀπὸ τῆς κοίλης, κοινωνέουσι δὲ πᾶσαι αἱ φλέβες καὶ διαρρέουσιν ἐς ἑωυτούς· αἱ μὲν γὰρ σφίσιν ἑωυταῖς ξυμβάλλουσιν, αἱ δὲ διὰ τῶν φλεβίων τῶν διατεταμένων ἀπὸ τῶν φλεβῶν, αἳ τρέφουσι τὰς σάρκας, ταύτῃ διαρρέουσι πρὸς ἑωυτάς.

'hollow' vein, has been established. We seem to have a duplicate system. The first pair of veins described would appear to be the vestiges of the two big veins of Diogenes of Apollonia, but they no longer go to the legs. They terminate in the testicles, and they are not connected with the heart. The second pair running from the heart seem to form a separate system which just serves the shoulders, but it is connected up, quite how is not clear, with the third pair, which run down from the neck into the hollow vein (the vein going through the heart) and passing from the midriff into the abdomen, send off a big branch to each leg, and also run branches coming off on each side, apparently up each flank into the shoulder vein. These branches represent the earlier hepatic and splenetic veins. The communications of these veins with each other may very well be based on anatomical observation.

The veins communicate very freely with one another, especially in certain regions of the body. Thus between the venous sinuses of the cranium, and between the veins in the neck, whose obstruction would be attended by imminent danger to the cerebral circulation, numerous anastomoses are found. Free communications also exist between the veins of the vertebral canal, and the veins composing the various plexuses in the abdomen and the pelvis.[1]

This treatise was not regarded by Littré as genuine, but it was included by him among those which bear the genuine stamp of the Hippocratean school.[2] And if some modern critics have thought that it was a product of the Cnidian school, all would be agreed in placing its date not later than the middle of the fourth century B.C. It is, incidentally, the treatise which begins with the famous sentence on which the 'circulationists' have laid such stress. 'To me, it seems that there is no beginning, first principle, or starting-point ($\dot{\alpha}\rho\chi\dot{\eta}$) of the body, but all things are equally beginning and end, for when a circle has been drawn, a beginning is not found.'[3]

Littré's comment on this passage is certainly intriguing:

Ideas like this, considering the ignorance in which people were of the anatomical and physiological conditions of the circulation, are certainly of great significance. This is the discovery of Harvey presented in the most formal manner. There is not one of the most advanced developments of contemporary medicine, which is not to be found in embryo in the medicine of the past. The knowledge of antiquity and that of today are fundamentally the same, in so far as they are made up of the same elements. What was only a shoot has become a robust branch. What was hidden under the bark

---

[1] Gray, *Anatomy* (27th edn.), p. 803. [2] Littré, i. 293, 355.
[3] *De locis in homine*, 1 : ἐμοὶ δοκέει ἀρχὴ μὲν οὐδεμία εἶναι τοῦ σώματος, ἀλλὰ πάντα ὁμοίως ἀρχὴ καὶ πάντα τελευτή. κύκλου γὰρ γραφέντος ἀρχὴ οὐχ εὑρέθη· καὶ τῶν νοσημάτων ἀπὸ παντὸς ὁμοίως τοῦ σώματος.

develops in the light of a single day. In science, as in everything else, nothing comes into being which was not once a seed.[1]

Littré then goes on to explain that the notion of the circulation was buried and neglected because the interests of the earlier physiologists, Aristotle for example, were concentrated on quite a different problem, the discovery of the heart as the centre of the vascular system. In these circumstances the intuition of the circulation with insufficient concrete evidence to back it was abandoned, and Littré regards this as a typical example of a process which has often taken place in the history of science, and evokes the complaint that the discovery of new facts often causes ancient doctrines of great value to be abandoned and so results really in a step backwards.[2]

This argument from the circle in the 'Hippocratic' writings, has, I am convinced, been taken too literally by many historians of ancient medicine. For our 'Hippocratic' author immediately goes on to remark that 'All diseases come likewise from all the body'. He seems to be concerned not at all with the motion of the blood, but with the much more fundamental conception of the body as an organic whole, a fact which is proved by the fact that when something goes wrong with one part of the body, all the other parts are affected, one of the prime discoveries of 'Hippocratic' medicine.

The author of this treatise also makes the vascular system start, as we have noted, in the head, and notes the pulsation of the blood vessels in the

[1] Littré, i. 222 f.: 'De telles idées, dans l'ignorance où l'on était des conditions anatomiques et physiologiques de la circulation, sont certainement d'une haute portée. C'est la découverte de Harvey pressentie de la manière la plus formelle. Il n'est pas un développement, le plus avancé de la médecine contemporaine, qui ne se trouve en embryon dans la médecine antérieure. Les connaissances antiques et les nôtres sont identiques au fond, en tant que composées des mêmes éléments: ce qui n'était qu'un bourgeon est devenu un robuste rameau; ce qui était caché sous l'écorce s'est développé à la lumière d'un jour. En science comme en tout autre chose rien n'est qui n'ait été en germe.'

[2] Ibid.: 'Tout prouve que les idées de cercle et de circulation n'ont été ni comprises ni poursuivies par les anciens physiologistes. Ils se sont obstinés à vouloir trouver une origine aux vaisseaux. Plus même l'anatomie est devenue exacte et a reconnu le trajet des veines et des artères et leur rapport avec le cœur, plus ils sont confirmés dans l'opinion que les vaisseaux devaient avoir un commencement. Il arrive, on le voit, que le progrès même de la science et les découvertes réelles ont pour effet de détruire des idées scientifiques d'une grande valeur. La pensée de la circulation est dans les livres hippocratiques. On l'y laisse pour poursuivre une théorie qui détourne évidemment les esprits de la recherche de la véritable condition des vaisseaux, du cœur, et du sang. D'exemples semblables, qui ne sont pas rares, proviennent ces plaintes souvent répétées, que la science rétrograde quand des faits de détail nouvellement aperçus brisent d'anciennes conceptions qui ont de la grandeur, et font perdre de vue des doctrines qui, nées d'une sorte d'intuition, et vraies dans le fond, manquent de toute démonstration. Aristote, qui avait beaucoup disséqué, fut conduit à faire partir du cœur les veines, mais en même temps il abandonna l'idée primitive de la constitution circulaire du corps animal. L'anatomie moderne n'admet pas, comme Aristote, que le cœur soit l'origine des vaisseaux sanguins, mais elle admet, comme les hippocratiques, que le corps organisé est un cercle sans commencement ni fin.'

temples, for which he gives what sounds to us today quite a preposterous explanation. Like the author of *On the nature of man,* he conceives the blood vessels as running down the neck in pairs from the top of the head, though he reduces their number.

And veins end in the crown of the head, going through the flesh [presumably of the scalp], keeping close to the bone. Two run from the top of the head straight down to where the eyebrows meet, and they terminate in the corner of the eyes. One runs from the crown of the head into the nose and splits up into the cartilage of each nostril. Another pair of 'veins' runs along the temples, between the temples and the ears, which press close to the eyes and are always pulsating. For these alone of all the veins do not supply blood, for the blood is turned away or shut off from them, and the blood which is turned away wishing to retreat, and that which has flowed in from above wishing to descend, the two streams pour and push against each other and by moving round each other create the pulsation in the veins . . . Two others, in between the ears, and the other veins just mentioned, go to the ears and press close upon them. Another pair of veins goes into the ears from the sutures of the bones of the skull.[1]

Then follows the passage already quoted, describing the two main veins into the kidneys.

It is not easy to make much sense out of the descriptions given in this treatise of the various blood vessels, for arteries and veins have not yet been distinguished, and no mention is made either of the heart or of the lungs.

We now pass to quite a different series of descriptions, which either implicitly or directly treat the heart as the centre of the vascular system. Three of these, the fragment *On the heart,* and the treatises *On nourishment* and *On the nature of the bones,* were among Kapferer's principal sources for his contention that Hippocrates was acquainted with the circulation of the blood.[2]

To deal first with the work *On the nature of the bones.* This is the longest account in the Hippocratic collection of the vascular system and, as Galen informs us,[3] originally had the title Περὶ φλεβῶν, *About the veins,*

---

[1] *De locis in homine,* 3 : φλέβες δὲ περαίνουσι μὲν ἐς τὴν κορυφὴν διὰ τῆς σαρκὸς ἔχουσαι πρὸς τὸ ὀστέον, φέρονται δὲ διὰ τῆς σαρκός, δύο μὲν ἐκ τῆς κορυφῆς κατ᾽ ἰθὺ ᾗ αἱ ὀφρύες ξυγκλείονται καὶ τελευτῶσιν ἐς τοὺς κανθοὺς τῶν ὀφθαλμῶν· μία ἀπὸ τῆς κορυφῆς ἐς τὴν ῥῖνα φέρεται καὶ σχίζεται ἐς τὸν χόνδρον τῆς ῥινὸς ἑκάτερον. ἄλλαι δύο φλέβες παρὰ τοὺς κροτάφους φέρονται ἐν μέσῳ τῶν κροτάφων καὶ τῶν ὤτων, αἳ πιέζουσι τὰς ὄψεις καὶ σφύζουσιν ἀεί· μοῦναι γὰρ αὗται οὐκ ἄρδουσι τῶν φλεβῶν. ἀλλ᾽ ἀποτρέπεται ἐξ αὐτῶν τὸ αἷμα· τὸ δ᾽ ἀποτρεπόμενον βουλόμενον ἀποχωρέειν, τὸ δ᾽ ἄνωθεν ἐπιρρέον βουλόμενον κάτω χωρέειν, ἐνταῦθα ὠθεύμενά τε καὶ ἀναχεόμενα πρὸς ἄλληλα καὶ κυκλεόμενα σφυγμὸν παρέχουσι τοῖσι φλεβίοισι . . . ἄλλαι δύο φλέβες ἐν μέσῳ τῶν ὤτων καὶ τῶν ἄλλων φλεβῶν αἳ φέρονται ἐς τὰ ὦτα καὶ πιέζουσι τὰ ὦτα. ἄλλαι δύο φλέβες ἐκ τῆς συγκλείσεως τοῦ ὀστέου ἐς τὰς ἀκοὰς φέρονται.

[2] See Abel, articles in *Hermes* and *Gesnerus,* op. cit.

[3] Galen, *Glossary,* K. xix. 128: ἐν τῷ περὶ φλεβῶν ὃ προσκεῖται τῷ μοχλικῷ.

though it was attached to the *Instruments of reduction*. It appears to be obviously a compilation of very different sources, including, as we have already noticed, two passages taken practically verbatim from other treatises in the *Corpus*, as well as one from Aristotle. As to its date, we can only make a 'guess bracket'. It was included in the list of Hippocrates' writings compiled by Bacchaeus of Tanagra, and must therefore have been written before 200 B.C., and it quotes (and cannot therefore be earlier than) Aristotle. But one section of it seems to be a complete treatise, and the quotation from Aristotle may well be a later addition. It is at any rate something of a hotch-potch, since it begins with a short section dealing very superficially with general anatomy, starting with the bones; hence its misleading title. This section does not appear to have any connection with the rest of the work. Taken as it stands in Littré's edition the work seems altogether confused, and though Kapferer[1] by rather arbitrarily rearranging the order of the various chapters attempts to make some anatomical sense out of it, the result is not, in my opinion, at all convincing. Moreover his anatomical interpretations, to a layman with some superficial acquaintance both with anatomy and with the Greek language, are, to say the least of it, hard to follow, requiring, as they do, such strange translations that the rearrangement of the chapters demanded cannot fail to appear improbable. It must, however, be noted that Sigerist, in a footnote to one of the pages in his chapter on the Hippocratic collection in the second (posthumous) volume of his history of medicine,[2] expresses the opinion that Kapferer made the most thorough study of Hippocratic anatomy and that his rearrangement of the chapters makes much more sense than the original. This would perhaps, as we shall see, not constitute an excessive claim. Nevertheless we shall content ourselves in our analysis with following the order of the traditional text, as transmitted by Littré.

Kapferer begins by transposing Chapter 11 to the head of the text. His reason for this operation is that it begins, like Chapter 1 in the traditional text, with a general description of the main classes of anatomical structures, describing the functions of the bones, tendons, or ligaments ($\nu\epsilon\hat{\upsilon}\rho\alpha$) as well as that of the 'veins'.[3] It also contains another passage which has been interpreted by the 'circulationists', including Kapferer, as one of the main supports of their hypothesis. It reads as follows:

The veins running all over the body provide *pneuma*, fluid, and movement. They all branch out from a single vein, but where this single vein begins, and where it ends, I do not know. For when a circle has come into being, you cannot find a beginning. But I will demonstrate where the branches of it begin and where in the body they end, and how this single vessel is co-ordinated with them (ὁμολογέει), and to what regions of the body they extend.[1]

Kapferer translates the phrase ὡς ἡ μία ταύτῃσιν ὁμολογέει as 'how the single vein with these branches reunites as a single vessel'[2]—a version which was very pertinently criticized by Diepgen,[3] who pointed out that the words cannot possibly bear this meaning, nor be taken to imply, as Kapferer would have it, a circulation of the blood. We must compare this use of the metaphor of circularity with the one just quoted from *Places in man*, where the author used the phrase, as we saw, not to hint at any circulation but to express, in a picturesque way, the notion of the body as an organism, no express reference being made to blood vessels. Here the 'Hippocratic' author certainly seems to be referring to the intercommunication of blood vessels, but there is no mention at all of their contents, except the general statement that *pneuma* and liquid flow through them to the various parts of the body. The heart is not mentioned at all. Kapferer maintains that Chapter 11 is the real introductory chapter to this treatise, since Chapter 1 is little other than a repetition of some of the passages contained in Chapter 11. He identifies the work with that promised in the treatise *On joints*, where 'Hippocrates' promised to produce a work in the form of a systematic treatise on the blood vessels and their connections,[4] a promise which, he maintains, is contained in almost identical words in the quotation we have just made from the eleventh chapter of the work *On the nature of bones*, which we are now discussing. In this connection it may be relevant to point out that the passage in the treatise *On joints*, which we have just quoted in a footnote, mentions both veins and arteries as different types of blood vessels, and the author

---

[1] *De natura ossium*, 11 : αἱ φλέβες διὰ τοῦ σώματος κεχυμέναι πνεῦμα καὶ ῥεῦμα καὶ κίνησιν παρέχονται, ἀπὸ μιᾶς πολλαὶ διαβλαστάνουσαι, καὶ αὕτη μὲν ἡ μία ὅθεν ἦρκται καὶ ᾗ τετελεύτηκεν οὐκ οἶδα. κύκλου γὰρ γεγενημένου ἀρχὴ οὐχ εὑρέθη. τὰς δ' ἀποφυάδας αὐτῆς ὅθεν ἦρκται καὶ ᾗ παύονται τοῦ σώματος, καὶ ὡς ἡ μία ταύτῃσιν ὁμολογέει, καὶ ἐν ὁποίοις τόποις τέτανται τοῦ σώματος, ἐγὼ δηλώσω.

[2] In his article, 'Der Blutkreislauf, seine Darstellung in den hippokratischen Schriften', *Hippokrates* (1937), pp. 697–9 he writes: 'Außer diesen Einzelbeschreibungen finden wir im Kap. II noch eine wichtige Stelle, an der der Blutkreislauf im allgemeinen geschildert wird. "Aus einer der einzigen (Ader) verzweigen sich viele; wo diese eine ausgeht und wo sie endigt, weiß ich nicht, denn an einem geschlossenen Kreis ist kein Anfang (bzw. kein Ende) zu finden. Von wo die Abzweigungen derselben im Körper ihren Ausgang nehmen und wo sie endigen und wie die eine (Ader) mit diesen (Abzweigungen) sich wieder vereinigt und an welchen Stellen des Körpers (diese Abzweigungen) ausgebreitet sind, werde ich kundtun." '

[3] P. Diepgen, op. cit., remarks: 'Es ist auch ganz willkürlich übersetzt, wenn Kapferer im Anschluß an diese Stelle, wo von den Verzweigungen dieser Ader die Rede ist, ὁμολογέει mit "sich wieder vereinigt" übersetzt, als ob der hippokratische Verfasser sagen wollte, daß die Verzweigungen zur Hauptader wieder zurückkehren. Es heißt nur, er wolle zeigen ὡς ἡ μία ταύτῃσιν ὁμολογέει : wie die eine (große Ader) diesen (Verzweigungen) homolog ist, also etwa zu ihnen paßt, mit ihnen einig ist, ein Ganzes bildet. Von einem Rücklauf ist nicht die Rede.'

[4] *De articulis*, 45: αἱ δὲ φλέβες καὶ ἀρτηριῶν κοινωνίαι ἐν ἑτέρῳ λόγῳ δεδηλώσονται, ὅσαι τε καὶ οἷαι, καὶ ὅθεν ὡρμημέναι, καὶ ἐν οἷοισιν οἷα δύνανται.

promises to tell us how many and of what kind they are, where they start from, and what functions they perform in what organs. This by itself would be sufficient to suggest a comparatively late date, not earlier than Praxagoras. Kapferer also cites a paragraph from the Dutch seventeenth-century anatomist De Waal in connection with this same chapter, to the effect that Hippocrates had anticipated the circulation and that it was his successors who failed to develop the theory and indeed obscured it, so that during the centuries which followed the circular motion of the blood was unknown.[1]

Kapferer's attempt to identify our treatise with the one promised in *On joints* carries little conviction, since, in spite of all his rearrangement, nothing like the systematic treatise there promised eventuates. Surely it would be much more reasonable to regard it, as Littré did, as an amalgam of at least five different elements,[2] and to leave the matter there. Chapters 11–19 were regarded by Littré as a separate work forming a comparatively coherent whole, one which was known to Galen. This would account quite satisfactorily for its introductory nature duplicating the matter contained in Chapter 1. And even Kapferer agrees that Chapters 12–19 are continuous.

To proceed, then, with our analysis. Chapter 1 starts with an outline of some of the bones which compose the skeleton, with the details of which we are not concerned. The author then proceeds to give a rather curious account of the disposal of liquids absorbed through the mouth.

The drink [goes?] through the pharynx and the oesophagus (στόμαχος); larynx to the lung and 'artery' and from these into the top of the bladder. Five lobes of the liver. And on the fourth lobe the gall lies, where its mouth leads [φέρει] to the diaphragm and heart and lung. A membrane encloses

---

[1] De Waal, *Ep. duae de motu chyli, etc.* appended to Thomae Bartholini *Anatomia*, etc. (The Hague, 1666), and reprinted in *Opera selecta Neerlandicorum de arte medica* iv (Amsterdam, 1922), 70 f.: 'Equidem ego satis mirari non possum, tot retroactis saeculis, hunc sanguinis motum ignotum fuisse, cum ejus varia nec levia indicia apud veteres inveniam.' De Waal then goes on to quote various passages from the *Hippocratic corpus*, the fragment from Diogenes of Apollonia which has come down to us in quotation by Aristotle and, after referring both to Aristotle's theory of sleep and to Plato's remarks on the movement of the blood in the *Timaeus*, concludes as follows: 'Qui hos consecuti sunt scriptores, non satis sanguinis motum excoluisse, imo hunc obscurasse suspicio est, quod ea quae praecedentes suis venis, hoc est venis et arteriis adscriberent, hi venis ut arteriis opponuntur iverint attributum; etiam Galenus, medicorum summus, omnibus restituendis in integrum non sufficeret, posteriores Graeci, ut et Arabi et Latini, nimis presse eum sequerentur aut describerent, unde suspicamur hunc sanguinis motum in hoc usque saeculum delituisse.'

[2] Littré i. 418 ff.; ix. 162 ff. Littré points out that in addition to the three quotations, the book contains a treatise on the blood vessels, which he identifies with the Περὶ φλεβῶν mentioned by Galen as the προσκείμενα τῷ μοχλικῷ in the form of Chapters 11–19, and another source or sources, comprising Chapters 4–7. These are of a later date than the προσκείμενα since they regard the blood vessels as all centred on or arising out of the heart, whereas the latter seems to regard them as beginning at the head rather after the manner of Diogenes of Apollonia.

the heart. Has large intestines larger than a dog. And they are attached to the part of the mesentery near the colon. The kidneys are attached to 'sinews' from the spine and the artery.

These cryptic notes may well puzzle us. They read like lecture notes, or even more like headings for a lecture. Kapferer insists that the word 'artery' where first mentioned means the pulmonary artery, which seems to me to be most improbable, if only because the pulmonary artery was called, as we shall see, a vein.[1] He also translates the word κύστις as 'Herzblase'[2] (the pericardial sack) which seems to me to be quite impossible. The most natural interpretation of the word 'artery' here would seem to be windpipe, though this too raises difficulties. How can the liquid pass from the throat via the lungs into the bladder? Some light may perhaps be thrown on this conundrum by the theory which was widely held, even in later times, that when we drink, some liquid, notwithstanding the closure of the epiglottis, manages to find its way into the lung. Indeed, one theory was that the liquid in the pericardial sack was maintained in this way, a notion which we shall find not only in Plato[3] but also in the fragment *On the heart*.[4] The use of the word artery without further qualification must refer to the descending aorta in the abdomen, which forms part of what is called by several authors the 'great artery'. The omission of the adjective in what looks like a series of notes needs no explanation.

Chapter 2 deals with the heart and the blood vessels. Here again we have the note-like style.

The fountain of the heart. A closely related vein stretches through the diaphragm, liver, spleen, kidneys into the hip; round the calf of the leg into the sole of the foot. And another from the heart under the armpits [and?] collar-bones [into] the throat, the head, the nose, the forehead, past the ears, the shoulders, and the part behind the midriff [μετάφρενον], i.e. the broad of the back,

---

[1] *De natura ossium*, 1 : ὀστέα χειρὸς εἴκοσι ἑπτά· ποδὸς εἴκοσι τέσσαρα· τραχήλου ἐς τὸν μέγαν ἑπτά· ὀσφύος πέντε· ῥάχιος εἴκοσι, κεφαλῆς ξὺν ὀπωπίοις ὀκτώ· ξύμπαντα ἐνενήκοντα ἕν, ξὺν ὄνυξιν ἑκατὸν ἕνδεκα. ἃ δ' ἡμεῖς αὐτοὶ ἐξ ἀνθρώπου ὀστέων κατεμάθομεν, σπόνδυλοι οἱ ἄνω τῆς κληῖδος ξὺν τῷ μεγάλῳ ἑπτά. οἱ δὲ κατὰ τὰς πλευράς, ὅσαι περ αἱ πλευραὶ δώδεκα. οἱ δὲ κατὰ κενεῶνας ἐκτός, ἐν ᾧ τὰ ἰσχία, ἐν τῇ ὀσφύϊ πέντε. τὸ δὲ σπέρμα οἷον κηρίον ἑκατέρωθεν τῆς κύστιος. ἐκ δ' αὐτῶν φλέβες ἑκατέρωθεν τοῦ οὐρητῆρος ἐς τὸ αἰδοῖον τείνουσι. ποτὸν διὰ φάρυγγος καὶ στομάχου· λάρυγξ ἐς πλεύμονα καὶ ἀρτηρίην· ἀπὸ δὲ τούτων ἐς ἄκρην κύστιν. ἥπατος πέντε λοβοί· ἐπὶ δὲ τοῦ τετάρτου ἐπίκειται ἡ χολή, ᾗ τὸ στόμα ἐπὶ φρένας καὶ καρδίην καὶ πλεύμονα φέρει. καρδίην ὑμὴν περίεστι. τὰ κῶλα ἔχει κυνὸς μείζω· ἤρτηται δὲ ἐκ τῶν μεσοκώλων. ταῦτα δὲ ἐκ νεύρων· ἀπὸ τῆς ῥάχιος ὑπὸ τὴν γαστέρα. νεφροὶ ἐκ νεύρων ἀπὸ ῥάχιος καὶ ἀρτηρίης.

[2] Kapferer, op. cit., p. 36: 'Von diesen [sc. fließt es] in die Herzblase.' (Sticker, in his translation of the *De natura ossium* in Kapferer's translation of the *Corpus*, simply omits the sentence.) The translation seems to me to be wholly unacceptable. As far as I am aware, the word κύστις is only used for the bladder or for the gall-bladder.

[3] *Timaeus*, 70 c: τὴν τοῦ πλεύμονος ἰδέαν ἐνεφύτευσαν, πρῶτον μὲν μαλακὴν καὶ ἄναιμον, εἶτα σήραγγας ἐντὸς ἔχουσαν οἷον σπόγγου κατατετρημένας, ἵνα τό τε πνεῦμα καὶ τὸ πῶμα δεχομένη, ψύχουσα, ἀναπνοὴν καὶ ῥᾳστώνην ἐν τῷ καύματι παρέχοι.

[4] See below, p. 85.

and past [διὰ] the chest and the belly through [διὰ] the forearm. And one through or past [διὰ] the armpit to the forearm, to the palm of the hand.[1]

This short paragraph reads not so much like notes taken *from* a lecture as notes written *for* one. As it is over two thousand years old, we must not be unduly surprised that in either case it should not seem very intelligible. It seems to trace two main vessels from the heart, one going downwards into the legs, and the other upwards into the neck and to the head, and then to return down the back, the chest, and the belly or perhaps through or past the belly of the forearm, an expression which would be rather difficult to justify or explain. The relation of this vessel to the one described as going past the armpit to the forearm is quite obscure. Kapferer with his accustomed temerity does not hesitate to slash at the Gordian knot. He translates the 'fountain of the heart' as 'der Herzausgang' and identifies the one which goes upwards with the ascending aorta. The second 'vein' he conveniently identifies with the arteria carotis communis and the third with the arteria subclavia, by dint of some rather curious translation.[2]

Chapter 3 deals entirely with an assembly of structures called nerves, which do not concern us here. I therefore transfer my literal translation to a footnote.[3]

Chapter 4 returns to the blood vessels, but Kapferer, for reasons which do not appear to have any philological or epigraphical justification,

---

[1] *De natura ossium*, 2: καρδίης πηγή· ξυγγενὴς φλὲψ τείνει διὰ φρενῶν, ἥπατος, σπληνός, νεφρῶν ἐς ἰσχίον· περὶ γαστεροκνημίην ἐπὶ τὸν ταρσόν. ἑτέρη δ' ἐκ καρδίης ὑπὸ μασχάλας, κληῖδας, σφαγάς, κεφαλήν, ῥῖνα, μέτωπον παρὰ τὰ ὦτα, ὤμους, μετάφρενον, στήθεα, γαστέρα διὰ πήχεος. ἡ δὲ διὰ μασχαλέων ἐπὶ πῆχυν, ἐπὶ ταρσόν.

[2] In his first article in *Hippokrates* (1937): 'Eine zweite, aber ausführliche Beschreibung der Blutgefäße vom und zum Herzen finden wir in der Schrift "Die Natur der Knochen". Dort wird im Kap. II zuerst die Aorta mit ihren Abzweigungen nach oben und unten wie folgt beschrieben: "Der Herzausgang: (aus ihm) zieht eine zugeordnete Ader durch das Zwerchfell, die Leber, die Milz, die Nieren zum Bein (≠ Aorta descendens), dagegen eine von zwei (Adern) vom Herzen her unten an ... die Kehle, den Kopf (≠ Arteria carotis commun.), die andere aber ... zum Arm, zur Handfläche (≠ Arteria subclavia)."' [Omissions Kapferer's.]

[3] *De natura ossium*, 3: νεύρων ἔκφυσις ἀπὸ τοῦ ἰνίου ἄχρι παρὰ ῥάχιν παρὰ ἰσχίον ἐς αἰδοῖα, ἐς μηρούς, πόδας, κνημάς, ἐς χεῖρας. ἀλλ' ἐς βραχίονας, τὰ μὲν ἐς σάρκας, τὰ δὲ παρὰ τὴν περόνην ἐς τὸν μέγαν δάκτυλον. τὰ δ' ἐκ τῶν σαρκῶν ἐπὶ τοὺς ἄλλους δακτύλους. ἀλλ' ἐς ὠμοπλάτην, στῆθος, γαστέρα, ὀστέοισι, ξυνδέσμοισι. ἀπὸ δὲ αἰδοίου παρ' ἀρχόν, κοτυληδόνα· τὸ μὲν ἄνωθεν μηροῦ, τὸ δὲ κάτωθεν ἐπὶ τὰ γούνατα, ἐντεῦθεν γούνατι ξυνταθὲν ἐπὶ τένοντα, πτέρναν, πόδας. τὸ δὲ ἐς περόνην· ἄλλα δ' ἐς τοὺς νεφρούς.

A literal translation of this chapter would read as follows: 'The outgrowth of "nerves" from the occiput to along the spine along the hip to the penis, to the thighs, the feet, the calves, to the hands. But [those going into?] the arms, some into the flesh, and some past the small bone of the radius to the thumb. And from the flesh to the other fingers. Others into the shoulder, the chest, the stomach, with bones and ligaments. And from the penis past the anus, and the socket of the thigh bone [?κοτυληδών]. One on the upper side of the thigh, and one on the lower side to the knees, from thence stretched over the knee, to the tendon [Achilles?], the heel, the feet. And the one that goes into the fibula [περόνη]. And others into the kidneys.'

Not a very illuminating note. The structures referred to seem to be nerves rather than sinews in some places, but *which* is far from clear.

entirely redistributes the order of the remaining chapters, while still, however, retaining the continuity of Chapters 12–19. He does this in order to arrive at what he conceives to be a more logical scheme, corresponding to the programme laid down in Chapter 11, which he places at the head of the treatise. In place of Chapter 4, which he relegates to the extreme end of the treatise to be followed only by the three chapters which are word-for-word translations from other works and must therefore be regarded as quotations (namely Chapters 8, 9, and 10), Kapferer transposes Chapters 12–19. Next, he places Chapters 5, 6, and 7, to be followed by Chapter 4, which he regards as a sort of appendix on the kidneys referring back to the theory of drinking expounded in Chapter 1 ; oblivious, it would seem, of the facts pointed out by Littré, going to show that these chapters are of much later date than Chapters 11–19. Finally, he places at the end of the treatise the three chapters taken word for word from other works: Chapter 8 from the third book of Aristotle's *History of animals*, or perhaps directly from Syennesis himself; Chapter 9 from the 'Hippocratic' *Nature of man*; and Chapter 10 from the second book of the *Epidemics*.[1]

Chapter 4 reads as follows:

And these veins are split on each side into two very big branches, one on this, and one on that, side of each kidney, and they open up into the kidneys. And the kidneys have the shape of the heart: they too have cavities. The kidney lies with its hollow parts turned towards the great veins. From which place the veins grow out of them which go to the bladder, the place where the drink was drawn into the kidneys through the veins. Since just as the water also seeps through the kidneys so does it through these inner parts which surround them, for the parts between the kidneys and the bladder are like a sponge, and from here the urine seeps in and is separated from the blood, wherefore it is red. For there are no other veins going into the kidneys, except the ones I have spoken of, nor is there, as far as I know, any other place where the drink could be collected.[2]

---

[1] Kapferer's order and schematization will be found on pp. 34 and 35 of the work under discussion. I have not thought it necessary to reproduce it. That the traditional text, as it appears in Littré, is confused may readily be granted, but that does not imply that Kapferer's rearrangement and emendations in any way lessen the confusion. Indeed they make confusion worse confounded. While we may agree that Chapter 4 appears to have little connection with Chapter 3, we must add that it does not follow any more logically as an appendix to Chapter 7, where Kapferer would like to place it. It looks much more like an isolated fragment from one of the earlier physiologists with rather primitive ideas about the structure of the human organs. For he likens the kidneys to the heart in shape and endows them with 'ventricles', and he appears to confuse the ureters with veins. His ideas of the seepage of liquid into the bladder is anything but clear.

[2] *De natura ossium*, 4: αὗται δὲ αἱ φλέβες ἐφ' ἑκάτερα διχῇ τὰ μέγιστα σχίζονται τὰ μὲν ἔνθεν τοῦ νεφροῦ ἑκατέρου, τὰ δ' ἔνθεν, καὶ διατέτρηνται ἐς τοὺς νεφρούς· καὶ εἶδος καρδίης οἱ νεφροὶ ἔχουσι· καὶ οὗτοι κοιλώδεες. ὁ δὲ νεφρὸς τὰ κοῖλα ἑωυτοῦ πρὸς τὰς φλέβας ἔχων κεῖται τὰς μεγάλας. ὅθεν ἐκπεφύκασιν ἐξ αὐτέου αἱ φλέβες αἱ ἐς κύστιν, ᾗ εἵλκετο τὸ ποτὸν διὰ τῶν φλεβῶν ἐς τοὺς νεφρούς. ἔπειθ' ὥσπερ καὶ διὰ τῶν νεφρῶν διηθεῖται τὸ ὕδωρ καὶ δι' αὐτέων τουτέων τῶν

Chapter 5, again, seems to have no connection either with Chapter 4 or with Chapter 2. It would appear to belong to an epoch much later than Diogenes of Apollonia. For in this chapter arteries and veins seem to be clearly distinguished. It cannot, therefore, be earlier than Praxagoras, and might, of course, be much later. Its opening sentence does not make it clear whether the author is talking about veins or arteries.

Those that stretch along the ribs run below each of the ribs, not on the headward side, but below them, and away from the 'artery'. Now the 'artery' there flowing under them gives out branches to the ribs. And one branch runs backwards from the thick one from the heart bending to the left. Then it [the artery] runs past the middle vertebrae up to the top of the ribs, not giving off branches to the ribs at equal intervals, to the right and to the left. Another one splits off on the right, which does give off branches at equal intervals, but higher up.[1]

Kapferer[2] thinks that it is arteries which are being referred to in the first sentence, and that the 'thick one' refers to the aorta, not to the vena cava which is commonly referred to as the thick vein. He also translates the words μέχρις ἄκρων πλευρέων as 'bis zu den äußersten (letzten) Rippen'. He is thus able to reproduce what he regards as a surprisingly accurate picture of the intercostal arteries. But can his translation of these words really be accepted? The Greek words can only mean one of two things, 'till the top of the ribs' or 'till the top ribs'. What Kapferer means by the phrase just quoted, 'the outermost [last] ribs', is not at all plain to me since neither Kapferer nor 'Hippocrates' gives any numbering. In any case the chapter simply cannot be integrated with the rest of the treatise.

Chapter 6 and Chapters 12–19, which form the work *On the veins* known to Galen, develop a description of the blood vessels which follows closely that of Diogenes, and recognizes no distinction between arteries and veins. Chapter 7, on the other hand, does separate them and is obviously based on a much later scheme of vascular knowledge.

Chapter 6 is quite short. It reads as follows:

And of the veins by each collar-bone, two go upwards and two go under the chest: and they throw off branches to the right and to the left. These

---

ἐντέρων ὧν ξυνεπακολουθεῖ· σπογγοειδὲς γάρ ἐστι τὸ ἀπ' αὐτέων ἐς τὴν κύστιν, καὶ ἐνταῦθα διηθούμενον καὶ ἀποκρινόμενον ἀπὸ τοῦ αἵματος τὸ οὖρον, διὸ δὴ ἐρυθρόν ἐστιν. οὐδὲ γὰρ ἐς τοὺς νεφροὺς ἦσαν ἄλλαι φλέβες ἢ αἱ εἴρηνται, οὐδ' ὅποι ἂν τὸ ποτὸν ξυντήκοιτο, ὅσον ἐγὼ οἶδα.

[1] Ibid., 5: αἱ παρὰ τὰς πλευρὰς κατατείνουσαι κάτωθεν εἰσὶν ἑκάστης τῶν πλευρέων, οὐ πρὸς κεφαλῆς, κατωτέρω δὲ καὶ ἀπὸ ἀρτηρίας. ἀρτηρίη μὲν οὖν εἶθ' ὑπορρεύσασα διαδιδοῖ τῇσι πλευρῇσι. ἀπὸ δὲ τῆς παχείης ἀπὸ καρδίης παλινδρομέει μία ἐς τὰ ἀριστερὰ ἐγκεκλιμένη. ἔπειτα ἡ μὲν διὰ μέσων σπονδύλων μέχρις ἄκρων πλευρέων πορεύεται, πλευρῇσιν οὐκ ἐξ ἴσου διαδιδοῦσα τῇσι δεξιῇσι, (καὶ) τῇσιν ἀριστερῇσι διασχίδας. ἄλλη ἴσας μὲν ἀνωτέρωθεν δὲ ἐν τοῖσι δεξιοῖσιν ἀποσχίζεται.

[2] Kapferer, op. cit., p. 48.

are rather more towards the neck. But two go more towards the heart, some to the right and some to the left. And from them [branches go?] along the ribs. And from them [branches split off?] like those from below, until they meet or mix with the one running backwards from the heart below.[1]

Kapferer here, with what justification I cannot imagine, translates 'veins' as 'arteries' and interprets the recurrent vein as the aorta. The justification for this would appear to be the fact that the first sentence of the next chapter speaks of 'this artery' and must therefore be taken to refer to the aorta.[2]

This chapter, 7, reads as follows:

From this artery the vessel flowing with blood [αἱμόρρους—an old expression which we have already met with in Alcmaeon] is separated [or branches off], for this reason, because it travels there on top through [or past] the heart; but in the parts below the ribs the so-called thick vein, the blood-flowing one, again sends off branches from itself, to the vertebrae. And here it keeps close to them [the vertebrae] and is not suspended any longer above them, as it is where it goes up through the liver. Now in the loins the artery runs on top and the blood-flowing vein underneath, the one which, coming from the liver through the diaphragm, runs on top of [or past] the right side of the heart up to the collar-bone, with no branches except where it communicates with the heart itself. Now the branches that split off from it run rather near the surface, but the part of it which goes through the ventricle of the heart, when it leaves the heart is located on the left side, running without branches towards the spine. It then runs in the opposite direction [presumably, that is, away from the spine] upwards to the upper parts of the body, up as far as the highest ribs. And it has offshoots running naturally along each rib up to the fastening of the chest, both on the right hand and on the left. And the straight section of it goes closer to the vertebrae than the path of the artery, and that of the vein from the liver. But in the part below the heart, the direction of its straight stretch is more towards the vertebrae than that of the artery, the second stretch, the one along or past the heart and turns down to the parts below the diaphragm which are adjoining the spine. From there go

---

[1] *De natura ossium*, 6: παρὰ δὲ κληῗδος ἑκατέρης τῶν φλεβῶν δύο μὲν ἄνω, δύο δὲ ὑπὸ τὸ στῆθος, αἱ μὲν ἐς δεξιά, αἱ δὲ ἐς ἀριστερὰ ἀπεσχίσθησαν ἀποσχίδες, πρὸς αὐχένος μὲν μᾶλλον αὗται· δύο δὲ πρὸς καρδίην μᾶλλον, αἱ μὲν ἐπὶ δεξιά, αἱ δ᾽ ἀριστερά· ἀφ᾽ ἑκατέρης παρὰ τὰς πλευράς. καὶ ἀπ᾽ αὐτέων ὥσπερ αἱ κάτω ἐσχίζοντο, μέχρις ὅτου ξυνέμιξαν τῇ κάτω παλινδρομησάσῃ ἀπὸ καρδίης.

[2] Kapferer, loc. cit.: 'Von den Adern an jedem Schlüsselbein (Art. subclav.) spalten sich Zweige nach oben (Art. vertebr.); zwei unter den Brustkorb (ae. mammar. int.), die einen in die rechte, die anderen in die linke Seite. Diese (nach oben) ziehen mehr am Nacken, zwei anderseits aber mehr nach dem Herzen. Von jeder einzelnen ziehen die einen Zweige nach rechts, die anderen nach links an den Rippen entlang (Rami intercostales). Sie spalten sich von ihnen geradeso ab wie die Adern unter sich abspalten, bis dorthin wo sie mit der unteren Ader, die vom Herzen entgegengesetzt läuft (Aorta thorac.), zusammenkommen.' Kapferer adds a note: 'Die Rami intercostales der vorderen inneren Brustwand anastomosen mit den Ae. intercostales der hinteren inneren Brustwand. Im Kap. vii wird diese Vereinigung genauer beschrieben.'

branches, each of them in a straight line through the bones and the flesh running into one another.[1]

Portions of this description are far from clear, but there can be no doubt that we are here dealing with an author who has advanced quite a long way beyond Diogenes. He has begun to make a distinction between two main systems of vessels, at any rate so far as the vena cava, the hollow or blood-flowing vein, and the artery, which is presumably the aorta. It is of course dangerous to make too wide inferences from a single paragraph or chapter. But we seem to be dealing with someone whose general topography of the vascular system is approximately correct in its main features. We may note in particular his accurate observation that in the abdomen the aorta descendens rides, before it divides, on top of the inferior vena cava; whereas in the thorax their relative positions are reversed, where the innominate vein overrides the arch of the aorta in the upper part of the thorax. Lower down in the thoracic cavity the aorta, of course, lies nearer to the surface of the chest. Kapferer, for reasons best known to himself, interprets the blood-flowing vein as the aorta, but this cannot possibly be correct, as the term seems to have been invented, possibly by Alcmaeon, precisely to distinguish the vena cava and its branches from the *pneuma*-carrying 'veins' which were supposed to contain less blood. Moreover it seems perfectly clear that the author is speaking of the hollow vein. The vein which comes from the liver through the diaphragm past the right side of the heart can surely be nothing else, since it was this which according to the 'Hippocratic' tradition, as we shall see later, was in direct communication with the right ventricle. Even more arbitrary is Kapferer's translation of the words στηθέος συνοκωχή,[2] which he renders as 'bis zum zusammentreffen mit (den Adern) der Brust' (the place where the blood vessels of the breast unite), adding in brackets the words '*rami intercostales*'. This is a mistranslation which might be cited as a *locus classicus* of the dangers of reading into an ancient text the findings of modern science. The word ξυνοκωχή, which

---

[1] *De natura ossium*, 7: ἡ δὲ αἱμόρρους ἀπὸ τῆς ἀρτηρίης ταύτης διὰ τοῦτο ἐσχίσθη ὅτι μετέωρος ἐνταῦθά ἐστι διὰ καρδίης πορευομένη. τὰ δὲ κάτω πλευρέων ἡ αἱμόρρους ἡ παχείη καλεομένη φλὲψ τοῖσι σφονδύλοισι αὖθις ἐφ' ἑωυτῆς διαδιδοῖ, καὶ ἐνταῦθα προσέχεται, καὶ οὐκ ἔτι κρέμαται ὥσπερ ἄνω δι' ἥπατος ἰοῦσα. ἔστι δὲ κατὰ μὲν ὀσφὺν ἄνω ἡ ἀρτηρίη, ὑποκάτω δὲ ἡ αἱμόρρους ἡ ἀπὸ τοῦ ἥπατος διὰ φρενῶν ἐλθοῦσα μετέωρος παρὰ τὰ ἐπιδεξιὰ τῆς καρδίης φέρεται ἄχρι κληΐδων ἁπλῆ, πλὴν ὅσον αὐτῇ τῇ καρδίῃ κοινωνέει. τὰ μὲν κατ' αὐτὴν σχιζόμενα ἐπιπολαιότερα, τὰ δὲ τὴν κοιλίην τῆς καρδίης διέχονται, ἔπειτα ἀπὸ τῆς καρδίης τὸ ἐπ' ἀριστερὰ κάθηται ἁπλῆ πρὸς ῥάχιν, ἢ παλινδρομέει ἐς μὲν τὸ ἄνω τοῦ σώματος ἄχρι τῶν ἀνωτάτων πλευρέων· καὶ ἀποσχίδας ἀφ' ἑωυτῆς ἔχει παρ' ἑκάστην πλευρὰν παρατεταμένας κατὰ φύσιν ἄχρι στήθεος συνοκωχῆς καὶ ἐπ' ἀριστερὰ καὶ ἐπὶ δεξιά. καὶ τὸ ἰθὺ αὐτέης πρὸς σφονδύλων μᾶλλόν ἐστι ἢ ὁ τῆς ἀρτηρίης τόνος, καὶ ὁ τῆς ἀπὸ τοῦ ἥπατος φλεβός· πρὸς δὲ τὸ κάτω μέρος τῆς καρδίης ὁ μὲν ἰθὺς τόνος ἀπ' αὐτέης πρὸς σφονδύλων μᾶλλόν ἐστιν ἢ ὁ τῆς ἀρτηρίης, ὁ δεύτερος, ὁ παρὰ καρδίην, καὶ ἐς τὰ κάτω μέρη φρενῶν ἐτράπετο, τὰ πρὸς ῥάχιος ἠρτημένα. ἐντεῦθεν δὲ ἀποσχίδες ἐς ἰθὺ ἕκασται ἐπιφέρονται, δι' ὀστέων καὶ σαρκῶν περαιωθεῖσαι ἀλλήλας.

[2] Kapferer, op. cit., p. 50.

I have translated 'fastening' cannot be anything but the sternum, the 'thing which holds the chest together'. He also has to assume quite arbitrarily a sudden change of subject from vena cava to aorta, where a straightforward reading of the text makes it quite plain that the author is dealing with the same blood vessel But enough of these misinterpretations. The important thing to note is that at the end of the chapter we are once more informed of branches running off the vena cava running into one another.

Chapters 8 and 9 are quotations which we have already mentioned: the first, from Aristotle,[1] the fragment from Diogenes of Apollonia quoted on p. 22; and the second the passage from the essay of Polybus or 'Hippocrates'[2] *On the nature of man.* The third quotation, that from the *Epidemics,*[3] which constitutes the tenth chapter, is also perhaps worth while reproducing textually.

And the liver vein, in its lower part in the loins up to the great vertebra, also gives off branches to the vertebrae. From there it rises up through the liver and the diaphragm to the heart, and from the heart it goes in a straight line to the collar-bone. From there, some branches go to the neck and some to the shoulder-blades, and some bend off downwards, turning off along the vertebrae and the ribs on the left side near the collar-bone, and on the right one to a certain place. And another bends off on both sides [of the vertebrae?] and another a little below, at the place where the first bent off, supplies the ribs, until it meets the one coming from the heart, bending away towards the left. And bending off downwards, it goes down towards the vertebrae, until it comes to the place where it began to come on top, giving off branches to all the other ribs, on this side and on that, branches that run along each of them, though it is a single vessel, running rather on the left side from the heart up to a certain point. Then it runs under the artery until it expends itself and comes to where the liver vein comes up to the surface. But before this, before it gets to this place, it splits into two near the last two ribs, and its two branches run along each side of the vertebrae and spend themselves. But the one that stretches upwards straight from the heart to the collar-bones is on top of the artery, just as along the loins it is below the artery. And from this there part down two into the liver, one vein to the gates, and the lobes, and the other to the rest of it, coming off close to it a little below the diaphragm. Now the diaphragm grows on to the liver, and it is not easy to separate them. And from the collar-bones two veins, one on each side, go under the chest into the belly. And whither they go from there, I do not yet know. And the diaphragm encircles the vertebra, the one under the ribs, where the kidney emerges from the artery. And arteries grow out of the kidney, one on each side, having the fashion of arteries. There somewhere the liver vein running backwards from the heart stops. And from the liver vein go the two biggest veins through the diaphragm, one on each side, near the surface, with many branches coming off them through

[1] Aristotle, *Hist. anim.* 3. 2.   [2] Hippocrates, *De natura hominis,* 11.
[3] *Epidemics,* ii. 10.

the diaphragm, and they grow on the upper side of the diaphragm, and these are rather more clearly visible.[1]

The rest of the chapter is devoted to a description of sinews or nerves, it is a little difficult to say which. This has nothing to do with the vascular system, and I must therefore relegate it to a footnote. The portion we have just quoted belongs to an epoch much later than Diogenes of Apollonia. It seems to represent a stage of knowledge intermediate between that of Praxagoras and that of Herophilus. The term *liver vein* seems, however, to recall an earlier period, that of the two main veins, the liver vein and the spleen vein, but the liver vein is clearly well on the way to becoming the thick or hollow vein, the main vein postulated by Aristotle as the trunk of all the veins. Our author seems to be acquainted with the heart as the focus of two different systems of blood vessels, and distinguishes clearly between the liver vein and the artery which is, of course, the aorta. But to attempt to identify his description in detail with anatomic facts does not seem very feasible. Two points of interest, however, are worth

[1] *De natura ossium*, 10: ἡ δὲ ἡπατῖτις ἐν ὀσφύϊ μέχρι τοῦ μεγάλου σπονδύλου κάτωθεν, καὶ σπονδύλοισι προσδιδοῖ, ἐντεῦθεν μετέωρος δι' ἥπατος καὶ διὰ φρενῶν ἐς καρδίην. καὶ ἥει μὲν εὐθεῖα ἐς κληῖδας· ἐντεῦθεν δὲ αἱ μὲν ἐς τράχηλον, αἱ δ' ἐπ' ὠμοπλάτας, αἱ δὲ ἀποκαμφθεῖσαι κάτω, παρὰ σπονδύλους καὶ πλευρὰς ἀποκλίνουσιν. ἐξ ἀριστερῶν μὲν μία ἐγγὺς κληῖδων, ἐκ δεξιῶν δὲ ἐπί τι αὐτὴ χωρίον. ἄλλη δὲ ἑκατέρωθεν ἀποκαμφθεῖσα, ἄλλη δὲ σμικρὸν κατωτέρω ἀποκαμφθεῖσα, ὅθεν μὲν ἐκείνη ἀπέλιπε, προσέδωκε τῆσι πλευρῆσι, ἔστ' ἂν τῇ ἐπ' αὐτέης τῆς καρδίης προστύχῃ ἐπικαμπτομένη ἐς τὰ ἀριστερά. ἀποκαμφθεῖσα δὲ κάτω ἐπὶ σπονδύλους καταβαίνει, ἔστ' ἂν ἀφίκηται ὅθεν ἤρξατο μετεωρίζεσθαι, ἀποδιδοῦσα τῇσι πλευρῇσι τῇσιν ἐπιλοίποις ἁπάσαις, καὶ ἔνθεν καὶ ἔνθεν ἀποσχίδας παρ' ἑκάστην διδοῦσα μία ἐοῦσα ἀπὸ μὲν τῆς καρδίης ἐπί τι χωρίον ἐν τοῖσιν ἀριστεροῖσιν μᾶλλον ἐοῦσα, ἔπειτα ὑποκάτω τῆς ἀρτηρίης, ἔστ' ἂν καταναλωθῇ, καὶ ἔλθη ὅθεν ἡ ἡπατῖτις ἐμετεωρίσθη. πρότερον δέ, πρὶν ἐνταῦθ' ἐλθεῖν, παρὰ τὰς ἐσχάτας δύο πλευρὰς ἐδιχώθη. καὶ ἡ μὲν ἔνθα, ἡ δ' ἔνθα τῶν σπονδύλων ἐλθοῦσα κατηναλώθη. ἡ δ' εὐθεῖα ἀπὸ καρδίης πρὸς κληῖδας τείνουσα ἄνωθεν τῆς ἀρτηρίης ἐστίν, ὥσπερ καὶ παρ' ὀσφὺν κάτωθεν τῆς ἀρτηρίης, καὶ ἀπὸ ταύτης ἀίσσει ἐς τὸ ἧπαρ, ἡ μὲν ἐπὶ πύλας καὶ λοβόν, ἡ δ' ἐς τὸ ἄλλο ἑξῆς ἀφωρμήκει σμικρὸν κάτωθεν φρενῶν. φρένες δὲ προσπεφύκασι τῷ ἥπατι, ἃς οὐ ῥάδιον χωρίσαι. δισσαὶ δ' ἀπὸ κληῖδων, αἱ μὲν ἔνθεν αἱ δ' ἔνθεν ὑπὸ στῆθος ἐς ἦτρον ὅποι δὲ ἐντεῦθεν, οὔπω οἶδα. φρένες δὲ κατὰ τὸν σπόνδυλον τὸν κάτω τῶν πλευρέων, ᾗ νεφρὸς ἐξ ἀρτηρίης ταύτῃ ἀμφιβεβηκυῖαι ἀρτηρίαι ἐκ τουτέου ἐκπεφύκασιν ἔνθεν καὶ ἔνθεν ἀρτηρίης τρόπον ἔχουσαι. ταύτῃ πῃ παλινδρομήσασα ἀπὸ καρδίης ἡ ἡπατῖτις ἔληγεν. ἀπὸ δὲ τῆς ἡπατίτιδος διὰ τῶν φρενῶν αἱ μέγισται δύο, ἡ μὲν ἔνθεν ἡ δὲ ἔνθεν φέρονται μετέωροι, πολυσχιδεῖς δὲ διὰ τῶν φρενῶν εἰσιν ἀμφὶ ταύτας, καὶ πεφύκασιν ἄνωθεν δὲ φρενῶν· αὗται δὲ μᾶλλόν τι ἐμφανέες.

The section devoted to what seems to be 'nerves' runs as follows: δύο δὲ παχεῖς τόνοι ἀπ' ἐγκεφάλου ὑπὸ τὸ ὀστέον τοῦ μεγάλου σπονδύλου ἄνωθεν, καὶ πρὸς τοῦ στομάχου μᾶλλον ἑκατέρωθεν τῆς ἀρτηρίης παρελθὼν ἑκάτερος εἰς ἑαυτὸν ἦλθεν ἴκελος ἑνί. ἔπειτα ᾗ σπόνδυλοι καὶ φρένες πεφύκασιν, ἐνταῦθ' ἐτελεύτων· καί τινες ἐνδοιαστοὶ πρὸς ἦπαρ καὶ σπλῆνα ἀπὸ τούτου τοῦ κοινωνήματος ἐδόκεον τείνειν. ἄλλος τόνος ἑκάτερωθεν ἐκ τῶν κατὰ κληῖδα σπονδύλων παρὰ ῥάχιν παρέτεινεν, ἐκ πλαγίου σπονδύλου, καὶ τῇσι πλευρῇσι ἀπένειμεν, ὥσπερ αἱ φλέβες, οὗτοι διὰ φρενῶν ἐς μεσεντέριόν μοι δοκέουσι τείνειν, ἐν δὲ τουτέοισι ἐξέλιπον, αὖθις δ' ὅθεν φρένες ἐξεπεφύκεσαν ἀπὸ τούτου συνεχέες ἐόντες, κατὰ μέσον κάτωθεν ἀρτηρίης τὸ δ' ἐπίλοιπον παρὰ σπονδύλους ἀπεδίδουν, ὥσπερ αἱ φλέβες, μέχρι κατηναλώθησαν πᾶν διελθόντες τὸ ἱερὸν ὀστέον.

The meaning of the word τόνος is far from clear; at first sight it looks much more like a sinew than a nerve, and is also used to denote a tendon. Kapferer translates it as 'nerve'. He sees in this description 'noch eine erstaunlich gute Schilderung des Verhanges der Stränge, nämlich des N vagus und des N sympathicus, die ist ein beredtes Zeugnis für die Sorgfalt der anatomischen Präparierung dieser nicht leicht zu verfolgenden Nerven'.

noticing. First, here too we seem to have a number of blood vessels inter-communicating. Secondly, the passage denotes an age of animal dissection. The liver is very hard to separate from the diaphragm, and our author is aware of the limitations of his knowledge, and hopes to discover more—'I do not yet know.'

Chapters 11–19 are identified by Littré with the treatise *On veins*, mentioned by Galen as being attached to the treatise *On levers*, or *Instruments of Reduction* as it has generally been called. This, as we have seen, would explain the duplication of Chapters 11 and 1. With the former we need not concern ourselves any further.

Chapter 12 begins quite abruptly:

This vein lies round the head, the middle part of it coming from the side. It is flat and thin and does not contain much blood. It sends many roots into the brain through the seams [of the skull], in the form of many slender little veins, and round the whole head it is like basket-work forming a network up to the forehead and the temples. And, itself, it is directed to the back of the head, on the outside by the skin of the spine. From there it goes down alongside of the external and internal veins, the ones in the throat. Beyond the ear it is joined by a branch from the chin, and stretches down on the outside, as a thick vein, and from it many veins branch off to the tongue. And this vein goes down past the collar-bone and under the shoulder-blade. And there a vein branches off from it, which goes through the ligament. [The Greek word is neuron, identified by Kapferer[1] with the brachial plexus.] It is a blood-flowing vein [αἱμόρρους] and contains a lot of blood, and is difficult to heal if it is broken or torn, for on one side of it is the flat ligament, and on the other, a cartilage [the cartilage of the first rib according to Kapferer], the space between them being occupied by it and the foam-like membrane. Now as the place has no flesh, the vein is easily broken, since there are no tissues growing round it. But if blood leaks into this part, it finds a wide empty space, and having no way of escape, solidifies and becomes hard. And when it gets hard, it produces illness. . . .

The vein which goes under the shoulder-blade buds off into many thin closely packed veins under the breasts, which cross one over another. And they go over the point of the shoulder and past the cartilage, but it dips below the surface and stretches into the arm, keeping the muscle on the left side. And it splits straightway near the shoulder and the upper part of the forearm. From there on it passes through the forearm, on both sides, and then again it goes through the wrist, from which it spreads through the whole hand, giving off many roots.[2]

[1] Kapferer, op. cit., p. 39.

[2] *De natura ossium*, 12: περὶ μὲν γὰρ τὴν κεφαλὴν κατὰ τὸ μέσον ἐκ πλαγίου περίκειται ἡ φλέψ, αὐτὴ πλατεῖα καὶ λεπτή, οὐ πολύαιμος. τῷ γὰρ ἐγκεφάλῳ κατὰ τὰς ἁρμονίας ἐνερρίζωκε πολλὰ καὶ λεπτὰ φλέβια, καὶ περὶ τὴν ὅλην κεφαλὴν ἐκτετάρσωται μέχρι τοῦ μετώπου καὶ τῶν κροτάφων. αὐτὴ δὲ ἀπιθύνεται ἐς τοὔπισθεν τῆς κεφαλῆς ἐκτὸς παρὰ τῆς ἀκάνθης τὸ δέρμα ἐντεῦθεν δὲ καθίεται παρὰ τὴν ἔξωθεν καὶ τὴν ἔσωθεν φλέβα τῶν ἐν τῇσι σφαγῇσι. πέρην δὲ τῆς ἀκοῆς ὑποσχισθεῖσα ἀπὸ τῆς γένυος ἔξωθεν τείνει παχεία. ἀπὸ δὲ ταύτης ἐς τὴν γλῶσσαν πολλαὶ καὶ λεπταί· πλὴν ἢ ὑπὸ τὴν γλῶσσαν ἢ ὑπὸ τοὺς γομφίους. αὐτὴ δὲ παχείη διὰ τῆς κληῖδος καθήκει ὑπὸ

The next chapter (13) seems to begin with a curious phrase, 'the ancient vein' (ἡ ἀρχαίη φλέψ). What this 'ancient vein' was has puzzled critics. But perhaps I may be permitted to propose an emendation. In spite of the fact that it was not suggested by so great a scholar as Littré, I cannot help feeling that for ἀρχαίη we should read παχείη, an alteration which implies only a small scribal error. This emendation would not, in my opinion, spoil the sense of the text. For though he appears to have rather a confused notion of its course, he is clearly referring to a vessel leading to the heart. Reading 'thick' for 'ancient', our text would run as follows: 'The thick vein, the one [that goes] along the spine and through the neck and the throat throws off from itself a vein into the heart, a very big one, with many mouths at the heart.'[1]

This sentence has caused quite a lot of difficulties for the critics. The phrase διὰ . . . τῆς σφαγῆς καὶ τοῦ βρόγχου seems fairly plain; though the word βρόγχος usually means the windpipe, it is also used for the throat generally. But the description of the vein as many-mouthed does not seem to fit any known anatomical conception, either of the cardiac approach of the vena cava or of the right auricle, which, as we have seen, was regarded by most Greeks as the terminal portion of the 'hollow' vein. It has been suggested, by Kapferer among others, that the word πολύστομος should be translated as 'big-mouthed', but this does not appear to have any parallel, with the possible exception of a passage from Heliodorus, quoted in Oribasius,[2] where it is applied to a fistula. The clause which follows also presents a puzzle.

And from there [the heart?] it channels [or 'there is a channel'] into the mouth, which is called the 'artery' through the lung. And it contains little

τὴν ὠμοπλάτην, καὶ ταύτῃ ἀπ' αὐτεῆς βεβλάστηκε φλὲψ διὰ τοῦ νεύρου τοῦ ὑπὸ τὴν ἐπωμίδα ἡ ἐπωμιδίη ὀνομαζομένη. αὐτὴ δὲ αἱμόρρους καὶ αἱματώδης καὶ δυσίητος ἢν ῥαγῇ ἢ σπασθῇ· τῇ μὲν γὰρ αὐτὴν νεῦρον περιέχει πλατύ, τῇ δὲ χόνδρος. τὸ δὲ μεταξὺ αὐτῶν αὐτή τε ξυνέχει καὶ ὑμὴν ἀφρώδης. ἀσάρκου οὖν ἐόντος τοῦ τόπου ῥηϊδίως ῥήγνυται, οὐκ ἔχουσα περιφύεσθαι σάρκας. ἤν τε ὑποδράμῃ τὸ αἷμα ἐς τοῦτο τὸ μέρος, ἐπιτυχὸν εὐρυχωρίης, οὐκ ἔχει ἀπαλλαγήν, ἀλλὰ σκληροῦται· σκληρωθὲν δὲ νοῦσον παρέχει. . . . ἡ δὲ ὑπὸ τὴν ὠμοπλάτην ἀποβεβλάστηκεν ὑπὸ τοῖσι μαζοῖσι πυκνῇσι καὶ λεπτῇσι καὶ ἐπηλλαγμένῃσι φλεψί· καὶ διὰ τῆς ἐπωμίδος παραλλάσσουσα τὸν χόνδρον, αὐτὴ νέρθεν ὑπονεμομένη ἐς τὸν βραχίονα τείνει, τὸν μῦν ἐν ἀριστερᾷ ἔχουσα. ἡ δὲ ἐξῆς σχίζεται αὐτὴ περὶ τὸν ὦμον καὶ τοῦ ἀγκῶνος τὴν ἄνω μοῖραν· τὸ δ' ἐντεῦθεν διαπέφυκε τοῦ ἀγκῶνος ἑκατέρωθεν, ἔπειτα αὖθις παρὰ τὸν καρπὸν τῆς χειρός· ἐντεῦθεν δὲ ἤδη ἀπορρέουσα δι' ὅλου ἀνὰ τὴν χεῖρα πολυπλανῶς ἐρρίζωται.

[1] Ibid., 13: ἡ δ' ἀρχαίη φλέψ, ἡ κειμένη παρὰ τὴν ἄκανθαν διὰ δὲ τοῦ μεταφρένου, τῆς σφαγῆς καὶ τοῦ βρόγχου ἐμπέφυκεν ἐς τὴν καρδίην ἀφ' ἑωυτῆς φλέβα εὐμεγέθεα πολύστομον κατὰ τὴν καρδίην. Kapferer would appear to adopt the same emendation, for he translates the phrase in question as 'Die (obere) Hauptader'. But in his article in the Münch. med. Wschr. he translates the passage with the text as it stands, 'Die alte Ader'.

[2] Oribasius, Coll. med. xliv. 20, 67 (Corp. Med. Graec. vi. 2. i): τῆς δὲ σύριγγος πολυστόμου καὶ μονοσχιδοῦς οὔσης πρότερον ἐκτέμνεσθαι πάντα τὰ φαινόμενα στόμια. Here there seems to be a contradiction in terms: it is difficult to see how a fistula can be both πολύστομος and μονοσχιδής. But the translation 'big-mouthed' does not seem to be suggested by the last words of the sentence which recommend the excision of all the apparent mouths.

blood and is full of breath or *pneuma*. For in the wide space and thin tissue of this organ there are many channels through the lung and it has [made] the others cartilaginous. Wherefore indeed into the channels which go through the lung some 'foreign bodies' are also carried, either in drink, or in the transit of the blood, since the veins are of this character, and the organ is like a sponge and can receive much liquid, since it grows upwards, for there is a law by which liquids entering are governed. Moreover not much blood is enclosed in these veins, and, because it does not flow swiftly, it does not drive out the bodies that fall into them. And when they are not brought up, but remain in the lung, a hard lump or stone is formed. And in this way the food that is drawn into the lung is lost, for this is the route that leads to the larynx and to the outside. But when the channels are blocked by the lump or calculus, quickness and difficulty of breathing arise, since [and here the text would seem to be corrupt—but the meaning would appear to be something like this] the lump cannot be blown out in the upward direction, and in the other, the channels are not adapted to pull it down. As a result of these conditions, diseases of these kinds arise, namely, asthma and dry 'consumptions'. And if in these circumstances the wet collecting in greater quantities prevails, so that the lung cannot condense and solidify it, it makes the lung rotten, as well as the parts near it, and empyemas and 'consumptions' or wasting diseases arise, though these illnesses may also arise from other causes.[1]

The first crux arising in this passage is connected with the word 'mouth' in the first sentence. Kapferer interprets this as meaning the mouth (ostium) of the heart.[2] He identifies the many-mouthed thick vein with the superior vena cava, and the mouths with the *ostium venosum dextrum*. From there, the right ventricle, the tube which channels into the mouth, is a combination of the pulmonary artery and the pulmonary vein, and the mouth is the left ostium, *ostium venosum sinistrum*. This combined vessel is called the 'artery through the lung', which contains little blood and much *pneuma*. Kapferer believes that the author is here describing the two kinds of vessels in the lungs, the blood vessels, and the cartilaginous air-vessels, the former being a tube which goes through the lung from the

---

[1] *De natura ossium*, 13: ἐντεῦθεν δὲ ἐς τὸ στόμα ἐσυρίγγωκεν ᾗπερ ἀρτηρίη διὰ τοῦ πλεύμονος ὀνομάζεται, ὀλίγαιμός τε καὶ πνευματώδης. ἐν γὰρ εὐρυχωρίῃ καὶ ἀραιώσει σπλάγχνου πολλαχῇ μὲν τοῦ πλεύμονος ὀχετεύεται χονδρώδεις δὲ τοὺς ἄλλους πεποίηται. διὸ δὴ καί τι ἐς ταύτας κατηνέχθη τὰς διόδους, τοῦ πλεύμονος τῶν ἀήθων, ἢ ἐν τῷ ποτῷ, ἢ ἐν τῇ τοῦ πνεύματός τε καὶ αἵματος διόδῳ, ἅτε τῶν φλεβῶν τοιουτέων ἐουσέων, καὶ τοῦ σπλάγχνου σπογγοειδέος πολύ τε ὑγρὸν δυναμένου δέξασθαι ἄνω τε πεφυκότος. τῶν γὰρ ἐσιόντων ὑγρῶν νόμος καθέστηκεν· ἔτι τε τὸ αἷμα διὰ τῶν φλεβῶν τουτέων οὐ πολὺ περισφίγγεται. καὶ οὐ ταχέως χωρέον οὐκ ἐξάγει τὰ ἐμπίπτοντα· οὐχ ὑπεξαγομένων δὲ αὐτῶν ἀλλ' ἐμμενόντων, γίνεται πῶρος. οὕτως δὲ ἀπολλύεται τὸ πλησιάζον τῆς τροφῆς, ταύτῃ ἐούσης τῆς προσαγωγῆς τοῦ λάρυγγος καὶ πρὸς τὰ ἔξω. ἐγκαταλαβομένων δὲ τῶν διόδων ὑπὸ τοῦ πώρου, ταχύπνοιά τε καὶ δύσπνοια ἴσχει τῇδε, μὴ δυναμένων τὴν φύσιν ἐξιέναι, τῇδε οὐκ εὐπόρως ἐχόντων κατασπᾶν. ἐκ δὴ τουτέων αἱ τοιαῦται νοῦσοι γίνονται οἷον ἄσθματα καὶ ξηραὶ φθινάδες. ἢν δὲ ἐν αὐτοῖσι ξυνιστάμενον πλέον τὸ ὑγρὸν κρατήσῃ, ὥστε μὴ δύνασθαι παχυνθὲν παγῆναι, καὶ σαπρὸν τὸν πλεύμονα ποιέει καὶ τὰ πλησιάζοντα, καὶ γίνονται ἔμπυοί τε καὶ φθινώδεες· γίνεται δὲ τὰ νουσήματα ταῦτα καὶ δι' ἄλλας αἰτίας.

[2] Kapferer, op. cit., p. 21.

right ventricle to the left ventricle.[1] To translate the word 'mouth' as 'cardiac ostium' does not seem to me to make any sense at all. The writer has just told us that a certain vein has many mouths into the heart, and then proceeds to inform us that from there are pipes to the mouth. To interpret this 'mouth' as the left *ostium* just makes nonsense of the passage. Moreover the use of the word σῦριγξ implies a windpipe and a pipe of some considerable length. It is quite inappropriate for the opening of a blood vessel into the heart. And the sentences which follow are concerned precisely with the passage of 'foreign bodies' in the shape of food and drink into the lung through the mouth. It seems to be quite clear that we are dealing here with a passage from a work which belongs to a very early stage in the development of anatomical knowledge. The writer has the vascular and bronchial systems hopelessly confused. He evidently regards the network of blood vessels and air-tubes in the lung as a single system, a not unnatural misconception perhaps for a pioneer. This brings us to the next point, the 'artery going through the lung'. This phrase cannot fail to suggest that he is referring to the windpipe, the object originally denoted by the word artery, though the existence of a new meaning to the term seems to be already implied. The hypothesis of Kapferer[2] that he is here referring to the pulmonary artery raises insuperable difficulties. In the first place, the pulmonary artery was

---

[1] In his article entitled 'Die Lungenvenen in der antiken Literatur', *Münch. med. Wschr.* (1955), pp. 673 ff. Kapferer translates the passages in question from Chapter 11 as follows: Die alte Ader, die längs der Wirbelsäule zwischen dem Rücken, der Kehlgegend und der Luftröhre (βρόγχος) hinzieht, läßt von sich eine sehr dicke Ader in das Herz wachsen [Vena cava sup.], mit vielen Ostien am Herzen [Ost. venos. dextr.]. Von hier (vom rechten Herzen) aber zieht sie röhrenartig in das (linke) Ostium [Ost. venos. sinist.]. Die wird Arterie durch die Lunge genannt, sie ist sowohl wenig bluthaltig als auch pneumareich. In dem weiten Raum und der Lockerheit des (Lungen-)Gewebes bildet sie nämlich an vielen Stellen der Lunge Kanäle [A. pulmonalis], knorplig aber hat sie sich die anderen [Kanäle] gebildet. Infolgedessen werden dann in diese Durchgänge der Lunge [Bronchien] auch manch unpassende Dinge, entweder beim Trinken oder beim Durchgang von Luft und Blut hinuntergeführt . . .

His comment on the chapter reads thus: 'In diesem Kapitel schildert also der Autor nacheinander treffend die beiden grundverschiedenen Kanäle durch die Lunge, einerseits die Art. pulmonalis vom rechten Herzen bis in das Ostium venos. sinist.; anderseits die knorpligen Kanäle, die Bronchien.'

A similar misconception, as we shall see, underlies his translation and interpretation of Chapter 19.

[2] Kapferer, op. cit., pp. 19–21. Kapferer begins, on grounds which I am unable to follow, to raise philological objections to the translation of 'the artery through the lung' as the windpipe: 'So sicher das Wort ἀρτηρίη in den Schriften *Die Anatomie* und *Die Siebenzahl* die Bedeutung der Luftröhre hat, ebenso sicher kann der Ausdruck ἀρτηρίη διὰ πνεύμονος in diesem Kapitel aus sprachlichen Gründen nicht "Luftröhre durch die Lunge" bedeuten. Ganz kurz vorher steht nämlich das Wort βρόγχος . . . Aus allen diesen Gründen [which I have not thought it worth while to reproduce—petat cui curae est] geht hervor, daß unter dem Ausdruck "Arterie durch die Lunge bezw. Arterie der Lunge" in allen drei Schriften [sc. the present treatise, the Περὶ ἀνατομῆς, and the Περὶ καρδίης] nicht die Luftröhre der Lunge, sondern die Arterie zu verstehen ist.'

regarded as a vein, and in the second, the description given of it, as rich in *pneuma* but containing little blood would appear, in the light of subsequent Greek theories, to point rather to the pulmonary vein. Moreover, these chapters, forming as they seem to do a separate continuous treatise, do not use the word artery to denote a blood vessel. Greek medicine, throughout its development, assumes a very close connection between the activity of breathing and the movements of the heart, and in some form or other postulated a connection between the heart and the lung which would permit air inhaled through the nose to be drawn into the heart. The pulmonary vein was regarded by Erasistratus and many others, including Galen, as the channel by which *pneuma* from the outer air reached the heart. There is therefore no very great difficulty in supposing that this artery through the lung is simply a conflation or confusion of the aorta, the pulmonary vein, and the bronchial tubes. This interpretation also explains our author's remark that 'It has made its other channels cartilaginous', which would otherwise be quite inexplicable, as well as the statement that because the blood flows too slowly it cannot carry away bits of food that have got into the lung, with the consequential diseases described.

The passage may also throw some light on the way in which the word *arteria* got its double meaning. The terms *arteria* and *bronchos* seem to have been originally more or less homonymous. A third term, *aorta*, as we have seen, was also used for the windpipe, according to Rufus. It would appear that the bronchial system and the arterial were by some early doctors considered as continuous. How else could the breath of life be distributed, as it must be, to the whole body? Moreover the heart was in communication with the lung through a vessel which was plainly different in texture from the hollow vein. Its texture, though not cartilaginous, was much more sinew-like, and a large sinew-like system of vessels went from the heart all over the body. The inference, before the interior of the heart and its vascular connections had been properly investigated, was irresistible. The two systems were a single complex.

Chapter 14 is devoted to the description of a 'large vein' with many branches which the writer seems to identify with one of the vessels described in the previous chapter. This would appear to be the artery through the lung in its continuation as the aorta, with which the pulmonary artery would appear to be hopelessly confused.

And from there [presumably the heart] this vein occupies the lung, and it stretches through the lobes, the two big ones which are turned inwards, under the diaphragm to the spine, white and sinewy, sending forth smaller but well-strung veins through the whole of the rest of the compact tissues of the body. And it forms a plexus round the vertebrae, with close-set little veins into the spinal marrow. And the other veins stretching through the body converge from all parts on to the spine, each of the veins uniting and bringing together its thinnest and simplest branches and discharging there. But the vein that extends itself through the network laid down brings them all to the same place together. And from there it sends roots into the kidneys near the false ribs in the form of thin threadlike veins. And going on from there it pulls its threads together and becomes thick and then near the anus it becomes sinewy, and pressing on the sphincter, it grows into the anus. It also sends out roots into the bladder, the testicles, and the prostate[s], in the form of a close network of thin, rigid, and thread-like branches.[1]

From there on [so the fifteenth chapter continues] its thickest and straightest branch turns back upon itself and forms a stalk which is the penis, and in its upward bend the branches of this vein rise up into these parts and through the womb and go upwards under the skin of the belly to meet those that go downwards, and they channel into each other. And the genital has growing through it thick veins and thin ones and closely set ones and twisted ones.[2]

According to Kapferer,[3] the author is to begin with describing the descending aorta, and this seems to be correct, since his characterization of the 'vein' as sinew- or tendon-like would fit the aorta better than the vena cava, the only other vessel which it could be supposed to be. But the description is not a very good one. The continuity with the trachea does however raise a point of some interest, which would explain Kapferer's identification of the 'artery' with the pulmonary artery. The 'sinewy' blood vessels were called arteries, just because their 'cartilage-like' tubes were considered much more like the trachea than like the veins. It is therefore just conceivable that our author saw a trachea-like tube coming out of the lung and going to the heart, and thought it was continuous with the windpipe. But since he makes no distinction between the right and

---

[1] De natura ossium, 14: ἐντεῦθέν τε ἡ φλὲψ αὕτη κατέχει τὸν πλεύμονα, καὶ διὰ τῶν λοβῶν τῶν δύο τῶν μεγάλων τῶν ἔσω τετραμμένων ὑπὸ τὰς φλέβας ἐπιτέταται τῇ ἀκάνθῃ λευκὴ καὶ νευρώδης, διαπέμπουσα φλέβια διὰ τοῦ ἄλλου σώματος πεπυκνωμένου, εὔτονα δέ, καὶ διά τε τῶν σφονδύλων πυκνοῖσι φλεβίοισι ἐς τὸν νωτιαῖον μυελὸν ἐγκισσεύεται. καὶ αἱ μὲν ἄλλαι φλέβες ἐν τῷ σώματι τεταμέναι, ἐκ πάντων τῶν μερῶν συντείνουσαι ἐς τὴν ἄκανθαν, τὸ λεπτότατον καὶ εἰλικρινέστατον ἑκάστη ξυνάγουσα ἐνταῦθ' ἐξερεύγεται. αὕτη δὲ ἡ ἐπιτεταμένη διὰ τῶν καθειμένων πλεκτανέων ἐς ταὐτὸ ξυνάγει· ἐντεῦθεν δὲ καὶ ἐς τοὺς νεφροὺς ἀπερρίζωται παρὰ τὴν νόθον πλευρὴν λεπτῇσι καὶ ἰνώδεσι φλεψί, καὶ τὸ ἐντεῦθεν ξυντείνουσα ξυμπεπύκνωται, ἔπειτα καὶ νενεύρωται πρὸς τὸν ἀρχὸν πιέσασα δὲ τοὺς ξυναγωγέας ἐμπέφυκεν αὐτῷ. τήν τε κύστιν καὶ τοὺς ὄρχιας καὶ τοὺς παραστάτας ἐρρίζωκε πολυπλόκοισι λεπτῇσί τε καὶ στερεῇσι καὶ ἰνώδεσι φλεψίν.

Note that the prostate was regarded as being two bodies. Galen informs us in the fourteenth book of his treatise, On the use of the parts, that Herophilus was the first to name them, calling them the gland-like protectors; cf. ibid., 11, K. iv. 190: καὶ πρῶτός γε Ἡρόφιλος, ἀδενοειδεῖς προστάτας, ἐκάλεσεν. Is it possible that the word παραστάτης was an earlier name for the same structure? It is difficult to believe that the chapter we are considering was written before Herophilus.

[2] De natura ossium, 15: ἐντεῦθεν αὐτῆς τὸ παχύτατον καὶ ἰθύτατον ἀνάπαλιν τραπὲν προσκεκαύληκεν ὅπερ ἐστὶν αἰδοῖον· ἐν δὲ τῇ ἀνακάμψει ἐνῆρται ἐς τὰ αὐτὰ ταῦτα καὶ διὰ τοῦ κτεινὸς ἄνω ὑπὸ τὸ δέρμα τῆς γαστρὸς ἐκ τῆς φλεβὸς αὐτέης ὡρμήκασι πρὸς τὰς κάτω φερούσας, αἳ ἐς ἀλλήλας ἐποχετεύονται· διαπεφύκασι δὲ διὰ τοῦ αἰδοίου φλέβες παχεῖαι, καὶ λεπταὶ καὶ πυκναὶ καὶ καμπύλαι.

[3] Kapferer, op. cit., pp. 41 f.

the left side of the heart, and does not mention that it has two ventricles, we cannot be at all certain. And the fact that he mentions that it contains little blood and a lot of *pneuma* definitely seems to imply the pulmonary vein. Nor is it easy to identify the plexus arrangements connected with the spine. These would appear to be connected with the theory, already known in the days of Alcmaeon, that the spinal marrow was the source of the seed, which must contain matter coming from every part of the body. The description of the vessels in the genitals is also rather intriguing. The bent or twisted veins suggest the testicle rather than the penis. Can the word αἰδοῖον be made to include both?

The rest of Chapter 15 is devoted to a description of the vascular system of the genitalia, which is of some interest:

In women it [the vein] is fastened round the womb, but in man it curls round the testicles. On account of its way of growing, this vein also contains most of the generative matter. For it is nourished from the most numerous and purest substances, and it contains little blood, though it is hollow [i.e. its lumen is large] and it has a thick sinew-like coat and is full of *pneuma*. When it is erected by the penis, it exercises pressure on the veins going down into the loins, and these, when pressed like a gourd used for cupping, discharge all their contents into the vein above. And matter from the other limbs of the body also flows together into this vein. But the largest part, as I have said, is collected from the marrow. And a sensation of pleasure is aroused, when this vein is filled with semen. For during the rest of the time it is habitually filled with little blood and *pneuma*, but when it is filled [with semen] and becomes hot, and the semen runs down into it, it grasps its contents tightly. And the *pneuma* it contains, and the pressure that has arisen, and the tension of the veins from all directions produce a tickling sensation.[1]

Chapter 16 deals with another vessel running from the head, or at any rate from the neck, down to the legs. This recalls one of the main vessels of Diogenes of Apollonia, since it goes right down the body to the soles of the feet, and then turns again upwards. The writer plunges *in medias res*. We are not even told to what vein he is referring.

And this vein produces a branch, going through or past the neck and the throat down along the spine, with many little veins that weave about the

[1] *De natura ossium*, 15: τῇσι δὲ θηλεῇσιν αὐτὴ ξυντείνει ἐς τὰς μήτρας, ἐς τὴν κύστιν καὶ ἐς τὴν οὐρήθρην. ἐντεῦθεν δὲ ἰθυπόρηκε, καὶ τῇσι γυναιξὶ μὲν περὶ τὰς μήτρας ἤρτηται, τοῖσι δὲ ἄρρεσι περὶ τοὺς ὄρχιας ἐσπείρωται. διὰ ταύτην τὴν φύσιν αὐτὴ ἡ φλὲψ καὶ τὰ γόνιμα πλεῖστα ξυλλαμβάνει· ἀπὸ γὰρ τῶν πλείστων καὶ εἰλικρινεστάτων μερῶν τρεφομένη, ὀλίγαιμός τε οὖσα καὶ κοίλη καὶ νευρόπαχυς καὶ πνευματώδης, ἐντεινομένη τε ὑπὸ τοῦ αἰδοίου, τὰ καθειμένα ἐς τὴν ἄκανθαν φλέβια βιάζεται, τὰ δὲ βιαζόμενα ὥσπερ σικύη ἐς ἑωυτὰ πάντα ἐκδιδοῖ ἐς τὴν ἄνω φλέβα· ξυλλείβεται δὲ καὶ ἐκ τῶν ἄλλων μελῶν τοῦ σώματος ἐς ταύτην· τὸ δὲ πλεῖστον, ὥσπερ εἴρηται, ἀπὸ τοῦ μυελοῦ ξυναλίζεται. ἡ δὲ ἡδονὴ τουτέῳ παραγίνεται τῆς φλεβὸς ταύτης πληρευμένης τῆς γονῆς. εἰωθυίης οὖν τὸν ἄλλον χρόνον ὑφαίμου τε εἶναι καὶ πνευματώδεος πληρευμένης τε καὶ θερμαινομένης, καὶ ξυρρέοντος κάτω τοῦ σπέρματος, περισφίγγει τὰ ἐν ἑωυτῇ. τὸ δὲ πνεῦμα τὸ ἐνεὸν καὶ ἡ παροῦσα βίη καὶ ἡ θερμότης καὶ τῶν φλεβίων πανταχόθεν ἡ ξυντονίη γαργαλισμὸν ἐμποιέει.

ribs. And it is closely intertwined crosswise through the tissues round the vertebrae, so as to be full of nourishment and full of blood. And it goes past the buttocks through the muscle hidden under the thigh. By the buttock, it bores a hole in the socket of the thigh-bone, near its head in a vein which provides respiration for the thigh, and it goes beyond the thigh past the bend of the knee. By the groin it puts forth another vein which has many roots close together, and is difficult to deal with. This vein, extending through the muscle, curls round the knee and sends out a pipe through the top of the shin-bone, which nourishes the marrow. It channels its way through the bottom of the shin-bone close to where the foot is fastened [to the leg]. But it [the main vessel] stretches through the great muscle of the thigh above the knee to the inside, going beneath the surface of the muscle of the calf, and is woven round the ankle on the inside, thick and full of blood. And from there it draws off a network of veins hard to distinguish, round the ankle and the tendon.[1]

Chapter 17 continues:

And it runs down under the sole of the foot, and from there, having woven together and thrust into the big toe a double vein full of blood, it bends up from the ankle under the skin, and becomes visible, having grown thick, along the outside of the ankle, and goes upwards past the spindle protruding at the front of the shin. And by the calf it makes a sort of sling. And from there it extends along the inside of the knee, and also throws out veins to the great muscle of the thigh, and along the inside of the great muscle of the thigh above the knee it weaves a porous or spongy vein. When this is diseased, it quickly collects a gall-like serous fluid. It also travels along by the inner hollow of the knee, and buds off into the hams a web of many veins, which going along by the lower sinews of the thigh, make their roots in the testicles and the anus. And by the sacred bone, they are extended round it in the form of thin united veins.[2]

---

[1] *De natura ossium*, 16: ἐκείνη δὲ ἀφ' ἑωυτῆς διέβλαστε, διά τε τοῦ μεταφρένου καὶ τῆς σφαγῆς παρὰ τὴν ἄκανθαν νεμομένη, πολλοῖσι φλεβίοισι τὰς πλευρὰς διαπέπλοχε· καὶ τοὺς σφονδύλους διὰ τῶν σαρκῶν ἐπηλλαγμένως ξυμπεπύκνωκεν, ὥστε τρόφιμός τε καὶ ἔναιμος εἶναι. αὐτὴ δὲ παρὰ τὸν γλουτὸν ἴεται διὰ τοῦ μυὸς ὑπὸ τῷ μηρῷ ὑποβρυχίη· πρὸς δὲ τοῦ γλουτοῦ τῇ κοτυλίδι τοῦ μηροῦ παρὰ τὴν κεφαλὴν ἐστετρύπηκε φλεβί, ἥπερ ἀναπνοὴν τῷ μηρῷ παρέχει· καὶ περᾷ τὸν μηρὸν παρὰ τὴν πρὸς τὸ γόνυ καμπήν. ἑτέρην δὲ παρὰ βουβῶνα καθῆκε πυκνόρριζον καὶ δυστράπελον. ἡ δὲ διὰ τοῦ μυὸς τείνουσα περί τε τὸ γόνυ ἐσπείρωται, καὶ διὰ τοῦ ὀστέου τοῦ κνημιαίου ἄκρου σεσυρίγγωκε φλέβα ἣ τρέφει τὸν μυελόν, καὶ ἐξοχετεύεται διὰ τοῦ νερτάτου τοῦ κνημιαίου, παρὰ τὴν ἔνδεσιν τοῦ ποδός. αὐτὴ δὲ διὰ τῆς ἐπιγουνίδος ἐς τὸ ἐντὸς διὰ τῆς κνήμης τοῦ μυὸς βρυχίη τέταται, καὶ ἐμπέπλοχε διὰ τοῦ σφυροῦ ἐντὸς παχέη καὶ ἔναιμος, καὶ ἐνταῦθα περὶ τὸ σφυρὸν καὶ τὸν τένοντα δυσκρίτους φλέβας μεμήρυκεν.

[2] Ibid., 17: αὐτὴ δὲ ὑποδεδράμηκε κάτωθεν τοῦ ποδὸς ὑπὸ τὸν ταρσόν· καὶ ἐνταῦθα διαπλέξασα καὶ ἐς τὸν μέγαν δάκτυλον ἐνερείσασα διπλῆν ἔναιμον φλέβα, ἄνωθεν ὑπὸ τὸ δέρμα ἐκ τοῦ ταρσοῦ ἀνακέκαμπται, καὶ πέφανται παχυνθεῖσα παρὰ τὸ ἐκτὸς τοῦ σφυροῦ, καὶ νέμεται ἄνω παρὰ τοῦ ἀντικνημίου τὴν ἀντιβεβλημένην κερκίδα· παρὰ δὲ τὴν γαστροκνημίην οἷον σφενδόνην πεποίηται· τὸ δ' ἐντεῦθεν τέταται παρὰ τοῦ γούνατος τὸ ἐντός. ἐπιβέβηκε δὲ καὶ τῇ ἐπιγουνατίδι φλέβας, καὶ κατὰ τὸ ἐντὸς τῆς ἐπιγουνατίδος ἐπίκοιλον ἐμπέπλεχε φλέβα. ἥν τις εἰ πονήσῃ τάχιστα ξυνάγει χολώδεα ἰχῶρα. διώρμηκε δὲ αὐτὴ κατὰ τὸ ἐντὸς καὶ κοῖλον τοῦ γούνατος· ἀποκεκάρπωκε δὲ καὶ ἐς τὰς ἰγνύας πολυπλόκους φλέβας, αἳ ἐντεῦθεν παρατείνουσαι κατὰ τὰ ὑποκάτω νεῦρα τοῦ μηροῦ κατερρίζωνται ἐς τοὺς ὄρχιας καὶ ἐς τὸν ἀρχόν, καὶ περὶ τὸ ἱερὸν δὲ ὀστέον λελεπτυσμέναι ἡνωμέναι περιτέτανται.

But [Chapter 18] the vein that comes from the inside of the knee along the inside of the thigh goes up into the groin and past the hip-bone and beyond it towards the spine, so that it has the muscle of the loin on the outside. Thick and broad, it rises up towards the liver. And throwing off sideways a bloodful vein settles into the kidney and the right lobe of the liver. And it goes passing underneath the liver and branches into the thick vein. This bends off and grows into the thick part of the liver. One part of it grows quite near the surface of that organ in which the gall-bladder is, and it has many roots and makes a network throughout the liver. The other part makes its channel through the interior of the liver. Two veins weave out between the two broad lobes [which, incredible though it may sound, Kapferer translates as *Muskellappen*!].[1] And one, passing through the top [of the liver?] and its skin, comes up from the navel. The other, pressing on the spine and the kidneys, anchors itself in the bladder and the genitals. When it begins to come up from the hip-joint to the belly, it sends out many veins, and it makes rings round the ribs and the vertebrae tying them to the spine, sending out these shoots as side growths, and it wraps itself round the intestines, and the belly. Now the veins that go up from the belly to the breasts and over the chin and the shoulder points entwine or run into each other. But the one that comes from the thick part of the liver and pipes off the gall goes upwards close to the spine and makes its way through the diaphragm. [Kapferer here adds 'into the right heart with many openings' (*Ostien*), a phrase not found in the text and derived (with a difference) from Chapter 13.] And the vein on the left side is in other respects rooted in the same manner as that on the right side, except that going up on the left side it does not throw off a branch into the liver, but grows into the spleen, by the head, which is in the thick part of it. From there it goes down into the interior of the spleen and makes a web of bloodful veins. Now the whole of the spleen is raised up from the omentum, and supplies it with blood by the veins that come from it. And these coming from the head of the spleen approach the spine and pass through the diaphragm.[2]

---

[1] Kapferer, op. cit., p. 46. Sticker, whose version of the *De nat. oss.* is given in vol. 16 of Kapferer's translation of the *Corpus*, simply translates them as *Leberlappen*.

[2] *De natura ossium*, 18 : ἡ δὲ ἀφιγμένη παρὰ τοῦ γούνατος τὸ ἐντὸς ἄνω παρὰ τοῦ μηροῦ τὸ ἐντὸς ἀνίεται ἐς τὸν βουβῶνα, καὶ διὰ τοῦ ἰσχίου πέρην πρὸς τὴν ἄκανθαν καὶ τὴν ψύαν ἐκτὸς ἔχουσα, παχεῖα καὶ πλατεῖα καὶ ἔναιμος, ἄνω ὤρεκται πρὸς τὸ ἧπαρ· καὶ διακραίην ἐκφύσασα ἔναιμον, κατέχει ἐς τὸν νεφρὸν (καὶ) τὸν δεξιὸν λοβὸν τὸν ἡπαταῖον. αὕτη δὲ ὑποκάτω τοῦ ἥπατος ὑπονησαμένη, ἀπέσχισται ἐς φλέβα παχέην. ἡ δ' ἀποκαμφθεῖσα ἐσπέφυκεν ἐς τὸ παχὺ τοῦ ἥπατος· καὶ τὸ μὲν αὐτῆς ἐπιπολάζον ἐπὶ τοῦ σπλάγχνου πέφυκεν, ἐν ᾧπερ ἡ χολή ἐστι, καὶ πολύρριζος καὶ διὰ τοῦ ἥπατος πεπλεκτανωμένη. τὸ δὲ διὰ τῶν ἐντὸς αὐτοῦ ὠχέτευται. δύο δὲ ἐκπεπλώκασι φλέβες μεταξὺ δύο λοβῶν τῶν πλατέων· καὶ μία μὲν διὰ τῶν κορυφῶν καὶ τοῦ δέρματος διασχοῦσα ἐκ τοῦ ὀμφαλοῦ ἀνῆκται· ἡ δὲ ἑτέρη πιέσασα ἐς τὴν ἄκανθαν καὶ ἐς τὸν νεφρὸν ἡγκυροβόληται ἐς τὴν κύστιν τε καὶ τὸ αἰδοῖον. ἐκ δὲ τοῦ ἰσχίου ἀρχομένη ἀνίεναι ἐπὶ τὸ ἧτρον, πολλὰς ἀπεπλάνησε φλέβας. καὶ τάς τε πλευρὰς καὶ τοὺς σφονδύλους ἐνεκρίκωσε πρὸς τὴν ἄκανθαν, καὶ ταύτας παραφυάδας ἐνεφλεβοτόμησε, καὶ τὰ ἔντερα καὶ τὴν νηδὺν ἐνειλίξατο. καὶ αἱ μὲν ἀπὸ τοῦ ἥτρου ἔς τε τοὺς μαζοὺς καὶ ὑπὲρ ἀνθερεῶνα καὶ τὰς ἀκρωμίας ἐπορεξάμεναι κατεπλάκησαν. ἡ δ' ἀφιγμένη παρὰ τὸ παχὺ τοῦ ἥπατος καὶ ἀποσυριγγώσασα τὴν χολὴν ἄνω ὑπὸ τὴν ἄκανθαν νέμεται διὰ τῶν φρενῶν ὁδὸν ποιησαμένη. ἡ δὲ ἐκ τῶν ἀριστερῶν φλέψ, τὰ μὲν ἄλλα τὴν αὐτὴν φύσιν ἐρρίζωται τῇ ἐν τοῖσι δεξιοῖσιν, ἐκ τῶν ἀριστερῶν ἐς τὸ ἧπαρ ἀνιοῦσα οὐκ ἐκβάλλει, ἀλλ' ἐς τὸν σπλῆνα ἐμπέφυκε κατὰ τὴν κεφαλὴν τὴν ἐν τῷ πάχει αὐτέου. ἐντεῦθεν δὲ κατεδύσατο ἐς τὸ ἐντὸς καὶ ἡραχνίωσε τοῦ σπληνὸς ἐναίμοισι φλεβίοισιν. ὁ δὲ ὅλος ἐκ τοῦ ἐπιπλόου αἰωρεῖται τοῖσιν ἐξ ἑωυτέου φλεβίοισιν

The last chapter (19) is devoted to a description of the two veins mentioned earlier, presumably our old friends the liver and the spleen vein, both of which seem to be conceived as passing under the lung with connections to the heart. The first sentence seems to follow on directly from the end of the eighteenth chapter but obviously does not fit.

From there on downwards [the word diaphragm with which chapter 18 ends would make nonsense] both the right and the left vein are drawn under the lung, and being full of blood they send irrigating channels into it. But the ones that go into the lung are thin and contain little blood, as the lung is naturally light of texture. They drain into the heart, as if they were milked by it, and form a bridle round its ears, and discharge into its ventricles. And the ones I have first mentioned also discharge into it. For it is situated in the narrow passage of the way through, just as if it were holding the reins of the whole body. Therefore, too, perceptions from all parts of the body are centred most of all in the thorax. And changes in complexion occur when it [the heart or the thorax?] tightens or loosens the veins. When it loosens them, the colour becomes red and beautiful and clear but when it constricts them, the complexion becomes pale and livid.[1]

The picture here presented reminds us in many ways of the description of the heart we saw in the *Timaeus*.[2] It is the knot of the blood vessels and the heart that is the centre of perception, though not explicitly of reason. The author, too, seems to be acquainted with two ventricles, though of this we cannot be altogether sure, and he appears to be acquainted with two other entrances to (or exits from?) the heart connected with Diogenes' liver and splenic veins, which are full of blood; as opposed to the veins coming to the auricles from the lungs, which contain less blood, though the heart does milk them. We seem here to have a considerable advance on earlier descriptions. Our author knows that both sides of the

ἐναιματώσας αὐτό. αἱ δὲ ἀπὸ τῆς κεφαλῆς τοῦ σπληνὸς πρὸς τὴν ἄκανθαν ἐγχρίπτουσαι, διὰ τῶν φρενῶν διωρμήκασιν.

[1] Ibid., 19: ἐντεῦθεν δὲ κάτω καὶ ἡ δεξιὴ καὶ ἡ ἀριστερὴ ὑπὸ τὸν πνεύμονα ἐλήλαται· αἱ δὲ ἐναίμονες ἐοῦσαι ὑπ' αὐτὸν ἐξοχετεύονται ἐς αὐτόν, ὀλίγαιμοι δὲ καὶ λεπταὶ αἱ ἀπὸ τοῦ πνεύμονος ἔσωθεν γενόμεναι, τῇ φύσει ἀραιοῦ ἐόντος, ἐς τὴν καρδίην, ἅτε ὑπ' αὐτέου ἐξαθελγόμεναι, ἐγκεχαλίνωνται περὶ τὰ ὦτα αὐτέης, καὶ ἐς τὰ κοῖλα τὰ ἐντὸς διερρυήκασιν. ἐμβάλλουσι δὲ καὶ αἱ πρότεραι καὶ αὗται ἐς αὐτήν· ἐν γὰρ στενοχωρίῃ τῆς διόδου ἐνίδρυται ὡς ἐκ παντὸς τοῦ σώματος τὰς ἡνίας ἔχουσα· διὸ καὶ παντὸς τοῦ σώματος περὶ τὸν θώρακα μάλιστά ἐστιν ἡ αἴσθησις. καὶ τῶν χρωμάτων αἱ μεταβολαὶ γίνονται ταύτης ἀποσφιγγούσης τὰς φλέβας καὶ χαλώσης. χαλώσης μὲν οὖν, ἐρυθρὰ τὰ χρώματα γίνεται καὶ εὔχροα καὶ διαφανέα· ξυναγούσης δέ, χλωρὰ καὶ πελιδνά. Here Kapferer characteristically tampers with the text, simply omitting the duplication of the veins and treating them as a single vessel: 'Von hier aus zieht sie, wohl ihr rechter, als auch ihr linker Ast.' His translation in the *Münch. med. Wschr.*, op. cit., gives the following rendering: 'Von hier unten (vom rechten Herzen) zieht die Ader, sowohl ihr rechter als auch ihr linker (Ast) unter die Lunge: sie (die Aeste) sind unter ihr blutvoll und bilden Kanäle an sie (Art. pulmon.). Wenig bluthaltig und dünn sind dagegen die Adern, die vom inneren der Lunge, die von Natur locker ist, in das Herz ziehen, weil sie von ihr ausgemolken werden ... sie dringen in seine Innenhöhlen (Vae. pulmonal.).'   [2] See above, p. 21.

heart are connected with the lungs, and that there are also quite separate connections between both sides of the heart and two systems of great blood vessels. Kapferer disregards these latter altogether, and quite perversely interprets the 'vessels full of blood' as the pulmonary arteries, and those with less blood as the pulmonary veins.

It is far from easy to arrive at any clear picture of the anatomical significance either of the isolated paragraphs, Chapters 4–7, or of the more coherent fragment, Chapters 11–19. Kapferer's identifications, many of which do such violence to the text, do not often appear to be even remotely probable. The Greek descriptions of the vessels are for the most part too vague, emanating from a period in which arteries and veins were not yet properly distinguished, and therefore only too easily confused, since by and large each kind of vessel follows roughly parallel courses. Ambiguity about the meaning of the term 'artery' increases the difficulty, since in the later portion of the treatise it would appear to be applied only to the tracheal system, all blood vessels being described by the term 'vein'. Arteries as blood vessels only appear in Chapter 5, Chapter 7, and the chapter (10) quoted from the *Epidemics*. Moreover the identifications made by Kapferer imply a much more intimate knowledge of human anatomy than can have been possible before, or even after, Alexandrian times, since even the most recent chapters in the treatise would appear to be almost certainly of a date before Herophilus. Confused as the text is, some of the sources, as Littré pointed out, can be identified quite clearly. The first seven are fairly obviously an assemblage of fragments varying in date, and quite clearly later than the concluding chapters. Two criteria of a provisional character for dating them may be adopted, by asking two simple questions. Do they regard the heart as the centre of the vascular system? If so, they are almost certainly later than Aristotle. Do they recognize a clear distinction between arteries and veins? If so, they must be later than Praxagoras, and may be later than Herophilus. Chapter 2 seems to suggest the heart as the starting-point of the great vessels, but makes no distinction between arteries and veins. Chapter 5 does. Chapter 6 does not, but it is too short to draw any conclusion as to its date. Chapter 7 is obviously post-Aristotelian and almost certainly also later than Praxagoras. The same considerations would appear to apply to the quotation from the *Epidemics* which constitutes the tenth chapter. On the other hand the basis of Chapters 11–19 is much nearer to that of Diogenes of Apollonia. We still have two more or less parallel main vessels, but there are certain modifications which denote considerable advance in anatomical knowledge. The existence of the sinewy vein is the foundation of the distinction between veins and arteries, and the last chapter seems to recognize that there are four vessels leading into the heart, two from the lungs via the auricles, and two from the big veins. Those leading from the lung are small without much blood—the pulmonary artery and pulmonary vein must have looked smaller than the aorta and the vena cava. But we are told nothing of the two ventricles of the heart, which do not yet appear to have been distinguished. The heart is definitely at the cross-roads of the vascular system, its focus. It has become the 'knot of the veins', as Plato describes it, even if this is only through the biggest branches which come off them. The arrangement, to my mind, is not entirely clear. The heart has become the centre, also, of perception (though we are not told of intelligence), and the seat of a curious kind of vasomotor system, though it is not clear whether this was supposed to be operated by the heart or the thorax. Of the heart's inner structure we are told nothing at all, and of the vessels leading to it what we are told is wrong, e.g. the many-mouthed opening of the branch of one of them. The accounts of the vessels communicating between the heart and the lung are confused, but the last chapter does seem to suggest that the writer had noted the pulmonary artery and the pulmonary vein, which he compares to reins.

Chapters 16–18 give a rather curious account of a vein which goes down from the neck to the leg and the foot, then turns back and goes upwards through the leg and the thigh, and finally empties itself into the vena cava. Kapferer, with some plausibility, identifies the downward path with the aorta and the arterial system, and the upward path with the venous, but as there is no certain indication of its starting-point, the identification must remain doubtful, to say the least of it. Moreover the beginning of the description looks more as if the author was dealing with the inferior vena cava rather than the descending aorta. In either case we get some sort of 'circular' connection established by certain blood vessels running into each other, such connections being mentioned in Chapter 6 as well as in the chapter borrowed from the *Epidemics*. But it would be quite misleading to interpret such connections with any knowledge of, or even guess at, the circulation of the blood as Harvey understood it. As Michler has pointed out, the fact that Hippocratic surgeons believed that when a vein was cut blood streamed out from both directions, completely disposes of the idea that they were acquainted with the circulation.[1]

In the treatise *On diseases* Book iv, which is separated by Littré from the treatise *On the nature of the infant* to which the manuscripts append it without any break, we find the doctrine definitely stated that the heart is the central point of the blood vessels, a doctrine which we shall find

---

[1] I am indebted for this observation to M. Michler's essay, 'Die hellenistische Chirurgie' (Habilitationschrift zu Erlangung der venia legendi, Faculty of Medicine, Hamburg, 1965), to which my attention was drawn by Professor Ackerknecht of Zürich, who kindly lent me the typescript of this dissertation.

repeated in the treatise *On fleshes* as well as in the fragmentary work *On the heart*. This doctrine had been clearly elaborated by Aristotle. In the first-mentioned treatise, 'Hippocrates' tells us:

The heart is the source or fountain of the blood. But in a sense the prime source of all humours is the belly, for they are all the products of things eaten or drunk. And I wish first to show how bile and blood and water [not, be it noted, black bile] and phlegm increase and decrease as the products of things eaten and drunk, in this fashion. The belly, when it is filled, is the source or fountain of all things in the body. But when it becomes empty, it draws sustenance from the body, which wastes away. And there are also four other sources or fountains, from which each of these humours flows to the body, when they receive them from the belly, and these, when they are empty, draw sustenance from the body. And the body itself draws them when the belly has something in it. Now the heart is the source of the blood, the head of the phlegm, the spleen of the water, and the place on the liver of the bile.[1]

This treatise also lays down the theory of physiological attraction, which will find its most mature development in Galen.

When a man eats or drinks anything which is like blood, the whole body draws it into itself, and the heart attracts or pulls into itself the blood-like substance . . . Now from the heart stretch thick veins, the ones named from throat-cutting the jugular, into which, if surplus arises, the blood-like substance is distributed, and these fill up and distribute it quickly to the head, and quickly to the body. And when a man eats or drinks something that is blood-like, at once the so-called jugular veins swell up and his face becomes red.

But if excess of blood-like substance is absorbed, no distress is caused in the heart, for the heart is a solid thing and dense or close-knit.[2]

In another passage in the same section, he expands upon this doctrine a little:

The head, the heart, and the spleen, each of them partake of all the fluids, unless a man is diseased. But each partakes most of its own proper fluid, the head of phlegm, the heart of blood, and the spleen of water. The veins take

---

[1] Hippocrates, *De morbis*, iv. 33 : ἐθέλω δὲ ἀποφῆναι πρῶτον πῶς ἡ χολὴ καὶ τὸ αἷμα καὶ ὁ ὕδρωψ καὶ τὸ φλέγμα πλέονα καὶ ἐλάσσονα γίνεται, ἀπὸ τῶν βρωμάτων καὶ τῶν πομάτων τρόπῳ τοιῷδε· ἡ κοιλίη τῷ σώματι πάντων πηγή ἐστι πλέη ἐοῦσα· κενεὴ δὲ γενομένη ἐπαυρίσκεται ἀπὸ τοῦ σώματος τηκομένου. εἰσὶ δὲ καὶ ἄλλαι πηγαὶ τέσσαρες, ἀφ' ὧν χωρέει τούτων ἕκαστον ἐς τὸ σῶμα, ἐπὴν αὗται ἀπὸ τῆς κοιλίης λάβωσι, καὶ αὗται ἐπὴν κενῶνται ἀπὸ τοῦ σώματος ἐπαυρίσκονται. ἕλκει δὲ καὶ αὐτὸ τὸ σῶμα, ἐπὴν ἡ κοιλίη τι ἔχῃ ἐν ἑωυτῇ· τῷ μὲν δὴ αἵματι ἡ καρδίη πηγή ἐστι, τῷ δὲ φλέγματι ἡ κεφαλή, τῷ δὲ ὕδατι ὁ σπλήν, τῇ δὲ χολῇ τὸ χωρίον τὸ ἐν τῷ ἥπατι.

[2] Ibid., 38 : ἐπήν τι πίῃ ἢ φάγῃ ὁ ἄνθρωπος ὅ τι ἐστὶν αἱματῶδες, ἕλκει μὲν καὶ τὸ σῶμα ἅπαν ἐς ἑωυτό, ἕλκει δὲ καὶ ἡ καρδίη τὸ αἱματῶδες ἐς ἑωυτήν . . . καὶ ἐξ αὐτέης παχεῖαι φλέβες τείνουσιν, αἱ σφάγιαι καλέομεναι, ἐς ἃς ταχέως ἢν πλέον προσγένηται διαδίδοται τὸ αἱματῶδες καὶ πιμπλά-μεναι κεῖναι τῇ κεφαλῇ καὶ τῷ σώματι διδόασιν ἐν τάχει, καὶ ἐπὴν τι φάγῃ ἢ πίῃ, ὅ τι ἐστὶν αἱμα-τῶδες, αὐτίκα αἱ σφάγιαι φλέβες ἀείρονται καὶ τὸ πρόσωπον ἐρυθέει. καὶ ἐπὴν πλέον εἰρύσῃ οὐ γίνεται τῇ καρδίῃ πόνος· στερεόν γάρ τι χρῆμα καὶ πυκνόν ἐστιν ἡ καρδίη.

up into themselves liquids other than blood as well, since they are thick and of a winding form, so that when they attract blood, they also attract each of the other liquids in succession. Now the jugular veins are near to the heart, and they are thick so that blood [and the other fluids] are quickly distributed into or by them, when the occasion arises. They distribute them to the rest of the body. At the same time the heart is close-knit and solid, so that it suffers no illness from the liquids. Illness caused by excess of liquid never occurs in the heart.[1]

The story of heart disease did not even begin to be worked out before the end of the seventeenth or indeed the end of the eighteenth century, and our author can only give us the most superficial account here of the vascular system and its function in the distribution of nourishment:

For there are veins throughout the whole of the body, some thicker and some thinner, many of them and set close together. And these, as long as a man remains alive, open and receive and send on the new liquid. But when he dies, they close up and become thin.[2]

In the treatise *On fleshes* which, as Sigerist has remarked, is haunted, perhaps under Eastern influence, by the number seven,[3] we find a 'philosophical' basis for the physiological doctrine, rather like the fragment from Diogenes of Apollonia. Only here the place of air is taken by 'the hot'—Heracleitus rather than Anaximenes. 'I think that what we call the hot is immortal, and thinks everything and sees everything and knows everything which is and which is to be',[4] words taken not literally but in the spirit from Diogenes. Then follows (Chapter 3) a description of the cosmic process which rather resembles in some ways that described by Empedocles, but with a difference:

When everything was confounded, the largest part of the hot went outwards, i.e. to the top periphery. And the ancients, I think, called it ether. And the second part went to the bottom. It is called earth, cold and dry, and having much movement. And in this there is much of the hot. And the

---

[1] Ibid., 40 : ἡ δὲ κεφαλὴ καὶ ἡ καρδίη καὶ ὁ σπλὴν μετέχουσι τῆς ἰκμάδος πάσης ἕκαστον, ἢν μή τι νοσέῃ. μετέχει πλείστων κατὰ φύσιν τὴν ἑαυτοῦ τῶν εἰρημένων, ἡ μὲν κεφαλὴ τοῦ φλέγματος, ἡ δὲ καρδίη τοῦ αἵματος, ὁ δὲ σπλὴν τοῦ ὕδατος. ἕλκουσι δὲ καὶ τῆς ἄλλης ἰκμάδος αἱ φλέβες ἐς ἑωυτάς, εὐρεῖαι καὶ παχεῖαι καὶ ἑλικοειδέες ἐοῦσαι, ὥστ᾽ ἐπὴν ἕλκωσιν ἕπεσθαι ἕτερον ἑτέρῳ τῆς ἄλλης ἰκμάδος, καὶ τῇ μὲν καρδίῃ πλησιάζουσιν αἱ σφάγιαι φλέβες, παχεῖαι μὲν οὖσαι, ἐς ἃς διαδίδοται ταχέως, ἐπὴν οἱ πλεῖον τοῦ καιροῦ προσγένηται. αἱ δὲ τῷ ἄλλῳ σώματι ἐκδιδόασι, καὶ ἅμα αὐτὴ ἡ καρδίη στερεὴ καὶ πυκνή ἐστιν, ὥστε μὴ νοσέειν ὑπὸ τῆς ἰκμάδος, καὶ τοῦτο νόσημα ἐν τῇ καρδίῃ οὐδὲν γίνεται.

[2] Ibid., 39 : φλέβες τε γάρ εἰσι διὰ παντὸς τοῦ σώματος, αἱ μὲν λεπτότεραι, αἱ δὲ παχύτεραι, πολλαὶ καὶ πυκναί· αὗται δὲ μέχρις οὗ ἂν ζώῃ ὁ ἄνθρωπος ἀνεώγασι καὶ δέχονταί τε καὶ ἀφίασι νεὸν ὑγρόν· ἐπὴν δὲ ἀποθάνῃ, ξυμμύουσι καὶ γίνονται λεπταί.

[3] Sigerist, op. cit. ii. 276.

[4] De carne, 2 : δοκέει δέ μοι ὁ καλέομεν θερμὸν ἀθάνατόν τε εἶναι καὶ νοέειν πάντα καὶ ὁρῆν καὶ εἰδέναι πάντα ἐόντα τε καὶ ἐσόμενα.

third part, that of the air, took the middle place being somewhat hot and wet. And the fourth part, which is nearest to the earth, is wettest and thickest.[1]

And when all these moved in circles, when all were confounded together, a lot of the hot was left in the earth in different places, in some large quantities, and in others less, and in others very little indeed, but taken all together, a lot. When, in the course of time the earth dried up under the influence of the hot, these elements collected and made rottennesses about them like tunics. And as the heating went on for a long time, whatever rottenness from the earth was fat and had least wet, burnt most quickly, and became bones, and whatever parts happened to be more gluey and had a share of the cold, could not, when they were heated, be burnt up, nor could they become part of the cold. They therefore took on a form different from the others and became solid tendons [νεῦρα] or sinews. For they did not have much of the cold in them. But the veins had a great deal of cold. And of this cold, the outer surface which was most glutinous was cooked by the hot, and became membrane, and the cold being overpowered by the hot, was dissolved, and for this reason became wet.[2]

Omitting further not too intelligible details, we come to the heart.

Now the heart has a lot of the glutinous and the cold, and being heated by the hot, it became hard flesh and tough,[3] enclosed in a membrane, and it was made hollow, but in a different way from the veins; and it is at the head of the vein, the most hollow one. For there are two hollow veins from the heart. One of them is called artery, and the other one, next to which the heart is, is called the hollow vein. And the heart has most of the hot where the hollow vein lies, and it is the treasury of the *pneuma*. And the other veins run into these two veins. And the most hollow vein, the one from the heart, runs through the whole body and down through the diaphragm, and there is a branch into the kidney. And in the loin it splits, and darts [ἀΐσσει] among the other parts to each leg. And it also runs above the heart towards the neck, a part of it to the right, and a part of it to the left. And from there it goes up to the head, and at the temples each branch splits. One could tell each of the veins by number, but

---

[1] *De carne*, 2 : τοῦτο οὖν τὸ πλεῖστον, ὅτε ἐταράχθη πάντα, ἐξεχώρησεν ἐς τὴν ἀνωτάτην περιφορήν, καὶ ὀνομῆναί μοι αὐτὸ δοκέουσιν οἱ παλαιοὶ αἰθέρα. ἡ δὲ δευτέρα μοῖρα κάτωθεν αὐτὴ καλέεται μὲν γῆ, ψυχρὸν καὶ ξηρὸν καὶ πουλὺ κινοῦν καὶ ἐν τουτέῳ ἔνι δὴ πουλὺ τοῦ θερμοῦ. ἡ δὲ τρίτη μοῖρα, ἡ τοῦ ἠέρος, μέσον χωρίον εἴληφε, θερμόν τι ὂν καὶ ὑγρόν. ἡ δὲ τετάρτη, ἡ τοῦ ἐγγυτάτω πρὸς τῇ γῇ, ὑγρότατόν τε καὶ παχύτατον.

[2] Ibid., 3 : κυκλεομένων δὲ τουτέων, ὅτε ξυνεταράχθη, ἀπελείφθη τοῦ θερμοῦ πουλὺ ἐν τῇ γῇ, ἄλλοθι καὶ ἄλλοθι, τὰ μὲν μεγάλα τὰ δὲ ἐλάσσω, τὰ δὲ καὶ πανὺ σμικρά, πλῆθος πολλά. καὶ τῷ χρόνῳ ὑπὸ τοῦ θερμοῦ ξηραινομένης τῆς γῆς, ταῦτα καταληφθέντα περὶ αὐτὰ σηπεδόνας ποιέει οἷόν περ χιτῶνας. καὶ πολλῷ χρόνῳ θερμαινόμενον, ὁκόσον μὲν ἐτύγχανεν ἐκ γαίης σηπεδόνος λιπαρόν τε ἐὸν καὶ ὀλίγιστον τοῦ ὑγροῦ ἔχον, τάχιστα ἐξεκαύθη καὶ ἐγένετο ὀστέα. ὁκόσα δὲ ἐτύγχανε κολλωδέστερα ἐόντα καὶ τοῦ ψυχροῦ μετέχοντα, ταῦτα δὲ θερμαινόμενα, οὐκ ἠδύνατο ἐκκαυθῆναι, οὐδὲ μὴν τοῦ ὑγροῦ γενέσθαι. διὰ τοῦτο εἰδέην ἀλλοιοτέρην ἔλαβε τῶν ἄλλων καὶ ἐγένετο νεῦρα στερεά. οὐδὲ γὰρ ἐνῆν πουλὺ τοῦ ψυχροῦ αὐτῷ. αἱ δὲ φλέβες τοῦ ψυχροῦ εἶχον πουλύ· καὶ τούτου τοῦ ψυχροῦ τὸ μὲν πέριξ ὅσον κολλωδέστατον ἦν, ὑπὸ τοῦ θερμοῦ ἐξοπτηθέν, μῆνιγξ ἐγένετο, τὸ δὲ ψυχρὸν ἐὸν κρατηθὲν ὑπὸ τοῦ θερμοῦ διελύθη καὶ ἐγένετο ὑγρὸν διὰ τοῦτο.

[3] The word here translated *tough* (γλίσχρος) in other connections means *viscous*: it is, as we shall see, generally applied to liquids, but is also used metaphorically as 'clinging'.

to put it in one sentence, from the hollow vein and the artery all the other veins in the body branch off. And the most hollow ones are those near the heart and the neck, and those in the head, and those below the heart as far as the hip-bone.[1]

And most [Chapter 6] of the hot is in the veins and in the heart, and for this reason the heart has *pneuma* because it is hotter than any other part in man. It is easy to get to know that it is the *pneuma* which nourishes the heart, through this fact, that the heart and the hollow veins are continually in motion. And most of the very hot is in the veins, and therefore the heart attracts *pneuma*, being the hottest part of man.[2]

Here follows an analogy drawn from combustion which must not be interpreted too closely in terms of modern chemical theory, though it is very tempting to try to do this.

If someone wishes to burn a fire in a building, when there is no wind blowing, the flame moves, sometimes more, sometimes less, and a lighted lamp moves in the same way, sometimes more and sometimes less, though no wind moves it which we are able to perceive as blowing. And the cold is food to the hot.[3]

The author then produces another analogy, drawn this time from the field of embryology, which has no direct interest for our present purposes, but is worth quoting because of the interesting sidelight it throws on one of the early theories of foetal respiration.

And the child in the belly, holding together its lips, sucks from the teats of the womb and draws nourishment and *pneuma* into its heart. For the condition of the child is hottest, when the mother is breathing in.[4]

---

[1] *De carne*, 5: ἡ δὲ καρδίη πουλὺ τοῦ κολλώδεος καὶ τοῦ ψυχροῦ ἔχει καὶ ὑπὸ τοῦ θερμοῦ θερμαινόμενον, κρέας ἐγένετο σκληρὸν καὶ γλίσχρον, καὶ μῆνιγξ περὶ αὐτήν, καὶ ἐκοιλώθη οὐχ ὥσπερ φλέβες, καί ἐστιν ἐπὶ τῆς κεφαλῆς τῆς φλεβὸς τῆς κοιλοτάτης. δύο γάρ εἰσι κοῖλαι φλέβες ἀπὸ τῆς καρδίης. τῇ μὲν ὄνομα ἀρτηρίη, τῇ δὲ κοίλη φλέψ, πρὸς ᾗ ἡ καρδίη ἐστίν. καὶ πλεῖστον ἔχει τοῦ θερμοῦ ἡ καρδίη, ᾗ ἡ κοίλη φλέψ, καὶ ταμιεύει τὸ πνεῦμα. πρὸς δὲ τούτοιν τοῖν φλεβοῖν ἄλλαι κατὰ τὸ σῶμα. ἡ δὲ κοιλοτάτη φλέψ, πρὸς ᾗ ἡ καρδίη, διὰ τῆς κοιλίης ἁπάσης διήκει καὶ διὰ τῶν φρενῶν, καὶ σχίζεται ἐς ἑκάτερον τῶν νεφρῶν. καὶ ἐπὶ τῇ ὀσφύι σχίζεται, καὶ ἀΐσσει ἐπί τε τὰ ἄλλα καὶ ἐς ἑκάτερον σκέλος, ἀτὰρ καὶ ἄνωθεν τῆς καρδίης πρὸς τῷ αὐχένι, τὰ μὲν ἐπὶ δεξιὰ τὰ δ' ἐπ' ἀριστερά· καὶ τότε ἐπὶ τὴν κεφαλὴν ἄγει καὶ ἐν τοῖς κροτάφοισι σχίζεται ἑκατέρη. ἔστι δὲ καὶ ἀριθμῷ εἰπεῖν τὰς φλέβας τὰς μεγίστας. ἑνὶ δὲ λόγῳ ἀπὸ τῆς κοίλης φλεβὸς καὶ ἀπὸ τῆς ἀρτηρίης αἱ ἄλλαι φλέβες ἐσχισμέναι εἰσὶ κατὰ πᾶν τὸ σῶμα· κοιλότατοι δὲ αἱ πρὸς τῇ καρδίῃ καὶ τῷ αὐχένι καὶ ἐν τῇ κεφαλῇ καὶ κάτωθεν τῆς καρδίης μέχρι τῶν ἰσχίων.

[2] Ibid., 6: καὶ τὸ θερμὸν πλεῖστον ἔνι τῇσι φλεψὶ καὶ τῇ καρδίῃ, καὶ διὰ τοῦτο πνεῦμα ἡ καρδίη ἔχει, θερμὴ ἐοῦσα μάλιστα τῶν ἐν τῷ ἀνθρώπῳ. ῥηΐδιον δὲ τοῦτο καταμαθεῖν, ὅτι τρέφον ἐστὶ τὸ πνεῦμα. ἡ καρδίη καὶ αἱ κοῖλαι φλέβες κινέονται αἰεί, καὶ τὸ θερμότατον πλεῖστον ἐν τῇσι φλεψί. καὶ διὰ τοῦτο πνεῦμα ἡ καρδίη ἕλκει, θερμὴ ἐοῦσα μάλιστα τῶν ἐν ἀνθρώπῳ.

[3] Ibid.: πῦρ εἴ τις θέλει καίειν ἐν οἰκήματι ὁκόταν ἄνεμος μὴ εἰσπνέῃ, φλὸξ κινέεται τοτὲ μὲν μᾶλλον, τοτὲ δ' ἧσσον, καὶ λυχνὸς καιόμενος τὸν αὐτὸν τρόπον κινέεται, τοτὲ μὲν μᾶλλον, τοτὲ δ' ἧττον ἀνέμου οὐδενὸς κινέοντος, ὅν τινα καὶ ἡμεῖς οἷοί τέ ἐσμεν γινώσκειν πνέοντα. καὶ τροφή ἐστι τῷ θερμῷ τὸ ψυχρόν.

[4] Ibid.: τὸ δὲ παιδίον ἐν τῇ γαστρὶ ξυνέχον τὰ χείλεα μύζει ἐκ τῶν μητρέων τῆς μητρὸς καὶ ἕλκει τὴν τροφὴν καὶ τὸ πνεῦμα τῇ καρδίῃ εἴσω. τοῦτο γὰρ θερμότατόν ἐστιν ἐν τῷ παιδίῳ ὅταν περ ἡ μήτηρ ἀναπνέῃ.

The author now returns to a description of the process by which the lung was formed.

The lung came into being next to the heart like this. The heart heating the most glutinous portion of the wet, quickly dried it up, so that it became like foam and full of pipes, with a lot of little veins in it. And it made the veins by this process. Whatever of the cold there was in the glutinous portion, this was melted by the hot and became liquid, and the membrane itself was made of the glutinous portion.[1]

The liver was formed as follows:

A large portion of the liquid was separated off with the hot without the glutinous and the fat parts. The cold overpowered the hot, and it became solidified. My proof of this is the following. When anyone sacrifices an animal, as long as the body remains warm, the blood stays liquid, but when it gets cold it coagulates. But if you shake it, it does not coagulate, for it is the fibres that are cold and glutinous.[2]

Finally, there is a short paragraph explaining the process of digestion:

For the veins that come from the belly and the intestines, into which food and drink are collected, when these materials have been heated, draw away the thinnest and wettest part. But the thickest part is left behind, and becomes dung in the lower intestines. But the veins pull the thinnest parts out of the belly, when the food has been made hot . . . And the nourishment when it comes to each part renders its contribution in the same shape or character as that part has, whatever it may be.[3]

Then follow descriptions of the formation of the spleen, the joints, the nails, the teeth, and the hair, with which we need not concern ourselves.

This, at first appearance rather fantastic, account is nevertheless of some importance. Following the method laid down by Empedocles, it attempts to interpret physiological events in terms of 'physics and chemistry', but the means at the writer's disposal are pitifully inadequate for this purpose, being confined to the four Empedoclean elements, earth, air, fire, and water, with their respective qualities of heat, cold, wetness,

---

[1] De carne, 7 : ὁ δὲ πνεύμων πρὸς τῇ καρδίῃ ἐγένετο ὧδε· τοῦ ὑγροῦ ὁκόσον ἦν κολλωδέστατον, ἡ καρδίη θερμαίνουσα ταχὺ ἐξήρανεν ὅκως περ ἀφρόν, καὶ ἐποίησε σηραγγῶδες, καὶ φλέβια πολλὰ ἐν αὐτέῳ. διὰ δὲ τοῦτο ἐποίησε τὰ φλέβια. ὁκόσον ἐν τῷ κολλώδει ἐνῆν ψυχρόν, τοῦτο μὲν ὑπὸ τοῦ θερμοῦ διετάκη καὶ ἐγένετο ὑγρόν· τὸ δὲ ἀπὸ τοῦ κολλώδεος αὐτὸς ὁ χιτών.

[2] Ibid., 8 : τὸ δὲ ἧπαρ ὧδε ξυνέστη· ξὺν τῷ θερμῷ πουλὺ τοῦ ὑγροῦ ἀποληφθὲν ἄνευ τοῦ κολλώδεος καὶ τοῦ λιπαροῦ ἐκράτησε τὸ ψυχρὸν τοῦ θερμοῦ, καὶ ἐπάγη. τεκμήριον δέ μοι τόδε· ὁκόταν σφάξῃ τις ἱερεῖον, τέως μὲν ἂν θερμὸν ᾖ, ὑγρόν ἐστι τὸ αἷμα· ἐπειδὰν δὲ ψυχθῇ, ἐπάγη. ἢν δέ τις αὐτὸ τινάσσῃ, οὐ πήγνυται· αἱ γὰρ ἶνές εἰσι ψυχραὶ καὶ κολλώδεες.

[3] Ibid., 13 : καὶ γὰρ αἱ φλέβες αἱ ἐκ τῆς νηδύος καὶ τῶν ἐντέρων, εἰς ἃ ξυλλέγεται τὰ σιτία καὶ τὰ ποτά, ἐπειδὰν θερμανθῇ ταῦτα ἕλκουσι τὸ λεπτότατον καὶ τὸ ὑγρότατον. τὸ δὲ παχύτατον αὐτέου καταλείπεται καὶ γίνεται κόπρος ἐν τοῖσιν ἐντέροις τοῖσι κάτω· τὸ δὲ λεπτότατον αἱ φλέβες ἕλκουσι καὶ τῶν ἐντέρων τῶν ἄνωθεν τῆς νήστιος, θερμαινομένων τῶν σιτίων . . . ἡ δὲ τροφὴ ἐπειδὰν ἀφίκηται ἐς ἕκαστον, τοιαύτην ἀπέδωκε τὴν εἰδέην ἑκάστου ὁκοῖά περ ἦν.

and dryness. But the attempt is made in a thorough-going fashion reminiscent almost of the nineteenth-century materialist. There is no irrelevant introduction of any 'spiritual principle' or of any theological agency, except for the first sentences of the treatise in which the hot has been endowed with the theological functions and qualities attributed by Diogenes of Apollonia to air. Moreover the writer has realized that the heart is the centre of the vascular system, of veins and arteries alike, a fact which seems to suggest a date rather later than Aristotle. And though there is a distinction between the two 'hollow' blood vessels, between the vena cava and the aortas which form the trunks from which all the vessels branch off, there is no clear distinction between two different kinds of blood vessel. The term artery is used once in the case of the aorta, but all the other vessels, arteries and veins alike, are called 'veins', including the branches of 'the artery'. It should be noted, too, that although the pulse is recognized, it is attributed to the 'veins' in general, which clearly indicates that, with the exception of the aorta (a term which our author does not use though it was known to Aristotle) veins and arteries were not yet distinguished. We are therefore almost certainly dealing with a physician before (the younger) Praxagoras.

Rüsche[1] points out, in agreement with Wellmann,[2] that the work should probably be dated before Diocles. It was therefore probably written in the first half of the fourth century B.C. From the point of view of this work, perhaps the most interesting feature of the treatise is the explanation given of the process of respiration. The heart is the seat of the innate heat, but this heat needs to be fed, and it is the cold *pneuma* drawn in from the atmosphere which feeds it. This is an interesting variation on the traditional theory which we shall meet in many places, that the innate heat needs to be cooled by the cold air breathed in. Here it is the cold air which as it were feeds the fire, a notion which sounds much more modern, though in fact it is not at all so. A somewhat similar theory is found in the treatise *On the nature of the child*; Rüsche quotes a passage which recalls the theory of respiration which we shall find again in Plato.[3]

Everything that is heated has *pneuma*. Now the *pneuma* breaks away and finds its path by itself and goes out. Now the part that is being heated itself draws into itself once more another bit of cold *pneuma* through its force . . . for all the hot is nourished by the moderately cold.[4]

[1] Rüsche, op. cit., p. 169.
[2] Wellmann, op. cit., p. 90. See also Fredrich, op. cit., pp. 139 f.
[3] See below, pp. 119 f.
[4] Hippocrates, *De natura pueri*, 1 : πάντα δὲ ὁκόσα θερμαίνεται πνεῦμα ἴσχει. τὸ δὲ πνεῦμα ῥήγνυσι καὶ ποιέει οἱ ὁδὸν αὐτὸ ἑωυτῷ καὶ χωρέει ἔξω· αὐτὸ δὲ τὸ θερμαινόμενον ἕλκει ἐς ἑωυτὸ αὖθις ἕτερον πνεῦμα ψυχρὸν διὰ τῆς ῥαγῆς, ἀφ' οὗ τρέφεται . . . πᾶν γὰρ τὸ θερμὸν τῷ ψυχρῷ τρέφεται τῷ μετρίῳ.

So far as the living organism is concerned, the hot principle, by which we 'live and move and have our being', can maintain itself only by feeding on its opposite, the cold. The soul seems to be just hot air. The notion of the vital spirit as the vaporization of the blood has not yet made its appearance. But the supreme principle is heat. A rather different metaphysic is found in the treatise *On regimen*, where the two principles composing the animal organism, including man, are fire and water.[1]

In the treatise miscalled *On nourishment* we find a much clearer distinction between veins and arteries, but here both systems are not centred in the heart. They start from different organs. The source or starting-point (ἀρχή) of the veins is the liver, that of the arteries the heart,[2] a doctrine which was to find its stoutest supporter in Galen. We find, too, what is perhaps the most famous of all the 'Hippocratic' sayings on which the case of the circulationists has been based. In Chapter 23 we read: 'There is one flowing together, one breathing together. All parts suffer together, both throughout the whole organism and in each part, what is in each part, according to its function.'[3]

This treatise is made up of a number of isolated statements. It is in the form of a collection of 'opinions' expressed in a somewhat Heracleitan manner. Indeed, a number of extracts from it have been included in Diels–Kranz's *Pre-Socratics*. But its origin has been pushed forwards by Diller[4] into the first century A.D. Diller admits that it was already included in the canon of Hippocrates' writings compiled by Erotion in the time of Nero, and that it was frequently quoted as genuine by Galen (Mehwaldt cites no less than twenty references),[5] even if, as some modern critics would suggest, his commentaries on it are spurious. It had been attributed to various authorities, Littré[6] informs us, to Thessalus, Philistion, and Phylotimus,[7] all writers comparatively near in date to Hippocrates. Littré[8] regards it as post-Aristotelian but old, by which he presumably

---

[1] Hippocrates, *De regimine*, i. 3: ξυνίσταται μὲν οὖν τὰ ζῷα τά τε ἄλλα πάντα καὶ ὁ ἄνθρωπος ἀπὸ δυοῖν, διαφόροιν μὲν τὴν δύναμιν, συμφόροιν δὲ τὴν χρῆσιν, πυρὸς καὶ ὕδατος.

[2] Hippocrates, *De alimento*, 31: ῥίζωσις φλεβῶν ἧπαρ· ῥίζωσις ἀρτηριῶν καρδίη· ἐκ τουτέων ἀποπλανᾶται ἐς πάντα αἷμα καὶ πνεῦμα, καὶ θερμασίη διὰ τούτων φοιτᾷ.

[3] Ibid., 23: ξύρροια μία, ξύμπνοια μία, ξυμπαθέα πάντα, κατὰ μὲν οὐλομελίην πάντα, κατὰ μέρος δὲ τὰ ἐν ἑκάστῳ μέρει μέρεα πρὸς τὸ ἔργον.

[4] H. Diller, 'Eine stoisch-pneumatische Schrift im Corpus Hippocraticum', *Arch. f. Gesch. d. Med.* xxix (1936).

[5] See his article, 'Galenus über echte und unechte Hippocratica', *Hermes* 44.

[6] Littré, i. 383.

[7] In a marginal note in Cod. Paris. 2145 and 2255, it is attributed to Thessalus or Herophilus, and according to Aulus Gellius (*N.A.* iii. 16), to Philistion or Pherecydes. See the article, 'Hippokrates', in Pauly–Wissowa, vol. viii. Mehwaldt had no doubt that Galen thought that it was genuine and saw no reason to doubt that the commentaries on it in the Galenic Corpus were also genuine.

[8] Littré, i. 382 f.: 'La composition n'en peut pas être placée avant Aristote et Praxagoras ... ce traité est fort ancien; car Glaucias, l'un des premiers commentateurs d'Alexandrie, l'a connu, ainsi que le prouve le témoignage de Galien.'

means late fourth century B.C. Diller is convinced on philological grounds (including certain of the expressions used, e.g. 'rooting of the veins' and other close coincidences of phrases with Aretaeus) that it was the work of a member of the Pneumatic school, though neither of the founder of the school, Athenaeus of Attalia, nor of Archigenes. Abel thinks that it was already in existence by the first century B.C. Whatever its actual date, there seems to be good reason to regard it as dating much later than Hippocrates, but to hang any theory on its very disconnected sentences, seems to me to be rather rash. Nor is the supposition of the Herakleitan character of its style at all convincing. It reads to me much more like my own headings of the notes for my lectures. We need not therefore devote to it any detailed analysis, but there are some interesting statements in it that deserve some comment. Chapter 29 tells us that the lungs attract to the body nourishment of the opposite nature to itself, whereas the other parts all attract nourishment of a like nature.[1] Chapter 36, that milk and blood are an excess, πλεονασμός (not περίττωμα), of nourishment.[2] The writer still uses the term vein in an indeterminate way, so as to denote both arteries and veins, since we can hardly suppose that he believed in the doctrine here stated in Chapter 48 that veins pulsate. He also informs us that both the pulsation of the veins and the respiration of the breath or *pneuma* vary with age and with the healthy and unhealthy condition of the body, of which they are indications, and ends this paragraph with a sentence stating that breath, too, is nourishment.[3] These statements afford a certain amount of matter for speculation as to the date, matter which points to somewhat contrary conclusions. For the indifferent use of veins for all blood vessels suggests a date certainly not later than Herophilus, while that concerning the pulse as a sign of health and disease, and the theory that pulse and respiration vary with age, have both been attributed to Herophilus, though they may be as old as Praxagoras. The identification of the function of *pneuma* with that of nourishment is a theory attributed by the author of the pseudo-Aristotelian treatise *On breath* to Aristogenes,[4] a physician whose date would appear to be in the second half of the fourth century B.C. The explanation of the difference between pus and pus-like discharges is of some interest. Pus, we are told, is that which comes from flesh, the pus-like fluid that which comes from blood and from other liquids. Pus is the nourishment of a wound, pus-like

[1] Hippocrates, *De alimento*, 29: πλεύμων ἐναντίην σώματι τροφὴν ἕλκει, τὰ δὲ ἄλλα πάντα τὴν αὐτήν.

[2] Ibid., 36: γάλα καὶ αἷμα τροφῆς πλεονασμός.

[3] Ibid., 48: φλεβῶν διασφύξιες καὶ ἀναπνοὴ πνεύματος καθ' ἡλικίην καὶ ξύμφωνα καὶ διάφωνα, καὶ νούσου καὶ ὑγιείης σημήϊα, καὶ ὑγιείης μᾶλλον ἢ νούσου, καὶ νούσου μᾶλλον ἢ ὑγιείης· τροφὴ γὰρ καὶ πνεῦμα.

[4] Aristotle, *De spiritu*, 2, 481ᵃˑ ᵇ: ἡ δ' ἐκ τῆς ἀναπνοῆς, ὥσπερ Ἀριστογένης οἴεται, καὶ τὸ πνεῦμα πεττόμενον οὐ τοῦ ἀέρος ἐν τῷ πνεύματι, τοῦτο δὲ εἰς τὰ ἀγγεῖα διαδίδοσθαι, τὸ περίττωμα πάλιν ἐκπέμπεσθαι, πλείους ἔχει τὰς ἀπορίας.

matter the nourishment of vein and artery (artery or windpipe?).[1] The real meaning of these notes is not by any means always clear, but it would appear that the writer is trying to distinguish pus from serous discharges, and we may therefore regard him perhaps as the author of the doctrine of laudable pus, which only received its final death-blow from Lister a century ago.

Passages from two other treatises must now be considered. The first is from the fragment *On anatomy*, which gives the following description of the heart, lungs, and blood vessels:

The windpipe [ἀρτηρίη] making its outgrowth from each [side of the?] pharynx, ends at the top of the lung; it is composed of concentric rings of the same shape lying on top of each other and touching each other. And the lung itself fills up, together with it, the thoracic cage. Seen from right to left, it has five projecting bulges, which they call lobes, ash-coloured, marked with hollow spots sharply defined, being by nature of ashen colour. And in the middle of them the heart is seated, being of a rather rounded shape in all animals. And from the heart many a bronchia [= artery?] goes down to the liver, and with the bronchia a vein called the big vein, through which 'the whole show' is nourished. Now the liver has a resemblance to all the other organs, but it is much bloodier than the others, having two projections which they call the gates lying on the right side. And from this [there is] a vein going slantwise to the parts below the kidneys. Now the kidneys in shape and colour are like apples. And from them there are rather oblique channels which lie on the top of the bladder.[2]

This little fragment has a vocabulary rather different from that of the rest of the *Hippocratic corpus*. Its use of two rather rare words, ὁμορρυσμίη and φαρύγγεθρον, may be noted, and above all, its use of the word βρογχίη for artery, for we can hardly suppose that the author intended us to regard the vessels going from the heart to the liver as windpipes or branches of the trachea. In this connection it should be remembered that Rufus of Ephesus said that the word *aorta*, like the word *artery* and the word *bronchia*, originally was applied to the tracheal system.[3] In this

---

[1] *De alimento*, 52 : πῦον τὸ ἐκ σαρκός· πυῶδες τὸ ἐξ αἵματος καὶ ἐξ ἄλλης ὑγρασίης· πῦον τροφὴ ἕλκεος· πυῶδες τροφὴ φλεβός, ἀρτηρίης.

[2] Hippocrates, *De anatomia*, L. viii. 538 : ἀρτηρίη ἐξ ἑκατέρου φαρυγγέθρου τὴν ἔκφυσιν ποιευμένη ἐς ἄκρον πνεύμονος τελευτᾷ κρίκοις ξυγκειμένη ὁμορυσμοῖς, τῶν περιηγέων ἀπτομένη κατ' ἐπίπεδον ἀλλήλων. αὐτὸς δὲ ὁ πνεύμων ξυνεξαναπληροῖ τὴν χέλυν, τετραμμένος ἐς τὰ ἀριστερά, πέντε ὑπερκορυφώσιας ἔχων, ἃς δὴ καλέουσι λοβούς, τεφρίνης χροιῆς τυχὼν στίγμασι ὀφρυόεσι κεκεντημένος, φύσει ἐὼν τενθρηνιώδης. μέσῳ δ' αὐτέῳ ἡ καρδίη ἐγκαθίδρυται στρογγυλωτέρη καθεστεῶσα πάντων ζῴων. ἀπὸ δὲ τῆς καρδίης ἐς ἧπαρ βρογχίη πολλὴ καθήκει, καὶ μετὰ βρογχίης φλὲψ μεγάλη καλευμένη, δι' ἧς οὖλον τὸ σκῆνος τρέφεται· τὸ δ' ἧπαρ ὁμορυσμίην μὲν ἔχει τοῖς ἄλλοις ἅπασιν, αἱμορρωδέστερον δὲ τῶν ἄλλων, ὑπερκορυφώσιας ἔχον δύο, ἃς καλέουσι πύλας, ἐν δεξιοῖς τόποις κειμένας· ἀπὸ δὲ τουτέου σκαληνὴ φλὲψ ἐπὶ τὰ κάτω νεφρῶν ἀποτείνουσα. νεφροὶ δὲ ὁμοιορυσμοὶ τὴν χροιὴν δὲ ἐναλίγκιοι μήλοισιν. ἀπὸ δὲ τουτέων ὀχετοὶ σκαληνοειδέες ἄκρην κορυφὴν κύστιος κεῖνται.

[3] Rufus, *De nominibus partium hominis*, Daremberg–Ruelle, p. 155 : τῆς δὲ τραχείας ἀρτηρίας (ὅλος ὁ πόρος) καλεῖται βρόγχος· αἱ δὲ εἰς τὸν πλεύμονα ἀποφύσεις βρογχίαι καὶ σήραγγες καὶ ἀορταί.

fragment, for what it is worth, we see a double system of blood vessels centred on the heart, with veins and arteries clearly distinguished, which suggests a date certainly after Praxagoras. It would be interesting to know from which school it originated.

The second passage is one containing an account of digestion and blood production in many respects similar to the one we have just quoted from the treatise *On nourishment*. It is found in the fourth book of the treatise *On diseases*, and begins as follows:

Now I will speak about blood, how and for what reasons it increases in the body. When a man drinks or eats anything that is blood-like the whole of the body draws it into itself . . . his face becomes red. And if the heart and the body receive more blood than is sufficient, from what has been eaten and drunk, and it is mixed with the other liquid, unless it is evacuated from the body, either by the belly or by the bladder, when it is mixed with the other fluid in the body, it produces pain or disease. . . . And these fountains or sources in the body which I have named, when they are full, always distribute their contents, but when they are empty, they are sustained by it. And so too does the belly work.[1]

The 'Hippocratic' works which we have so far considered tell us really very little about the heart, almost nothing about its anatomy, and still less about the way it works. In the treatise *On the heart*, though it would appear to be only a fragment, we find a much more accurate piece of anatomical description, so accurate indeed that Wellmann was convinced that it was based on dissection of the human as opposed to the animal heart.[2] Indeed it contains a passage the most natural interpretation of which would definitely support this idea. Its inclusion in the *Hippocratic corpus*, though comparatively late, was, it would appear, accepted by Galen, and the earliest reference to it which has come down to us is in Plutarch.[3] The date of its composition is far from clear. Littré[4] naturally thought that it was obviously later than Aristotle, since its

---

[1] *De morbis*, iv. 38: νῦν δὲ ἐρέω περὶ αἵματος ὅκως τε καὶ διότι πλεῖον γίνεται ἐν τῷ σώματι. ἐπήν τι πίῃ ἢ φάγῃ ὁ ἄνθρωπος ὅ τι ἐστὶν αἱματῶδες, ἕλκει μὲν καὶ τὸ σῶμα ἅπαν ἐς ἑωυτό (see above, p. 74, n. 2) . . . τὸ πρόσωπον ἐρευθέει. προσγενομένου δὲ τῇ καρδίῃ καὶ τῷ σώματι τοῦ αἵματος πλείονος τοῦ ἱκανοῦ ἀπὸ τῶν βρωτῶν καὶ τῶν ποτῶν καὶ μισγομένου τῷ ἄλλῳ ὑγρῷ, ἢν μὴ ἀπ' αὐτοῦ ἐξέλθῃ κατὰ τὴν κοιλίην ἢ κατὰ τὴν κύστιν, μιγὲν τῇ ἄλλῃ ἰκμάδι ἐν τῷ σώματι πόνον παρέχει. . . . (39) τὰς δὲ πηγὰς ἃς ὠνόμασα αὗται τῷ σώματι ὁκόταν πλήρεες ἔωσιν ἀεὶ ἐπιδιδόασιν· ὁκόταν δὲ κεναί, περιίστανται ἀπ' αὐτοῦ· οὕτω δὲ καὶ ἡ κοιλίη ποιέει.

[2] Wellmann, op. cit., p. 94.

[3] Plutarch does not mention the treatise by name, but in *Quaest. conv.* vii. 1 he cites Hippocrates as supporting the theory mentioned in the *Timaeus*, that some of the proceeds of things drunk pass down the windpipe into the lung, and the only 'Hippocratic' treatise in which this theory is stated is the *De corde*. Plutarch's reference, quoted by Wellmann, op. cit., p. 100, is as follows: ἔτι δὴ τῶν μαρτύρων τῷ Πλάτωνι προσκαλοῦμαι Φιλιστίωνά τε τὸν Λοκρὸν . . . καὶ Ἱπποκράτην καὶ Δέξιππον τὸν Ἱπποκράτειον· οὗτοι γὰρ οὐχ ἑτέραν ὁδόν, ἀλλ' ἣν Πλάτων, ὑφηγοῦνται τοῦ πόματος.

[4] Littré, i. 203.

basic assumption is that the heart is the centre of the vascular system, a fact which Aristotle himself claimed to have discovered. Later critics, like Abel,[1] agree to this on philological grounds, but suggest that the knowledge of the valves in the heart which it displays points to a date after Erasistratus. Fredrich,[2] on the other hand, disagreed with Littré's post-Aristotelian dating, and regarded it as coming from the time of Diocles of Carystus. He maintained this early date on the grounds that it does not display the influence of the clearly marked distinction between arteries and veins first laid down by Praxagoras, nor of his doctrine that the arteries contained only *pneuma* and not also blood. Wellmann[3] regards it as emanating from the Sicilian school and showing the influence of Philistion of Locri. He points out that the Cnidian and Sicilian schools worked in close conjunction in their cardiocentric theory and in their inauguration of anatomical studies, mentioning the tradition which attributed the distinction between arteries and veins to Euryphon, an earlier contemporary of Hippocrates. F. R. Hurlbutt[4] agrees with Wellmann's attribution to the Sicilian school, and would place it after Diocles, 'when the investigation of the human body really began'. This would at any rate make it fairly certain that it cannot be earlier than the generation or two after Hippocrates. But it would still place it several generations before the great Alexandrians. But if we can trust the tradition that it was Erasistratus who first described the valves in the heart accurately, a tradition accepted by Galen, we shall have to consider that it was written after his time.

The most detailed recent discussion of its date is that given in Abel's article in *Hermes*, published in 1958. Abel argues on philological grounds, the details of which need not concern us, that the authorship must be Hellenistic, and some considerable time after Aristotle. But in view of the quite small percentage of Greek literature which has survived, more especially in the field of medicine, I cannot look upon such arguments as compelling any absolute conclusion. So many authors must have been lost completely, surviving neither in quotation nor in doxographies or references, that we cannot reach anything like certainty. Abel insists that on stylistic grounds the *De corde* could not possibly have been written by a contemporary of Diocles. With much more cogency he argues that the author's knowledge of the valves of the heart is so accurate as to compel us to place him either in the lifetime of Erasistratus, or even later. This would leave his use of the word 'vein' for all blood vessels unexplained. He even

---

[1] Abel, *Hermes* lxxxvi, p. 196.   [2] Fredrich, op. cit., p. 77.

[3] *Fragmente*, pp. 95–107.

[4] Hurlbutt, Translation of the Peri Kardies and Introduction in *Bull. Hist. Med.* 7 (1939), pp. 104 ff. See also the article by J. Bidez and G. Lebouc, *Revue étud. grecques* 57 (1944), 7 ff., in which Philistion is simply treated as the author, without any convincing evidence.

calls the ventricle of the heart itself a 'vein' in one place. We must therefore assume that the word was still used, at any rate for some time after
Herophilus and Erasistratus, as a general word for any vessel containing
blood. A rather similar ambiguity exists with respect to the German word
Ader, which is of course derived from the Latin *arteria*, and by itself
unqalified means *vein*. Finally the curious passage on human dissection
which the treatise contains is, as we shall see, more easily explained if we
regard it as the fragment of a work of the Alexandrian school. Yet its
inclusion in the *Hippocratic corpus* still requires explanation, particularly
the fact that Galen, who quotes it anonymously, did not condemn it as
spurious. Moreover its rather curious conception of the aorta and its
valve does not fit in exactly with any Alexandrian doctrine that has been
reported to us.

In addition to doubts about its date, there have also been doubts about
its content. For its text is not at all easy to interpret in more than one
passage. Thus some authorities, such as Diepgen and Diller, maintain that
the writer knew only two of the heart's valves, those closing the aorta and
the pulmonary artery; while others, including both Kapferer and Abel,
are of the opinion, which seems to me to be really quite incontestable,
that he was also acquainted with, and indeed describes, the atrio-
ventricular valves. It is therefore incumbent upon us to examine the text
in some detail. The author begins by describing the shape and colour of
the heart. Its shape is like that of a pyramid, and its colour is dark red.[1]
It is a very strong muscle, strong not because it is like a sinew or tendon,
but because of the thickness of its texture.[2] In this connection it is perhaps
interesting to observe the conjunction of the facts described in almost
identical terms in a modern textbook: Gray's section on the heart begins,
'The heart is a hollow muscular organ of a somewhat conical form';[3] and,
secondly, the fact that Galen, as we shall see later,[4] denied that the heart
is a muscle. The author is also acquainted with the pericardial sack and
the pericardial fluid: 'It has a smooth tunic, which contains a little liquid
with the appearance of urine.' The reason for this liquid is that it enables
the heart to jump with great force in safety. Its chief purpose is to prevent
over-heating. The heart absorbs and drinks this liquid, it takes it up and
consumes it, sipping drink from the lung.[5] The author presents an
experimental proof of this fact. If you give a pig a drink of water, dyed
blue or scarlet, and cut its throat immediately after it has drunk it, you

---

[1] Hippocrates, *De corde*, 1: καρδίη σχῆμα μὲν ὁκοίη πυραμὶς χροίην δὲ κατακορὴς φοινικέα.
[2] Ibid., 4: ἡ καρδίη μῦς ἐστι κάρτα ἰσχυρὸς οὐ τῷ νεύρῳ ἀλλὰ πιλήματι σαρκός.
[3] Gray, op. cit., p. 669.   [4] See below, p. 270.
[5] *De corde*, 1: περιβλέπεται χιτῶνα λειὸν καὶ ἔστιν ἐν αὐτέῳ ὑγρὸν σμικρὸν ὁποῖον οὖρον, ὥστε
δόξεις ἐν κύστει τὴν καρδίην ἀνατρέφεσθαι. γεγένηται δὲ τούτου ἕνεκα, ὅκως ἅλληται ῥωσκομένως
ἐν φυλακῇ. ἔχει δὲ τὸ ὕγρασμα ὁκόσον μάλιστα καὶ πυρευμένη ἄκος. τοῦτο δὲ τὸ ὑγρὸν διορροῖ
ἡ καρδίη πίνουσα ἀναλαμβανομένη καὶ ἀναλίσκουσα λάπτουσα τοῦ πνεύμονος τὸ ποτόν.

will see that some of the dyed water has entered the windpipe.[1] The small amount of water that passes into the lung puts the windpipe in good condition. Though water in any quantity causes troublesome coughing, a little of it lubricates the windpipe and is returned to the outer air with the breath. But a small portion of this liquid gets into the pericardium.[2] We have here another version of the theory we shall find reproduced by Plato, that part of the liquid drunk through the mouth bypasses the epiglottis and gets into the lung. Here, in addition to an attempted experimental proof, we have a typically Hellenic functional or teleo-logical explanation of this phenomenon, which was denied, incidentally, by Erasistratus, but still maintained by Galen.[3]

This teleological explanation of the pericardial fluid and its origin is also found in the *Timaeus*,[4] the medical doctrines of which were supposed to have been derived by Plato from his friend Philistion of Locri, a fact which was regarded by Wellmann as one of the reasons for looking on the *De corde* as a product of the Sicilian school.

[The heart] has two bellies, separate, but contained in a single envelope, one on this side and the other on that. They are not at all like each other, for the one on the right lies on its mouth, i.e. face-downwards, being joined on to the other vein.[5]

Littré not unnaturally found difficulties in making sense of the last two words, and therefore simply deleted the word *vein*, though it has been retained by Bidez and Lebouc,[6] but Hurlbutt in his translation follows Littré in omitting it. It is not at all easy to determine to what extent the author of this fragment was able to distinguish clearly between the two types of blood vessel, though he does seem to have known the distinction in character between the vena cava and the aorta and pulmonary artery, since he refers to both of these as aortas. And he is very well acquainted with the difference between the two ventricles. The right is 'more capacious' than the left and much more relaxed, and it does not reach the apex of the heart; it is of considerable depth, and as if it had been sewn on from the outside. The left ventricle lies nearly underneath it, and

---

[1] *De corde*, 2 : σημήϊον τοῦτο· ἢν γάρ τις κυάνῳ ἢ μίλτῳ φόρυξας ὕδωρ δοίη δεδιψηκότι πάνυ πιεῖν, μάλιστα δὲ συΐ, τὸ γὰρ κτῆνος οὐκ ἔστιν ἐπιμελὲς οὐδὲ φιλόκαλον, ἔπειτα δὲ εἰ ἔτι πίνοντος ἀνα-τέμνοις τὸν λαιμόν, εὕροις ἂν τοῦτον κεχρωσμένον τῷ ποτῷ.

[2] Ibid.: οὔκουν ἀπιστητέον ἡμῖν περὶ τοῦ ποτοῦ εἰ εὐτρεπίζει τὴν σύριγγα τῷ ἀνθρώπῳ. ἀλλὰ πῶς ὕδωρ ἀναιδὲς ἐνορουῦν ὄχλον καὶ βῆχα πουλλήν; οὕνεκα, φημί, ἀπαντικρὺ τῆς ἀναπνοῆς φέρεται. τὸ γὰρ διὰ τῆς ῥύμης ἐσρέον, ἅτε παρὰ τυτθὸν ἴον, οὐκ ἐνίσταται τῇ ἀναφορῇ τοῦ ἠέρος, ἀλλά τινα καὶ λείην ὁδόν οἱ παρέχει ἡ ἐπίτεγξις.

[3] See below, p. 394.   [4] See below, p. 119.

[5] *De corde*, 4: καὶ δύο γαστέρας ἔχει διακεκριμένας ἐν ἑνὶ περιβόλῳ, τὴν μὲν ἔνθα, τὴν δ' ἔνθα. οὐδὲν ἐοίκασιν ἀλλήλοισιν, ἡ μὲν γὰρ ἐν τοῖσι δεξιοῖσι ἐπὶ στόμα κέεται, ὁμιλέουσα τῇ ἑτέρῃ φλεβί.

[6] Bidez and Lebouc, op. cit. It is translated as 'another vein' which does not seem to be an accurate rendering of the words τῇ ἑτέρῃ φλεβί, besides leaving our problem unsolved.

nearly in line towards the left breast, where the beat of the heart is also visible. It has a thick wall, and lies embedded in a pit or trench. Its shape is like a mortar. It is softly enclosed by the lung, which surrounds it, and tempers the excess of heat. For the lung is by nature cold, being cooled by the intake of breath.[1] The insides of both ventricles are rough, and as it were somewhat eaten into or corroded, the left more so than the right. For the innate heat is not in the right, so that it is not surprising that the left ventricle's wall is tougher, since it breathes in air unmixed. Its wall was made thicker to guard against the strength of the heat.[2]

Besides bellies the heart also has ears. These auricles are described as follows:

And near the place where the veins grow out there are cavernous soft bodies bestriding the ventricles, which are called the ears, but they do not have any holes like ears, for they do not hear noises, but they are the instruments by which nature gets hold of the air. And I think they are the creation of a good craftsman. He foresaw that the heart would be a solid body, owing to the thick felty nature of its wall, which would not attract matter. So he placed beside it bellows like those the braziers have for their furnaces. It is through these auricles that the heart gets hold of its air. For you can see the two ventricles, that is the whole heart, tossing together, but the auricles blow out and collapse quite separately.[3]

The valves are described in the following terms:

The mouths [of the ventricles] are not visible, unless you cut off the tops of the auricles and the top of the heart. If you do this, two mouths will become visible in each ventricle. For the thick vein springing from one of them misleads the sight, if it is cut open. These ventricles [not mouths] are the fountains of man's nature, and from them run the rivers throughout the body by which the 'scene' is irrigated. These rivers too bring life to man, and when they dry up a man dies.[4]

[1] De corde, 4: ἀτὰρ ἥδε καὶ πάμπαν εὐρυκοίλιος καὶ λαγαρωτέρη πολλῷ τῆς ἑτέρης. οὐδὲ τῆς καρδίης νέμεται τὴν ἐσχατίην, ἀλλ᾽ ἐγκαταλείπει τὸν οὐραχόν, καὶ στερεόν καί ἐστιν ὥσπερ ἔξωθεν προσερραμμένη. ἡ δ᾽ ἑτέρη κέεται ὑπένερθεν μὲν μάλιστα, καὶ κατ᾽ ἰθυωρίην μάλιστα μὲν μαζῷ ἀριστερῷ, ὅπη καὶ διασημαίνει τὸ ἅλμα. (5) περίβολον δ᾽ ἔχει παχὺν καὶ βόθρον ἐμβεβόθρωται, τὸ εἶδος εἴκελον ὅλμῳ. ἀλλὰ γὰρ ἤδη καὶ τοῦ πνεύμονος ἐνδύεται μετὰ προσηνίης, καὶ κολάζει τὴν ἀκρασίην τοῦ θερμοῦ περιβαλλομένη. ὁ γὰρ πνεύμων φύσει ψυχρός· ἀτὰρ καὶ ψυχόμενος τῇ εἰσπνοῇ.

[2] Ibid., 6: ἄμφω γε μὴν δασεῖαι τὰ ἔνδον καὶ ὥσπερ ὑποδιαβεβρωμέναι, καὶ μᾶλλον τῆς δεξιῆς ἡ λαιή. τὸ γὰρ ἔμφυτον πῦρ οὐκ ἐν τῇ δεξιῇ, ὥστε οὐ θαῦμα τρηχυτέρην γενέσθαι τὴν λαιὴν ἐσπνέουσαν ἀκρήτου. ταύτῃ καὶ πάχετον ἐνδεδόμηται φυλακῆς εἵνεκα τῆς ἰσχύος τοῦ θερμοῦ.

[3] Ibid., 8: ἀγχοῦ δὲ τῆς ἐκφύσιος τῶν φλεβῶν σώματα τῇσι κοιλίῃσι ἀμφιβεβήκασι μαλθακὰ σηραγγώδεα, ἃ κλῄσκεται μὲν οὔατα· τρήματα δ᾽ οὐκ ἐστὶν οὐάτων. ταῦτα γὰρ οὐκ ἐνακούουσιν ἰαχῆς, ἔστι δ᾽ ὄργανα τοῖσιν ἡ φύσις ἁρπάζει τὸν ἠέρα. καίτοι δοκέω τὸ ποίημα χειρώνακτος ἀγαθοῦ. κατασκεψάμενος γὰρ σχῆμα στερεόν ἐσόμενον τὸ σπλάγχνον διὰ τὸ πιλητικὸν τοῦ ἐγχύματος, ἔπειτα πᾶν ἐὸν (πάνυ οὐκ) ἑλκτικόν, παρέθηκεν αὐτέῳ φύσας, καθάπερ τοῖσι χοάνοισιν οἱ χαλκέες, ὥστε διὰ τουτέων χειροῦται τὴν πνοήν. τὴν μὲν γὰρ καρδίην ἴδοις ἂν ῥιπταζομένην οὐλομελῆ, τὰ δ᾽ οὔατα κατ᾽ ἰδίην ἀναφυσώμενά τε καὶ ξυμπίπτοντα.

[4] Ibid., 7: στόματα δ᾽ αὐτέοισι οὐκ ἀνεώγασιν, εἰ μή τις ἀποκείρει τῶν οὐάτων τὴν κορυφήν (τὴν καρδίην), καὶ τῆς καρδίης τὴν κεφαλήν. ἢν δ᾽ ἀποκείρῃ φανήσεται καὶ δισσὰ στόματα ἐπὶ

The two 'outlet' valves, the aorta and the pulmonary, are the only ones which are described in the fragment of the treatise that has come down to us. So in Chapter 10 we are told:

The rest of the argument is concerned with the invisible membranes of the heart.... For there are membranes and other threads [reading with Unger, ἄλλαι ἶνες] like spiders' webs in the ventricles, which stretch across and bind together the mouths in all directions. They throw off fibres into the solid wall of the heart. These seem to me to be the hinges or braces of the organ and the beginnings of the aortas. There is a pair of aortas, and their doors have been designed with three membranes to each of them, going round the edges like the segments of a circle, which when they come together close the mouths which are the limits or starting-points of the aorta. [Bidez–Lebouc with Unger read: 'gates' instead of 'limits', a not at all improbable emendation.][1]

Kapferer believes that this chapter (10) describes both sets of valves, the inlet valves, which he calls *Cuspidalklappen*, and the semi-lunar valves which close the openings of the two aortas, the pulmonary valve and the aorta proper, as it is now called. Notwithstanding the fact that the author, after describing the valves and their attachments growing out of the solid wall of the heart, expressly states that they are the beginning of the aortas, Kapferer insists that it is the 'inlet' valves, the tricuspid and the mitral, that he is referring to, though he admits that it is the semi-lunar valves that are referred to in the following sentence. With typical perverse ingenuity, he goes on to explain that the author is acquainted with the two circulations carrying the blood from the right side of the heart to the left.[2]

δυσὶ γαστέροιν. ἡ γὰρ παχείη φλὲψ ἐκ μιῆς ἀναθέουσα πλανᾷ τὴν ὄψιν, ἢν ἀνατμηθῇ. αὗται γὰρ πηγαὶ φύσιος ἀνθρώπου, καὶ οἱ ποταμοὶ ἐνταῦθα (ἐντεῦθεν) ἀνὰ τὸ σῶμα τοῖσιν ἄρδεται τὸ σκῆνος· οὗτοι δὲ καὶ τὴν ζωὴν φέρουσι τῷ ἀνθρώπῳ, κἢν αὐανθέωσι, ἀπέθανεν ὤνθρωπος.

[1] De corde, 10: λοιπός ἐστιν ὁ λόγος ὁ τῆς καρδίης ὑμένες ἀφανέες, ἔργον ἀξιαπηγητότατον. ὑμένες γὰρ καὶ ἄλλαι ἶνες ἐν τῇσι κοιλιῇσι ὁκοῖον ἀράχναι διαπετέες ζωσάντες πάντῃ τὰ στόματα κτηδόνας ἐμβάλλουσιν ἐς τὴν στερεὴν καρδίην. οὗτοί μοι δοκέουσιν οἱ τόνοι τοῦ σπλάγχνου καὶ τῶν ἀγγείων ἀρχαὶ τῇσιν ἀορτῇσιν. ἔστι δ' αὐτέων τόνοι τοῦ σπλάγχνου καὶ τῶν ἀγγείων, ἀρχαὶ τῇσιν ἀορτῇσιν· ἔστι δὲ αὐτέων ζεῦγος αἱ θύραισι μεμηχάνηνται, τρεῖς ὑμένες ἑκάστῃ περιφερέες ἐξ ἄκρου περ ὁκόσον ἡμίτομα κύκλου. οἵ τε ξυνιόντες θαυμάσιον ὡς κλείουσι τὰ στόματα τῶν ἀορτέων πέρας (πυλάς).

[2] Kapferer, *Hippokrates* (1937), op. cit.: 'Wir haben hier eine sehr gute Beschreibung der beiden Eingangspforten des Herzens mit ihren Cuspidalklappen vor uns. Der nächste Satz bringt dann die ebenso gute Darstellung der beiden Herzausgänge mit ihren Semilunarklappen.' [After giving his rendering specially designed to suit his purpose:] 'Es gibt ferner von diesen Oeffnungen ein Paar, etc.' [Kapferer proceeds:] 'Diese beiden Sätze über zwei "Aorten" geben uns zweifellos eine nach echt hippokratischer Art einheitlich zusammengefaßte Betrachtung des Gefäßverlaufs. Der Autor belegt die beiden Blutgefäße, die aus den Ventrikeln in den Körper und von dem Körper in die Ventrikel zurückführen, mit dem Wort "Aorten" und bezeichnet dabei, ganz entsprechend unserer heutigen Auffassung, die beiden Semilunarklappen als "der Aorten unteres Ende" und die beiden Cuspidalklappen als "obere Enden der Aorten". Kein Zweifel, der Autor kennt die zwei vom Herzen zum Herzen verlaufenden Kreisbögen der Blutgefäße.'

We now come to a passage which has given rise to a great deal of controversy, since it raises the question of human dissection in its most acute form. The author appears to have had a fairly intimate acquaintance with the heart: he knows the valves, though he describes only two of them, and he has some notion of the chordae tendineae; in fact his knowledge seems, as Wellmann recognized, to have been based on the human, not the animal, heart. Bidez and Lebouc point out that his description of the position of the heart with reference to the lungs and the thorax is more accurate than that of Galen based on the dissection of the monkey.[1]

If a man, knowing the ancient order [rule] or custom, removes the heart of a dead man and folds the membranes to, neither can water get into the heart, nor air, if blown against them, particularly in the case of the left, for they were here designed more surely and rightly so, since the mind of man grows in the left ventricle, and rules over the rest of the soul or life-principle.[2]

This brings us up against the question whether before the foundation of the Alexandrian school human dissection was possible, a question on which historians of Greek medicine have held very different opinions. Was it, for example, possible, as Wellmann would seem to imply, in Sicily in the days of Philistion? Lebouc, without producing any confirmatory evidence, maintains that Philistion, like Alcmaeon, did dissect human bodies and justified this procedure by citing the ancient Egyptian practice, since Cnidians Chrysippus and Eudoxus, his pupils, had visited Egypt before coming to Syracuse. But would it not be simpler to suppose that the fragment is, if not Alexandrian, at any rate later in date than Herophilus and Erasistratus? According to the ancient Egyptian practice the principal organs including the heart were removed from the body and embalmed separately in Canopic jars. It is surely more than a mere coincidence that it was in Alexandria that the dissection of human bodies under the early Ptolemies became a regular, albeit a short-lived, practice of the medical school. It seems to me to be hardly probable that a Sicilian physician of the first half of the fourth century B.C. could have appealed to Egyptian practice to justify human dissection, and even more improbable that a local Sicilian rule or custom could have existed to be invoked.

---

[1] Bidez and Lebouc, op. cit. Lebouc's comment on Chapter 4: 'Cette description du cœur dans son ensemble est parfaite: elle expose avec précision l'aspect de l'organe en place, après l'ablation du plastron sternal. Dès à présent, on peut affirmer qu'il s'agit du cœur humain. La remarque que l'organe tout entier est reporté du côté gauche en fait foi. C'est la station verticale, qui faisant s'appuyer le cœur sur le diaphragme plutôt que sur le plastron sternal, a produit un déplacement vers la gauche. Le fait est contrasté par Galien, qui, étudiant de l'anatomie chez les singes, place le cœur au milieu de la cage thoracique.'

[2] De corde, 10: καὶ τὴν καρδίην ἀποθανόντος ἤν τις ἐξεπιστάμενος τὸν ἀρχαῖον κόσμον ἀφελών, τῶνδε τὸν μὲν ἀποστερήσει (ἀποστήσῃ) τὸν δ' ἐπανακλίνῃ, οὔτε ὕδωρ ἂν διέλθοι ἐς τὴν καρδίην, οὔτε φῦσα ἐμβαλλομένη, καὶ μᾶλλον τῶν τῆς ἀριστερῆς· τοίγαρ ἐμηχανήθησαν ἀτρεκέστερον κατὰ δίκην. γνώμη γὰρ ἡ τοῦ ἀνθρώπου πέφυκεν ἐν τῇ λαιῇ κοιλίῃ, καὶ ἄρχει (ἀρχὴ) τῆς ἄλλης ψυχῆς.

To return to the *De corde*. It might have been thought that after the brilliant description of the heart and its valves, we should have been told something about the way in which it worked. But here we are doomed to disappointment. It is impossible to elicit from the text any consistent account of how the ensemble functions, largely because of the mistaken connections assumed by ancient Greek medicine between the vascular and the respiratory systems. In a passage we have just quoted, the auricles are likened to bellows blowing air from the lungs into the ventricles, but it would appear that this is true only of the left auricle, for in a later passage the account of the administration of air to the right ventricle is quite different. The need for air of the two ventricles is not the same: the left, which contains the innate heat, needs much more air to cool it than the right.

For this reason I say that veins operate the breathing in of air into the left ventricle and an artery into the other, for the soft vessel has greater power of attraction and is more elastic.[1]

Kapferer's interpretation of this passage is quite astonishingly unlikely. He asks us to recognize in the vessels mentioned the venae pulmonales, which is easy enough; but the artery is the vena cava, justifying this misreading on the ground that φλέψ and ἀρτηρίη in the Hippocratic vocabulary are words having the same meaning and can refer to either type of vessel.[2]

The part of the text which follows is obviously corrupt and has been variously emended since the days of Littré, but the general idea which the author is trying to convey seems to be clear enough. It was necessary that the surrounding tissues of the heart should be cooler than the heart, hence the necessity of breathing in air (reading μᾶλλον with Littré rather than μεῖον with Unger), but since there is less heat in the right ventricle, the air supply for it can be delivered by a less ready instrument, in order to avoid the danger of what heat there is in the right ventricle being entirely overcome or destroyed by the cold air coming in from the lungs.[3] The idea apparently being that the pulmonary artery which supplies

---

[1] *De corde*, 9: διὰ τοῦτο δέ φημι καὶ φλέβια μὲν ἐργάζεται τὴν ἀναπνοὴν ἐς τὴν ἀριστερὴν κοιλίην, ἀρτηρίη δὲ ἐς τὴν ἄλλην. τὸ γὰρ μαλακὸν ἑλκτικώτερον καὶ ἐπιδόσιας ἔχει (ἔχον).

[2] Kapferer, op. cit.: 'Hieraus erkennen wir unschwer die in den linken Ventrikel einmündenden Venae pulmonales und die in den rechten Ventrikel führende Vena cava. Allerdings ist die hippokratische Nomenklatur für uns befremdlich, weil wir meinen, das Wort ἀρτηρίη dürfe nur für eine Arterie gebraucht werden. In den hippokratischen Schriften werden aber die Bezeichnungen ἀρτηρίη und φλέψ wahllos gebraucht, so daß man mit Recht von einer verworrenen Nomenklatur sprechen kann.'

[3] *De corde*, 9: Littré reads: ἔχρη δὲ ἡμῖν μᾶλλον τὰ ἐπικείμενα τῆς καρδίης διαψύχεσθαι· βέβλαπται (MSS. βεβλημα, βεβλήματα) ἔς τι γὰρ τὸ θερμὸν ἐν τοῖσι δεξιοῖσιν, ὥστε διὰ τὴν πάθην οὐκ ἔλαβεν εὐπετὲς ὄργανον, ἵνα μὴ πάμπαν κρατηθῇ ὑπὸ τοῦ ἐσιόντος. Bidez and Lebouc read ἔχρη δὲ ἡμῖν μεῖον τὰ ἐπικείμενα τῆς καρδίης διαψύχεσθαι ἐπιβλήματα, ἐστὶ γὰρ θερμὸν οὐκ ἐν τοῖσι δεξιοῖσι, κτλ.

blood to the lungs also conveys a little air from them to the right ventricle. And for this reason the pulmonary valve is not quite air-tight. A little air enters the right ventricle through it. For there the hot is controlled or mastered by the service of the cold.[1] Here there is no mention of the auricle at all, and how the air passes from the pulmonary artery into the bellows of the auricle is a complete mystery.[2] It is to be noted that both the aorta and the pulmonary artery are spoken of simply as the artery in different passages, and that they are also referred to as aortas.

The peculiar feature of the physiology presented in the *De corde* is that although it represents the left ventricle of the heart as containing only air and no blood, it does not adopt the theory formulated by Praxagoras that the whole of the arterial system contains only air, or its derivative *pneuma*. The fact of the empty left ventricle, which may very well have been known in the time of Alcmaeon, is cited as an experimental datum. If you cut an animal's throat and let it bleed to death, and then open up the left ventricle, you will find it quite empty, except for a little serum and yellow bile; but the right ventricle and the artery, i.e. the aorta, are full of blood. The author seems to have been fascinated by the notion of the left ventricle as the seat of the soul and the intelligence and the innate heat. It is this lofty function which is ultimately the reason for the heart's valves, at any rate that closing the aorta.[3] For the left ventricle does not contain any blood, though the right ventricle and the (great) artery do. Its function is too lofty for it to receive its nourishment from so coarse a substance as blood, no food fit for a commander. But some nourishment it must have. This is in fact ultimately derived from blood, by a sort of fractional distillation which produces a pure and light-like 'super-essence' which it draws from the blood nearest to it, presumably that in the aorta, by sending out its rays.[4] To understand this statement, it must be remembered that one of the most common early Greek theories of sight was that the form or visible shape of the object was carried to the brain, not by rays

---

[1] Ibid., 12: τὸ δ' αὖ φερόμενον ἐκ τῆς δεξιῆς ζυγοῦται μὲν καὶ τοῦτο τῇ συμβολῇ τῶν ὑμένων, πλὴν οὐ κάρτα ἔθρωσκεν ὑπ' ἀσθενείης· ἀλλ' ἀνοίγεται μὲν ἐς πνεύμονα, ὡς αἷμα παρασχεῖν αὐτέῳ ἐς τὴν τροφήν, κλείεται δὲ ἐς τὴν καρδίην (οὐχ) ἁρμῷ ὅκως ἐσίῃ μὲν ὁ ἠήρ, οὐ πανὺ δὲ πουλύς. ἀσθενὲς γὰρ ἐνταῦθα τὸ θερμὸν δυναστευόμενον χρήματι ψυχροῦ. τὸ αἷμα γὰρ οὔκ ἐστι τῇ φύσει θερμόν, οὐδὲ γὰρ ἄλλο τὸ ὕδωρ, ἀλλὰ θερμαίνεται, δοκέει δὲ τοῖσι πολλοῖσι φύσει θερμόν.

[2] Can it be that the notion of the right auricle as a bellows has just been abandoned and that 'artery' here means the windpipe?

[3] *De corde*, 11: ἀποσφαγέντος τοῦ ζῴου, σχισθείσης τῆς ἀριστερῆς κοιλίης ἐρημίη φαίνεται πᾶσα πλὴν ἰχωρός τινος καὶ χολῆς ξανθῆς, καὶ τῶν ὑμενέων περὶ ὧν ἤδη μοι πέφανται. ἡ δὲ ἀρτηρίη οὐ λειφαιμοῦσα, οὐδὲ ἡ δεξιὴ κοιλίη. τουτέῳ μὲν οὖν τῷ ἀγγείῳ κατ' ἐμὸν νόον ἤδε πρόφασις τῶν ὑμένων.

[4] Ibid.: τρέφεται δὲ οὔτε σιτίοισιν οὔτε ποτοῖσιν ἀπὸ τῆς νηδύος, ἀλλὰ καθαρῇ καὶ φωτοειδεῖ περιουσίῃ γεγονυίῃ ἐκ τῆς διακρίσεως τοῦ αἵματος. εὐπορέει δὲ τὴν τροφὴν ἐκ τῆς ἔγγιστα δεξαμένης τοῦ αἵματος, διαβάλλουσα τὰς ἀκτῖνας καὶ νεμομένη ὥσπερ ἐκ νηδύος καὶ ἐντέρων τὴν τροφὴν οὐκ ὂν κατὰ φύσιν. ὅκως δὲ μὴ ἀνακωχῇ τὸ σιτίον τὰ ἐνεόντα ἐν τῇ ἀρτηρίῃ ἐν ζάλῃ ἐόν, ἀποκλείει τὴν ἐπ' αὐτὴν κέλευθον. ἡ γὰρ μεγάλη ἀρτηρίη βόσκεται τὴν γαστέρα καὶ τὰ ἔντερα καὶ γέμει τροφῆς οὐχ ἡγεμονικῆς.

emitted by the object reaching the retina, but by rays emitted by the eye, bringing back as it were the object's form.[1] The idea of the light-like super-essence being brought back to the left ventricle by rays emitted from it is, according to Wellmann, derived from Diocles. In support of this derivation he cites a passage from a Latin author whom he identifies with Vindicianus, which he believes to be a doxographical fragment representing the doctrine of the 'second Hippocrates' from Carystus.[2]

The resemblance of the passage in Vindicianus to that of the *De corde* is certainly on the face of it rather striking, but as Wellmann himself states in a footnote, the similarity with Stoic doctrine is obvious, and our author may very well have derived his conception from this source. This would once more point to a Hellenistic not a fourth-century Sicilian origin for our fragment. The experimental proof of the bloodless left ventricle combined with a bloodful aorta also raises difficulties. Abel points out that this is not in accordance with experimental evidence, since in fact not only the left ventricle but the whole main arterial system should have been found without blood for physiological reasons, since after death, he explains, the vasoconstrictor centres governing these arteries are strongly stimulated by the increase of carbon dioxide and the lack of oxygen in the blood, with the result that the blood is drawn into the veins. The aorta should therefore have been found empty.[3] The phenomenon of empty arteries in dead bodies had been noted very early by Greek physicians and may perhaps lie at the root of the distinction already found in Alcmaeon between 'veins' and 'blood-flowing veins' which we have already noted.[4] Why then does the author of the *De corde*

---

[1] Cf. Jablonski, 'Die Theorie des Sehens im griechischen Altertum bis auf Aristoteles', *Arch. f. Gesch. d. Med.* xxiii (1930): 'Nach den Pythagoreern . . . ging aus den Augen etwas, ἡ ὄψις hervor, die Dinge berührend und ihre Form und Farben erfassend. Martin (*Études sur le Timée de Platon*) übersetzt mit *feu invisible*, unsichtbares Feuer, und diese Übertragung erscheint berechtigt angesichts der Weiterbildung, welche die übernommene pythagoreische Lehre bei den Stoikern erfuhr. Die Stoiker bezeichneten den durch die Augen entsandten unsichtbaren Strom, bald als ὄψεως ἀκτῖνες πυρικαί, des Gesichtes feurige Strahlen, bald als ὁρατικὸν πνεῦμα, Seh-hauch. Es muß sich also um ein dünnes, feurig-luftartiges Fluidum halten; seine Strahlen erzeigten, nach den Stoikern eine Art Spannung in einem Luftkegel, dessen Basis auf dem Objekt, und dessen Spitze auf der Pupille lag, und diese Luft diente durch Rückwirkung auf das Auge als Vermittler zwischen Organ und Objekt.'

[2] Wellmann, *Fragmente*, pp. 3 f. and 105. The passage cited from Vindicianus (cap. 17) reads as follows: 'Sic enim supradicto exemplo ignei splendoris seu radii ex partibus loci in corde constituti, in quo anima consistit, usque ad omnes fines corporis nostri supervenit et consensus in illis partibus fiet, in quibus etiam irruentia perficiuntur.' Op. cit., p. 219.

[3] Abel, *Gesnerus* 15 (1958), op. cit., note 11 to p. 86. 'Das Phenomen der post-mortalen Blutleere ist nicht nur im linken Ventrikel, sondern im gesamten Arteriensystem zu beobachten. Die Erscheinung erklärt sich daher, daß bei Eintritt des Todes, das Vasokonstriktorencentrum durch Kohlensäureanreicherung und Sauerstoffmangel stark erregt wird. Um so bemerkenswerter ist es daß im *de corde* die Bluthaltigkeit der Aorta betont wird' (*Hermes* 86, note 4 to p. 205).

[4] See above, p. 8.

go out of his way to tell us that it is not lacking in blood? He is, of course, trying to produce evidence for his theory of the function of the aortal valve, which he conceives as being that of preventing the blood from entering the left ventricle. Is he therefore faking the evidence to prove his theory? It may not be necessary to adopt quite so drastic an assumption. He may, on finding that the aorta of a living animal contained blood, and opening up the left ventricle and finding it empty and the valve closed, have assumed that it still contained blood. Or again, he might have opened up the aorta very soon after death and found some blood in it. For it would seem that the emptying of the arterial system of blood at death is not an instantaneous happening.

A recent series of experiments carried out by a Swedish pathologist in Uppsala may perhaps throw a little light on this problem. Fåhraeus, in a paper entitled 'Empty arteries' delivered to the Fifteenth International Congress of the History of Medicine held in Madrid in 1957, gives an account of a number of autopsies made at least twenty-four hours after death. He says that on introducing a cannula connected with a mano-meter into the carotid or femoral artery, one finds a negative pressure of a few millimetres to one decimetre. If you now begin the autopsy and open the thoracic cage, the pressure immediately rises to zero, owing to the absorption of air by the arteries. He believes that the explanation of this negative pressure is the following. Pressure in the arteries becomes negative because after death part of the arterial system dilates. This dilation cannot take place in the big arteries, it must therefore be the little arteries that dilate and draw (*aspirent*) a certain quantity of blood from the big arteries. This phenomenon varies with the age of the person. The height of the negative pressure increases sharply from the ages of 18 to 70, and then remains pretty constant.

Our Swedish doctor's findings may perhaps help to explain this apparent paradox, but cannot remove the inconsistencies which we have noted in the account of the *De corde* to which we have already drawn attention, namely the abandonment of the bellows theory in the case of the right auricle. Our author has to get some *pneuma* or air from the lungs into the right ventricle, and he seems to be aware that the right auricle introduces blood not air into the right ventricle. The right ventricle, like the left, has an aorta, but it leads only to the lung through a 'mouth' closed, like that of the other aorta, by a semi-lunar valve. He is therefore reduced to the rather desperate expedient of making the pulmonary valve insufficient, and assuming a two-way traffic of blood one way and air the other along the pulmonary artery. It is interesting to note in this connection that Galen is driven to a similar expedient in the case of the mitral valve, which has at one and the same time to draw air into the left ventricle, and expel waste products through it back into the lung.[1] It should be noted, too, that the doctrine here stated of the function of the pulmonary artery as feeding the lung was also adopted by Galen, and was perhaps the principal reason why he failed to discover the pulmonary circulation.

It is certainly difficult for us to make much sense of the description given in this fragment of the way in which the heart works. Perhaps we should be a little better off in this respect if we possessed the whole treatise, which can hardly have failed to give an account of the atrio-ventricular valves. As it is we can only guess how the cardio-vascular system was supposed to work, and the most important piece of evidence is missing. How, for example, does blood get from the right ventricle into the aorta, since it would not appear to be possible for it to pass through the heart or through the lungs. And what happens to the air which is received by the left ventricle? We know its function, which is to cool the innate heat; does it return to the outer atmosphere via the lung, and if so how much? When the left ventricle contracts, what happens to the aortal valve? Does it open and expel air or *pneuma* into the aorta and the arterial system? For if it does not, there would not seem to be any reason for its existence. All these are mysteries to which we have no key. One point, however, is perhaps worth noting. In the fragment as we have received it, no mention is made of *pneuma*; what comes into the heart via the lungs is just air. Does this point to an early date for its composition, before the doctrine of *pneuma* had been properly developed? And what is the character of this pure and light-like super-essence? Is it the prototype of the exhalation from the blood which Galen regards as one of the constituents of the psychic *pneuma*?[2] To these questions the fragmentary nature of the treatise does not permit us to give any definite answer. But it is perhaps worth while examining a little more closely the fragment of Vindicianus, which was incorporated from the Brussels MS.[3] into the sixteenth-century edition of Octavius Horatianus by Count Neuenar. The text of this fragment, reproduced in Wellmann,[4] purports to be an account of Diocles' doctrine of the nature of the semen. Diocles[5] regards the heart as the seat of the intelligence and combines this with the theory of the double respiration of lungs and skin by which the heart receives its air from alternate sources. And as air is drawn to the heart from all over the body, so the 'ray' of the power of sensation sent out from that portion of the heart in which the soul resides reaches out to all the borders of the

[1] See below, pp. 307 f.
[2] See below, p. 370.
[3] The manuscript is one of Theodore Priscian, cod. Bruxell., Nr. 1342–50.
[4] *Fragmente*, pp. 208–34.
[5] The passage in question is only introduced by 'inquit' like many others, but Wellmann was convinced that the 'he' referred to is Diocles.

body, and a consciousness takes place in those parts in which inrushing data are also put together or perfected. There is one single power of sensation in the heart, which is transmitted to the soul, but the sense channels through which sensations are brought in are different, but it would appear that sense data are not impressed mechanically from the outside. They are brought in by the sensitive power of the soul, and it is the rational soul seated in the high places of the heart which accomplishes or perfects all the senses. The light by which we see comes from the soul via the heart, and rushing in upon the visible object apprehends or seizes its image.[1] And the nurture of this power, according to the *De corde*, is provided by the super-essence distilled from the blood brought in by the soul or intelligence through its 'rays'. The difficulties of accounting for consciousness in terms of matter, whether in the heart or in the brain, are nothing new.

It would hardly appear that this 'Dioclean' theory of the heart's nourishment can supply us with any conclusive evidence for the date of the treatise whose fragment we have been examining. It seems to me to be more reasonable to suppose that, even if it were ultimately traceable to some Sicilian source, it can hardly have been composed earlier than the lifetime of Erasistratus. Galen, though he never cites it by name, was almost certainly acquainted with it,[2] and the fact that he never mentions it as belonging to the *Hippocratic corpus*, into which it was certainly a later if not the latest entrant, would seem to point to a late date.

Galen is quite clear that it was Erasistratus who discovered the valves of the heart. Had they been described so fully by some earlier author he would have mentioned it, and nothing could surely have pleased him better than to discover that they had been known to Hippocrates himself. That the author was not of the school of Erasistratus is also quite clear, for Erasistratus and Herophilus, his elder contemporary, both insist that the brain not the heart is the seat of consciousness. It would therefore seem very unlikely that he was an Alexandrian, but he may well have been one of the earlier Pneumatists, a fragment of whose treatise was finally incorporated into a late revision of the *Corpus*.

---

[1] See the passage from Vindicianus quoted above in footnote 2 to p. 92, and the following extracts from par. 19: 'Cum ex corde sensifica virtus limpida atque splendens ad oculos pervenit infusa per humorem vitreum . . . exinde rursum redit ad sphaeram, hoc est ultimam interius tunicam, quam Graeci κρυσταλλοειδῆ vocant. . . . Tunc tenuans atque splendificans sphaeram ad eius centrum ac mediam partem, quam appellamus facoidem, confugit. Exinde ad pupillam omnis concidens celerrimo lapsu per eius raritates accipit casum tamquam ex suffecto secundam sphaeram a vertice ad tenuam pupillae viam conducta. Atque irruens visibilibus rebus, hoc est quas videmus, earum facit apprehensionem. . . . Accedit etiam quod secum plurimum luminis ex anima trahat (atque) ex corde perfecto in similitudine radii per visificas vias irruat et ab hoc corpore in aerem cadens longo itinere non intereat.'

[2] Galen's 'quotation' may after all perhaps not have come from the *De corde* at all, but from an unknown source which both he and the author used.

The fragmentary nature of this essay and its consequent obscurity make it difficult, to say the least of it, to endorse the extraordinary judgement of Kapferer that it affords clear proof of Hippocrates' complete anticipation of Harvey's discovery.[1] Here I must add a short parenthesis. In this study I have dealt only with what we may call professional medical literature. But as was suggested to me by Mr. J. Fettes when this chapter had already gone to press, if the circulation of the blood had been postulated by any medical writer, the idea would have become public knowledge among educated persons and familiar to all philosophers, orators, and dramatists. One would therefore expect to find some casual references or allusions to it scattered about Greek literature. Had Hippocrates really propounded it, could Aristophanes have refrained from poking fun at it, or Aristotle failed to cite its teleological significance? And if Galen, could Lucian have failed to mention it? As far as I know, there is not a single passage in any non-medical work which could be taken even remotely to refer to it. And indeed, in medical literature, if we may be permitted to include certain passages in the *Timaeus* in this category, the nearest I can think of, *sed quanto proximus intervallo*, is the passage discussed in the next chapter, about the blood rushing through the limbs.

[1] In his introduction to his translation of the *De corde* (vol. 16, p. 59), Kapferer remarks: 'Was die Physiologie des Herzens betrifft, so sind die Schilderungen seiner Druck- und Saugefunktionen und die Funktion der Herzohren hervorgehoben. Das gröste Interesse aber erweckt die Schilderung des Blutkreislaufs . . . Mit anderen Worten, der Autor sieht ganz klar die zwei vom Herzen und zum Herzen sich spannenden Kreisbogen der Blutgefäße. Der Blutkreislauf war also bereits ca. 400 vor Christ bekannt.'

3 · AFTER HIPPOCRATES

W E have now examined all the principal passages in the *Hippocratic corpus* which deal with the heart and the vascular system. After our analysis of the various theories found in them, can we conclude as Littré appears to have done that they show any acquaintance with the circulation of the blood as it has been understood since the days of Harvey? The answer must, in my opinion, be definitely 'no'. Though we found in many places accounts of blood vessels running into one another, the work of the heart as a propulsive organ is practically ignored. No description of it at all or of its chambers is to be found, except in the much later fragment, the *De corde*. The heart is recognized as being in continual motion, and as being at the cross-roads of two systems of great vessels. Arguments as to the meaning of the passage on the circle which has no beginning will not carry us to any certain conclusion, and can be explained most simply by the notion that the various blood vessels ran into each other, as indeed some of the veins and arteries do. Nor can any case for a knowledge of the circulation be deduced from the famous passage already quoted from the treatise *On nourishment* about the 'one flowing together, one breathing together', which seems to be a general reference to the principle that the body is an organism, not a description of the circulation of any fluids within it. How much then did the physicians of the generations immediately following the death of Hippocrates, those of the second half of the fourth and the beginning of the third century B.C., really know about the heart and the vascular system? Our answer to this question must, of course, depend on our general ideas about the date of the principal works of the *Hippocratic corpus*. Without subscribing to the nihilism of Edelstein or attempting to make pronouncements on the genuineness of particular treatises, it would appear to be safe to assume that of the principal works both Books i and iii of the *Epidemics* and the *Prognostics* were probably written before the end of the fifth century B.C., as Kudlien,[1] in agreement with Deichgräber,[2] maintains;

[1] See his article, 'Hippokrates', in the Kleines Pauly–Wissowa, p. 1169.
[2] Deichgräber, 'Die Epidemien und das Corpus Hippocraticum', *Abh. Preuß. Akad. Wiss.* (Jahrg. 1933).

while quite a number of other treatises can be placed, with a more than fair degree of probability in the earliest years of the fourth century B.C., such as the works on *Joints* and *Fractures* and possibly some of the other surgical treatises and parts of the *Aphorisms*, *Airs*, *waters*, *and places*, *The nature of man*, and *On the sacred disease* are placed by Deichgräber rather earlier than by Kudlien, who would defer them to the second half of the fourth century B.C., together with *Regimen*, *Regimen in acute diseases*, and *The art*. The gynaecological works, which are Cnidian, as well as the first three books *On diseases* may very well belong to the early half of the century, while the work *On fleshes* is placed by Deichgräber at the end of the period of the sophists. Temkin's survey[1] suggests that before the century was ended, indeed perhaps by the middle of it, a systematic body of medical doctrine, both of aetiology and treatment, to which the school of Cnidos as well as that of Cos had contributed, had come into existence based upon the pathology of the four humours, a systematic body which did not, of course, exclude a great deal of diversity of opinion on many points. That there were alternative theories of the causes of disease in the schools both of Cos and of Cnidos is shown by the fragment of Menon's treatise in the Anonymous Londoner as well as the fragments of the Anonymous Parisian,[2] but the evidence for their origin and implications is too slight for any dogmatic conclusions. With regard to the heart, the state of knowledge which had been attained is far from clear, but we might perhaps without too much risk of inaccuracy construct a picture, on the following lines, of the state of medical knowledge in this field at the time when the Alexandrian school was founded. Before 300 B.C. they had already discovered that the heart had four chambers, two of which were usually thought of as the terminal processes of blood vessels, i.e. the pulmonary vein (the vein-like artery), and the 'hollow' vein (the vena cava). They knew, too, that there were two main trunks of vessels coming out of the heart, one on the right side and the other on the left, from which all the other blood vessels in the body, except those in the lungs, were derived. And they knew that these trunks had a different appearance, and that all the blood vessels in the body, except those in the lungs, were derived from one or the other. They knew that each of these great vessels ran both upwards and downwards, and that their main trunks forked both above and below the heart, one branch going to the right and the other to the left, and that these forks provided the vessels running into the limbs above and below the heart, those above leading to the arms and the neck and the head, and those below to the legs. They also had some acquaintance with the portal system, and realized that the

---

[1] Temkin, 'Der systematische Zusammenhang im Corpus Hippocraticum', *Kyklos*, Bd. I (1928).
[2] AMG (1895), 532 ff.

liver was connected with the heart by one of the great vessels. They were also aware of vessels connecting the heart with the lungs quite separate from the great vessels. And if their conception of these vessels was far from accurate, before condemning them for their errors we must remember that they had only animals to work on, and that they had little or no technical tradition to help them since they were the first pioneers in this field. And for the pioneer unfurnished with any specialized instruments, except those evolved for the metallurgical techniques of jewellery and ornamentation, the confused connections of different kinds of tubes and strings, membranes, ligaments, tendons, and what have you, drenched with blood and excrements, must have made early dissection, and still more vivisection, most bewildering—a confused amalgam which must at first have taken a prolonged effort to sort out.

The fact remains, however, that *grosso modo* the Greeks of the fourth century B.C. had arrived at a surprisingly correct picture, both of the main organs and of the vascular system. They made some very large mistakes, and their ignorance of certain individual organs was by modern standards colossal. Of the contents of the skull, for example, it was practically complete, except for the fact that the brain was enveloped by membranes. Its connection with the spinal marrow had been assumed, according to one theory, and Alcmaeon had probably observed some and guessed others of the nervous connections between the brain and the eyes, the ears, and the tongue, and had assumed its position as the seat of consciousness. But the nervous system was to wait for its discovery for the Alexandrians; its functions being performed by the endings of the vascular system. For Aristotle its chief function is to act as a cooling gland, cooling being as we shall see a most essential function, and in this capacity it is also essential for producing sleep. But even after the Alexandrian discoveries of the nervous system, many physicians continued, in particular the pneumatic school, to uphold the candidature of the heart for the primacy of the organs and the seat of consciousness.

It may be doubted whether the inhabitants of ancient India or of contemporary China arrived at anything like as accurate a conception of the structure of the human body and of the way it works as the Greeks of the fifth and fourth centuries B.C., to say nothing of the post-Alexandrian physicians of Hellenistic times. To evaluate their failures as well as their successes, one must bear in mind the fact that before the days of Herophilus and Erasistratus, that is the third century B.C., most of their knowledge must have been derived from animals. Most, but it would, I believe, be incorrect to say 'all'. Some time before the end of the fourth century B.C., when the principal surgical works of the *Hippocratic corpus* had almost certainly been written, some very curious pathological facts about the human body had been discovered, such as the existence of tubercular cavities in the lungs, which the Greek physicians called φύματα. Thus, in the treatise *On joints*, we are told that hunchbacks, where the hump is above the diaphragm, have reduced narrow pointed chests, and their malformation makes them hold themselves in a way which causes constriction in the gullet and makes breathing difficult. Hence they are apt to have 'hard and unripened "tubercles" [φύματα] in their lungs'.[1] The production of 'tubercles' in the lungs is also referred to in the first book of the treatise *On diseases.*

A 'tubercle' [φῦμα] is formed in the lung in this manner, whenever phlegm or bile collects, and suppurates. As long as it is still rather raw, it causes slight pain and a dry cough. But when it is fully ripened, sharp pain before and behind supervenes, and feverish heat and violent coughing occur. Now if it ripens very quickly, and the contents of the abscess when it bursts are wholly spewed up, and the cavity which contained them falls in and dries out, complete health is re-established. But if it bursts quickly and ripens and is brought up, but the cavity is not able to dry out completely, the tubercle multiplies the pus spontaneously and the result is fatal.[2]

This passage and the 'Hippocratic' state of knowledge of the disease have been summarized by Pagel in his textbook *Pulmonary tuberculosis* in the following sentences:

As early as the Hippocratic writings (fifth and fourth centuries B.C.) symptomatology and pathology of phthisis were highly developed. Here we meet the attempt at explaining scientifically the arresting phenomenon of 'phthisis'. It was linked with a definite anatomical entity; a *cavity* forming in the lung by softening of a solid *focus*. This, the so-called '*phyma*', unlike an ordinary abscess, tends to slow development and progress. Drying out and collapse of the cavity (*koilia, vomica*) means spontaneous cure; continued 'catarrh', i.e. flow of mucus from the head into the lung, when it is subject to putrefaction, keeps the cavity open, maintains disease, and is attended by haemoptysis, purulent sputum, fever, phthisis, diarrhoea, and death.[3]

---

[1] Hippocrates, *De articulis*, 41 : καὶ ὅσοισιν ἂν ᾖ ἀνωτέρω τῶν φρενῶν τὸ κῦφος, τούτοισι μὲν αἵ τε πλευραὶ οὐκ ἐθέλουσι ἐς τὸ εὐρὺ αὔξεσθαι, ἀλλὰ ἐς τοὔμπροσθεν, τὸ δὲ στῆθος ὀξὺ γίνεται, ἀλλ' οὐ πλατύ, αὐτοί τε δύσπνοοι γίνονται καὶ κερχνώδεες· ἧσσον γὰρ εὐρυχωρίην ἔχουσιν αἱ κοιλίαι αἱ τὸ πνεῦμα δεχόμεναι καὶ προπέμπουσαι. καὶ γὰρ δὴ καὶ ἀναγκάζονται κατὰ τὸν μέγαν σπόνδυλον λορδὸν καὶ αὐχένα ἔχειν, ὡς μὴ προπετὴς ᾖ αὐτοῖσι ἡ κεφαλή· στενοχωρίην μὲν οὖν πολλὴν τῇ φάρυγγι παρέχει καὶ τοῦτο ἐς τὸ ἔσω ῥέπον· καὶ γὰρ τοῖσιν ὀρθοῖσι, φύσει δύσπνοιαν παρέχει τοῦτο τὸ ὀστέον, ἢν ἔσω ῥέψῃ, ἔστ' ἂν ἀναπιεχθῇ. δι' οὖν τὸ τοιοῦτον σχῆμα ἐξεχέβρογχοι οἱ τοιοῦτοι τῶν ἀνθρώπων μᾶλλον φαίνονται ἢ οἱ ὑγιέες· φυματίαι τε ὡς ἐπὶ τὸ πολὺ κατὰ τὸν πλεύμονά εἰσιν οἱ τοιοῦτοι σκληρῶν φυμάτων καὶ ἀπέπτων.

[2] Hippocrates, *De morbis*, i. 19 : φῦμα δὲ γίνεται ἐν πλεύμονι ὁκόταν φλέγμα ἢ χολὴ ξυστραφῇ, σήπεται, καὶ ἕως μὲν ἂν ἔτι ὠμότερον ἔῃ, ὀδύνην τε παρέχει λεπτὴν καὶ βῆχα ξηρήν· ὁκόταν δὲ πεπαίνηται, ὀδύνη γίνεται καὶ πρόσθεν καὶ ὄπισθεν ὀξέη, καὶ θερμαὶ λαμβάνουσι καὶ βὴξ ἰσχυρή· καὶ ἢν μὲν ὅτι τάχιστα πεπανθῇ καὶ ῥαγῇ καὶ ἄνω τράπηται τὸ πύον, καὶ ἀναπτυσθῇ πᾶν, καὶ ἡ κοιλίη ἐν ᾖ τὸ πύον ἐνί, προσπέσῃ τε καὶ ἀναξηρανθῇ, ὑγιὴς γίνεται παντελῶς· ἢν δὲ ῥαγῇ μὲν ὅτι τάχιστα καὶ πεπανθῇ καὶ ἀνακαθαίρηται, ἀποξηρανθῆναι δὲ παντάπασιν μὴ δύνηται, ἀλλ' αὐτὸ ἀφ' ἑαυτοῦ τὸ φῦμα ἀναδίδῳ τὸ πύον, ὀλέθριον τοῦτο.

[3] W. Pagel, F. A. H. Simmons, Norman Macdonald, and E. Nassau, *Pulmonary Tuberculosis*, 4th edn., p. 3.

It seems a little difficult to believe that these pathological changes in the lung could have been obtained purely from animal dissection, e.g. from a post-mortem dissection of cases of bovine tuberculosis. Another case of a pathological phenomenon contained in the *Corpus*, observed this time in both animals and man, to which Dr. Pagel drew my attention, is that of hydatid cysts in the lungs of oxen, dogs, and pigs, which seems to imply a systematic dissection, since the author of the treatise *On internal affections* speaks of dissecting these φύματα and evacuating their liquid which he specifies as water. He also expresses the opinion that these cysts occur even more frequently in men than in the beasts of the field, on account of man's unhealthy diet.[1] Whether the opinion here expressed is a mere piece of guesswork or founded on human autopsy is not stated, but it seems to me to be rather difficult to suppose that it is founded upon mere conjecture. The author evidently regards these cysts as a special form of 'tubercle'.

There are also two special passages to which Edelstein has drawn attention. Both of these come from the treatise *On joints*.[2] These and several more loci could be adduced which suggest knowledge which could only have been gained from actual dissection of human corpses. That such a practice was general cannot, however, be assumed. The view most generally accepted is that human dissection was not practised in Hippocrates' lifetime, or in the two generations after his death. But

[1] Hippocrates, *De affect. intern.* 24: γίνεται δὲ (ὕδερος) καὶ ἢν φύματα ἐν τῷ πλεύμονι ἐμφυῇ καὶ πλησθῇ ὕδατος καὶ ῥαγῇ ἐς τὰ στήθεα. ὡς δὲ γίνεται ἀπὸ φυμάτων ὕδερος, τόδε μοι μαρτύριον καὶ ἐν βοΐ καὶ ἐν κυνὶ καὶ ἐν ὑΐ· μάλιστα γὰρ τῶν τετραπόδων ἐν τούτοισι γίνεται φύματα ἐν τῷ πλεύμονι ἅπερ ἔχει ὕδωρ. διαταμὼν δ᾽ ἂν γνοίης τάχιστα τοιαῦτα· ῥεύσεται γὰρ τὸ ὕδωρ. δοκεῖ δὲ καὶ ἐν τῷ ἀνθρώπῳ ἐγγίνεσθαι τοιαῦτα πολὺ μᾶλλον ἢ ἐν προβάτοισιν, ὁκόσῳ καὶ τῇ διαιτῇ ἐπινούσῳ χρεόμεθα μᾶλλον.

[2] Edelstein, *Die Geschichte der Sektion in der Antike* (Berlin, 1932). The first of these reads as follows (Loeb, trs. Withington) and is taken from the first chapter. The writer is dealing with a dislocation of the shoulder-joint and remarks: 'Suppose one laid bare the point of the shoulder and the fleshy parts of the arm, and also denuded it at the part where the muscle is attached, and laid bare the tendon stretching along the armpit and collar-bone to the chest, the head of the humerus would be seen to have a strongly marked projection forwards though not dislocated. For the head of the humerus is naturally inclined forwards, while the rest of the bone is curved outwards.'

εἴ τις τοῦ βραχίονος ψιλώσειε μὲν τῶν σαρκῶν τὴν ἐπωμίδα, ψιλώσειε δὲ ᾗ ὁ μῦς ἀνατείνει, ψιλώσειε δὲ τὸν τένοντα τὸν κατὰ τὴν μασχάλην τε καὶ τὴν κληῖδα πρὸς τὸ στῆθος ἔχοντα, φαίνοιτο ἂν ἡ κεφαλὴ τοῦ βραχίονος ἐς τοὔμπροσθεν ἐξέχουσα ἰσχυρῶς, καίπερ οὐκ ἐκπεπτωκυῖα· πέφυκε γὰρ ἐς τοὔμπροσθεν προπετὴς ἡ κεφαλὴ τοῦ βραχίονος· τὸ δ᾽ ἄλλο ὀστέον τοῦ βραχίονος ἐς τὰ ἔξω καμπύλον.

The second passage is taken from Chapter 46 and deals with the dislocation of the spine, as the result of some heavy weight falling upon it. 'So, then the impossibility of reducing such a dislocation either by succussion or by any other method is obvious, unless after cutting open the patient, one inserted the hand into the body cavity and made pressure from within outwards. One might do this with a corpse, but hardly with a living patient.'

ὥστε δὴ οὐδ᾽ ἐμβαλεῖν οἷόν τε πρόδηλον τὸν τοιοῦτον οὔτε κατασείσει οὔτε ἄλλῳ τρόπῳ οὐδενί, εἰ μή τις διαταμὼν τὸν ἄνθρωπον, ἔπειτα ἐσμασάμενος ἐς τὴν κοιλίην, ἐκ τοῦ ἔσωθεν τῇ χειρὶ ἐς τὸ ἔξω ἀντωθέοι· καὶ τοῦτο νεκρῷ μὲν οἷόν τε ποιεῖν, ζῶντι δ᾽ οὐ πάνυ.

argument from isolated statements of this kind is far from satisfactory, so far so, indeed, that the more eminent historians of ancient Greek medicine have failed to agree. Thus in the history of medicine edited by Neuburger and Pagel, von Töply, the author of the section on anatomy in the second volume, comes very decidedly to the conclusion that the anatomic knowledge of this period was not based on the dissection of human corpses, a judgement which he bases on purely anatomical grounds.[1] Julius Pagel on the other hand, in his *Introduction to the history of medicine*, stated that it may be assumed as a certainty that the corpses of criminals, and bodies found deserted on the wayside were in fact dissected.[2] Fuchs in the first volume of Neuburger and Pagel's compilation, in a chapter called *The state of medical knowledge in the Hippocratic writings*, seemed inclined to agree rather with Pagel than with von Töply. He came to the conclusion that the descriptions of the vertebrae, the diaphragm, the sinews, ligaments, etc., and the nerves show that these could not have been derived from monkeys but must have been obtained from human bodies.[3] Neuburger himself, while agreeing that no systematic human dissection was permitted, came to the conclusion that eminent physicians availed themselves, where and when they could, of the opportunity of dissecting human bodies in the case of barbarians and traitors, which he assumes were exempt

[1] Ritter von Töply, in Puschmann's *Handbuch der Geschichte der Medizin*, ed. M. Neuburger and J. Pagel, ii. 175 (Jena, 1902): 'Die Frage, ob die Griechen Anatomie von Menschenleichen geübt haben, ist vielfach — zu vielfach von Anatomen mit philologischen, von Philologen mit anatomischen Bewerenmitteln — erörtert worden. Eine genauere Durchsicht der Stellen, welche als Stütze für eine solche Annahme hervorgezogen worden sind, insbesonders aber auch das Eingehen auf die thatsächlichen anatomischen Errungenschaften des Corpus, führen zu der Überzeugung, daß die Anatomie des Corpus Hippocrat. auf gelegentlichen Beobachtungen, wie solche am Krankenbette ergeben, auf Zergliederung von Tieren, zum Teil auf reinen Hypothesen beruht, keineswegs aber auf Zergliederung von Menschenleichen.'

[2] Julius Pagel, *Einführung in die Geschichte der Medizin* (Berlin, 1898), p. 77: 'Es ist vor allem als sicher anzunehmen, daß die Leichen von Verbrechern und auf der Straße gefundenen Todten, zur Sektion kamen. Die Griechen haben auch zootomische Übungen vorgenommen.'

[3] R. Fuchs, 'Die Heilkunde in den hippokratischen Schriften', in Puschmann's *Handbuch der Geschichte der Medizin* i. 236 f.: 'Die anatomischen Kenntnisse gewannen die Asklepiaden auf mannigfache Weise: durch mündliche und schriftliche Überlieferungen, durch Zuschauen bei Opfern und Hausschlachtung, durch den Verkehr in der Palästra, durch Verletzungen im Felde und im Frieden, durch Betrachtung der angeschwemmten und unbeerdigten Leichen und Leichenresten, und durch Thieranatomie . . . Und wie steht es mit der Anatomie der Menschenleichen? Die hypothetische Form, in der *de art. rep. I* vom Präpariren des Humerus gesprochen wird, beruht zweifellos auf exakter Kenntnis, und die genaue Beschreibung der Wirbel (der "Zahnwirbel"), der Wirbelsäule, des Zwerchfells und der Bänder, Sehnen- und Nervenstränge setzt unbedingt voraus, daß der Verfasser dieses Alles nicht am Affen, wie später Galenus, sondern am Menschen selbst beobachtet hat. Mag auch die Lage der inneren Eingeweide mangelhaft beschrieben sein, (Aristot. *de part. an.* 1, 16) um so klarer ist die Kenntnis der Osteologie und Histologie, namentlich der Extremitäten. Es ist freilich richtig, daß die Vorschrift der sofortigen Beerdigung Gefallener, und der Abscheu vor dem Todten, Religion und Aberglaube eine *planmäßig* ausgeführte Sektion von Leichen hemmte, doch konnten alle diese Hindernisse weder gelegentlich Einblicke in geöffnete Körperhöhlen, noch partielle Untersuchungen rein anatomischer Art völlig ausschließen.'

from the religious sanctions attached to corpses.[1] Littré, as Temkin
has noted, decided that the physicians of the Hippocratic age must have
dissected human bodies,[2] though Sprengel denied this. But the important point Temkin makes is that like Sigerist he maintains that an
exact knowledge gained from dissection was not the foundation of
Hippocratic medicine,[3] and it would be most misleading to interpret
statements like the famous sentence that 'The nature of the body is the
beginning or principle of reasoning in medicine' as implying anything at
all like the modern concept of anatomy as the foundation of medical
knowledge.[4]

In the generations immediately following the death of the historical
Hippocrates there were two physicians about whom we have a fair
degree of knowledge although none of their writing has survived, who
refused to accept the theory of Alcmaeon and the author of the *Sacred
disease*, and continued to maintain the primacy of the heart, namely
the 'Second Hippocrates', Diocles of Carystos, and Praxagoras of Cos.
The dates of both these are far from certain, and that of Diocles, as we
have already noted, has been the subject of some controversy. Wellmann[5]
connected him closely with Philistion and the Sicilian school and placed
his *floruit* about 380 B.C. Jaeger,[6] on the other hand, insisted that he
was a pupil of Aristotle who lived between 320 and 260 B.C., a date which
Kudlien[7] regards as much too late. He looks upon him as a contemporary
of Plato rather than of Aristotle, and would place his *floruit* about 360 B.C.
Praxagoras was by tradition a somewhat younger contemporary of Diocles,
and was reported to be the teacher of Herophilus. There were at least

---

[1] M. Neuburger, *Geschichte der Medizin* (Stuttgart, 1906) i, 221. 'Von einer planmäßigen
Sektion menschlicher Leichen konnte bei den strengen religiösen Vorschriften, welche sofort
Beerdigung geboten, bei dem abergläubischen Abscheu vor dem toten keine Rede sein. Wie
wohl nicht einwandsfrei bewiesen, so doch nicht ganz abzuweisen ist dagegen die Annahme,
daß einzelne hervorragende Forscher, wenn sich die seltene Gelegenheit darbot, auch vor
der Untersuchung menschlicher Körper, oder wenigstens Körperteile (namentlich Knochen)
nicht zurückschreckten, und dieselbe zur Korrektur der herrschenden Anschauungen ver-
wendet. Die Wahrscheinlichkeit dieser Annahme ergibt sich, abgesehen von manchen
Erzählungen der antiken Autoren, insbesondere aus der der Überlieferung, daß die Leichen
von Barbaren, Vaterlandsverrätern, Verbrechern, dem Bannkreis der religiösen Satzungen
entzogen waren, und daher ebenso wie die zufällig angeschwämmten Leichenteile, die
Neugier wissenschaftlicher Forscher reizen könnten.'

[2] Littré, iii. 542 f.   [3] Sigerist, *Antike Heilkunde*, p. 40.

[4] Temkin, op. cit.: 'Wie Sigerist vorgehoben hat . . . bildet die Anatomie im heutigen
Sinne einer exakten Zergliederung nicht die Grundlage der griechischen Medizin, zumindest
soweit es ihren hippokratischen Abschnitt betrifft. Es sind sehr viele Stellen im Corpus so
gedeutet worden, als ob ein anatomisches Studium analog dem modernen gefördert würde.'

[5] Wellmann, *Fragmente*.

[6] Werner Jaeger, *Diokles von Karystos* (Berlin, 1938), pp. 55–9, paragraph entitled 'Diokles,
Schüler des späten Aristoteles'.

[7] F. Kudlien, 'Probleme von Diokles von Karystos', *Arch. f. Gesch. d. Med.* xlvii (1963),
456 ff. See also the article by F. Heinemann, 'Diokles von Karystos und der prophylaktische
Brief an König Antigonus', *Mus. Hel.* 12 (1955).

three physicians of Cos known by that name, one of whom was by tradition a pupil of Hippocrates; the 'great' Praxagoras was almost certainly
his grandson. Steckerl,[1] who follows Jaeger's dating for Diocles, places
his *floruit* about 300 B.C., but this would appear to be rather too late.
Of Diocles' doctrines Wellmann has given an extensive account based
largely on a fragment of a manuscript of Theodor Priscianus in Brussels,
which is an obvious insertion. Wellmann believed that the author of
this doxographical fragment was Priscianus' master, Vindicianus the
comes archiatrorum at the end of the fourth century A.D., a contemporary of
Saint Augustine, and that the physician whose doctrine is described in it
at some length is Diocles. This ascription has been accepted generally, by
Rusche, for example, and the opinions expressed in it agree remarkably
well with those attributed to Diocles by the Anonymous Parisian.[2]

If we can believe the tradition reported by Wellmann, Diocles is
reported to have assigned the 'leading part', 'like Empedocles and Aristotle and the sect of the Stoics' to the heart.[3] This may be correct enough
as implying the cardio-centric view, though the word ἡγεμονικόν is bound
to sound a little suspect as a Stoic interpolation. He was also, it would
appear, acquainted with the fact that the heart had two chambers, and
regarded the left ventricle as the seat of the innate heat and the innate
pneuma, though he does not seem to have used that expression himself but
is reported as using the expression 'psychic *pneuma*'. According to Wellmann, his doctrine was largely derived from Empedocles, but whereas
Empedocles regarded the blood round the heart as the vehicle of the
intelligence, Diocles substituted for the blood the psychic *pneuma*,[4] an
expression of which we shall hear much more, going forth from the heart,
a doctrine closely related also to that of Diogenes of Apollonia, for whom
the soul, as we have already noted, was air.[5] This doctrine of *pneuma* was
probably first put forward by Philistion.[6] Diocles, unlike Praxagoras,

---

[1] F. Steckerl, *The Fragments of Praxagoras of Cos and his School* (Leiden, 1958), p. 2.

[2] Wellmann, *Fragmente*, pp. 3–14.

[3] That is, assuming the correctness of his emendation of the passage from Theodoret,
22. 6, which would substitute 'Aristotle and Diocles' for an otherwise unknown Aristocles
in the list of those who regard the heart as the seat of the governing principle. The statement as
emended reads as follows: Ἐμπεδοκλῆς δὲ καὶ Ἀριστο(τέλης, Διο)κλῆς καὶ τῶν Στωικῶν ἡ
ξυμμορία τὴν καρδίαν ἀπεκλήρωσαν τούτῳ (τῷ ἡγεμονικῷ).
See Wellmann, *Fragmente*, p. 14.

[4] Ibid., p. 15: 'Der Unterschied zwischen seiner Lehre und der von Empedokles besteht
darin, daß er auf das Pneuma übertrug, was jener vom Blut aussagte: nicht das Blut, so
lautet sein Dogma, sondern das vom Herz ausgehende πνεῦμα ψυχικόν ist der Träger der
Vernunft.' Cf. AMG (1894), fr. 5, quoted below, p. 105, n. 2. Wellmann on the suggestion
of Diels also emended, as we have noted, another passage substituting Diocles for Diogenes
in Aetius/Plutarch: Διοκλῆς ἐν τῇ ἀρτηριακῇ κοιλίᾳ τῆς καρδίας, ἥτις ἐστὶ πνευματικὴ (εἶναί
φησι τὸ ἡγεμονικὸν τὸ τῆς ψυχῆς).

[5] See above, pp. 20 ff.

[6] See above, pp. 19 f., 38.

held that the arteries as well as the veins (he does not seem to have been acquainted with the distinction) contained both blood and *pneuma*— a theory which is also found, as we have seen, in several treatises of the *Hippocratic corpus*.[1] He also regarded the heart as the source or fountain of blood. But he agrees that headaches may be dangerous, not because the brain is the seat of the intelligence, but because headaches are due to obstructions in the hollow veins of the head which may in turn affect the heart from which the psychic *pneuma* issues.[2] The Cnidian–Sicilian theory is quite different from that contained in the Coan treatises, with its doctrine of the primacy of the brain and the direct inhalation of *pneuma* or air from the nose into the brain. But it would appear that Diocles may have made some concession to the Alcmaeonic theory of the primacy of that organ, if we can still regard, as Wellmann did, the Brussels fragment of Vindicianus as really reproducing Diocles' teaching. Here we find a rather peculiar doctrine which does assign to the brain a function which is connected with the mediation both of perception and of intelligence. Dealing with the *phrenetica passio* disease, which is accompanied by delirium, he says that this is due to a tumour in the heart, which cuts off the blood-supply and normal heat, by which the brain provides perception and intelligence. There are two sides to the brain: the right half provides sensation and the left half intelligence. And beneath the brain is the heart, with its two ears or auricles, for it is always on the watch hearing and understanding.[3] This doctrine, if indeed it be Diocles', represents an interesting compromise, an attempt to maintain the primacy of the heart while acknowledging the physiological importance of the brain. The brain supplies the contents both of sensation and of intelligence, but it is the heart at the centre which hears and understands. But the doctrine of the heart's auricles we find here is expressly repudiated in the *De corde*. It must also be noted that this

[1] See above, pp. 40 f., 43 f.

[2] AMG (1894), fr. 5: Διοκλῆς τὴν κεφαλαίαν φησὶ γίνεσθαι περὶ τὰς κοίλας καὶ βυθίους φλέβας τῆς κεφαλῆς ἐμφράξεως γενόμενης. γίνεσθαι δὲ αὐτὴν ἐπικίνδυνον ἐὰν τὸν ἡγέμονα τοῦ σώματος συνδιαθῇ, τῇ καρδίᾳ ἀφ' ἧς τὸ ψυχικὸν πνεῦμα τοῦ σώματος ὥρμηται κατ' αὐτήν.

[3] See Para. 44 of the *Brussels fragment* which reads as follows: 'Freneticam passionem, inquit, fieri tumore in corde effecto, et suffocato sanguine seu calore consuetudinario, ex quo cerebrum sensum et intellectum praebet. Aliud est enim quo intelligitur, aliud quo sentitur. Sic itaque duo cerebra sunt in capite constituta, unum quod intellectum dat, aliud quod sensum praebet idque quod in dextra parte jacet, ab eo sentitur, a sinistro vero intelligitur: ob hoc sub ea parte subjacente corde et semper vigilante audiente et intelligente, quia et aures habet ad audiendum, quod est pericardia habet ventres, id est receptacula sanguinis et spiritus singulis in partibus secundum aures, nunc ex venis promere sanguinem, nunc ex arteria spiritum, ut graece dicimus ἀρτηρία μικρὸν μὲν (τὸ) αἷμα, πολὺ δὲ τὸ πνεῦμα, αἱ δὲ φλέβες πολὺ ἔχουσι (τὸ) αἷμα, μικρὸν δὲ τὸ πνεῦμα. Id est, arteria multum habet spiritum et modicum sanguinem, venae autem multum habent sanguinem et modicum spiritum' (Wellmann, *Fragmente*, p. 234).

The theory of the auricles as hearing is, as we have noted, denied both in the *De corde* and in the *De morbo sacro*.

doctrine of the origin of phrenitis does not agree with that attributed to Diocles by the Anonymous Parisian, who in fragment 1 tells us that Diocles regarded phrenitis as an inflammation of the diaphragm.[1] But the compromise doctrine which we have just examined, be it Diocles' or no, is almost certainly the invention of some fourth-century physician before the foundation of the Alexandrian medical school.

For Diocles, as for Philistion, the purpose of respiration is, as Galen informs us,[2] a 'sort of cooling' of the innate heat. Both of them adopted the idea, first mooted by Empedocles, of respiration through the 'pores', which they combined with that of respiration through the nose, mouth, throat, and lungs. The reciprocal action of the different currents of air derived from these two sources is also described by Plato, who no doubt obtained the idea from Philistion. When the air drawn into the lungs in breathing in is expelled in breathing out, the air from the outside that has been brought in through the 'pores' is expelled; when the air drawn into the lungs is expelled by breathing out, the air from the outside is drawn in through the 'pores'.[3] Diocles was therefore acquainted with vessels connecting the heart and the lungs. As a consequence of this double form of respiration, so another passage from Vindicianus informs us, both arteries and veins contain both blood and *pneuma*. But the 'thick' artery has much *pneuma* and comparatively little blood, while the 'thick' vein has much blood and comparatively little *pneuma*.[4] This passage would suggest that Diocles, even if he was not acquainted with the difference between arteries and veins as such, had already distinguished the vena cava from the aorta. We do know that he had inherited this doctrine from his father Archidamus, who was also a physician.[5]

By the middle of the fourth century B.C., the importance of the *pneuma* was recognized equally by those who assigned the primacy to the brain and those who assigned it to the heart. But they conceived its function in a rather different manner. Thus the author of *On the sacred disease* makes the brain the first centre of distribution, not the heart. For the head not the heart is the starting-point of the blood vessels which are the instruments of respiration. The nature of the *pneuma* is also conceived differently.

[1] AMG (1894), fr. 1: ὁ δὲ Διοκλῆς φλεγμονὴν τοῦ διαφράγματός φησιν εἶναι τὴν φρενῖτιν, ἀπὸ τόπου καὶ οὐκ ἀπὸ ἐνεργείας τὸ πάθος καλῶν, συνδιατιθεμένης καὶ τῆς καρδίας. ἔοικε γὰρ καὶ οὗτος τὴν φρόνησιν περὶ ταύτην ἀπολείπειν.

[2] Galen, *De usu resp.* 1, K. iv. 471, quoted below, p. 112, n. 2.

[3] Plato, *Timaeus*, 79 b and c. See below, pp. 119 f.

[4] See the passage from Vindicianus, Wellmann, *Fragmente*, p. 228, fragm. cap. 32: 'Hunc [sc. aerem] adducit [sc. anima] non solum per nares, verum etiam per totum corpus officio commutato. Quando enim per nares inferius adducitur, per fauces ad pulmonem fertur, exinde pars cordi, pars thoraci transmittitur. Tunc impletis locis inductus aer per vias totius corporis insensuales totus egeritur. Quando autem ex pulmone atque corde et ventre redditur, rursum per fauces reciprocus fertur ad narium atque oris vias: tunc via servata rursum per totam corporis superficiem inducitur per eiusmodi qui per supradictas vias exierit.'

[5] Jaeger, op. cit., p. 215.

For the author of *On the sacred disease* it seems to be just air; for the Sicilian school and their cardio-centric colleagues in western Greece, it has become something rather different, a product of air and blood with its own peculiar character, a very special form of 'steam' or 'vapour'. We may therefore, I think, agree with Rüsche[1] in seeing in Diocles one of the founders of the theory of the vital spirit as the ἀναθυμίασις of the blood which was to play such an important part in the pneumatic theory of the Stoics, and received its final development in the theories of the pneumatic school, and finally in the physiology of Galen. The relation between the innate heat and the *pneuma* breathed in, or taken in with the food and developed inside the body, is not always easy to grasp, since it has to be inferred from the disconnected passages concerning the aetiology of various diseases affecting the consciousness contained in the fragments of the Anonymous Parisian of Fuchs. The cause of these diseases was referred by Diocles to some kind of obstruction to the *pneuma* caused either by phlegm which congealed the blood by cooling it,[2] or by over-heating which also caused a thickening of the blood,[3] or by boiling which was responsible for the causation of 'mania', a form of over-heating which did not result in any thickening of the blood.[4] From these fragments, Rüsche has deduced that according to Diocles the vaporization (*Verdünstung* or *Blutverdampfung*) could take two forms, a normal one which he calls the finer ἀναθυμίασις, and an abnormal excessive form of 'boiling' which caused madness. He points out that the idea of ἀναθυμίασις may very well have been derived from Heracleitus, who, according to a fragment from Aetius, taught that the world-soul was a vaporization of the wet things in the cosmos, while the soul of animals was a similar vaporization of the wet things in the environment and in their bodies.[5] Diocles is not reported to have used the word ἀναθυμίασις in this connection, though Vindicianus does report him as using it in connection with the disease jaundice.[6] The notion of vapour being given off by blood is also

---

[1] Rüsche, op. cit., pp. 151–64.

[2] e.g., lethargy, as in AMG (1894), fr. 2: Διοκλῆς δὲ τοῦ περὶ τὴν καρδίαν καὶ τὸν ἐγκέφαλον ψυχικοῦ πνεύματος κατάψυξιν ἡγεῖται εἶναι καὶ τοῦ ταύτῃ συνοίκου αἵματος πῆξιν.

[3] e.g., a particular kind of melancholy called *windy*. See Galen, *De locis affectis*, iii. 10, K. viii. 186 f.: τοὺς δὲ φυσώδεις καλουμένους ὑπολαμβάνειν δεῖ πλεῖον ἔχειν τὸ θερμὸν τοῦ προσήκοντος ἐν ταῖς φλεψὶ ταῖς ἐκ τῆς γαστρὸς τὴν τροφὴν δεχομέναις, καὶ τὸ αἷμα πεπαχύνθαι τούτων. δηλοῖ γὰρ ὅτι μέν ἐστιν ἔμφραξις περὶ ταύτας τὰς φλέβας, τὸ μὴ καταδέχεσθαι τὸ σῶμα τὴν τροφήν, ἀλλ' ἐν τῇ γαστρὶ διαμένειν ἀκατέργαστον.

[4] AMG (1894), fr. 17: ὁ δὲ Διοκλῆς ζέσιν τοῦ ἐν τῇ καρδίᾳ αἵματός φησιν εἶναι χωρὶς ἐμφράξεως γινομένην, διὰ τοῦτο γὰρ μηδὲ πυρετοὺς ἔπεσθαι· ὅτι δὲ ἡ ζέσις γίνεται τοῦ αἵματος δηλοῖ ἡ συνήθεια, τοὺς γὰρ μανιώδεις τεθερμάνθαι φαμέν.

[5] Aetius iv. 3: Ἡράκλειτος τὴν μὲν τοῦ κόσμου ψυχὴν ἀναθυμίασιν ἐκ τῶν ἐν αὐτῷ ὑγρῶν (ἔλεγεν) τὴν δὲ ἐν τοῖς ζῴοις ἀπὸ τῆς ἐκτὸς καὶ τῆς ἐν αὐτοῖς ἀναθυμιάσεως ὁμογενῆ (D–K, vol. i, 147).

[6] Vindicianus, cap. 37 of the fragment in Wellmann, *Fragmente*, p. 232: 'Ictericum inquit fieri, qui apud nos auriginosus seu arquatus vocatur, nam vulgo morbum regium vocant, (fit) obtruso meatu qui ad ventrem ducit ex eo, qui ad fellis folliculum tendit. Suspicatur

to be found in the 'Hippocratic' treatise *On breaths*, but here there is no notion corresponding to the psychic *pneuma* attached to it. The vapour formed by the blood in fevers is the cause of perspiration. To Diocles too may be attributed, even if he was not its inventor, the distinction between two grades of *pneuma* in the body, the natural and the psychic. The former, which is also associated with the natural heat, is responsible for the vegetative functions such as digestion and growth, the latter for the animal functions such as voluntary or appetitive movement and thought.[1]

The theory of the primacy of the heart and its function as the seat of the intelligence had a prominent representative in Diocles' younger contemporary Praxagoras of Cos,[2] the son of Nicarchos and the master of Herophilus of Calchedon, who is usually regarded as the founder of the school of Alexandria, which came into being during the reign of the first Ptolemy who ruled Alexandria from 323 to 285 B.C.

None of Praxagoras' works has survived. We must depend therefore on quotations and doxography for our knowledge of his teaching. He is very important for our purposes because of two doctrines attributed to him, namely the distinction of arteries and veins as separate systems, and the theory that arteries contained no blood, only *pneuma*.[3] The first of these has indeed been attributed to Euryphon of Cnidos[4] and is also contained, as we have noted, in implicit form in one of the fairly early treatises of the *Hippocratic corpus*, the essay *On fleshes*, which recognizes two main blood vessels emerging from the heart, the one called the artery, and the other the hollow vein.[5] The date of this work is by no means certain, but Wellmann considers that Diocles must have known it, and Deichgräber, who produced the most recent edition, considered it to be a work belonging to the period of the sophists,[6] which would seem to place it before Aristotle. Aristotle himself does not know the term *artery* as applied to a blood vessel, but he does use the term *aorta* for the vessel

enim, si quid in sanguine fuerit acrius factum, hoc per spirationem tenuem, quam graece ἀναθυμίασιν vocamus, ad jecoris ferri vesicam, quam fel appellamus, etc.'

[1] Rüsche, op. cit., pp. 163 f. See also the quotation from Galen's *Isagoge* below, p. 217, n. 1.

[2] Kurt Bardong, following Jaeger's date for Diocles, places his *floruit* about 300 B.C., a dating in which he is supported by Steckerl in his *Praxagoras*. But Kudlien would appear to place him a little earlier.

[3] See Galen, *De dignoscendis pulsibus*, iv. 2, K. viii. 941 : τὸ μέν γε τοῦ Πραξαγόρου καὶ θαυμαστὸν ἴσως σοι φανεῖται· μηδὲ γὰρ περιέχεσθαι λέγων ἐν ἀρτηρίαις τοὺς χυμοὺς ὅμως ἐκ τῶν σφυγμῶν ἰδέας τινὰς αὐτῶν ἀναλογίζεσθαι πειρᾶται.

This theory of bloodless arteries was also held by his father Nicarchus, as Galen tells us (*De plenitudine*, 11, K. vii. 573).

[4] Caelius Aurelianus, *De morbis chronicis*, ii. 10: 'Differentias etiam fluoris sanguinis veteres quaesierunt. Et quidam aiunt unam solam esse vel intelligi, hoc est, vulnerationis, ut Themison libro tardarum passionum. Alii vero eruptiones, ut Hippocrates, Euryphon. Sed Hippocrates solarum venarum, Euryphon vero etiam arteriarum.'

[5] See the passage quoted above, p. 36, n. 3.

[6] Deichgräber, op. cit., p. 4: 'Der Verfasser von περὶ σαρκῶν gehört dem Zeitalter der Sophistiker.'

we still call by that name; and aorta, Rufus of Ephesus informs us, was another word for the 'artery' or windpipe. It is generally assumed that the clear recognition of two distinct systems of blood vessels was due to Praxagoras, and he is also credited with the use, if not the invention, of the term *thick artery* as a vessel corresponding to the ancient term *thick vein*.[1] The anatomical difference between the two types of blood vessel was first fully described by his pupil Herophilus, in a fashion which eliminated finally all confusion between them. The second of these doctrines, that of the air-filled arteries, was really one of the tragical mistakes in the history of Greek medicine, a mistake which more almost than any other prevented the discovery of the circulation. Praxagoras was also credited, on what Galen regarded as insufficient evidence, with the discovery of the pulse. He seems to have mixed this up with certain phenomena of a nervous rather than a cardiac origin, attributing to arterial action not only παλμός a word usually translated *palpitation*, but also 'trembling' τρόμος, and 'spasm' σπασμός.[2] What Praxagoras actually meant by these words is far from clear. He is reported to have regarded them as an affection (πάθος) of the arteries—no mention of the heart.[3] Indeed, it looks as if we are dealing with a condition which has no cardiac implications and may very well have been attributed to arteries because the blood vessels had been regarded as performing the functions of the not-yet isolated nervous system. In the matter of the presidency of the organs, Praxagoras followed the teaching of the Cnidian rather than that of the Coan school, assigning it to the heart rather than to the head, with the result that he was forced to postulate rather fantastic notions about maladies which gave rise to mental symptoms. Delirium (φρενῖτις) was attributed by him to inflammation of the heart,[4] and 'apoplexy', which included what we now call a stroke, was also looked upon by him as of cardiac origin. It was

---

[1] AMG (1894), fr. 3: ἐπιληψίας αἰτία. Πραξαγόρας περὶ τὴν παχεῖαν ἀρτηρίαν φησὶ γίνεσθαι κτλ. Also ibid., fr. 4: ἀποπληξίας αἰτία. Πραξαγόρας καὶ Διοκλῆς περὶ τὴν παχεῖαν ἀρτηρίαν γίνεσθαι κτλ.

[2] See Galen, *De tremore, palpitatione, convulsione, et rigore*, i, K. vii. 584: Ἐπειδὴ Πραξαγόρας ὁ Νικάρχου τά τε ἄλλα τῆς ἰατρικῆς ἐν τοῖς ἀρίστοις γενόμενος ... οὐκ ὀρθῶς μοι δοκεῖ περί τε σφυγμοῦ καὶ παλμοῦ καὶ σπασμοῦ καὶ τρόμου γιγνώσκειν, ἀρτηριῶν μὲν ἅπαντα νομίζων εἶναι πάθη, διαφέρειν δὲ ἀλλήλων μεγέθει. See also K. vii. 598: Πραξαγόρας δὲ καὶ ταῖς ἀρτηρίαις ἀνατίθησι σφυγμόν. ὥσπερ ἀμέλει καὶ παλμὸν καὶ τρόμον καὶ σπασμὸν ἀρτηριῶν πάθη· καὶ σφυγμὸν μὲν ἐν τῷ κατὰ φύσιν ἔχειν· παλμὸν δὲ καὶ τρόμον καὶ σπασμὸν ἀλλήλων μὲν διαφέρειν μεγέθει, κινήσεις δὲ εἶναι παρὰ φύσιν.

[3] Galen, *De differentiis pulsuum*, iv. 3, K. viii. 723: Πραξαγόραν οὐκ ὀρθῶς ἀποφηνάμενον ἀρτηριῶν πάθος εἶναι καὶ παλμὸν καὶ τρόμον καὶ σπασμόν, οὐ γένει διαφέροντα τῆς σφυγμώδους ἐν αὐτοῖς κινήσεως, ἀλλὰ μεγέθει. Cf. *De plac. Hipp. et Plat.* vi. 6, K. v. 561: οὐκ οἶδ' ὅπως αὐτῶν ἐν τῷδε Πραξαγόρας τε καὶ Φιλότιμος ὁμολογήσαντες τἄλλα, καὶ νομίζουσι τὸ πάμπαν ἐξ ἑαυτῶν σφύζειν τὰς ἀρτηρίας.

[4] AMG (1894), fr. 1: φρενίτιδος αἰτία ... Πραξαγόρας δὲ φλεγμονὴν τῆς καρδίας εἶναί φησι τὴν φρενῖτιν, ἧς καὶ τὸ κατὰ φύσιν ἔργον φρόνησιν οἴεται εἶναι. ὑπὸ δὲ τῆς φλεγμονῆς ταρασσομένην τὴν καρδίαν τοῦδε τοῦ πάθους συστατικὴν γίνεσθαι.

caused by cold and thick phlegm obstructing the aorta (παχείη ἀρτερίη), so that not even the smallest amount of *pneuma* was able to pass through it.[1] So, too, paralysis was caused by cold and thick phlegm getting into the vessels growing out of the heart and the 'thick' artery, through which voluntary motion is transmitted to the body.[2] What is more, Praxagoras is taken to task by Galen for stating that he found the origin of the nerves in the heart—a doctrine which is also to be found in the Aristotelian writings. Here Galen definitely accuses Praxagoras of dishonesty:

For this man since he never saw any nerve growing out of the heart, and being envious of the reputation of Hippocrates, wanted at all cost to deprive the brain of its rule over the nerves, and had the impudence to tell a big lie, saying that the arteries, as they got further [from the heart] were divided into smaller and smaller branches, became narrower, and grew into nerves. For though their body was indeed nerve-like, it was still hollow, and as it became more divided in the animal, the lumen became so small that its coats collapsed upon each other, with the result that from the first place where this had happened, from thereon, the vessel had clearly become a nerve.[3]

Apart from Galen's characteristic attempt to show up in the worst light physicians with whose doctrines he disagreed, the passage is of some interest, since it shows how confused the notions of the nervous system were in the generations immediately after Hippocrates. Without attributing dishonesty to Praxagoras, we are still bound to admit that he made a bad blunder in supposing that the heart was the centre of the nervous system. As to the nerves in the heart, we can hardly credit him with the discovery of the atrio-ventricular bundle, or even that of the cardiac plexus, which might have lent some appearance of plausibility to his aetiology of mania, which was caused, he thought, by a swelling of 'the seat of wisdom', the heart, adding a rider to the effect that it was a disease that did not have fever as one of its consequences, because outward swellings do not give rise to fevers.[4] This rider was, apparently, in agreement with the teachings of the 'Hippocratic' school. For we are informed

---

[1] AMG (1894), fr. 4: Πραξαγόρας καὶ Διοκλῆς περὶ τὴν παχεῖαν ἀρτηρίαν γίνεσθαί φασι τὸ πάθος ὑπὸ φλέγματος ψυχροῦ καὶ παχέος ὡς μήδ' ἐν αὐτῇ οὐχ ὁτιοῦν πνεῦμα παραπνεῖσθαι.

[2] Ibid., fr. 20: Πραξαγόρας δὲ καὶ Διοκλῆς ὑπὸ παχέος καὶ ψυχροῦ φλέγματος περὶ τὰς ἀποφύσεις τὰς ἀπὸ καρδίας καὶ τῆς παχείας ἀρτηρίας γινόμενον, δι' ὧνπερ ἡ κατὰ προαίρεσιν κίνησις ἐπιπέμπεται τῷ σώματι.

[3] Galen, De plac. Hipp. et Plat. i. 6, K. v. 188: οὗτος γὰρ ὁ ἀνὴρ ἐπειδὴ μηδὲν ἑώρα νεῦρον ἐκφυόμενον τῆς καρδίας, ἐφιλοτιμεῖτο δὲ πρὸς Ἱπποκράτην καὶ πάντως ἐβούλετο τὸν ἐγκέφαλον ἀφελέσθαι τῆς τῶν νεύρων ἀρχῆς, οὐ σμικρὸν ἀπετόλμησε ψεύσασθαι τὰς ἀρτηρίας φάμενος ἐν τῷ προιέναι καὶ κατασχίζεσθαι στενὰς γενομένας εἰς νεῦρα μεταβάλλειν. τοῦ γὰρ σώματος αὐτῶν ὑπάρχοντος νευρώδους μὲν ἀλλὰ κοίλου καὶ κατὰ τὴν ἐπὶ πλέον ἐν τῷ ζῴῳ σχίσιν οὕτω γινομένων μικρῶν τῶν κοιλοτήτων, ὡς ἐπιπίπτειν ἀλλήλοις τοὺς χιτῶνας, ὁπόταν τοῦτο πρῶτον γένηται, νεῦρον ἤδη φαίνεσθαι τὸ ἀγγεῖον.

[4] AMG (1894), fr. 17: Πραξαγόρας τὴν μανίαν γίνεσθαί φησιν κατ' οἴδησιν τῆς καρδίας. οὗπερ καὶ τὸ φρονεῖν εἶναι δεδόξακε. μὴ ἐπιγίνεσθαι δὲ αὐτῇ πυρετοὺς διὰ τὸ μηδὲν [ἐπὶ] τὰ ἐκτὸς οἰδήματα ποεῖν πυρώσεις.

by the Anonymous Parisian that Hippocrates thought that mania was due
to the (yellow) bilification and heating of the thought-*pneuma* in the
brain, a purely local occurrence since it did not produce fever as a
consequence.[1] A rather interesting sidelight to Praxagoras' doctrine was
noted by Wellmann, who observes that he also gives a cardio-centric
physiological explanation of religious frenzy, quite in the spirit of the
nineteenth century. Here again the Anonymous Parisian is our in-
formant. He attributes to Praxagoras, who, he tells us, was the only one of
the ancients to mention this phenomenon, the theory that this too was
concerned with the heart and the 'thick artery'. It is due to bubbles rising
up from the feet. By these bubbles various parts of the body are affected.
The possessed sometimes make violent movements with their hands,
which they 'throw about', and sometimes with their head.[2] Bubbles also
appear in his account of the causes of epilepsy, which he thought was
caused by the collection in the 'thick artery', the aorta, of phlegmatic
humours (he recognized many more humours than the 'Hippocratic'
four), which bubbled up and blocked the passage of the psychic *pneuma*
from the heart, and shook and convulsed the body. When the bubbles
subsided, the fit ceased.[3] A similar theory of blockage was also held by
Diocles.[4] The theory of epilepsy being due to blockage of the *pneuma* is
very similar to that put forward by the author of *On the sacred disease*, only
the blockage takes place not in the brain but in the heart. But there were
several important points on which Praxagoras differed from Diocles. One
of these was the doctrine of innate heat. He believed, Galen tells us, all
heat in the animal body to be acquired from without,[5] presumably from
the digestion of ingested foodstuffs, and it would appear, if we may trust
the fragment from Phylotimus who was his pupil, bubbles to be produced
in the process of digestion.[6] We are also told by Galen that Praxagoras

---

[1] Ibid.: Ἱπποκράτης δὲ κατὰ τὴν ἐγχόλωσιν καὶ πύρωσιν τοῦ ἐν τῷ ἐγκεφάλῳ νοεροῦ πνεύματος συνίστασθαι τὴν μανίαν φησίν. εἶναι δὲ ταύτην τοπικὴν διὰ τὸ πυρετοὺς μὴ ἐπιφέρειν.
Wellmann (*Fragmente*, p. 21, n. 1) refers, in this connection, to 'Hippocrates' *De morbo
sacro*, 14, though 'Hippocrates' is referring there not to mania but to epilepsy.

[2] AMG (1894), fr. 19: Πραξαγόρας τοῦ ἐνθεαστικοῦ πάθους μόνος τῶν ἀρχαίων ἐμνήσθη,
φάσκων περὶ τὴν καρδίαν αὐτὴν εἶναι καὶ τὴν παχεῖαν ἀρτηρίαν. γίνεσθαι δὲ καὶ τῶν πομφολύγων
ἐπανάστασιν ποσί· διὰ τούτων γάρ, φησίν, ἐπανακοινοῦται ἄλλοτε ἄλλη· ὁτὲ μὲν τὰς χεῖρας, ὁτὲ
δὲ τὴν κεφαλὴν ῥιπτοῦνται.

[3] Ibid., fr. 3: Πραξαγόρας περὶ τὴν παχεῖαν ἀρτηρίαν φησὶ γίνεσθαι φλεγματικῶν χυμῶν συ-
στάντων ἐν αὐτῇ· οὓς δὴ πομφολυγουμένους ἀποκλείειν τὴν δίοδον τοῦ ἀπὸ καρδίας ψυχικοῦ
πνεύματος καὶ οὕτω τοῦτο κραδαίνειν καὶ σπᾶν τὸ σῶμα· πάλιν δὲ κατασταθεισῶν [καταρραγεισῶν
Wellmann] τῶν πομφολύγων παύεσθαι τὸ πάθος.

[4] Ibid.: Διοκλῆς δὲ καὶ αὐτὸς ἔμφραξιν περὶ τὸν αὐτὸν τόπον οἴεται.

[5] Galen, *De trem. palp. convuls. et rig.* 6, K. vii. 614: ἐγὼ μὲν γὰρ εἶπον τοῦ κατὰ φύσιν
θερμοῦ πάθος εἶναι τὸ ῥῖγος, ἵνα μή τις τοῦ ἔξωθεν νομίσας εἰρῆσθαι, καταψεύδεσθαί με δόξειεν
Ἐρασιστράτου καὶ Πραξαγόρου καὶ Φιλοτίμου καὶ Ἀσκληπιάδου καὶ μυρίων ἄλλων, ὅσοι τὸ θερμὸν οὐκ ἔμφυτον ἀλλ' ἐπίκτητον εἶναι νομίζουσι.

[6] Quoted by Steckerl, op. cit., p. 115: τοῖς δὲ νύκτωρ ψυχρὸν πίνουσι καταψύχει τούς τε
πρότερον εἰρημένους τόπους πάντας καὶ τὴν τροφὴν ἐν ἀκμῇ μάλιστα οὖσαν τοῦ θερμαίνεσθαι

regarded the power of pulsation possessed by the arteries not as being transmitted by the heart but as an independent power of movement possessed by them even when removed from the body,[1] and that he looked upon the strengthening of the soul, but not like Asclepiades its generation, as the purpose of respiration, differing on this point from Diocles, who regarded its function as being the cooling of the innate heat.[2] One more point from Galen's account of his teaching should be noted. The *pneuma* which activates the body is not just atmospheric air. It has become denser and is 'rather steam-like'.[3]

From these tantalizingly discrete fragments, Steckerl has attempted to reconstruct the whole jigsaw puzzle of a physiological theory. His ingenious suggestions are certainly most entertaining, but to my mind they do not carry much conviction. Steckerl sees in the bubbles the key to his problems. The innate *pneuma*-like heat has no existence, the warmth that the inspired air receives comes from the body, from the bubbles produced by digestion with its heat-producing process.

For Praxagoras the soul obviously was nothing other than the *pneuma*, or even better, the *pneuma* in the heart. He must have conceived the soul as a mixture of the air which enters the body, and of the air which is inclosed in the bubbles, and which will be released from them. In reality, the soul is a continuous mixture and exchange between the air from outside and the air from inside.[4]

The bubbles which arise in the system of the veins are somehow transferred to the arteries—neither Steckerl nor Praxagoras tells us how —where they become responsible not only for warming and mixing with the in-breathed atmospheric air to form the *pneuma*, but also for the pulse, which Praxagoras is supposed by some historians to have been the first to distinguish in the arteries as opposed to the veins, the expansion of the arteries in the pulse-beat being brought about by the bursting of the bubbles. Praxagoras thus connected the kinds of pulse with the kinds of bubbles produced in the manufacture of the humours in the process of digestion.

καὶ τὴν ἕψησιν κωλύει καὶ τὴν τροφὴν ζέουσαν καὶ τὰς ἐν αὐτῇ πομφόλυγας γινομένας ταπεινοῖ καὶ καθίστησιν εἰς ἕδραν, καὶ τὴν διαλελυμένην καὶ τετηκυῖαν τῆς τροφῆς ποιεῖ παχυτέραν. The quotation comes from Oribasius, *Coll. med.* v. 22, C.M.G. vi. i, p. 151.

[1] *De plac. Hipp. et Plat.* vi. 7, K. v. 561: ἀπεσχίσθησαν δ' οὖν οὐκ οἶδ' ὅπως αὐτῶν ἐν τῷδε Πραξαγόρας τε καὶ Φιλότιμος [Φιλότιμος] ὁμολογήσαντες τἄλλα, καὶ νομίζουσι τὸ πάμπαν ἐξ ἑαυτῶν σφύζειν τὰς ἀρτηρίας, ὥστε καὶ εἰ σάρκα τις ἐκτεμὼν ζῴου καταθείη παλλομένην ἐπὶ τῆς γῆς, ἐναργῶς ὁρᾶσθαι καὶ τὴν κίνησιν τῶν ἀρτηριῶν.

[2] Galen, *De usu resp.* 1, K. iv. 471: τί ποτε οὖν τηλικοῦτόν ἐστι τὸ παρὰ τῆς ἀναπνοῆς ἡμῖν χρηστόν; ἆρά γε τῆς ψυχῆς αὐτῆς ἐστι γένεσις, ὡς Ἀσκληπιάδης φησίν; ἢ γένεσις μὲν οὐχί, ῥῶσις δέ τις, ὡς τοῦ Νικάρχου Πραξαγόρας; ἢ τῆς ἐμφύτου θερμασίας ἀνάψυξίς τις, ὡς Φιλιστίων τε καὶ Διοκλῆς ἔλεγον.

[3] Galen, *De sanguine in arteriis*, 2, K. iv. 707: Πραξαγόρας μὲν οὖν καὶ παχυμερέστερον αὐτὸ καὶ ἱκανῶς ἀτμῶδες εἶναί φησιν.

[4] Steckerl, *Praxagoras*, p. 21.

Praxagoras connected the pathological variations of the pulse with bubbles. It would be a natural consequence of his conception for him to have thought that the normal movement of the arteries, the normal pulse, is caused by bubbles which arise in the normal course of digestion.[1]

A very pretty theory, but had it really been Praxagoras', I cannot help wondering how it was that Praxagoras' bubbles evaded the attention of ancient doxographers, not to mention Galen, who could hardly have resisted the temptation to make fun of it. Moreover, how can the digestive bubbles get to the aorta at all? They are contained in the veins, and the only connections between veins and arteries are the capillaries, the invention of which is not by tradition attributed to Praxagoras.

The modern inquirer will no doubt be compelled to ask himself how any intelligent layman, let alone physician, could have embraced, even in the fourth century B.C., these two doctrines of the bloodless arteries and the heart-centred consciousness. As to the first of them, we have already noted the paradox that the bloodless arteries were a discovery of the dissecting table, made before any clear distinction between the two types of blood vessel had been arrived at. Moreover, almost everywhere upon the exterior surface of the body it is the veins not the arteries that are plainly visible. Nor is the confusion of the arterial with the nervous system so unintelligible in a primitive physiology. What kept the body alive was *pneuma*. This came from without, being drawn into the lungs, which were filled with many very small tubes, some containing air and some blood, and they were visibly connected with the heart. Now the act of respiration must have a purpose very intimately connected with the maintenance of life. When a man died, not only did he stop breathing, but his heart stopped beating, and all his movements ceased. Therefore what keeps him alive and able to move must be the *pneuma*. The empty arterial system discovered in the dissected body must contain something, for nature abhors a vacuum; and according to some Greek 'philosophers' a vacuum, being nothing, cannot exist—as all but that eccentric Democritus would be forced on cross-examination to admit. The arteries must therefore contain something, even if they look empty, and that something is air or some substance derived from air, which we call *pneuma*.

Nor is the notion of the heart as the seat of consciousness altogether absurd. Strong emotions can and do sometimes produce disturbances in the heart-beat as well as changes in the rate of respiration, and emotions are often accompanied by various visceral sensations. Moreover these cardiac and respirational changes may be accompanied by changes in the movements of the diaphragm. Ancient usage among the Greeks had

[1] Ibid., p. 23.

somehow connected the diaphragm with the mind.[1] φρήν is the singular of φρένες which cannot, I am convinced, really be identified with the lungs, as one modern scholar has suggested, even in Homer. The diaphragm, whose philology is so closely connected with the notion of the mind, also seems to have become a third candidate for the presidency of the body, but it obtained only a small minority vote. It included among its supporters Ariston, the pupil of the Aeginetan Petron, who, as the Anonymous Parisian informs us, considered it, as it were, the temple of the body.[2] Emotions are not 'felt' *in* the brain, and its only outward physiological activity which could be observed was the secretion of phlegm, which obviously came down from the brain into the nose and the bronchial system. Moreover its grey-whitish appearance made it look of much less vital importance than the heart or the liver.

In this connection it is interesting to compare some of the conclusions arrived at by the physicians of ancient Egypt many centuries earlier, and set down in the papyrus *Ebers*. They too, like Praxagoras, the Cnidians,

[1] This connection survived till quite late in Greek medical thought. Thus the Anonymous Parisian tells us that Diocles regarded φρενῖτις, a disease the main characteristic of which was delirium, as an inflammation of the diaphragm. See AMG (1894), fr. 1: ὁ δὲ Διοκλῆς φλεγμονὴν τοῦ διαφράγματός φησιν εἶναι τὴν φρενῖτιν ἀπὸ τόπου καὶ οὐκ ἀπ' ἐνεργείας τὸ πάθος καλῶν, συνδιατιθεμένης καὶ τῆς καρδίας. ἔοικε γὰρ καὶ οὗτος τὴν φρόνησιν περὶ ταύτην ἀπολείπειν. A vestige of this doctrine can still be found in Galen, who distinguishes the visceral from the cerebral form.

[2] See AMG (1894), fr. 10, where the author tells us about the cause of 'cardiac syncope', which is the result of an inflammation of the 'mouth' of the stomach. The ancients did not think this was a direct affliction of the heart, but that it occurred when principal organs, especially the mouth of the stomach, were inflamed. Now the mouth of the stomach was called καρδία, so that it came to be considered an affliction of the heart itself by some of them which occurred when the *pneuma* lost its tension and was dissolved like incense in contact with fire. The fragment ends quite inconsequentially with the saying attributed to Ariston, and mentions quite incidentally that Ariston regarded the diaphragm as the temple of the body. This passage, which raises certain points which we shall treat at some length in a later chapter (see below, pp. 431–41), reads as follows: συγκοπῶν αἰτία καρδίας. ὀνομαστὶ μὲν τοῦ πάθους οἱ παλαιοὶ οὐκ ἐμνήσθησαν ὡς καθ' αὑτὸ γινομένου, ἐπιγινομένου δὲ κυρίοις τόποις φλεγμαίνουσι, μάλιστα δὲ στομάχῳ, ὅπερ καλεῖται καρδία, δι' ὅπερ τινὲς καρδίας ὑπέλαβον τὸ πάθος γίνεσθαι δ' αὐτὸ ὑπὸ φλεγμονῆς ἐκτονιζομένου τοῦ πνεύματος καὶ λυομένου καθάπερ λιβανώτου τῷ πυρὶ ὁμιλήσαντος· ἐστὶ τοίνυν αὕτη ἡ τοῦ σώματος ἕξις, συμβαίνει δὲ μάλιστα ἐπὶ στομάχῳ πεπονθότι, ἐπεὶ καθάπερ νεὼς τοῦ σώματος ὑπόζωμα ὑπάρχει, ὥς φησιν Ἀρίστων ὁ ἀπὸ Πέτρωνος. Quoted by Wellmann (*Fragmente*, p. 16), who inserts the word τὸ between σώματος and ὑπόζωμα. The interesting suggestion has been made to me that νεὼς should really be νεώς, the diaphragm being compared to the brace of a ship. This would appear to make good sense, and for all we know may have been Ariston's view, but it does nothing to explain the mental connotation of φρήν. The author of *On the sacred disease* puts the duplicity of meaning down to mere accident: cf. cap. 20: Αἱ δὲ φρένες ἄλλως οὔνομα ἔχουσι τῇ τύχῃ κεκτημένον καὶ τῷ νόμῳ, τῷ δ' ἐόντι οὐκ, οὐδὲ τῇ φύσει. (Jones, Loeb edition.) H. Grensemann (Berlin, 1968) reads τὸ δ' ἐὸν οὔ [τῇ φύσει] and numbers the chapter, 17. But 'Hippocrates' does seem to suggest that some of his contemporaries or predecessors, or at any rate laymen, did regard the diaphragm as the organ of knowledge, and admits that both the diaphragm and the heart can 'feel': ἀνάγκη δὲ καὶ ἀνιώμενον φρίσσειν τε τὸ σῶμα καὶ συντείνεσθαι καὶ ὑπερχαίροντα ταὐτὸ τοῦτο πάσχειν. διότι ἡ καρδίη αἰσθάνεταί τε μάλιστα καὶ αἱ φρένες, τῆς μέντοι φρονήσιος οὐδετέρῳ μέτεστιν, ἀλλὰ πάντων τούτων αἴτιος ὁ ἐγκέφαλός ἐστιν.

and the Sicilians, regarded the heart as the seat of the intelligence. Grapow, in his work on ancient Egyptian medicine, reproduces a passage from this papyrus in a translation by H. Junker.[1]

It is the fact that the heart and the tongue rule over all the limbs, according to the doctrine that the heart is in each body and the tongue in each mouth of all Gods, men, and beasts. Inasmuch as the heart thinks whatsoever it will, and the tongue commands all that it wills. The seeing of the eyes, the hearing of the ears, the breathing of the nose, they bring tidings to the heart. It is the heart which brings into being each act of intelligence, and the tongue it is which repeats what is thought by the heart. And so all works are performed, and all handiwork, the doing of the hands, the going of the feet, the movement of all the limbs, according to its command.

The heart was also considered by the Egyptians to be the centre of the vascular system, and its beating and the pulse had been discovered. It could be felt in places all over the body, because 'All limbs possess its vessels, that is, the heart speaks out of the vessels of every limb'.[2] They knew, too, something of the significance of an abnormal pulse, but their conception of the vascular system seems to have been extremely crude and primitive. They thought that the heart was the centre of all the channels of the body, channels that conveyed not only blood, but also air, urine, and faeces. The word *mt*, translated *vessel*, whose hieroglyphic symbol was an erect penis, could mean artery, vein, tendon, muscle, windpipe, and nerve; its connotation being a good deal more inclusive than the Greek *neuron*. The function of most of these *mt* was to bring air from the nose via the heart to all the portions of the body. So in the papyrus Ebers we read: 'As to the breath which enters the nose, it enters into the heart and the lungs, and these give to the whole body.'

The similarity to the Greek theory we have just described appears almost startling, and it would be interesting to discover if any connection between the two can be established, similar to that worked out by Steuer and Saunders on the theory propounded by the school of Cnidos on 'residues' as the principal cause of disease, which they trace back to the ancient Egyptian theory of *whdw*, a faecal derivative, as the principal morbific agency.[3]

For Diocles, as we have seen, the seat of the intelligence is still the heart, but the fragment of Vindicianus quoted above on p. 105 seems to suggest that he postulated a very special connection between the heart and the brain. The theory of the primacy of the brain may well have originated in Magna Graecia, and Pythagoras, if we may trust Diogenes

---

[1] See H. Grapow, *Grundriß der Geschichte der Medizin der alten Ägypter* (Berlin, 1954–9), i. 64.

[2] Papyrus Ebers 99, quoted by Sigerist, op. cit. i. 349 ff.

[3] Steuer and Saunders, *Ancient Egyptian and Cnidian Medicine* (University of California Press, 1959).

Laertius, adopted the theory in a special form by separating the different portions of the soul, placing the reason in the brain, and the emotions in the heart, an arrangement in which he was followed by another philosopher, Plato. The doctrine of the primacy of the heart did not go unchallenged in medical circles on the western side of the Adriatic. Philolaus of Croton, the Pythagorean contemporary of Plato, defended the main thesis of his compatriot Alcmaeon by placing the seat of reason in the brain. At the same time, he regards the heart as the seat of the vital principle of *psyche*, which we have so often to mistranslate as soul, and of sense perception, the navel as that of the 'vegetable' functions of growth and nutrition, and the genitals as in a sense the starting-point ($\dot{a}\rho\chi\dot{\eta}$) of all these powers, since it is from the seed that all alike spring.[1] These views, attributed to him by a late doxographer, the author of the Anonymous Londoner, seem in many respects to agree with those expressed in the *Timaeus*. Philistion, on the other hand, borrowed not from Alcmaeon but from Empedocles some of his most important principles. He took over his theory of the four elements, fire, air, water, and earth, each of them endowed with a single quality, heat, cold, wetness, or dryness,[2] not with the two qualities which were to become the mainstay of the 'Hippocratic' doctrine embraced and expounded by Galen. These four elements make up the human body. He also adopted Empedocles' theory of 'poral' respiration in addition to that through the throat and lungs,[3] in contrast to the doctrine of the 'Hippocratic' treatise *On the sacred disease*. His theory of disease is closely bound up with that of respiration. Disease must be attributed to three general categories of causes, (1) the elements, (2) the condition of the body, (3) the external environment, a classification not unlike that found in the 'Hippocratic' treatise *On airs, waters, and places*. Category (1) embraces diseases caused by excess or deficiency of the prime elementary qualities, (2) is concerned with the circulation of the *pneuma*. When the whole body is properly aerated, and the *pneuma* can pass in and out all over the body without hindrance, health ensues. This implies proper respiration through both the nostrils and the 'pores'. Category (3) embraces factors like climate, excess or deficiency of heat and cold and sudden changes of temperature, as well as improper feeding,

---

[1] See D–K, vol. 1, 413: καὶ τέσσαρες ἀρχαὶ τοῦ ζῴου τοῦ λογικοῦ, ὥσπερ καὶ Φιλόλαος ἐν τῷ περὶ φύσεως λέγει, ἐγκέφαλος, καρδία, ὀμφαλός, αἰδοῖον. κεφαλὰ μὲν νόου, καρδία δὲ ψυχᾶς καὶ αἰσθήσιος, ὀμφαλὸς δὲ ῥιζώσιος καὶ ἀναφύσιος τοῦ πρώτου, αἰδοῖον δὲ σπέρματος καταβολᾶς τε καὶ γεννήσιος. ἐγκέφαλος δὲ (σημαίνει) τὰν ἀνθρώπω ἀρχάν, καρδία δὲ τὰν ζῴου, ὀμφαλὸς δὲ τὰν φυτοῦ, αἰδοῖον δὲ τὰν ξυμπάντων. πάντα γὰρ ἀπὸ σπέρματος καὶ θάλλοντι καὶ βλαστάνοντι.

[2] *Anonymus Londinensis*, xx. 24, J. 81: Φιλιστίων δ' οἴεται ἐκ δ' ἰδεῶν συνεστάναι ἡμᾶς, τοῦτ' ἔστιν ἐκ δ' στοιχείων· πυρός, ἀέρος, ὕδατος, γῆς· εἶναι δὲ ἑκάστου δυνάμεις, τοῦ μὲν πυρὸς τὸ θερμόν, τοῦ δὲ ἀέρος τὸ ψυχρόν, τοῦ δὲ ὕδατος τὸ ὑγρόν, τῆς δὲ γῆς τὸ ξηρόν.

[3] Ibid.: ὅταν γὰρ φησὶν εὐπνοῇ ὅλον τὸ σῶμα καὶ διεξῇ ἀκωλύτως τὸ πνεῦμα, ὑγίεια γίνεται· οὐ γὰρ μόνον κατὰ τὸ στόμα καὶ τοὺς μυκτῆρας ἡ ἀναπνοὴ γίνεται, ἀλλὰ καὶ καθ' ὅλον τὸ σῶμα.

indigestible or rotten, decayed food, and, finally, wounds.[1] Philistion, who, incidentally, was regarded by some people in Galen's time as the author of the 'Hippocratic' treatise *On healthy diet*,[2] was as we have seen a friend of Plato. He is mentioned in the philosopher's second *Epistle*, where Plato asks Dionysius, whose physician he was, to allow him to pay a visit to Athens.[3] Philistion was also one of the first promoters of the theory that the function of respiration was to cool the heart's innate heat.

The question now arises how far the physiological doctrines laid down by the astronomical expert in the *Timaeus* represent Plato's own views, and how far, too, they are an accurate representation of Philistion's opinions. This is a question to which I do not feel myself competent to give any considered answer. Nor is it really relevant to our purpose. For us it is sufficient to note that these theories were being discussed in Plato's circle.

Plato's physiological pronouncements are almost all of them to be found in that notoriously difficult dialogue the *Timaeus*, and some, if not most, of them have been traced by Wellmann to Philistion. But long before writing the *Timaeus*, Plato had in the *Republic* divided the soul of man into three parts, the rational, the 'spirited', and the appetitive. The problem of justice was solved by regarding it as the functioning of these three parts in accordance with their natural order of integration, the control of the appetitive by the reasonable assisted by the spirited element. In the *Timaeus*, Plato gives us the physiological setting to this tripartite arrangement. Like Philolaus and Philistion, he accepts the heart as the seat of the emotions, but his chief concern is to separate the immortal from the mortal parts of the soul. The immortal part resides in the head, the mortal in the belly. The head, being spherical and the sphere the most perfect of all geometrical forms, is the most appropriate organ for the immortal reason[4]—a characteristically Hellenic argument which we shall find perpetuated in the cosmology, though not, curiously enough,

---

[1] Ibid.: τὰς δὲ νόσους γίνεσθαι πολυτρόπως κατ' αὐτόν, ὡς δὲ τύπῳ καὶ γενικώτερον εἰπεῖν τριχῶς. ἢ γὰρ παρὰ τὰ στοιχεῖα ἢ παρὰ τὴν τῶν σωμάτων διάθεσιν ἢ παρὰ τὰ ἐκτός. παρὰ μὲν οὖν τὰ στοιχεῖα, ἐπειδὰν πλεονάσῃ τὸ θερμὸν καὶ τὸ ὑγρόν, ἢ ἐπειδὰν μεῖον γένηται καὶ ἀμαυρὸν τὸ θερμόν . . . παρὰ δὲ τὰ ἐκτὸς γ' ἢ γὰρ ὑπὸ τραυμάτων καὶ ἑλκῶν ἢ ὑπὸ ὑπερβολῆς θάλπους, ψύχους, τῶν ὁμοίων, ἢ ὑπὸ μεταβολῆς θερμοῦ εἰς ψυχρὸν ἢ ψυχροῦ εἰς θερμὸν ἢ τροφῆς εἰς τὸ ἀνοίκειον καὶ διεφθορός.

[2] Galen, *Hipp. de acut. morb. vict. comment.* I. xvii, K. xv. 455: εἰ γὰρ καὶ μὴ Ἱπποκράτους ἐστὶν ἐκεῖνο τὸ βιβλίον, ἀλλ' Εὐρυφῶντος ἢ Φιλιστίωνος ἤ τινος ἄλλου τῶν παλαιῶν. Cf. *Comment. in Hipp. aphorism.*, K. xviiiA. 9: εἰ δὲ τῷ διαιτητικῷ τῷ ὑγιεινῷ τῷ Ἱπποκράτει μὲν ἐπιγεγραμμένῳ καὶ αὐτῷ, τοῖς δ' ἀποξενοῦσιν αὐτό, τισὶ μὲν εἰς Φιλιστίωνα, τισὶ δ' εἰς Ἀρίστωνα, τισὶ δ' εἰς Φερεκύδην ἀναφέρουσι . . .

[3] Plato, *Epistle* 2, 314 e: Φιλιστίωνι δέ, εἰ μὲν αὐτὸς χρῇ, σφόδρα χρῶ, εἰ δὲ οἷόν τε, Σπευσίππῳ χρῆσον καὶ ἀπόπεμψον. δεῖται δὲ σοῦ καὶ Σπεύσιππος. ὑπέσχετο δέ μοι καὶ Φιλιστίων, εἰ σὺ ἀφίῃς αὐτόν, ἥξειν προθύμως Ἀθήναζε.

[4] Plato, *Timaeus*, 44 d: τὰς μὲν δὴ θείας περιόδους δύο οὔσας, τὸ τοῦ παντὸς σχῆμα ἀπομιμησάμενοι περιφερὲς ὄν, εἰς σφαιροειδὲς σῶμα ἐνέδησαν, τοῦτο ὃ νῦν κεφαλὴν ἐπονομάζομεν, ὃ θειότατόν τ' ἐστὶ καὶ τῶν ἐν ἡμῖν πάντων δεσποτοῦν.

in the physiology of Aristotle his pupil, which was to haunt European physical thinking until the days of Kepler. Lest the divine portion of the soul should be polluted more than is absolutely necessary, the gods separated the head from the lower parts of the body by the isthmus of the neck. The mortal part of the soul is divided into two, just as the belly is separated from the thorax by the diaphragm. The superior mortal portion of the soul resides in the thorax, for the heart is the seat of the spirited part, while the lower, the appetitive, has its seat in the belly.[1]

This tripartite division of the soul was modified by Aristotle in functional or biological terms into a division between the vegetable, animal, and reasoning functions, and is no doubt the ancestral model of the tripartite arrangement attributed to Galen, whose doctrine was interpreted by his Arabic and medieval European successors as entailing the existence of three kinds of spirit, the natural, the animal, and the psychic, though some doubt has recently been thrown on the idea that Galen himself did actually teach the existence of a natural spirit.[2] His own division of physiological 'powers' corresponds fairly closely to Aristotle's division of the faculties.

But to return to Plato. Like Philistion he regards the body as made up of four elementary bodies, earth, air, fire, and water, each with their special quality or 'power'. How these elements were formed by different kinds of geometrical figures, and how they were mixed by 'God' to form the various parts of the body, need not concern us here. Except for mathematics, Plato does not seem to have had any great interest in physical science, but some of the physiological doctrines which he records are worth noting, if only because they throw some light on contemporary medical thinking. Like Philistion, Timaeus is acquainted with the system of bronchial tubes and of some vascular connection between the heart and the lungs, which were conceived by Plato as having a double purpose, that of cooling the innate heat resident in the heart, and that of moderating the passion of anger. Hence the gods:

placed the heart, the knot of the veins and the source or fountain of the blood that races through the limbs, was set in the place of guard, that when the might of passion was roused by reason making proclamation of any wrong

---

[1] Plato, *Timaeus*, 69 d : διὰ ταῦτα δὴ σεβόμενοι μιαίνειν τὸ θεῖον, ὅ τι μὴ πᾶσα ἦν ἀνάγκη, χωρὶς ἐκείνου κατοικίζουσιν εἰς ἄλλην τοῦ σώματος οἴκησιν τὸ θνητόν, ἰσθμὸν καὶ ὅρον διοικοδομήσαντες τῆς κεφαλῆς καὶ τοῦ στήθους, αὐχένα μεταξὺ τιθέντες ἵνα εἴη χωρίς. ἐν δὲ δὴ τοῖς στήθεσι καὶ τῷ καλουμένῳ θώρακι τὸ τῆς ψυχῆς θνητὸν γένος ἐνέδουν. καὶ ἐπειδὴ τὸ μὲν ἄμεινον αὐτῆς τὸ χεῖρον ἐπεπεφύκει, διοικοδομοῦσι τοῦ θώρακος αὖ τὸ κύτος . . . τὰς φρένας διάφραγμα εἰς τὸ μέσον αὐτῶν τιθέντες. τὸ μετέχον οὖν τῆς ψυχῆς ἀνδρείας καὶ θυμοῦ . . . κατῴκισαν ἐγγυτέρω τῆς κεφαλῆς μεταξὺ τῶν φρενῶν τε καὶ αὐχένος.
Ibid., 70 d : τὸ δὲ σιτίων καὶ ποτῶν ἐπιθυμητικὸν τῆς ψυχῆς καὶ ὅσων ἔνδειαν διὰ τὴν τοῦ σώματος ἴσχει φύσιν, τοῦτο εἰς τὰ μεταξὺ τῶν τε φρενῶν καὶ τοῦ πρὸς τὸν ὀμφαλὸν ὅρου κατῴκισαν.
[2] Notably by O. Temkin; see his article, 'On Galen's pneumatology', *Gesnerus* 8 (1951), 180–9.

assailing them from without or being perpetrated by the desires within, quickly the whole power of feeling in the body, perceiving these commands and threats, might obey and follow through every turn and alley, and thus allow the principle of the best to have command in all of them. But the gods, fore-knowing that the palpitation of the heart in the expectation of danger and the swelling and excitement of passion was caused by fire, formed and implanted as a supporter to the heart the lung, which was in the first place soft and bloodless, and also had within hollows like the pores of a sponge, in order that, by receiving the breath and the drink, it might give coolness and the power of respiration and alleviate the heat. Wherefore they cut the air-channels leading to the lung, and placed the lung about the heart as a soft mattress, that, when passion was rife within, the heart, beating against a yielding body, might be cooled and suffer less, and might thus become more ready to join with passion in the service of reason.[1]   (trs. Jowett.)

With regard to respiration, Plato thus adopts the double process of Empedocles and Philistion, which he explains as follows:

Since there is no such thing as a vacuum into which any of these things which are moved can enter, and the breath is carried from us into the external air, the next point is, as will be clear to everyone, that it does not go into a vacant space, but pushes its neighbour out of its place, and that which is thrust out in turn drives out its neighbour; and in this way everything of necessity at last comes round to that place from whence the breath came forth, and enters in there, and following the breath, fills up the vacant space; and this goes on like the rotation of a wheel, because there can be no such thing as a vacuum. Wherefore also the breast and the lungs, when they emit the breath, are replenished by the air which surrounds the body and which enters in through the pores of the flesh and is driven round in a circle; and again the air which is sent away and passes out through the body forces the breath inwards through the passage of the mouth and nostrils. Now the origin of this movement may be supposed to be as follows. In the interior of every animal the hottest part is that which is around the blood and the veins; it is in a manner an internal fountain of fire, which we compare to the network of a creel, being woven all of fire and extended through the centre of the body, while the outer parts are composed of air. Now we must admit that heat naturally proceeds outwards

---

[1] *Timaeus*, 70 a–d: τὴν δὲ δὴ καρδίαν ἅμμα τῶν φλεβῶν καὶ πηγὴν τοῦ περιφερομένου κατὰ τὰ πάντα μέλη σφοδρῶς αἵματος εἰς τὴν δορυφορικὴν οἴκησιν κατέστησαν ἵνα ὅτε ζέσειε τὸ τοῦ θυμοῦ μένος, τοῦ λόγου παραγγείλαντος, ὥς τις ἄδικος περὶ αὐτὰ γίγνεται πρᾶξις ἔξωθεν ἢ καί τις ἀπὸ τῶν ἔνδοθεν ἐπιθυμιῶν, ὀξέως διὰ πάντων στενωπῶν πᾶν, ὅσον αἰσθητικὸν ἐν τῷ σώματι τῶν τε παρακελεύσεων καὶ ἀπειλῶν αἰσθανόμενον γίγνοιτο ἐπήκοον καὶ ἕποιτο πάντῃ καὶ τὸ βέλτιστον οὕτως ἐν αὐτοῖς πᾶσιν ἡγεμονεῖν ἐφ. τῇ δὲ δὴ πηδήσει τῆς καρδίας ἐν τῇ τῶν δεινῶν προσδοκίᾳ καὶ τῇ τοῦ θυμοῦ ἐγέρσει, προγιγνώσκοντες, ὅτι διὰ πυρὸς ἡ τοιαύτη πᾶσα ἔμελλεν οἴδησις γίγνεσθαι τῶν θυμουμένων, ἐπικουρίαν αὐτῇ μηχανώμενοι, τὴν τοῦ πλεύμονος ἰδέαν ἐνεφύτευσαν, πρῶτον μὲν μαλακὴν καὶ ἄναιμον, εἶτα σήραγγας ἐντὸς ἔχουσαν οἷον σπόγγου κατατετρημένας, ἵνα τό τε πνεῦμα καὶ τὸ πῶμα δεχομένη, ψύχουσα ἀναπνοὴν καὶ ῥᾳστώνην ἐν τῷ καύματι παρέχοι. διὸ δὴ τῆς ἀρτηρίας ὀχετοὺς ἐπὶ τὸν πλεύμονα ἔτεμον, καὶ περὶ τὴν καρδίαν αὐτὸν περιέστησαν οἷον ἅλμα μαλακόν, ἵν᾿ ὁ θυμὸς ἡνίκα ἐν αὐτῇ ἀκμάζοι, πηδῶσα εἰς ὑπεῖκον καὶ ἀναψυχομένη, πονοῦσα ἧττον μᾶλλον τῷ λόγῳ μετὰ θυμοῦ δύναιτο ὑπηρετεῖν.

to its own place and to its kindred element, and as there are two exits for the heat, the one through the body, and the other through the mouth and the nostrils, when it moves towards the one, it drives round the air at the other, and that which is driven round falls into the fire and becomes warm, and that which goes forth is cooled. But when the heat changes its place, and the particles at the other exit grow warmer, the hotter air inclining in that direction and carried towards its native element, fire, pushes round the air at the other; and this being effected in the same way and communicating the same impulse, a circular swaying to and fro is produced by the double process, which we call inspiration and expiration.[1]

The physics of this process of pushing round (περίωσις) sound rather strange to modern ears, but this theory played an important part in the physiological explanations of classical Greek medicine, and was, as we shall see, one of the factors which prevented their discovery of the circulation. Concerning the blood vessels themselves, Plato has little new to tell us. His general scheme seems to be derived from Diogenes of Apollonia, but it is less complete. The gods irrigated the body by providing it with channels.

In the first place, they cut two hidden channels or veins down the back where the skin and the flesh join, which answered severally to the right and left side of the body. These they let down along the backbone, so as to have the marrow of generation between them, where it was most likely to flourish, and in order that the stream coming down from above might flow freely to the other parts, and equalize the irrigation. In the next place, they divided the veins about the head, and interlacing them, they sent them in opposite directions; those coming from the right did they send to the left of the body, and those from the left, they diverted towards the right, so that they and the skin might together form a bond which should fasten the head to the body.

[1] *Timaeus*, 79 a : πάλιν δὲ τὸ τῆς ἀναπνοῆς ἴδωμεν πάθος, αἷς χρώμενον αἰτίαις τοιοῦτον γέγονεν, οἷόνπερ τὰ νῦν ἐστιν. ὧδ' οὖν ἐπειδὴ κενὸν οὐδέν ἐστιν, εἰς ὃ τῶν φερομένων δύναιτ' ἂν εἰσελθεῖν τι, τὸ δὲ πνεῦμα φέρεται παρ' ἡμῶν ἔξω, τὸ μετὰ τοῦτο ἤδη παντὶ δῆλον, ὡς οὐκ εἰς κενόν, ἀλλὰ τὸ πλησίον ἐκ τῆς ἕδρας ὠθεῖ. τὸ δ' ὠθούμενον ἐξελαύνει τὸ πλησίον ἀεί, καὶ κατὰ ταύτην τὴν ἀνάγκην πᾶν περιελαυνόμενον εἰς τὴν ἕδραν ὅθεν ἐξῆλθε τὸ πνεῦμα, εἰσιὸν ἐκεῖσε καὶ ἀναπληροῦν αὐτὴν ξυνέπεται τῷ πνεύματι, καὶ τοῦτο ἅμα πᾶν οἷον τροχοῦ περιαγομένου γίγνεται διὰ τὸ κενὸν μηδὲν εἶναι. διὸ δὴ τὸ τῶν στηθῶν καὶ τὸ τοῦ πλεύμονος ἔξω μεθιὲν τὸ πνεῦμα πάλιν ὑπὸ τοῦ περὶ τὸ σῶμα ἀέρος, εἴσω διὰ μανῶν τῶν σαρκῶν δυομένου καὶ περιελαυνομένου, γίγνεται πλῆρες. αὖθις δὲ ἀποτρεπόμενος ὁ ἀὴρ καὶ διὰ τοῦ σώματος ἔξω ἰὼν εἴσω τὴν ἀναπνοὴν περιωθεῖ κατὰ τὴν τοῦ στόματος καὶ τὴν τῶν μυκτήρων δίοδον. τὴν δ' αἰτίαν τῆς ἀρχῆς αὐτῶν θετέον τήνδε· πᾶν ζῷον ἑαυτοῦ τἀντὸς περὶ τὸ αἷμα καὶ τὰς φλέβας θερμότητα ἔχει, οἷον ἐν ἑαυτῷ πηγήν τινα ἐνοῦσαν πυρός· ὃ δὴ καὶ προσηκάζομεν τῷ τοῦ κύρτου πλέγματι, κατὰ μέσον διατεταμένον ἐκ πυρὸς πεπλέχθαι πᾶν, τὰ δ' ἄλλα, ὅσα ἔξωθεν, ἀέρος. τὸ θερμὸν δὴ κατὰ φύσιν εἰς τὴν αὑτοῦ χώραν ἔξω πρὸς τὸ ξυγγενὲς ὁμολογητέον ἰέναι. δυοῖν δὲ ταῖν διεξόδοιν οὔσαιν, τῆς μὲν κατὰ τὸ σῶμα ἔξω, τῆς δὲ αὖ κατὰ τὸ στόμα καὶ τὰς ῥῖνας, ὅταν μὲν ἐπὶ θάτερα ὁρμήσῃ, θάτερα περιωθεῖ· τὸ δὲ περιωσθὲν εἰς τὸ πῦρ ἐμπίπτον θερμαίνεται, τὸ δ' ἐξιὸν ψύχεται. μεταβαλλούσης δὲ τῆς θερμότητος καὶ τῶν κατὰ τὴν ἑτέραν ἔξοδον θερμοτέρων γιγνομένων πάλιν ἐκείνη ῥέπον αὖ τὸ θερμότερον μᾶλλον, πρὸς τὴν αὑτοῦ φύσιν φερόμενον, περιωθεῖ τὸ κατὰ θάτερα· τὸ δὲ τὰ αὐτὰ πάσχον καὶ τὰ αὐτὰ ἀνταποδιδὸν ἀεί, κύκλον οὕτω σαλευόμενον ἔνθα καὶ ἔνθα ἀπειργασμένον ὑπ' ἀμφοτέρων τὴν ἀναπνοὴν καὶ ἐκπνοὴν γίγνεσθαι παρέχεται.

since the crown of the head was not encircled by sinews; and also in order that the sensations from both sides might be distributed over the whole body.[1]

As we have already noted, Plato makes some advance on Diogenes in that he recognizes the heart as the focal point of the blood vessels and describes it as the source or fountain of the blood which moves about the body, but it would be a great mistake to attach too much significance to his picturesque phrases. The blood 'racing through the limbs' does not pursue any circular course. Of the heart itself, Plato gives us no anatomical description, either of its chambers, or of its functioning; and as Abel has pointed out, he is far from guessing that the heart is the cause of the movement of the blood.[2] Among the functions of the blood vessels he appears to include the transmission of sensations, no doubt through the agency of the *pneuma* introduced into them by the two-fold Empedoclean process of respiration; and Kapferer has even attempted to attribute to him if not the discovery of, at any rate an acquaintance with, the nervous system.[3]

When we pass to Aristotle, we find ourselves in a very different world from that of the *Timaeus*, even though on one point of capital importance it is Aristotle not Plato who backed the wrong horse. For Aristotle (see Fig. 4), unlike his master, regarded the heart, not the brain, as the seat of consciousness, impressed, no doubt, by the fact that the heart is the organ from which all the blood vessels arise, a conception much more definite than that which we have noted of the heart as the 'knot of the veins' found in the *Timaeus*. For Aristotle, as for Plato, there is no clear distinction between arteries and veins;[4] both are called φλέβες, and the surprising

---

[1] Ibid., 77 c–e: τὸ σῶμα αὐτὸ ἡμῶν διωχέτευσαν τέμνοντες οἷον ἐν κήποις ὀχετοὺς ἵνα ὥσπερ ἐκ νάματος ἐπιόντος ἄρδοιτο. καὶ πρῶτον μὲν ὀχετοὺς κρυφαίους ὑπὸ τὴν ξύμφυσιν τοῦ δέρματος καὶ τῆς σαρκὸς δύο φλέβας ἔτεμον νωτιαίας, δίδυμον, ὡς τὸ σῶμα ἐτύγχανε δεξιοῖς τε καὶ ἀριστεροῖς ὄν. ταύτας δὲ καθῆκαν παρὰ τὴν ῥάχιν, καὶ τὸν γόνιμον μεταξὺ λαβόντες μυελόν, ἵνα οὗτός τε ὅτι μάλιστα θάλλοι, καὶ ἐπὶ τἆλλα εὔρους ἐντεῦθεν ἅτε ἐπὶ κάταντες ἡ ἐπίχυσις γενομένη παρέχοι τὴν ὑδρείαν ὁμαλήν. μετὰ δὲ ταῦτα σχίσαντες περὶ τὴν κεφαλὴν τὰς φλέβας καὶ δι' ἀλλήλων ἐναντίας πλέξαντες διεῖσαν, τὰς μὲν ἐκ τῶν δεξιῶν ἐπὶ τὰ ἀριστερὰ τοῦ σώματος, τὰς δ' ἐκ τῶν ἀριστερῶν ἐπὶ τὰ δεξιὰ κλίναντες, ὅπως δεσμὸς ἅμα τῇ κεφαλῇ πρὸς τὸ σῶμα εἴη μετὰ τοῦ δέρματος, ἐπειδὴ νεύροις οὐκ ἦν κύκλῳ κατὰ κορυφὴν περιειλημμένη, καὶ δὴ καὶ τὸ τῶν αἰσθήσεων πάθος ἵν' ἀφ' ἑκατέρων τῶν μερῶν εἰς ἅπαν τὸ σῶμα εἴη διαδιδόμενον.

[2] See his article, 'Plato und die Medizin seiner Zeit', *Gesnerus* 14, p. 104. The 'nerves' mentioned in the passage quoted in the footnote above are, of course, as Jowett correctly translated them, sinews, not, *pace* Kapferer, nerves.

[3] In his translation of the *Timaeus*.

[4] Aristotle seems to use the word φλέψ indifferently to mean both arteries and veins, e.g. in the *Parts of animals* and also in the *History of animals*, but he makes a clear distinction between the 'big vein' and the 'aorta', though he uses the name φλέψ for the branches of the latter as well as those of the former. The word *artery* is only used to designate the windpipe. The *De spiritu*, which does show an Erasistratean distinction between the two kinds of blood vessel and indeed reproduces Erasistratus' three-fold skein of veins, arteries, and nerves, can hardly be counted as a genuine work. See the Introduction to the Loeb edition by W. S. Hett, p. 484.

The most striking instance of his ignorance of the new meaning of the term *artery* is perhaps the passage in the *De respiratione*, 480, where he speaks of all the veins throbbing, and throbbing simultaneously with each other. See below, p. 163.

thing is that his knowledge of the anatomy of the heart is curiously inaccurate. He was, of course, not a physician, though the son of one, and he himself informs us that he practised dissection of animals, but his description of the hearts of larger animals contains some surprising mistakes. Yet even here he would appear to mark an important stage in the advance of physiological knowledge. He seems, if Littré is correct, to have been the first of the Greek scientists we know to have placed on record the fact that the heart consists of more than one chamber, and that there are two main trunks of blood vessels, one arising from the right side of the heart, and the other from the left from which all the blood vessels in the body branch off; in other words, he was the first to lay down quite unambiguously the fact that the heart is the centre of the vascular system. It is more than just a meeting-point and more than a mere fountain. It is the ἀρχὴ καὶ πηγή, the starting-point of the blood vessels, and the starting-point of all of them, for all are in continuous connection with it, just as all bones are in continuous connection with the spine. There are no isolated bones or blood vessels. Isolated blood vessels could not retain their blood, for it is the heat from the heart which keeps the blood liquid. Moreover, blood that is separated from the heart decays.[1] Aristotle conceives the system of blood vessels as a double-trunked tree springing from a common root. All vessels (except those of the lungs) are connected either with the vena cava, the 'hollow' or 'big' vein, or with the aorta, and both vena cava and aorta have their origin in the heart.[2] That Aristotle had dissected many different animal hearts and that he was, as far as the animal kingdom was concerned, a competent comparative anatomist, can hardly be doubted. He expressly refers to the difficulty of distinguishing the chambers of the hearts of very small animals, and he tells us quite a lot about the technique of dissection, as we shall see presently. It therefore comes to us as something of a shock when he states that the hearts of the largest animals (including of course man) have three chambers or ventricles.[3] His description of the heart's position with respect to the

---

[1] Aristotle, De partibus animalium, 2. 9, 654ᵃ32–ᵇ13: ἔχει δ' ὁμοίως ἥ τε τῶν ὀστῶν καὶ ἡ τῶν φλεβῶν φύσις. ἑκατέρα γὰρ αὐτῶν ἀφ' ἑνὸς ἠργμένη συνεχής ἐστι, καὶ οὔτ' ὀστοῦν ἐστιν αὐτὸ καθ' αὑτὸ οὐδέν, ἀλλ' ἢ μόριον ὡς συνεχοῦς ἢ ἁπτόμενον καὶ προσδεδεμένον, ἵνα χρῆται ἡ φύσις καὶ ὡς ἑνὶ καὶ συνεχεῖ καὶ ὡς δυσὶ καὶ διῃρημένοις πρὸς τὴν κάμψιν. ὁμοίως δὲ καὶ φλὲψ οὐδεμία αὐτὴ καθ' αὑτήν ἐστιν, ἀλλὰ πᾶσαι μόριον μιᾶς εἰσιν. . . . εἴτε φλὲψ ἦν τις κεχωρισμένη καὶ μὴ συνεχὴς πρὸς τὴν ἀρχήν, οὐκ ἂν ἔσωζε τὸ ἐν αὐτῇ αἷμα. ἡ γὰρ ἐκείνης θερμότης κωλύει πήγνυσθαι, φαίνεται δὲ καὶ σηπόμενον τὸ χωριζόμενον. ἀρχὴ δὲ τῶν μὲν φλεβῶν ἡ καρδία, τῶν δ' ὀστῶν ἡ καλουμένη ῥάχις.

[2] Aristotle, De historia animalium, 3. 3, 513ᵃ16–22: ἔχει δὲ τοῦτον τὸν τρόπον ἡ τῶν φλεβῶν φύσις. δύο φλέβες εἰσὶν ἐν τῷ θώρακι κατὰ τὴν ῥάχιν ἐντός, ἔστι δὲ κειμένη αὐτῶν ἡ μὲν μείζων ἐν τοῖς ἔμπροσθεν, ἡ δ' ἐλάττων ὄπισθεν ταύτης, καὶ ἡ μὲν μείζων ἐν τοῖς δεξιοῖς μᾶλλον, ἡ δ' ἐλάττων ἐν τοῖς ἀριστεροῖς, ἣν καλοῦσί τινες ἀορτὴν ἐκ τοῦ τεθεᾶσθαι καὶ ἐν τοῖς τεθνεῶσιν τὸ νευρῶδες αὐτῆς μόριον. αὗται δ' ἔχουσι τὰς ἀρχὰς ἀπὸ τῆς καρδίας.

[3] De part. an. 3. 4, 666ᵇ22–3: κοιλίας δ' ἔχουσιν αἱ μὲν τῶν μεγάλων ζῴων τρεῖς, αἱ δὲ τῶν ἐλασσόνων δύο. De hist. an. 3. 3, 513ᵃ27–30: ἔχουσι δ' αἱ καρδίαι πᾶσαι μὲν κοιλίας ἐν αὑταῖς,

lungs is perhaps not quite so clear as that of Plato, though he goes into it at some length, not only in animals but also in man.

The heart lies above the lung, at the point where the windpipe divides into two, and has a fat thick membrane, where it is attached to the great vein and the aorta. And it lies with its pointed end upon the aorta. This end of it lies towards the chest in all animals which have a chest. And in all animals, whether they have a chest or not, the pointed end of the heart is always forwards, though this fact may very likely escape observation owing to some change in position while dissection is in progress. The rounded end of the heart is at the top. The pointed end is very largely fleshy and firm in texture, and there are 'nerves' or 'sinews' in its cavities. In animals other than man, which have a chest, its position is in the middle of the chest, but in man it is somewhat over to the left, inclined slightly from the division of the breasts towards the left breast in the upper part of the chest. Further, the heart is not large, and its shape as a whole is not elongated but roundish, except of course that it is pointed at the end.[1]   (trs. Peck.)

Between the right and the left ventricle, Aristotle inserts a third middle cavity or chamber, the exact position of which is not easy to identify or to visualize.

As I have already said, it has three cavities, the largest being on the right side, the smallest on the left, and the medium-sized one in the middle. All of them, even the two small ones, have a connection with the lung, and this is quite clearly visible in respect of one of them. Below, at the place of attachment from or to the largest cavity, there is a connection to the great blood vessel, and from the middle cavity there is a connection to the aorta.[2]

Thus it would appear that Aristotle considered that only one of the ventricles, the right and biggest one, was *visibly* connected with the lung. He does not actually tell us which, but we must assume that this visible connection could be none other than the pulmonary artery, which emerges

---

ἀλλ' αἱ μὲν τῶν σφόδρα μικρῶν ζῴων μόλις φανερὰν τὴν μεγίστην ἔχουσι, τὰ δὲ μέσα τῷ μεγέθει τῶν ζῴων καὶ τὴν ἑτέραν, τὰ δὲ μέγιστα τὰς τρεῖς.

[1] De hist. an. 1. 17, 496ᵃ4–19: ἡ δὲ καρδία ἔχει μὲν τρεῖς κοιλίας, κεῖται δ' ἀνωτέρω τοῦ πνεύμονος κατὰ τὴν σχίσιν τῆς ἀρτηρίας. ἔχει δ' ὑμένα πιμελώδη καὶ παχύν, ᾗ προσπέφυκε τῇ φλεβὶ τῇ μεγάλῃ καὶ τῇ ἀορτῇ. κεῖται δ' ἐπὶ τῇ ἀορτῇ κατὰ τὰ ὀξέα. κεῖται δὲ τὰ ὀξέα κατὰ τὸ στῆθος ὁμοίως ἁπάντων τῶν ζῴων, ὅσα ἔχει στῆθος. πᾶσι δ' ὁμοίως καὶ τοῖς ἔχουσι καὶ τοῖς μὴ ἔχουσι τοῦτο τὸ μόριον εἰς τὸ πρόσθεν ἔχει ἡ καρδία τὸ ὀξύ. λάθοι δ' ἂν πολλάκις διὰ τὸ μεταπίπτειν διαιρουμένων. τὸ δὲ κυρτὸν αὐτῆς ἐστιν ἄνω. ἔχει δὲ τὸ ὀξὺ σαρκῶδες ἐπὶ πολὺ καὶ πυκνόν, καὶ ἐν τοῖς κοίλοις αὐτῆς νεῦρα ἔνεστιν. κεῖται δὲ τὴν θέσιν ἐν μὲν τοῖς ἄλλοις κατὰ μέσον τὸ στῆθος, ὅσα ἔχει στῆθος, τοῖς δ' ἀνθρώποις ἐν τοῖς ἀριστεροῖς μᾶλλον, μικρὸν τῆς διαιρέσεως τῶν μαστῶν ἐγκλίνουσα εἰς τὸν ἀριστερὸν μαστὸν ἐν τῷ ἄνω μέρει τοῦ στήθους. καὶ οὔτε μεγάλη, τὸ θ' ὅλον αὐτῆς εἶδος οὐ πρόμηκές ἐστιν ἀλλὰ στρογγυλώτερον. πλὴν τὸ ἄκρον εἰς ὀξὺ συνῆκται.

[2] Ibid., 496ᵃ19–27: ἔχει δὲ κοιλίας τρεῖς, ὥσπερ εἴρηται, μεγίστην μὲν τὴν ἐν τοῖς δεξιοῖς. ἐλαχίστην δὲ τὴν ἐν ἀριστεροῖς, μέσην δὲ μεγέθει τὴν ἀνὰ μέσον. ἁπάσας δ' ἔχει, καὶ τὰς δύο μικράς, εἰς τὸν πνεύμονα τετρημένας, κατάδηλον δὲ κατὰ μίαν τῶν κοιλιῶν. κάτωθεν δ' ἐκ τῆς προσφύσεως κατὰ μὲν τὴν μεγίστην κοιλίαν ἐξήρτηται τῇ μεγάλῃ φλεβὶ [πρὸς ἣν καὶ τὸ μεσεντέριόν ἐστι], κατὰ δὲ τὴν μέσην τῇ ἀορτῇ.

from the great ventricle on the right. This passage, which I have reproduced in Dr. Peck's translation, requires rather careful examination, if
only because of the peculiar word used for the connections between the
ventricles and the lung, which does not appear at first sight at all appropriate for describing blood vessels. Its literal rendering would be
'perforated into', an expression which is far from clear—a subject which
we shall discuss at greater length later in this chapter. Nor is it any
clearer to what he is referring when he speaks of the smaller connections.
For in the next paragraph he goes on to state:

> Passages also lead into the lung from the heart, and they divide off just as
> the windpipe does, running all over the lung, and accompanying those which
> come from the windpipe. Those from the heart are uppermost. There is no
> common passage, but in virtue of their contact, they receive the breath and
> convey it to the heart, one passage leading to the right cavity and the other to
> the left.[1]

Are these passages the pulmonary veins, while the connections mentioned
in the previous paragraph are the pulmonary arteries? This would
still leave unsolved the problem of the connection with the lung of the
third ventricle, for all three are connected with it. Incidentally, may we
regard Aristotle as having anticipated Leonardo da Vinci in his
insistence that the vascular and bronchial systems are not continuous?[2]
Much must depend upon the interpretation which we give to the word
synapsis, which Dr. Peck translates as *contact*. The most natural interpretation seems to me to be that the terminal branches of the bronchioles
and the pulmonary veins coincide but are not actually continuous. We
shall meet this problem again in Galen.[3]

Aristotle, unlike Plato, knows that the lungs contain a lot of blood. He
also seems to know that the superior vena cava and the pulmonary artery
both emerge from the right ventricle, his biggest. The connecting vessel
coming out of this conveys blood to the lung, and it would appear to be
quite separate from the passages mentioned in the following paragraphs,
which convey air to the heart; for these, be it noted, connect the lungs
with both the outside ventricles, i.e. the right and the left, but not the
middle ventricle. Nor is there any hint of a pulmonary circulation. The
blood which flows from the heart to the lung would appear to have only

---

[1] *De hist. an.* I. 17, 496ᵃ28–33: φέρουσι δὲ καὶ εἰς τὸν πνεύμονα πόροι ἀπὸ τῆς καρδίας, καὶ
σχίζονται τὸν αὐτὸν τρόπον ὅνπερ ἡ ἀρτηρία, κατὰ πάντα τὸν πνεύμονα παρακολουθοῦντες τοῖς ἀπὸ
τῆς ἀρτηρίας. ἐπάνω δ' εἰσὶν οἱ ἀπὸ τῆς καρδίας πόροι. οὐδεὶς δ' ἐστὶ κοινὸς πόρος, ἀλλὰ διὰ τὴν
σύναψιν δέχονται τὸ πνεῦμα καὶ τῇ καρδίᾳ διαπέμπουσιν. φέρει γὰρ ὁ μὲν εἰς τὸ δεξιὸν κοῖλον
τῶν πόρων, ὁ δ' εἰς τὸ ἀριστερόν.

[2] Leonardo da Vinci, Q. ii. 1ʳ: 'It seems impossible that any air can penetrate into the
heart through the trachea.' K. D. Keele, *Leonardo da Vinci on Movement of the Heart and Blood*
(London, 1952), p. 50.

[3] See below, p. 308.

one function, that of nourishment. For Aristotle, nourishment is all-important. The viscera are merely deposits left by the current of blood flowing outward from the heart in the blood vessels.[1] We thus have the arrangement that the great ventricle and the smallest ventricle as well as the middle one are connected with the lungs. The middle ventricle is also connected with the aorta.

In the *De somno et vigilia*, we find a rather different arrangement. Here it is the left or smallest, not the middle, ventricle which is connected with the aorta, the middle cavity only being directly connected with the other two.[2] This, as Platt has observed,[3] is the Aristotelian theory criticized by Galen. As to the three ventricles, the largest is on top, while the smallest on the left would be the lowest. The right ventricle is much larger than the other two, the middle one being somewhat larger than the smallest. All three ventricles in the account given in the *History of animals* are connected with the lungs, but it is not at all clear whether this also holds good of the arrangement envisaged in the *De somno*, which does not deal with the connections between the heart and the lungs at all; but presumably the scheme outlined in the great biological works is assumed, since we have no indication to the contrary, even if the relation between the three ventricles is rather different. The problem then is to try to envisage how he arrived at this triple connection. The only suggestion that I have been able to arrive at is that he observed the division of the pulmonary veins, two going to each lung, and concluded that their two branches emerged from different ventricles. This would seem to fit his general scheme without too much difficulty.

Of the three ventricles, the right contains the most blood and the most heat, and the left the least, while the middle one contains a middling portion of both. But it contains the purest blood, since it is the source or principle ($\dot{\alpha}\rho\chi\dot{\eta}$) of the blood in the other two. Moreover, the middle ventricle is practically motionless, and the blood which it contains is intermediate between that in the other two, as regards both its amount and the heat which it contains (I had almost yielded to the temptation of saying the temperature), because the source or fountain must remain as calm as possible, and this condition is only secured when the blood is pure, and when it is middling both in capacity and in heat.[4]

---

[1] *De part. an.* 2. 1, 647ᵇ1–4: αἱματικὴ γὰρ ἡ φύσις πάντων αὐτῶν διὰ τὸ τὴν θέσιν ἔχειν ἐπὶ πόροις φλεβικοῖς καὶ διαλήψεσιν. καθάπερ οὖν ῥέοντος ὕδατος ἰλύς, τἆλλα σπλάγχνα τῆς διὰ φλεβῶν ῥύσεως τοῦ αἵματος προχεύματά ἐστιν.

[2] *De somno et vigilia*, 3, 458ᵃ15–19: παντὸς δὲ τοῦ αἵματος ἀρχή, ὥσπερ εἴρηται καὶ ἐνταῦθα καὶ ἐν ἄλλοις, ἡ καρδία. τῶν δ' ἐν τῇ καρδίᾳ ἑκατέρας τῆς θαλάμης κοινὴ ἡ μέση. ἐκείνων δ' ἑκατέρα δέχεται ἐξ ἑκατέρας τῆς φλεβός, τῆς τε μεγάλης καλουμένης καὶ τῆς ἀορτῆς.

[3] A. Platt, 'Aristotle on the heart', in C. Singer, *Studies in the History and Method of Science*, (Oxford, 1921), 2. 520–32.

[4] *De part. an.* 3. 4, 667ᵃ1–6: τούτων δὲ πλεῖστον μὲν αἷμα καὶ θερμότατον ἔχουσιν αἱ δεξιαί . . . ἐλάχιστον δὲ καὶ ψυχρότατον αἱ ἀριστεραί· μέσον δ' αἱ μέσαι τῷ πλήθει καὶ θερμότητι, καθαρώτατον

The problem of Aristotle's third ventricle has exercised many critics from the days of Galen onwards, among them no less distinguished persons than Vesalius and Thomas Henry Huxley, not to mention continental historians of anatomy, like von Töply, and more recently the short-lived Dr. Mühsam, who propounded a new theory on this subject. All of these, even Huxley, have been rather hard put to it to explain how the Father of comparative anatomy, if we may so call him, could have arrived at this curious conclusion, which to a superficial inspection seems such an elementary mistake. But perhaps the most interesting feature in the situation is the fact that the explanations given even in modern times do not agree with one another. And none of them, in my opinion, appears to be wholly convincing.

Galen, impressed no doubt by the fact that the right ventricle is more capacious than the left and possibly realizing some of the consequences of Aristotle's method of dissection (which involved death by strangulation after the animal had been kept a long time without food[1]— a procedure which left the right auricle and right ventricle gorged with blood and the left side of the heart empty), thought that he mistook the right ventricle to consist of two separate chambers, basing his explanation, as Platt observed,[2] on the description given in the *De somno et vigilia* rather than that found in the *History*, or the *Parts of animals*.

The body of the heart [Galen tells us in his work *On the dissection of veins and arteries*] has two arteries which spread round over it, one of which, the bigger one, covers the largest portion of its area, while the other is distributed chiefly over that area where Aristotle thought the third ventricle is situated. This ventricle is really a portion of the right ventricle, that part which lies in the flat or broad part of the heart. It is not a third separate ventricle. And from it grows out the vein which splits up into the lung, whose coat is the same as that of the artery [i.e. the pulmonary artery].[3]

This arrangement seems a little difficult to envisage, since we must, I suppose, assume that the lower half of the right ventricle was still the largest, the left ventricle being the middle one; though this does not seem consistent with his statement that the smallest ventricle is on the left; nor

δέ. δεῖ γὰρ τὴν ἀρχὴν ὅτι μάλιστα ἠρεμεῖν, τοιαύτη δ' ἂν εἴη καθαροῦ τοῦ αἵματος ὄντος, τῷ πλήθει καὶ θερμότητι μέσου.

[1] *De hist. an.* 3. 3, 513ᵃ13–14, where Aristotle remarks that the only method of making veins visible in dissection is to combine strangulation with starvation: χαλεπῆς δ' οὔσης, ὥσπερ εἴρηται, τῆς θεωρίας, ἐν μόνοις τοῖς ἀποπνιγομένοις τῶν ζῴων προλεπτυνθεῖσιν ἔστιν ἱκανῶς καταμαθεῖν.

[2] Platt, op. cit., p. 523.

[3] Galen, *De ven. et art. diss.* 9, K. ii. 817: καὶ μέντοι καὶ δι' αὐτὸ τὸ τῆς καρδίας σῶμα περιχεομένας ἐν κύκλῳ δύο ἀρτηρίας ἔχει, τὴν μὲν ἑτέραν, τὴν μείζω, τὸ πλεῖστον αὐτῆς διαπλέκουσαν, τὴν δὲ ἑτέραν εἰς ἐκεῖνα μάλιστα διανεμομένην, ἔνθα τὴν τρίτην ἐνόμιζεν εἶναι κοιλίαν ὁ Ἀριστοτέλης. αὕτη δέ ἐστιν ἡ κατὰ πλατὺ τῆς καρδίας μόριον οὖσα τῆς δεξιᾶς, οὐκ ἄλλη τρίτη τις. πέφυκε δ' ἐξ αὐτῆς εἰς τὸν πνεύμονα κατασχιζομένη φλέψ, ἧς ὁ χιτὼν ὁ αὐτός ἐστι τῷ τῆς ἀρτηρίας.

can we accept Platt's view that the left ventricle was the largest, and the lower part of the right ventricle the middle one, seeing that in the *History of animals* Aristotle is quite certain that the largest ventricle is the right, and the smallest that on the left, with the middle-sized one between them.[1]

Vesalius, on the other hand, thought that Aristotle regarded the left ventricle as consisting of two chambers, being misled by the flap of the mitral valve in his dissection into thinking it constituted a third chamber, a pardonable error when compared with his other mistaken opinion that the number of ventricles depended on the size of the species.[2]

Huxley, whose opinion was followed by Ogle in his edition of the *Parts of animals*, took the view that Aristotle thought that the left auricle was the smallest ventricle, the left ventricle his middle ventricle, and the right ventricle his biggest ventricle. He based this opinion on observations from dissecting animals which had died from suffocation, an overdose of chloroform for example.

If anyone will lay open the thorax of a dog or rabbit which has been killed by chloroform, he will at once see why Aristotle adopted this view. For the inferior vena cava, the right auricle, and the superior vena cava, and the innominate vein, distended with blood seem to form one column to which the heart is attached as a sort of appendage. This column is, as Aristotle says, vein above and vein below, the upper and lower divisions being connected διὰ τοῦ κοιλοῦ τοῦ μέσου—or by means of the intervening cavity or chamber— which is the right auricle.

But when from the four cavities of the heart recognized by us moderns, one is excluded, there remain three—which is just what Aristotle says. The solution of the difficulty is in fact as absurdly simple as that presented by the egg of Columbus . . . The three cavities are just those which remain if the right auricle is omitted . . . For in a suffocated animal the 'right cavity' which is directly connected with the great vein and is obviously the right ventricle, being distended with blood, will look much larger than the middle cavity, which, since it gives rise to the aorta, can only be the left ventricle. And this again will appear larger than the thin and collapsed left auricle, which must be Aristotle's left cavity inasmuch as this cavity is said to be connected by πόροι to the lung.[3]

Huxley's solution is admirably simple, but unfortunately too simple to account for all the facts. Later tradition, and in all probability that of

[1] See the passage quoted above, p. 123, n. 2.

[2] The passage cited in this connection by Platt, op. cit., from the *De fabrica corporis humani*, vi. 12, reads as follows: 'Caeterum iste in sinistro cordis ventriculo ad septi eminentissimam sedem atque ad magnae arteriae orificium ascensus post dextram orificii venalis arteriae membranam, inter dissecandum latens conscendensque, Aristoteli imposuit, ut inibi tertium cordis ventriculum constituerit, illum arteriae principium esse recensens. Quod sane multo minus incusandum venerit, quam quod ventriculorum cordis numerum pro animalium mole variari scripserit.'

[3] T. H. Huxley, 'On certain errors respecting the structure of the heart attributed to Aristotle', *Nature*, 21 (London) (1880), 1–5.

Aristotle's own time, looked upon the auricles as part of the blood vessels, their terminal processes, not, with the exception of Herophilus and his school, as part of the heart itself, as Huxley was also well aware. His explanation of the reasons why Aristotle treated the two auricles differently does not really sound very convincing. He says:

The reason why Aristotle considered the left auricle to be part of the heart, while he merged the right auricle in the great vein, is obviously the small relative size of the venous trunks and their sharper demarcation from the auricles.

It seems to me to be a rather unsatisfactory argument to maintain that the gorged right auricle should be excluded from the heart, while the small left auricle should be included in it. But Huxley is able to give a rather more convincing explanation of Aristotle's remark that in animals of medium size only two of the ventricles are perceptible.[1]

If the left chamber is so small a thing as the auricle, that is why Aristotle could not make it out in animals of intermediate size. If the left ventricle is the middle chamber, that is why Aristotle says that the aorta comes from the middle chamber. And should it be objected that he says his middle chamber is much smaller than the right one, the answer is that it really would appear to be, in an animal which had been suffocated. And the right auricle is entirely ignored by him, because in a suffocated animal, it would appear to be part of the vena cava.

Aristotle's description of the vessels leading out of the heart and their mutual relations is very difficult to follow, especially where the lungs are concerned, and Huxley has some difficulty in reconciling his description of the vessel 'which is obviously the pulmonary artery' as a branch of the great vein.

However this difficulty also disappears if we reflect that in Aristotle's way of looking at the matter, the line of demarcation between the great vein and the heart coincides with the right auriculo-ventricular aperture; and that inasmuch as the conical prolongation of the right ventricle which leads to the pulmonary artery lies close in front of the auricle, its base may very easily (as the figure shows) be regarded as part of the general opening of the great vein into the right ventricle. In fact it is clear that Aristotle, having failed to notice the valves of the heart did not distinguish the part of the right ventricle from which the pulmonary artery arises from the proper trunk of the artery on the one hand, and from the right auricle on the other. Thus the root, as we may call it, of the pulmonary artery and the right auricle taken together are spoken of as 'part of the great vein which extends upwards', and as the vena azygos was one branch of this, so 'the vein to the lung' was another branch of it. But the latter branch being given off close to the connection of the great vein

---

[1] *De hist. an.* 3. 3, 513^{a}27–30, quoted above, p. 122, n. 3.

with the ventricle, was also counted as one of the two πόροι by which the heart (that is to say the right ventricle, the left ventricle, and the left auricle of our nomenclature) communicates with the lung.

Huxley does not include among his citations the account of the *De somno et vigilia*, in which the aorta is made to emerge from the left ventricle, which in this treatise (which is not, after all, concerned except incidentally with the heart) is not stated to be the smallest. Nor is he able to explain the statements made in the *History of animals*, both in the first and in the third book, that all three ventricles are connected with the lung.[1] The connection of the middle ventricle, from which the aorta emerges, with the lung remains an unresolved puzzle which Huxley is unable to account for in a satisfactory manner. He can only tell us:

I can only imagine then, that so far as this passage applies to the left ventricle, it merely refers to the indirect communication of that cavity with the vessels of the lungs through the left auricle.

But the use of the words τετρημένας, συντέτρηνται seems to me to imply quite clearly a direct connection. And the notion that Aristotle believed the pulmonary artery to be a branch of the great vein strikes me as rather unlikely in view of the fact that he recognizes the structural difference of the great vein from the aorta with such precision. It was no doubt this fact which led D'Arcy Thompson to propound quite a different interpretation of the meaning of Aristotle's text. Whereas Ogle, quite independently of Huxley, arrived at the notion that the third ventricle was really the left auricle,[2] D'Arcy Thompson thought that Galen had reached the correct conclusion in supposing that Aristotle's mistake was to divide the right ventricle into two compartments. He could not possibly have regarded the pulmonary artery as a branch of the great vein. He is puzzled by the fact that Aristotle in his description of the great vessels connected with the heart mentions only two, the aorta and the great vein. Neither the pulmonary artery nor the pulmonary veins are clearly described.

A chief cause of difficulty in interpreting the whole account is the lack of precise reference to the pulmonary artery. We should have expected two great sinewy tubes of equal size running side by side and leading, one from one, and one from the other side of the heart to have been indicated clearly above all other landmarks: but of the two great vessels connected with the heart, one is the aorta, and the other . . . is undoubtedly the vena cava; the pulmonary artery must be included under or indicated in connection with one or other of these two.

[1] *De hist. an.* 1. 17, 496ᵃ22–4: ἁπάσας δ᾽ ἔχει, καὶ τὰς δύο μικράς, εἰς τὸν πνεύμονα τετρημένας, κατάδηλον δὲ κατὰ μίαν τῶν κοιλιῶν. Cf. ibid. 3. 3, 513ᵃ35–6: συντέτρηνται μέντοι πᾶσαι αὗται πρὸς τὸν πνεύμονα, ἀλλ᾽ ἄδηλοι [αἱ τρήσεις add. Dittmeyer] διὰ σμικρότητα τῶν πόρων πλὴν μιᾶς.
[2] See his note on the *Parts of Animals* 3. 4 (666ᵇ22) in vol. 5 of the Oxford Translation of Aristotle (ed. Smith and Ross, 1912).

We may on the one hand argue (as Huxley and others have done) that the pulmonary artery, connected as it is with the right side of the heart, was associated by Aristotle with the veins that are likewise connected with that side; and so that his great vessel corresponds to the superior and inferior venae cavae together with the right auricle, that the largest chamber was the right ventricle, that it was in this ventricle that the blood 'broadens its channel as a river widening into a lake', and that the pulmonary artery was that by which the great blood vessel comes out as a blood vessel again . . .

This brings Aristotle's description into close agreement with the facts, but it is nevertheless difficult to accept for the following reasons:

1. It is hard to suppose that Aristotle knew or believed the venae cavae and pulmonary artery to be in such close a connection, or was aware that the venous circulation of the blood was continued directly through the heart into the pulmonary circulation;

2. To include the pulmonary artery in Aristotle's enumeration of the veins is to lose the force of his well-marked distinction between the sinewy texture of artery and the membranous texture of vein;

3. The aorta is not 'much narrower' than the pulmonary artery, but as near as may be of the same size;

4. We are afterwards told that the aorta and its branches follow the whole course already ascribed to the veins, including therefore a distribution to the lungs.

It seems to me much more likely that the pulmonary artery and the aorta, both alike empty of blood in the dead subject and so similar in texture and appearance to one another, and so plainly different from the veins, were together spoken of as 'the aorta', in other words, as the arterial system: though this hypothesis will force us to admit that Aristotle did not detect the simple fact of these two vessels communicating with opposite sides of the heart . . .

According to this view, the great vein which passes through the heart and is continued again is simply the vena cava, whose inferior and superior portions meet 'as in a reservoir' in the right auricle, and are thereby attached to the right ventricle, the largest of cavities. The part of the great vein above the heart includes the pulmonary veins (their distinctness from the superior vena cava and their communication with the other auricle being overlooked); and these veins stretch away to the lung and to the point of its attachment to the artery, while the other portion, that is to say the superior vena cava itself, goes on towards the backbone and splits into the two innominate veins from which come the jugular and sub-clavian branches. With all this system of veins an arterial system, the pulmonary artery and the branches of the aorta, runs parallel.[1]

As to the third ventricle, D'Arcy Thompson remarks:

Galen suggests that Aristotle's middle cavity was a portion of the right chamber. I am inclined to accept this hypothesis as a partial solution of the

---

[1] D'Arcy Thompson, note to the passage in *Hist. an.* 3. 3, 513[a]30 ff., in the Oxford translation, vol. 4 (1910).

riddle, and to suppose that this was the middle chamber in which διάκρισις took place, that part of the aorta or arterial system now known as the pulmonary artery opening into it.

Plain to be seen as the aorta is elsewhere, it is concealed in the immediate neighbourhood of the heart by the pulmonary artery, which is the most conspicuous of all vessels.

Finally, D'Arcy Thompson calls attention to the well-known passage in the *Hippocratic corpus* in the *De carnibus* which Poschenrieder regards as being post-Aristotelian,[1] describing the two main blood vessels, the aorta and the great vein. This treatise, which follows Aristotle pretty closely, gives us 'no possible opportunity to suppose that the pulmonary artery was ever associated with the venous system'.

We may also add, that were the pulmonary artery not as naturally associated with the aorta as the arteries are easy to distinguish from the veins, the view could never have arisen that the veins sprang from the liver and the arteries from the heart.

D'Arcy Thompson's view that Aristotle regarded the term *aorta* as applying to the arterial system as such, and not merely to what we now call the aorta, may perhaps receive some measure of support from the *De corde*, where in one passage the author speaks of two aortae, meaning quite clearly the pulmonary artery and the aorta proper.[2] But it does not seem to me that D'Arcy Thompson's interpretation can be successful, as he himself recognizes, in making anatomical sense of Aristotle's text. The connection of his first cavity with the lungs remains difficult to explain as he realized, even if we do regard the branch from the great vein to the lung as representing the pulmonary veins rather than the pulmonary arteries. Nor are we any better off in making sense of the passage where Aristotle is made to say that the (great) vein stretches through the heart into the aorta, whichever way we interpret that word. Huxley took the passage to mean 'stretches toward the aorta', and I suggest later that a possible translation would be 'on to', though this is not a very satisfactory rendering of the word εἰς. There may however be something to say for the idea that Aristotle may have been aware of a double system of blood vessels in the lung, though there is no explicit mention of the two systems of 'roots' accompanying the ramifications of the trachea. We do however

---

[1] Franz Poschenrieder, *Die naturwissenschaftlichen Schriften des Aristoteles in ihrem Verhältnis zu den Büchern der hippokratischen Sammlung* (Programm der königlichen Studienanstalt Bamberg, I, 1887), p. 25: 'Bedenkt man nun, daß Aristoteles Hist. an. III c 3 ausdrücklich versichert, seine Ansicht über den Ausgangspunkt der Adern sei etwas Neues, berücksichtigt man ferner, daß die von dem Hippokratiker gebotene Beschreibung der Blutgefäße gegenüber jener ausführlichen des Aristoteles doch mehr als Auszug aus letzterer erscheint, so kommt man zu dem Schlusse, daß die Schrift *De carnibus* nacharistotelischen Ursprungs sein müsse.'

[2] 'Hippocrates', *De corde*; see the passage quoted above, p. 88, n. 1.

know that Aristotle did not share the view of Praxagoras and Erasistratus that the pulmonary veins contained, like the arteries in general, only air or *pneuma*, since he informs us that all the ventricles of the heart contain blood. But we must not be misled into thinking that he had any inkling of a pulmonary transit.

Aubert and Wimmer, the German editors of the *History of animals*, in the middle of the last century propounded quite a different solution. They thought that Aristotle made the two auricles into his third ventricle by simply disregarding the existence of the auricular septum. This, they contended, would agree with Aristotle's account of the relative sizes of the three cavities, the two auricles combined being the largest, the right ventricle the middle cavity, and the left ventricle the smallest.[1] But this appears to me to be most unlikely. It does not seem to me at all probable that he should have done this in view of the gorged and swollen right auricle and the thin and empty left auricle; moreover the connections with the lung do not work out correctly, for the middle cavity would be connected with the lung it is true, but the left cavity, the left ventricle, would only communicate with the lung indirectly, through the middle ventricle.

Dr. Erich Mühsam, in a posthumously published essay,[2] propounded yet another solution to the puzzle of the third ventricle. His theory was that Aristotle's largest ventricle represented the whole of the right side of the heart, auricle and ventricle combined, the left ventricle being the middle cavity, and the smallest cavity being the left auricle. He accepted the notion that the pulmonary artery and vena cava emerged from the cavity as a single channel in Aristotle's opinion. The superior vena cava and pulmonary artery emerge from the right auricle-ventricle as a combined great vein (*ungeteilte und große Ader*) and run as such to the proximity of the lung and the attachment of the aorta to the pericardium. There the vena cava parts from the pulmonary artery and throws off the azygos vein. This hypothesis does nothing to diminish Thompson's objection that Aristotle could never have confused the great vein with the pulmonary artery. Nor does it help to solve the problem of the connection of all three ventricles with the lung; for here the left ventricle is devoid of direct connection with it.

---

[1] H. Aubert and Fr. Wimmer, *Aristoteles'* De animalium Historia etc. . . . *Thierkunde, kritischberichtigter Text mit deutscher Übersetzung, etc.* (Leipzig, 1868), note to vol. 1, p. 319: 'Daß Aristoteles nur die Herzhöhlen erkannte, während doch das Herz zwei Vorhöfen und zwei Kammern bei den Säugethieren besitzt, kann nur darauf beruhen, daß er die Scheidewand der Vorhöfe übersah. Dieser Annahme schließen sich die folgenden Angaben am besten an, und hier ist wohl der Irrthum am ersten zu erwarten. Die μεγίστη würde also den beiden Vorhöfen, die μέση der rechten Kammer, die ἐλαχίστη der linken Kammer gleichzusetzen sein: damit würden auch die Angaben über die Größenverhältnisse harmonieren.'

[2] E. Mühsam, 'Zur Lehre vom Bau und Bedeutung des menschlichen Herzes im klassischen Altertum', *Janus* 15 (1910), 797–831.

Perhaps after all, it might be simpler to accept the fact that Aristotle just made a mistake, without puzzling too long over the reason why he did so, or the exact nature of the mistake itself.[1]

Aristotle's descriptions of the heart and the blood vessels, though they show (as Littré was perhaps the first modern scholar to indicate, and Huxley recognized) a very important step forward, representing as they do very great progress on his predecessors, need not, indeed cannot, be construed into correctness. We must therefore content ourselves with reproducing the relevant texts. There may, however, be some sense in reminding ourselves that Aristotle, Father of comparative anatomy though he was, had interests so widely spread over the whole field of knowledge that perfect accuracy in all of them is hardly to be expected. Moreover, it is difficult to resist the temptation to relate his anatomical doctrine of the three ventricles to one of his fundamental philosophical principles, the doctrine of the mean, which dominated Hellenic ethics no less than Greek aesthetics. Aristotle, indeed, seems to us almost obsessed with the notion, and made it the principle not only of virtue, but also of good constitutional government. We may therefore perhaps be excused for suspecting that he did not always obey strictly the principle laid down by the great French physiologist Claude Bernard, to take extreme precaution not to find what you are looking for. Moreover Aristotle, no less than Plato, was dominated by a teleological conception of nature. Nature does nothing superfluous or without a purpose,[2] and since there are two principal ἀρχηγοί blood vessels, it was better that their sources should be separate also. But this would have meant that the two main blood vessels contained separately two different kinds of blood. But though its qualities vary somewhat in the different parts of the body, blood is only of one kind. It was therefore better that there should be a middle ventricle as the original source of the blood in the other two, for it was better that there should be one source rather than many.[3] This teleological argument

[1] Galen, who is anxious to excuse him though fully conscious of the enormity of the error, reminds us that Aristotle was not after all a 'professional' anatomist, working as a full-time specialist in this field. If men like Marinus, who have devoted their entire lives to this study, can still make mistakes, an error can be pardoned to the pioneer amateur. See De anat. admin. vii. 10, K. ii. 621: καὶ θαυμαστὸν οὐδέν, ἄλλα τε πολλὰ κατὰ τὰς ἀνατομὰς Ἀριστοτέλη διαμαρτεῖν, καὶ ἡγεῖσθαι, τρεῖς ἔχειν κοιλίας ἐπὶ τῶν μεγάλων ζώων τὴν καρδίαν. ὅτι μὲν οὖν ἀγύμναστος ὢν ἐν ταῖς ἀνατομαῖς ἐσφάλη περὶ τὴν τῶν μορίων εὕρεσιν, οὔτε θαυμάζειν χρή, καὶ συγγιγνώσκειν αὐτῷ προσήκει. ὅπου γὰρ οἱ τὸν ὅλον ἑαυτῶν βίον ἀναθέντες τῇ θεωρίᾳ ταύτῃ, καθάπερ ὁ Μαρῖνος, ἥμαρτον πολλά, τί χρὴ νομίζειν συμβαίνειν τοῖς ἐξαίφνης μὲν ἐπ' αὐτὴν ἐλθοῦσι;

[2] Aristotle, De part. an. 4. 11, 691ᵇ4: οὐδὲν γὰρ ποιεῖ περίεργον ἡ φύσις.

[3] Ibid., 3. 4, 666ᵇ23-33: δεῖ γὰρ εἶναι τόπον τινὰ τῆς καρδίας καὶ ὑποδοχὴν τοῦ πρώτου αἵματος . . . διὰ δὲ τὸ τὰς ἀρχηγοὺς φλέβας δύο εἶναι, τήν τε μεγάλην καλουμένην καὶ τὴν ἀορτήν, ἑκατέρας δ' οὔσης ἀρχῆς τῶν φλεβῶν, καὶ διαφορὰς ἐχουσῶν . . . βέλτιον καὶ τὰς ἀρχὰς αὐτῶν κεχωρίσθαι. τοῦτο δ' ἂν εἴη διφυοῦς ὄντος τοῦ αἵματος καὶ κεχωρισμένου. διόπερ ἐν οἷς ἐνδέχεται, δύ' εἰσὶν ὑποδοχαί. ἐνδέχεται δ' ἐν τοῖς μεγάλοις. τούτων γὰρ ἔχουσι καὶ αἱ καρδίαι μέγεθος. ἔτι δὲ βέλτιον τρεῖς εἶναι τὰς κοιλίας, ὅπως ᾖ μία ἀρχὴ κοινή.

is supported by another, which to modern ears seems very strange. The heart's position is in the ruler's place, in the middle, rather higher than lower, and rather in front than behind. For in man, as in all other animals, the most honourable organ is put by nature in the most honourable position, unless she is prevented from doing so. The clearest proof of this is found in man. Nature therefore intends that all the necessary organs should be in the middle. The lower portion of this middle region is the digestive tract. But limbs in animals grow in many different positions, for they are not necessary to life; so that when they are removed, the animal can still go on living; as well as when they have an extra one.[1]

These typically metaphysical arguments were inspired by two main considerations. The heart with the blood that it contains is the first organ to be formed in the embryo,[2] and it is the only organ which contains its own blood supply. The blood contained in all the others is supplied by and contained in the blood vessels. Indeed, in some respects Aristotle seems inclined to treat the heart as being part of the blood vessels, in one place indeed he calls it a part of them,[3] and he insists that its character is 'vein-like', that is, of the same kind as the blood vessels.[4] Finally, we cannot take leave of Aristotle's anatomical description of the heart without mentioning his other famous feature, the bone in the heart, a somewhat contradictory peculiarity, since it does not appear to have any connection with the spine. Aristotle tells us that none of the hearts that he has examined has a bone, except those of horses and a certain kind of ox. In these creatures the heart, owing to its great size, is provided with a bone in order to give it support.[5] We shall meet this bone again in Galen, who explains its real anatomical nature.[6]

As a final note of credit to Aristotle's observation we may add that he correctly observed the sulci which he compares with seams.[7]

---

[1] De part. an. 3. 4, 665ᵇ18–27: ἔχει δὲ καὶ ἡ θέσις αὐτῆς ἀρχικὴν χώραν. περὶ μέσον γάρ, μᾶλλον δ' ἐν τῷ ἄνω ἢ κάτω καὶ ἔμπροσθεν ἢ ὄπισθεν. ἐν τοῖς γὰρ τιμιωτέροις τὸ τιμιώτερον καθίδρυκεν ἡ φύσις, οὗ μή τι κωλύει μεῖζον. ἐμφανέστατον δὲ τὸ λεχθέν ἐστιν ἐπὶ τῶν ἀνθρώπων, βούλεται δὲ καὶ ἐν τοῖς ἄλλοις ὁμολόγως ἐν μέσῳ κεῖσθαι τοῦ ἀναγκαίου σώματος, τούτου δὲ πέρας ᾗ τὰ περιττώματα ἀποκρίνεται. τὰ δὲ κῶλα πέφυκεν ἄλλοις ἄλλως, καὶ οὐκ ἔστι τῶν πρὸς τὸ ζῆν ἀναγκαίων, διὸ καὶ ἀφαιρουμένων ζῷσιν. δῆλον δ' ὡς οὐδὲ προστιθέμενα φθείρει.

[2] Ibid., 666ᵃ20: ἐν γὰρ τοῖς ἐμβρύοις εὐθέως ἡ καρδία φαίνεται κινουμένη τῶν μορίων.

[3] De hist. an. 3. 3, 513ᵃ22–5, where, speaking of the 'great vein' and the aorta, he says: αὗται δ' ἔχουσι τὰς ἀρχὰς ἀπὸ τῆς καρδίας. διὰ μὲν γὰρ τῶν ἄλλων σπλάγχνων, ᾗ τυγχάνουσι τείνουσαι, ὅλαι δι' αὐτῶν διέρχονται σωζόμεναι καὶ οὖσαι φλέβες, ἡ δὲ καρδία ὥσπερ μόριον αὐτῶν ἐστι, καὶ μᾶλλον τῆς ἐμπροσθίας καὶ μείζονος. De part. an. 3. 4, 665ᵇ31–3: ὥσπερ δ' ἐλέχθη, διὰ μὲν τῶν ἄλλων σπλάγχνων διέχουσιν αἱ φλέβες, διὰ δὲ τῆς καρδίας οὐ διατείνει φλέψ. ὅθεν καὶ δῆλον ὅτι μόριον καὶ ἀρχὴ τῶν φλεβῶν ἐστιν ἡ καρδία.

[4] De part. an. 3. 4, 665ᵇ16–17: καὶ ἡ φύσις αὐτῆς φλεβώδης ὡς ὁμογενοῦς οὔσης.

[5] Ibid., 666ᵇ18–21: ἔστι δ' ἀνόστεος πάντων ὅσα καὶ ἡμεῖς τεθεάμεθα, πλὴν τῶν ἵππων καὶ γένους τινὸς βοῶν. τούτοις δὲ διὰ τὸ μέγεθος οἷον ἐρείσματος χάριν ὀστοῦν ὕπεστι, καθάπερ καὶ τοῖς ὅλοις σώμασιν.   [6] See below, p. 280.

[7] De part. an. 3. 4, 667ᵃ7–9: ἔχουσι δὲ καὶ διάρθρωσίν τινα αἱ καρδίαι παραπλησίαν ταῖς ῥαφαῖς. οὐκ εἰσὶ δὲ συναφεῖς ὡς τινος ἐκ πλειόνων συνθέτου, ἀλλὰ καθάπερ εἴπομεν, διαρθρώσει μᾶλλον.

Aristotle's doctrine of the origin of blood is not altogether easy to understand. Though he, of course, agrees with the doctrine that blood is produced from the intake of food and drink, and that it is consumed by the organs and the tissues, he gives us no clear indication of how the transformation is brought about. The original or first blood, τὸ πρῶτον αἷμα, comes into being in the heart, and it is only in that organ that the final stages of sanguinification take place. Blood flows from the heart to the other parts of the body, it does not come to the heart from elsewhere.[1] No circulation for the Master of those that Know. We have already noted that Aristotle was acquainted with two varieties of blood, a purer or cleaner variety, and one less clean. For the blood in the right ventricle is the hottest—a theory very different from the one inherited by Galen, perhaps from Diocles, in which it is the left ventricle which is the seat of the *pneuma* and of the innate heat. The cleanest as well as the best blood is found in the middle ventricle and it is cooler than that in the right, and hotter than that in the left. But the attempt to link the differing kinds of blood with the arterial and venous systems is not really feasible. For though in the *De partibus animalium*, as we have seen, he argues that the two kinds of blood vessels have different characters because they carry different kinds of blood,[2] in the *De somno* we are told that the two kinds of blood have different locations in the body. The blood in the head is the rarest and purest, while that in the lower parts of the body is thick and turbid.[3] A somewhat similar account is also found in the *History of animals*, where the blood in the lower parts is thicker and blacker.[4] The two kinds of blood in the *De somno* are separated off from each other in the middle ventricle, which does not communicate directly with either the vena cava or the aorta. We may well ask why the purest blood should go to the brain, since according to Aristotle the brain is a less honourable organ than the heart, and plays quite a subordinate part in his physiological scheme, as an organ of refrigeration and for the secretion of phlegm. The answer Aristotle gives to this question is that to temper the heat and boiling in the heart, the brain must have a moderate amount of heat which is supplied by the blood vessels in the meninges, which are not

[1] Ibid., 666ᵃ3–9: ἐν ταύτῃ γὰρ μόνῃ τῶν σπλάγχνων καὶ τοῦ σώματος αἷμα ἄνευ φλεβῶν ἐστι, τῶν δ' ἄλλων μορίων ἕκαστον ἐν ταῖς φλεψὶν ἔχει τὸ αἷμα. καὶ τοῦτ' εὐλόγως. ἐκ τῆς καρδίας γὰρ ἐποχετεύεται (καὶ) εἰς τὰς φλέβας, εἰς δὲ τὴν καρδίαν οὐκ ἄλλοθεν. αὕτη γάρ ἐστιν ἀρχὴ καὶ πηγὴ τοῦ αἵματος ἢ ὑποδοχὴ πρώτη. But in the *De somno* we have rather a different picture. Here in the *De somno*, 3, 456ᵇ2–5 the products of digestion seem to be transformed into blood: τῆς μὲν οὖν θύραθεν τροφῆς εἰσιούσης εἰς τοὺς δεκτικοὺς τόπους γίνεται ἡ ἀναθυμίασις εἰς τὰς φλέβας, ἐκεῖ δὲ μεταβάλλουσα ἐξαιματοῦται καὶ πορεύεται ἐπὶ τὴν ἀρχήν.

[2] See the passage quoted above, p. 125, n. 5.

[3] *De somno*, 3, 458ᵃ13–19: ἐστὶ δὲ λεπτότατον μὲν αἷμα καὶ καθαρώτατον τὸ ἐν τῇ κεφαλῇ, παχύτατον δε καὶ θολερώτατον τὸ ἐν τοῖς κάτω μέρεσιν . . . τῶν δ' ἐν τῇ καρδίᾳ ἑκατέρας τῆς θαλάμης κοινὴ ἡ μέση . . . ἐν δὲ τῇ μέσῃ γίνεται ἡ διάκρισις.

[4] *De hist. an.* 3. 19, 521ᵃ2–5: ἔχει δὲ λεπτότατον μὲν αἷμα καὶ καθαρώτατον ἄνθρωπος . . . καὶ ἐν τοῖς κάτω δὲ μορίοις ἢ ἐν τοῖς ἄνω παχύτερον τὸ αἷμα καὶ μελάντερον.

few and large but small and multitudinous, and contain only thin and clear, not thick and turbid blood.[1] Moreover, another function of the brain is to produce sleep, which is caused by the vaporization of the products of digestion, their cooling in the brain, and their descent in a dense mass.[2] Sleep in all blooded animals is a physiological necessity, the brain therefore exists in order to preserve the organism as a whole.[3]

Before the Alexandrian school did its great anatomical work of discovery, Greek physicians had already worked out, largely under the influence of the Cnidian school, some idea of the heart as distributing blood mixed with *pneuma* to the various organs of the body through the blood vessels, and it was Praxagoras, the master of Herophilus, who had distinguished the system of arteries from that of the veins, a distinction not yet realized by Aristotle, though he had apparently known that all the blood vessels are derived from two main trunks rising out of different chambers of the heart. But Aristotle seems to have had only the most superficial notions of how the heart works. That it beats or 'jumps' had been noted, and that this beating was continuous throughout life, but this was only very vaguely associated with the propulsion of the blood, as we shall have reason to observe presently. With the interior structure of the organ his acquaintance was very superficial. The valves, for example, are nowhere mentioned.

To understand his conception of the way the heart, the most important organ of the body, functions, we must examine briefly his ideas about what blood is, what it does, and how it is produced. To take the latter first, Peck has explained the process as follows:[4]

Having received its first stage of concoction in the stomach, the nourishment passes to the heart, where, as we should expect, it undergoes the most important stage of its conception, and is thereby turned into blood, the 'ultimate nourishment' for the whole body. It is probable that, in Aristotle's view, an important

---

[1] *De part. an.* 2. 7, 652ᵇ27–33: ὁ μὲν οὖν ἐγκέφαλος εὔκρατον ποεῖ τὴν ἐν τῇ καρδίᾳ θερμότητα καὶ ζέσιν. ἵνα δὲ καὶ τοῦτο τὸ μόριον τυγχάνῃ μετρίας θερμότητος, ἀφ' ἑκατέρας τῆς φλεβός, τῆς τε μεγάλης καὶ τῆς καλουμένης ἀορτῆς, τελευτῶσιν αἱ φλέβες εἰς τὴν μήνιγγα τὴν περὶ τὸν ἐγκέφαλον. πρὸς δὲ τὸ τῇ θερμότητι μὴ βλάπτειν, ἀντὶ μὲν μεγάλων (καὶ) ὀλίγων πυκναὶ καὶ λεπταὶ φλέβες περιέχουσιν αὐτόν. ἀντὶ δὲ θολεροῦ καὶ παχέος αἵματος λεπτὸν καὶ καθαρόν.
Cf. *De somno*, 3, 458ᵃ5–8: πρὸς δὲ τὸ καταψύχεσθαι καὶ μὴ δέχεσθαι ῥᾳδίως τὴν ἀναθυμίασιν συμβάλλεται καὶ ἡ λεπτότης καὶ ἡ στενότης τῶν περὶ τὸν ἐγκέφαλον φλεβῶν.

[2] *De somno*, 3, 456ᵇ17–24: ἀλλὰ γάρ, ὥσπερ εἴπομεν, οὐκ ἔστιν ὁ ὕπνος ἀδυναμία πᾶσα τοῦ αἰσθητικοῦ, ἀλλ' ἐκ τῆς περὶ τὴν τροφὴν ἀναθυμιάσεως γίνεται τὸ πάθος τοῦτο. ἀναγκαῖον γὰρ τὸ ἀναθυμιώμενον μέχρι τοῦ ὠθεῖσθαι, εἶτ' ἀντιστρέφειν καὶ μεταβάλλειν καθάπερ εὔριπον. τὸ δὲ θερμὸν ἑκάστου τῶν ζῴων πρὸς τὸ ἄνω πέφυκε φέρεσθαι. ὅταν δ' ἐν τοῖς ἄνω τόποις γένηται, ἀθρόον πάλιν ἀντιστρέφει καὶ καταφέρεται. διὸ μάλιστα γίνονται ὕπνοι ἀπὸ τῆς τροφῆς.
Cf. *De part. an.* 2. 7, 653ᵃ11–16: ποιεῖ δὲ καὶ τὸν ὕπνον τοῖς ζῴοις τοῦτο τὸ μόριον τοῖς ἔχουσιν ἐγκέφαλον, τοῖς δὲ μὴ ἔχουσιν τὸ ἀνάλογον. καταψῦχον γὰρ τὴν ἀπὸ τῆς τροφῆς τοῦ αἵματος ἐπίρρυσιν, ἢ καὶ διά τινας ὁμοίας αἰτίας ἄλλας, βαρύνει τε τὸν τόπον, διὸ τὴν κεφαλὴν καρηβαροῦσιν οἱ ὑπνώσσοντες, καὶ κάτω ποιεῖ τὸ θερμὸν ὑποφεύγειν μετὰ τοῦ αἵματος.

[3] Ibid., 652ᵇ6–7: ὑπάρχει δὲ τοῖς ζῴοις πρὸς τὴν τῆς φύσεως ὅλης σωτηρίαν.

[4] See his introduction to the Loeb edition of the *Generation of animals*, par. 63.

part of this process was the pneumatization of the blood, i.e. the charging of it with σύμφυτον πνεῦμα and with the special 'movement' requisite to enable it (a) to maintain the being of the animal, and (b) to supply its growth.

The physiological process of digestion is explained *inter alios locos* in the *Parts of animals*, in a paragraph which compares the essential nature of nutrition in both plants and animals.

Since everything that grows must take food, and all nourishment comes from the wet and the dry [i.e. from solids and liquids], the digestion of these and their transformation takes place through the power of the hot substance [or as we should say heat]. Therefore, if for no other reason, all animals and plants must possess in themselves a natural source of heat . . . Now in animals the first visible processing of food is through the mouth and the parts that are in it, which perform the necessary function of dividing food. But this division is in no way the cause of digestion as such, but only of good digestion. For the division of the food into small pieces makes the operation of heat easier. For the operation of the upper and the lower belly effects digestion through the agency of the natural heat. And just as the mouth and the part continuous with it which they call the oesophagus in those animals which have it conveys the undigested or unprocessed food into the stomach, so there must be also other passages [Peck] through which the body receives its food as from a manger, from the stomach and from the intestinal system. But plants get their nourishment already processed from the earth through their roots—that is why plants have no waste products, for they make use of the soil and the heat inside it instead of a belly . . . The mouth having done its duty hands on the food to the stomach [and intestines] where it undergoes another processing . . . for veins stretch along the whole of the abdomen, beginning at the bottom of the mesentery right up to the stomach.[1]

This explains Aristotle's postulation of the big vein stretching all along the intestines, which we shall meet with in his description of the branches of the 'great vein'. Presumably this branch is not connected with the

---

[1] *De part. an.* 2. 3, 650ª3–32: ἐπεὶ δ' ἀνάγκη πᾶν τὸ αὐξανόμενον λαμβάνειν τροφήν, ἡ δὲ τροφὴ πᾶσιν ἐξ ὑγροῦ καὶ ξηροῦ, καὶ τούτων ἡ πέψις γίνεται καὶ ἡ μεταβολὴ διὰ τῆς τοῦ θερμοῦ δυνάμεως, καὶ τὰ ζῷα πάντα καὶ τὰ φυτά, κἂν εἰ μὴ δι' ἄλλην αἰτίαν, ἀλλὰ διὰ ταύτην ἀναγκαῖον ἔχειν ἀρχὴν θερμοῦ φυσικήν . . . ἡ μὲν γὰρ πρώτη φανερὰ τοῖς ζῴοις λειτουργία διὰ τοῦ στόματος οὖσα καὶ τῶν ἐν τούτῳ μορίων, ὅσων ἡ τροφὴ δεῖται διαιρέσεως. ἀλλ' αὕτη μὲν οὐδεμιᾶς αἰτία πέψεως, ἀλλ' εὐπεψίας μᾶλλον. ἡ γὰρ εἰς μικρὰ διαίρεσις τῆς τροφῆς ῥᾴω ποιεῖ τῷ θερμῷ τὴν ἐργασίαν. ἡ δὲ τῆς ἄνω καὶ τῆς κάτω κοιλίας ἤδη μετὰ θερμότητος φυσικῆς ποιεῖται τὴν πέψιν. ὥσπερ δὲ καὶ τὸ στόμα τῆς ἀκατεργάστου τροφῆς πόρος ἐστί, καὶ τὸ συνεχὲς αὐτῷ μόριον ὃ καλοῦσιν οἰσοφάγον, ὅσα τῶν ζῴων ἔχει τοῦτο τὸ μόριον, ἕως εἰς τὴν κοιλίαν, οὕτω καὶ ἄλλους δεῖ πόρους εἶναι, δι' ὧν ἅπαν λήψεται τὸ σῶμα τὴν τροφήν, ὥσπερ ἐκ φάτνης, ἐκ δὲ τῆς κοιλίας καὶ τῆς τῶν ἐντέρων φύσεως. τὰ μὲν γὰρ φυτὰ λαμβάνει τὴν τροφὴν κατειργασμένην ἐκ τῆς γῆς ταῖς ῥίζαις — διὸ καὶ περίττωμα οὐ γίνεται τοῖς φυτοῖς. τῇ γὰρ γῇ καὶ τῇ ἐν αὐτῇ θερμότητι χρῆται ὥσπερ κοιλία . . . ἡ μὲν γὰρ τοῦ στόματος ἐργασία παραδίδωσι τῇ κοιλίᾳ, παρὰ δὲ ταύτης ἕτερον ἀναγκαῖον λαμβάνειν, ὅπερ συμβέβηκεν. αἱ γὰρ φλέβες κατατείνονται διὰ τοῦ μεσεντερίου παράπαν, κάτωθεν ἀρξάμεναι μέχρι τῆς κοιλίας.

portal system, for unlike Galen, Aristotle does not seem to regard the liver as playing any part in the manufacture of blood. The natural heat which is responsible for this process of concoction must not be confused with the element fire. It is the so-called hot substance which, as we shall see, is identified with the connate or innate *pneuma*, a much more subtle substance than the fire which is one of the four elements of the sublunary world. And the ultimate product of concoction is not blood but semen, though blood is its principal artefact. The great bulk of food ingested is thus turned into blood: this explains why the blood diminishes in quantity when no food is taken and increases when it is, and why bad food creates bad blood and good, good. Blood is the ultimate nourishment and that is its *raison d'être*.[1]

The formation of the various parts from the blood is described in the second book of the *Generation of animals*.

The coming into being of the uniform parts takes place through cooling and heating, for some things are solidified by cold and some by heat . . . Now nourishment oozes through the veins and the channels in the various parts, just as water does through the unfired pots of earthenware, and so forms or brings into being flesh or its equivalent, which is congealed by the cold, and therefore dissolved or liquefied by heat. And the excessively earthy parts of the nourishment as it wells up, having little wetness and heat become cooled, and as the fluid evaporates with the hot principle, these become hard and earthy in appearance turning into nails, horns, hoofs, and beaks . . . But sinews and bones are formed by the internal heat, as the dampness dries up. Wherefore bones like earthenware cannot be dissolved by fire . . .[2]

At each stage of this formative process residues are produced in the form of waste products, which are useless and are therefore excreted. But there are also useful residues produced by a further concoction of nutriment or the blood itself. These useful residues are semen in the male,[3]

---

[1] *De part. an.* 2. 3, 650ᵃ34–ᵇ3 : φανερὸν ὅτι τὸ αἷμα ἡ τελευταία τροφὴ τοῖς ζῴοις τοῖς ἐναίμοις ἐστί, τοῖς δ᾽ ἀναίμοις τὸ ἀνάλογον. καὶ διὰ τοῦτο μὴ λαμβάνουσί τε τροφὴν ὑπολείπει τοῦτο καὶ λαμβάνουσιν αὐξάνεται, καὶ χρηστῆς μὲν οὔσης ὑγιεινόν, φαύλης δὲ φαῦλον. ὅτι μὲν οὖν τὸ αἷμα τροφῆς ἕνεκεν ὑπάρχει τοῖς ἐναίμοις, φανερὸν ἐκ τούτων καὶ τῶν τοιούτων.

[2] *De gen. an.* 2. 6, 743ᵃ3–19 : ἡ δὲ γένεσίς ἐστι τῶν ὁμοιομερῶν ὑπὸ ψύξεως καὶ θερμότητος. συνίσταται γὰρ καὶ πήγνυται τὰ μὲν ψυχρῷ τὰ δὲ θερμῷ . . . διὰ μὲν οὖν τῶν φλεβῶν καὶ τῶν ἐν ἑκάστοις πόρων διαπιδύουσα ἡ τροφή, καθάπερ ἐν τοῖς ὠμοῖς κεραμίοις τὸ ὕδωρ, γίνονται σάρκες ἢ τὸ ταύταις ἀνάλογον, ὑπὸ τοῦ ψυχροῦ συνιστάμεναι, διὸ καὶ λύονται ἀπὸ πυρός. ὅσα δὲ γεηρὰ λίαν τῶν ἀνατελλόντων, ὀλίγην ἔχοντα ὑγρότητα καὶ θερμότητα, ταῦτα ἐξατμίζοντος τοῦ ὑγροῦ μετὰ τοῦ θερμοῦ γίνεται σκληρὰ καὶ γεώδη τὴν μορφήν, οἷον ὄνυχες καὶ κέρατα καὶ ὁπλαὶ καὶ ῥύγχη . . . ὑπὸ δὲ τῆς ἐντὸς θερμότητος τά τε νεῦρα καὶ τὰ ὀστᾶ γίνεται, ξηραινομένης τῆς ὑγρότητος. διὸ καὶ ἄλυτά ἐστι τὰ ὀστᾶ ὑπὸ τοῦ πυρός, καθάπερ κέραμος.

[3] Ibid., 1. 19, 726ᵇ3–11 : ἐπεὶ δὲ καὶ ἡ γονὴ περίττωμά ἐστι τροφῆς καὶ τῆς ἐσχάτης, ἤτοι αἷμα ἂν εἴη ἢ τὸ ἀνάλογον ἢ ἐκ τούτων τι . . . τὸ δὲ σπέρμα πεφθὲν μὲν ἀλλοιότερον ἀποκρίνεται τοῦ αἵματος, ἄπεπτον δ᾽ ὄν, καὶ ὅταν τις προσβιάζηται πλεονάκις χρώμενος τῷ ἀφροδισιάζειν, ἐνίοις αἱματῶδες ἤδη προελήλυθεν, φανερὸν ὅτι τῆς αἱματικῆς ἂν εἴη περίττωμα τροφῆς τὸ σπέρμα, τῆς εἰς τὰ μέρη διαδιδομένης τελευταίας.

and milk and menstrual blood in the female.[1] Semen contains the vital principle of *pneuma*, which, though it is defined in one passage as hot air, is as we shall see a much more subtle substance. Its physical foam-like character is conferred on it by *pneuma*; hence too the appropriateness of the name Aphrodite conferred upon the goddess of love.[2] Menstrual blood too is a concoction of nutriment. It is analogous to semen, but it provides the material as opposed to the form of the living embryo.[3] At the moment of conception it is 'set' by the semen entering the womb, as milk is turned into junket by rennet.[4] Milk too has the same nature as menstrual blood,[5] and is employed differently in two stages. Man is the only animal in which the period of gestation varies. Infants are born at any time from seven to ten months after conception.[6] Milk must therefore be available in a useful form at seven months. In the earlier stages of pregnancy this particular residue is used up in the formation of the embryo; when, however, this is reaching its final stages less of it is used up and more of it remains as a residue, since it is now only used for the small degree of intra-uterine growth taking place after the completion of the embryo.[7] Hence its accumulation in the mother's breasts.

Now the process of concoction by the innate, or connate, heat, whose principal seat or location is in the heart, is the fundamental process of metabolism and something more. For the power of concoction conferred by the innate heat is also responsible for the differentiation of the sexes. In the creatures that reproduce spontaneously or asexually from the proceeds of nutrition, it is heat which supplies the principle of fetation.[8] And

---

[1] Ibid., 727ᵃ2–4: ὅτι μὲν οὖν ἐστὶ τὰ καταμήνια περίττωμα, καὶ ὅτι ἀνάλογον ὡς τοῖς ἄρρεσιν ἡ γονή, οὕτω τοῖς θήλεσι τὰ καταμήνια, φανερόν.

[2] Ibid., 2. 2, 735ᵇ37–736ᵃ21: ἔστι μὲν οὖν τὸ σπέρμα κοινὸν πνεύματος καὶ ὕδατος, τὸ δὲ πνεῦμά ἐστι θερμὸς ἀήρ . . . αἴτιον δὲ τῆς λευκότητος τοῦ σπέρματος ὅτι ἐστὶν ἡ γονὴ ἀφρός, ὁ δ' ἀφρὸς λευκόν . . . ἔοικε δὲ οὐδὲ τοὺς ἀρχαίους λανθάνειν ἀφρώδης ἡ τοῦ σπέρματος οὖσα φύσις. τὴν οὖν κυρίαν θεὸν τῆς μίξεως ἀπὸ τῆς δυνάμεως ταύτης προσηγόρευσαν.

[3] Ibid., 1. 19, 727ᵇ31–3: ὅτι μὲν οὖν συμβάλλεται τὸ θῆλυ εἰς τὴν γένεσιν τὴν ὕλην, τοῦτο δ' ἐστὶν ἐν τῇ τῶν καταμηνίων συστάσει, τὰ δὲ καταμήνια περίττωμα, δῆλον.

[4] Ibid., 2. 4, 739ᵇ20–5: ὅταν δὲ συστῇ ἡ ἐν ταῖς ὑστέραις ἀπόκρισις τοῦ θήλεος ὑπὸ τῆς τοῦ ἄρρενος γονῆς, παραπλήσιον ποιούσης ὥσπερ ἐπὶ τοῦ γάλακτος τῆς πυετίας. καὶ γὰρ ἡ πυετία γάλα ἐστὶ θερμότητα ζωτικὴν ἔχον, ἣ τὸ ὅμοιον εἰς ἓν ἄγει καὶ συνίστησι, καὶ ἡ γονὴ πρὸς τὴν τῶν καταμηνίων φύσιν ταὐτὸ πέπονθεν.

[5] Ibid., 739ᵇ25: ἡ γὰρ αὐτὴ φύσις ἐστὶ γάλακτος καὶ καταμηνίων.

[6] Ibid., 4. 4, 772ᵇ6–9: διὰ δὲ τοῦτο καὶ τοὺς τῆς κυήσεως χρόνους μόνῳ τῶν ζῴων ἀνωμάλους εἶναι συμβέβηκεν. τοῖς μὲν γὰρ ἄλλοις εἷς ἐστὶν ὁ χρόνος, τοῖς δ' ἀνθρώποις πλείους. καὶ γὰρ ἑπτάμηνα καὶ δεκάμηνα γεννῶνται καὶ κατὰ τοὺς μεταξὺ χρόνους.

[7] Ibid., 4. 8, 776ᵃ26–ᵇ4: τὸ μὲν γὰρ πρῶτον ἡ τοῦ τοιούτου περιττώματος ἀπόκρισις εἰς τὴν τῶν ἐμβρύων ἀναλίσκεται γένεσιν· πάντων δ' ἡ τροφὴ τὸ γλυκύτατον καὶ πεπεμμένον . . . τελεουμένων δὲ τῶν κυημάτων πλέον τὸ περίττωμα περιγιγνόμενον, ἔλαττον γὰρ τὸ ἀναλισκόμενον, καὶ γλυκύτερον, οὐκ ἀφαιρουμένου ὁμοίως τοῦ εὐπέπτου· οὐ γὰρ ἔτι εἰς πλάσιν τοῦ ἐμβρύου γίγνεται ἡ δαπάνη, ἀλλ' εἰς μικρὰν αὔξησιν, ὥσπερ ἑστηκὸς ἤδη διὰ τὸ τέλος ἔχειν τὸ ἔμβρυον. ἔστι γάρ τις καὶ κυήματος τελείωσις . . . εἰς δὲ τὸν ἄνω τόπον καὶ τοὺς μαστοὺς συλλέγεται . . .

[8] Ibid., 3. 9, 762ᵇ6–8: δεῖ δὴ λαβεῖν ὅτι καὶ ἐν τοῖς ζῴοις τοῖς γεννῶσιν ἐκ τῆς εἰσιούσης

in those reproducing sexually, it is also heat which supplies the superior power of concoction which characterizes the semen as opposed to the menstrual blood. For it is the semen which provides the principle of movement and the form, whereas the menstrual blood only provides the matter. The blood of the male is therefore hotter than that of the female.[1] The difference of the sexes is essentially reduced to a difference in this power of concoction. The male is of course for Aristotle, as for all Hellenes, the more perfect form of humanity, and a female child is formed when the formative principle is unable to gain complete mastery over its material and is unable, through deficiency of the vital heat, to effect complete concoction and to transform the material provided by the mother into its own proper form, that is the male form. When this occurs, then of necessity the material is changed into the 'opposite' or female form.[2] And since the two sexes differ in power and capacity, they also differ in the instruments which they possess. Indeed this instrumental difference entails a difference in their whole make-up, as is shown in the case of eunuchs who assume the exterior characteristics of the opposite sex.[3] Masculinity is a principle (ἀρχή). The male is male by virtue of a certain ability, and the female female through an absence of that ability, namely the ability to effect the concoction of the ultimate nourishment, the blood. And the reason for this ability or its absence lies in the part of the body which contains the principle of the natural heat, that is, the heart. The ultimate source of sex is therefore the heart in animals which have blood, or its counterpart in those which do not.[4] Moreover, the blood of the two sexes also differs. Given equality in health and age, the blood of the female is thicker and blacker, women have less blood on the surface of the body and more inside. Moreover, the human female has more

τροφῆς ἡ ἐν τῷ ζῴῳ θερμότης ἀποκρίνουσα καὶ συμπέττουσα ποιεῖ τὸ περίττωμα, τὴν ἀρχὴν τοῦ κυήματος.

[1] De gen. an. 4.1, 765ᵇ8–18: ἀλλ' ἐπὶ τὸ ἄρρεν καὶ τὸ θῆλυ διώρισται δυνάμει τινὶ καὶ ἀδυναμίᾳ— τὸ μὲν γὰρ δυνάμενον πέττειν καὶ συνιστάναι τε καὶ ἐκκρίνειν τὸ σπέρμα ἔχον ἀρχὴν τοῦ εἴδους ἄρρεν. λέγω δ' ἀρχὴν οὐ τὴν τοιαύτην ἐξ ἧς ὥσπερ ὕλης γίνεται τοιοῦτον οἷον τὸ γεννῶν, ἀλλὰ τὴν κινοῦσαν πρώτην ... ἔτι εἰ πᾶσα πέψις ἐργάζεται θερμῷ, ἀνάγκη καὶ τῶν ζῴων τὰ ἄρρενα τῶν θηλέων θερμότερα εἶναι. διὰ γὰρ ψυχρότητα καὶ ἀδυναμίαν πολυαιμεῖ κατὰ τόπους τινὰς τὸ θῆλυ μᾶλλον.

[2] Ibid., 766ᵃ18–22: ὅταν γὰρ μὴ κρατῇ ἡ ἀρχὴ μηδὲ δύνηται πέψαι δι' ἔνδειαν θερμότητος μηδ' ἀγάγῃ εἰς τὸ ἴδιον εἶδος τὸ αὐτοῦ, ἀλλὰ ταύτῃ ἡττηθῇ, ἀνάγκη εἰς τοὐναντίον μεταβάλλειν. ἐναντίον δὲ τῷ ἄρρενι τὸ θῆλυ, καὶ ταύτῃ ᾗ τὸ μὲν ἄρρεν τὸ δὲ θῆλυ. ἐπεὶ δ' ἔχει διαφορὰν ἐν τῇ δυνάμει, ἔχει καὶ τὸ ὄργανον διαφέρον.

[3] Ibid., 766ᵃ24–8: ἑνὸς δὲ μορίου ἐπικαίρου μεταβάλλοντος ὅλη ἡ σύστασις τοῦ ζῴου πολὺ τῷ εἴδει διαφέρει. ὁρᾶν δ' ἔξεστιν ἐπὶ τῶν εὐνούχων, οἳ ἑνὸς μορίου πηρωθέντος τοσοῦτον ἐξαλλάττουσι τῆς ἀρχαίας μορφῆς καὶ μικρὸν ἐλλείπουσι τοῦ θήλεος τὴν ἰδέαν.

[4] Ibid., 766ᵃ30–ᵇ3: εἰ οὖν τὸ μὲν ἄρρεν ἀρχή τις καὶ αἴτιον, ἔστι δ' ἄρρεν ᾗ δύναταί τι, θῆλυ δὲ ᾗ ἀδυνατεῖ, τῆς δὲ δυνάμεως ὅρος καὶ τῆς ἀδυναμίας τὸ πεπτικὸν εἶναι ἢ μὴ πεπτικὸν τῆς ὑστάτης τροφῆς, ὃ ἐν μὲν τοῖς ἐναίμοις αἷμα καλεῖται, ἐν δὲ τοῖς ἄλλοις τὸ ἀνάλογον, τούτου δὲ τὸ αἴτιον ἐν τῇ ἀρχῇ καὶ τῷ μορίῳ τῷ ἔχοντι τὴν τῆς φυσικῆς θερμότητος ἀρχήν, ἀναγκαῖον ἄρα ἐν τοῖς ἐναίμοις συνίστασθαι καρδίαν, καὶ ἢ ἄρρεν ἔσεσθαι ἢ θῆλυ τὸ γινόμενον, ἐν δὲ τοῖς ἄλλοις γένεσιν οἷς ὑπάρχει τὸ θῆλυ καὶ τὸ ἄρρεν τὸ τῇ καρδίᾳ ἀνάλογον.

blood than any other female animal, and her catamenia are more abundant. With the exception of the disease called flux, women have less diseases connected with the blood than men. Few women suffer from varicose veins, haemorrhoids, or nose-bleeding, and if any of these occur, their menstrual discharge becomes worse, i.e. less plentiful.[1]

Blood also differs in quantity and appearance according to age. In very young animals it is serous (ichor-like) and plentiful; in the old, thick, black, and scanty; in the prime of life of intermediate quality. The blood of the old coagulates quickly, even when it is near the surface—a thing which does not take place in the young. Serum (ichor) is unconcocted blood, either because it has not yet been 'cooked', or because it has been transformed.[2] Changes in the serous character of the blood fluid seem to have interested Aristotle. If blood becomes too watery, animals (and people) become ill, because it is too ichorous and turns into serum, so that some people have actually been known to sweat a blood-like liquid. And in certain cases the blood, when it comes out of the body, does not congeal at all, or only here and there, in separated places. In sleep the blood in the exterior portions of the body decreases, so that even when animals are pricked, it does not flow out in the usual way. Now blood is formed from the concoction of serum, and fat from the concoction of blood.[3]

In all blooded animals blood is the most essential and universal part. It is not acquired from without but is present in all from the outset, in all those who are not decaying or undergoing dissolution.[4] It is the only fluid which remains in every part of the body as long as they are alive. Further, it is first formed in the heart before the body as a whole has become articulated.[5] All the blood is always found in a container, the so-called blood vessels, and in no other organ except the heart itself. Blood,

[1] De hist. an. 3. 19, 521ᵃ22–31 : τὸ δὲ τῶν θηλειῶν πρὸς τὸ τῶν ἀρρένων διαφέρει. παχύτερόν τε γὰρ καὶ μελάντερόν ἐστιν, ὁμοίως ἐχόντων πρὸς ὑγίειαν καὶ ἡλικίαν, ἐν τοῖς θήλεσιν, καὶ ἐπιπολῆς μὲν ἔλαττον ἐν τοῖς θήλεσιν, ἐντὸς δὲ πολυαιμότερα. μάλιστα δὲ καὶ τῶν θηλέων ζῴων γυνὴ πολύαιμον, καὶ τὰ καλούμενα καταμήνια γίγνεται πλεῖστα τῶν ζῴων ταῖς γυναιξίν. νενοσηκὸς δὲ τοῦτο τὸ αἷμα καλεῖται ῥοῦς. τῶν δ' ἄλλων νοσηματικῶν ἧττον μετέχουσιν αἱ γυναῖκες. ὀλίγαις δὲ γίνεται ἰξία καὶ αἱμορροῖς καὶ ἐκ ῥινῶν ῥύσις. ἐὰν δέ τι συμβαίνῃ τούτων τὰ καταμήνια χείρω γίγνεται.

[2] Ibid., 521ᵃ32–ᵇ3 : διαφέρει δὲ κατὰ τὰς ἡλικίας πλήθει καὶ εἴδει τὸ αἷμα· ἐν μὲν γὰρ τοῖς πάμπαν νέοις ἰχωροειδές ἐστι καὶ πλέον, ἐν δὲ τοῖς γέρουσι παχὺ καὶ μέλαν καὶ ὀλίγον, ἐν ἀκμάζουσι δὲ μέσως. καὶ πήγνυται ταχὺ τὸ τῶν γερόντων, κἂν ἐν τῷ σώματι ᾖ ἐπιπολῆς· τοῖς δὲ νέοις οὐ γίγνεται τοῦτο. ἰχὼρ δ' ἐστὶν ἄπεπτον αἷμα, ἢ τῷ μήπω πεπέφθαι ἢ τῷ διωρῶσθαι.

[3] Ibid., 521ᵃ12–18 : ἐξυγραινομένου δὲ λίαν νοσοῦσιν. γίγνεται γὰρ ἰχωροειδές, καὶ διοροῦται οὕτως ὥστε ἤδη τινὲς ἰδίαν αἱματώδη ἱδρῶτα. καὶ ἐξίον ἐνίοις οὐ πήγνυται παντελῶς ἢ διωρισμένως καὶ χωρίς. τοῖς δὲ καθεύδουσιν ἐν τοῖς ἐκτὸς μέρεσιν ἔλαττον γίγνεται τὸ αἷμα, ὥστε καὶ κεντουμένων μὴ ῥεῖν ὁμοίως. γίγνεται δὲ πεττομένων ἐξ ἰχῶρος μὲν αἷμα, ἐξ αἵματος δὲ πιμελή.

[4] Ibid., 520ᵇ10–12 : περὶ δ' αἵματος ὧδε ἔχει. τοῦτο γὰρ πᾶσιν ἀναγκαιότατον καὶ κοινότατον τοῖς ἐναίμοις καὶ οὐκ ἐπικτητόν, ἀλλ' ὑπάρχει πᾶσι τοῖς μὴ φθειρομένοις.

[5] Ibid., 521ᵃ7–10 : καὶ ἔστι τῶν ὑγρῶν μένον καθ' ἅπαν τὸ σῶμα τοῖς ζῴοις καὶ ἀεὶ ἕως ἂν ζῇ, τὸ αἷμα μόνον. πρῶτον δὲ γίγνεται τὸ αἷμα ἐν τῇ καρδίᾳ τοῖς ζῴοις καὶ πρὶν ἢ ὅλον διηρθρῶσθαι τὸ σῶμα.

when it is touched, does not give rise to any sensation in any animal, any more than the excrements in the belly, or the brain, and the marrow.[1] Wherever you cut the flesh in a living animal, blood appears, unless the flesh has become corrupted. Blood naturally has a sweet taste, if it is healthy, and its colour is red. But if it is spoiled, either naturally or through disease, it is rather black. The best blood is neither too thick nor too thin, unless it has deteriorated, either naturally or through disease. In a living animal it is always liquid and hot, but when it is separated from the body, it congeals in all animals except the deer, the gazelle, and other animals of a similar character. But the blood of all other animals congeals, unless the fibres are removed. That of the bull is the quickest of all animals to congeal.[2] This is because bull's blood is very fibrous. Now fibres are not contained in the blood of all animals. They are the earthy part of the blood, and the blood of deer and of gazelles does not have fibres; that is why it does not congeal. Bulls, on the other hand, have thick fibres in profusion and are the earthiest of animals, and therefore subject to fits of passion.[3]

Blood, though it is classed by Aristotle as one of the uniform parts of the body (ὁμοιομέρη), was not regarded by him as uniform throughout the organism, still less as uniform in different species of animals. Its qualities vary. It can be thick or thin, clear or muddy in different degrees, and, as we have already noted, in some animals its qualities vary in different parts of the body.[4] The thicker and warmer it is, the more it produces strength, and the thinner and colder, the more it gives rise to powers of sensation and intelligence. The same considerations

---

[1] De hist. an. 3. 19, 520ᵇ12–17 : πᾶν δ' αἷμά ἐστιν ἐν ἀγγείῳ ἐν ταῖς καλουμέναις φλεψίν, ἐν ἄλλῳ δ' οὐδενὶ πλὴν ἐν τῇ καρδίᾳ μόνον. οὐκ ἔχει δ' αἴσθησιν τὸ αἷμα ἀπομένων ἐν οὐδενὶ τῶν ζῴων, ὥσπερ οὐδ' ἡ περίττωσις ἡ τῆς κοιλίας· οὐδὲ δὴ ὁ ἐγκέφαλος οὐδ' ὁ μυελὸς οὐκ ἔχει αἴσθησιν ἀπομένων.

[2] Ibid., 520ᵇ17–27 : ὅπου δ' ἄν τις διέλῃ τὴν σάρκα, γίγνεται αἷμα ἐν ζῶντι, ἐὰν μὴ διεφθαρμένη ἡ σὰρξ ᾖ. ἔστι δὲ τὴν φύσιν τὸ αἷμα τόν τε χυμὸν ἔχον γλυκύν, ἐάν περ ὑγιὲς ᾖ, καὶ τὸ χρῶμα ἐρυθρόν. τὸ δὲ χεῖρον ἢ φύσει ἢ νόσῳ μελάντερον. καὶ οὔτε λίαν παχὺ οὔτε λίαν λεπτὸν τὸ βέλτιστον, ἐὰν μὴ χεῖρον ᾖ διὰ φύσιν ἢ διὰ νόσον. καὶ ἐν μὲν τῷ ζῴῳ ὑγρὸν καὶ θερμὸν ἀεί, ἐξιὸν δ' ἔξω πήγνυται πάντων πλὴν ἐλάφου καὶ προκὸς καὶ εἴ τι ἄλλο τοιαύτην ἔχει φύσιν. τὸ δ' ἄλλο αἷμα πήγνυται, ἐὰν μὴ ἐξαιρεθῶσιν αἱ ἶνες. τάχιστα δὲ πήγνυται τὸ τοῦ ταύρου αἷμα πάντων.

[3] De part. an. 2. 4, 650ᵇ14–18 : τὰς δὲ καλουμένας ἶνας τὸ μὲν ἔχει αἷμα τὸ δ' οὐκ ἔχει, οἷον τῶν ἐλάφων καὶ προκῶν. διόπερ οὐ πήγνυται τὸ τοιοῦτον αἷμα ... αἱ δ' ἶνες γῆς εἰσιν ... (650ᵇ33–651ᵃ5) τὰ δὲ πολλὰς ἔχοντα λίαν ἶνας καὶ παχείας γεωδέστερα τὴν φύσιν ἐστὶ καὶ θυμώδη τὸ ἦθος καὶ ἐκστατικὰ διὰ θυμόν. θερμότητος γὰρ ποιητικὸν ὁ θυμὸς τὰ δὲ στερεὰ θερμανθέντα μᾶλλον θερμαίνει τῶν ὑγρῶν· αἱ δ' ἶνες στερεὸν καὶ γεῶδες, ὥστε γίνονται οἷον πυρίαι ἐν τῷ αἵματι καὶ ζέσιν ποιοῦσιν ἐν τοῖς θυμοῖς. διὸ οἱ ταῦροι καὶ οἱ κάπροι θυμώδεις καὶ ἐκστατικοί. τὸ γὰρ αἷμα τούτων ἰνωδέστατον, καὶ τὸ τοῦ ταύρου τάχιστα πήγνυται πάντων.

[4] Ibid., 2. 2, 647ᵇ10–13, 29–36. τῶν δ' ὁμοιομερῶν μορίων ἐν τοῖς ζῴοις ἐστὶ τὰ μὲν μαλακὰ καὶ ὑγρά, τὰ δὲ σκληρὰ καὶ στερεά· ὑγρὰ μὲν ... οἷον αἷμα, ἰχώρ ... αὐτῶν δὲ τούτων αἱ διαφοραὶ πρὸς ἄλληλα τοῦ βελτίονος ἕνεκέν εἰσιν, οἷον τῶν τε ἄλλων καὶ αἵματος πρὸς αἷμα. τὸ μὲν γὰρ λεπτότερον τὸ δὲ παχύτερον καὶ τὸ μὲν καθαρώτερόν ἐστι τὸ δὲ θολερώτερον, ἔτι δὲ τὸ μὲν ψυχρότερον τὸ δὲ θερμότερον, ἔν τε τοῖς μορίοις τοῦ ἑνὸς ζῴου—τὸ γὰρ ἐν τοῖς ἄνω μέρεσι πρὸς τὰ κάτω μόρια διαφέρει ταύταις ταῖς διαφοραῖς—καὶ ἑτέρῳ πρὸς ἕτερον ...

apply to the functional equivalent of blood in bloodless animals, and serve to explain why bees, for example, are more intelligent than many animals that possess blood. Best of all animals are those whose blood is hot, thin, and clear, for these have both courage and intelligence.[1]

We have now dealt with the principal passages in Aristotle's biological works dealing with blood. They show the fruits of quite extensive observation and perhaps experiment, though it is difficult to reconcile either of these with some of his statements, such as the denial of the existence of 'fibres' in the blood of deer, and the assertion that it does not congeal at all. If great Homer may be permitted to nod, there seems to be no reason to deny this privilege to Aristotle. We can pass on then, without further ado, to his exposition of the double system of blood vessels. To examine in some detail the descriptions of the topographical courses of the venous and the arterial systems is certainly worth while, in order to show not so much his errors as the considerable advances made since the Hippocratic age. We have already noted some interesting features of his technique of dissection. In the third book of the *History of animals*, before describing the blood vessels, he gives us some notes about the difficulties of dissection. In the bodies of dead animals the nature of the most important 'veins' is difficult to perceive, because as soon as they are emptied of blood they collapse. Presumably this would apply, for example, to animals sacrificed as well as to others whose throats had been cut. But these vessels become visible when the animal has been strangled after being previously starved.[2] He goes on to describe the two principal vessels in the thorax running inside along the spine, the larger one the superior vena cava and the smaller the aorta, the first of these being in front and the latter behind.[3] For, as he tells us in his book on the *Parts of animals*, just as the right side is superior to and hotter than the left, so the front is superior to the back. The former is easier to see, and all blooded animals have it plainly visible, but the latter and its branches are difficult to see in some

---

[1] Ibid., 648ᵃ3–11: ἔστι δ' ἰσχύος μὲν ποιητικώτερον τὸ παχύτερον αἷμα καὶ θερμότερον, αἰσθητικώτερον δὲ καὶ νοερώτερον τὸ λεπτότερον καὶ ψυχρότερον. τὴν αὐτὴν δ' ἔχει διαφορὰν καὶ τὸ ἀνάλογον ὑπάρχον πρὸς τὸ αἷμα. διὸ καὶ μέλιτται καὶ ἄλλα τοιαῦτα ζῷα φρονιμώτερα τὴν φύσιν ἐστὶν ἐναίμων πολλῶν, καὶ τῶν ἐναίμων τὰ ψυχρὸν ἔχοντα καὶ λεπτὸν αἷμα φρονιμώτερα τῶν ἐναντίων ἐστίν. ἄριστα δὲ τὰ θερμὸν ἔχοντα καὶ λεπτὸν καὶ καθαρόν. ἅμα γὰρ πρός τ' ἀνδρείαν τὰ τοιαῦτα καὶ πρὸς φρόνησιν ἔχει καλῶς.

[2] *De hist. an.* 3. 2, 511ᵇ10–23: ἐπεὶ δ' ἀρχῇ ἔοικεν ἡ τοῦ αἵματος φύσις καὶ ἡ τῶν φλεβῶν, πρῶτον περὶ τούτων λεκτέον ἄλλως τ' ἐπειδὴ καὶ τῶν πρότερον εἰρηκότων τινὲς οὐ καλῶς λέγουσιν. αἴτιον δὲ τῆς ἀγνοίας τὸ δυσθεώρητον αὐτῶν. ἐν μὲν γὰρ τοῖς τεθνεῶσι τῶν ζῴων ἄδηλος ἡ φύσις τῶν κυριωτάτων φλεβῶν διὰ τὸ συμπίπτειν εὐθὺς ἐξιόντος τοῦ αἵματος μάλιστα ταύτας· ἐκ τούτων γὰρ ἐκχεῖται ἀθρόον ὥσπερ ἐξ ἀγγείου. καθ' αὑτὸ γὰρ οὐδὲν ἔχει αἷμα, πλὴν ὀλίγον ἐν τῇ καρδίᾳ ἀλλὰ πᾶν ἐστιν ἐν ταῖς φλεψίν, ἐν δὲ τοῖς ζῶσιν ἀδύνατόν ἐστι θεάσασθαι πῶς ἔχουσιν, ἐντὸς γὰρ ἡ φύσις αὐτῶν. ὥσθ' οἱ μὲν ἐν τεθνεῶσι καὶ διῃρημένοις τοῖς ζῴοις θεωροῦντες τὰς μεγίστας ἀρχὰς οὐκ ἐθεώρουν, οἱ δ' ἐν τοῖς λελεπτυσμένοις σφόδρα ἀνθρώποις ἐκ τῶν τότε ἔξωθεν φαινομένων τὰς ἀρχὰς τῶν φλεβῶν διώρισαν.

[3] See the passage from the same chapter quoted p. 122, n. 2.

animals or even invisible. The 'large vein' has precedence over the aorta, and all blood vessels are branches of one or the other, and they spread throughout the whole body, because blood is the matter of the body.[1] The character of the two great vessels is distinct. The 'big vein' has a texture resembling that of a membrane or skin, while the aorta, which is narrower, is very like a sinew or tendon.[2] Its character, though somewhat similar, is also distinct from that of the windpipe, the ἀρτηρία or φάρυγξ, which is called cartilaginous.[3]

Aristotle, as we have seen, has made great advances in the knowledge of the heart, as compared with the contemporaries of Hippocrates. However inexplicable his error on the third ventricle, he has grasped the fact that the two bigger ventricles are the roots of the two main trunks of blood vessels, and he is reasonably correct on their relative positions. He knows that viewed from the front, the vena cava superior and its main branches lie on top of the aorta in the thorax, and he has noted that the convexity of the vena cava's curve lies to the right side.[4] He has also noted the difference in the texture of the coats of the two main vessels. But when it comes to the connections of the greater blood vessels with the chambers of the heart, we are on much less solid ground.

The description of the 'great vein' and its branches, particularly its relation to the heart, raises a number of difficulties. According to Peck's translation in the Loeb edition, it reads as follows:

Now the great blood vessel is attached to the largest cavity, i.e. the one which is uppermost and on the right side, then it runs through the middle cavity and reappears as a blood vessel again, as though the cavity were part of it like a lake formed by the blood. The aorta is attached to the middle cavity, though the arrangement is dissimilar—the connection here is by a much narrower pipe.[5]

The connection of the great vein with the middle cavity, i.e. the third or middle ventricle, has never been explained satisfactorily, since the

---

[1] *De part. an.* 3. 5, 667ᵇ32–668ᵃ3: δύο δ' εἰσὶ διὰ τὸ τὰ σώματα εἶναι διμερῆ τῶν ἐναίμων τε καὶ πορευτικῶν. ἐν πᾶσι γὰρ τούτοις διώρισται τὸ ἔμπροσθεν καὶ τὸ ὄπισθεν καὶ τὸ δεξιὸν καὶ τὸ ἀριστερὸν καὶ τὸ ἄνω καὶ τὸ κάτω. ὅσῳ δὲ τιμιώτερον καὶ ἡγεμονικώτερον τὸ ἔμπροσθεν τοῦ ὄπισθεν, τοσούτῳ καὶ ἡ μεγάλη φλὲψ τῆς ἀορτῆς. ἡ μὲν γὰρ ἐν τοῖς ἔμπροσθεν, ἡ δ' ἐν τοῖς ὄπισθεν κεῖται, καὶ τὴν μὲν ἅπαντ' ἔχει τὰ ἔναιμα φανερῶς, τὴν δ' ἔνια μὲν ἀμυδρῶς ἔνια δ' ἀφανῶς.

[2] *De hist. an.* 3. 3, 513ᵇ7–11 : καὶ ἔστιν ἡ μὲν μεγάλη φλὲψ ὑμενώδης καὶ δερματώδης, ἡ δ' ἀορτὴ στενοτέρα μὲν ταύτης, σφόδρα δὲ νευρώδης. καὶ ἀποτεινομένη πόρρω πρὸς τὴν κεφαλήν, καὶ πρὸς τὰ κάτω μόρια στένη τε γίγνεται καὶ νευρώδης πάμπαν.

[3] *De part. an.* 3. 3, 664ᵃ35: ἡ δὲ καλουμένη φάρυγξ καὶ ἀρτηρία συνέστηκεν ἐκ χονδρώδους σώματος.

[4] Gray, op. cit., p. 827. Cf. *De hist. an.* 3. 3, 513ᵃ18–20: ἔστι δὲ κειμένη αὐτῶν ἡ μὲν μείζων ἐν τοῖς ἔμπροσθεν, ἡ δ' ἐλάττων ὄπισθεν ταύτης, καὶ ἡ μὲν μείζων ἐν τοῖς δεξιοῖς μᾶλλον, ἡ δ' ἐλάττων ἐν τοῖς ἀριστεροῖς, ἣν καλοῦσί τινες ἀορτήν.

[5] *De hist. an.* 3. 3, 513ᵇ1–6: ἡ μὲν οὖν μεγάλη φλὲψ ἐκ τῆς μεγίστης ἤρτηται κοιλίας τῆς ἄνω καὶ ἐν τοῖς δεξιοῖς, εἶτα διὰ τοῦ κοίλου τοῦ μέσου τείνασα γίγνεται πάλιν φλέψ, ὡς οὔσης τῆς κοιλίας μορίου τῆς φλεβὸς ἐν ᾧ λιμνάζει τὸ αἷμα. ἡ δ' ἀορτὴ ἀπὸ τῆς μέσης· πλὴν οὐχ οὕτως ἀλλὰ κατὰ στενοτέραν σύριγγα πολλῷ κοινωνεῖ.

aorta is also attached to it in this passage, which does not appear to make any sense. But it seems fairly clear, as Huxley noted, that what Aristotle was describing when he speaks of the 'reappearance as a blood vessel' is the junction by the right auricle of the superior vena cava with the inferior vena cava. And since Aristotle shows no acquaintance with the valves of the heart, he may very well have looked upon even the right ventricle as a mere extension of the vena cava. It is the 'middle ventricle' which raises difficulties. Huxley seems to have made a distinction between the κοῖλον and the κοιλία. The latter he regards as referring to the right auricle which is intermediate between the upper and the lower parts of the 'great vein' and is not a part of the heart at all. We could also by a slight textual alteration, reading διὰ μέσου τοῦ κοίλου for διὰ τοῦ κοίλου τοῦ μέσου, avoid the chief anatomical absurdity of the passage as it now stands, making the vein run through the middle of the ventricle, which amounts to regarding the ventricle itself as a part of the vena cava. This will not help to solve the question of the third ventricle, but it will make some anatomical sense. It should be observed that a little lower down Aristotle expressly contrasts the 'great vein' with the aorta; the latter comes out of the heart, the former runs through it. But this statement rests only on a textual emendation. For the next sentence has also given rise to difficulties. 'Thus the blood vessel passes through the heart and it extends into the aorta from the heart.' The attempt to envisage this as referring to the ductus arteriosus may be dismissed, and Peck simply secludes the last clause,[1] adding in a footnote: 'This statement is incorrect and inconsistent with Aristotle's account.'[2] Almost the same desperate words are used by D'Arcy Thompson. 'This passage has been a stumbling-block to all interpreters and brings confusion into the whole Aristotelian account of the vascular system. The statement is contrary to fact, and even the construction is under suspicion.' Yet, as Aubert and Wimmer (the Teubner editors) point out, all the principal manuscripts support it. A number of alternative readings have been proposed by various scholars, none of which can be considered as more than a guess obviously designed to rescue us from a physiological dilemma imposed by our modern knowledge. The emendation ἡ δ' ἀορτή makes good anatomical sense, but one cannot help trying to make some sense of the passage as it stands. The word εἰς does not necessarily imply any anastomosis of the great vein with the aorta, so we may be permitted to translate it as *on to*—Huxley rendered it *towards*. Nor can we absolutely rule out

[1] Ibid., 513ᵇ6: καὶ ἡ μὲν φλὲψ διὰ τῆς καρδίας, ἡ δ' ἀορτὴ ἀπὸ τῆς καρδίας τείνει. ἡ δ' ἀορτή is an emendation of εἰς δὲ τὴν ἀορτήν. Peck's Loeb text reads: καὶ ἡ μὲν φλὲψ διὰ τῆς καρδίας, †εἰς δὲ τὴν ἀορτὴν ἀπὸ τῆς καρδίας† τείνει. εἰς δὲ τὴν ἀορτήν is the reading of the principal manuscripts. Dittmeyer conjectured εἰς δὲ τὴν ἀορτὴν ⟨πόρος⟩; Sylburg and others conjectured ἡ δ' ἀορτή; D'Arcy Thompson conjectured ἡ δ' ἀορτὴ εἰς τὴν ἀριστεράν.
[2] Peck, loc. cit.

the possibility that Aristotle did believe that such an anastomosis existed. We know too little of his ideas on the movements of the blood to be completely certain.

The remainder of the paragraph is devoted to a description we have just quoted in a footnote of the differing textures of the two main blood vessels, the great vein and the aorta, which shows that the differentiation of veins from arteries was beginning to be made, at any rate in the case of the main trunks. Aristotle then reverts to the description of the first of these vessels.

First, then, there is a part of the great blood vessels which runs from the heart towards the lung and the 'synapsis' of the aorta; this is a large and undivided blood vessel. But two parts split off from it, one towards the lung, and the other towards the backbone and the last vertebra of the neck.[1]

(trs. Peck.)

From this it seems clear that Aristotle, as Mühsam and before him Huxley pointed out, looked upon the pulmonary artery as a branch of the vena cava, which perhaps sounds a little queer to us moderns; but, as Huxley observes,

the canal which leads from the right cavity of the heart to the lung is without doubt the pulmonary artery. But it may be said that in this case Aristotle contradicts himself, inasmuch as . . . a vessel which is obviously the pulmonary artery is described as a branch of the great vein. However this difficulty also disappears, if we reflect that in Aristotle's way of looking at the matter, the line of demarcation between the great vein and the heart coincides with the right auriculo-ventricular aperture; and that inasmuch as the conical prolongation of the right ventricle which leads to the pulmonary artery lies close in front of the auricle, its base may very easily be regarded as part of the general opening of the great vein into the right ventricle.[2]

The 'synapsis' of the aorta is also ambiguous. Peck translates the word as 'attachment', but I cannot help suspecting that Aristotle is here alluding to the aortic arch, through or under which the pulmonary trunk travels before dividing off to the lungs; or he may be referring to the junction of the ascending and the descending aorta. On the other hand he may merely be referring to the ligamentum arteriosum. The two parts which split off from it are the pulmonary artery and a vessel by which he may be attempting to describe the azygos vein, as a later sentence would appear to demonstrate.

---

[1] *De hist. an.* 3. 3, 513ᵇ11–16: τείνει δὲ πρῶτον μὲν ἄνω ἀπὸ τῆς καρδίας τῆς μεγάλης φλεβὸς μόριον πρὸς τὸν πνεύμονα καὶ τὴν σύναψιν τῆς ἀορτῆς, ἄσχιστος καὶ μεγάλη οὖσα φλέψ. σχίζεται δ' ἀπ' αὐτῆς μόρια δύο, τὸ μὲν ἐπὶ τὸν πνεύμονα, τὸ δ' ἐπὶ τὴν ῥάχιν καὶ τὸν ὕστατον τοῦ τραχήλου σφόνδυλον.   [2] Huxley, loc. cit.

And the blood vessel which runs to the vertebra of the neck and the backbone extends back again alongside the backbone. This is the blood vessel mentioned by Homer in the passage where he says:

'All that vein he severed through
which to the neck runs right along the back.'

And from this blood vessel there run small blood vessels along each rib and to each vertebra, and at the vertebra above the kidneys the blood vessel divides into two.[1]

(trs. Peck.)

I have translated the words παρὰ τὴν πλευράν as *along*, not as Peck does *past*, each rib. It seems to me that Aristotle is here almost certainly referring to the posterior intercostal veins, which run into the azygos vein on the right side. He seems too to have some inkling of the hemiazygos vein in his reference to the division of the vessel at the vertebra above the kidney. But not too much importance should be attached to these attempted identifications.[2]

Aristotle now returns, after describing the pulmonary artery and its ramifications in the lung, to the great vein itself.

Above these, from that part of the vein which extends from the heart, the whole vein divides into two directions. The one set leads off to the sides and the collar-bones. They then go through the armpits, extending in men to the arms, in four-footed animals into the front legs, in birds into the wings, and in fishes into the pectoral fins. Now the beginning portions of these veins where they first divide are called the jugular. And where they divide into the neck (away from the great vein), they run alongside of the 'artery' (the one of the lung). If these are pressed from the outside, sometimes men fall down unconscious, without choking, with their eyes closed. This is the course they take: keeping the windpipe between them, going right up to the ears, where the lower jaws join up with the skull. From that point, they split into four, that is two on each side, one branch on each side bending backwards, which goes down the neck and through the shoulder and joins up with the former branch, mentioned earlier, of the vein near the bend of the arm, while the other part terminates in the hand and the fingers.[3]

[1] De hist. an. 3. 3, 513ᵇ24–31: ἡ δ' ἐπὶ τὸν σφόνδυλον τοῦ τραχήλου τείνουσα φλὲψ καὶ τὴν ῥάχιν πάλιν παρὰ τὴν ῥάχιν τείνει· ἣν καὶ Ὅμηρος ἐν τοῖς ἔπεσιν εἴρηκε ποιήσας·

ἀπὸ δὲ φλέβα πᾶσαν ἔκερσεν,
ἥ τ' ἀνὰ νῶτα θέουσα διαμπερὲς αὐχέν' ἱκάνει.

ἀπὸ δὲ ταύτης τείνουσι παρά τε τὴν πλευρὰν ἑκάστην φλέβια καὶ πρὸς ἕκαστον τὸν σφόνδυλον, κατὰ δὲ τὸν ὑπὲρ τῶν νεφρῶν σφόνδυλον σχίζεται διχῇ.

[2] See Gray, op. cit., pp. 827 f. The description of the bifurcation of the azygos vein is, of course, far from accurate, but as a first approximation it is very good. There can be little doubt about this identification.

[3] De hist. an. 3. 3, 513ᵇ33–514ᵃ14: ὑπεράνω δὲ τούτων ἀπὸ τῆς ἐκ τῆς καρδίας τεταμένης πάλιν ἡ ὅλη σχίζεται εἰς δύο τόπους. αἱ μὲν γὰρ φέρουσιν εἰς τὰ πλάγια καὶ τὰς κλεῖδας, κἄπειτα διὰ τῶν μασχαλῶν τοῖς μὲν ἀνθρώποις εἰς τοὺς βραχίονας, τοῖς δὲ τετράποσιν εἰς τὰ πρόσθια σκέλη τείνουσι, τοῖς δ' ὄρνισιν εἰς τὰς πτέρυγας, τοῖς δ' ἰχθύσιν εἰς τὰ πτερύγια τὰ πρανῆ. αἱ δὲ ἀρχαὶ τούτων τῶν φλεβῶν, ᾗ σχίζονται τὸ πρῶτον καλοῦνται σφαγίτιδες. ᾗ δὲ σχίζονται εἰς τὸν αὐχένα (ἀπὸ τῆς μεγάλης φλεβός), παρὰ τὴν ἀρτηρίαν τείνουσιν (τὴν τοῦ πνεύμονος) ὧν ἐπιλαμβανομένων ἐνίοτε ἔξωθεν ἄνευ πνιγμοῦ καταπίπτουσιν οἱ ἄνθρωποι μετ' ἀναισθησίας, τὰ βλέφαρα

This description is not absolutely clear, since it does not show how distinctly Aristotle recognized the two bifurcations of the 'great vein', that of the vena cava into the right and left innominate veins and the bifurcation of these into the subscapular and internal jugular, since he seems to regard the branches of the first bifurcation as the jugular veins, though this may be merely a matter of customary terminology, and the doubt I have expressed due rather to his ambiguity of description; since it is perhaps a little unlikely that he should have made this topographical error. In a rather confused way he is aware of the existence of two jugular veins, though his description of the external jugular vein is hopelessly incorrect.

His description of the veins of the head is quite inadequate. Dealing with the internal jugular vein and its connections he says:

And from the place by each ear [that is, presumably, the place where the vein he has just described turns down to descend through the neck] another single branch extends towards the brain, and splits up into many thin little veins into the meninx, as it is called, which envelops the brain. Now the brain itself in all animals is bloodless, and neither any big nor any small vein ends in it. And of the other branches that split off from this vein, some surround the head in a circle, while others terminate in the sense organs and the teeth in the form of very slender little veins.[1]

The idea of the bloodless brain, which seems so absurd to us, was of course a very natural conclusion from its external appearance, which also inspired the notion perhaps of its refrigerating function as the source of phlegm.

Aristotle also describes the course of the great vein below the heart in some detail. Much of what he tells us is fantastically inaccurate and cannot be related to any of the known courses of the blood vessels, even supposing a failure to distinguish an artery from a vein. He has however grasped quite correctly that both the inferior vena cava and the abdominal aorta divide into two main iliac branches and that the relative position of the two vessels changes, the aorta in the abdomen riding at its fork over, i.e. on top of, the vena cava.

συμβεβληκότες. οὕτω δὲ τείνουσαι καὶ μεταξὺ λαμβάνουσαι τὴν ἀρτηρίαν φέρουσι μέχρι τῶν ὤτων, ᾗ συμβάλλουσιν αἱ γένυες τῇ κεφαλῇ. πάλιν δ' ἐντεῦθεν εἰς τέτταρας σχίζονται φλέβας, ὧν μία μὲν ἐπανακάμψασα καταβαίνει διὰ τοῦ τραχήλου καὶ τοῦ ὤμου, καὶ συμβάλλει τῇ πρότερον ἀποσχίσει τῆς φλεβὸς κατὰ τὴν τοῦ βραχίονος καμπήν, τὸ δ' ἕτερον μόριον εἰς τὴν χεῖρα τελευτᾷ καὶ τοὺς δακτύλους. The translation of this passage is my own, and I have purposely translated the word *artery* before the first bracket in inverted commas, because here it obviously means *windpipe*, and the bracketed words are an obvious scribal insertion.

[1] *De hist. an.* 3. 3, 514ᵃ15–22: μία δ' ἑτέρα ἀφ' ἑκατέρου τοῦ περὶ τὰ ὦτα ἐπὶ τὸν ἐγκέφαλον τείνει, καὶ σχίζεται εἰς πολλὰ καὶ λεπτὰ φλέβια εἰς τὴν καλουμένην μήνιγγα τὴν περὶ τὸν ἐγκέφαλον. αὐτὸς δ' ὁ ἐγκέφαλος ἄναιμος πάντων ἐστί, καὶ οὔτε μικρὸν οὔτε μέγα φλέβιον τελευτᾷ εἰς αὐτόν. τῶν δὲ λοιπῶν τῶν ἀπὸ φλεβὸς ταύτης σχισθεισῶν φλεβῶν αἱ μὲν τὴν κεφαλὴν κύκλῳ περιλαμβάνουσιν, αἱ δὲ εἰς τὰ αἰσθητήρια ἀποτελευτῶσι καὶ τοὺς ὀδόντας λεπτοῖς πάμπαν φλεβίοις.

His description of the blood vessels below the heart runs as follows:

The part of the great vein which is below the heart runs perpendicularly downwards through the midriff, and it is attached to the aorta and to the spine by slack membrane-like channels [πόροι]. And from it a short but broad vein stretches through the liver, from which many fine branches extend into the liver and are lost to sight. And there are two branches from the vein through the liver, of which one terminates in the midriff, the so-called diaphragm. The other turns upwards and goes up through the armpit into the right arm and joins up with the other veins at the inside of the bend. For this reason when doctors lance this vein, patients are relieved of certain pains round the liver. And from its left side there is a small but thick vein to the spleen, the branches of which disappear into it. Another part divides off from the big vein to the left and goes up in the same way to the left arm.[1]

The short but broad vein to the liver was, as we shall see, to play an important part in the physiology of Galen. What Aristotle meant by the 'vein through the liver' is not at all clear, since the description that he gives of the portal system suggests that he thought that the vein passed right through the liver. He tells us that it sends out many small branches into the liver, but he nowhere explains that all these invisible little veinules reunite at the 'gates' to form the portal vein.[2] For Galen, as for the author of the 'Hippocratic' treatise On nourishment, the liver is the root of the veinous system, not the heart; and for Erasistratus and Galen the liver is the place where the blood is made.[3] Not so for Aristotle.[4] For him it is only a kind of filter to purify the blood of the 'residue' bile which exists for no definite biological purpose, but is merely an 'off-scouring'. The healthy liver is sweet, whereas bile is bitter.[5] The reason of the

[1] Ibid., 3. 4, 514ᵃ29–ᵇ8: τὸ δ' ὑποκάτω τῆς καρδίας μέρος τῆς μεγάλης φλεβὸς τείνει μετέωρον διὰ τοῦ ὑποζώματος, συνέχεται δὲ καὶ πρὸς τὴν ἀορτὴν καὶ πρὸς τὴν ῥάχιν πόροις ὑμενώδεσι καὶ χαλαροῖς. τείνει δ' ἀπ' αὐτῆς μία μὲν διὰ τοῦ ἥπατος φλὲψ βραχεῖα μὲν πλατεῖα δέ. ἀφ' ἧς πολλαὶ καὶ λεπταὶ εἰς τὸ ἧπαρ ἀποτείνουσαι ἀφανίζονται. δύο δ' ἀπὸ τῆς διὰ τοῦ ἥπατος φλεβὸς ἀποσχίσεις εἰσίν, ὧν ἡ μὲν εἰς τὸ ὑπόζωμα τελευτᾷ καὶ τὰς καλουμένας φρένας, ἡ δὲ πάλιν ἐπανελθοῦσα διὰ τῆς μασχάλης εἰς τὸν βραχίονα τὸν δεξιὸν συμβάλλει ταῖς ἑτέραις φλεψὶ κατὰ τὴν ἐντὸς καμπήν. διὸ ἀποσχαζόντων τῶν ἰατρῶν ταύτην ἀπολύονταί τινων πόνων περὶ τὸ ἧπαρ. ἐκ δὲ τῶν ἀριστερῶν αὐτῆς μικρὰ μὲν παχεῖα δὲ φλὲψ τείνει εἰς τὸν σπλῆνα, καὶ ἀφανίζεται τὰ ἀπ' αὐτῆς φλέβια εἰς τοῦτον. ἕτερον δὲ μέρος ἀπὸ τῶν ἀριστερῶν τῆς μεγάλης φλεβὸς ἀποσχισθὲν τὸν αὐτὸν τρόπον ἀναβαίνει ἐπὶ τὸν ἀριστερὸν βραχίονα.

[2] Ibid., 1. 17, 496ᵇ29–31: προσπέφυκε δὲ τῇ μεγάλῃ φλεβὶ τὸ ἧπαρ, τῇ δ' ἀορτῇ οὐ κοινωνεῖ. διὰ γὰρ τοῦ ἥπατος διέχει ἡ ἀπὸ τῆς μεγάλης φλεβὸς φλέψ, ᾗ αἱ καλούμεναι πύλαι εἰσὶ τοῦ ἥπατος.

[3] See above, p. 80; for Erasistratus, below, p. 197; and for Galen, below, p. 325.

[4] De part. an. 3. 4, 666ᵃ24–34: ὑπάρχει δὲ καὶ τὸ ἧπαρ πᾶσι τοῖς ἐναίμοις. ἀλλ' οὐθεὶς ἂν ἀξιώσειεν αὐτὸ ἀρχὴν εἶναι οὔτε τοῦ ὅλου σώματος οὔτε τοῦ αἵματος . . . ἐπεὶ οὖν ἀνάγκη μὲν θάτερον τούτων ἀρχὴν εἶναι, μή ἐστι δὲ τὸ ἧπαρ, ἀνάγκη τὴν καρδίαν εἶναι καὶ τοῦ αἵματος ἀρχήν.

[5] Ibid., 3. 12, 673ᵇ24–8: διόπερ ἔνια καὶ οὐκ ἔχει χολὴν τῶν ζωοτόκων. τὸ γὰρ ἧπαρ συμβάλλεται πολὺ μέρος πρὸς εὐκρασίαν τοῦ σώματος καὶ ὑγίειαν. ἐν μὲν γὰρ τῷ αἵματι μάλιστα τὸ τούτων τέλος, τὸ δ' ἧπαρ αἱματικώτατον μετὰ τὴν καρδίαν τῶν σπλάγχνων.

Cf. ibid., 4. 2, 677ᵃ11–30: ἀλλ' ἔοικεν ἡ χολή, καθάπερ καὶ ἡ κατὰ τὸ ἄλλο σῶμα γινομένη περίττωμά τί ἐστιν ἢ σύντηξις, οὕτω καὶ ἡ ἐπὶ τῷ ἥπατι χολὴ περίττωμα εἶναι καὶ οὐχ ἕνεκά τινος, ὥσπερ καὶ ἡ ἐν τῇ κοιλίᾳ καὶ ἐν τοῖς ἐντέροις ὑπόστασις. καταχρῆται μὲν οὖν ἐνίοτε ἡ φύσις εἰς τὸ

'sweetness' of the liver was not to be elucidated till the nineteenth century, in the work of Claude Bernard. Another point which calls for elucidation is the use of the term πόρος for the connections or attachments of the great vein to the aorta and the spine. Did Aristotle regard these channels as being filled with blood, or did he look upon them as solid processes? The latter would to us appear to be more probable, yet he has just used the same word to describe connections between the heart and the lungs. In this connection it might perhaps be relevant to remember that the word πόρος appears to have been used by Alcmaeon to describe the optic nerve.

The account of the blood vessels or 'veins' in the intestines and the omentum does not seem to show any but the most superficial acquaintance with anatomical fact.

There are still further branches which divide off from the great vein, one to the omentum, and one to the so-called pancreas. And from this branch many veins extend through the mesentery. All these end up in a single big vein, which extends along or past the whole intestine and the stomach as far as the oesophagus, and round these parts many veins divide off from it. Now as far as the kidneys the great vein and the aorta both run single and undivided. But from here on they run more closely attached to the spine and split into two, each forming as it were the letter *lambda*; and the great vein now runs rather behind the aorta.[1]

Aristotle now proceeds to describe the abdominal aorta, having told us earlier that above the heart the branches of this smaller main trunk divide off from it in the same way as those which branch off the great vein; the only difference is that it and its branches are of much smaller diameter.[2] Here too there is some obscurity about the attachments. The aorta is more firmly attached to the spine near the heart, by small

ὠφέλιμον καὶ τοῖς περιττώμασιν, οὐ μὴν διὰ τοῦτο δεῖ ζητεῖν πάντα ἕνεκα τίνος. . . . ὅσοις μὲν οὖν ἡ τοῦ ἥπατος σύστασις ὑγιεινή ἐστι καὶ ἡ τοῦ αἵματος φύσις γλυκεῖα ἡ εἰς τοῦτ' ἀποκρινομένη, ταῦτα μὲν ἢ πάμπαν οὐκ ἴσχει χολὴν ἐπὶ τοῦ ἥπατος, ἢ ἔν τισι φλεβίοις, ἢ τὰ μὲν τὰ δ' οὔ. διὸ καὶ τὰ ἥπατα τὰ τῶν ἀχόλων εὔχρω καὶ γλυκερά ἐστιν ὡς ἐπίπαν εἰπεῖν, καὶ τῶν ἐχόντων χολὴν τὸ ὑπὸ τῇ χολῇ τοῦ ἥπατος γλυκύτατόν ἐστιν. τῶν δὲ συνισταμένων ἐξ ἧττον καθαροῦ αἵματος τούτου ἐστὶν ἡ χολὴ τὸ γινόμενον περίττωμα. ἐναντίον τε γὰρ τῇ τροφῇ τὸ περίττωμα βούλεται εἶναι καὶ τῷ γλυκεῖ τὸ πικρόν, καὶ τὸ αἷμα γλυκὺ τὸ ὑγιαῖνον. φανερὸν οὖν ὅτι οὔ τινος ἕνεκα, ἀλλ' ἀποκάθαρμά ἐστιν ἡ χολή.

[1] *De hist. an.* 3. 4, 514ᵇ10–19: ἔτι δ' ἄλλαι ἀπὸ τῆς μεγάλης φλεβὸς ἀποσχίζονται, ἡ μὲν ἐπὶ τὸ ἐπίπλοον, ἡ δ' ἐπὶ τὸ καλούμενον πάγκρεας. ἀπὸ δὲ ταύτης πολλαὶ φλέβες διὰ τοῦ μεσεντερίου τείνουσιν. πᾶσαι δ' αὗται εἰς μίαν φλέβα μεγάλην τελευτῶσιν, παρὰ πᾶν τὸ ἔντερον καὶ τὴν κοιλίαν μέχρι τοῦ στομάχου τεταμένην. καὶ περὶ ταῦτα τὰ μόρια πολλαὶ ἀπ' αὐτῶν σχίζονται φλέβες.

μέχρι μὲν οὖν τῶν νεφρῶν μία οὖσα ἑκατέρα τείνει, καὶ ἡ ἀορτὴ καὶ ἡ μεγάλη φλέψ. ἐνταῦθα δὲ πρός τε τὴν ῥάχιν μᾶλλον προσπεφύκασι καὶ σχίζονται εἰς δύο ὡσπερεὶ λάμβδα ἑκάτερα, καὶ γίγνεται εἰς τοὔπισθεν μᾶλλον ἡ μεγάλη φλὲψ τῆς ἀορτῆς.

[2] *Ibid.*, 514ᵃ23–6: τὸν δ' αὐτὸν τρόπον καὶ τὰ τῆς ἐλάττονος φλεβός, καλουμένης δ' ἀορτῆς, ἔσχισται μέρη, συμπαρακολουθοῦντα τοῖς τῆς μεγάλης. πλὴν ἐλάττους οἱ πόροι καὶ τὰ φλέβια πολλῷ ἐλάττω ταύτης ἐστὶ τῶν τῆς μεγάλης φλεβός.

sinewy little veins. Except for the liver and the spleen, the branches of the aorta in the mesentery and the omentum also follow those of the great vein.

The aorta is most closely attached to the spine near the heart. The attachment takes the form of small, sinew-like little veins. The aorta when it emerges from the heart is a vessel of very large diameter, but as it proceeds it becomes narrower and more sinew-like. And veins extend from the aorta to the mesentery, just as they do from the great vein, except that they are much smaller in size, for they are narrow and thread-like, and terminate in fine complicated thread-like little veins. But there is no vein which extends from the aorta to the liver and the spleen.

Now divisions from each of these two great vessels extend to each flank, and they both attach themselves to the bone. And veins run from the great vein and from the aorta into the kidneys. Only they do not go into the cavity but spend themselves in the body of the kidneys. Now from the aorta two other channels, strong and continuous, go into the bladder, and there are others which come out of the hollow of the kidneys, which have no connection with the great vein. To the middle of each kidney a hollow sinew-like vein is attached which extends along the spine itself through the narrows. Then each of them disappears into the flank or hip-joint, but further on they become visible again as their course runs against the hip-bone. And their endings attach themselves to the penis in males and to the womb in females. But from the big vein there is no branch leading to the womb, but there are many, closely packed from the aorta.[1]

It might appear, at first sight, that he has confused the ureters with some branch of the aorta, but in his account of the bladder he carefully distinguishes the channels leading from the kidneys to the bladder from the ones that come from the aorta by the fact that they have no blood in

---

[1] Ibid., 514ᵇ19–515ᵃ6: προσπέφυκε δ' ἡ ἀορτὴ μάλιστα τῇ ῥάχει περὶ τὴν καρδίαν. ἡ δὲ πρόσφυσίς ἐστι φλεβίοις νευρώδεσι καὶ μικροῖς. ἔστι δ' ἡ ἀορτὴ ἀπὸ μὲν τῆς καρδίας ἀγομένη εὖ μάλα κοίλη, προϊοῦσα δ' ἐστὶ στενοτέρα καὶ νευρωδεστέρα. τείνουσι δὲ καὶ ἀπὸ τῆς ἀορτῆς εἰς τὸ μεσεντέριον φλέβες ὥσπερ αἱ ἀπὸ τῆς μεγάλης φλεβός, πλὴν πολλῷ λειπόμεναι τῷ μεγέθει. στεναὶ γάρ εἰσι καὶ ἰνώδεις, λεπτοῖς δὲ καὶ ποικίλοις καὶ ἰνώδεσι τελευτῶσι φλεβίοις. εἰς δὲ τὸ ἧπαρ καὶ τὸν σπλῆνα οὐδεμία τείνει ἀπὸ τῆς ἀορτῆς φλέψ.

αἱ δὲ σχίσεις ἑκατέρας τῆς φλεβὸς τείνουσιν εἰς τὸ ἰσχίον ἑκάτερον, καὶ καθάπτουσιν εἰς τὸ ὀστοῦν ἀμφότεραι. φέρουσι δὲ καὶ εἰς τοὺς νεφροὺς ἀπό τε τῆς μεγάλης φλεβὸς καὶ τῆς ἀορτῆς φλέβες, πλὴν οὐκ εἰς τὸ κοῖλον ἀλλ' εἰς τὸ σῶμα καταναλίσκονται τῶν νεφρῶν. ἀπὸ μὲν οὖν τῆς ἀορτῆς ἄλλοι δύο πόροι φέρουσιν εἰς τὴν κύστιν, ἰσχυροὶ καὶ συνεχεῖς. καὶ ἄλλοι ἐκ τοῦ κοίλου τῶν νεφρῶν, οὐδὲν κοινωνοῦντες τῇ μεγάλῃ φλεβί. ἐκ μέσου δὲ τῶν νεφρῶν ἑκατέρου φλὲψ κοίλη καὶ νευρώδης ἐξήρτηται, τείνουσα παρ' αὐτὴν τὴν ῥάχιν διὰ τῶν στενῶν. εἶτα εἰς ἑκάτερον τὸ ἰσχίον ἀφανίζεται ἑκατέρα πρῶτον, ἔπειτα δῆλαι γίγνονται πάλιν διατεταμέναι πρὸς τὸ ἰσχίον. καθάπτουσι δὲ πρὸς ⟨τὴν κύστιν καὶ⟩ τὸ αἰδοῖον τὰ πέρατα αὐτῶν ἐν τοῖς ἄρρεσιν, ἐν δὲ τοῖς θήλεσι πρὸς τὰς ὑστέρας. τείνει δ' ἀπὸ μὲν τῆς μεγάλης φλεβὸς οὐδεμία εἰς τὰς ὑστέρας, ἀπὸ δὲ τῆς ἀορτῆς πολλαὶ καὶ πυκναί.

But in the *Generation of animals* we are told rather a different story. Both the great vein and the aorta appear to send out little veins which terminate in the womb. Cf. *De gen. an.* 2. 4, 738ᵃ9–12: τοῖς μὲν οὖν θήλεσι περὶ τὸν τῶν ὑστερῶν τόπον, σχιζομένων ἄνωθεν τῶν δύο φλεβῶν τῆς τε μεγάλης καὶ τῆς ἀορτῆς, πολλαὶ καὶ λεπταὶ φλέβες τελευτῶσιν εἰς τὰς ὑστέρας ...

them. While the latter were described as strong and continuous, the ureters themselves are described as 'vigorous' (νεανικοί), aptly rendered by Peck as 'sturdy'.[1] This duplication must, I fear, remain something of a mystery. With the course of the main vessels connected with the iliac artery and the iliac vein, Aristotle shows a general acquaintance, in so far as he realizes that they form the blood vessels running down the thigh and the leg, but his description of the criss-crossing through the groin and the thighs remains very obscure. Was he trying to describe the rather complicated intertwinings of the iliac veins and arteries and their derivatives? What he says about them runs as follows:

And from the aorta and the great vein, where they divide, other branches also come off, some of them large and hollow to begin with, going first to the buttocks, and then through the legs ending up in the feet and the toes. And others run back [i.e. in the opposite direction?] through the buttocks and the thighs going cross-wise, the one from the left side over to the right, and the one from the right side over to the left, and they join the other veins in the hams.[2]

The description of the blood vessels given in the treatise on the *Parts of animals* follows in general along the same lines as that in the *History*, but here we are given a short account of the blood's physiological functions as the ultimate form of nourishment. The course of the veins must be extended over the whole body; blood must go through every part and be everywhere, since every portion of the body is composed of it.[3] Then follows the well-known comparison of the vascular system with, first, an irrigation system for a garden, and, secondly, the laying out of materials on the site of the construction of a house.

The system of blood vessels resembles the arrangement of watercourses in gardens which are constructed of a single source or spring and divided up into many channels, each branching into many more, so that they supply water to every part. It also resembles the arrangements whereby, in the construction of houses, stones are placed all along the line-plan of the foundations. This is because the plants in a garden grow out of water—the material of which they are composed—while the foundations of a house are built up out of stones.

---

[1] *De part. an.* 3. 9, 671ᵇ13–18: ὁ δ' ἀπὸ τῆς φλεβὸς τείνων πόρος οὐκ εἰς τὸ κοῖλον τῶν νεφρῶν καταταλευτᾷ, ἀλλ' εἰς τὸ σῶμα καταναλίσκεται τῶν νεφρῶν. διόπερ ἐν τοῖς κοίλοις αὐτῶν οὐκ ἐγγίνεται αἷμα, οὐδὲ πήγνυνται τελευτώντων. ἐκ δὲ τοῦ κοίλου τῶν νεφρῶν φέρουσι πόροι ἄναιμοι εἰς τὴν κύστιν δύο νεανικοί, ἐξ ἑκατέρου εἷς, καὶ ἄλλοι ἐκ τῆς ἀορτῆς ἰσχυροὶ καὶ συνεχεῖς.

[2] *De hist. an.* 3. 4, 515ᵃ6–13: τείνουσι δ' ἀπὸ τῆς ἀορτῆς καὶ τῆς μεγάλης φλεβὸς σχιζομένων καὶ ἄλλαι, αἱ μὲν ἐπὶ τοὺς βουβῶνας πρῶτον μεγάλαι καὶ κοῖλαι, ἔπειτα διὰ τῶν σκελῶν τελευτῶσιν εἰς τοὺς πόδας καὶ τοὺς δακτύλους. καὶ πάλιν ἔτεραι διὰ τῶν βουβώνων καὶ τῶν μηρῶν φέρουσιν ἐναλλάξ, ἡ μὲν ἐκ τῶν ἀριστερῶν εἰς τὰ δεξιά, ἡ δ' εἰς τὰ ἀριστερὰ ἐκ τῶν δεξιῶν. καὶ συνάπτουσι περὶ τὰς ἰγνύας ταῖς ἑτέραις φλεψίν.

[3] *De part. an.* 3. 5, 668ᵃ10–13: συνισταμένων δὲ τῶν μορίων ἐκ τοῦ αἵματος καθάπερ εἴπομεν, εὐλόγως ἡ τῶν φλεβῶν ῥύσις διὰ παντὸς τοῦ σώματος πέφυκεν. δεῖ γὰρ καὶ τὸ αἷμα διὰ παντὸς καὶ παρὰ πᾶν εἶναι, εἴπερ τῶν μορίων ἕκαστον ἐκ τούτου συνέστηκεν.

In the same way nature channels blood through the body, since blood is the material of all its parts. This is quite clearly shown in persons who are very emaciated, for there is nothing to be seen in their bodies but the veins, just as, when they dry up, the leaves of vines or fig trees or such like, leave nothing else to be seen except their veins. The reason for this is that the blood and its equivalent the sap are *potentially* the body, that is, the flesh or its vegetable counterpart. Now just as in irrigation works the largest channels stay put, while the smallest quickly disappear beneath the flood, only to re-appear when it subsides, so in the body, the largest veins persist, but the smallest ones *actually* become flesh, though *potentially* they are none the less veins. Therefore as long as flesh remains flesh, wherever it is cut, blood runs out. Nevertheless without veins there can be no blood, even if no vein, not even the smallest, is visible, just as in irrigation systems the channels are invisible until the flooding has subsided.[1]

The blood vessels decrease progressively until they become so small that the diameter of their lumen is insufficient to permit the blood to pass along them. But even if blood cannot pass through, sweat is able to do so, when the body is thoroughly heated, and the veins open their mouths wider. In certain cases the sweat excreted has a blood-like character. This is due to bad bodily condition, when the blood has become watery due to lack of concoction owing to the scantiness of the heat in the little veins, which is insufficient to effect concoction. Now this scantiness is relative to the quantity of food ingested, or to its indigestible character.[2]

A passage now follows describing, rather more succinctly than the equivalent paragraphs in the *History of animals*, the respective courses of the great vein and the aorta.

[1] Ibid., 668ᵃ14–ᵇ1 : ἔοικε δ' ὥσπερ ἔν τε τοῖς κήποις αἱ ὑδραγωγίαι κατασκευάζονται ἀπὸ μιᾶς ἀρχῆς καὶ πηγῆς εἰς πολλοὺς ὀχετοὺς καὶ ἄλλους ἀεὶ πρὸς τὸ πάντῃ μεταδιδόναι, καὶ ἐν ταῖς οἰκοδομίαις παρὰ πᾶσαν τὴν τῶν θεμελίων ὑπογραφὴν λίθοι παραβέβληνται, διὰ τὸ τὰ μὲν κηπευ-όμενα φύεσθαι ἐκ τοῦ ὕδατος, τοὺς δὲ θεμελίους ἐκ τῶν λίθων οἰκοδομεῖσθαι, τὸν αὐτὸν τρόπον καὶ ἡ φύσις τὸ αἷμα διὰ παντὸς ᾠχέτευκε τοῦ σώματος, ἐπειδὴ παντὸς ὕλη πέφυκε τοῦτο. γίνεται δὲ κατάδηλον ἐν τοῖς μάλιστα καταλελεπτυσμένοις. οὐθὲν γὰρ ἄλλο φαίνεται παρὰ τὰς φλέβας, καθάπερ ἐπὶ τῶν ἀμπελίνων τε καὶ συκίνων φύλλων καὶ ὅσ' ἄλλα τοιαῦτα. καὶ γὰρ τούτων αὐαι-νομένων φλέβες λείπονται μόνον. τούτων δ' αἴτιον ὅτι τὸ αἷμα καὶ τὸ ἀνάλογον τούτῳ δυνάμει σῶμα καὶ σάρξ ἢ τὸ ἀνάλογόν ἐστιν. καθάπερ οὖν ἐν ταῖς ὀχεταίαις αἱ μέγισται τῶν τάφρων διαμένουσιν, αἱ δ' ἐλάχισται πρῶται καὶ ταχέως ὑπὸ τῆς ἰλύος ἀφανίζονται, πάλιν δ' ἐκλειπούσης φανεραὶ γίνονται, τὸν αὐτὸν τρόπον καὶ τῶν φλεβῶν αἱ μὲν μέγισται διαμένουσιν, αἱ δ' ἐλάχισται γίνονται σάρκες ἐνεργείᾳ, δυνάμει δ' εἰσὶν οὐδὲν ἧσσον φλέβες. διὸ καὶ σωζομένων τῶν σαρκῶν καθ' ὁτιοῦν αἷμα ῥεῖ διαιρουμένων. καίτοι ἄνευ μὲν φλεβὸς οὐκ ἔστιν αἷμα, φλέβιον δ' οὐδὲν δῆλον, ὥσπερ ἐν τοῖς ὀχετοῖς αἱ τάφροι πρὶν ἢ τὴν ἰλὺν ἐξαιρεθῆναι.

[2] Ibid., 668ᵇ1–13 : ἐκ μειζόνων δ' εἰς ἐλάσσους αἱ φλέβες ἀεὶ προέρχονται ἕως τοῦ γενέσθαι τοὺς πόρους ἐλάσσους τῆς τοῦ αἵματος παχύτητος· δι' ὧν τῷ μὲν αἵματι δίοδος οὐκ ἔστι, τῷ δὲ περιττώματι τῆς ὑγρᾶς ἰκμάδος, ὃν καλοῦμεν ἱδρῶτα, καὶ τοῦτο διαθερμανθέντος τοῦ σώματος καὶ τῶν φλεβίων ἀναστομωθέντων. ἤδη δέ τισιν ἱδρῶσαι συνέβη αἱματώδει περιττώματι διὰ καχεξίαν, τοῦ μὲν σώματος ῥυάδος καὶ μανοῦ γενομένου, τοῦ δ' αἵματος ἐξυγρανθέντος δι' ἀπεψίαν, ἀδυνατού-σης τῆς ἐν τοῖς φλεβίοις θερμότητος πέσσειν δι' ὀλιγότητα. εἴρηται γὰρ ὅτι πᾶν τὸ κοινὸν γῆς καὶ ὕδατος παχύνεται πεσσόμενον, ἡ δὲ τροφὴ καὶ τὸ αἷμα μικτὸν ἐξ ἀμφοῖν. ἀδυνατεῖ δὲ πέσσειν ἡ θερμότης οὐ μόνον διὰ τὴν αὑτῆς ὀλιγότητα ἀλλὰ καὶ διὰ πλῆθος καὶ ὑπερβολὴν τῆς εἰσφερομένης τροφῆς.

In their upper parts the great vein and the aorta are some distance away from one another, but lower down they change their respective positions and hold the body together. For as they descend they split in two in accordance with the divergence of the legs. And one of them [sc. the great vein] from being in front now runs behind, while the other [sc. the aorta] which was behind now runs in front; and[1] they come together to form a single structure. For just as in plaited objects intertwining produces greater coherence, so the front parts of the body are bound to the back parts by this intertwining of the veins. A similar thing happens above the heart.[1]

This notion of the blood vessels as forming a framework to hold the body together is also found in the treatise *On the generation of animals*, where they are compared to κάναβοι, a word which may mean either the wooden framework round which modellers moulded their wax or plaster, or, so Liddell and Scott tell us, a mannikin or rough drawing of the human frame. As Peck observes, the former would certainly appear to be the more appropriate translation in this case.[2]

So much for the main blood vessels of which Aristotle's account represents an enormous advance on that of Diogenes of Apollonia, indeed quite a fair first approximation to the anatomical truth. It is when we come to examine his theory of the vascular connections between the lungs and the heart that we find ourselves on much less clearly mapped territory. The lungs are, as we have already noted, connected with all three ventricles of the heart by passages, which in the case of two of them are not clearly distinguishable owing to their small size.[3] These passages are something of a puzzle. Assuming the 'visible' passage connecting the great ventricle with the lung to be the pulmonary artery, it is not easy to understand how the other set of vessels connecting lung and heart, the pulmonary veins, could be called difficult to see on account of their smallness. Aristotle was, of course, aware that there were two systems of vessels forming an arrangement not unlike the branches of a tree in the lungs, one of which contained air and the other blood. Did he know also of another similar system, which we call today the pulmonary veins? For he tells us that if you blow down the windpipe the passage of air into the heart is perfectly clear in the case of the larger animals,[4] in spite of the fact that there is no direct connection with the blood vessel leading from

---

[1] *De part. an.* 3. 5, 668ᵇ20–8 : διεστῶσαι δ' ἄνωθεν ἥ τε μεγάλη φλὲψ καὶ ἡ ἀορτή, κάτω δ' ἐναλλάσσουσαι συνέχουσι τὸ σῶμα. προϊοῦσαι γὰρ σχίζονται κατὰ τὴν διφυΐαν τῶν κώλων, καὶ ἡ μὲν ἐκ τοῦ ἔμπροσθεν εἰς τοὔπισθεν προέρχεται, ἡ δ' ἐκ τοῦ ὄπισθεν εἰς τὸ ἔμπροσθεν καὶ συμβάλλουσιν εἰς ἕν. ὥσπερ γὰρ ἐν τοῖς πλεκομένοις ἐγγίνεται τὸ συνεχὲς μᾶλλον, οὕτω καὶ διὰ τῆς τῶν φλεβῶν ἐναλλάξεως συνδεῖται τῶν σωμάτων τὰ πρόσθια τοῖς ὄπισθεν. ὁμοίως δὲ καὶ ἀπὸ τῆς καρδίας ἐν τοῖς ἄνω τόποις συμβαίνει.

[2] *De gen. an.* 2. 6, 743ᵃ1–3 : ἐκ δὲ τῆς καρδίας αἱ φλέβες διατέτανται καθάπερ οἱ τοὺς κανάβους γράφοντες ἐν τοῖς τοίχοις· τὰ γὰρ μέρη περὶ ταύτας ἐστίν, ἅτε γινόμενα ἐκ τούτων.

[3] See the passage from *De hist. an.*, quoted p. 123, n. 2.

[4] *De hist. an.* 1., 16, 495ᵇ14 : φυσωμένης δὲ τῆς ἀρτηρίας ἐν ἐνίοις μὲν οὐ κατάδηλον ποιεῖ, ἐν δὲ τοῖς μείζοσι τῶν ζῴων δῆλον ὅτι εἰσέρχεται τὸ πνεῦμα εἰς αὐτήν.

the heart.[1] Yet these vessels do receive the breath and convey it to the heart. It is not at all clear whether these passages (πόροι) are the same as the visible connection or a different set of tubes, but it seems probable that they are. If so, the existence of the pulmonary veins as opposed to or differentiated from the pulmonary arteries must have escaped Aristotle's observation. This indeed seems to me to be almost certain, since an examination of his description of the lungs does not suggest any acquaintance with a double set of blood vessels in the lung itself. Yet we cannot be too confident on this point, for if the branches of the aorta follow the same course as those of the 'great vein', there should be a branch of the aorta corresponding to the pulmonary artery, though this is nowhere mentioned. Some light might perhaps have been thrown upon this problem if the work on *Dissections*, which he mentions more than once, had survived. As it is, we must try to make what sense we can out of the descriptions given in the surviving biological works.

Aristotle seems to have looked upon the lungs, or rather the lung (for he regards it as a single organ),[2] as a sort of inflatable sack supplied with air through the bronchial system, the branches of which he characterizes as cartilaginous.[3] The windpipe divides first into two, one branch going into what we should describe as each lung, and each branch divides into progressively smaller and smaller branches or pipes, the ends of which are not closed but constitute an orifice (τρῆμα). The lung has empty spaces between these vessels into which the air is drawn through the windpipe when a creature breathes in. These empty spaces have cartilage-like 'germinations' coming off at an acute angle, and from these 'germinating' branches there are 'perforations' which pervade the whole lung, as each branch opens up into progressively smaller ones. Along each branch and offshoot of the windpipe there runs a corresponding branch of the 'vein', which extends from the heart into the lung, so that there is no part of the lung which does not contain a veinule and the perforated end of a bronchiole, the terminations of which are too small to be seen, and in this complex arrangement of vessels the branches of the vein are always above those of the windpipe. And though there is no common passage, the heart draws breath or *pneuma* through the blood vessels into the heart.[4]

---

[1] Ibid., 496ª, a passage quoted p. 124.

[2] Ibid., 1. 16, 495ᵇ33–ᵇ5: θέλει γὰρ εἶναι διμερὴς ὁ πνεύμων ἐν ἅπασι τοῖς ἔχουσιν αὐτόν. ἀλλ' ἐν μὲν τοῖς ζωοτόκοις οὐχ ὁμοίως ἡ διάστασις φανερά, ἥκιστα δ' ἐν ἀνθρώπῳ . . . ἐν δὲ τοῖς ῳοτόκοις . . . πολὺ τὸ μέρος ἑκάτερον ἀπ' ἀλλήλων ἔσχισται, ὥστε δοκεῖν δύο ἔχειν πνεύμονας.

[3] Ibid., 495ª23–4: ἔστι δ' ἡ μὲν ἀρτηρία χονδρώδης τὴν φύσιν καὶ ὀλίγαιμος πολλοῖς λεπτοῖς φλεβίοις περιεχομένη.

[4] Ibid., 495ᵇ8–12: φυσωμένης δὲ τῆς ἀρτηρίας διαδίδωσιν εἰς τὰ κοῖλα μέρη τοῦ πνεύμονος τὸ πνεῦμα. ταῦτα δὲ διαφύσεις ἔχει χονδρώδεις εἰς ὀξὺ συνηκούσας· ἐκ δὲ τῶν διαφύσεων τρήματα διὰ παντός ἐστι τοῦ πνεύμονος, ἀεὶ ἐκ μειζόνων εἰς ἐλάττω διαδιδόμενα.

Cf. ibid. 3. 3, 513ᵇ17–23: ἡ μὲν οὖν ἐπὶ τὸν πνεύμονα τείνουσα φλὲψ εἰς διμερῆ ὄντ' αὐτὸν διχῆ σχίζεται πρῶτον. εἶτα παρ' ἑκάστην σύριγγα καὶ ἕκαστον τρῆμα τείνει, μείζων μὲν παρὰ τὰ μείζω,

In making this précis I have deliberately departed in one place from the translation of the text of the *History of animals*, both of D'Arcy Thompson and of Peck, who translate the word διάφυσις as *division* in the passage quoted in p. 155, n. 4, where Aristotle is made to say of the hollow parts of the lung: 'These parts have divisions, consisting of gristle, which meet in a point; and from the divisions there are "apertures" running through the whole of the lung, breaking up into smaller and smaller ones.'[1] What these gristly or cartilaginous divisions in the lung can be supposed to be, I have not been able to imagine, but if we look at some of the other meanings given in Liddell and Scott, we may perhaps see a little daylight. The first meaning there given is 'germination', in a citation from Theophrastus,[2] and the derivation from διαφύω is also stated. Another meaning is adduced from 'Hippocrates', where it is made to signify the point or line of separation between the stalk and the branch.[3] There would therefore appear to be ample justification for regarding these 'divisions' as points of bifurcation between branches of the 'artery'. The next crux concerns the meaning of this much-used word τρήματα. This must, I think, refer to the bronchioles, which are also in other passages referred to as pipes, σύριγγες. It looks to me as if the word ἀρτηρία was applied only to the windpipe and its main branches, the word σύριγξ to the smaller branches, and the word τρῆμα to the air tubes corresponding to the invisible terminations of the bronchioles through which the air is drawn into the hollow parts of the lung.

The words used by Aristotle to describe the various tubes in the lung were submitted by Huxley to a careful examination.[4] He refuses to accept the translation of 'divisions' or 'partitions' for the word διαφύσεις, or that of 'perforations' or 'openings' for the word τρήματα, which are used by Aubert and Wimmer in their translation.[5]

I cannot think that by διαφύσεις and τρήματα in this passage Aristotle meant either partitions or openings in the ordinary sense of the word. For in Book III, cap. 3, in describing the 'vein which goes to the lung' (the pulmonary artery) he says that it 'extends alongside each tube (σύριγξ) and each passage (πόρος), the larger beside the larger and the smaller beside the smaller, etc., so that no part can be found from which a passage (πόρος) and a vein are absent'. It is plain that by σύριγγες Aristotle means the bronchi

---

ἐλάττων δὲ παρὰ τὰ ἐλάττω, οὕτως ὥστε μηδὲν εἶναι μόριον λαβεῖν ἐν ᾧ οὐ τρῆμά τ' ἔνεστι καὶ φλέβιον· τὰ γὰρ τελευταῖα τῷ μεγέθει ἄδηλα διὰ τὴν μικρότητά ἐστιν, ἀλλὰ πᾶς ὁ πνεύμων φαίνεται μεστὸς ὢν αἵματος.

[1] Cf. the passage from *De hist. an.* I. 17, quoted above.
[2] Theophrastus, *Hist. Plant.* 81. 6.
[3] Hippocrates, *On the eight-month child*, 10.   [4] Huxley, op. cit.
[5] 'Diese aber haben knorpelige Scheidewände, welche unter spitzen Winkeln zusammentreten, und aus ihnen führen Oeffnungen durch die ganze Lunge, indem sie sich immer kleiner verzweigen.'

and so many of their larger divisions as obviously contain cartilages, and that by his διαφύσεις χονδρώδεις he describes the same thing, and if this be so, then the τρήματα must be the smaller bronchial canals in which the cartilages disappear. In every part of the lung there is an air-tube derived from the τραχεῖα and other tubes derived from the πόροι which lead from the heart to the lung. Their applied walls constitute the thin synapses through which the air passes out of the air-tubes into the πόροι or blood vessels by transudation or diffusion, for there is no community between the cavities of the air-tubes and the cavity of the canals, that is to say, no opening from one to the other.

The general scheme thus described by Huxley seems to be clear enough, though I am a little uncertain as to some of the details. Huxley speaks of diffusion and transudation, neither of which are mentioned as such by Aristotle. My conception of the mechanism is slightly different. The transfer of the in-breathed air from the air-tubes to the blood vessels appears to me to take place rather through their open ends which co-incide. This conception we shall meet with again in Galen. But the general idea of the inflated bag as applying to the lung seems to me to be plain enough.

From these hollow parts the air passes via the 'veins' into the heart. This raises two queries. Did Aristotle believe that through the pulmonary arteries blood passed in one direction from the heart to the lung, while *pneuma* passed in the other from the lung to the heart, or did he postulate a separate set of channels to carry air or *pneuma* to one, presumably the leftmost and smallest ventricle? It has generally been assumed that the blood vessel described as being a visible connection of the lung with one of the ventricles was the pulmonary artery, e.g. by Huxley and Mühsam, but D'Arcy Thompson thought that Aristotle probably regarded the aorta and the pulmonary artery as a single system,[1] which seems to me to be rather improbable. Symmetry would seem to require a blood vessel corresponding to the pulmonary artery to connect the lung with the left ventricle, but unfortunately there is the evidence of Aristotle's own description of the invisibility of the connection between the lungs and two similar ventricles against this assumption. We have already noted that we find surprisingly little accurate information about the heart and its vascular connections in the *Hippocratic corpus*, with the exception of the fragment *On the heart*. In the treatise *On the nature of bones*, the 'old' or 'thick' vein sends off a thick branch into the heart 'with many mouths', πολύστομον.[2] It is perhaps important to consider that the anatomical knowledge of the beginning of the fourth century B.C. was, for the most part, still quite incredibly crude. The 'Hippocratic' treatise which we

---

[1] See his note to the passage in 513ª in the Oxford translation of the *History of Animals*, quoted above, p. 130.

[2] See above, p. 63.

have just cited begins with that cryptic chapter which contains the words, 'drink through the pharynx and the oesophagus, the larynx into the lung, and the windpipe and from these into the top of the bladder',[1] stating apparently a doctrine which Aristotle himself takes the trouble to refute. The idea that drink goes down the windpipe is absurd. The windpipe does nothing but take in breath and emit it. When any matter, solid or fluid, goes into it by mistake, it causes choking and distressful coughing.[2] He thus by implication refutes the theory put forward by Plato in the *Timaeus*, which we have already mentioned,[3] as well as the view which was expressed in the 'Hippocratic' treatise. This, he tells us, is proved by the following facts. There is no passage leading from the lung into the stomach, and there is no doubt where any vomited fluids come from. It is also clear that the fluids we drink do not collect directly in the bladder; they go first to the stomach, a fact that is proved by the appearance of wine dregs in fluid evacuated from it.[4]

There is little to tell us how Aristotle actually conceived the motion of the blood in the body. In the treatise *On sleep*, which gives us the most logical account of the physiology of the three ventricles, we are told that the middle ventricle is connected, how he does not tell us, with the other two, of which one, the largest presumably, the right ventricle, is connected with the 'great vein' and the other, the smallest, with the aorta. We are also told that each of the outside ventricles receives blood from the 'great vein' and the aorta respectively. Where does this blood come from and where is it made? The heart is, as we have seen from the other treatises *passim*, the starting-point and the fountain of blood, and the middle ventricle is the source of the blood in the other two, as we have already noted. But in the *De somno*, we have rather a different account. Blood is, in the ultimate resort, produced out of the food and drink ingested by the animal, and this transformation takes place in the 'veins' which lead from the stomach and intestines to the heart.[5] We are told in the *History of animals* of a large vein running the whole length of the

[1] See above, p. 53.

[2] *De hist. an.* 1. 16, 495ᵇ16–19: ἡ μὲν οὖν ἀρτηρία τοῦτον ἔχει τὸν τρόπον, καὶ δέχεται μόνον τὸ πνεῦμα καὶ ἀφίησιν, ἄλλο δ' οὐδὲν οὔτε ξηρὸν οὔθ' ὑγρόν, ἢ πόνον παρέχει, ἕως ἂν ἐκβήξῃ τὸ κατελθόν.

[3] See above, pp. 86, 119.

[4] *De part. an.* 3. 3, 664ᵇ4–17: ἐὰν γάρ τι παρεισρυῇ ξηρὸν ἢ ὑγρὸν εἰς τὴν ἀρτηρίαν, πνιγμοὺς καὶ πόνους καὶ βῆχας χαλεπὰς ἐμποιεῖ. ὃ δὴ καὶ θαυμάσειεν ἄν τις τῶν λεγόντων ὡς ταύτῃ τὸ ποτὸν δέχεται τὸ ζῷον· συμβαίνει γὰρ φανερῶς τὰ λεχθέντα πᾶσιν οἷς ἂν παραρρυῇ τι τῆς τροφῆς. πολλαχῇ δὲ γελοῖον φαίνεται τὸ λέγειν ὡς ταύτῃ τὸ ποτὸν εἰσδέχεται τὰ ζῷα. πόρος γὰρ οὐδείς ἐστιν εἰς τὴν κοιλίαν ἀπὸ τοῦ πλεύμονος, ὥσπερ ἐκ τοῦ στόματος ὁρῶμεν τὸν οἰσοφάγον. ἔτι δ' ἐν τοῖς ἐμέτοις καὶ ναυτίαις οὐκ ἄδηλον πόθεν τὸ ὑγρὸν φαίνεται πορευόμενον. δῆλον δὲ καὶ ὅτι οὐκ εὐθέως εἰς τὴν κύστιν συλλέγεται τὸ ὑγρόν, ἀλλ' εἰς τὴν κοιλίαν πρότερον· τὰ γὰρ τῆς κοιλίας περιττώματα φαίνεται χρωματίζειν ἡ ἰλὺς τοῦ μέλανος οἴνου.

[5] *De somno*, 3, 456ᵇ2–5, quoted above, p. 135, n. 1.

intestines and the stomach connecting up with the 'great vein',[1] and the existence of a corresponding branch of the aorta is, of course, implied, though this will be of much smaller lumen than the one leading into the 'great vein'. For the aorta, according to the *De somno*, is connected with the smallest, i.e. the leftmost, ventricle. The middle ventricle is where the two kinds of blood, the thick and 'muddy' and the 'light and clear', are separated. Putting these two accounts together, we seem to arrive at the following picture. The nutritive elements of ingested food and drink which have been cooked up in the stomach and intestines, through the influence of the connate heat conveyed through the 'veins' from the heart, are carried, while undergoing this transformation, to the heart, where they receive their final elaboration, being turned into blood, it would appear, in the two exterior ventricles, whose contents are passed on to the middle ventricle, where the separation of the two kinds of blood takes place. These two kinds must not be identified with what we today call arterial and venous blood, for though there are two different kinds of main blood vessels, the membrane-like stemming from the 'great vein' and the sinew-like stemming from the aorta, each system conveys both kinds of blood, since the two kinds are located in the upper and the lower portions of the body respectively, i.e. above and below the heart.[2] The difference between the blood in the two systems of blood vessels seems to be merely one of temperature, for the blood in the ventricle communicating with the aorta, be it the middle ventricle or the left, is cooler than that of the right ventricle, or at any rate contains less heat.[3] But difference in temperature would also appear to be responsible for the fractional distillation resulting in the two kinds of blood.

Sleep comes when the fluid and semi-solid [σωματοειδές] substances are brought upwards by the heat, or hot substance, through the veins to the head. When that which has been brought upwards is no longer able to rise further, owing to its volume or quantity, it pushes the hot back again and flows downwards . . . the brain . . . is the coldest portion of the body . . . and just as moisture vaporized by the heat of the sun, when it reaches the upper regions condenses owing to their coldness, and becomes liquid, collecting in drops and returning to the earth as rain, so when the heat carries the vaporized products of digestion to the head, the portion of these which resembles a residue condenses into phlegm—hence catarrhs seem to come down from the head—while the nutritious and healthy portions are carried downwards in condensed form and cool the hot . . .

Awakening occurs when digestion is completed and when the heat has been concentrated into a small space in large quantities drawn from the periphery and has gained the upper hand, and the more solid-like blood has been separated from the cleanest or most pure.[4]

---

[1] See above, p. 137.   [2] See above, p. 135.   [3] See above, p. 135.
[4] *De somno*, 3, 457ᵇ20–458ᵃ12 : γίνεται γὰρ ὁ ὕπνος . . . τοῦ σωματώδους ἀναφερομένου ὑπὸ τοῦ

This ingenious explanation concerning the heaviness of the limbs in after-dinner sleep has implications which include a two-way traffic of blood in both main systems wholly unreconcilable with even the slightest knowledge of the valves. The coldness of the brain, incidentally, also serves to perform another function. The more accurate of the sense organs are situated in the head because they need the cleanest and apparently the coldest blood, since heat in the blood 'knocks out' (ἐκκόπτει) by its motion the activity of sensation.[1]

For Aristotle, as we have already noted, the heart not the head was the principal organ of the body. In accordance with his view that it is the seat of consciousness and the source of motion,[2] he endows it with a large quantity of nerves or sinews—the two have not yet become distinguished. The existence of 'nerves' in the heart follows logically from the fact that it is the origin of all motions in the body. For all movements are performed either by pulling or by letting go.[3] Moreover, in the De spiritu we are told that that which serves the purpose of movement seems to be not the bones, but rather the νεῦρα or what corresponds to them, i.e. that in which the pneuma which causes movement primarily resides, since even the belly moves and the heart has 'nerves' (neura).[4] Here once more the ambiguity of the Greek vocabulary of the period becomes manifest in connection with the meaning of the word neuron. Galen, as we have already seen, rebukes Praxagoras for having seen in the heart a lot of

θερμοῦ διὰ τῶν φλεβῶν πρὸς τὴν κεφαλήν. ὅταν δὲ μηκέτι δύνηται, ἀλλὰ τῷ πλήθει ὑπερβάλλῃ τὸ ἀναχθέν, πάλιν ἀνταπωθεῖ καὶ κάτω ῥεῖ ... πάντων δ' ἐστὶ τῶν ἐν τῷ σώματι ψυχρότατον ὁ ἐγκέφαλος ... ὥσπερ οὖν τὸ ἀτμίζον ὑγρὸν ὑπὸ τῆς τοῦ ἡλίου θερμότητος, ὅταν ἔλθῃ εἰς τὸν ἄνω τόπον, διὰ τὴν ψυχρότητα αὐτοῦ καταψύχεται καὶ συστὰν καταφέρεται γενόμενον πάλιν ὕδωρ, οὕτως ἐν τῇ ἀναφορᾷ τοῦ θερμοῦ πρὸς τὸν ἐγκέφαλον ἡ μὲν περιττωματικὴ ἀναθυμίασις εἰς φλέγμα συνέρχεται — διὸ καὶ οἱ κατάρροι φαίνονται γιγνόμενοι ἐκ τῆς κεφαλῆς — ἡ δὲ τρόφιμος καὶ μὴ νοσώδης καταφέρεται συνισταμένη καὶ καταψύχει τὸ θερμόν ... ἐγείρεται δ' ὅταν πεφθῇ καὶ κρατήσῃ ἡ συνεωσμένη θερμότης ἐν ὀλίγῳ πολλὴ ἐκ τοῦ περιεστῶτος, καὶ διακριθῇ τό τε σωματωδέστερον αἷμα καὶ τὸ καθαρώτατον.

[1] De part. an. 2. 10, 656ᵃ37–ᵇ6: ἡ δ' ὄψις πᾶσι τοῖς ἔχουσιν εὐλόγως ἐστὶ περὶ τὸν ἐγκέφαλον· ὁ μὲν γὰρ ὑγρὸς καὶ ψυχρός, ἡ δ' ὕδωρ τὴν φύσιν ἐστίν. τοῦτο γὰρ τῶν διαφανῶν εὐφυλακτότατόν ἐστιν. ἔτι δὲ τὰς ἀκριβεστέρας τῶν αἰσθήσεων διὰ τῶν καθαρώτερον ἐχόντων τὸ αἷμα μορίων ἀναγκαῖον ἀκριβεστέρας γίνεσθαι· ἐκκόπτει γὰρ ἡ τῆς ἐν τῷ αἵματι θερμότητος κίνησις τὴν αἰσθητικὴν ἐνέργειαν.

[2] Ibid., 2. 1, 647ᵃ24–31: τῆς δ' αἰσθητικῆς δυνάμεως καὶ τῆς κινούσης τὸ ζῷον καὶ τῆς θρεπτικῆς ἐν ταὐτῷ μορίῳ τοῦ σώματος οὔσης ... ἀναγκαῖον τὸ ἔχον πρῶτον μόριον τὰς τοιαύτας ἀρχάς, ᾗ μέν ἐστι δεκτικὸν πάντων τῶν αἰσθητῶν, τῶν ἁπλῶν εἶναι μορίων, ᾗ δὲ κινητικὸν καὶ πρακτικόν, τῶν ἀνομοιομερῶν. διόπερ ἐν μὲν τοῖς ἀναίμοις τὸ ἀνάλογον, ἐν δὲ τοῖς ἐναίμοις ἡ καρδία τοιοῦτόν ἐστιν.

[3] Ibid., 3. 4, 666ᵇ14–17: ἔχει δὲ καὶ νεύρων πλῆθος ἡ καρδία, καὶ τοῦτ' εὐλόγως· ἀπὸ ταύτης γὰρ αἱ κινήσεις, περαίνονται δὲ διὰ τοῦ ἕλκειν καὶ ἀνιέναι· δεῖ οὖν τοιαύτης ὑπηρεσίας καὶ ἰσχύος.

[4] De spiritu, 8, 485ᵃ5–8: οὐκ ἂν δόξειε κινήσεως ἕνεκα τὰ ὀστᾶ, ἀλλὰ μᾶλλον τὰ νεῦρα ἢ τὰ ἀνάλογον, ἐν ᾧ πρώτῳ τὸ πνεῦμα τὸ κινητικόν, ἐπεὶ καὶ ἡ κοιλία κινεῖται καὶ ἡ καρδία νεῦρα ἔχει. Though the author of this treatise was not Aristotle himself, we may perhaps assume that here at least he was reproducing Aristotle's doctrine?

non-existent 'nerves' growing out of it, and Aristotle by implication is guilty of the same crime, though he is excused of any dishonesty. We must ask ourselves therefore what they did see. Since *neuron* has been used to denote the cord of a sling, the string of a lyre, and a bow-string as well as a tendon or sinew, it does not need much imagination to conjecture that on dissecting some of the larger animal hearts both Aristotle and Praxagoras may have been struck by the sinew-like attachments of the valves, the musculi papillares and the chordae tendineae, as indeed Galen himself suggests in the case of the former.[1] Or did they regard the muscular fibres of the heart itself as nerves? The latter would appear to be the most probable hypothesis, for Aristotle at any rate, since the word μῦς is not used by him at all, and the word νεῦρον is defined in the *Generation of animals* as meaning the structure which holds the parts of the animal together:[2] its essential character is 'toughness' or 'stickiness?' (τὸ γλίσχρον). The starting-point (ἀρχή) of the sinews is the heart, and the heart itself has sinews in its largest ventricle, while the aorta so-called is a sinew-like vein, especially its final terminations, which are no longer hollow, but have the power of stretching (τάσις) which sinews have where they end up in the joints of the bones.[3] The sinews do not however constitute, like the blood vessels, a single continuous system; they are scattered about the body round the joints and the bones. Particularly large ones are those responsible for the act of jumping, and another double sinew called the tendon, and the ones that are of assistance in feats of strength, the ἐπίτονος, a term used by Plato in the *Timaeus* for the great sinews of the shoulder and the arms. All the bones are bound together by sinews except those of the head, which are joined together by sutures.[4] Sinews can be split lengthwise but not crosswise and each has a great power of being stretched.[5] Aristotle also recognizes as distinct

---

[1] *De plac. Hipp. et Plat.* i. 10, K. v. 206: ἐμοὶ μὲν δοκεῖ τὰς ὑπὸ Ἡροφίλου νευρώδεις διαφύσεις ὠνομασμένας αὐτὰς οὐ νευρώδεις ἀλλ' ἄντικρυς εἰρηκέναι νεῦρα.

[2] *De gen. an.* 737ᵃ36–ᵇ4: πάντα δὲ τὰ σώματα συνέχει τὸ γλίσχρον· ὅπερ καὶ προϊοῦσι καὶ μείζοσι γιγνομένοις ἡ τοῦ νεύρου λαμβάνει φύσις, ἥπερ συνέχει τὰ μόρια τῶν ζῴων, ἐν μὲν τοῖς οὖσα νεῦρον, ἐν δὲ τοῖς τὸ ἀνάλογον.

[3] *De hist. an.* 3. 5, 515ᵃ27–33: τὰ δὲ νεῦρα τοῖς ζῴοις ἔχει τόνδε τὸν τρόπον. ἡ μὲν ἀρχὴ καὶ τούτων ἐστὶν ἀπὸ τῆς καρδίας. καὶ γὰρ ἐν αὐτῇ ἡ καρδία ἔχει νεῦρα ἐν τῇ μεγίστῃ κοιλίᾳ, καὶ ἡ καλουμένη ἀορτὴ νευρώδης ἐστὶ φλέψ, τὰ μέντοι τελευταῖα καὶ παντελῶς αὐτῆς· ἄκοιλα γάρ ἐστι, καὶ τάσιν ἔχει τοιαύτην οἵαν περ τὰ νεῦρα, ᾗ τελευτᾷ πρὸς τὰς κάμπας τῶν ὀστῶν.

[4] *Ibid.*, 515ᵃ33–ᵇ14: οὐ μὴν ἀλλ' οὐκ ἔστι συνεχὴς ἡ τῶν νεύρων φύσις ἀπὸ μιᾶς ἀρχῆς ὥσπερ αἱ φλέβες ... τὰ δὲ νεῦρα διεσπασμένα περὶ τὰ ἄρθρα καὶ τὰς τῶν ὀστῶν ἐστι κάμψεις ... μέγιστα δὲ μέρη τῶν νεύρων τό τε περὶ τὸ μόριον τῆς ἄλσεως κύριον—καλεῖται δὲ τοῦτο ἰγνύα—καὶ ἕτερον νεῦρον διπτυχές, ὁ τένων, καὶ τὰ πρὸς τὴν ἰσχὺν βοηθητικά, ἐπίτονός τε καὶ ὠμιαία. τὰ δ' ἀνώνυμα περὶ τὴν τῶν ὀστῶν κάμψιν. πάντα γὰρ τὰ ὀστᾶ, ὅσα ἁπτόμενα πρὸς ἄλληλα σύγκεινται, συνδέδενται νεύροις, καὶ περὶ πάντα ἐστὶ τὰ ὀστᾶ, πλῆθος νεύρων. πλὴν ἐν τῇ κεφαλῇ οὐκ ἔστιν οὐδέν, ἀλλ' αἱ ῥαφαὶ αὐτῶν τῶν ὀστῶν συνέχουσιν αὐτήν. Cf. Plato, *Timaeus* 84 e, where ἐπίτονος is used for the great sinews of the shoulder and arm.

[5] *Ibid.*, 515ᵇ15–16: ἔστι δ' ἡ τοῦ νεύρου φύσις σχιστὴ κατὰ μῆκος, κατὰ δὲ πλάτος ἄσχιστος καὶ τάσιν ἔχουσα πολλήν.

from sinews certain things called fibres, which he carefully distinguishes from the fibres in the blood of some animals. These are intermediate between sinews and 'veins' and some of them are filled with *ichor*, a serous fluid which is an imperfectly concocted form of blood. They extend from the sinews to the 'veins' and vice versa.[1]

The idea that arteries should terminate in muscles (he tells us nothing of the terminations of the veins, i.e. the blood vessels branching off from the 'great' vein), even if anatomically incorrect, was an essential conclusion following the premiss of the heart as the chief organ of the body and the seat of consciousness. For before the nervous system had been discovered by the Alexandrians, the vascular system was the only instrument by which the heart could command the organism. For the heart was the seat of the connate heat and the connate breath, σύμφυτον πνεῦμα, which was ultimately responsible for all movement. A similar theory appears to have been held by both Praxagoras and Diocles of Carystus, according to Wellmann,[2] who cites a passage from the Anonymous Londoner to the effect that they taught that paralysis was due to the blocking of the ducts or branches coming from the heart and the great artery, i.e. the aorta, through which voluntary action is transmitted to the body.[3]

Dismissing Galen's indignation at the notion of nerves in the heart, we see that for Aristotle, as for the author of the 'Hippocratic' *De corde*, the heart is essentially a muscle, and the function of muscles is to move or to be moved. There are three principal types of motion in which the heart itself is concerned. It has three modes of action, which are not always properly distinguished, namely palpitation, heart-beat and pulse, and respiration.[4] The first of these is due to a violent compression of the heat in the heart due to a chilling caused by residues or excrements or by a chilling colliquescence, such as may occur in the disease called the twitch (παλμός) or in other diseases as well as in fright. For persons suffering from fright are chilled in their upper parts, while the heat retreating and collecting itself makes the leap or palpitation, through being compressed into a small space, with the result that sometimes animals die through fear or through the incidence of diseases.[5]

---

[1] *De hist. an.* 3. 6, 515ᵇ27–30: αἱ δ' ἶνές εἰσι μεταξὺ νεύρου καὶ φλεβός. ἔνιαι δ' αὐτῶν ἔχουσιν ὑγρότητα τὴν τοῦ ἰχῶρος, καὶ διέχουσιν ἀπό τε τῶν νεύρων πρὸς τὰς φλέβας καὶ ἀπ' ἐκείνων πρὸς τὰ νεῦρα.   [2] Wellmann, *Fragmente*, p. 12.

[3] See AMG (1894), fr. 20: Πραξαγόρας δὲ καὶ Διοκλῆς ὑπὸ παχέος καὶ ψυχροῦ φλέγματος περὶ τὰς ἀποφύσεις τὰς ἀπὸ καρδίας καὶ τῆς παχείας ἀρτηρίας γενομένου, δι' ὧνπερ ἡ κατὰ προαίρεσιν κίνησις ἐπιπέμπεται τῷ σώματι.

[4] Aristotle, *De resp.* 20, 479ᵇ17–19: τρία ἐστὶ τὰ συμβαίνοντα περὶ τὴν καρδίαν, ἃ δοκεῖ τὴν αὐτὴν φύσιν ἔχειν, ἔχει δ' οὐ τὴν αὐτήν, πήδησις καὶ σφυγμὸς καὶ ἀναπνοή.

[5] Ibid., 479ᵇ19–26: πήδησις μὲν οὖν ἐστι σύνωσις τοῦ θερμοῦ διὰ κατάψυξιν περιττωματικὴν ἢ συντηκτικήν, οἷον ἐν τῇ νόσῳ τῇ καλουμένῃ παλμῷ καὶ ἐν ἄλλαις δὲ νόσοις, καὶ ἐν τοῖς φόβοις δέ· καὶ γὰρ οἱ φοβούμενοι καταψύχονται τὰ ἄνω, τὸ δὲ θερμὸν ὑποφεῦγον καὶ συστελλόμενον ποεῖ

The normal beating of the heart, which, as we can see, takes place continuously, may be compared with swellings that throb to the accompaniment of pain owing to a pathological change in the blood. This throbbing goes on until the abscess or swelling has been concocted and turned into pus and evacuated. The phenomenon is like boiling. For boiling occurs when a fluid is vaporized by heat. For it expands owing to its increase in volume. Now in the case of an abscess, if there is no dissipation by exhalation, the liquid becomes thicker, and relief is obtained by the evacuation of the putrefaction; in that of boiling, the excess volume of liquid overflows its container. But in the heart, the expansion of the liquid continuously taking place as the result of feeding, under the influence of heat produces the heart-beat, since the expanded liquid rises to the furthest wall of the heart. And this is taking place continuously without interruption. For the liquid is continuously flowing into the heart out of which the blood is constituted. For it is first fashioned or manufactured in the heart. And this is plainly visible in the first stages of the process of generation. For the heart is clearly seen to contain blood before the differentiation of the blood vessels has taken place. For this reason pulsation or heart-beat takes place more in the young than in the old, for there is more vaporization in the young. All the 'veins' pulsate, and all do so at the same time, since they are connected with the heart which is continuously in motion, so that they too are always in motion, moving simultaneously with the heart.[1]

The relation between the heart-beat and respiration needs rather careful examination. Both heart-beat and pulse are the result of the vaporization of foodstuffs after digestion through the agency of the connate heat which is principally resident in the right ventricle. The application of heat to a liquid to turn it into air or vapour entails an increase in its volume, for the air occupies more space, as is explained in the De caelo. This is proved by the fact that liquids subjected to heat often burst their

τὴν πήδησιν, εἰς μικρὸν συνωθούμενον οὕτως ὥστ' ἐνίοτ' ἀποσβέννυσθαι διὰ φόβον τὰ ζῷα καὶ ἀποθνήσκειν διὰ φόβον καὶ διὰ πάθος νοσηματικόν.

[1] De resp. 19, 479ᵇ26–480ᵃ13 : ἡ δὲ συμβαίνουσα σφύξις τῆς καρδίας, ἣν ἀεὶ φαίνεται ποιουμένη συνεχῶς, ὁμοία φύμασίν ἐστιν, ἣν ποιοῦνται κίνησιν μετ' ἀλγηδόνος διὰ τὸ παρὰ φύσιν εἶναι τῷ αἵματι τὴν μεταβολήν. γίνεται δὲ μέχρις ἂν πυωθῇ πεφθέν. ἔστι δ' ὅμοιον ζέσει τοῦτο τὸ πάθος· ἡ γὰρ ζέσις γίνεται πνευματουμένου τοῦ ὑγροῦ ὑπὸ τοῦ θερμοῦ· αἴρεται γὰρ διὰ τὸ πλείω γίνεσθαι τὸν ὄγκον. παῦλα δ' ἐν μὲν τοῖς φύμασιν, ἐὰν μὴ διαπνεύσῃ, παχυτέρου γινομένου τοῦ ὑγροῦ, σῆψις, τῇ δὲ ζέσει ἡ ἔκπτωσις διὰ τῶν ὁριζόντων. ἐν δὲ τῇ καρδίᾳ ἡ τοῦ ἀεὶ προσιόντος ἐκ τῆς τροφῆς ὑγροῦ διὰ τῆς θερμότητος ὄγκωσις ποιεῖ σφυγμόν, αἰρομένη πρὸς τὸν ἔσχατον χιτῶνα τῆς καρδίας. καὶ τοῦτ' ἀεὶ γίνεται συνεχῶς, ἐξ οὗ γίνεται ἡ τοῦ αἵματος φύσις· πρῶτον γὰρ ἐν τῇ καρδίᾳ δημιουργεῖται. δῆλον δ' ἐν τῇ γενέσει ἐξ ἀρχῆς· οὔπω γὰρ διωρισμένων τῶν φλεβῶν φαίνεται ἔχουσα αἷμα. καὶ διὰ τοῦτο σφύζει μᾶλλον τοῖς νεωτέροις τῶν πρεσβυτέρων· γίνεται γὰρ ἡ ἀναθυμίασις πλείων τοῖς νεωτέροις. καὶ σφύζουσιν αἱ φλέβες πᾶσαι, καὶ ἅμα ἀλλήλαις, διὰ τὸ ἠρτῆσθαι ἐκ τῆς καρδίας. κινεῖ δ' ἀεί· ὥστε κἀκεῖναι ἀεί, καὶ ἅμα ἀλλήλαις, ὅτε κινεῖ.

Steckerl, as we have noted, would identify these φύματα with 'bubbles', but it seems to me that they are more like abscesses.

containers.[1] This increase in volume of the liquid contents of digestion causes the push against the walls of the heart which swells and then subsides, for the process of respiration, by drawing cold air into the heart, quenches the excess of heat which caused the swelling. For respiration takes place when the heat in the heart, the initiator (ἀρχή) of nourishment, undergoes an increase. When this increase takes place, and the heart's contents expand, it is raised up. The organ which surrounds it, the lungs, must therefore also expand. Both lungs and heart are rather like bellows. The lungs on expanding draw in cold air from the outside, which eliminates the excess of the heart's heat, with the result that both heart and lungs subside, and the air is expelled, the air breathed out being hot owing to the heat with which it comes in contact in the lungs, which is derived ultimately from the heart.[2] The actual meaning of the text in this passage taken from the De respiratione is by no means easy to grasp, but this, according to Rüsche, is its general significance, and I have no doubt that he is right.[3]

The connection between heart-beat and respiration here established puts the traditional doctrine in a rather crude form, since it would appear on the face of it to establish a one to one relation between pulse-rate and rate of drawn breaths, which it is somewhat difficult to believe that Aristotle could have believed to be the case. Moreover, this doctrine is expressly controverted in the De spiritu which, though not by Aristotle, appears to reproduce his teaching on the heart-beat. The author recognizes quite clearly, as some of his predecessors or contemporaries did not, that heart-beat and pulse were quite separate from the movement of breathing, and he attributes the 'pulse which is found primarily and in the first place in the heart' to the expansion of the 'gasified', as we might perhaps call it, contents of the liquid entrapped in the heart, which as it were blows out (ἐκπνευματούμενον) its contents against its walls.[4] There

[1] Aristotle, De caelo, 3. 7, 305ᵇ11–16: ὅταν δ᾽ ἐξ ὕδατος ἀὴρ γένηται, πλείω καταλαμβάνει τόπον· τὸ δὲ λεπτομερέστερον ἐν πλείονι τόπῳ γίγνεται. φανερὸν δὲ τοῦτό γε καὶ ἐν τῇ μεταβάσει· διατμιζομένου γὰρ καὶ πνευματουμένου τοῦ ὑγροῦ ῥήγνυται τὰ περιέχοντα τοὺς ὄγκους ἀγγεία διὰ τὴν στενοχωρίαν.

[2] De resp. 21, 480ᵃ16–25: ἡ δ᾽ ἀναπνοὴ γίνεται αὐξανομένου τοῦ θερμοῦ, ἐν ᾧ ἡ ἀρχὴ ἡ θρεπτική. καθάπερ γὰρ καὶ τἆλλα δεῖται τροφῆς κἀκεῖνο καὶ τῶν ἄλλων μᾶλλον· καὶ γὰρ τοῖς ἄλλοις ἐκείνο τῆς τροφῆς αἴτιόν ἐστιν. ἀνάγκη δὲ πλέον γινόμενον αἴρειν τὸ ὄργανον. δεῖ δ᾽ ὑπολαβεῖν τὴν σύστασιν τοῦ ὀργάνου παραπλησίαν μὲν εἶναι ταῖς φύσαις ταῖς ἐν τοῖς χαλκείοις· οὐ πόρρω γὰρ οὔθ᾽ ὁ πνεύμων οὔθ᾽ ἡ καρδία πρὸς τὸ δέξασθαι σχῆμα τοιοῦτον· διπλοῦν δ᾽ εἶναι τὸ τοιοῦτον· δεῖ γὰρ ἐν τῷ μέσῳ τὸ θρεπτικὸν εἶναι τῆς φυσικῆς δυνάμεως. See also 480ᵃ25–ᵇ12, quoted below, p. 169, n. 3.

[3] Rüsche, op. cit., pp. 220 ff.

[4] De spiritu, 4, 482ᵇ29–483ᵃ3: ὁ δὲ σφυγμὸς ἴδιός τις παρὰ ταύτας, τῇ μὲν ἂν δοκῶν εἶναι κατὰ συμβεβηκός, εἴπερ, ὅταν ἐν ὑγρῷ πλῆθος ᾖ θερμότητος, ἀνάγκη τὸ ἐκπνευματούμενον διὰ τὴν ἐναπόληψιν ποιεῖν σφυγμόν, ἐν τῇ ἀρχῇ δὲ καὶ καὶ πρῶτον, εἴπερ τοῖς πρώτοις σύμφυτον· ἐν γὰρ τῇ καρδίᾳ μάλιστα καὶ πρῶτον, ἀφ᾽ ἧς καὶ τοῖς ἄλλοις ... ὅτι δ᾽ οὐδὲν πρὸς τὴν ἀναπνοὴν ὁ σφυγμός, σημεῖον· ἐάν τε γὰρ πυκνὸν ἐάν τε ὁμαλὸν ἐάν τε σφοδρὸν ἢ πρᾶον ἀναπνέῃ τις, ὅ γε σφυγμὸς ὅμοιος καὶ ὁ αὐτός.

does not seem to be any suggestion of any independent action of the walls of the blood vessels themselves of the kind which later Galen was to attribute to the arteries. This account of the 'pneumatization' of the heart's contents as they are being turned into blood, to which Peck draws attention in Appendix B to his edition of the *Generation of animals*, does not afford us much more than a sidelight on the nature of that rather mysterious entity the 'connate breath'. What, for example, is its relation to the *pneuma* absorbed or taken in by the heart in the act of respiration? For as we have seen, Aristotle maintains that air does pass from the lungs to the heart, though through what passages we are not clearly informed. Aristotle seems to have been one of the earlier authorities, even if not the first, to attribute to respiration the double function, which was to be adopted in a more developed form by Galen, of cooling the innate heat in the heart and 'nourishing' the vital or psychic spirit,[1] one of whose constituents at any rate was a vaporization of the blood.

The role assigned by Aristotle to the 'connate *pneuma*', so conveniently abbreviated by Peck as *ΣΠ*, was of fundamental physiological importance. Not only was it responsible for the differentiation of the parts of the developing embryo,[2] it was also the vehicle of the innate heat and the instrument of the generative soul. And it was at the same time the channel by which sensations reached the heart, and the instrument by which the soul or vital principle effected the pushing and pulling entailed in the movement of the limbs. This pushing and pulling Aristotle tries to explain by the physical nature of *pneuma* itself, which to us today seems quite unintelligible.

To reproduce Peck's translation of the passage in *De motu animalium*, cap. 10:

Now the functions of movement are thrusting and pulling, so that the organ of movement must be able to increase and contract. And the nature of spirit has these qualities; for when it contracts it is without force, and one and the same cause gives it force and enables it to thrust, and it possesses weight as compared with the fiery element, and lightness as compared with the contrary elements. Now that which is to create movement without causing alteration must be of this kind; for the natural bodies overcome one another according as one of them prevails, the light being conquered and borne down by the heavier and the heavy borne up by the lighter.[3]

He is here clearly envisaging the *pneuma* as a material cause, just as he does in the passage quoted below, where he defined it as 'hot air'; but it is a very special kind of matter. Its heat is not to be equated with that of the sublunary element fire. The sperm which conveys the formal element,

---

[1] See below, p. 337.
[2] *De gen. an.* 2. 6, 741^{b}37: διορίζεται δὲ τὰ μέρη τῶν ζῴων πνεύματι.
[3] Loeb edition, p. 475.

which is the soul, to the menstrual blood in conception, is itself a compound of water and hot air.[1]

But it would appear that the power or faculty of every soul (that is, the nutritive and the sensitive) is associated with some other body, one more divine than the so-called elements. And as one soul differs from another in glory or honour, so this substance also differs. In all cases an animal's seed contains that which makes it reproductive, the so-called hot substance. But this is not fire nor any power of that character, but the *pneuma* which is embraced in the sperm and its foam-like substance, which is analogous to the element of which the stars are composed (aether). That is why fire reproduces no animal, nor do we see any animal being put together in substances that are being burnt, or in fluid or solid (wet or dry) substances. But the heat of the sun, as well as that of animals, does effect generation, and not only that contained in sperm, but also in the case of any other residue which happens also to contain the principle of life.[2]

The element of which the stars are composed is of course eternal, capable neither of generation nor corruption,[3] but the analogy does not extend to the immortality of the animal soul. The 'soul', which we may perhaps retranslate as the 'principle of life', is the 'form' of the body, that which makes it what it is, for 'matter' is as such wholly indeterminate, a pure potentiality; all the specific characteristics of a 'thing' being conferred on it by the form, a dead eye being an eye only in name, that is, it is a different thing from a live one.[4] So too the form of the heart varies with, and indeed determines, the psychic characteristics of an animal. Thus:

The differences of hearts in respect of size, big or small, and consistency, hard or soft, also tend to influence their characters in some respects. Creatures which are dull of perception have a hard and close-knit heart, while those whose perceptions are more sensitive tend to have a softer heart. Those that have large hearts are cowardly, while those whose hearts are small or of medium size tend to be more courageous. This is because the condition which gives

---

[1] *De gen. an.* 2. 2, 735^b37–736^a1 : ἔστι μὲν οὖν τὸ σπέρμα κοινὸν πνεύματος καὶ ὕδατος, τὸ δὲ πνεῦμά ἐστι θερμὸς ἀήρ.

[2] Ibid., 2. 3, 736^b29–737^a5 : πάσης μὲν οὖν ψυχῆς δύναμις ἑτέρου σώματος ἔοικε κεκοινωνηκέναι καὶ θειοτέρου τῶν καλουμένων στοιχείων· ὡς δὲ διαφέρουσι τιμιότητι αἱ ψυχαὶ καὶ ἀτιμίᾳ ἀλλήλων, οὕτω καὶ ἡ τοιαύτη διαφέρει φύσις. πάντων μὲν γὰρ ἐν τῷ σπέρματι ἐνυπάρχει, ὅπερ ποιεῖ γόνιμα εἶναι τὰ σπέρματα, τὸ καλούμενον θερμόν. τοῦτο δ' οὐ πῦρ οὐδὲ τοιαύτη δύναμίς ἐστιν, ἀλλὰ τὸ ἐμπεριλαμβανόμενον ἐν τῷ σπέρματι καὶ ἐν τῷ ἀφρώδει πνεῦμα καὶ ἡ ἐν τῷ πνεύματι φύσις, ἀνάλογον οὖσα τῷ τῶν ἄστρων στοιχείῳ. διὸ πῦρ μὲν οὐθὲν γεννᾷ ζῷον, οὐδὲ φαίνεται συνιστάμενον ἐν πυρουμένοις οὔτ' ἐν ὑγροῖς οὔτ' ἐν ξηροῖς οὐθέν· ἡ δὲ τοῦ ἡλίου θερμότης καὶ ἡ τῶν ζῴων οὐ μόνον ἡ διὰ τοῦ σπέρματος, ἀλλὰ κἄν τι περίττωμα τύχῃ τῆς φύσεως ὂν ἕτερον, ὅμως ἔχει καὶ τοῦτο ζωτικὴν ἀρχήν.

[3] *De caelo*, 1.

[4] *De gen. an.* 2. 1, 735^a : οὔτε γὰρ ψυχὴ ἐν ἄλλῳ οὐδεμία ἔσται πλὴν ἐν ἐκείνῳ οὗ ἐστιν· οὔτε μόριον ἔσται μὴ μετέχον, ἀλλ' ἢ ὁμωνύμως, ὥσπερ τεθνεῶτος ὀφθαλμός.

rise to fear is their normal state, namely coldness, for they do not have the quantity of heat proportionate to the size of their heart, the amount they possess being small and therefore very dim in that large space. Their blood is therefore rather cold. Now the animals that have large hearts are the hare, the deer, the mouse, the hyena, the donkey, the leopard, and the marten, and almost all others which are visibly cowardly or those whom fear makes mischievous. The same considerations more or less apply to the veins and to the ventricles. For large veins and large ventricles are both cold. For just as a fire of a given size produces less heat in a large than in a small house, so it is with their organic heat.[1]

The innate heat is, as we have already noted, one of the essential conditions of life as such. It is, as it were, the motive force (sensu moderno) responsible for all the physiological activities of all living things, plants and animals alike. The prime function of all physiological processes is therefore the preservation of this innate heat, which in all blooded animals resides in the heart. Now this problem of preservation was conceived by Aristotle and by almost all of the Greek physicians in the centuries to come, in a way which to our ideas, based on the laws of thermodynamics fundamental to modern physics, must appear a bit odd. The crux of the problem was not how to produce enough heat to keep the animal alive, but how to prevent the innate heat from burning up the whole organism. It was essentially a problem of cooling. In plants the nutriment drawn from the cold earth and the surrounding air was able to look after its preservation in all but excessively cold winters, for the nutriment drawn through the roots has a cooling effect just as the entry of food into the human organism does at the beginning.[2] But in warm-blooded animals there has to be a special organ to discharge this office, namely the lung. Food and drink have, it would appear, a double function, the growth and upkeep of the various tissues, and the employment or spending of the innate heat which is responsible for 'cooking' the ingesta. At any rate, when this heat is not employed in cooking ingested food, owing to fasting, the animal or plant consumes itself, the 'natural'

---

[1] De part. an. 3. 4, 667ª11–28: αἱ διαφοραὶ τῆς καρδίας κατὰ μέγεθός τε καὶ μικρότητα καὶ σκληρότητά τε καὶ μαλακότητα τείνουσί πη καὶ πρὸς τὰ ἤθη· τὰ μὲν γὰρ ἀναίσθητα σκληρὰν ἔχει τὴν καρδίαν καὶ πυκνήν, τὰ δ' αἰσθητικὰ μαλακωτέραν καὶ τὰ μὲν μεγάλας ἔχοντα τὰς καρδίας δειλά, τὰ δ' ἐλάσσους καὶ μέσας θαρραλεώτερα· τὸ γὰρ συμβαῖνον πάθος ὑπὸ τοῦ φοβεῖσθαι προϋπάρχει τούτοις διὰ τὸ μὴ ἀνάλογον ἔχειν τὸ θερμὸν τῇ καρδίᾳ, μικρὸν δ' ὂν ἐν μεγάλοις ἀμαυροῦσθαι, καὶ τὸ αἷμα ψυχρότερον εἶναι. μεγάλας δὲ τὰς καρδίας ἔχουσι λαγώς, ἔλαφος, μῦς, ὕαινα, ὄνος, πάρδαλις, γαλῆ, καὶ τἆλλα σχεδὸν πάνθ' ὅσα φανερῶς δειλὰ ἢ διὰ φόβον κακοῦργα. παραπλησίως δὲ καὶ ἐπὶ τῶν φλεβῶν καὶ ἐπὶ τῶν κοιλιῶν ἔχει. ψυχραὶ γὰρ αἱ μεγάλαι φλέβες καὶ κοιλίαι. ὥσπερ γὰρ ἐν μικρῷ καὶ μεγάλῳ οἰκήματι τὸ ἴσον πῦρ ἧσσον ἐν τῷ μείζονι θερμαίνει, οὕτω κἀν τούτοις τὸ θερμόν.

[2] De juventute et senectute, 6, 470ª19–24: ἐπεὶ δὲ πᾶν ζῷον ἔχει ψυχήν, αὕτη δ' οὐκ ἄνευ φυσικῆς ὑπάρχει θερμότητος, ὥσπερ εἴπομεν, τοῖς μὲν φυτοῖς ἡ διὰ τῆς τροφῆς καὶ τοῦ περιέχοντος ἱκανὴ γίνεται βοήθεια πρὸς τὴν τοῦ φυσικοῦ θερμοῦ σωτηρίαν. καὶ γὰρ ἡ τροφὴ ποιεῖ κατάψυξιν εἰσιοῦσα, καθάπερ καὶ τοῖς ἀνθρώποις τὸ πρῶτον προσενεγκομένοις.

or innate heat consuming its container.[1] The essential functions of the animal soul are nutrition, sensation, and, as we have seen, 'voluntary' movement, i.e. movement inspired by desire (ἐπιθυμία), and each of these functions requires heat, the innate heat contained in *pneuma*[2] and the heart. The higher up an animal is in the scale of nature, the more heat it possesses, and the more honourable its soul.[3] These functions are all concentrated in a single centre in the higher animals, and this centre can only be the heart, the seat of the natural heat. All the senses must have a common place of perception (κοινὸν αἰσθητήριον) and this can only be the heart.[4]

Among the physiological functions which have their origin or starting-point in the heart, was, as we saw,[5] the process of breathing. Aristotle's explanation of the process of respiration is as follows: The maintenance of life and the possession of soul depend on a certain degree or kind of heat. For digestion, through which nourishment is made available, cannot take place without heat and life.[6]

And without the faculty of nutrition, the other faculties of the soul cannot exist . . . nor can that faculty or power exist without natural fire . . . Now there are two ways in which this fire can be destroyed . . . It can be quenched, or it can die out. Quenching is effected by means of its opposite, cold; but dying out is due to excess of heat. Thus an animal can die by excess of cold, and also from excess of heat. Unless it receives food, it wastes away or dries up. Hence some arrangements are necessary to protect it from this form of destruction. Nature therefore invented breathing for this purpose.[7]

Now the cause of respiration is the lung, which is spongy and full of pipes. And it has more blood than any other organ, and the blood that it contains needs to be cooled quickly, for the balance of the innate heat [here called the

---

[1] *De longitudine vitae*, 5, 466ᵇ28–33: τροφὴν δὲ μὴ λαμβάνοντα καὶ τὰ φυτὰ καὶ τὰ ζῷα φθείρονται· συντήκει γὰρ αὐτὰ ἑαυτά· ὥσπερ γὰρ ἡ πολλὴ φλὸξ κατακαίει καὶ φθείρει τὴν ὀλίγην, τῷ τὴν τροφὴν ἀναλίσκειν, οὕτω τὸ φυσικὸν θερμὸν τὸ πρῶτον πεπτικὸν ἀναλίσκει τὴν ὕλην ἐν ᾗ ἐστιν.

[2] *De resp.* 8. 474ᵃ25–8: εἴρηται πρότερον ὅτι τὸ ζῆν καὶ ἡ τῆς ψυχῆς ἕξις μετὰ θερμότητός τινός ἐστιν· οὐδὲ γὰρ ἡ πέψις, δι' ἧς ἡ τροφὴ γίνεται τοῖς ζῴοις, οὔτ' ἄνευ ψυχῆς οὔτ' ἄνευ θερμότητός ἐστιν· πυρὶ γὰρ ἐργάζεται πάντα.

[3] Ibid., 13, 477ᵃ14–17: διὰ τί δὲ τοῦτο τὸ μόριον ἔχουσιν ἔνια, καὶ διὰ τί τὰ ἔχοντα δεῖται ἀναπνοῆς, αἴτιον τοῦ μὲν ἔχειν ὅτι τὰ τιμιώτερα τῶν ζῴων πλείονος τετύχηκε θερμότητος· ἅμα γὰρ ἀνάγκη καὶ ψυχῆς τετυχηκέναι τιμιωτέρας.

[4] *De juv.* 3, 469ᵃ2–14: φανερὸν τοίνυν ὅτι μίαν μέν τινα ἐργασίαν ἡ τοῦ στόματος λειτουργεῖ δύναμις, ἑτέραν δ' ἡ τῆς κοιλίας περὶ τὴν τροφήν· ἡ δὲ καρδία κυριωτάτη, καὶ τὸ τέλος ἐπιτίθησιν. ὥστ' ἀνάγκη καὶ τῆς αἰσθητικῆς καὶ τῆς θρεπτικῆς ψυχῆς ἐν τῇ καρδίᾳ τὴν ἀρχὴν εἶναι τοῖς ἐναίμοις . . . ἀλλὰ μὴν τό γε κύριον τῶν αἰσθήσεων ἐν ταύτῃ τοῖς ἐναίμοις πᾶσιν· ἐν τούτῳ γὰρ ἀναγκαῖον εἶναι τὸ πάντων τῶν αἰσθητηρίων κοινὸν αἰσθητήριον· δύο δὲ φανερῶς ἐνταῦθα συντεινούσας ὁρῶμεν, τήν τε γεῦσιν καὶ τὴν ἁφήν, ὥστε καὶ τὰς ἄλλας ἀναγκαῖον.

[5] See above, pp. 163 f.   [6] *De resp.* 7, 474ᵃ25–8, quoted above n. 2.

[7] Ibid., 474ᵇ10–24: τὰς μὲν οὖν ἄλλας δυνάμεις τῆς ψυχῆς ἀδύνατον ὑπάρχειν ἄνευ τῆς θρεπτικῆς . . . ταύτην δ' ἄνευ τοῦ φυσικοῦ πυρός . . . φθορὰ δὲ πυρός, ὥσπερ εἴρηται πρότερον, σβέσις καὶ μάρανσις. σβέσις μὲν ἡ ὑπὸ τῶν ἐναντίων· διόπερ ἀθρόον τε ὑπὸ τῆς τοῦ περιέχοντος ψυχρότητος . . . ἡ δὲ μάρανσις διὰ πλῆθος θερμότητος· καὶ γὰρ ἂν ὑπερβάλλῃ τὸ πέριξ θερμόν, καὶ τροφὴν ἐὰν μὴ λαμβάνῃ, φθείρεται τὸ πυρούμενον, οὐ ψυχόμενον ἀλλὰ μαραινόμενον. ὥστ' ἀνάγκη γίνεσθαι κατάψυξιν, εἰ μέλλει τεύξεσθαι σωτηρίας· τοῦτο γὰρ βοηθεῖ πρὸς ταύτην τὴν φθοράν.

fire of life] is delicate, and it is able to enter all parts of the body, owing to the quantity of blood and the heat which it carries. Now air is able to perform the work of cooling, because it also is thin and light by nature, and can quickly penetrate all the parts of the body to cool them. But water has the opposite quality. From this it is obvious why animals which have blood in their lung breathe most. For the warmer animal needs more cooling, and at the same time the breathed air goes to the source of heat in the heart quite easily.[1]

The heart is the source of the movement of the lung, which owing to its size provides a large space for the air to enter.[2] The lungs are rather like bellows in a smithy, and the heart corresponds to the hearth.[3] When air enters into them, they expand, and the chest expands likewise. This is visibly the case, as we can see that when people breathe in they expand the thorax, and when their chest expands, the air must be drawn in from the outside as it is in bellows, and since it is cold, it cools and quenches the excessive heat of the innate fire. When it has quenched it, it necessarily subsides; and as it subsides, the air goes out. When it comes in, it is cold, but when it returns it is warm, owing to its contact with the heat that is in the lungs. For the air falls into many pipes, like channels in the lung, alongside of which veins are extended, so that the whole lung seems filled with blood. And the return of the air is called expiration. And this process goes on continually, as long as the animal keeps alive. The lungs keep moving continually.[4] Philistion and the Sicilian

[1] Ibid., 15, 478ª11–25: διὰ τί δὲ τὰ ἔχοντα δέχεται τὸν ἀέρα καὶ ἀναπνέουσι, καὶ μάλιστα αὐτῶν ὅσα ἔχουσιν ἔναιμον, αἴτιον τοῦ μὲν ἀναπνεῖν ὁ πνεύμων σομφὸς ὢν καὶ συρίγγων πλήρης. καὶ ἐναιμότατον δὴ μάλιστα τοῦτο τὸ μόριον τῶν καλουμένων σπλάγχνων. ὅσα δὴ ἔχει ἔναιμον αὐτό, ταχείας μὲν δεῖται τῆς καταψύξεως διὰ τὸ μικρὰν εἶναι τὴν ῥοπὴν τοῦ ψυχικοῦ πυρός, εἴσω δ' εἰσιέναι διὰ παντὸς διὰ τὸ πλῆθος τοῦ αἵματος καὶ τῆς θερμότητος. ταῦτα δ' ἀμφότερα ὁ μὲν ἀὴρ δύναται ῥᾳδίως ποιεῖν· διὰ γὰρ τὸ λεπτὴν ἔχειν τὴν φύσιν διὰ παντὸς τε καὶ ταχέως διαδυόμενος διαψύχει· τὸ δ' ὕδωρ τοὐναντίον. καὶ διότι δὴ μάλιστ' ἀναπνέουσι τὰ ἔχοντα τὸν πνεύμονα ἔναιμον, ἐκ τούτων δῆλον· τό τε γὰρ θερμότερον πλείονος δεῖται τῆς καταψύξεως, ἅμα δὲ καὶ πρὸς τὴν ἀρχὴν τῆς θερμότητος τῆς ἐν τῇ καρδίᾳ πορεύεται τὸ πνεῦμα ῥᾳδίως.

[2] De part. an. 3. 6, 669ª14–17: τοῦ δ' ἀναπνεῖν ὁ πλεύμων ὄργανόν ἐστι, τὴν μὲν ἀρχὴν τῆς κινήσεως ἔχων ἀπὸ τῆς καρδίας, ποιῶν δ' εὐρυχωρίαν τῇ εἰσόδῳ τοῦ πνεύματος διὰ τὴν αὐτοῦ σομφότητα καὶ τὸ μέγεθος.

[3] De resp. 21, 480ª20–3: δεῖ δ' ὑπολαβεῖν τὴν σύστασιν τοῦ ὀργάνου παραπλησίαν μὲν εἶναι ταῖς φύσαις ταῖς ἐν τοῖς χαλκείοις, οὐ πόρρω γὰρ οὔθ' ὁ πνεύμων οὔθ' ἡ καρδία πρὸς τὸ δέξασθαι σχῆμα τοιοῦτον.

[4] Ibid., 480ª25–ᵇ12: αἴρεται μὲν οὖν πλεῖον γενόμενον, αἰρομένου δ' ἀναγκαῖον αἴρεσθαι καὶ τὸ περιέχον αὐτὸ μόριον. ὅπερ φαίνονται ποιεῖν οἱ ἀναπνέοντες· αἴρουσι γὰρ τὸν θώρακα διὰ τὸ τὴν ἀρχὴν τὴν ἐνοῦσαν αὐτῷ τοῦ τοιούτου μορίου ταὐτὸ τοῦτο ποιεῖν· αἰρομένου γὰρ, καθάπερ εἰς τὰς φύσας, ἀναγκαῖον εἰσρεῖν τὸν ἀέρα τὸν θύραθεν, καὶ ψυχρὸν ὄντα καὶ καταψύχοντα σβεννύναι τὴν ὑπεροχὴν τὴν τοῦ πυρός. ὥσπερ δ' αὐξανομένου ᾔρετο τοῦτο τὸ μόριον, καὶ φθίνοντος ἀναγκαῖον συνίζειν, καὶ συνίζοντος ἐξιέναι τὸν ἀέρα τὸν εἰσελθόντα πάλιν, εἰσιόντα μὲν ψυχρὸν ἐξιόντα δὲ θερμὸν διὰ τὴν ἀφὴν τοῦ θερμοῦ τοῦ ἐνόντος ἐν τῷ μορίῳ τούτῳ, καὶ μάλιστα τοῖς τὸν πνεύμονα ἔναιμον ἔχουσιν· εἰς πολλοὺς γὰρ οἷον αὐλῶνας ἐμπίπτειν τὰς ἐν τῷ πνεύμονι, ὧν παρ' ἑκάστην παρατέτανται φλέβες, ὥστε δοκεῖν ὅλον εἶναι τὸν πνεύμονα πλήρη αἵματος. καλεῖται δ' ἡ μὲν εἴσοδος τοῦ ἀέρος ἀναπνοή, ἡ δ' ἔξοδος ἐκπνοή. καὶ ἀεὶ δὴ τοῦτο γίνεται συνεχῶς, ἕως περ ἂν ζῇ καὶ κινῇ τοῦτο τὸ μόριον συνεχῶς. καὶ διὰ τοῦτο ἐν τῷ ἀναπνεῖν καὶ ἐκπνεῖν ἐστι τὸ ζῆν.

school,[1] followed by Plato in the *Timaeus*, had assumed that the windpipe is not absolutely dry inside, and had regarded the small portion of
liquid which the lung receives from the process of drinking as one of the
factors in the process of cooling. But Aristotle will have none of this. The
windpipe receives no liquid, only air. The heart is entirely air-cooled.

The physics and chemistry of this process of cooling are not at all easy
to understand. On several occasions in trying to explain it, Aristotle
introduces the comparison of the flame, in which it would seem natural to
regard the air as a substance nourishing the flame, but this is precisely
what it is not. He is very careful to refute the theory, of some of his contemporaries perhaps, that respiration exists for nutritional purposes, on
the supposition that the internal fire is nourished by breath, respiration
adding fuel to the fire,[2] exhalation taking place when the fire has been
fully fed. In combating this argument, he appears to depart somewhat
from his theory of the nature of the innate heat, which he hints may be
generated from food,[3] though in another passage, which we have already
examined, he implies that the digestion of food uses up heat:[4] moreover

[1] See Plutarch, *Quaest. conv.* VII, Q. i, Πρὸς τοὺς ἐγκαλοῦντας Πλάτωνι τὸ ποτὸν εἰπόντι
διὰ τοῦ πλεύμονος ἐξιέναι, Loeb ed. vol. ix (1969), pp. 14 f.: ἔτι δὴ τῶν μαρτύρων τῷ
Πλάτωνι προσκαλοῦμαι, Φιλιστίωνά τε τὸν Λοκρόν, εὖ μάλα παλαιὸν ἄνδρα καὶ λαμπρὸν ἀπὸ τῆς
τεχνῆς ὑμῶν γενόμενον, καὶ Ἱπποκράτην καὶ Διώξιππον τὸν Ἱπποκράτειον· οὗτοι γὰρ οὐχ
ἑτέραν ὁδὸν ἀλλ' ἣν Πλάτων ὑφηγοῦνται τοῦ πόματος. ἥ γε μὴν πολυτίμητος ἐπιγλωττὶς οὐκ
ἔλαθε τὸν Διώξιππον, ἀλλὰ περὶ ταύτην φησὶ τὸ ὑγρὸν ἐν τῇ καταπόσει διακρινόμενον εἰς τὴν
ἀρτηρίαν ἐπιρρεῖν, τὸ δὲ σίτιον εἰς τὸν στόμαχον ἐπικυλινδεῖσθαι· καὶ τῇ μὲν ἀρτηρίᾳ τῶν
ἐδωδίμων μηδὲν παρεμπίπτειν, τὸν δὲ στόμαχον ἅμα τῇ ξηρᾷ τροφῇ καὶ τῆς ὑγρᾶς ἀναμιγνύμενόν
τι μέρος ὑποδέχεσθαι· πιθανὸν γάρ ἐστι· τὴν μὲν γὰρ ἐπιγλωττίδα τῆς ἀρτηρίας προκεῖσθαι
διάφραγμα καὶ ταμιεῖον, ὅπως ἀτρέμα καὶ κατ' ὀλίγον διηθῆται τὸ ποτόν, ἀλλὰ μὴ ταχὺ μηδ'
ἄθρουν μηδ' ἐπιρρακτὸν ἀποβιάζηται τὸ πνεῦμα καὶ διαταράττῃ ... μαρτύρων μὲν οὖν ἅλις. ὁ δὲ
λόγος τῷ Πλάτωνι πρῶτον ἐκ τῆς αἰσθήσεως ἔχει τὴν πίστιν· τῆς γὰρ ἀρτηρίας τρωθείσης οὐ
καταπίνεται τὸ ὑγρόν, ἀλλ' ὥσπερ ὀχετοῦ διακοπέντος ἐκπῖπτον ἔξω καὶ ἀποκρουνίζον ὁρᾶται,
καίπερ ὑγιοῦς καὶ ἀκεραίου τοῦ στομάχου μένοντος.
It is not at all clear from this passage how much liquid Dioxippus thought went down
into the lung. Nor is Plato's conception in the *Timaeus* much clearer on this point. See Cornford,
Plato's Cosmology (London, 1937), note 1 to p. 284. Galen, in his treatise *On the doctrines of Hippocrates and Plato*, viii. 8, K. v. 713 ff., refuses to believe that Plato thought that the whole of
the drink swallowed went into the lungs, as this was plainly absurd. He therefore interprets
the passage in *Timaeus*, 70 c, quoted in the footnote to p. 119, as meaning only that a small
quantity goes into the lungs. εἰ μὲν οὖν ἡγεῖται Πλάτων ἅπαν τὸ πόμα καταπίνειν ἡμᾶς εἰς
τὸν πνεύμονα, δίκαιός ἐστι καταγιγνώσκεσθαι προφανέστατον πρᾶγμα μὴ γιγνώσκων· εἰ δὲ μέρος τι
τοῦ πόματος ἡγεῖται διὰ τῆς τραχείας ἀραχείας ἀρτηρίας παρωθούμενον εἰς τὸν πνεύμονα καταφέρεσθαι, τῶν ἐνδεχομένων τι λέγει. If, however, we compare *Tim.* 70 c with the other passages
in which this subject is dealt with, namely those in 72 e, 78 a–b, and 91 a, it certainly looks
as if Plato thought that the larger part of what we drink passes via the lungs into the bladder.
Or perhaps we should say, not Plato, but Timaeus. That this was a doctrine held by some
of the earlier physicians of the Hippocratic age seems to be suggested by the passage from the
beginning of the *De ossium natura*, which we have already quoted in the previous chapter.

[2] *De resp.* 6, 473ª3–6: ἀλλὰ μὴν οὐδὲ τροφῆς γε χάριν ὑποληπτέον γίνεσθαι τὴν ἀναπνοήν,
ὡς τρεφομένου τῷ πνεύματι τοῦ ἐντὸς πυρός, καὶ ἀναπνέοντος μὲν ὥσπερ ἐπὶ πῦρ ὑπέκκαυμα ὑπο-
βάλλεσθαι, τραφέντος δὲ τοῦ πυρὸς γίνεσθαι τὴν ἐκπνοήν.

[3] Ibid., 473ª10–12: ἔπειτα καὶ τὸ γίνεσθαι θερμὸν ἐκ τοῦ πνεύματος τίνα χρὴ τρόπον λέγειν,
πλασματῶδες ὄν; μᾶλλον γὰρ ἐκ τῆς τροφῆς τοῦτο γινόμενον ὁρῶμεν.   [4] See above, p. 164.

his account of the final extinction of the fire of life is not at all easy to understand. Having made the distinction between natural and violent death, he tells us that ultimately they are due to the same cause, for in both cases hot substance is extinguished through the lack of ability to obtain its proper food. In this process the opposite, by checking its concoction, prevents it from attaining nourishment. The wasting away of old age is explained in words which must strike the modern ear rather strangely.

Sometimes the fire wastes away or dies out, when too much heat has been accumulated owing to the failure to breathe and to cool it. For in this way the excess of heat developed quickly consumes the food, and finishes up by consuming it before the process of vaporization (which turns the food into blood) has taken place. Wherefore not only does a smaller fire fade out in the presence of a larger one, but the flame of a lamp placed in a larger flame automatically is consumed or burnt up like any other combustible substance. The reason for this is that the larger flame gets hold of the food available, before the smaller one can get access to it. But the fire continues burning and spreading like a river with such a speed that the extinction of the smaller flame is not noticed.[1]

This not very helpful analogy is supplemented by another. If the innate heat is to be preserved, there must be some cooling down in its source. This can be illustrated by the damping down of coals. When they are covered all over with a lid which we call a 'choke', they are very soon quenched, but if the lid is put on and taken off in quick succession they remain alive for a long time. And banking up a fire preserves it, for the air is not prevented entirely from getting at it, though the banking protects the fire by preventing the surrounding air generating so much heat that it is extinguished.[2] The result of the ageing of the animal produces rather a paradoxical effect. For, in spite of the fact that old age means a great diminution in the quantity of the innate heat, it is excess of

---

[1] *De juv.* 5, 469ᵇ23–470ᵃ5: συμβαίνει δ' ἀμφοτέρας διὰ ταὐτὸ γίνεσθαι τὰς φθοράς· ὑπολειπούσης γὰρ τῆς τροφῆς, οὐ δυναμένου λαμβάνειν τοῦ θερμοῦ τὴν τροφήν, φθορὰ γίνεται τοῦ πυρός. τὸ μὲν γὰρ ἐναντίον παῦον τὴν πέψιν κωλύει τρέφεσθαι· ὀτὲ δὲ μαραίνεσθαι συμβαίνει, πλείονος ἀθροιζομένου θερμοῦ διὰ τὸ μὴ ἀναπνεῖν μηδὲ καταψύχεσθαι· ταχὺ γὰρ καὶ οὕτω καταναλίσκει τὴν τροφὴν πολὺ συναθροιζόμενον τὸ θερμόν, καὶ φθάνει καταναλίσκον πρὶν ἐπιστῆναι τὴν ἀναθυμίασιν. διόπερ οὐ μόνον μαραίνεται τὸ ἔλαττον παρὰ τὸ πλεῖον πῦρ, ἀλλὰ καὶ αὐτὴ καθ' αὑτὴν ἡ τοῦ λύχνου φλὸξ ἐντιθεμένη πλείονι φλογὶ κατακαίεται, καθάπερ ὁτιοῦν ἄλλο τῶν καυστῶν. αἴτιον δ' ὅτι τὴν μὲν οὖσαν ἐν τῇ φλογὶ τροφὴν φθάνει λαμβάνουσα ἡ μείζων φλὸξ πρὶν ἐπελθεῖν ἑτέραν, τὸ δὲ πῦρ ἀεὶ διατελεῖ γινόμενον καὶ ῥέον ὥσπερ ποταμός, ἀλλὰ λανθάνει διὰ τὸ τάχος.

[2] Ibid., 470ᵃ5–15: δῆλον τοίνυν ὡς εἴπερ δεῖ σῴζεσθαι τὸ θερμόν ... δεῖ γίνεσθαί τινα τοῦ θερμοῦ τοῦ ἐν τῇ ἀρχῇ κατάψυξιν. παράδειγμα δὲ τούτου λαβεῖν ἔστι τὸ συμβαῖνον ἐπὶ τῶν καταπνιγομένων ἀνθράκων· ἂν μὲν γὰρ ὦσι περιπεπωμασμένοι τῷ καλουμένῳ πνιγεῖ συνεχῶς, ἀποσβέννυνται ταχέως· ἂν δὲ παρ' ἄλληλά τις ποιῇ πυκνὰ τὴν ἀφαίρεσιν καὶ τὴν ἐπίθεσιν, μένουσι πεπυρωμένοι πολὺν χρόνον. ἡ δὲ κρύψις σῴζει τὸ πῦρ· οὔτε γὰρ ἀποπνεῖν κωλύεται διὰ μανότητα τῆς τέφρας, ἀντιφράττει τε τῷ πέριξ ἀέρι πρὸς τὸ μὴ σβεννύναι τῷ πλήθει τῆς ἐνυπαρχούσης αὐτῷ θερμότητος.

heat which ultimately causes death.[1] Apparently he thought that the flame of life became so dim that even a little overheating, due to the induration of the ageing lung, was sufficient to extinguish it.[2]

The influence of Aristotle thus tended to reinforce the theory of the refrigerating function of breathing, which was to haunt Greek medicine throughout classical times, and its corollary, the emphasis on the respiratory function of the heart itself, which was to prove a great obstacle to the envisagement of any notion of the circulation. Unfortunately, the treatise *On respiration* throws no light on the problem of Aristotle's conception of the pulmonary vascular arrangements. *Pneuma* enters the heart from the lungs, but we do not know by what passages or into which of the three ventricles, nor whether he thought that there was a separate set of tubes to convey air to the heart. Nor are we able to elicit any clear idea of what Aristotle conceived this *pneuma* to be. Was it just hot air perpetually replaced by cold air drawn in through the mouth and the windpipe from the outer atmosphere, and heated by the blood and in the heart by the natural or innate heat? As Hett remarks, one cannot avoid the conclusion that 'obviously it is not the same thing as ordinary breath. The epithet σύμφυτον is usually attached to make the distinction clear; but it is often omitted. One might have supposed that πνεῦμα is peculiar to living organisms but in the *Generation of animals* (762ᵃ20) we are told that "water is present in earth, and πνεῦμα in water, and soul-heat in all πνεῦμα, so that in a sense all things are full of soul".'[3] The last expression is, of course, an adaptation of Thales' famous dictum that all things are full of gods, πάντα πλήρη θεῶν. The occasion of Aristotle's remark is the explanation of spontaneous generation of certain of the animal creatures, namely Testacea.

Looking back on Aristotle's teaching on the heart and its functions, we cannot help being struck by the fact that the greatest scientist of his age—indeed one of the greatest of all time—should have embraced the theory that the heart was the principal organ and the seat of the principle

---

[1] *De resp.* 17, 479ᵃ7–15: ἡ δ' ἀρχὴ τῆς ζωῆς ἐκλείπει τοῖς ἔχουσιν, ὅταν μὴ καταψύχηται τὸ θερμὸν τὸ κοινωνοῦν αὐτῆς. καθάπερ γὰρ εἴρηται πολλάκις, συντήκεται αὐτὸ ὑφ' αὑτοῦ. ὅταν οὖν τοῖς μὲν ὁ πνεύμων τοῖς δὲ τὰ βράγχια σκληρύνηται, διὰ χρόνου μῆκος ξηραινομένων τοῖς μὲν τῶν βραγχίων τοῖς δὲ τοῦ πλεύμονος, καὶ γινομένων γεηρῶν, οὐ δύναται ταῦτα τὰ μόρια κινεῖν οὐδ' αἴρειν καὶ συνάγειν. τέλος δὲ γινομένης ἐπιτάσεως καταμαραίνεται τὸ πῦρ.

[2] Ibid., 479ᵃ21–8: οὐδενὸς γὰρ βιαίου πάθους αὐτοῖς συμβαίνοντος τελευτῶσιν, ἀλλ' ἀναίσθητος ἡ τῆς ψυχῆς ἀπόλυσις γίνεται παντελῶς. καὶ τῶν νοσημάτων ὅσα ποιοῦσι τὸν πλεύμονα σκληρὸν ἢ φύμασιν ἢ περιττώμασιν, ἢ θερμότητος νοσηματικῆς ὑπερβολῇ, καθάπερ ἐν τοῖς πυρετοῖς, πυκνὸν τὸ πνεῦμα ποιοῦσι διὰ τὸ μὴ δύνασθαι τὸν πλεύμονα μακρὰν αἴρειν ἄνω καὶ συνίζειν· τέλος δ' ὅταν μηκέτι δύνωνται κινεῖν, τελευτῶσιν ἀποπνεύσαντες.

[3] See Hett's edition and translation of the *Parva naturalia* in the Loeb series, Introduction to the essay *On length and shortness of life*, p. 391. The passage in the *De gen. an.* 3. 12, reads as follows: γίνεται δ' ἐν γῇ καὶ ἐν ὑγρῷ τὰ ζῷα καὶ τὰ φυτὰ διὰ τὸ ἐν γῇ μὲν ὕδωρ ὑπάρχειν, ἐν δ' ὕδατι πνεῦμα, ἐν δὲ τούτῳ παντὶ θερμότητα ψυχικήν, ὥστε τρόπον τινὰ πάντα ψυχῆς εἶναι πλήρη.

of life, of sensation, and the emotions, when the alternative doctrine of the brain as the organ responsible for all cognitive processes had already been worked out, not only by Alcmaeon, but also by the 'Hippocratic' school.[1] His mistaken, but not patently absurd, notion of the brain as the source of phlegm, the humour generally recognized by contemporary physicians as cold, badly misled him. Perverse as a cardio-centric doctrine must seem to us today, it merits something more than a summary dismissal. For Aristotle, it appeared a logical deduction from observed fact. The primacy of the heart rests ultimately upon the evidence of the senses. In embryos the heart can be seen to be moving as soon as they are formed, just like a living creature, before any of the other parts.[2] The heart in blooded animals (as well as the liver) is visible as soon as they are formed at all. In eggs, it is visible as soon as the third day, just the size of a pin's head, and small hearts are visible in aborted embryos.[3] We have already quoted passages from the *History of animals* where it is shown that the heart is the first part to be formed and straightway has blood in it.[4] It is also the last to die. 'The heart is the place where life fails last of all: and we find universally that what is the last to be formed is the first to fail, and the first to be formed is the last to fail.'[5]

As a coda to what we may perhaps be permitted to call Aristotle's cardial symphony, there is one passage which may appear of some interest. This is the paragraph in which he states the fact that sacrificial animals often show signs of disease in various organs, but never in the heart, and the conclusions which he draws from this observation. The passage in question has been interpreted since Daremberg, in more than one way. Daremberg[6] interpreted it to mean that, since in sacrificial animals no

---

[1] See above, pp. 39 f.

[2] *De part. an.* 3. 4, 666ᵃ19-22: οὐ μόνον δὲ κατὰ τὸν λόγον οὕτως ἔχειν φαίνεται, ἀλλὰ καὶ κατὰ τὴν αἴσθησιν. ἐν γὰρ τοῖς ἐμβρύοις εὐθέως ἡ καρδία φαίνεται κινουμένη τῶν μορίων καθάπερ εἰ ζῷον, ὡς ἀρχὴ τῆς φύσεως τοῖς ἐναίμοις οὖσα.

[3] Ibid., 665ᵃ33-ᵇ2: συνισταμένων γὰρ εὐθέως τῶν ἐναίμων, καὶ πάμπαν ὄντων μικρῶν, ἔνδηλα γίνεται ἡ καρδία τε καὶ ἧπαρ· φαίνεται γὰρ ἐν μὲν τοῖς ᾠοῖς ἐνίοτε τριταίοις οὖσι στιγμῆς ἔχοντα μέγεθος, πάμμικρα δὲ καὶ ἐν τοῖς ἐκβολίμοις τῶν ἐμβρύων.

[4] See above, p. 134, n. 2.

[5] *De gen. an.* 2. 5, 741ᵇ15-21: γίγνεται δὲ πρῶτον ἡ ἀρχή. αὕτη δ᾽ ἐστὶν ἡ καρδία τοῖς ἐναίμοις, τοῖς δ᾽ ἄλλοις τὸ ἀνάλογον, ὥσπερ εἴρηται πολλάκις. καὶ τοῦτο φανερὸν οὐ μόνον κατὰ τὴν αἴσθησιν, ὅτι γίνεται πρῶτον, ἀλλὰ καὶ περὶ τὴν τελευτήν· ἀπολείπει γὰρ τὸ ζῆν ἐντεῦθεν τελευταῖον, συμβαίνει δ᾽ ἐπὶ πάντων τὸ τελευταῖον γινόμενον πρῶτον ἀπολείπειν, τὸ δὲ πρῶτον τελευταῖον.

[6] Daremberg, *Œuvres anatomiques et physiologiques de Galien* (Paris, 1854), i. 400, n. 3. 'Dans le traité *Des maladies* liv. IV ... on lit que la substance du cœur est dure et dense, de telle sorte qu'elle n'est pas lésée par l'humeur, et que le cœur n'est pas sujet aux maladies. Aristote, *De part. anim. III, iv*, ... développe ainsi cette proposition "Seul de tous les viscères, et en général de toutes les parties du corps, le cœur n'est pas sujet à des maladies qui aient le temps de devenir graves; et ce n'est pas sans cause, car si le principe est lésé, quel moyen a-t-il de venire en aide ... aux autres parties ... qui sont sous sa dépendance. La preuve que le cœur ne contacte aucune affection, c'est que sur aucun des animaux immolés pour les sacrifices on ne voit dans ce viscère nulle trace des maladies qui attaquent les autres. Les reins et le foie sont souvent farcis de calculs, de tubercules (φυμάτων), et de petites pustules

signs of disease in the heart are ever to be seen while their other organs show many such signs, the heart as such is not susceptible to disease. We have already noted a similar doctrine in the *Hippocratic corpus*, where its freedom from disease is attributed to the thickness or close-knit character of its flesh.[1] Peck,[2] on the other hand, as well as Ogle,[3] interprets it as meaning that the heart is unable to tolerate the slightest form of disease, which does not to me appear to make so much biological sense. I have therefore translated it as follows:

Of all organs and parts of the body, the heart alone is not susceptible to and has not to undergo any serious disease, and this is readily understood. For if the source were destroyed [or as Peck translates it, ailing], there is no place from which assistance could be sent to the other parts which are dependent upon or connected with it. And the proof that the heart is never affected by disease is that in none of the victims offered in sacrifices has any affection of the heart been observed, such as those which have been seen in the other organs. For the kidneys are often seen to be full of stones, growths, and little abscesses. The same applies to the liver and the lung, and more particularly to the spleen. Many different affections are to be visible in or about them but least of all do they show up, in the case of the lung, near the windpipe and in the case of the liver near the place where it joins up with the great vein. And this is easy to understand. For in these places they are in closest communication with the heart. But in those animals which die of disease or of some of these afflictions, when they are dissected pathological conditions are clearly visible near or around the heart.[4]

The point at issue turns on our meaning given to the words ὑποφέρει and ἐπιδέχεσθαι, and that given to the preposition περί at the end of the

(δοθιήνων) ; il en est de même du poumon et surtout de la rate. Beaucoup d'autres affections se rencontrent dans ces organes; mais elles sont plus rares pour le poumon au voisinage de l'artère, et pour le foie à son point de jonction avec la grande veine, et cela avec raison, car c'est par ces pointes que ces deux viscères sont le plus en rapport avec le cœur. Mais chez tous les animaux qui meurent de maladies et chez qui se présentent ces affections, nous avons trouvé, en les disséquant, des états morbides du côté du cœur." '

[1] See above, p. 75.   [2] Loeb translation, pp. 245–6.
[3] Oxford translation (vol. 5), 667ᵃ.
[4] *De part. an.* 3. 4, 667ᵃ32–ᵇ12 : μόνον δὲ τῶν σπλάγχνων καὶ ὅλως τῶν ἐν τῷ σώματι μορίων ἡ καρδία χαλεπὸν πάθος οὐδὲν ὑποφέρει, καὶ τοῦτ' εὐλόγως· φθειρομένης γὰρ τῆς ἀρχῆς οὐκ ἔστιν ἐξ οὗ γένοιτ' ἂν βοήθεια τοῖς ἄλλοις ἐκ ταύτης ἠρτημένοις. σημεῖον δὲ τοῦ μηθὲν ἐπιδέχεσθαι πάθος τὴν καρδίαν τὸ ἐν μηδενὶ τῶν θυομένων ἱερείων ὦφθαι τοιοῦτον πάθος περὶ αὐτὴν ὥσπερ ἐπὶ τῶν ἄλλων σπλάγχνων. οἵ τε γὰρ νεφροὶ πολλάκις φαίνονται λίθων μεστοὶ καὶ φυμάτων καὶ δοθιήνων καὶ τὸ ἧπαρ, ὡσαύτως δὲ καὶ ὁ πλεύμων, μάλιστα δ' ὁ σπλήν. πολλὰ δὲ καὶ ἕτερα παθήματα συμβαίνοντα περὶ αὐτὰ φαίνεται, ἥκιστα δὲ τοῦ μὲν πλεύμονος περὶ τὴν ἀρτηρίαν, τοῦ δ' ἥπατος περὶ τὴν σύναψιν τῇ μεγάλῃ φλεβί, καὶ τοῦτ' εὐλόγως· ταύτῃ γὰρ μάλιστα κοινωνοῦσι τῇ καρδίᾳ. ὅσα δὲ διὰ νόσον καὶ τοιαῦτα πάθη φαίνεται τελευτῶντα τῶν ζῴων, τούτοις ἀνατεμνομένοις φαίνεται περὶ τὴν καρδίαν νοσώδη πάθη.

Surely the simplest solution to the problem we are discussing would be to assume that all the manuscripts have omitted the word οὐ before φαίνεται in the last sentence. But this bold assumption may seem to the scholar too much like cutting the knot rather than attempting to untie it.

paragraph. Both Peck and Ogle take the first two of these words to mean 'cannot withstand' or 'cannot put up with'—perfectly correct translations, but they do not seem to me to make good sense in this context. For Aristotle goes on to argue that if anything went wrong with the heart, then no animal could survive other diseases in other parts of the body, an argument which appears to me to be quite inconsistent with the notion of the heart being unable to endure or resist disease. As to the pathological conditions observed in post-mortem examinations, all that Aristotle seems to me to be telling us is that in the organs specially mentioned, the liver and the lung, they are not visible in the parts nearest to the heart; the implication being, so I would imagine, that the heart itself was surrounded by a fence of immunity. I am therefore unable to accept the arguments put forward by Ogle in his footnote to the translation of this passage, where he remarks:

Daremberg represents Aristotle as saying that the heart is not liable to disease, or at any rate less liable than other organs, just as Galen said that it was made of hard flesh and could not be injured. But, in fact, Aristotle says nothing of the kind, but merely states what is fairly true, viz., that diseases of the heart are more certainly fatal and less consistent with apparent good health than diseases in the other parts, so that when a victim, i.e. an animal supposed to be of good health, is sacrificed, its heart is never found diseased, though such is frequently the case when an animal dies of malady.

It seems to me to be at least possible that Aristotle accepted the notion held by some, if not most, contemporary physicians concerning the insusceptibility of the heart to disease, which would fit very well with his theory of the heart as the ἀρχή, we might also say the arx or citadel, of the vital spirit.

The easiest, if not the most correct, solution of our problem would be to follow the suggestion made in my footnote. Otherwise we should have to assume that Aristotle is indulging in a rather obscure and imperfectly presented argument. The fact that the heart cannot put up with any disease seems a curious way of explaining the absence of pathological cardiac symptoms in sacrificed animals, especially as he lays particular stress on the fact that if it were attacked by disease it could not offer any assistance to the neighbouring organs. What he may have been explaining is that once any disease has reached the heart it is always fatal. But the implication of the heart sending assistance to its neighbouring or dependent organs, the use of the word βοήθεια which might be quite properly translated as *reinforcements*, would on the face of it suggest that the heart is the strongest of the organs, not the weakest.[1]

[1] In preparing this account of Aristotle's doctrine, I have omitted to take any general account of the obviously spurious treatise *De spiritu*, which, though it shows some acquaintance with Aristotle's teaching, is a most confused and confusing piece of argumentation.

As its translator in the Loeb edition, W. S. Hett, pointed out in his Introduction, the author seems to confuse the bronchial with the arterial system quite unintelligibly. He uses the word ἀρτηρία without qualification for windpipe and blood vessel, with the result that it is impossible, for me at any rate, to understand his physiological system. Some of his ideas on the vascular system are perhaps worth a passing glimpse. He mentions a theory according to which the bronchial system is connected with the arterial through a passage by which *pneuma* passes in respiration from the windpipe into the belly and out again, and that this is perceptible by the senses. 483ᵃ18–23 : τὸ δὲ πνεῦμα τὸ ἐκ τῆς ἀναπνοῆς φέρεσθαι μὲν εἰς τὴν κοιλίαν, οὐ διὰ τοῦ στομάχου—τοῦτο μὲν γὰρ ἀδύνατον—ἀλλὰ πόρον εἶναι παρὰ τὴν ὀσφύν, δι᾽ οὗ τὸ πνεῦμα τῇ ἀναπνοῇ φέρεσθαι ἐκ τοῦ βρογχίου εἰς τὴν κοιλίαν καὶ πάλιν ἔξω· τοῦτο δὲ τῇ αἰσθήσει φανερόν.

Our author does not accept this theory, but his ideas appear to be even more fantastic. There are three motions of the *pneuma* in the 'artery' namely, respiration, pulsation, and thirdly that which introduces and acts upon food. Cap. 4, 482ᵇ14–17 : ἐπεὶ δὲ τρεῖς αἱ κινήσεις τοῦ ἐν τῇ ἀρτηρίᾳ πνεύματος, ἀναπνοή, σφυγμός, τρίτη δ᾽ ἡ τὴν τροφὴν ἐπάγουσα καὶ κατεργαζομένη, λεκτέον ὑπὲρ ἑκάστης καὶ ποῦ καὶ πῶς καὶ τίνος χάριν.

We are also told that veins and 'arteries' are joined to each other—once more the ambiguity of the word συνάπτειν—and that this is perceptible to the senses, the reason for this arrangement being that the wet has need of *pneuma* and the *pneuma* need of the wet. 483ᵇ35–484ᵃ4 : τὰς δὲ φλέβας καὶ τὰς ἀρτηρίας συνάπτειν εἰς ἀλλήλας καὶ τῇ αἰσθήσει φανερὸν εἶναι. τοῦτο δ᾽ οὐκ ἂν συμβαίνειν, εἰ μὴ ἐδεῖτο καὶ τὸ ὑγρὸν πνεύματος καὶ τὸ πνεῦμα ὑγροῦ, τῷ θερμὸν εἶναι ἐν νεύρῳ καὶ ἀρτηρίᾳ καὶ φλεβί.

It would appear from another passage, however, that veins alone contain blood, and 'arteries' air. In a passage strongly reminiscent of the threefold tissues of Erasistratus, he tells us that the skin is made up of vein, 'artery', and 'nerve' or 'sinew', another ambiguity which we have already met with. When pricked it bleeds, it also has τάσις, translated by Hett as elasticity, while the 'artery' provides it with 'transpiration', for it alone carries *pneuma*. 483ᵇ15–18 : τὸ δὲ δέρμα ἐκ φλεβὸς καὶ νεύρου καὶ ἀρτηρίας, ἐκ φλεβὸς μὲν ὅτι κεντηθὲν αἷμα ἀναδίδωσιν, ἐκ νεύρου δὲ ὅτι τάσιν ἔχει, ἐξ ἀρτηρίας δὲ ὅτι διαπνοὴν ἔχει. μόνον γὰρ δεκτικὸν πνεύματος ἡ ἀρτηρία.

Finally, he also gives us the bubble theory of the pulse. Pulsation is quasi-accidental, since when there is much heat in a liquid, that which is evaporated must cause pulsation due to the trapping of air within. This would not seem to be consistent with the theory that 'arteries' contain only air. In another place we are told that the pulse and respiration have no connection, and that the pulse does not seem to have any purpose at all—a most un-Aristotelian conception. But he insists that it is found chiefly and primarily in the heart from which it is communicated to the other organs, and that it is visible already in the egg, i.e. before birth.

4 · THE ALEXANDRIANS

T HE next great stage in the development of knowledge took place in Alexandria about the beginning of the third century B.C. Here for a short time under the earlier Ptolemies, dissection of the human body was permitted to form a regular part of medical training, possibly as an indirect result of closer acquaintance with the traditional ancient Egyptian practice of embalming and mummification, which entailed the removal of the internal organs from the bodies of the dead and their separate pickling in the so-called Canopic jars. The two great Greek physicians who were the pioneers of human dissection were Herophilus and Erasistratus, whose respective affiliations with the schools of Cos and Cnidos can be traced. Unfortunately their works have joined the greater portion of ancient Greek literature which has perished, owing to the destruction of the great library at Alexandria. We know them only in isolated quotations and reports of their doctrines found either in later physicians, such as Rufus of Ephesus and, particularly, Galen, or in historians of medicine such as Celsus and the later doxographers like Aetius, Oribasius, and Caelius Aurelianus.

Recent research has thrown some doubt on the traditionally accepted version of the development of the Alexandrian school. That Herophilus practised human dissection in Alexandria is scarcely to be doubted, but the association of Erasistratus with Alexandria has been seriously questioned. About eighty years ago, Susemihl,[1] in his important *History of Greek Literature in the Hellenistic Age*, maintained that there was not a trace of evidence that Erasistratus had worked in Alexandria at all, though later, under the influence of Max Wellmann, he modified this rather startling assertion. Quite recently Mr. P. M. Fraser,[2] in an article of great erudition published in an Italian journal, has revived Susemihl's thesis. In opposition to Wellmann, Fraser also maintains that the evidence does not suggest that he practised human anatomy,[3] a conclusion I am unable to accept. Galen's report of his comparisons between the human

[1] F. Susemihl, *Gesh. d. gr. Lit. in d. Alexandriner Zeit* (Leipzig, 1891), p. 800, n. 129.
[2] P. M. Fraser, 'The career of Erasistratus of Ceos', in *Rendiconti*, Classe di Lettere, Istituto Lombardo—Accademia di Scienze e Lettere 103 (Milan, 1969), 518–37.
[3] Ibid., 532.

and the animal brain, and of his reference to his description of the valves of the heart, which he tells us Herophilus described rather carelessly, seem to me to imply human dissection. Moreover Celsus brackets Erasistratus with Herophilus as a vivisector of human beings, and Celsus cannot be taken as a witness of no, or even little, weight. Celsus says:

> Moreover, as pains, and also various kinds of diseases arise in the more internal parts, they (the rational school) hold that no one can apply remedies for these who is ignorant about the parts themselves; hence it becomes necessary to lay open the bodies of the dead and to scrutinise their viscera and intestines. They hold that Herophilus and Erasistratus did this in the best way by far, when they laid open men whilst still alive—criminals received out of prison from the kings—and whilst these were still breathing, observed parts which beforehand nature had concealed, their position, colour, shape, size, arrangement, hardness, softness, smoothness, relation, processes, and depressions of each, and whether any part is inserted into or is received into another.[1]

Fraser, though not affirming the incorrectness of Celsus' statement, denies that it entails any implication that Herophilus and Erasistratus both worked in the same place, and finds no difficulty in accepting the possibility that human dissection (and vivisection?) could have been permitted in Antioch, where tradition agrees that Erasistratus at one time practised, as well as in Alexandria.[2] This appears to me highly improbable. As far as I am aware, there is no evidence whatever that human dissection was practised anywhere else in Hellenistic times except in Alexandria. It was only in Egypt that the successors of Alexander the Great ruled over a people accustomed to systematic surgical intervention in the treatment of the human corpse. I have therefore followed Wellmann in including Erasistratus among the Alexandrians. A detailed examination of Fraser's arguments and evidence lies outside the scope of this essay. So to Herophilus we return.

With the details of Herophilus' anatomical discoveries, which covered the whole human body, we need not be concerned; Dobson has collected nearly everything which has survived.[3]

Herophilus may be regarded with some measure of probability as the discoverer of the nervous system, and his general contributions to the ancient Greek knowledge of the organs of the body, especially the sexual

---

[1] Celsus, *De medicina*, Prooemium (Loeb ed., tr. W. G. Spencer, vol. i, pp. 12 f.) : 'Praeterea haec, cum in interioribus partibus et dolores et morborum varia genera nascantur, neminem putant his adhibere posse remedia, qui ipsas ignoret. Ergo necessarium esse incidere corpora mortuorum, eorumque viscera atque intestina scrutari; longeque optime fecisse Herophilum et Erasistratum, qui nocentes homines a regibus ex carcere acceptos vivos inciderint, considerarintque etiamnum spiritu remanente ea, quae natura ante clausisset, eorumque positum, colorem, figuram, magnitudinem, ordinem, duritiem, mollitiem, levorem, contactum, processus, deinde singulorum et recessus, et sive quid inseritur alteri, sive quid partem alterius in se recipit.'   [2] Fraser, art. cit., p. 531.

[3] J. F. Dobson, 'Herophilus of Alexandria', *Proc. R. Soc. Med.* 18 (1925), 19 ff.

organs, were important, if Galen's judgement is correct. But here we are chiefly concerned with his discoveries dealing with the vascular system. These were of great significance, even if his knowledge of the detailed construction of the heart and its valves was much less perfect than that of his younger contemporary Erasistratus. Herophilus established once and for all the anatomical distinction between arteries and veins. He was the first to point out that the coats of the arteries were much thicker than those of the veins, six times as thick, so Galen informs us; and he recognized quite clearly that the vessel leading from the right ventricle to the lung was an artery, not a vein—a fact which had, indeed, already been observed by the time of Aristotle, who did not, however, have any clear notion of the distinction. Since at least from the time of his master Praxagoras onwards, all vessels emerging from the right ventricle appear to have been called veins while those emerging from the left ventricle were called arteries, Herophilus named what we know today as the pulmonary artery the artery-like vein, and what we call the pulmonary vein the vein-like artery.[1] He also noted the fact that in a dead body, the veins if emptied of blood collapse, while the arteries do not.[2]

No description by Herophilus of the heart and its structure has survived, and the accounts given by Galen and other authorities are too fragmentary for us to form any coherent picture of his discoveries. That he had some acquaintance with the valves of the heart is clearly implied by Galen, but his description of them was regarded by Galen as inadequate. (He definitely categorized it as careless, in contrast with that of Erasistratus, which he describes as accurate.[3]) Herophilus had evidently dissected hearts, for Galen attributes to him the term *sinew* or nerve-like process for the 'rims' or 'edges' of the membranes of the 'mouths' of the heart[4] (papillary muscles, or chordae tendineae, or perhaps the tendon of the infundibulum?). In another passage however, in the Galenic? treatise *On the best sect*, we are told that Asclepiades, in criticizing Erasistratus,

[1] Galen, *De usu partium*, vi. 10, K. iii. 445: οὐ γὰρ δὴ μάτην οὐδ' ὡς ἔτυχεν ἡ πάντα σοφὴ φύσις ὥσπερ οὐδ' ἄλλο οὐδὲν ἐποίησεν ἐν ἅπασι τοῖς ζῴοις, οὕτως οὐδ' ἐπὶ τοῦ πνεύμονος· ἐνήλλαξε γὰρ τῶν ἀγγείων τοὺς χιτῶνας, ἀρτηριώδη μὲν ἐργασαμένη τὴν φλέβα, φλεβώδη δὲ τὴν ἀρτηρίαν. ἐν μὲν γὰρ τοῖς ἄλλοις ἅπασι μορίοις τῆς ἴσης ἀρτηρίας τῇ φλεβὶ τὸ πάχος τῶν χιτώνων οὐκ ἴσον, ἀλλ' εἰς τοσοῦτον ἄρα διενήνοχεν, ὡς Ἡρόφιλος ὀρθῶς ἐστοχάσθαι δοκεῖ, τὴν ἀρτηρίαν τῆς φλεβὸς ἐξαπλασίαν ἀποφηνάμενος εἶναι τῷ πάχει. κατὰ δὲ τὸν πνεύμονα μόνον ἁπάντων ὀργάνων τε καὶ μορίων ἡ μὲν ἀρτηρία φλεβός, ἡ δὲ φλὲψ ἀρτηρίας ἔσχε χιτῶνας.

Cf. Rufus of Ephesus, *De nom. part.*, D–R, 162: Ἡρόφιλος δὲ ἀρτηρίαν τὴν φλέβα τὴν παχυτάτην καὶ μεγίστην ἀπὸ τῆς καρδίας καλεῖ φερομένην ἐπὶ τὸν πλεύμονα· ἔχει γὰρ ὑπεναντίως τῷ πλεύμονι πρὸς τἆλλα. αἱ μὲν φλέβες ἐνταῦθα ἐρρωμέναι καὶ ἐγγυτάτω τὴν φύσιν ἀρτηριῶν· αἱ δὲ ἀρτηρίαι ἀσθενεῖς καὶ ἐγγυτάτω τὴν φύσιν φλεβῶν.

[2] Galen, *De differentiis pulsuum*, iv. 10, K. viii. 747: βούλεται γὰρ (Ἡρόφιλος), ὥσπερ ἐπὶ τῶν τεθνεώτων ὁρᾶται, διεστὼς ὁ χιτὼν τῆς ἀρτηρίας, οὕτω κἀπὶ τῶν ζώντων ὅσον ἐφ' ἑαυτῷ διεστάναι.

[3] Galen, *De dogm. Hipp. et Plat.* i. 10, K. v. 206: τῶν ἐπὶ τοῖς στόμασι τῆς καρδίας ὑμένων, ὑπὲρ ὧν Ἐρασίστρατος μὲν ἀκριβῶς ἔγραψεν, Ἡρόφιλος δ' ἀμελῶς.

[4] Ibid.: ἐμοὶ μὲν δοκεῖ τὰς ὑπὸ Ἡροφίλου νευρώδεις διαφύσας ὠνομασμένας, αὐτὰς οὐ νευρώδεις ἀλλ' ἄντικρυς εἰρηκέναι νεῦρα. πέρατα δ' ἐστὶ ταῦτα τῶν ἐπὶ τοῖς στόμασι τῆς καρδίας ὑμένων.

stated that Herophilus, though he had dissected many hearts, never saw
the valves.[1] In contrast both to Erasistratus and to Galen, Herophilus
regarded the auricles as part of the heart, not merely as the terminal
processes of the vena cava and the pulmonary vein, which, incidentally,
has no valves. Galen appears to imply that Herophilus' theory would add
two to the number of the heart's valves. Thus he tells us : 'If anyone were
to regard the auricles as parts of the heart increasing the number of
cardiac orifices as did Herophilus, he would differ from Erasistratus and
me. For we have declared that for the four vessels of the heart there are
only four orifices' (trs. Singer).[2] If Herophilus actually did make this
mistake, this could perhaps in part be explained by assuming that he
regarded the lowest valve of the vena cava as another 'mouth', though
a similar structure could hardly be postulated in the pulmonary vein. On
the controversial question of the origin of the venous system—heart or
liver—Herophilus seems to have been an agnostic,[3] but he definitely
repudiated the conception of his master Praxagoras and his younger contemporary Erasistratus that the arteries contained only *pneuma*.[4] Indeed,
he attributed to the arteries, if we can trust the Anonymous Londoner, the
predominating role among the blood vessels. Not only do they distribute
pneuma with the blood stream, they also distribute nourishment, and that
even more plentifully than the veins, which were regarded by the majority
of Greek physicians, including the Anonymous Londoner himself, as the
principal distributors. For even if, so he tells us, arteries are externally
as large as veins, their coats being four times as thick, the internal dimension of their lumen is much smaller.[5] Herophilus, however, disagreed with
the view that veins were the largest distributors of nourishment, because

---

[1] Galen, *De optima secta*, 2, K. i. 109: ὥσπερ ἀμέλει καὶ Ἀσκληπιάδης περὶ τῶν ἐπιπεφυκότων
τῇ καρδίᾳ ὑμένων διαλεγόμενος Ἐρασίστρατον πλανᾶσθαί φησιν. Ἡρόφιλον γὰρ πολλὰ ἀνατετμη-
κότα μὴ ἑωρακέναι.

[2] Galen, *De anat. admin.* vii. 11, K. ii. 624: εἰρήσεται δὲ καὶ ὅτι τὰ τῆς καρδίας ὦτα τῶν
κοιλιῶν αὐτῆς ἐκτός ἐστιν, εἰ δέ τις αὐτὰ μέρη τοῦ σπλάγχνου θέμενος, ὥσπερ Ἡρόφιλος, ἐπὶ
πλεῖον ἐξέτεινε τὸν ἀριθμὸν τῶν στομάτων καὶ ταύτῃ διαφωνεῖν Ἐρασιστράτῳ τε καὶ ἡμῖν εἰρηκόσι
δ' τὰ πάντα εἶναι στόματα τῶν κατὰ τὴν καρδίαν ἀγγείων τεττάρων.

[3] Galen, *De plac. Hipp. et Plat.* v. 5, K. v. 543: ἀπορεῖν ὑπὲρ ἀρχῆς ἔφησεν, ὡς Ἡρόφιλος.

[4] Galen, *De sanguine in arteriis*, 8, K. iv. 731: ὥσθ' ὅταν ἀπορῶσι πῶς εἰς ὅλον τὸ σῶμα
παρὰ τῆς καρδίας κομισθήσεται τὸ πνεῦμα, πεπληρωμένων αἵματος τῶν ἀρτηριῶν, οὐ χαλεπὸν
ἐπιλύσασθαι τὴν ἀπορίαν αὐτῶν, μὴ πέμπεσθαι φάντας ἀλλ' ἕλκεσθαι, μήτ' ἐκ καρδίας μόνης,
ἀλλὰ πανταχόθεν, ὡς Ἡροφίλῳ τε καὶ πρὸ τούτου Πραξαγόρᾳ καὶ Φιλοτίμῳ καὶ Διοκλεῖ κα
Πλειστονίκῳ καὶ Ἱπποκράτει καὶ μυρίοις ἑτέροις ἀρέσκει. At first sight it might seem a little odd
to find Praxagoras in this company, since he believed that the arteries contained only *pneuma*,
but Galen is arguing that unlike Erasistratus he too believed that *pneuma* was distributed,
not by the physical pressure of the heart, but by a sort of physiological attraction.

[5] *Anonymus Londinensis*, xxviii, J. 110: ἀξιολογώτεραι δέ εἰσιν τῶν ἀρτηριῶν αἱ φλέβες ἐν αἷς εἰκότως πλείων γενήσεται ἡ ἀνάδοσις, καὶ εἰ ἴσαι εἰσὶν κατὰ τὸ μέγεθος αἱ ἀρτηρίαι ταῖς φλεψίν—φέρε γὰρ
οὕτως ἔχειν—εἰ δ' οὖν ἴσαι, αἱ μὲν ἀρτηρίαι μείζονες οὖσαι κατὰ τὴν περιοχὴν αὐτὸ μόνον φανή-
σονται τῷ τε τετραχίτωνες εἶναι καὶ συνεστάναι ἐξ εὐρώστων τῶν χιτώνων. αἱ δὲ φλέβες, ἀσθενέ-
στεραι ὑπάρχουσαι κατὰ τὴν περιοχὴν τῷ μονοχίτωνες εἶναι ὅμως εὐρυκοιλιώτεραί εἰσιν τῶν
ἀρτηριῶν.

he thought that though arteries and veins had equal powers of absorbing food, the amount of it yielded to the tissues by the arteries was greater on account of their power of pulsation which the veins do not possess. The extra pressure, or push, provided by pulsation makes the actual nutritional yield of the arteries the greater.[1]

The fragments of Herophilus which have survived tell us nothing about his theory of the way the heart works, nor of its relation to the movement of the blood, but one question, which was to interest and even perhaps puzzle Galen, though he treats it rather superciliously, was raised by Herophilus. If the arteries are full of blood, how can they also distribute *pneuma*? Herophilus adopted, according to Galen, the traditional theory which he attributes also to Praxagoras and Diocles, among others, that *pneuma* was not propelled by the heart at all, but attracted into the arteries, pulled into them not only from the heart but from all directions by the process of their expansion in the pulse—a theory which we shall have to deal with at length when examining Galen's views. It was Erasistratus, we shall see, who first understood the action of the heart's ventricles as a pump, most clearly in the case of the left ventricle, which he looked upon as a sort of air-pump, sending out with each systole a puff of *pneuma* into the aorta and the arteries, none of which contained, normally, any blood. Herophilus, on the other hand, seems to have adopted the theory of Empedocles that both heart and arteries draw in *pneuma*, not only through the lungs but also through the pores from the surface of the skin. But of Herophilus' ideas on the relation between the two substances, blood and *pneuma*, in the arteries we have no direct knowledge, any more than of his conception of the heart's functions. A fragment from the late doxographer Caelius Aurelianus (fifth century A.D.) does, however, give us an interesting piece of information, namely that Herophilus recognized the phenomenon of heart failure, in that he attributed sudden deaths, for which no cause could be found, to the paralysis of that organ.[2]

A fairly detailed description of Herophilus' theory of the pulse has come down to us through the reports of Rufus of Ephesus and of Galen. His teaching differed quite explicitly from that of his master Praxagoras. Praxagoras, who, as we have already noted, first clearly distinguished the arteries from the veins though he does not appear to have defined their

---

[1] Ibid.: ὁ μέντοι γε Ἡρόφιλος ἐναντίως διείληφεν· οἴεται γὰρ πλείονα μὲν γίνεσθαι ἀνάδοσιν ἐν ταῖς ἀρτηρίαις . . . ἥσσονα δὲ ἐν ταῖς φλεψὶ διὰ δύο ταῦτα· ᾗ μέν, ἐπειδήπερ ἀμφότεραι μὲν ὀρεκτικῶς ἔχουσι τῆς τροφῆς, ἥ τε φλὲψ καὶ ἡ ἀρτηρία, ἐπεὶ δὲ κατ' ἴσον ὀρέγονται τροφῆς, κατ' ἴσον καὶ ἡ ἀνάδοσις εἰς αὐτὰς γενήσεται. δεύτερον δὲ αἱ μὲν ἀρτηρίαι, φησίν, συστέλλονταί τε καὶ διαστέλλονται τόν τε σφυγμὸν ἀποδιδόασιν, αἱ δὲ φλέβες οὔτε διαστέλλονται οὔτε σφυγμωδῶς κεινοῦνται, ἐπεὶ τοιγάρτοι αἱ μὲν ἀρτηρίαι σφυγμωδῶς κεινοῦνται, αἱ δὲ φλέβες οὐ κεινοῦνται σφυγμωδῶς, ταύτῃ ἐπὶ τῶν ἀρτηριῶν διὰ τὴν ὦσιν ἐκείνην εὔλογον πλείονα γίνεσθαι τὴν ἀνάδοσιν ἤπερ ἐπὶ τῶν φλεβῶν διὰ τὴν εἰρημένην αἰτίαν.

[2] Caelius Aurelianus, *De morbis chronicis*, ii. 1: 'Repentinam mortem, nulla ex manifesta causa venientem, fieri inquit paralysi cordis.'

anatomical difference, was, it would appear, the first Greek physician to restrict pulsation to the arteries as opposed to the veins.[1] He asserted, so Galen tells us, that the power of pulsation possessed by the arteries was quite independent of the heart, though the heart itself also possessed this power. It would appear, too, that he tried to prove this fact experimentally, for he stated that if one cut a piece of flesh out of a living animal and threw it on the ground, one would actually see the arteries moving— a statement for which he is severely called to task by Galen, who argues that if a ligature tied round an artery in a living animal is sufficient to stop it pulsating on the distal side, it is ridiculous to suppose that the piece of an artery severed entirely from the body would continue to pulsate.[2] Herophilus did not accept this theory of independent pulsation of arteries, but maintained, as Galen did after him, that they received the power of pulsation from the heart,[3] though he did not interpret this transmission of power, like Erasistratus, in mechanical terms. A further point on which Herophilus differed from his teacher was the relation between the different kinds of cardiac and arterial movements and the actual pulse. Praxagoras regarded 'palpitation' (παλμός), 'tremor' (τρόμος), and 'spasm' (σπασμός) as differing from the pulse and from one another only quantitatively.[4] In order to understand the point at issue, it will be necessary to inquire a little more fully into the meaning of these four terms παλμός, τρόμος, σπασμός, and σφυγμός. After the discovery of the arterial pulse as one of the great 'constants' of physiological behaviour, the word σφυγμός very quickly came to be restricted to the heartbeat and the pulse in its modern sense. What then did Praxagoras, Herophilus, and after them Galen mean by the other three terms? The word παλμός, 'palpitation', had been used by Aegimius of Elis, or the author of a book attributed to him, very much as Praxagoras and Hero-

[1] See F. Steckerl, *The Fragments of Praxagoras of Cos and his School* (Leiden, 1958), p. 22.

[2] Galen, *De differentiis pulsuum*, iv. 2, K. viii. 702: ἔτι δὲ μείζων ἄλλη διαφορὰ τοῖς ἰατροῖς ἐκ παλαιοῦ περὶ τῶν ἀρτηριῶν ἐγένετο, τινῶν μὲν ἡγουμένων αὐτὰς ἐξ ἑαυτῶν σφύζειν, σύμφυτον ἐχούσας ὁμοίως τῇ καρδίᾳ τὴν τοιαύτην δύναμιν, ὧν ἐστι καὶ ὁ Πραξαγόρας.

De plac. Hipp. et Plat. vi. 7, K. v. 561: ἀπεσχίσθησαν δὲ οὖν, οὐκ οἶδα ὅπως, αὐτῶν (πολλῶν τε καὶ δοκίμων ἀνδρῶν) ἐν τῷδε Πραξαγόρας τε καὶ Φιλότιμος, ὁμολογήσαντες τἆλλα καὶ νομίζουσι τὸ πάμπαν ἐξ ἑαυτῶν σφύζειν τὰς ἀρτηρίας, ὥστε καὶ εἰ σάρκα τις ἐκτεμὼν ζῴου καταθείη παλλομένην ἐπὶ τῆς γῆς, ἐναργῶς ὁρᾶσθαι τὴν κίνησιν τῶν ἀρτηριῶν ... χρὴ δ' οἶμαι, γιγνώσκεσθαι ... δὲ καὶ ὡς, εἰ μόνην ἐκτέμοις ἀρτηρίαν, οὐ κινεῖται, καθάπερ οὐδ' εἰ βρόχῳ διαλάβοις ἔτι συνημμένην τῇ καρδίᾳ· καίτοι θαυμαστὸν ἡνίκα μέν ἐστιν ἔξω τοῦ ζῴου, μὴ μόνον τῆς καρδίας, ἀλλὰ καὶ τῆς τῶν ἄλλων μορίων ἀφηρημένης συμπνοίας, ἀκωλύτως σφύζειν αὐτήν, ἡνίκα δὲ συνῆπται πᾶσιν, ἄσφυκτον γίγνεσθαι.

[3] Galen, *De diff. puls.* iv. 2, K. viii. 702 f.: ἐνίων δὲ σφύζειν μὲν αὐτοῦ τοῦ χιτῶνος αὐτῶν διαστελλομένου τε καὶ συστελλομένου, καθάπερ ἡ καρδία, τὴν δύναμιν δὲ οὐκ ἐχουσῶν σύμφυτον ᾗ δρῶσιν, ἀλλὰ παρὰ καρδίαν λαμβανουσῶν· ἧς γνώμης ἔχεται καὶ Ἡρόφιλος.

[4] Rufus of Ephesus, *Synopsis de pulsibus*, 2, quoted below, p. 184, n. 2. Cf. Galen, *De trem. palp. convuls. et rig.* 1, K. vii. 584: ἐπειδὴ Πραξαγόρας ὁ τοῦ Νικάρχου τά τε ἄλλα τῆς ἰατρικῆς ἐν τοῖς ἀρίστοις γενόμενος, ἔν τε τοῖς περὶ φύσιν λογισμοῖς δεινότατος, οὐκ ὀρθῶς μοί δοκεῖ περί τε σφυγμοῦ καὶ παλμοῦ καὶ σπασμοῦ καὶ τρόμου γινώσκειν, ἀρτηριῶν μὲν ἅπαντα νομίζων εἶναι πάθη, διαφέρειν δὲ ἀλλήλων μεγέθει.

philus had used the word σφυγμός to cover all movement of the arteries;[1] but Galen uses it frequently to cover movements which are not connected with the vascular system. παλμός can occur in any part which is capable of being distended, as an unnatural expansion, including, besides the arteries and the heart, the bladder, the womb, the intestines, the spleen, and the liver, as well as the diaphragm. When it occurs in the arteries and the heart, it is a movement different from, and additional to, or contrary to, the pulse.[2] It is not a phenomenon peculiar to the organs subject to the control of the will.[3] It differs from pulsation in that it is caused by an 'explosion' of the *pneuma* and can take place in all parts of the body, while the pulse is the activation of a peculiar power or faculty, and takes place only in the arteries[4]—and, of course, the heart. According to Galen's definition, it is clear that 'tremor' and 'spasm' have nothing at all to do with the vascular system as such. Tremor, like paralysis, spasm, and numbness, is a spoiling of, or injury to, a voluntary activity[5]—the misfunctioning of a movement normally carried out by the nerves and the muscles, of a kind which may also occur sometimes in 'palpitation'.[6] It is due to a failure in strength of the carrying and moving faculty, the failure to sustain the movement of a limb against the force of gravity. For each limb having weight, tends of itself to fall and needs the activity of nerves and muscles to sustain it, as it were, like wings.[7] Spasm, on the other hand, is the involuntary movement of a muscle normally subject to the control of the will, a condition due to a pathological state of the motor nerve.[8]

[1] Galen, De diff. puls. i. 2, K. viii. 498: ὁ δὲ τὸ περὶ παλμῶν ἐπιγεγραμμένον Αἰγιμίου βιβλίον συνθείς, εἴτ' αὐτὸς ἦν ὁ Ἡλεῖος Αἰγίμιος εἴτ' ἄλλος τις, ἰδίως κέχρηται τῷ ὀνόματι, καὶ πολὺ παρὰ τὸ τῶν ἄλλων οὐκ ἰατρῶν μόνον, ἀλλὰ καὶ ἰδιωτῶν ἔθος, ἅπασαν ἀρτηριῶν κίνησιν παλμὸν ὀνομάζει. ἡ δὲ Πραξαγόρου καὶ Ἡροφίλου χρῆσις ἔτι καὶ εἰς τάδε κρατεῖ· σφυγμὸν γὰρ οὗτοι πᾶσαν ἀρτηριῶν κίνησιν τὴν αἰσθητὴν καλοῦσι.

[2] Galen, Comment. in Hipp. de humor. ii. 33, K. xvi. 335: ἐστὶ γὰρ παλμὸς διαστολὴ παρὰ φύσιν, ἥπερ γίνεσθαι πέφυκεν ἐν ἅπασι τοῖς μορίοις, ὅσα γε διαστέλλεσθαι πέφυκε ... συμπίπτει δὲ παλμὸς μὴ μόνον κατὰ τὴν καρδίαν, ἀλλὰ καὶ κατὰ γαστέρα καὶ κύστιν καὶ μήτραν, ἔντερά τε καὶ σπλῆνα καὶ ἧπαρ καὶ διάφραγμα. ὅταν δὲ ταῖς ἀρτηρίαις καὶ τῇ καρδίᾳ συμπίπτῃ, ἑτέρα τις κίνησις ἐν αὐταῖς γίνεται παρὰ τὸν σφυγμόν.

[3] Ibid.: οὔτ' οὖν τῆς προαιρετικῆς δυνάμεως οὔτε τῶν προαιρετικῶν ὀργάνων ἴδιόν ἐστι τὸ πάθος, ὥσπερ ὁ τρόμος τε καὶ ὁ σπασμός, ἀλλὰ πᾶσι τοῖς σώμασιν ἐγγίγνεται τοῖς διαστέλλεσθαι δυναμένοις.

[4] Galen (?), De pulsibus ad Antonium, K. xix. 637 sq.: τί διαφέρει παλμὸς σφυγμοῦ; ὅτι ὁ μὲν παλμὸς δι' ἔκπτωσιν τοῦ πνεύματος γίνεται καὶ ἐν παντὶ τῷ σώματι· ὁ δὲ σφυγμὸς ἐνεργείᾳ δυνάμεως κινεῖται καὶ ἐν ἀρτηρίαις μόναις.

[5] Galen, De symptomatum causis, ii. 2, K. vii. 149: προαιρετικῆς μὲν οὖν ἐνεργείας βλάβη παράλυσίς τε καὶ σπασμὸς καὶ τρόμος καὶ νάρκη.

[6] Galen, De trem. palp. convuls. et rig. 2, K. vii. 585–6: ἀλλ' ἥ γε διὰ τῶν μυῶν τε καὶ τῶν νεύρων γινομένη (κίνησις) καθ' ἣν καὶ τὰς χεῖρας καὶ τὰ σκέλη κινοῦμεν ἐν τρόμοις καὶ σπασμοῖς καὶ ῥίγεσι νοσώδεσιν, ἐνίοτε δὲ καὶ τοῖς παλμοῖς φαίνεται. πάντα γὰρ τὰ τοιαῦτα παθήματα πλημμελεῖς κινήσεις εἰσὶ τῶν αὐτῶν ὀργάνων, ἀφ' ὧν ὑγιαινόντων αἱ καθ' ὁρμὴν ἐπιτελοῦνται κινήσεις.

[7] Ibid., 3 (586): ὁ τρόμος μὲν οὖν γίνεται τῆς ὀχούσης καὶ κινούσης τὸ σῶμα δυνάμεως ἀρρωστία. οὐ γὰρ ἐξ ἑαυτῶν δήπου τὰ μόρια τῶν ζῴων οὕτως ὄντα βαρέα καὶ κάτω φέρεσθαι πεφυκότα, τὰς εἰς ἅπαντα τόπον ἔχει κινήσεις, ἀλλ' ἡ διὰ τῶν νεύρων τοῖς μυσὶν ἀπὸ τῆς ἀρχῆς ἐκπεμπομένη δύναμις οἷον ὄχημά τι καὶ πτέρωμα τῆς κινήσεως αὐτοῖς ἐστιν.

[8] Ibid., 8, K. vii. 639: πασῶν γὰρ τῶν καθ' ὁρμὴν κινήσεων ἐπιτελουμένων διὰ τῶν μυῶν ὅταν

Praxagoras' identification of all three of these physiological phenomena with the motion of the arteries immediately becomes intelligible when we remember that he believed that the arterioles terminated in nerves, both alike being vehicles for *pneuma*, the agency through which the movement of the muscles was effected. Herophilus distinguished the pulse from palpitation[1] and from tremor and spasm, while still maintaining that σφυγμός included all the motions of the arteries, but he avoided, if Rufus' account is correct, Galen's rather anomalous conception of palpitation as a motion of the arteries separate from, or additional to, the pulse.[2] Herophilus' theory seems to have been a variant of one of the doctrines of the 'Hippocratic' tradition, according to a statement in the pseudo-Galenic treatise, *De animi erroribus*, which informs us that the ancient physicians confined the term σφυγμός only to perceptible movements of the arteries, and that Hippocrates was the first to apply it to all arterial movements.[3] Herophilus regarded παλμός as a pathological affection of the muscles, and τρόμος as an affection of the nerves, for which he is criticized by Galen.[4] On the relation between the heartbeat and the pulse neither Herophilus nor Galen appears to have propounded any intelligible explanation, in contrast to Erasistratus whose mechanical interpretation we shall shortly examine. But the real importance of his pulse-lore lies in the fact that Herophilus was, it would appear, the first to distinguish the pulse as a specific physiological reaction, and to recognize its importance as a clinical sign in diagnosis and prognosis, quite independently of any consideration of the movement of the heart or the condition of the brain or of the cerebral membranes, which were regarded

ἐπὶ τὰς ἑαυτῶν κεφαλὰς ἀνελκόμενοι συνεπισπάσωνται τῶν μορίων ἕκαστον εἰς ὃ καταπεφύκασιν, ἐπειδὰν γένηταί τι πάθος εἰς τάσιν αὐτοὺς ἄγον, ἀκολουθεῖ τούτῳ κίνησις, ὁμοία μὲν τῇ κατὰ φύσιν ἀβούλητος δέ, καὶ καλεῖται τὸ πάθος σπασμός.

[1] Galen, De diff. puls. iv. 2, K. viii. 716: τὸν Ἡρόφιλον εὕροις ἂν εὐθὺς ἐν ἀρχῇ τῆς περὶ σφυγμῶν πραγματείας διορίζοντα σφυγμὸν παλμοῦ.

[2] Rufus, Synopsis de pulsibus, 2, D–R, p. 220: ὡμοίωται δὲ τῷ σφυγμῷ ὅ τε παλμὸς καὶ ὁ σπασμὸς καὶ ὁ τρόμος· καὶ γὰρ καὶ ταῦτα δοκεῖ τισιν οὕτω γίγνεσθαι ὥσπερ καὶ ὁ σφυγμὸς ἔκ τε διαστολῆς καὶ συστολῆς. διαφορὰ δὲ ἐν αὐτοῖς ὑπάρχει πλείστη· Πραξαγόρας μὲν οὖν ὑπέλαβε ταῦτα ἀλλήλων διαφέρειν ποσότητι, οὐκέτι δὲ ποιότητι· γίγνεσθαι γὰρ ἐκ μὲν τοῦ σφυγμοῦ μᾶλλον αὐτοῦ περὶ τὴν κίνησιν ἐπιταθέντος τὸν παλμόν, ἐκ δὲ τοῦ παλμοῦ τὸν τρόμον ... ὁ δὲ Ἡρόφιλος ἀκριβέστερον ἐπιστήσας τῷ τόπῳ ἐν ποιότητι μᾶλλον αὐτῶν τὰς διαφορὰς εὗρεν. γίγνεσθαι γὰρ τὸν σφυγμὸν περὶ μόνας ἀρτηρίας καὶ καρδίαν, τὸν δὲ παλμὸν καὶ τὸν σπασμὸν καὶ τὸν τρόμον περὶ μύας τε καὶ νεῦρα· καὶ τὸν μὲν σφυγμὸν συγγεννᾶσθαι τῷ ζῴῳ καὶ συναποθνήσκειν, ταῦτα δ' οὔ· καὶ τὸν μὲν σφυγμὸν πληρουμένων τε καὶ κενουμένων τῶν ἀρτηριῶν, ταῦτα δ' οὔ.

[3] Galen (?), De animi erroribus, 8, K. iv. 804: φλέβας μὲν γὰρ καὶ τὰς ἀρτηρίας ἐκάλουν οἱ παλαιοί ... οὐδέπω δὲ πᾶσαν ἀρτηριῶν κίνησιν ὠνόμαζον σφυγμὸν ἀλλὰ μόνον τὴν αἰσθητὴν αὐτὴν αὐτῷ τῷ ἀνθρώπῳ πάντως οὖσαν σφοδράν. Ἱπποκράτης δέ, ὡς καὶ πρῶτος ἄρξας τοῦ μετὰ ταῦτα κρατήσαντος ἔθους εἴρηκέ που σφυγμὸν ἁπασῶν τῶν ἀρτηριῶν τὴν κίνησιν, ὁποία τις ἂν εἴη.

[4] Galen, De trem. palp. convuls. etc. 5, K. vii. 594: ἀλλ' εἴτε μυῶν ἐστι πάθος μόνον ὁ παλμός, ὡς Ἡρόφιλος ἐνόμιζεν. Ibid., K. vii. 605: καὶ μέμφομαί γε ἐνταῦθα Πραξαγόρᾳ καὶ Ἡροφίλῳ, τῷ μὲν ἀρτηριῶν πάθος εἰπόντι τὸν τρόμον, Ἡροφίλῳ δὲ φιλοτιμουμένῳ δεῖξαι περὶ τὸ νευρῶδες αὐτὸ γένος ἀεὶ συνιστάμενον ... ὁ δὲ Ἡρόφιλος ἠπατήθη τὸ τῆς δυνάμεως πάθος ἀναφέρων τοῖς ὀργάνοις.

as being in motion by some physicians.[1] And though he is accused by Galen of a want of clarity in his exposition and of undue prolixity,[2] there can be little doubt that his description of the different classes of pulse and their qualities and variations formed the basis of the teaching of the later physicians, notably Archigenes, Rufus, and Galen, who built upon the foundations which he had laid.[3]

We can thus envisage three stages in the evolution of Greek pulse-lore. Before the discovery of the distinction between veins and arteries, the throbbing of certain blood vessels and the beat of the heart must have been observed from very early times. Hearts leaped up long before Wordsworth, and in Homer they even reached the mouth, as is shown in the case of Andromache's anticipation of Hector's death.[4] According to a passage from 'Hippocrates' quoted by Galen,[5] patients whose 'veins' throbbed in their elbows were liable to madness and quick-tempered, while those patients in which they are motionless are stupid. The term *pulse* seems to have been applied at this stage only to those movements of the blood vessels which were sufficiently pronounced to be perceptible to the patient himself. Hence the term σφυγμός, which rapidly became equally applicable to a movement perceptible by the physician. But in Hippocrates' time this perceptible pulse would appear to have often been looked on as a pathological symptom. Galen tells us that the ancient physicians applied the terms σφύζειν and σφυγμός only to the perceptible throbbing of inflamed, but never of healthy, parts of the body, throbbings perceptible to a patient himself, a usage which Erasistratus at one time seems also to have adopted.[6] Hippocrates was the first medical writer to

---

[1] Galen, *De diff. puls.* iv. 2, K. viii. 717: φαίνεται γὰρ ὁ ἀνὴρ οὗτος ('Ηρόφιλος) ἅπασαν ἀρτηριῶν κίνησιν ἣν ὁρῶμεν ἐξ ἀρχῆς ἡμῖν ἕως τέλους ὑπάρχουσαν, ὀνομάζων σφυγμόν, ἐξ οὗ καὶ τὰς διαγνώσεις τῶν παρόντων καὶ τὰς προγνώσεις τῶν ἐσομένων ποιούμεθα, μηδὲν τοῦ κατὰ τὴν καρδίαν ἢ τὸν ἐγκέφαλον ἢ τὰ τὰς μήνιγγας δεόμενοι σφυγμοῦ.

[2] Ibid., iv. 3, K. viii. 724: ἀλλ' ὡς ἔθος 'Ηροφίλῳ δι' ἑρμηνείας ἀσαφοῦς ... ὥστε εἰ μνημονεύω νῦν αὐτῆς 'Ηροφίλου ῥήσεως, ἣν ἐν ἀρχῇ τοῦ πρώτου περὶ σφυγμοῦ ἔγραψεν, ἢ τῶν εἰρημένων τοῖς ἀπ' αὐτοῦ, μέγεθος ἑνὸς βιβλίου γενήσεται.

[3] Ibid., ii. 7, K. viii. 602: Ἀρχιγένης δέ, τούτου γὰρ πρώτου δίκαιον μνημονεύειν, μετά γε τὸν 'Ηρόφιλον, ἐπιφωνήσαντας τὸν "Ομηρον.

οἶος πέπνυται, τοὶ δὲ σκιαὶ ἀΐσσουσιν.

[4] Homer, *Iliad* xxii. 452:   ἐν δ' ἐμοὶ αὐτῇ
στήθεσι πάλλεται ἦτορ ἀνὰ στόμα, νέρθε δὲ γοῦνα
πήγνυται . . .

[5] Galen, *De animi moribus*, 8, K. iv. 803: ἀλλ' ἀρκεῖ παραγράψαι δείγματος ἕνεκα τήνδε τὴν λέξιν αὐτοῦ ('Ιπποκράτους) ὧν ἡ φλὲψ ἡ ἐν ἀγκῶνι σφύζει, μανικοὶ καὶ ὀξύθυμοι, ὧν δ' ἂν ἀτρεμέῃ, τυφώδεις. The passage from 'Hippocrates' referred to is *Epidem.* ii, sect. 5 (L. v. 131): οὗ ἂν ἡ φλὲψ ἡ ἐν τῷ ἀγκῶνι σφύζῃ, μανικὸς καὶ ὀξύθυμος· ᾧ δ' ἂν ἀτρεμέῃ, τυφώδης.

[6] Galen, *De diff. puls.* iv. 2, K. viii. 716: ὡσαύτως οὖν ὅταν ἀναγνῶμεν ἔν τινι τῶν παλαιῶν ἰατρῶν βιβλίῳ, σφύζειν τὸ φλεγμαῖνον μόνον μόριον, ἢ τὴν ἐπὶ φλεγμονῇ κίνησιν, τῶν ἀρτηριῶν σφυγμὸν ὀνομάζοντας μόνην, ἐπὶ δὲ τοῦ κατὰ φύσιν ἔχοντος τοῦ σώματος οὐδέποτε χρωμένους τῇ προσηγορίᾳ, λογιζόμεθα μὴ πᾶσαν ἀρτηριῶν κίνησιν, ἀλλ' ἤτοι τὴν μεγάλην καὶ σφοδρὰν ἢ τὴν αἰσθητικὴν αὐτῷ τῷ κάμνοντι, προσαγορεύεσθαι σφυγμόν. οὕτω δὲ δοκεῖ τῇ προσηγορίᾳ τοῦ σφυγμοῦ κεχρῆσθαι καὶ ὁ 'Ερασίστρατος.

use the term, but he does not appear to have developed any theory about it, or made any clinical use of it.[1]

With Praxagoras' working out of the distinction between veins and arteries and his discovery that only arteries pulsate, a great step forward has been made, but the pulse has not yet been divested of its pathological character, which was connected with the theory that arteries ended in nerves, hence the attribution of 'tremor' and 'spasm' to the arteries. It is only with Herophilus, who was also the discoverer of the nervous system, that we come to a clear differentiation and classification of the pulse as we understand it today. Unfortunately, owing to the loss of his works, it is not possible to establish the exact nature of Herophilus' contribution. As Marx pointed out over a century ago, Galen's accounts of Herophilus' doctrines are so mixed up with his own opinions that it is in many cases almost impossible to decide with any certainty how much of them represent the Alexandrian's doctrine and how much his own.[2]

According to Galen, Herophilus divided the differences in the pulse into four kinds, according to size, speed, strength, and rhythm, and also by a sort of cross-division according to differences of order and disorder, regularity and irregularity.[3] The pulse he regarded as the distension or pushing apart (διαστολή) and the contraction or συστολή of the walls of the heart and arteries, terms which have survived until the present day. The first of these he regarded as an active process, the second as the return of the heart walls to their original position or state.[4] His notion was founded on the observation that since in dead bodies the walls of the arteries are not found collapsed, but still have a perceptible lumen, their natural condition in life is similar. The activity of distension or diastole is the function of the vital faculty, for a strong pulse is due to strength of the vital faculty in the arteries,[5] or rather, perhaps, to a combination of

---

[1] Galen, De diff. puls. i. 2, K. viii. 497: πρῶτος μὲν οὖν ἁπάντων ὧν ἴσμεν Ἱπποκράτης τό τε ὄνομα τοῦ σφυγμοῦ γράφει καὶ τὴν ἐν αὐτῷ τεχνὴν οὐκ ἀγνοεῖν ἔοικεν, οὐ μὴν οὔτ' ἐπὶ πλέον ἐξειργάσατο τοῦτο τὸ μέρος τῆς τέχνης, οὔτ' ἐπὶ πάσης ἀρτηριῶν κινήσεως τοὔνομα φέρει. παραπλήσιον δέ τι φαίνεται ποιεῖν αὐτῷ καὶ ὁ Ἐρασίστρατος.

[2] See Marx, Herophilus (Karlsruhe, 1838), pp. 40 f. : 'Wenn wir die von ihm hierüber verfaßte Schrift besäßen, würden wir wahrscheinlich die Ueberzeugung gewinnen, daß die Hauptsätze der Puls-lehre von ihm ausgefunden, und die späteren Griechen wenig Wesentliches hinzugefügt worden sey. Dieses läßt sich aus den ausführlichen Abhandlungen des Galens über den Puls schliessen, wo er indeßen sein und des Herophilus Ansichten so durch einander gemischt hat, daß die Abtrennung dieser, von was dem Letzten alleine gehört, sehr schwierig ist.'

[3] Galen, De diff. puls. ii. 10, K. viii. 625 : Ἡρόφιλος κατὰ γένος τὰς ἄλλας διαφορὰς τῶν σφυγμῶν ἐκθέμενος οὕτως· μέγεθος, τάχος, σφοδρότης, ῥυθμός, ἀσυζύγως κατ' εἶδος τάξεως ἐμνήσθη καὶ ἀταξίας ὁμαλότητός τε καὶ ἀνωμαλίας.

[4] Ibid. iv. 10, K. viii. 747: ἐὰν γὰρ ἀκριβῶς ἔπηται τοῖς Ἡροφίλου δόγμασιν, ἡ συστολὴ μὲν ἐνέργεια τῶν ἀρτηριῶν ἐστιν, ἡ διαστολὴ δὲ εἰς τὴν οἰκείαν τε καὶ φυσικὴν κατάστασιν τοῦ σώματος αὐτῶν ἐπάνοδος. βούλεται γάρ, ὥσπερ ἐπὶ τῶν τεθνεώτων ὁρᾶται διεστὼς ὁ χιτὼν τῆς ἀρτηρίας, οὕτω κἀπὶ τῶν ζώντων ὅσον ἐφ' ἑαυτῷ διεστάναι.

[5] Ibid. iii. 2, K. viii. 645: Ἡρόφιλος μὲν γάρ φησι ῥώμην τῆς κατὰ τῆς ἀρτηρίας ζωτικῆς δυνάμεως αἰτίαν εἶναι σφοδροῦ σφυγμοῦ.

the vital and the psychic or 'animal' faculties according to Chrysermus.[1] A somewhat similar explanation is given, as we shall see presently, of the movement of the lungs in respiration.

The pattern of the pulse movements seems to have been Herophilus' chief interest. It was their temporal rhythm which he was the first to analyse in a rather complicated and to us not entirely intelligible scheme of musical analogies. The passage from Galen which is one of our authorities for this quasi-musical arrangement runs as follows:

Herophilus moreover has written concerning the time intervals of systole and diastole, and reduced their proportions into rhythms varying in accordance with age. For just as musicians arrange the time lengths of notes comparing 'rise' (ἄρσις) and 'fall' (θέσις) with each other according to determinate time intervals, so also Herophilus, regarding 'rise' as analogous to diastole and 'fall' as analogous to systole, began his examination with the new-born child. He postulated a quasi-atomic minimum perceptible time unit, the interval occupied by the expansion of the infant's artery, and he also says that the systole or contraction is measured by an equal time unit, but he makes no clear definition of either of the periods of quiet.[2]

This passage, the meaning of which at first sight might seem to be anything but clear, is explained by a passage from Rufus of Ephesus as implying a rhythmical division into the 'feet' of the classical metres. 'Herophilus', Allbutt tells us,[3] 'distinguished certain cardiac rhythms as characteristic of periods of life. The rhythm of infancy, he said, was a pyrrhic (‿ ‿), of adolescence, a trochee (– ‿), of middle life, a spondee (– –), of old age, an iambus (‿ –).' According to the interpretation given by Rufus, Herophilus based his conception of rhythm on the metrical scheme invented by Aristoxenus, a peripatetic philosopher and musician who flourished at the beginning of the third century B.C. and propounded the notion of 'feet' composed of long and short syllables.[4] Herophilus was

[1] Ibid. iv. 10, K. viii. 744: τῷ δὲ ὑπὸ ζωτικῆς καὶ ψυχικῆς δυνάμεως γίνεσθαι τὸν σφυγμὸν ὑπὸ Χρυσέρμου λελεγμένῳ προσέθηκεν ὁ Ἡρακλείδης τὸ πλειστοδυναμούσης, ἐπειδὴ καὶ ἄλλα τινὰ συντελεῖν εἰς τὴν τῶν σφυγμῶν γένεσιν ὁ Ἡρόφιλος αὐτός φησι καὶ πάντες οἱ ἀπ' αὐτοῦ κληθέντες Ἡροφίλειοι.

[2] Galen, Synopsis de pulsibus, 12, K. ix. 463 f.: γέγραπται μὲν οὖν καὶ Ἡροφίλῳ τὰ κατὰ τοὺς χρόνους μετὰ τῆς διαστολῆς τε καὶ συστολῆς ἕνεκα τῶν ἡλικιῶν εἰς ῥυθμοὺς ἀνάγοντι τὸν λόγον. ὥσπερ γὰρ ἐκείνους οἱ μουσικοὶ κατά τινας ὡρισμένας χρόνων τάξεις συνιστῶσι παραβάλλοντες ἀλλήλαις ἄρσιν καὶ θέσιν, οὕτως καὶ Ἡρόφιλος ἀνάλογον μὲν ἄρσει τὴν διαστολὴν ὑποθέμενος, ἀνάλογον δὲ θέσει τὴν συστολὴν τῆς ἀρτηρίας, ἀρξάμενος ἀπὸ τοῦ νεογενοῦς παιδίου τὴν τήρησιν ἐποιήσατο, πρῶτον χρόνον αἰσθητὸν ὑποθέμενος ἐν ᾧ διαστελλομένην εὕρισκε τὴν ἀρτηρίαν, ἴσον δ' αὐτῇ καὶ τὸν τῆς συστολῆς εἶναί φησιν, οὐ πάνυ τι διοριζόμενος ὑπὲρ ἑκατέρας τῶν ἡσυχιῶν.

[3] Allbutt, op. cit., p. 312.

[4] The surviving works of Aristoxenus were edited by Bartels, Aristoxeni elementorum rhythmicorum fragmenta (Bonn, 1854). Aristoxenus' definition is given on p. 6: ἀκόλουθον δὲ ἐστὶ τοῖς εἰρημένοις καὶ αὐτῷ τῷ φαινομένῳ τὸ λέγειν τὸν ῥυθμὸν γίνεσθαι ὅταν ἡ τῶν χρόνων διαίρεσις τάξιν τινὰ λάβῃ ἀφωρισμένην. His notion of the 'long' and 'short' foot is explained as follows: ὥρισται δὲ τῶν ποδῶν ἕκαστος ἤτοι λόγῳ τινὶ ἢ ἀλογίᾳ τοιαύτῃ, ἥτις δὲ λόγων γνωρίμων τῇ

the first to apply this idea to the time measurement of the two movements of contraction and expansion of the arteries.[1] There were two main kinds of pulse rhythm, one in which the two movements of systole and diastole were of equal length, the other in which their length was unequal. Now the difference between the time intervals taken up by the two movements could be 'rational' or 'irrational'. It was rational if the proportion between the time intervals occupied by the two movements could be expressed in terms of whole numbers of the minimal perceptible time intervals, the 'first time', i.e. if one interval was two or three times as long as the other; irrational if it could only be expressed in terms of fractions of these minimal time intervals, e.g. diastole occupies, say, two, and systole five, seven, or nine, or eleven.[2] Aristoxenus only conceived of three elementary types of rhythm, spondee, trochee, and iambus, but Herophilus had the notion of much longer 'feet'. Thus he conceived conditions in which systole could, in old age, occupy a time interval equal to as many as ten of the 'first times'.[3] He thought that the fastest pulse in adult life occupied three of these, and refused, according to Galen, to recognize as possible one which merely occupied two. But Rufus tells us that in the case of the new-born infant, the pulse of which was very 'short', he thought that systole and diastole were both so quick that they could not properly be distinguished; the infantile pulse therefore could only be called irrational, since the two movements had no ratio to each other. Its size was so small that it felt like a pinprick.[4] Rufus therefore regarded it as a 'pyrrhic' (∪ ∪), but Galen tells us that he regarded the pulse of the new-born child as having an equal rhythm.[5] With adolescence, Rufus continues, it becomes a trochee, composed of three 'first times', the movement of diastole taking up two of these and that of systole one. At the prime of life it is a spondee, which occupies four 'first times', each of the two

αἰσθήσει ἀνὰ μέσον ἔσται. γένοιτο δὲ τὸ εἰρημένον ὧδε· καταφανὲς εἰ ληφθείησαν δύο πόδες, ὁ μὲν ἴσον τὸ ἄνω τῷ κάτω ἔχων, καὶ δίσημον ἑκάτερον, ὁ δὲ τὸ μὲν κάτω δίσημον τὸ δὲ ἄνω ἥμισυ· τρίτος δέ τις ληφθείη ποὺς παρὰ τούτους, τὴν μὲν βάσιν ἴσην αὐτοῖς ἀμφοτέροις ἔχων, τὴν δὲ ἄρσιν μέσον μέγεθος ἔχουσαν τῶν ἄρσεων, ὁ γὰρ τοιοῦτος ποὺς ἄλογον μὲν ἕξει τὸ ἄνω πρὸς τὸ κάτω· ἔσται δ' ἡ ἀλογία μεταξὺ δύο λόγων γνωρίμων τῇ αἰσθήσει, τοῦ τε ἴσου καὶ τοῦ διπλασίου.

[1] Galen, De diff. puls. iii. 2, K. viii. 913: Ἡρόφιλος πρῶτός τινα πρὸς αἴσθησιν ὑποτίθεται χρόνον, ᾧ τοὺς ἄλλους μέτρων ἢ δυοῖν ἢ καὶ τριῶν ἢ πλειόνων εἶναι φάσκει.

[2] See Wellmann, 'Die pneumatische Schule', Philologische Untersuchungen 14 (1895), 190 ff.

[3] Galen, De praesag. ex puls. 3, K. ix. 278: εἴπερ γὰρ ἡγεῖταί ποτε (Ἡρόφιλος) δύνασθαι γενέσθαι συστολὴν ἐπὶ τῶν γεγηρακότων ἄχρι δὴ τῶν δέκα πρώτων χρόνων ἐκτεταμένην, εὔδηλός ἐστι τῆς ὄντως συστολῆς ἀναισθήτως ἔχειν.

[4] Rufus, Synopsis de pulsibus, D–R, p. 224: τῶν μὲν οὖν ἀρτιγενῶν παίδων ὁ σφυγμὸς ὑπάρχει βραχὺς παντελῶς καὶ οὐ διωρισμένος ἔν τε τῇ συστολῇ καὶ τῇ διαστολῇ. τοῦτον τὸν σφυγμὸν Ἡρόφιλος ἄλογον συνεστάναι φησίν. ἄλογον δὲ καλεῖ τὸν σφυγμὸν τὸν μὴ ἔχοντα πρός τινα ἀναλογίαν· οὔτε γὰρ διπλάσιον οὔτε τὸν ἡμιόλιον οὔτε ἕτερόν τινα λόγον ἔχει οὗτος, ἀλλά ἐστι βραχὺς παντελῶς καὶ τῷ μεγέθει βελόνης κεντήματι ὁμοίως ἡμῖν ὑποπίπτει.

[5] Galen, Synop. lib. de puls. 12, K. ix. 465: καθ' ὅσον μὲν οὖν δι' ἴσου τὸν τοῦ ῥυθμοῦ σφυγμὸν εἶναί φησιν ἐπὶ τῶν ἀρτιγενῶν ὁ Ἡρόφιλος, κατὰ τοσοῦτο διαγιγνώσκειν ἔδοξέ μοι τὴν ἀρχὴν τῆς συστολῆς.

movements occupying two. Past the prime of life, in old age, the pulse once more occupies only three time intervals, but now the movement of diastole takes up only one of these while that of systole takes up two, and these intervals are longer.[1]

The important thing to remember is that what Herophilus and his successors called rhythm applies only to the single pulse-beat; it is not concerned at all with the pattern of successive beats. Galen, who as we have seen criticizes Herophilus for not distinguishing clearly between the time intervals of the movements of diastole and systole and the pauses of quiescence which follow each of these movements, implies that without some elementary knowledge of musical theory Herophilus' doctrine of the pulse cannot be understood, and he criticizes his followers the Herophilians as evolving a theory of rhythm which was quite useless for the purpose of clinical prediction.[2] But he insists that Herophilus himself invented his theory of rhythm precisely for this purpose.[3] He admits, however, that his theory of rhythm is difficult to interpret, not, as we have seen, altogether without reason. The 'ambiguity' of Herophilus' definition of rhythm is criticized by Galen in the following terms:

It is, however, difficult to discover what he means by rhythm. Is it the proportion of the time taken by expansion only to the time taken by contraction only, or does he include in it also the intervals of quiescence following both these movements? And for this reason not even those who are named after him Herophilians agree on what he really taught about this. For a reading of his text does not clearly demonstrate either of these alternatives, nor does the actual nature of the facts provide sufficiently certain evidence. If now we adhere to one of these alternatives, we shall, following the musicians, add the time taken by the periods of quiescence to that taken by the above-mentioned

---

[1] Rufus, op. cit., D–R, pp. 224 f.: προβαινούσης δὲ τῆς ἡλικίας καὶ τοῦ σώματος εἰς αὔξησιν ἐρχομένου, καὶ ὁ σφυγμὸς πρὸς λόγον μεγεθύνεται, πρὸς λόγον τὴν διαστολὴν τῆς συστολῆς λαμβάνων πλατυτέραν· ὅτε λοιπόν ἐστιν αὐτοῖς καὶ ἐφαρμόσαι πρὸς ἀπόδειξιν τοῦ ποδισμοῦ τῆς γραμματικῆς. ὁ μὲν γὰρ πρῶτος ἐπὶ τῶν ἀρτιγενῶν παίδων εὑρισκόμενος σφυγμὸς ῥυθμὸν λήψεται τὸν τοῦ βραχυσυλλάβου, καὶ γὰρ ἐν τῇ διαστολῇ καὶ τῇ συστολῇ βραχὺς ὑπάρχει, καὶ διὰ τοῦτο δίχρονος νοεῖται. ὁ δὲ τῶν πρὸς αὔξησιν ὄντων ἀναλογεῖ τῷ τε παρ' ἐκείνοις ποδὶ τροχαίῳ. ἔστι δὲ οὗτος τρίχρονος, τὴν μὲν διαστολὴν ἐπὶ δύο χρόνους λαμβάνων, ἐπὶ ἕνα δὲ συστολήν. ὁ δὲ τῶν ἀκμαζόντων ταῖς ἡλικίαις ἐν ἀμφοτέροις ἴσος ὑπάρχει, ἔν τε τῇ διαστολῇ καὶ τῇ συστολῇ, συγκρινόμενος τῷ καλουμένῳ σπονδείῳ ὃς τῶν δισυλλάβων ποδῶν μακρότητός ἐστιν. ἔστιν οὖν συγκείμενος ἐκ χρόνων τεσσάρων. τοῦτον τὸν σφυγμὸν Ἡρόφιλος διὰ ἴσου καλεῖ. ὁ δὲ τῶν παρακμαζόντων καὶ σχεδὸν ἤδη γερόντων καὶ αὐτός ἐκ τριῶν συγκεῖται, τὴν συστολὴν τῆς διαστολῆς διπλῆν παραλαμβάνων καὶ χρονιωτέραν.

[2] Galen, De dignosc. puls. iii. 3, K. viii. 871 f.: διὰ τοῦτο γοῦν καὶ περὶ τῶν ῥυθμῶν ὅσα μὲν ἐχρῆν αὐτοὺς ἔτι παῖδας ὄντας ἐν τοῖς τῆς μουσικῆς διδασκαλείοις ἐκμαθεῖν, ταῦτ' οὐδόλως εἰς τὰ τῆς ἰατρικῆς συγγράμματα φέρουσι, τὸ τῶν ὀψιμαθῶν πάθημα πάσχοντες, οὐδὲ σιωπῆσαι δυνάμενοι κἂν ἑτέρας ᾖ τεχνῆς. πῶς δ' ἀπὸ ῥυθμοῦ δεῖ σημειοῦσθαι, οὐκέτ' οὐδεὶς ἔγραψεν αὐτῶν, ἀλλ' Ἡρόφιλός γε τὴν ἐναντίαν ὁδὸν ἰὼν αὐτοῖς, παραλείπει μὲν ἃ παρὰ τοῖς μουσικοῖς ἐχρῆν μεμαθηκέναι τὸν ἀξίως τῆς τεχνῆς πεπαιδευμένον, ὡς ἐπισταμένοις δ' αὐτοῖς διαλέγεται, τὸ χρήσιμον εἰς τὴν ἰατρικὴν ἐξ αὐτῶν λαμβάνων.

[3] Ibid., K. viii. 911: αὐτὸς δὲ ὁ Ἡρόφιλος πολλαχόθι μὲν ῥυθμῶν εἰς τὰς προγνώσεις μνημονεύει.

movements. But if, for the purpose of prognosis, we compare only the times taken by the movements, we shall reckon the times taken by the periods of quiescence separately.[1]

That the latter alternative would appear to have been Herophilus' own doctrine we can gather from another passage, where Galen tells us that according to Herophilus it was precisely in comparison of the times taken by the movements of diastole and systole themselves that the degree of illness of the patient could be measured.[2]

Herophilus was also credited by Markellinos, a physician of the first century A.D. with the first attempt we know of to count the pulse, i.e. the number of successive beats per unit of time, by means of a water-clock. Markellinos, who probably lived in the second half of the first century some time between Archigenes and Galen (for he quotes the former but does not mention the latter), gives in his treatise on the pulse an account of Herophilus' teaching on the relation of the pulse to fever.

Herophilus demonstrated that a man has fever whenever his pulse becomes more frequent, larger, and more forceful, to the accompaniment of great internal heat. If the pulse loses its forcefulness and its magnitude, an alleviation of the fever takes place. Now the increased frequency of the pulse is the first symptom of the beginning of a fever, and continues until its final disappearance. Herophilus therefore, as the result of his confidence in the belief that the frequency of the pulse could be measured and was a reliable symptom, prepared a water-clock, made to contain a given quantity of water, in accordance with the figures settled for the natural pulse corresponding to each age. And going to the patient's bedside, he used to place the water-clock in position, and take hold of the patient's wrist. And in so far as a larger number of pulse-beats occurred during the set period determined by the time required to fill (or as we might say to empty) the water-clock, than the natural number, this proved that the pulse was by so much the more frequent than the natural, that is to say, the patient had more or less fever.[3]

---

[1] Galen, De dignoscend. puls. iii. 3, K. viii. 911–12 : χαλεπὸν μὴν ἐξευρεῖν τί ποτε καὶ λέγει τὸν ῥυθμόν, ἀρά γε τὸν λόγον τὸν τῆς διαστολῆς μόνον χρόνου πρὸς τὸν τῆς συστολῆς μόνης, ἢ καὶ αὐτὸν τῆς ἑπομένης ἑκατέρᾳ τῶν κινήσεων ἠρεμίας προσνέμει. καὶ διὰ τοῦτο οὐδὲ τοῖς ὑπ' αὐτοῦ κληθεῖσιν 'Ηροφιλείοις ὁμολογεῖται, τί ποθ' ὑπὲρ αὐτῶν φρονεῖ δεόντως. οὔτε γὰρ ἡ λέξις αὐτοῦ θάτερον ἐνδείκνυται σαφῶς, οὔθ' ἡ τῶν πραγμάτων φύσις ἱκανὴ πιστώσασθαι. εἰ μὲν οὖν τὴν ἑτέραν τῶν δοξῶν φυλάττωμεν ἑπόμενοι τοῖς μουσικοῖς, τοὺς τῶν ἡσυχιῶν χρόνους προσθήσομεν τοῖς τῶν προηγουμένων κινήσεων· εἰ δὲ τὴν εἰς τὰς προγνώσεις χρείαν τὴν κίνησιν τῇ κινήσει παραβάλλοντες ἰδίᾳ τὸν τῶν ἡσυχιῶν χρόνον ἐπισκεψόμεθα.

[2] Galen, Synop. lib. de puls. 14, K. ix. 470: ἐν δὲ τῷ παραβάλλειν τὸν χρόνον τῆς διαστολῆς τῷ χρόνῳ τῆς συστολῆς, ὡς 'Ηρόφιλος ἠξίου, τὸ μὲν ὅτι παρὰ φύσιν ὁ κάμνων ἔχει δύνατόν ἐστι γνωσθῆναι. Cf. Pliny, Nat. Hist. xi. 89: 'Arteriarum pulsus in cacumine maxime membrorum evidens index fere morborum, in modulos certos legesque metricas per aetates—stabilis aut citatus aut tardus—descriptus ab Herophilo medicinae vate miranda arte: nimiam propter subtilitatem desertus, observatione tamen crebri aut languidi ictus gubernacula vitae temperat.'

[3] Markellinos, De pulsibus, xi (ed. Schoene, Festschrift zur 49. Versammlung deutscher Philologen und Schulmänne, Basel, 1907, pp. 448–71) : ὁ δὲ 'Ηρόφιλος πυρέσσειν ἀπεφήνατο τὸν ἄνθρωπον, ὁπόταν πυκνότερος καὶ μείζων ἢ καὶ σφοδρότερος ὁ σφυγμὸς γένηται μετὰ πολλῆς θερμασίας ἔνδον, εἰ

It is not easy to believe that this story is a complete invention, either of Markellinos or of some predecessor, though from the technical point of view it can hardly fail to arouse some suspicions, since it is anything but easy to envisage how this pulse-counter could have been calibrated with any degree of accuracy for the various age-groups. Can we admit the possibility of an apparatus something like the egg-boiling sand-glass of today, using water instead of sand? The proof that the instrument can hardly have been a success would seem to be implied in the fact that no one else has ever been reported to have used one. We can therefore, if we like, look upon Herophilus as an unsuccessful predecessor of Floyer, but the intuitive counting of the pulse-rate was probably more accurate.

Herophilus did, however, lay down the main categories which most of his successors elaborated. The size of the pulse, considered as measurable in three dimensions, the distinction between speed and frequency, and the notions of regularity and irregularity. It is interesting also in this connection to note that the subtleties of measurement which he was the first to invent were not universally accepted. Agathinus, for example, the tutor of Archigenes, denied that the contraction of the artery could be felt at all.[1] But though the doctrines of Herophilus were generally condemned by most of his successors as over-subtle so far as his musical interpretation of rhythm was concerned,[2] he did give names to certain pulse patterns which were adopted by most of his successors. These were named after their supposed resemblance to the gait of certain animals, the 'gazelling', the 'anting', and the 'worming'. Unfortunately the treatise which Galen tells us he was going to write on Herophilus' doctrine of the pulse has not survived, if it was ever written.[3]

The theory of the pulse which Herophilus invented and his successors developed, seems to have been a rather curious mixture of sense-percepts and rational interpretation. He believed, as Galen also did, that the pulse

μὲν οὖν προαπαλλάξειε τὴν σφοδρότητα καὶ τὸ μέγεθος, ἔνδοσιν τοῦ πυρετοῦ λαμβάνοντος. τὴν δὲ πυκνότητα τῶν σφυγμῶν ἀρχομένων τε τῶν πυρετῶν πρώτην συνίστασθαι καὶ συμπαραμένειν μέχρι τῆς τελείας αὐτῶν λύσεως λέγει. οὕτω δὲ τῇ πυκνοσφυξίᾳ τὸν Ἡρόφιλον θαρρεῖν, λόγος ὡς, βεβαίῳ σημείῳ χρώμενος, ὥστε κλεψύδραν κατασκευάσαι χωρητικὴν ἀριθμοῦ ῥητοῦ τῶν κατὰ φύσιν σφυγμῶν ἑκάστης ἡλικίας, εἰσιόντα τε πρὸς τὸν ἄρρωστον καὶ τιθέντα τὴν κλεψύδραν ἅπτεσθαι τοῦ πυρέσσοντος· ὅσῳ δ' ἂν πλείονες παρέλθοιεν κινήσεις τῷ σφυγμῷ παρὰ τὸ κατὰ φύσιν εἰς τὴν ἐκπλήρωσιν τῆς κλεψύδρας, τοσούτῳ καὶ τὸν σφυγμὸν πυκνότερον ἀποφαίνειν, τοῦτ' ἔστι πυρέσσειν ἢ μᾶλλον ἢ ἧττον.

[1] Galen, De dignosc. puls. i. 3, K. viii. 786: Ἀγαθίνου τοίνυν λέγοντος ἀναίσθητον εἶναι τὴν συστολὴν τῆς ἀρτηρίας, Ἡροφίλου δὲ διὰ παντὸς ὡς ὑπὲρ αἰσθητῆς διαλεγομένου.

[2] Cf. Pliny, Nat. Hist. xxix. 4: 'Dissederuntque hae scholae et omnes eas damnavit Herophilus in musicos pedes venarum pulsu descripto per aetatum gradus. Deserta deinde et haec secta est, quoniam necesse erat in ea litteras scire.'

[3] See Galen, De praesag. ex puls. ii. 3, K. ix. 279, where he refers to a writing of his own on the pulse-lore of Herophilus, which must, surely, be more than the account given in Chapter 12 of his synopsis of his own writings on the pulse: τὰ δ' ἐξ ὧν ἰδίᾳ γράψομεν ὑπὲρ τῆς τοῦ Ἡροφίλου περὶ τοὺς σφυγμοὺς τέχνης.

was caused by a contraction and an expansion of the arteries, both of which could be felt directly and measured in time, and that between these two movements there were two perceptible intervals, during which the coats of the arteries remained motionless. The pulse pattern was therefore a quadripartite affair involving besides the times taken by diastole and systole and their relative proportions to each other, the relation of these to the two periods of quiescence.[1] Herophilus was criticized by Galen for his failure to distinguish these four elements sufficiently clearly, but he was, Galen admits, the first person to apply time units to the measurement of the actual perception of the arterial movements of diastole and systole.[2] To what extent he recognized in theory the intervals between these two movements is far from certain. Galen tells us that he confused them, he does not say that he denied their existence. In the ages which were to follow, these intervals of quiescence became important, since they were looked upon as determining the frequency, as opposed to the speed, of the pulse.[3] Galen criticizes Herophilus' arrangement of the pulse-beat into metric feet in two passages of considerable length, which are perhaps worth quoting in full: In the *De praesagitione ex pulsibus*, Chapter 3, he tells us that Herophilus wrote at length on this matter, but that he treated it rather in the manner of one describing observations and experiments than in the manner of one expounding a logical method. For he wrote an account detailing the pulse-rhythms that generally occur in each age-group, but in the first place, he did not tell us anything about the natural condition of the patients on whom he made his observations. Moreover, from his teaching it is clear that he is both confused and inarticulate, because he fails to distinguish the time interval of diastole from that of the period of quiescence. For if he really thinks that time taken by the systole of old men can be extended to the length of ten times the smallest time units, it is clear that he cannot have perceived the length of the actual diastole. For though systole sometimes takes a shorter time than diastole, and it also, as he wrote, sometimes takes longer, it can never be, as he thinks, five times as long, it can only be just a little longer.[4]

[1] See below, pp. 402 ff.
[2] Galen, De dignosc. puls. iii. 3, K. viii. 913: Ἡρόφιλος πρῶτός τινα πρὸς αἴσθησιν ὑποτίθεται χρόνον, ᾧ τοὺς ἄλλους μετρῶν ἢ δυοῖν ἢ καὶ τριῶν ἢ καὶ πλειόνων εἶναι φάσκει.
[3] Galen, De diff. puls. ii. 7, K. viii. 512: μεταβῶμεν δ᾽ ἐπὶ τοὺς αἰσθάνεσθαι φάσκοντας τῆς συστολῆς βραδύτητα μὲν καὶ τάχος ὁμοίως ἐκείνοις ἐν τῷ τῆς διαστολῆς χρόνῳ τιθεμένους, ἤδη δὲ κἂν τῷ τῆς συστολῆς, οὐ μὴν τήν γε πυκνότητα καὶ τὴν ἀραιότητα, καὶ τὸν ῥυθμὸν ἔθ᾽ ὡσαύτως ἐκείνοις, ἀλλὰ τὴν μὲν πυκνότητα καὶ ἀραιότητα κατὰ τὰς ἠρεμίας ἑκατέρας, τὸν ῥυθμὸν δὲ κατὰ τὸν τῆς διαστολῆς χρόνον ἅμα τῷ τῆς μετ᾽ αὐτὴν ἡσυχίας παραβαλλόμενον τῷ τῆς συστολῆς ἅμα τῷ τῆς μετ᾽ αὐτὴν ἠρεμίας.
[4] Galen, De praesag. ex puls. ii. 3, K. ix. 278: ἐξῆς δ᾽ ἐστὶν ἐπί γε τῇ τάξει τοῦ λόγου περὶ ῥυθμῶν διελθεῖν, ὑπὲρ ὧν Ἡροφίλῳ μὲν ἐπὶ πλέον εἴρηται, τήρησίν τινα καὶ ἐμπειρίαν ἱστοροῦντι μᾶλλον ἢ λογικὴν μέθοδον ἐκδιδάσκοντι. τοὺς γὰρ καθ᾽ ἑκάστην ἡλικίαν ὡς τὸ πολὺ φαινομένους

A similar charge of ambiguity is brought by Galen in his *Synopsis of his own works on the pulse*, which seems to bring out the difference between the various views current in Galen's time on the nature of the pulse-rhythm. These differences depend largely on the question of how much of the movements both of diastole and of systole could be directly perceived by the fingers. For those who consider the systole of the arteries to be imperceptible to the fingers, the rhythm of the beat is divided into just two periods, that of the perceived motion of expansion of the artery, the diastole, which was generally though not universally regarded as perceptible, when the artery in diastole hits our touch, and the remaining interval before the next 'beat', which is composed of (a) the period of quiescence between expansion and contraction, (b) the movement of contraction itself, (c) the period of quiescence following the systole, which is, of course, as imperceptible as the systole itself, and (d) the beginning of the movement of diastole, which is not perceptible to the fingers. This school of thought divides the pulse movement into beat and interval, a theory favoured by the Empirics, and determines the frequency or rareness of the pulse by the size of the interval, just as it measures the speed, as opposed to the frequency, of the beat by its quickness or slowness. Now, in so far as Herophilus says that the rhythm of the pulse of the newly-born child is measured by equal time intervals, he seems to me to that extent to distinguish the beginning of the systole from the quiescence; but in so far as he prolongs the systole of old men's arteries into ten of his 'first periods', he no longer maintains this distinction, but determines diastole by the perceived motion which we distinguish as the beat on our fingers; but he identifies systole with the whole of the interval during which we can feel no motion.[1]

ῥυθμοὺς τῶν σφυγμῶν ἔγραψε, πρῶτον μὲν οὐδ' ἐφ' ὧν τινων φύσεων ἐτήρησεν αὐτοὺς οὐδὲν ἡμῖν εἰπών· εἶτ' ἐξ αὐτῶν ὧν διδάσκει δῆλον ὅτι συγκέχυταί τε καὶ ἀδιάρθρωτός ἐστι περὶ τὴν τῆς συστολῆς καὶ τῶν ἠρεμιῶν διάγνωσιν. εἴπερ γὰρ ἡγεῖταί ποτε δύνασθαι γενέσθαι συστολὴν ἐπὶ τῶν γεγηρακότων ἄχρι δὴ τῶν δέκα πρώτων χρόνων ἐκτεταμένην, εὔδηλός ἐστι τῆς ὄντως συστολῆς ἀναισθήτως ἔχων. αὕτη γὰρ ἐνίοτε μὲν ὀλιγοχρονιωτέρα τῆς διαστολῆς ἐστιν, ἐνίοτε δ' ἰσόχρονός ἐστιν, ὁτὲ δέ, ὡς ἐκεῖνος γράφει, πολυχρονιωτέρα μέν, οὐ μὴν ὡς οἴεται πενταπλασίων, ἀλλὰ βραχεῖ τινι μείζων.

[1] Galen, *Synops. libb. de puls.* 12, K. ix. 464: οὕτως καὶ Ἡρόφιλος ἀνάλογον μὲν ἄρσει τὴν διαστολὴν ὑποθέμενος, ἀνάλογον δὲ θέσει τὴν συστολὴν τῆς ἀρτηρίας, ἀρξάμενος ἀπὸ τοῦ νεογενοῦς παιδίου τὴν τήρησιν ἐποιήσατο, πρῶτον χρόνον αἰσθητὸν ὑποθέμενος ἐν ᾧ διαστελλομένην εὕρισκε τὴν ἀρτηρίαν, ἴσον δ' αὐτῇ καὶ τὸν τῆς συστολῆς εἶναί φησιν, οὐ πάνυ τι διοριζόμενος ὑπὲρ ἑκατέρας τῶν ἡσυχιῶν. οἷς γὰρ ἀναίσθητός ἐστιν ἡ τῆς ἀρτηρίας συστολή, τούτοις εἰς δύο χρόνους τοὺς πάντας ὁ ῥυθμὸς τοῦ σφυγμοῦ μερίζεται, τόν τε τῆς αἰσθητῆς κινήσεως, ἡνίκα πλήττει τὴν ἀφὴν ἡμῶν ἡ ἀρτηρία διαστελλομένη, καὶ τὸ λοιπὸν ἅπαντα συγκείμενον ἔκ τε τῆς ἐκτὸς ἠρεμίας καὶ τῆς μετ' αὐτὴν συστολῆς, καὶ τῆς ἐπ' ἐκείνῃ πάλιν ἠρεμίας καὶ τῶν πρώτων τῆς διαστολῆς, ἅπερ ἐστὶν ἀναίσθητα καὶ αὐτά. καὶ διὰ τοῦτο εἰς πληγὴν καὶ διάλειμμα μερίζουσι τὸν σφυγμόν, ἐν τῷ τοῦ διαλείμματος ποσῷ πυκνότητα καὶ ἀραιότητα τιθέμενοι, καθάπερ ἐν τῷ τῆς πληγῆς τάχος καὶ βραδύτητα. καθ' ὅσον μὲν οὖν δι' ἴσου τὸν τοῦ ῥυθμοῦ σφυγμὸν εἶναί φησιν ἐπὶ τῶν ἀρτιγενῶν ὁ Ἡρόφιλος, κατὰ τοσοῦτο διαγινώσκειν ἔδοξέ μοι τὴν ἀρχὴν τῆς συστολῆς. καθ' ὅσον δὲ πάλιν ἄχρι δέκα χρόνων τῶν πρώτων ἐκτείνει τὴν συστολὴν τῆς τῶν γερόντων ἀρτηρίας, κατὰ τοσοῦτο

These distinctions appear to the layman as rather over-refined, but Herophilus apparently regarded them as important, since he thought that any variation in the proportionate time of diastole to systole from the pattern proper to each age-group was a measure of the extent of disease. All these discussions imply a subtlety of perception which it would be interesting to compare with modern experience, with modern descriptions of the findings of digital manipulation compared with the curves traced by the sphygmograph. The first point to be considered is that Herophilus regarded the arterial contraction and expansion as something quite independent of the liquid or gaseous (pneumatic) content of either the heart or the arteries themselves, or indeed of the actual motion of the heart's muscles. The second point is that it is the active power of expansion of the arteries themselves which is regarded as the essential phenomenon of the pulse, and this is what the fingers are supposed to feel, the perceptibility of the contraction being, even according to Galen, much less certain.[1]

Herophilus' doctrine of the characteristic normal pulse varying according to age in the rhythm of the single beat has not, so far as I am aware, received any confirmation in modern teaching. But the characteristic frequency, as distinguished from 'speed', of the pulse has been considered in modern times to vary according to sex and age. Thus according to the table reproduced in Ewart, the normal frequency of the adult pulse is 72 beats a minute in the male and 80 in the female. In the foetus it varies from 140 to 150, at birth and during the first year from 130 to 140, at five years of age from 90 to 94. At about fifteen the normal adult pulse-rate is attained, and remains more or less constant till the age of fifty. From then onwards a slight increase begins to take place. At eighty the average normal pulse is about 79, and from eighty to ninety years of age about 80 plus. These figures do not exclude very large variations in the healthy individual's normal pulse-rate. But the doctrine of quiescent intervals between pulse-waves so dear to Galen, if not to Herophilus himself, is incorrect. 'There is no real pause in normal pulses, since one pulse-wave does not terminate till the ensuing one begins.'[2]

Herophilus' doctrine of the relation of the heart-beat to the pulse is not at all clear. Both heart and arteries 'pulsate', and the arteries have their own power of pulsation, i.e. of contraction and expansion. But this power is not an independent physiological inborn tendency (σύμφυτον) as Praxagoras thought. The arteries receive it from the heart. It would appear that Herophilus, no less than Galen, regarded the expansion and

μηκέτι διαγινώσκειν, ἀλλὰ τὴν διαστολὴν ταῖς αἰσθηταῖς κινήσεσι γνωρίζειν, ἃς ἐκ τοῦ πλήττεσθαι τοὺς δακτύλους ἡμῶν διαγινώσκομεν, τὴν συστολὴν δὲ πᾶν τὸ λοιπὸν τίθεσθαι καθ' ὃ κινήσεως οὐκ ᾐσθάνετο.

[1] See below, p. 405.   [2] Ewart, Heart Studies I (London, 1894), 78.

contraction of the arteries as a continuation or extension, as it were, of the expansion and contraction of the ventricles which takes place simultaneously; whereas Erasistratus, and Rufus also, were aware that the expansion of the arteries coincides in time with the contraction, not the expansion, of the ventricles, and vice versa.[1] This rather elementary error of Herophilus and Galen was, as we shall see, one of the factors which made it difficult for those who made it to arrive at the conception of the circulation. And though Erasistratus was not misled by it, his adoption of the theory of Praxagoras that the arteries contained only *pneuma* was equally effective in preventing him from arriving at it.

Though none of his works has survived, we are rather better informed about the doctrines of Erasistratus, largely through the numerous citations of his teachings in the work of Galen, who though he has been held to imply, wrongly in my opinion, that already in his day Erasistratus' works had been lost,[2] quotes a large number of passages from them as if they were still available.[3] He was a pupil of the younger Cnidian Chrysippus, though he also studied for some time under Praxagoras of Cos. On one point of fundamental importance he followed the Coan, rather than the Cnidian, tradition. He regarded the brain, not the heart, as the directing organ of the body. He also adopted the theory first worked out by Praxagoras that the arteries contained not blood but *pneuma*.[4] He has sometimes been regarded, for example by Wellmann, as the Father of comparative anatomy, since he dissected both animals and human corpses,[5] and in two fields he made important advances on the discoveries of his older contemporary Herophilus: namely (*a*) in the anatomy of the heart, and (*b*) in that of the brain and the nervous system. It is chiefly with the former that we shall here be concerned. Galen, no

---

[1] Galen, *De diff. puls.* iv. 1, K. viii. 702–3: ἔτι δὲ μείζων ἄλλη διαφορὰ τοῖς ἰατροῖς ἐκ παλαιοῦ περὶ τῶν ἀρτηριῶν ἐγένετο, τινῶν μὲν ἡγουμένων αὐτὰς ἐξ ἑαυτῶν σφύζειν, σύμφυτον ἐχούσας ὁμοίως τῇ καρδίᾳ τὴν τοιαύτην δύναμιν, ὧν ἐστι καὶ Πραξαγόρας, ἐνίων δὲ σφύζειν μὲν αὐτοῦ τοῦ χιτῶνος αὐτῶν διαστελλομένου τε καὶ συστελλομένου, καθάπερ ἡ καρδία, τὴν δύναμιν δὲ οὐκ ἐχουσῶν σύμφυτον ἧ τοῦτο δρῶσιν, ἀλλὰ παρὰ καρδίαν λαμβανουσῶν· ἧς γνώμης ἔχεται καὶ Ἡρόφιλος· Ἐρασιστράτῳ δὲ οὐδέτερον ἀρέσκει, βούλεται γὰρ ἔμπαλιν τῆς καρδίας τὰς ἀρτηρίας σφύζειν, ἐκείνης μέν, ὅτε διαστέλλεται πληρουμένης τῇ πρὸς τὸ κενούμενον ἀκολουθίᾳ, τῶν δὲ ἀρτηριῶν ὅτε πληροῦνται διαστελλομένων, πληροῦσθαι δὲ αὐτὰς τοῦ παρὰ καρδίας ἐπιπεμπομένου πνεύματός φησιν.

[2] Galen, *De venae sectione*, 5, K. xi. 221: ἐγὼ μὲν οὖν εἰ καὶ μηδὲν ἐσῴζετο Ἐρασιστράτου βιβλίον, ἀλλ' ἤδη πάντα ἀπολώλει, καθάπερ τὰ Χρυσίππου κινδυνεύει παθεῖν, τοῦτο τοῖς μαθηταῖς ἂν αὐτοῦ μᾶλλον ἐπίστευσα περὶ τοῦ διδασκάλου λέγουσιν ἢ τοῖς μήτ' Ἐρασίστρατον αὐτὸν ἰδοῦσί ποτε μήτε μαθητὴν αὐτοῦ. Thus, e.g., Kühn or his indexer: see index, XX. 228: 'Ejus librorum nullus jam supererat Galeni tempore.'

[3] Galen, *De nat. fac.* i. 17, K. ii. 71: ὅτι δὲ καὶ ὁ Ἐρασίστρατος οὕτως ἐγίγνωσκεν, οἱ τὸ πρῶτον ἀνεγνωκότες αὐτοῦ σύγγραμμα τῶν καθόλου λόγων ἐπίστανται.

[4] Galen, *De usu partium*, vi. 17, K. iii. 492: ὅσοι ταῖς ἀρτηρίαις οὐδ' ὅλως αἵματος μεταδιδόασι, ὥσπερ καὶ ὁ Ἐρασίστρατος. Cf. *De foetuum formatione*, 3, K. iv. 664: ἢ διὰ τῆς μεγάλης ἀρτηρίας ἐχούσης αἷμα καὶ αὐτῆς, οὐχ ὡς Ἐρασίστρατος οἴεται μόνον πνεῦμα. And ibid., 671: κατὰ γὰρ τὰς ἀρτηρίας Ἐρασίστρατος μὲν οὐδ' ὅλως οἴεται περιέχεσθαι τὸν χυμὸν τοῦτον (αἷμα)

[5] Wellmann, 'Erasistratus', in *RE* vi.

friend of his or of his doctrines, records that he was the first person to give an accurate account of the valves of the heart. Indeed he tells us that he himself could not give a better one.[1] He understood quite clearly how they worked. Unlike Herophilus, he did not regard the auricles as part of the heart, but following the older tradition looked upon them as the terminations of the vena cava and the vein-like artery, the pulmonary vein.[2] Like Aristotle, he regarded the heart as the starting-point of the whole vascular system, arteries and veins alike—a point on which he is rebuked by Galen, in a long passage in the treatise *On the opinions of Hippocrates and Plato*.[3] He also seems to have invented rather than discovered the capillary system, which he inferred to exist as forming connections between the arteries and the veins, for these capillaries were too small to be visible, they were only to be seen by the eye of reason— thus anticipating Harvey by more than 1,800 years. His doctrine on the capillaries is summed up by Galen, in the treatise *On phlebotomy, against Erasistratus*, in the following terms:

Arteries and veins, the vessels carrying respectively *pneuma* and blood, are each successively divided up into a great number of smaller and smaller branches, and are spread to all the parts of the body, so that there is no part in which their terminations are not present. They end up in such small vessels, the mouths of which are joined, that the blood contained [in the veinlets] is held up or prevented from passing. And for this reason, since the mouths of the veinlets and arterioles are continuous, being alongside each other, the blood remains within the bounds of the venous system, and in health never penetrates into the vessels of the arterioles. But if such penetration should take place, disease must of necessity follow.[4]

In spite of his assumption of these interconnections, and in spite of his knowledge of the valves of the heart, their structure, and the principles on which they worked, as a kind of pump with both intake and outlet

---

[1] Galen, *De usu pulsuum*, 5, K. v. 166: αἰτία δὲ αἱ τῶν ὑμένων ἐπιφύσεις, ὑπὲρ ὧν αὐτάρκως Ἐρασιστράτου διαλεγομένου, περιττὸν ἡμᾶς νῦν γράφειν. Cf. the passage from the *De dogm. Hipp. et Plat*. i. 10, quoted above, p. 179, n. 3.

[2] See the passage from Galen's *De anatom. administ*. vii. 11, quoted above, p. 180, n. 2.

[3] Galen, *De plac. Hipp. et Plat*. vi. 6, K. v. 548 sq.: ἀλλὰ τό γε νῦν εἶναι προκείμενον, ὡς ὑφ' οὗ τρέφεται τὰ σύμπαντα μέλη τοῦ ζῴου, τοῦτ' ἐξ ἥπατος, οὐκ ἐκ τῆς καρδίας ὁρμᾶται, δείξειν ἐπαγγέλλομαι τῶν ἐξ ἀνατομῆς φαινομένων ἀρχὴν τῷ λόγῳ ποιησάμενος, ὃ μάλιστα μάχεται τοῖς Ἐρασιστρατείοις, οἳ νῦν ἡμῖν ἐροῦσιν, ὡς παράδοξά τε καὶ καινὰ κατασκευάζουσιν.

[4] Galen, *De venae sectione*, 2, K. xi. 153: ἀρέσκει δὲ αὐτῷ ('Ερασιστράτῳ) πνεύματος μὲν ἀγγεῖον εἶναι τὴν ἀρτηρίαν, αἵματος δὲ τὴν φλέβα· σχιζόμενα δ' ἀεὶ τὰ μείζω τῶν ἀγγείων εἰς ἐλάττονα μὲν τὸ μέγεθος, ἀριθμὸν δὲ πλείω· καὶ πάντῃ τοῦ σώματος ἐνεχθέντα, μηδένα γὰρ εἶναι τόπον ἔνθα μὴ πέρας ἀγγείου κείμενον ὑπάρχει, εἰς οὕτω σμικρὰ πέρατα τελευτᾶν, ὥστε τῇ μύσει τῶν ἐσχάτων στομάτων κρατούμενον ἐντὸς αὐτῶν ἴσχεσθαι τὸ αἷμα. καὶ διὰ τοῦτο καίτοι παρακειμένων ἀλλήλοις τοῦ στόματος τοῦ τε τῆς φλεβὸς καὶ τῆς ἀρτηρίας, ἐν τοῖς ἰδίοις ὅροις μένειν τὸ αἷμα μηδαμόθι τοῖς τοῦ πνεύματος ἐπεμβαῖνον ἀγγείοις. μέχρι μὲν δὴ τοῦδε νόμῳ φύσεως διοικεῖσθαι τὸ ζῷον· ἐπεὶ δέ τις αἰτία βίαιος ἐκ τῶν φλεβῶν εἰς τὰς ἀρτηρίας τὸ αἷμα μεταχθῆναι, αὐτὸ νοσεῖν ἀναγκαῖον ἤδη.

valves,[1] Erasistratus still failed to arrive at the notion of a circulation. This was because he adopted the theory propounded by Praxagoras, and adumbrated, it would appear, even earlier by the Cnidian school,[2] that the left side of the heart and the arteries which had their origin in the left ventricle contained only *pneuma*, a substance derived from the atmospheric air. This conception led, as Galen was only too ready to point out, to a number of physiological contradictions. One of these has been examined and explained by a recent commentator, Lonie.[3] Erasistratus, as we have seen, regarded the heart as a kind of double pump, the right ventricle distributing blood to all parts of the body via the veins, and the left ventricle distributing *pneuma*.[4] Blood is primarily produced from the products of digestion in the liver, though what this process of blood production is, Erasistratus, according to Galen, cannot tell us at all, since he leaves the whole of this activity unexplained.[5] The blood formed in the liver is transmitted by the vena cava to the right ventricle of the heart, where it receives its final elaboration,[6] and from the heart it is distributed, by the contraction of the right ventricle, into the veins and to the whole body through them, just as *pneuma* is distributed by the left ventricle through the arteries.

In this connection, it is worth while quoting Galen's account of Erasistratus' description of the valves in greater detail.

At the mouth of the vena cava there are three membranes, in shape arranged like the barb of an arrow, wherefore some of the Erasistratans have called them, I believe, the three-cusped membranes, and at the mouth of the vein-like artery, for thus I call the divided vessel leading from the left ventricle of the heart into the lungs, there are membranes of a very similar shape, but not the same number. For only two membranes grow out of its mouth. But the other mouths each of them have three membranes, all of which are shaped like the letter sigma. According to Erasistratus' description of the phenomenon, one of the mouths evacuates blood to the lungs, and the other *pneuma* to the whole of the animal body. In his opinion, these membranes perform at alternate times opposite services to the heart. The ones that are attached to the vessels leading matter into the heart from the outside are rotated by the entrance of the matter, so as to provide, by opening inwards towards the heart, an unimpeded passage into the heart's ventricles. For, he says, the matters do not automatically run in on their own, as if they were poured into

---

[1] Galen, *De plac. Hipp. et Plat.* vi. 6, K. v. 548: εἴρηται δὲ τὸ φαινόμενον ὑπὲρ Ἐρασιστράτου κατὰ τὴν τῶν πυρετῶν πραγματείαν, ὡς ὑμένες ἐπιπεφύκασι τοῖς στόμασι τῶν ἀγγείων, οἷς εἰς ὑπηρεσίαν ὑλῶν εἰσαγωγῆς τε καὶ αὖθις ἐξαγωγῆς ἡ καρδία προσχρῆται.

[2] See above, p. 37.   [3] I. M. Lonie, *Bull. Hist. Med.* 38 (1964).

[4] Galen, K. v. 551: μὴ τοίνυν πέμπεσθαι λέγετε (Ἐρασιστράτειοι) τῷ παντὶ σώματι παρὰ τῆς καρδίας αἷμα καὶ πνεῦμα.

[5] Ibid., 553: εἰκότως μὲν οὖν ἀσαφὴς ἡ γνώμη τἀνδρός ἐστιν, ἡ περὶ τῶν φλεβῶν, οὐδὲν εἰπόντος ὑπὲρ αἵματος γενέσεως, ἀλλ' ὅλην ταύτην παραλιπόντος ἄσκεπτον τὴν ἐνέργειαν.

[6] Ibid., 550: τὸ προπαρεσκευάσθαι μὲν ἐν τῷ ἥπατι τὸ αἷμα, φέρεσθαι δὲ ἐντεῦθεν εἰς τὴν καρδίαν, ἀπολειφόμενον ἐνταῦθα τὸ λεῖπον τῆς οἰκείας ἰδέας εἰς ἀκριβῆ τελειότητα.

a non-living vessel, but the heart itself expanding like a smith's bellows, draws the matter in through its expansion. Membranes are also attached to the vessels which lead matter out of the heart, and he considers that they undergo a contrary process. For they turn from the inside outwards, so as to open the mouths of the vessels under the pressure of the matter flowing out, on the occasion when the heart distributes matter. But for all the rest of the time they firmly close the mouths of the vessels, and do not permit any of the matter which has been expelled to return. So too the membranes on the mouths of the vessels which lead matter into the heart close their mouths when the heart contracts, so as not to permit any of the matter which has been drawn into the heart to flow backwards through them to the outside.[1]

It is clear from this description that Erasistratus must have been acquainted with the pulmonary artery and its function of conveying blood from the right ventricle to the lung, but what he thought happened to the blood so conveyed we do not know. It may very well be that he thought, as Galen did after him, that it conveyed nutriment to the lungs and that most of it was consumed in this way. Some historians indeed have supposed that he may have anticipated Servetus and Ibn-an Nafis in discovering the pulmonary circulation, but this has been shown by Dobson to be incorrect.[2] The relevant passage from Galen, which has given rise to this misinterpretation, occurs in his treatise *On the affected parts*, where he is discussing certain morbid affections of the lung, criticizing Erasistratus' theory of the spitting of blood and pus coming from the lung, a subject on which Erasistratus had apparently written a book, and the sources of the matter brought up. Erasistratus wrote as follows:

From the artery lying along the spine there are branches—vessels running along each rib, to the right and to the left. These split up into many branches

---

[1] Galen, *De plac. Hipp. et Plat.* vi. 6, K. v. 548 sq.: εἰσὶ δ' ἐπὶ μὲν τῷ στόματι τῆς κοίλης φλεβὸς τρεῖς (s.c. ὑμένες) ἀκίδων γλωχῖσιν ὁμοιότατοι τὴν σύνταξιν, ὅθεν οἶμαι καὶ τριγλώχινας ἔνιοι τῶν Ἐρασιστρατείων ἐκάλεσαν αὐτούς· ἐπὶ δὲ τῆς ἀρτηρίας τῆς φλεβώδους (οὕτω δὲ ὀνομάζω τὴν ἐκ τῆς ἀριστερᾶς κοιλίας τῆς καρδίας εἰς τὸν πνεύμονα κατασχιζομένην) ὁμοιότατοι μὲν τὸ εἶδος, ἀριθμῷ δ' οὐκ ἴσοι· μόνῳ γὰρ τούτῳ τῷ στόματι δυοῖν ὑμένων ἐπίφυσίς ἐστι, τῶν δ' ἄλλων στομάτων ἑκατέρῳ τρεῖς ὑμένες εἰσὶν ἅπαντες σιγμοειδεῖς. ἐξάγει δ' ὡς Ἐρασίστρατός φησιν ἐξηγούμενος τὸ φαινόμενον, ἑκάτερον μὲν τῶν στομάτων αἷμα μὲν εἰς τὸν πνεύμονα ἕτερον αὐτῶν, πνεῦμα δ' εἰς ὅλον τὸ ζῷον ἕτερον· τὸν τῶν ὑμένων, ὡς ἐκείνῳ δοκεῖ, πρὸς ἐναντίας ὑπηρεσίας τῇ καρδίᾳ χρόνον, ἀμοιβαῖς ἐγκαίροις ὑπαλλαττομένας, τοὺς μὲν ἐπὶ τοῖς εἰσάγουσιν τὰς ὕλας ἀγγείοις ἐπιπεφυκότας ἔξωθεν ἔσω φερομένους, ἀνατρέπεσθαι μὲν ὑπὸ τῆς εἰσόδου τῶν ὑλῶν, ἀναπίπτοντας δ' εἰς τὰς κοιλότητας τῆς καρδίας ἀνοιγνύντας τὰ στόματα παρέχειν ἀκώλυτον τὴν φορὰν τοῖς εἰς τὴν αὐτὴν ἑλκομένοις· οὐ γὰρ δὴ αὐτομάτως γε τὰς ὕλας εἰσθεῖν φησι, ὡς εἰς ἄψυχόν τινα δεξαμένην, ἀλλ' αὐτὴν τὴν καρδίαν διαστελλομένην, ὥσπερ τὰς τῶν χαλκέων φύσας, ἐπισπᾶσθαι πληροῦσαν τῇ διαστολῇ. ἐπὶ δὲ τοῖς ἐξάγουσιν ἀγγείοις τὰς ὕλας ἐλέγομεν ἐπικεῖσθαι, καὶ τοὐναντίον ἡγεῖσθαι πάθος πάσχειν. ἔσωθεν γὰρ ἔξω ῥέποντας ἀνατρεπομένους μὲν ὑπὸ τῶν ἐξιόντων ἀνοιγνύναι τὰ στόματα, καθ' ὃν ἂν ἡ καρδία λόγον ἐχορήγει τὰς ὕλας· ἐν τῷ λοιπῷ παντὶ κλείειν ἀκριβῶς τὰ στόματα, μηδ' ἐνίας τῶν ἐκπεμφθέντων ἐπανέρχεσθαι συγχωροῦντας, οὕτως δὲ καὶ τοῖς ἐπὶ τοῖς εἰσάγουσι, ὅταν ἡ καρδία συστέλληται κλείειν τὰ στόματα, μηδὲν τῶν ἑλχθέντων ὑπ' αὐτῆς αὖθις ἔξω παλινδρομεῖν ἐπιτρέποντας.

[2] Dobson, 'Erasistratus', *Proc. R. Soc. Med.* 20 (1927), Sec. Hist. Med., 825–32.

spreading into the adjacent places and finally end by becoming invisible. Now when there is an infiltration of blood into these arteries, it sometimes makes its way up the hollow artery [the aorta] into the places round or near the lung, and along the attachments by which the lung is attached to the artery along the spine. For by this vessel also there is a way up into the lung for the infiltrated blood. And how it comes to be brought up has already been described.[1]

Galen, not without some reason, regards this description as deliberately obscure, since it leaves completely unexplained how the blood goes from the great artery, the aorta, into the lung, using a purposely obscure phrase, 'the places round the lung', instead of simply saying 'the lung'.[2] Even more obscure is his description of the 'attachments' by which the passage of the blood is effected. If they are sinew- or fibre-like processes, they cannot contain blood, since blood must be carried in vessels. There would have, therefore, to be blood vessels leading from the artery which carry blood into the lung. But this function is performed not by the aorta, but, as the followers of Erasistratus say, the artery placed beneath the lung, q.e.a.[3] Without the survival of Erasistratus' text it is not possible to make any conclusive judgement on the validity of this account. It is clear, however, that Erasistratus is only dealing with a morbid process arising under special conditions. There can be no question of any anticipation of the pulmonary circulation. What Galen seems to be accusing Erasistratus about appears to be the hypothesis of a non-existent connection between the aorta and the lung, in addition to the pulmonary artery.[4]

---

[1] Galen, *De locis affectis*, v. 3, K. viii. 311 f.: κατὰ δὲ τὸν αὐτὸν τρόπον εὔλογον γίγνεσθαι καὶ τὰς ἐκ τοῦ θώρακος αἵματός τε καὶ πύου πτύσεις ἐφ᾽ ὧν Ἐρασίστρατος ζητῶν τὰς ὁδοὺς ἀπίθανα γράφει κατὰ τὸ περὶ τῆς ἀναγωγῆς τοῦ αἵματος βιβλίον ἐν τῇδε τῇ ῥήσει. ἡ δὲ ὁδὸς ἐπὶ τὴν ἀναγωγὴν τοῖς ἀπὸ τούτων τῶν τόπων ἀναφερομένοις τοιαύτη τις γίνεται· ἀπὸ τῆς παρὰ τὴν ῥάχιν κειμένης ἀρτηρίας ἀποφύσεις εἰσὶν ἀγγείων παρ᾽ ἑκάστην πλευράν, ὁμοίως ἔκ τε τῶν δεξιῶν καὶ τῶν ἀριστερῶν· αὗται δ᾽ εἰς τοὺς πλησίον τόπους ἐπὶ πλεῖον σχιζόμεναι εἰς ἄδηλα τῇ αἰσθήσει ἀποτελευτῶσιν· ὅταν οὖν γίγνηταί τις εἰς ταύτας τὰς ἀρτηρίας παρέμπτωσις αἵματος, κατὰ τὴν κοίλην ἀρτηρίαν ἐνίοτε λαμβάνει τὴν ἀναφορὰν ἐπὶ τοὺς περὶ τὸν πνεύμονα τόπους καὶ κατὰ τὰς προσφύσεις, αἷς ὁ πνεύμων προσπέφυκεν τῇ ἀρτηρίᾳ κατὰ τὴν ῥάχιν· γίγνεται γάρ τις καὶ ταύτῃ τῶν παρεμπεπτωκότων ἐπάνοδος εἰς τὸν πνεύμονα, ἐκ δὲ τοῦ πνεύμονος, ὅπως εἰς τὴν ἀναγωγὴν ἐπανέρχεται, πρότερον εἴρηται.

[2] Ibid., 312: ὅπως δὲ γίγνεται καὶ κατὰ τίνας συμφύσεις, οὐκέτι οὐδ᾽ ἐνταῦθα προσέθηκεν ... διὸ καὶ μᾶλλον ἄν τις ἡγήσαιτο μοχθηρὸν εἶναι τὸν λόγον, ὑποπτευθέντα καὶ αὐτῷ τῷ Ἐρασιστράτῳ τοιοῦτον ὑπάρχειν. ἑκών γ᾽ οὖν φαίνεται λέξεσιν ἀσαφέσιν κεχρῆσθαι, χάριν τοῦ δόξαι τι λέγειν, καίτοι λέγων μηδέν ... ἀλλὰ καὶ κατ᾽ αὐτὸ τοῦτο τὸ φάναι, τοὺς περὶ τὸν πνεύμονα τόπους, ἐνὸν εἰπεῖν τὸν πνεύμονα, δῆλός ἐστιν ἑκὼν ἐπιταράττων τὸν λόγον.

[3] Ibid., 314: οὐδὲ γὰρ ἐνταῦθα τίνας λέγει προσφύσεις ἐδήλωσεν. καὶ γὰρ ἐὰν δι᾽ ὑμένων ἤ τινων ἰνωδῶν σωμάτων γίγνονται, πλέον οὐδὲν ὡς πρὸς τὴν τοῦ περιεχομένου κατὰ τὴν μεγάλην ἀρτηρίαν αἵματος εἰς τὸν πνεύμονα φοράν· ἐκφύεσθαι γάρ τινα δεῖ τῆς ἀρτηρίας ἀγγεῖα, δι᾽ ὧν εἰς τὸν πνεύμονα παραγενήσεται τὸ αἷμα.

[4] Erasistratus, we must remember, was possibly at one time a disciple of the Peripatetic school and, if D'Arcy Thompson's suggestion is correct, the aorta of which Erasistratus was speaking was not what we call the aorta but the pulmonary artery.

Galen, as Lonie has pointed out, accuses Erasistratus of maintaining that the blood is distributed through the venous system by the right ventricle, through the pulmonary artery. Whether Erasistratus really did hold this theory we have no method of judging. We can, in the last resort, if we refuse to believe this, only suppose that Galen has misunderstood him. Erasistratus certainly knew that blood was distributed by the pulmonary artery to the lung, but how did it pass from the lung to the rest of the venous system? Did he suppose that there was a connection of some sort between the pulmonary artery and the superior vena cava or, like Mühsam's version of Aristotle's theory, that the pulmonary artery and the vena cava emerged from the heart as a single vessel? Galen is on firm ground when he points out that in order to distribute blood to the venous system, the right ventricle would have to have another 'mouth', since the 'mouth' opening from the left auricle opens inwards, and the 'mouth' which opens outwards leads only to the lungs. And no such 'mouth' exists.[1] For, according to Galen, veins have their origin not in the heart but in the liver. There would therefore have to be another trunk emerging from the heart, from which all veins branched off.[2] It seems probable that Erasistratus himself had realized that the theory of the right ventricle as a blood pump did not work satisfactorily, for, as we shall see later, he was compelled to call in another principle, that of the *horror vacui*, to explain the distribution of the blood to the tissues.

Galen, too, was up against the same problem, for he too believed that blood was produced in the liver, and from there went to the right ventricle. And his solution of the problem of its distribution seems no more plausible than that of his Alexandrian predecessor whom he criticizes so sharply. Indeed, he is led into an absurdity which Erasistratus was at any rate able to avoid, that of the two-way traffic of material through the imperfectly functioning mitral valve.[3]

But Erasistratus' adoption of the theory of the bloodless arteries led him into even greater difficulties. For, since the arteries are filled only with *pneuma*, he had to explain the fact, confirmed by universal experience, that if you cut an artery or pricked it, blood always spurted out. This he thought he was able to do by recourse to the physical theories of his contemporary, Strato of Lampsacus, surnamed *Physicus*, who is credited with the invention of the principle of the *horror vacui*. Strato, the successor of Theophrastus as the head of Aristotle's school the Lyceum, was tutor to Ptolemy Philadelphus, and Erasistratus had, according to one tradition,

---

[1] Galen, *De dogm. Hipp. et Plat.* vi. 6, K. v. 551: δείξατε οὖν ἡμῖν ἕτερον ἀγγεῖον ἐξάγον ἐκ τῆς καρδίας τουτὶ τὸ κοσμηθὲν αἷμα καὶ διανεμόμενον εἰς ἅπαντα τὰ σώματα, καθάπερ ἡ ἀρτηρία τὸ πνεῦμα.

[2] Ibid.: πέμπτον δ' ἄλλο στόμα οὐκ ἔχει κατὰ τὴν καρδίαν, ᾧ τὸ ἐξ ἥπατος ἀφικόμενον εἰς αὐτὴν αἷμα πρὸς ὅλον ἀποπέμψει τὸ σῶμα.

[3] See below, pp. 393 ff.

himself attended Theophrastus' lectures.[1] Strato's theory, which, since his works have perished, has survived only in reconstructions[2] based largely on the assumption that it is that reproduced in the introduction to Hero of Alexandria's *Pneumatika*, seems to have attempted a compromise between the atomic theory of Democritus and the Aristotelian physics of the four (or five) elements. Strato, though he accepts the four elementary bodies, air, fire, water, and earth, regards these as in a sense derivative. Like the Stoics after him, it was the four primary qualities, heat, cold, dryness, and wetness, which he looked upon as the ἀρχαί or στοιχεῖα (first principles or elements).[3] Though, according to another authority, it is fire, or the hot substance, which he regarded as the cause of all things.[4] Unlike Democritus but like Aristotle, he conceived the physical universe, indeed space itself, as a limited whole, outside of which even a vacuum or empty space does not exist,[5] and he defines a vacuum as the interval between the container and the contained.[6] He agrees, however, with Epicurus as against Aristotle, that all bodies have weight, and that they therefore move naturally towards the centre of the limited cosmos, the heavier bodies in this centripetal movement displacing the lighter. The universe thus consists of a series of concentric spheres, earth the lowest, water above it, air above that, and fire, the lightest, above all three.[7] Bodies are not made up of solid individual particles, as Democritus and Epicurus postulated, they are, in theory at least, infinitely divisible, but in practice they exist, it would seem, in very small (mostly) invisible particles.[8] These particles do not move about in a

---

[1] Galen, *De sanguine in arteriis*, 7, K. iv. 729: θαυμάζω δ' ὑμῶν, ὦ Ἐρασιστράτειοι, πῶς ὑμνοῦντες ἑκάστοτε τὸν Ἐρασίστρατον τά τ' ἄλλα καὶ ὡς Θεοφράστῳ συνεγένετο.

[2] For my account of Strato's doctrines I am chiefly indebted to Wehrle, *Die Schule des Aristoteles*, Heft v (Basel, 1950), Diels's monograph, *Ueber das physikalische System des Straton, Sitzungsberichte der Berl. Akademie* (1893), and H. B. Gottschalk's 'Strato of Lampsacus, some texts', *Proceedings of the Leeds Philosophical and Literary Society*, Literary and Historical Section, 9, vi (1965), 95–182.

[3] Pseudo-Galen, *De hist. philos.* 5, K. xix. 244: Ἡρακλείδης ὁ Ποντικὸς καὶ Ἀσκληπιάδης ὁ Βιθυνὸς ἀναρμόστους ὄγκους τὰς ἀρχὰς ὑποτιθέντες τῶν ὅρων . . . Στράτων δὲ ὁ φυσικὸς ἐπωνομασμένος τὰς ποιότητας.

Cf. Sextus Empiricus, *Hypotyposes*, iii. 37: Στράτων δὲ ὁ φυσικὸς τὰς ποιότητας (ἀρχὰς εἶναι εἶπεν).

[4] Epiphanius, *Adversus Haereses* iii. 33: Στράτων ἐκ Λαμψαχοῦ τὴν θερμὴν οὐσίαν ἔλεγεν αἰτίαν πάντων ὑπάρχειν.

[5] Theodoretus, *Graecarum affectionum curatio*, v. 14: ὁ δὲ Στράτων ἔμπαλιν ἔξωθεν μὲν (τοῦ παντὸς) μηδὲν εἶναι κενόν, ἔνδοθεν δὲ δυνατὸν εἶναι.

[6] διάστημα τοῦ περιέχοντος καὶ τοῦ περιεχομένου.

[7] Simplicius, *In Aristot. de coelo comment.*, pp. 267–8 (Heiberg): ταύτης δὲ γεγόνασι τῆς δόξης μετ' αὐτὸν Στράτων τε καὶ Ἐπίκουρος, πᾶν σῶμα βαρύτητα ἔχειν νομίζοντες καὶ πρὸς τὸ μέσον φέρεσθαι, τῷ δὲ τὰ βαρύτερα ὑφιζάνειν τὰ ἧττον βαρέα ὑπ' ἐκείνων ἐκθλίβεσθαι βίᾳ πρὸς τὸ ἄνω, ὥστε εἴ τις ὑφείλε τὴν γῆν, ἐλθεῖν ἂν τὸ ὕδωρ εἰς τὸ κέντρον, καὶ εἴ τις τὸ ὕδωρ, τὸν ἀέρα, καὶ εἰ τὸν ἀέρα, τὸ πῦρ.

[8] Diels, op. cit., quotes a passage cited in Sextus Empiricus, *Adversus Mathematicos*, τὰ σώματα καὶ τοὺς τόπους εἰς ἄπειρον τέμνεσθαι. He remarks that this τέμνεσθαι was not κατὰ τὸ αἰσθητόν but only κατὰ τὸ λόγῳ θεωρητόν, i.e. δυνάμει, not ἐνεργείᾳ.

vacuum, it is the vacuum which moves about in them. There are two views, Hero tells us, about the nature of the vacuum. Some say that such a thing does not exist at all, others, whose opinion he adopts, say that there is no continuous vacuum in nature, but that vacua, in little pieces or bits, are scattered all over particles of air, water, fire, and earth, and all other bodies.[1] Strato thought that these vacua existed in all bodies except 'adamant' (diamond?), which cannot be burned because of its exceedingly dense texture, so close that even the smallest particles of the lightest element, fire, could not find any vacuoles by which to enter, but had therefore to remain on its surface, with the consequence that it receives no heat, since the particles cannot enter into it. But in the case of air, the next lightest element, the particles are all pressed tightly against each other, but they do not absolutely fit, so that there are empty spaces between them. They are like the grains of sand upon the beach.[2] This last simile, with its implication of a lack of continuity, might appear to suggest something more like the atoms of Democritus, but Simplicius in a passage in *Physica* 603, quoted by Diels, makes it clear that what Strato was trying to insist on was the lack of continuity, not in the particles but in the vacuoles they contain. A continuous vacuum cannot exist, since whenever any body moves or is moved, another body immediately takes its place, according to the law of 'the following up into the vacated space' (πρὸς τὸ κενούμενον ἐπακολουθίᾳ), which constitutes the principle of the *horror vacui*.[3] These vacuoles inside the smallest particles, the discontinuous empty spaces, have an important part to play in

[1] Hero Alexandrinus, *Pneumatica*, i, Prooemium (ed. Schmidt, Leipzig, 1899, p. 4) : πρὸ δὲ τῶν λέγεσθαι μελλόντων πρῶτον περὶ κενοῦ διαληπτέον· οἱ μὲν γὰρ τὸ καθόλου μηδὲν εἶναι κενὸν (λέγουσι), οἱ δὲ ἄθρουν μὲν κατὰ φύσιν μηδὲν εἶναι κενόν, παρεσπαρμένον δὲ κατὰ μικρὰ μόρια τῷ ἀέρι καὶ τῷ ὑγρῷ καὶ (τῷ) πυρὶ καὶ τοῖς ἄλλοις σώμασιν οἷς μάλιστα συμφέρεσθαι προσήκει.

[2] Ibid., p. 6: οὐχ ὑποληπτέον οὖν ἐν τοῖς οὖσι κενοῦ τινα φύσιν ἀθρόαν αὐτὴν καθ᾽ ἑαυτὴν ὑπάρχειν, παρεσπαρμένον δὲ κατὰ μικρὰ μόρια, τῷ τε ἀέρι καὶ τῷ ὑγρῷ καὶ τοῖς ἄλλοις σώμασιν, εἰ μὴ ἄρα τὸν ἀδάμαντα μόνον μὴ κοινωνεῖν ⟨εἴποι τις⟩ τῇ τοῦ κενοῦ φύσει, διὰ τὸ μήτε πύρωσιν ἐπιδέχεσθαι μήτε διακόπτεσθαι, τυπτόμενον δὲ εἰς τοὺς ἄκμονας καὶ τὰς σφύρας ὅλον ἐνδύεσθαι. τοῦτο δὲ αὐτῷ παρακολουθεῖ διὰ τὴν συνεχῆ πυκνότητα. τὰ γὰρ τοῦ πυρὸς σώματα παχυμερέστερα ὄντα τῶν ἐν τῷ λίθῳ κενῶν, οὐ παρεισέρχεται, ἀλλὰ μόνον ἐπιψαύει τῆς ἐκτὸς ἐπιφανείας. διόπερ μὴ προκατεισδύνοντα ἐντὸς καθάπερ ἐπὶ τῶν ἄλλων σωμάτων, οὐδὲ δέχεται θερμότητα. τὰ δὲ τοῦ ἀέρος σώματα συνερείδει μὲν πρὸς ἄλληλα, οὐ κατὰ πᾶν δὲ μέρος ἐφαρμόζει, ἀλλ᾽ ἔχει τινὰ διαστήματα μεταξὺ κενά, καθάπερ ἡ ἐν τοῖς αἰγιάλοις ψάμμος.

[3] Ibid., p. 28: διὸ καὶ καταχρηστικῶς μηδὲν εἶναι κενὸν ⟨ἄθρουν⟩ λέγομεν βίας τινὸς μὴ παρεισελθούσης, ἀλλὰ πάντα πλήρη εἶναι ἤτοι ἀέρος ἢ ὑγροῦ ἢ ἄλλης τινὸς οὐσίας· καθ᾽ ὁπόσον δ᾽ ἄν τι τούτων ἐγχωρῇ, κατὰ τοσοῦτον ἕτερον ἐπακολουθοῦν τὸν κενούμενον ἀναπληροῖ τόπον. καὶ ὅτι κενὸν μὲν ἄθρουν οὐκ ἔστι κατὰ φύσιν, βίας τινὸς μὴ παρεισελθούσης, καὶ πάλιν ὅτι οὐκ ἔστι ποτὲ τὸ παράπαν κενόν, παρὰ φύσιν δὲ γινόμενον. Cf. Simplicius, *In Phys.*, p. 693: ὁ μέν τοι Λαμψακηνὸς Στράτων δεικνύναι πειρᾶται ὅτι ἔστι τὸ κενὸν διαλαμβάνον τὸ πᾶν σῶμα ὥστε μὴ εἶναι συνεχές, λέγων ὅτι οὐκ ἂν δι᾽ ὕδατος ἢ ἀέρος ἢ ἄλλου σώματος ἐδύνατο διεκπίπτειν τὸ φῶς, οὐδὲ ἡ θερμότης οὐδὲ ἄλλη δύναμις οὐδεμία σωματική. πῶς γὰρ ἂν αἱ τοῦ ἡλίου ἀκτῖνες διεξέπιπτον εἰς τὸ τοῦ ἀγγείου ἔδαφος; εἰ γὰρ τὸ ὑγρὸν μὴ εἶχε πόρους, ἀλλὰ βίᾳ διέστελλον αὐτὸ αἱ αὐγαί, συνέβαινεν ὑπερεκχεῖσθαι τὰ πλήρη τῶν ἀγγείων, καὶ οὐκ ἂν αἱ μὲν τῶν ἀκτίνων ἀνεκλῶντο πρὸς τὸν ἄνω τόπον, αἱ δὲ κάτω διεξέπιπτον.

Strato's explanation of physical phenomena. They are made to account for the propagation of light and heat and for the action of other forces, including the electric shock of the sting-ray.[1]

The relation of Erasistratus' doctrine of the *horror vacui* to that of Strato has not been universally accepted.[2] Wellmann, for example, thought that his teaching was derived from Chrysippus who, he believed, also held this theory, and derived it from Philistion the physician from whom Plato borrowed it to explain the theory of respiration by περίωσις, reproduced in the *Timaeus*, which we have already examined.[3] But, as Gottschalk has pointed out,[4] the two theories are not really identical. The attribution of Erasistratus' theory of inflammation which Wellmann attributed to Chrysippus is not supported by any adequate evidence, and even if he did believe that inflammation was due to infiltration of blood from the venous system via the capillaries into the *pneuma*-containing arteries, we cannot assume that he thought this process was brought about by the *horror vacui*. The difference between Plato's theory of περίωσις and that described by Hero and attributed to Strato is explained by Gottschalk as follows:

The idea of the *horror vacui* is that whenever a vacuum is created the surrounding matter is *pulled* in (ἐπισπᾶται) owing to the power of the void, in order to fill it, that of περίωσις, that the surrounding matter is *pushed* in to make room for another body.

Gottschalk thinks that Hero's theory was ultimately derived from the consideration of the process of sucking up a liquid through a tube and that Hero probably obtained his knowledge of the theory from Ctesibius, a third-century Alexandrian engineer who may have known Strato personally. In this connection one must also remember that Galen, when expounding Erasistratus' quasi-atomic theory, makes no mention of

[1] Hero, op. cit., p. 26: φέρεται δὲ καὶ τὸ φῶς τὸ ἕτερον διὰ τοῦ ἑτέρου· ὅταν γάρ τις πλείους ἄψῃ λύχνους, ἅπαντα φωτίζεται μᾶλλον, τῶν αὐγῶν πάντῃ φερομένων δι' ἀλλήλων. ἀλλὰ μὴν καὶ διὰ χαλκοῦ καὶ σιδηροῦ καὶ τῶν ἄλλων ἁπάντων διεκπίπτει σωμάτων, καθάπερ καὶ τὸ ἐπὶ τῆς νάρκης τῆς θαλασσίας γινόμενον.

[2] Wellmann, 'Zur Geschichte der Medizin im Alterthum', *Hermes* 35 (1900), remarks in a footnote to p. 377: 'Damit fällt meines Erachtens auch der von H. Diels a. a. o. geführte Nachweis, daß Erasistratus die seiner Lehre von den Synanastomosen zu Grunde liegende Vacuumtheorie dem Straton verdanke. Der Weg auf dem Chrysipp zu dieser Theorie, die er doch ohne Zweifel gleichfalls vertrat, gelangt war, ist ein anderer. Man wird sich erinnern daß Plato im *Timaeos* (79, 80) in der von ihm ausführlich gehaltenen Darstellung des Athmungsprozesses hervorhebt, daß dieser Vorgang auf den *horror vacui* beruhe. Nun geht aber, wie ich an anderer Stelle nachweisen werde, die platonische Erklärung des Athmungsprozesses auf Philistion zurück: folglich ist diese Vacuumlehre schon vor Chrysipp in ärztlichen Kreisen verbreitet gewesen. Chrysipp hatte, wenn er, wie später nachgewiesen wird, mit dem Enkel des großen Knidiers identisch ist, physikalisches Interesse; er schreib ψυσικὰ θεωρήματα nach Diogenes Laertius, VIII, 89.' [3] See above, pp. 119 f.

[4] Gottschalk, 'Strato of Lampsacus, some texts', *Proc. Leeds Phil. & Lit. Soc.*, September 1965, p. 132.

Strato. The Strato whom he associates with Erasistratus is not the 'philosopher' but a doctor disciple. But Galen lived after all nearly five hundred years after Strato, whose works may have been, if not already lost, at least almost totally forgotten. Incidentally the pseudo?-Galenic *History of philosophy*, though it mentions Strato the 'philosopher' in several places, makes no mention of the theory of the *horror vacui*. That Erasistratus did in fact derive this theory from Strato must, I think, be accepted, all the more so since the quasi-atomic theory of 'simple' bodies attributed to him by Galen in the *Natural faculties* can hardly have any other origin.[1] And Strato's 'determinism' would appear to have exercised a strong influence on his thinking.

Erasistratus, whose attitude to physiological problems was in many ways the most modern of the ancient medical theorists, was the first to apply the physical law of the *horror vacui* to the explanation of physiological processes, thus making the first adventure, however unsuccessful, in biophysics. He also attempted to apply Strato's notion of the character of small particles to the constituents of the human body. His explanation of why a wounded artery bleeds sounds today quite fantastic, particularly in a physician who had a fairly correct notion of the pumping mechanism of the heart. But his adoption of Praxagoras' theory of the *pneuma*-containing arteries really left him with no alternative. He was forced to conclude that when an artery is cut, the first thing which happens is that the *pneuma* it contains escapes unperceived. This creates a vacuum in the artery, and the vacuum draws blood into it from the veins through the unseen capillaries, through the synastomoses of the venules with the arterioles, and the blood then comes spurting out through the cut.[2] This process of infiltration of blood from the venous into the arterial system, which Galen calls in one place 'the dogma of infiltration', was found by Erasistratus and his school to have many possible applications. It was used by them to form the basis of their aetiological theory of disease, and to explain not only inflammation, for without infiltration

---

[1] See below, pp. 218 f.

[2] Galen, *De usu partium*, vi. 17, K. iii. 492: ὅτι μὲν οὖν ἀρτηρίας εἴ τις ἐπικαίρους τε καὶ πολλὰς ἅμα τρώσειεν, ἐκκενοῦται δι' αὐτῶν αἷμα ὡμολόγηται σχεδὸν ἅπασι· καὶ διὰ τοῦτο καὶ ὅσοι ταῖς ἀρτηρίαις οὐδ' ὅλως αἵματος μεταδιδόασιν, ὥσπερ καὶ ὁ Ἐρασίστρατος, οὐδὲν ἧττον ὁμολογοῦσιν αὐτὰς καὶ οὗτοι συνανεστομῶσθαι ταῖς φλεψίν. *De venae sectione*, 3, K. xi. 154: ἐπὶ τραύμασι δὲ φλεγμονὴν αἰτιᾶται μέν, κἀνταῦθα τὴν παρέμπτωσιν ἐκ τῶν φλεβῶν εἰς τὰς ἀρτηρίας τοῦ αἵματος, αὐτῆς δὲ τῆς παρεμπτώσεως αἰτίαν εἶναί φησι τὴν πρὸς τὸ κενούμενον ἀκολουθίαν. ὅταν γὰρ τῶν ἐν τῷ τετρωμένῳ μέρει διαιρεθεισῶν ἀρτηριῶν ἐκχυθῇ, κατὰ τὴν τρῶσιν ἅπαν τὸ πνεῦμα καὶ κίνδυνος ᾖ κενὸν γενέσθαι τόπον, ἕπεσθαι κατὰ τὰς συναναστομώσεις τὸ αἷμα, τοῦ κενουμένου πνεύματος τὴν βάσιν ἀναπληροῦντος. Cf. *Anonymus Londinensis*, xxvi, J. 103: πρὸς ὃν λόγον ἀπολογοῦνται οἱ Ἐρασιστράτειοι λέγοντες, διότι διαιρέσεως γενομένης κατὰ τὰς ἀρτηρίας κενοῦται τὸ αἷμα κἀπορεῖ τῶν ἐκεῖ φλεβῶν . . . τότε γὰρ συνεστομοῦσθαί τε τὰς φλέβας εἰς τὰς ἀρτηρίας καὶ τὸ ἔνον οὕτω μὴ δύνασθαι κενὸν ἀθρόον ἀπολείπεσθαι τόπον μετὰ τὴν πνεύματος κένωσιν. παρεμπίπτειν γὰρ τὸ αἷμα ἐκ τῶν φλεβῶν εἰς τὰς ἀρτηρίας· διὰ μέντοι τῶν ἀρτηριῶν ἀπορεῖν ἐκ τούτων ὡς διὰ καλάμων ἔξω.

inflammation cannot occur,[1] but all manner of diseases as well, since all forms of fever ultimately have their origin in inflammation. The excess of blood is its most common cause, because it distends the walls of the veins and forces open the mouths of the capillary veins, their anastomoses with the arterioles which had previously been shut, and so allows blood to flow into the arteries, where it collides with and resists the *pneuma* pumped into them by the left ventricle of the heart. This collision is the fever, while the penetration of the blood into the arterioles is inflammation.[2] So inflammation is by definition fever, according to the pseudo?-Galenic *History of philosophy*, where we are told that Erasistratus defined fever as the movement of infiltration of the blood into the vessels of the *pneuma*, an infiltration which takes place involuntarily. Then follows a rather unusually picturesque simile which makes one inclined to feel that it is genuinely Erasistratus':

Just as when no breath [ἄνεμος] stirs it, the sea is calm, but when a violent unnatural gale blows upon it, the whole of it is in revolution, so also in the body, when the blood is stirred into motion, it infiltrates into the vessels of the *pneumata* [Erasistratus recognized two forms of *pneuma*] and creates fever and heats up the whole body.[3]

This passage is, however, difficult to reconcile with the rather better authenticated quotation from the *Introduction*, where we are told that whereas the ancient physicians thought that fever was in and by itself a disease, Erasistratus regarded it merely as a symptom or accompaniment, an opinion which is attributed in the *History of philosophy* to Diocles.[4] The *Introduction* also informs us that Erasistratus, speaking generally, assigned one single cause to all diseases, namely this process

---

[1] Galen, *De usu partium*, vi. 17, K. iii. 493: διδάσκει γοῦν αὐτὸς Ἐρασίστρατος ἐπιμελῶς ἡμᾶς, ὡς οὐχ ἐνδέχεται γενέσθαι φλεγμονὴν ἄνευ τοῦ παρεμπεσεῖν ποτε ἐκ τῶν φλεβῶν εἰς τὰς ἀρτηρίας αἷμα.

[2] Galen, *Comment. in Hipp. de nat. hom.* ii. 10, K. xv. 159: καθάπερ Ἐρασίστρατος ἐπὶ φλεγμονῇ γίνεσθαι βουλόμενος ἅπαντας τοὺς πυρετούς. Cf. *De venae sectione*, 3, K. xi. 153 f.: ἐπεὶ δέ τις αἰτία βίαιος ἐκ τῶν φλεβῶν εἰς τὰς ἀρτηρίας τὸ αἷμα μεταχθῆναι αὐτὸ νοσεῖν ἀναγκαῖον ἤδη. αἰτίας δὲ καὶ ἄλλας τινὰς καὶ οὐδεμιᾶς ἐλάττω τὸ πλῆθος εἶναι τοῦ αἵματος, ὑφ' οὗ διατείνεσθαι μὲν τὸν χιτῶνα τῆς φλεβὸς ἀναστομοῦσθαι δὲ τὰ πρότερον μεμυκότα πέρατα, μεταχεῖσθαι δὲ εἰς τὰς ἀρτηρίας τὸ αἷμα, κἀντεῦθεν τῷ παρὰ καρδίας φερομένῳ πνεύματι προσκόπτον καὶ ἐνιστάμενον, ἀλλοιοῦντι τὴν ἐκείνου κίνησιν ἡνίκ' ἂν ἐγγὺς ᾖ, καὶ κατ' εὐθὺ τῆς ἀρχῆς, καὶ τοῦτ' εἶναι τὸν πυρετόν. ὠθούμενόν τε ὑπ' αὐτοῦ πρόσω σφηνοῦσθαι κατὰ τὰ πέρατα τῶν ἀρτηριῶν καὶ τοῦτ' εἶναι τὴν φλεγμονήν. οὕτω μὲν ἐπὶ πλήθει φλεγμονὴν ἐργάζεται τῷ λόγῳ τῷδε.

[3] Galen (?), *De hist. philos.* 39, K. xix. 342–3: Ἐρασίστρατος ὁρίζεται τὸν πυρετὸν κίνημα αἵματος παρεμπεπτωκότος εἰς τὰ τοῦ πνεύματος ἀγγεῖα ἀπροαιρέτως γινόμενον καθάπερ ἐπὶ τῆς θαλάσσης, ὅταν μηδὲν κινῇ αὐτὴν πνεῦμα ἠρεμεῖ, ἀνέμου δὲ ἐμπνέοντος βιαίου παρὰ φύσιν, τότε ἐξ ὅλης κυκλεῖται, οὕτω καὶ ἐν τῷ σώματι ὅταν κινηθῇ τὸ αἷμα, ἐμπίπτει μὲν εἰς τὰ ἀγγεῖα τῶν πνευμάτων, πυρούμενον δὲ θερμαίνει τὸ ὅλον σῶμα.

[4] Galen, *Introductio sive medicus*, 13, K. xiv. 729: τὸν μὲν οὖν πυρετὸν οἱ παλαιοὶ πάθος αὐτὸν καθ' αὐτὸν ἡγοῦνται· Ἐρασίστρατος δὲ καὶ τῶν νεωτέρων τινὲς ἐπιγένημα. Cf. *De hist. philos.* 39, K. xix. 343: Διοκλῆς δέ φησιν ἐπιγένημα εἶναι τὸν πυρετόν.

of infiltration,[1] thus exhibiting a tendency to universal extrapolation which has not been altogether unknown in later members of his profession.

The theory of infiltration encountered, as might be expected, a more than usually indignant refutation on the part of Galen, not only in his general comprehensive treatises on anatomy and physiology, but also in two other specially written essays, the one *On blood in the arteries* and the other *On venesection*, which practice Erasistratus had the courage to oppose, following in this the teaching of his master Chrysippus. With the details of Galen's rather dreary and oft-repeated refutation we need not concern ourselves, but one rather typical piece of argument taken from the latter is perhaps worth examining for the light that it throws on the nature of physiological reasoning in Hellenistic circles, even if its inaccurate physics cause us to smile. Galen raises the obvious commonsense objections to Erasistratus' theory of arterial bleeding, namely, first, that the process of the escape of *pneuma* is not perceptible by the senses, and secondly, that whenever arteries are pricked even with the smallest instrument or weapon, blood spurts out at once, which, on Erasistratus' theory, it should not do, since the escape of *pneuma* from a tiny opening must take some time. Some time must therefore elapse before the arteries could begin to bleed.[2] He then puts Erasistratus in the witness-box, as it were, and submits him to a long cross-examination. If *pneuma* does escape from a cut artery, it must do so either *proprio motu*, or because it is pushed out by something. On these alternatives the school of Erasistratus is divided, some holding one, some the other. Taking the first, that of the 'automatic' escape of arterial *pneuma*, this must be due, they will tell you, to the fact that *pneuma* is less dense and composed of less heavy particles than the surrounding atmosphere, something like the aether, the matter of the celestial bodies, or because it is in some other way hotter.[3] But neither of these conditions can be true, for according to Erasistratus the *pneuma* is constituted by the air drawn into the body through the windpipe and the bronchial tubes in the lungs, the 'first arteries', and from the lungs into the heart and so into the other arteries. On its way through the body it must encounter moist substances, and probably therefore become thicker and more like a soft solid (ἀπαλωδέστερον). It does, indeed, become hotter, but this implies that it becomes

[1] *Introductio sive medicus*, 13, K. xiv. 728: κατὰ δὲ Ἐρασίστρατον καὶ Ἀσκληπιάδην, ὡς ἐπίπαν μίαν αἰτίαν ἐπὶ πάσης νόσου, καθ᾽ ὃν μὲν ἡ παρέμπτωσις εἰς τὰς ἀρτηρίας τοῦ αἵματος.

[2] Galen, *An in art. nat. sang. cont.* 2, K. iv. 707: γελοῖον δ᾽ ἴσως ποιοῦμεν ἐξ ἑτέρων αὐτὸ συλλογιζόμενοι, παρὸν αὐτοὺς ὑπομνῆσαι τῶν ἀρτηριῶν, ἐξ ὧν ὅταν ἀθρόον ἐξακοντίζηται τὸ αἷμα σαφῶς ἐκφυσώμενον φαίνεται· ὡς γὰρ θερμότερον οὕτω καὶ ἀτμωδέστερον τὸ κατὰ τὰς ἀρτηρίας αἷμα· οὐ μὴν αὐτός γε καθ᾽ ἑαυτὸν ἀτμός, ἢ ἀήρ, ἢ αἰθήρ, ἢ ὅλως πνεῦμα περιεχόμενον ἐν αὐτῷ φαίνεται. καὶ γὰρ εἰ τῇ λεπτοτάτῃ βελόνῃ διατρήσαιο ἀρτηρίαν, εὐθὺς ἐξακοντίζεται τὸ αἷμα.

[3] Ibid., 706: ἢ γὰρ τοῦτο πάντη δήπου λεπτομερέστερον, οἷον τὸ αἰθεριῶδες, ἢ ἄλλως πως θερμότερον εἶναι φήσουσιν αὐτὸ τοῦ περιέχοντος ἡμᾶς ἀέρος.

'steamier', and therefore its escape from the artery would become perceptible and would not be instantaneous. Praxagoras said that it was denser, or composed of bigger particles than the atmospheric air, but Erasistratus himself made no pronouncement on any difference in density. Judging, however, from his other statements, one would guess that in his opinion, the *pneuma* was not at all a 'rare' substance. For he says that the cavities of the muscles and the walls of the arteries are dilated when they are filled with it, which would be impossible if it were really a rarer substance than the atmospheric air, since it could in that case no longer be contained by these vessels. Moreover, why does it not blow out, as it does in wounds of the chest, the thorax, the peritoneum, and the pharynx?[1]

Furthermore, if we assume that a vacuum is created and that the *pneuma* is sufficiently rare to escape instantly, *pneuma* would not only be evacuated from the severed artery, but from the whole arterial system as well, if we assume, as Erasistratus did, that *pneuma* is a continuous substance, which like a good Stratonist he should have done.[2] Moreover, the complete evacuation of all the *pneuma* in the body would have to take considerable time, at any rate in the case of all but the biggest wounds.[3] Indeed, according to the logic of Erasistratus' theory of the *horror vacui*, not only all the blood but all the *pneuma* should also be evacuated even from the smallest wound. The smallest arterial perforation would therefore be sufficient to empty the body completely of the vital spirit and therefore to cause death. The theory therefore entails a double absurdity, when compared with the facts, for a wound made by a small prick does not, in fact, empty the whole body of blood, nor does the animal so wounded die.[4]

[1] Ibid., 706–7: λεπτομερέστερον μὲν οὖν οὐκ ἂν εἴη τὸ κατὰ τὰς ἀρτηρίας πνεῦμα τοῦ περιέχοντος ἡμᾶς ἀέρος, ὡς ἡ γένεσις αὐτοῦ διδάσκει. γίγνεται γὰρ κατὰ τὸν Ἐρασίστρατον ἐκ τοῦ περιέχοντος ἡμᾶς ἀέρος εἴσω τοῦ σώματος, εἰς μὲν τὰς κατὰ πνεύμονα πρώτας ἀρτηρίας ἐλθόντος, ἔπειτα δὲ εἰς τὴν καρδίαν καὶ τὰς ἄλλας. εἰς ὅσον οὖν ὑγροτέροις ὁμιλεῖ σώμασιν, εἰς τοσοῦτο εἰκὸς αὐτὸ παχυμερέστερόν τε καὶ ἀπαλωδέστερον γίνεσθαι· θερμότερον δὲ γίνεται, ἀλλ᾽ ὡς ἀτμὸς ἄνω φερόμενον οὔτε ἀφανῆ τὴν κένωσιν οὔτε οὕτως ὠκεῖαν ἕξει. Πραξαγόρας μὲν οὖν καὶ παχυμερέστερον αὐτὸ καὶ ἱκανῶς ἀτμῶδες εἶναί φησιν, Ἐρασίστρατος δέ, ὅπῃ μὲν ἔχει πάχους, οὐ διώρισεν, ἐξ ὧν δ᾽ ὑπὲρ αὐτοῦ λέγει τεκμήραιτ᾽ ἄν τις, οὐδαμῶς αὐτὸ προσήκειν εἶναι λεπτόν. τάς τε γὰρ ἀρτηρίας ὑπ᾽ αὐτοῦ πληρουμένας διαστέλλεσθαί φησι καὶ τὰς τῶν μυῶν κοιλίας ὡσαύτως, οὐδετέρου δὴ τούτων γίγνεσθαί ποτ᾽ ἂν δυνηθέντος, εἰ λεπτομερὲς ἀκριβῶς ὑπῆρχεν· οὐ γὰρ δὴ ἴσχεσθαί γε τὸ τοιοῦτο μᾶλλον ἐν τοῖς σώμασιν, ἀλλ᾽ ἐκπέμπεσθαι πρέπει. τί ποτ᾽ οὖν ἐκφυσώμενον οὐ φαίνεται παραπλησίως τῷ κατὰ τὰς ἐκ τοῦ θώρακος τε καὶ τοῦ περιτοναίου καὶ τῆς φάρυγγος τρώσεις;

[2] Ibid., 708: εἰ γὰρ συνεχὲς αὐτῷ πάντως ἐστὶ τὸ κατὰ τὰς ἀρτηρίας πνεῦμα, καὶ οὕτως εὐκίνητόν τε καὶ λεπτὸν ὡς ἐν ἀκαρεῖ χρόνῳ κενοῦσθαι ῥᾳδίως, οὐ τὸ μὲν ταῖς διαιρουμέναις ἀρτηρίαις, κενωθήσεται μόνον, τὸ δ᾽ ἐν ἄλλαις ἁπάσαις μενεῖ.

[3] Ibid.: ἐχρῆν δ᾽, οἶμαι, καὶ εἰ μὴ διὰ τοῦ μεγάλου τραύματος, ἀλλὰ γοῦν τοῦ μετρίου, μὴ ταχέως μηδ᾽ ἀναισθήτως, ἀλλ᾽ ἐν χρόνῳ πλείονι κενοῦσθαι τὸ πνεῦμα.

[4] Ibid., 708–9. Galen argues that on Erasistratus' principle of the *horror vacui* all the blood would have to be evacuated from the body, once the blood has been drawn in through the anastomoses, to be followed by all the *pneuma*: q.e.a. ἐν αὐτῇ οὖν πρώτως κίνδυνος τοῦ κενὸν

Nor will the alternative hypothesis that *pneuma* escapes through the arterial wound because it is pushed by the heart make Erasistratus' theory any more credible.[1] Moreover, other objections to it can be raised. Erasistratus taught that under normal conditions the 'mouths' of the last and smallest veins were closed; what about the arterioles? Are they firmly closed or are they (as in fact they are) only partially closed? In neither case does it necessarily follow that a vacuum is created when an artery is cut. For when the *pneuma* is evacuated, it is possible that the vessel would collapse and close itself—a 'third alternative' proposed by Asclepiades.[2] And even if we assume that the 'mouth' does remain open, a vacuum need not be produced. Take the analogy of a reed or pipe. When we blow down it, even supposing it to have a certain degree of natural elasticity, we only cause it to expand up to the limits of this elasticity. When we stop blowing, it contracts again to its natural dimensions. It is only the extra air which we have blown in which escapes. So, too, in the case of the arteries, on Erasistratus' theory. When they are contracted, they still contain a certain amount of *pneuma*, and when more *pneuma* is sent into them from the heart, this over-fills the arteries and makes them expand thus effecting their diastole at the moment of the issue of *pneuma* from the heart. When the *pneuma* passes on, the arteries contract to their original volume in their systole. And in this process there is really no necessity for the infiltration of blood.[3]

γενέσθαι τόπον, εἰ μὴ τῆς οὐσίας πληρώσειε τὴν χώραν τοῦ μεταλαμβανομένου πνεύματος· καὶ διὰ τοῦτο ἐξ ἀνάγκης ἔπεται τὸ διὰ τῶν συναναστομώσεων, ὡς αὐτός φησιν, αἷμα τῇ πρὸς τὸ κενούμενον ἀκολουθίᾳ, καὶ τοῦτο ὥσπερ προδεδεμένον τῷ κατὰ τὰ πέρατα τῶν ὑστάτων ἀρτηριῶν πνεύματι, πρῶτον μὲν ἅπαντος τοῦ ἄλλου αἵματος, ὕστατον δὲ παντὸς τοῦ κατὰ τὰς ἀρτηρίας πνεύματος κενωθήσεται. δύο οὖν ἄτοπα μέγιστα συμβήσεται κατὰ τὸν λόγον, πρότερον μὲν τὸ διὰ τοῦ κατὰ τὴν βελόνην τρήματος ἅπαν ἐκκενοῦσθαι τὸ κατὰ τὰς ἀρτηρίας πνεῦμα ταχέως οὕτως ὥστε λαθεῖν, δεύτερον δὲ τὸ ζῆν ἔτι τὸ ζῷον, ἅπαντος τοῦ ζωτικοῦ πνεύματος ἐκκενουμένου.

[1] Galen, *An in art. nat. sang. cont.* 3, 709: ὡς οὐδ᾽ εἰ παρὰ τῆς καρδίας θλιβούσης ἐπιπέμποιτο τὸ πνεῦμα ταῖς ἀρτηρίαις πιθανὸν οὐδ᾽ οὕτως ἐστὶ τὸ τῆς παρεμπτώσεως δόγμα.

[2] Ibid., 709–10: πότερον τὸ εἰς ἔσχατον πεφυκέναι συστέλλεσθαι τὰς ἀρτηρίας, ὥσπερ καὶ τὰς φλέβας, ἤ, ὅπερ ἀληθές ἐστι, μέχρι τινός; ἔστω τὸ πρότερον, τὸ εἰς ἔσχατον, ἵνα μηδὲν παραλείπηται. ἀλλ᾽ εἰ τοῦτο, μοχθηρὸς ὁ λόγος ἔσται καὶ ἀπέραντος μᾶλλον παρὰ τὸ τῆς διαιρέσεως ἐλλειπές. οὐκέτι γὰρ ἔξεστι λέγειν, κενουμένου τοῦ πνεύματος ἤτοι κενὸς ἔσται τόπος ἀθρόος, ἢ τὸ συνεχὲς ἀκολουθήσει. ἀλλ᾽ ὑπομνήσωμεν αὐτόν, ὡς καὶ τρίτον ἐστὶ παραλειπόμενον ἐν τῇ διαιρέσει, τὸ κενούμενον ἀγγεῖον συσταλήσεται ... οὕτως μὲν οὖν μοχθηρὸς ὁ τῆς παρεμπτώσεως ἐπιδειχθήσεται λόγος, εἰ τέλεως ἡ ἀρτηρία συστέλλοιτο. This 'third alternative' was in fact put forward by Asclepiades. See Galen, *De nat. fac.* ii. 1, K. ii. 75: ἀλλ᾽ ὅ γ᾽ Ἀσκληπιάδης οὐ δυοῖν θάτερόν φησιν, ἀλλὰ τριῶν ἕν τι χρῆναι λέγειν ἐπὶ τοῖς κενουμένοις ἀγγείοις ἔπεσθαι, ἢ κενὸν ἀθρόως τόπον ἢ τὸ συνεχὲς ἀκολουθήσειν, ἢ συστέλλεσθαι τὸ ἀγγεῖον.

[3] Galen, op. cit., K. iv. 710: εἰ δὲ μέχρι ποσοῦ τινος, ἐκεῖνος αὖθις ὁ λόγος ἀποδειχθήσεται μοχθηρὸς ἐὰν τὸ κατὰ τοὺς ἁπαλοὺς καλάμους ἀναμνησθῶμεν φαινόμενον, οὓς ἐμφυσῶντες ἐπὶ τοσοῦτον αὐτοὺς διαστέλλομεν, ἐφ᾽ ὅσον πεφύκασιν· εἶτ᾽ αὖθις ἐκκενοῦται κατὰ τὸ πέρας ὁ ἀὴρ τοσούτος, εἰς ὅσον ὁ κάλαμος πέφυκε συστέλλεσθαι· πλέον γὰρ ἂν ὁ κάλαμος οὔτ᾽ ἐκτείνοιτο φυσώντων, οὔτ᾽ αὖ συστέλλοιτο. ὅσον γὰρ ἐνεφυσήσαμεν, τοσοῦτ᾽ ἀναγκαῖον κενοῦσθαι μόνον. ὅσον δ᾽ ἔφθανεν ἀέρος περιέχεσθαι, καὶ πρὶν ἡμᾶς ἐμφυσῆσαι, τοῦθ᾽ ὑπομένειν ἀναγκαῖον. οὕτως οὖν ἔχει καὶ κατὰ τὰς ἀρτηρίας. περιέχεται μὲν γάρ τι πνεῦμα, καὶ συνεσταλμένων αὐτῶν, ἐπιπέμπεται δ᾽ ἕτερον ὑπὸ τῆς καρδίας πληρούσης, καὶ τοῦτο ἐπιπληροῖ μὲν αὐτῶν τὰς κοιλίας, παρ᾽

Another typical argument against the theory of infiltration is given by Galen in his great physiological treatise *On the use of parts*. It is cast in a characteristically teleological form, though Erasistratus set little store by teleology, even if he formally admitted it. Erasistratus and his followers, Galen argues, admit the existence of synastomoses between the capillary venules and arterioles, but in the light of their doctrine of *pneuma*-filled arteries, what purpose could these anastomoses serve? Did nature produce them just accidentally, or did she in fact make a mistake in creating them? For according to Erasistratus' theory of infiltration in accordance with the principle of the *horror vacui*, these anastomoses are so far from producing any benefit to the organism that their only effect can be to produce a great deal of damage in the form of disease.[1]

With Galen's further arguments on the inconsistencies and absurdities of Erasistratus' theories on *pneuma*-filled arteries and infiltration of blood into the capillaries, we need not concern ourselves any further, except to point out that Galen was not content merely to expose bad argument. As we shall see below,[2] he also produced experimental evidence that arteries normally contained blood. Before leaving this rather barren territory, we must however note that Galen's controversial attitude to Erasistratus' theories had been anticipated by the Anonymous Londoner, who spends quite a lot of space in refuting the arguments, not so much of Erasistratus himself as of his followers, in defence of the theory of arterial bleeding *per horrorem vacui*.

Much of this discussion seems today mere quibbling, but one argument cited was later also refuted by Galen, who also maintained, as we have just noted, that severing an artery would not cause a vacuum through the escape of *pneuma* because the severed artery will still retain part of its air.[3] The Anonymous Londoner will not accept Asclepiades' 'third

ὃν χρόνον ἐξέρχεται, καὶ τὴν διαστολὴν ἐργάζεται, κενουμένων δὲ συστέλλεσθαι πάλιν, εἰς ὅσον ἐξ ἀρχῆς ἐπιτρέψει· οὐκ οὖν οὐκέτι οὐδὲ κατὰ τοῦτον τὸν λόγον οὐδεμία τῆς τοῦ αἵματος παρεμπτώσεως ἀνάγκη.

[1] Galen, *De usu partium*, vi. 17, K. iii. 492 f.: οὐδὲν ἧττον ὁμολογοῦσιν αὐτὰς καὶ οὗτοι συναναστομῶσθαι ταῖς φλεψίν. εἶτα, καίτοι τεχνικῶς ὑπὸ τῆς φύσεως οἰόμενοι κατεσκευάσθαι πάντα, καὶ μάτην μηδέν, οὐκ αἰσθάνονται τὰς ἀναστομώσεις ταύτας ὁμολογοῦντες εἰκῆ γεγονέναι. καίτοι γε μικρὸν ἂν ἦν μόνον τοῦτο, μάτην αὐτὰς κατεσκευάσθαι, καὶ μηδὲν ἐκπορίζειν τῷ ζῴῳ χρηστόν. ἀλλὰ τὸ τούτου δεινότερον, ὅπερ οὐκ ἂν ἔτι μικρὸν οἰηθείη τις εἶναι τῆς φύσεως ἁμάρτημα, τὸ πρὸς τῷ μηδὲν ὠφελεῖν ἔτι καὶ βλάπτειν τὰ μέγιστα, καὶ τοῦτ' ἐξ ἀκολουθίας προσίενται· διδάσκει γοῦν αὐτὸς Ἐρασίστρατος ἐπιμελῶς ἡμᾶς, ὡς οὐκ ἐνδέχεται γενέσθαι φλεγμονὴν ἄνευ τοῦ παρεμπεσεῖν ποτε ἐκ τῶν φλεβῶν εἰς τὰς ἀρτηρίας αἷμα.

[2] See below, p. 268, n. 1.

[3] *Anonymus Londinensis*, xxvi sq., J. 104: τὰ ἡμέτερα σώματα τοῖς ἀσυμπτώτοις ἔοικε σώμασιν ὡς σίφωσί τε καὶ καλάμοις· ὡς γὰρ οὗτοι καταχθέντες ἢ τρυπηθέντες οὐκ ἀποκρίνουσι τὸ ἐν αὐτοῖς περιεχόμενον πνεῦμα οὐδὲ κενοὶ γίνονται τούτου, ἀλλ' ἐμμένον ἔχουσιν ἐν αὐτοῖς, οὕτως καὶ ἐπὶ τῶν ἀρτηριῶν διαιρεθεισῶν οὐ πάντως κενωθήσεται τὰ [ἐντὸς] τοῦ πνεύματος, ἀλλ' ἐμμενεῖ ἐν ταῖς ἀρτηρίαις καὶ μετὰ τὴν διαίρεσιν, ὥσπερ κἀπὶ τῶν ἐκτός.

alternative' of collapsing arteries when emptied of *pneuma* on the ground that it is physiologically incorrect, though it looks as if some of the Herophilians adopted it, arguing that the vascular system is like a bladder filled with liquid and inflated. When you prick it, it lets out both. So too the arteries when severed let blood escape through but not out of themselves. Presumably this explanation was to account not only for the bleeding but also for its eventual cessation, but the text is far from clear, though the author points out that here again the formation of the Stratonian 'continuous vacuum' is quite inconsistent. Even if we admit that simile, when a bladder collapses on the evacuation of its contents no continuous vacuum is formed, and, according to their argument, when an artery is severed it should just have collapsed after the escape of the air without any vacuum-produced secretion or irruption of blood.[1]

But to return to Erasistratus. Of his description of the vascular system, beyond the facts we have mentioned, very little has survived. But it would be reasonable to suppose that *grosso modo* it was fairly accurate. He accepted Herophilus' distinction between arteries and veins and their different anatomical structure. Indeed, as we shall see, he rather over-accentuated this difference, making it a primary elemental factor. Since his knowledge was derived from human dissection, it was probably a great improvement on that of his pre-Alexandrian forerunners, but of the details we know nothing. Wellmann[2] made a list of the arteries and veins mentioned in citations from his works, but this really tells us very little. The blood vessels mentioned include the following: the aorta, and the ascending aorta with its thoracic branches right and left, the hepatic arteries, the arteries of the stomach, and the artery-like vein the pulmonary artery, the vena cava and the hepatic vein which opens into it, the azygos vein, the portal vein, and the vein-like artery the pulmonary vein. Galen would certainly have called him to task if he had been seriously at fault in his description of the main blood vessels, and he does so in the case that we have just examined, concerning the source of the blood which enters the windpipe from the pleural cavity as

---

[1] *Anonymus Londinensis*, xxvii, J. 106 : φασὶν οἱ Ἐρασιστράτειοι, οὐκ ἔοικε τὰ ἡμέτερα σώματα τοῖς ἀσυμπτώτοις σώμασιν, ἃ κυρίως κατωνόμασται, ἀλλὰ ἀσκῷ ἐνπεπληρωμένῳ ὑγροῦ καὶ ἐμπεπνευμα-τωμένῳ [ωσο.νον] ὃς τρωθεὶς ἀποκρείνει δι' αὐτοῦ τό τε πνεῦμα καὶ ὑγρόν, ἅμα δὲ καὶ ἐξ ἑαυτοῦ· οὕτως καὶ αἱ ἀρτηρίαι διαιρεθεῖσαι αἷμα, οὐκ ἐξ αὐτῶν δέ· πρὸς δὲ καὶ τοῦτ' εἴποιμεν, διότι οὐ τοῖς οὖσι συμπτώτοις ἔοικεν τὰ ἡμέτερα σώματα, ὥς φασιν πταίοντες, ἀλλὰ τοῖς ὑπάρχουσιν ἀσυμπτώτοις, ὡς ταῦτα δῆλα ἐπὶ τῶν τελευτῶν· κατὰ γὰρ τὰ ὑμένια εὑρίσκονται αἱ ἀρτηρίαι ἀσύμπτωτοι. ἀλλ' οὗτοι σύμπτωτοι, εἰ τοιγάρτοι ταῦτα τοῦτον ἔχει τὸν τρόπον, μοχθηροὶ φαίνονται καὶ κατὰ ταῦτα οἱ Ἐρασιστράτειοι. εἶτα φέρε δὲ καὶ οἰκειοῦντες μὴ τοῖς ἀσυμπτώτοις, ἀλλὰ τοῖς εὐσυμπτώτοις ὡς ἀσκοῖς, ἵνα καὶ αὐτοῖς συναγορεύωμεν, λέγωμεν, ὡς ἐπὶ τοῦ ἀσκ[οῦ τοῦ ἐνόντος κενωθέντος ἐπισύμπτωσις γίνεται, καὶ οὐχὶ κενὸς ἀθρόυς τόπος]. ἀλλὰ ἐχρῆν καὶ ἐπὶ τῆς διαιρέσεως τῶν ἀρτηριῶν μετὰ τὴν κένωσιν τοῦ πνεύματος ἐπισυμπείπτειν ταύτας. ἐπισυμπειπτουσῶν δὲ αὐτῶν οὐκ ἂν ἐγίνετο κενὸς ἀθρούς οὐδὲ παρέμπτωσις αἵματος οὐδὲ ἀπόκρισις τούτου οὐδέ γε κένωσις.

[2] See his article on 'Erasistratus' in *RE*.

a consequence of a wound in the thorax. Here, in the course of the argument, he throws an incidental light on Erasistratus' real understanding of the propulsive power of the heart's muscle. According to Erasistratus' own theory blood could not possibly reach the lung via the aorta, since the blast of the *pneuma* from each heartbeat, stronger than the most violent winds, would be sufficient to scatter it through the arterial system all over the body.[1]

We shall perhaps be able to understand better how Erasistratus just missed Harvey's discovery if we examine his doctrines concerning *pneuma* a little more closely. *Pneuma* or air is constantly being absorbed from the outer atmosphere and drawn into the heart via the throat, the windpipe, and the bronchi or 'first arteries', which are connected with the vein-like arteries, the pulmonary veins in the lungs. In this connection it is interesting to note that Erasistratus' doctrine of the direct absorption of *pneuma* by the heart via the lungs led him to maintain a quite incorrect corollary, again inspired by what we might call iatrophysical reasoning. He took the view that when the breath is held, the heart is unable to draw *pneuma* from the lungs because the respiratory organs then maintain their internal volume unchanged. If now the heart were to absorb any *pneuma* while the volume of the thorax, an enclosed space, is unchanged, a vacuum would have to be created, which on Strato's principles would be impossible. Hence, in spite of every effort to do so, the heart is unable to get any *pneuma* and the animal chokes.[2] This corollary, Galen points out, is not in accordance with the facts. When we hold our breath, the heart still goes on expanding and contracting. Erasistratus' main thesis that arteries contain only *pneuma*, drawn directly into the heart via the lungs, is once more criticized by Galen on teleological grounds in an argument which has perhaps been lent some degree of undreamed relevance by modern evolutionary theory. If the arteries contain only *pneuma*, the double system of pipes

---

[1] Galen, *De locis affectis*, v. 3, K. viii. 315–16: ἡ δὲ μετάληψις τοῦ αἵματος ἦν ἐκ τῆς μεγάλης ἀρτηρίας εἰς τὸν πνεύμονα γίγνεσθαί φασιν, οὐκ ὀρθῶς φαίνεται λεγομένη. πρῶτον μὲν γὰρ εἰς μεγάλην ἀρτηρίαν ἐκ τῶν μεσοπλευρίων ἀδύνατον ἐνεχθῆναι τὸ αἷμα, παλινδρομήσει γὰρ αὐτίκα συνελαυνόμενον ὑπὸ τοῦ πνεύματος, ὃ παρὰ τῆς καρδίας διὰ τῆς μεγάλης ἀρτηρίας εἰς ταύτας ἐπιπέμπεται . . . βούλεται γὰρ εἰς τὴν ἀρτηρίαν ταύτην ἐνθλιβόμενον ὑπὸ τῆς καρδίας τὸ πνεῦμα, διασῶζον τῆς βολῆς τὴν ῥύμην, εἰς ὅλον φέρεσθαι τὸ σῶμα διὰ τῶν ἀπ' ἐκείνης πεφυκυιῶν ἀρτηριῶν· ὡς κατὰ μίαν ἔνθλιψιν τῆς ἀρτηρίας ἐξικνεῖσθαι μέχρι τῶν κατὰ τοὺς πόδας ἄκρων τὴν φορὰν τοῦ πνεύματος, ὑπὲρ τοὺς σφοδροτάτους ἀνέμους τὸ τῆς φορᾶς τάχος εἶναι βουλόμενος.

[2] Galen, *De usu resp.* 2, K. iv. 473: ἀλλὰ πρὸς τοῦθ' ὁ Ἐρασίστρατός φησιν ὅτι μηδ' ἕλκειν δύναται τὸν ἐκ τοῦ πνεύμονος ἀέρα κατὰ τὴν τῆς ἀναπνοῆς ἐπίσχεσιν ἡ καρδία· φυλάττεσθαι γὰρ τῶν ἀναπνευστικῶν ὀργάνων τὸν ἴσον ὄγκον τῆς διαστάσεως ἐν ταῖς τοιαύταις καταστάσεσιν. εἴπερ οὖν εἵλκυσέ τι μέρος ἀέρος ἡ καρδία, κενὸς ἂν ὁ τοῦ καταληφθέντος ἐγένετο τόπος. τοῦτο δὲ ἐγένετο ἀδύνατον· ἵν' οὖν μὴ γένηται ἀδύνατον, οὐδὲ μεταλήψεσθαί φησι τὴν ἀρχήν· δεῖ γὰρ ἵνα τι μεταληφθῇ, μὴ μόνον εἶναι τὸ ἕλξον, ἀλλὰ καὶ τὸ μεταδιδοῦν. οὐ μεταδίδωσιν δὲ ὁ θώραξ, τὸν ἴσον ὄγκον τῆς διαστάσεως φυλάττων, οὐδ' οὖν οὐδ' ἡ καρδία δύναται μεταλαμβάνειν, ἀλλ' ἐπιχειρεῖ μὲν ὡς ἔμπροσθεν ἀνύει δ' οὐδέν, κἀντεῦθεν τὸ πνίγεσθαι.

in the lung conveying only air seems a useless duplication. Nature does not indulge in such superfluous luxuries.[1]

The fate of the *pneuma* continually being absorbed also requires investigation. The heart distributes continually and in great force the *pneuma* to the arterial system, which ends in capillary arterioles which synanastomose with the blood-containing venules. Why then, if plethora of blood may force that liquid into the arterial capillaries, does not the pressure of *pneuma*, constantly being pumped by the left ventricle from the air drawn in by respiration, force back the blood into a very small portion of the venous system? What happens to the *pneuma* which is constantly being supplied? Erasistratus, it would appear, adopted like many of his predecessors the theory of double respiration invented by Empedocles. Most of the *pneuma* taken in by respiration is returned in expiration through the lung, but some is also returned to the outer air through the skin via the 'pores', though exactly how this process worked we are not informed. The Anonymous Londoner who is our chief authority does not tell us whether Erasistratus thought that some of the arterioles were directly connected with the pores, or whether the *pneuma* conveyed to the arterioles on the surface of the skin merely leaked through. The latter would appear to be more in accordance with his description.

Now *pneuma* is drawn in from the outside by the mouth and the nostrils and is carried through the rough artery, the windpipe, into the lung and the heart and also the thorax . . . and from these places it is carried into the separate arteries, and it is also carried into the cavities. And similarly also into all the pores in the whole of the body. Then it runs through the natural pores in the flesh to the outside environment. The largest part of it is exhaled through the mouth and the nostrils [*desunt aliqua*]. Now more than what is breathed in, is breathed out through these parts, I mean, through the mouth and the nostrils, which is perhaps something of a paradox. For how is it possible for more to be breathed out than is breathed in since some of what is breathed in is expended in the body? But this is not really a paradox, because in the same way that some of that which is breathed in is allotted to the body, something is also added from the body to the *pneuma*, more in fact than is absorbed by it. And this makes the volume of the *pneuma* sent out the greater.[2]

---

[1] Galen, *De usu partium*, vii. 8, K. iii. 537: εἰ γὰρ δὴ κἀκεῖναι (λεῖαι ἀρτηρίαι) τελέως εἰσὶν αἵματος ἄμοιροι, καθάπερ αἱ τραχεῖαι ἀρτηρίαι — τοῦτο γὰρ Ἐρασίστρατος ὑπολαμβάνει — τί οὐκ εὐθὺς εἰς τὴν καρδίαν αἱ τραχεῖαι περαίνουσι; διὰ τί δὲ φλεβῶν ἀποβλαστήματα μικρὰ ταῖς μὲν τραχείαις ἐμφύεται, ταῖς λείαις δ' οὐκ ἐμφύεται; μάτην γὰρ οὕτως ἡ μηδὲν εἰκῇ δημιουργοῦσα φύσις.

[2] *Anonymus Londinensis*, xxiii, J. 89: ἕλκεται τοιγάρτοι τὸ πνεῦμα ἔξωθεν ὑπὸ τοῦ στόματος καὶ τῶν μυκτήρων, καὶ διὰ τῆς τραχείας ἀρτηρίας φέρεται εἰς πνεύμονα καὶ καρδίαν, ἔτι δὲ θώρακα· διηθεῖται δὲ καὶ εἰς κοιλίαν ὀλίγον διὰ τοῦ στομάχου καθ' ἡμᾶς, οὐ μὴν δὲ κατὰ τὸν Ἐρασίστρατον. ἀπὸ τούτων δὴ τῶν τόπων φέρεται εἰς τὰς κατὰ μέρος ἀρτηρίας. φέρεται δὲ καὶ εἰς τὰ κοιλώματα· ὡς ὁμοίως δὲ καὶ εἰς τὰ καθ' ὅλον τὸ σῶμα ἀραιώματα, εἶτα διεκθεῖ διὰ τῶν ἐν τῇ σαρκὶ φυσικῶν ἀραιωμάτων εἰς τὸ ἐκτός. τὸ δὲ πλεῖον ἐκπνεῖται διά τε τοῦ στόματος καὶ τῶν μυκτήρων. καὶ δὴ τοῦ

Since we are not told what portions of the body contribute to make these additions to the exhaled *pneuma*, nor is any information given about its nature, it would certainly be quite fanciful to regard Erasistratus as the predecessor of Lavoisier.

So far as the left ventricle and *pneuma* are concerned, Erasistratus is able to give a reasonably plausible account of the heart as a pump. It is when we come to the right ventricle that his troubles, as we have already noted, begin. Here serious difficulties at once arise. The venous system contains all the blood, and its starting-point is the heart, not the liver. The function of the blood is to nourish all the tissues. How, then, is it distributed to them? Not through the pulmonary artery, since that carries blood only to the lungs. Blood, we saw, receives its first stage of sanguinification in the liver which works on the products of digestion, and passes by the hepatic vein into the vena cava and the right ventricle of the heart; but not all of it, so it seems, enters into the heart, only enough to feed the lungs, a doctrine which appears in a modified form also in Galen.[1] The distribution of blood-nutriment to the various tissues has therefore to be explained by factors quite unconnected with the contraction of the right ventricle. The first of these is, as we might expect, the *horror vacui*, the application of which is bound up with Erasistratus' theory of nutrition and growth. Unlike Hippocrates and Aristotle, Erasistratus refuses to interpret nutrition as a 'vital' process. Growth and nutrition are interpreted in a purely mechanical fashion. Digestion is merely the division or attrition of foodstuffs into their quasi-atomic components by the stomach muscles activated by *pneuma* absorbed from the environment, not a process of 'cooking' brought about by the innate heat.[2] The products of digestion finished off in the heart are distributed by the veins. Nutrition is in essence the replacement of worn parts by particles of blood, and here the *horror vacui* plays an important

εἰσπνεομένου πλεῖον ἐκπνεῖται διὰ τούτων τῶν τόπων, λέγω δὲ διὰ στόματος καὶ μυκτήρων, ὅπερ ἐστὶν ἴσως παράδοξον. πῶς γὰρ οἷόν τ' ἐστὶν πλεῖον ἐκπνεῖσθαι, καίτοι γε ἀπὸ τοῦ εἰσπνεομένου ἀναλουμένου τινὸς εἰς τὰ σώματα; ἀλλ' οὐκ ἔστιν παράδοξον· ὃν γὰρ τρόπον κατατάσσεταί τι εἰς τὰ σώματα ἀπὸ τοῦ εἰσπνεομένου, τὸν αὐτὸν τρόπον καὶ τῷ πνεύματί τινα προστίθεται ἀπὸ τῶν σωμάτων καὶ πλείονά γε, ἅτινα καὶ πλεῖον ἀποτελεῖ τὸ ἐκπεμπόμενον πνεῦμα.

[1] Galen, *De nat. fac.* ii. 1, K. ii. 77: μόνη γὰρ αὕτη (καρδία) τῶν μεθ' ἧπαρ εἰς τὴν δεξιὰν αὑτῆς κοιλίαν ἕλκει τὴν τροφήν, εἶτα διὰ τῆς φλεβὸς τῆς ἀρτηριώδους ἐκπέμπει τῷ πνεύμονι. τῶν δὲ ἄλλων οὐδὲν οὐδ' αὐτὸς ὁ Ἐρασίστρατος ἐκ καρδίας βούλεται τρέφεσθαι διὰ τὴν ὑμένων ἐπίφυσιν. For Galen's modified form of this doctrine, which adds the blood passing through the pores of the septum into the left ventricle, see below, pp. 323 ff.

[2] Galen (?), *Definitiones*, xcix, K. xix. 372 f.: τὰς πέψεις τῆς τροφῆς Ἱπποκράτης μὲν ὑπὸ τοῦ ἐμφύτου θερμοῦ φησι γίνεσθαι, Ἐρασίστρατος δὲ τρίψει καὶ λειώσει καὶ περιστολῇ τῆς γαστρὸς καὶ ἐπικτήτου πνεύματος ἰδιότητι. Cf. Galen, *Comment. in Hipp. de aliment.* ii. 7, K. xv. 247–8: ὁ δ' Ἐρασίστρατος γελοῖός τε καὶ ἀμαθής ἐστι. σαφῶς γὰρ Ἀριστοτέλους λέγοντος τὴν πέψιν ἑψήσει παραπλήσιον ὑπάρχειν, ὅπως τοῦτο λέγεται, οὐχ οἷός τε ἦν εἰδέναι. φησὶ γὰρ οὐκ εἰκὸς εἶναι τὴν πέψιν παραπλήσιον τυγχάνειν τῇ ἑψήσει τῇ ἐλαφρὰν ἐχούσῃ θερμασίαν, ὥσπερ ἀεὶ πῦρ καὶ φλόγα ὑποθεῖναι τῇ γαστρὶ ὥσπερ καὶ λέβητι, ἢ ἄλλως αὐτῆς ἀλλοιῶσαι τὰ σιτία μὴ δυναμένης.

part.[1] It appears that the vacuum created by the wearing draws the blood into the otherwise empty space. The theory is not in this form consistent, since blood is perfected in the heart and therefore all of it must at some stage pass from the heart's right ventricle into the venous system by a channel different from that of the pulmonary artery—if we can trust Galen's account. Whatever the explanation of this inconsistency, it is quite clear that Erasistratus endeavoured to explain this, as well as other physiological phenomena, in terms of mechanics. He was in fact the first iatro-physicist, and it is not a mere coincidence that it was Borelli who tried at the end of the seventeenth century to revive, albeit in a somewhat different form, his theory of muscular contraction.[2]

Galen takes the strongest exception to his attempt to interpret growth and nourishment as purely mechanical processes, since this would involve the denial of his most dearly held principle, the conception of nature's artistic skill. Galen accuses him of imagining that animals grow like webs, ropes, sacks, or baskets, each of which has woven on to its margins additions of material similar to that of which it is composed.[3] This interpretation of Erasistratus, coming as it does from a hostile source, must be suspected of incompleteness, if not of inaccuracy, but it is to a large extent confirmed by the Anonymous Londoner, who sums up Erasistratus' theory of nutrition as follows:

Since our organs or bodies are subjected to continual wastage, unless some method of replacement existed, they would perish only too easily. Nature therefore contrived to solve this problem for animals through the inter-action of three factors, appetites, foodstuffs, and powers [of assimilation and nutrition], appetite to pick up food, and food to replace wastage, and powers or faculties to deal with the foodstuffs. Now appetite would have been quite useless if there had not been any foodstuffs, nor would foodstuffs have been of any use unless there were also faculties to deal with them. So nature provided as materials food and *pneuma*. For those two are the principal things which an animal always needs, as Erasistratus has told us.[4]

[1] Galen, *De nat. fac.* i. 16, K. ii. 63 f.: οὐ γὰρ ἤρκεσεν αὐτῷ μόνον εἰπεῖν ὅτι διὰ φλεβῶν, ἀλλὰ καὶ πῶς, ἐπεξῆλθεν ὅτι τῇ πρὸς τὸ κενούμενον ἀκολουθίᾳ.

[2] See below, pp. 232 f.

[3] Galen, *De nat. fac.* ii. 3, K. ii. 87: ἀλλ' οὐδὲ τοῦτο Ἐρασίστρατος οἶδεν, ὁ τὴν τέχνην τῆς φύσεως ὑμνῶν, ἀλλ' οὕτως αὐξάνεσθαι τὰ ζῷα νομίζει καθάπερ τινὰ κρησέραν ἢ σειρὰν ἢ σάκκον ἢ τάλαρον, ὧν ἑκάστῳ κατὰ τὸ πέρας ἐπιπλεκομένων ὁμοίων ἑτέρων τοῖς ἐξ ἀρχῆς αὐτὰ συν-τιθεῖσιν ἡ πρόσθεσις γίνεται.

[4] *Anonymus Londinensis*, xxii, J. 87: τούτων δὴ οὕτως ἐχόντων καὶ ἀποφορὰς συνεχοῦς γινομένης ἀπὸ τῶν ἡμετέρων σωμάτων, εἴπερ ἀντὶ τῶν ἀποφερομένων μὴ ἐγένετο εἰς τὰ σώματα πρόσθεσις, κἂν διεφθείρετο ῥαϊδίως τὰ σώματα. ὅθεν ἡ φύσις ἐμηχανήσατο ὀρέξεις τε τοῖς ζῴοις καὶ ὕλην καὶ δυνάμεις, ὀρέξεις μὲν εἰς τὸ τὴν ὕλην αἱρεῖσθαι, ὕλην δὲ εἰς ἀναπλήρωσιν τῶν ἀποφερομένων, δυνάμεις μέντοι γε εἰς διοίκησιν τῆς ὕλης· καὶ γὰρ οὐδὲν ὄφελος ἦν ὀρέξεως, εἰ μὴ ὕλη παρῆν. οὐδὲ μὴν ὕλης ὄφελος ἦν, εἰ μὴ δυνάμεις παρῆσαν αἱ διοικονομοῦσαι. ἀλλὰ γὰρ ὕλην ὑπεβάλετο τροφήν τε καὶ πνεῦμα· δύο γὰρ πρῶτα καὶ κυριώτατά ἐστιν, οἷς διοικεῖται τὸ ζῷον, ὥς φησιν ὁ Ἐρασί-στρατος.

The replacement of worn parts takes place through the capillary veins, the thin and simple ultimate branches of the venous system. The deposit of the nutritive matter into the empty space created by wear takes place in accordance with the *horror vacui*, the particles of blood being attracted sideways through the walls of the capillary veins.[1] Erasistratus, however, does not seem to have been entirely satisfied with this explanation, nor did he feel that the principle of the *horror vacui* could by itself explain all the movements of the blood in the venous system. Galen hints that he was forced to recognize two other propulsive forces. The stomach or belly can exert a forward pressure on the veins, and the veins themselves are capable of exerting a kind of peristaltic action which pushes their contents forward, a notion which according to Galen would make the *horror vacui* quite superfluous.[2] But even as assisted by the peristaltic process, the vacuum principle does not afford, according to Galen, at all a satisfactory explanation. The pressure of the stomach, we must assume, can only work on the mesentery and the portal systems, pushing the contents of the digestive tract into the liver. The vacuum created by the diastole of the right ventricle could only suck the blood prepared in the liver up the vena cava into the right ventricle. This would leave the peripheral vacua all over the body to move the rest of the blood. Quite apart from the dubious physics of Erasistratus' theory of the movement of the blood, there was one anatomical fact which, had it been discovered, would have made nonsense of the whole physiological scheme which he had inherited and developed, namely the existence of the valves in the veins. Though it is true this discovery has been attributed to Hippocrates by two modern Greek physicians,[3] it is not possible to take this claim at all seriously. It seems fairly certain that Erasistratus, had he discovered them, would have understood their significance, though

---

[1] Galen, *De nat. fac.* ii. 6, K. ii. 105: τοῖς ἐσχάτοις τε καὶ ἁπλοῖς λεπτοῖς τε καὶ στενοῖς οὖσιν, ἐκ τῶν παρακειμένων ἀγγείων ἡ πρόσθεσις συμβαίνει εἰς τὰ κενώματα τῶν ἀπενεχθέντων κατὰ τὰ πλάγια τῶν ἀγγείων ἑλκομένης τῆς τροφῆς καὶ καταχωριζομένης. Incidentally, Galen, while accepting this process of nutrition as more or less accurate, disagrees on the mechanism of distribution. For him, as we shall see below, the distributing force is the attractive power of the organ which effects the deposit of the nutriment, not the *horror vacui*. He also accuses Erasistratus of inconsistency in his application of the Stratonian principle, since according to Strato only vacua of a visible size could be filled by the filling up of empty space, whereas Erasistratus has assumed that the venules are too small to be visible, being perceptible only to the eye of reason, like Strato's vacua scattered about inside the smallest bodies, which were not subject to the principle of the *horror vacui*. See ibid., 99: ἐπὶ γὰρ τῶν αἰσθητῶν μόνων, οὐκ ἐπὶ τῶν λόγῳ θεωρητῶν ἔχει τὴν δύναμιν, ὡς αὐτὸς Ἐρασίστρατος ὁμολογεῖ διαρρήδην, οὐ περὶ τοιούτου κενοῦ φάσκων ἑκάστοτε ποιεῖσθαι τὸν λόγον, ὃ κατὰ βραχὺ παρέσπαρται τοῖς σώμασιν, ἀλλὰ περὶ τοῦ σαφοῦς καὶ αἰσθητοῦ καὶ ἀθρόου καὶ μεγάλου καὶ ἐναργοῦς καὶ ὅπως ἂν ἄλλως ὀνομάζειν ἐθέλοις.

[2] Ibid., ii. 1, K. ii. 76: καθ' ἕτερον δ' αὖ τρόπον, εἰ καὶ ἀληθὴς εἴη, περιττή, τῆς μὲν κοιλίας ἐνθλίβειν ταῖς φλεψὶ δυναμένης, ὡς αὐτὸς ὑπέθετο, τῶν φλεβῶν δ' αὖ περιστέλλεσθαι τῷ ἐνυπάρχοντι καὶ προωθεῖν αὐτό.

[3] Pezopoulos and Lamera, op. cit., p. 4.

as to that, some doubt must still persist, seeing that neither Fabricius nor Canano really grasped their function.[1] And if we recognize that it was Praxagoras' theory which was principally responsible for the fact that he never reached the idea of a circulation, we must also remember that his own theory of nutrition made assurance doubly sure that he would never reach that goal. For his general physiological notion of what we today call metabolism made the idea of any circulation of the blood quite superfluous and indeed unmeaning. Blood was just nature's material for replacements, the idea that it should wander about returning to its source would have been utterly meaningless. It was also the material for growth, a process which, as Galen did not fail to point out, could not be explained by the theory of the *horror vacui*. For this principle could only provide for the replacement of something which had actually disappeared and was disappearing continually; it could scarcely be invoked to account for a process of addition to the existing volume of the body, or even for the case of a man putting on weight after emaciation, when the parts replaced are much greater than the current wear and tear.[2]

But what exactly the elements were, presumably derived from Strato, out of which Erasistratus constructed the animal body is really far from clear. In the treatise entitled *Introduction or the doctor*, which has been regarded by most modern critics as spurious,[3] Galen (?) embarks on a historical discussion of the various theories which have been held concerning the elements of which the body is composed, including those of Hippocrates and Erasistratus.

Now man, according to Hippocrates, who follows the natural scientists, is composed of the four primary cosmic elements, fire, air, water, and earth— man being made up not of these as such, but of bodies compounded of them. And when he dies, he dissolves into these first elements, as Hippocrates himself said. And it is necessary for each of these first elements to return to its own nature, when a man dies, the dry to the dry, the cold to the cold, the wet to the wet, and the hot to the hot. And such also is the nature of all other animals. They all come into being and perish in the same way. For their nature is put together from the above-mentioned principles or factors, and ends, as I have explained, in the same way. For each turns back into the elements from

---

[1] K. J. Franklin, 'Valves in the veins. An historical survey', *Proc. R. Soc. of Med.* 21 (1928), 4.

[2] Galen, *De nat. fac.* ii. 6, K. ii. 103–4: πῶς οὖν ἡ πρὸς τὸ κενούμενον ἀκολουθία τρέφειν ἀδύνατός ἐστι τὸν οὕτω διακείμενον; ὅτι τοσοῦτον ἀκολουθεῖν ἀναγκάζει τῶν συνεχῶν, ὅσον ἀπορρεῖ. τοῦτο δ' ἐπὶ μὲν τῶν εὐεκτούντων ἱκανόν ἐστιν εἰς τὴν θρέψιν, ἴσα γὰρ ἐπ' αὐτῶν εἶναι χρὴ τοῖς ἀπορρέουσι τὰ προστιθέμενα· ἐπὶ δὲ τῶν ἐσχάτως ἰσχνῶν καὶ πολλῆς ἀναθρέψεως δεομένων, εἰ μὴ πολλαπλάσιον εἴη τὸ προστιθέμενον τοῦ κενουμένου, τὴν ἐξ ἀρχῆς ἕξιν ἀναλαβεῖν οὐκ ἄν ποτε δύναιτο.

[3] Cf. the proofs of its spurious character adduced by H. Schoene, *Schedae philol. f. H. Usener* (1891), 88; and E. Issel, 'Questiones Sextianae et Galenicae', *Diss. Marburg* (1917); both cited by Diller in his article, 'Zur Hippokratische Auffassung des Galen', *Hermes* 68 (1933), heft 2.

which it was composed, even so as Homer says, 'but may you all become water and earth', demonstrating their dissolution into these. But they also say that man is composed of four secondary substances, more closely resembling the human character or nature, namely the four humours, blood, phlegm, yellow bile, and black bile. Wherefore in the first development of the foetus the embryo is put together from the seed and the [menstrual] blood of the mother, which penetrates through the urachus. And in these materials were present the four humours. And man, once he has been formed, is composed of three compound bodies, namely liquids, solids, and airs. And these Hippocrates calls containers, contents, and energizers. Containers are the solid parts, bones, tendons, and ligaments, veins and arteries, out of which the whole complex of tissues, muscles, and different kinds of flesh, and the whole bulk of the body is woven, and their internal and external concretions. The contents are the liquids carried about in all the different vessels and distributed all over the body, which Hippocrates calls the above-mentioned four humours . . . The energizers are the airs or breaths. There are, according to the ancients, two kinds of breath or *pneuma*, the animal and the natural.

. . . Now Erasistratus regards as principles and elements of the whole body the threefold plait of vessels, nerves, and veins and arteries, and he omits the liquids and the *pneumas*. Because he says, that an animal is regulated or managed by two sorts of matter, namely, blood as nourishment, and *pneuma* as co-operating with and putting into action its natural [i.e. mechanical?] activities. But he does not include these among the first principles [ἀρχάς]. And there are also many other kinds of tissues [σώματα], such as the brain, the marrow, and all the bones. Now he has the audacity to call the brain and the marrow deposits of nourishment [παρέγχυμα], just as he does the fat and the tissues of the liver, the spleen, and the lung. But bones he could not call 'deposits' of nourishment, nor could he maintain that they are woven from the above-mentioned three kinds of vessels.[1]

---

[1] Galen (?), *Introductio*, 9, K. xiv. 695–8: συνέστηκε τοίνυν ὁ ἄνθρωπος ἀκολούθως τοῖς φυσικοῖς καθ' Ἱπποκράτην ἐκ τῶν κοσμικῶν τῶν πρώτων στοιχείων, ἐκ πυρὸς καὶ ἀέρος καὶ ὕδατος καὶ γῆς· οὐχ ὡς ἐκ τούτων αὐτῶν, ἀλλὰ ἐκ τῶν ἀναλόγων αὐτοῖς συνεστῶτος τοῦ ἀνθρώπου. ἐν δὲ τῷ διαλύεσθαι εἰς ταῦτα τὰ πρῶτα ἀναλύεται, καθὼς αὐτός ὁ Ἱπποκράτης ἔφη· καὶ πάλιν ἀνάγκη ἀποχωρέειν εἰς τὴν ἑωϋτοῦ φύσιν ἕκαστον, τελευτῶντος τοῦ ἀνθρώπου, τό τε ξηρὸν πρὸς τὸ ξηρὸν καὶ τὸ ψυχρὸν πρὸς τὸ ψυχρὸν καὶ τὸ ὑγρὸν πρὸς τὸ ὑγρὸν καὶ τὸ θερμὸν πρὸς τὸ θερμόν. τοιαύτη δὲ καὶ τῶν ζώων ἐστὶν ἡ φύσις καὶ τῶν ἄλλων ἁπάντων. γίνεταί τε ὁμοίως πάντα καὶ τελευτᾷ ὁμοίως. συνίσταται γὰρ αὐτῶν ἡ φύσις ἀπὸ τούτων τῶν εἰρημένων καὶ τελευτᾷ κατὰ τὰ εἰρημένα εἰς τὸ αὐτό. ὅθεν περ συνέστηκεν ἕκαστον, ἐνταῦθα καὶ ἀπεχώρησεν. καθὰ καὶ Ὅμηρος ἔφη,

Ἀλλ' ὑμεῖς μὲν πάντες ὕδωρ καὶ γαῖα γένοισθε,

δηλῶν τὴν εἰς ταῦτα διάλυσιν. ὡς δὲ ἐκ τῶν δευτέρων καὶ ἐγγὺς ὄντων τῇ ἀνθρωπίνῃ φύσει, ἐκ τῶν τεσσάρων χυμῶν, αἵματος καὶ φλέγματος καὶ χολῆς ξανθῆς τε καὶ μελαίνης συνεστάναι φασὶ τὸν ἄνθρωπον, διότι ἐν τῇ πρώτῃ διαπλάσει τοῦ ἐμβρύου, ἐκ τε τοῦ γόνου καὶ τοῦ παρὰ τῆς μητρὸς ἐπιρρέοντος αἵματος διὰ τοῦ οὐραχοῦ ἡ σύστασις γίνεται τοῦ τικτομένου. ἐν δὲ τούτοις ἦσαν οἱ τέσσαρες χυμοί. οἱ δὲ ἐκ τῶν τριῶν καὶ συνθέτων τὸν ἤδη γεννώμενον ἄνθρωπον ἐκ τῶνδέ φασι συγκεῖσθαι, ἔκ τε τῶν ὑγρῶν καὶ ξηρῶν καὶ πνευμάτων. καλεῖ δὲ αὐτὰ Ἱπποκράτης ἴσχοντα, ἰσχόμενα, καὶ ἐνορμῶντα. ἴσχοντα μὲν οὖν ἐστιν ὅσα στερεά, ὀστᾶ καὶ νεῦρα καὶ φλέβες καὶ ἀρτηρίαι, ἐξ ὧν οἵ τε μύες καὶ αἱ σάρκες καὶ πᾶς ὁ τοῦ σώματος ὄγκος πέπλεκται τῶν τε ἐντὸς καὶ τῶν ἐκτὸς τὰ συγκρίματα. ἰσχόμενα δέ ἐστι τὰ ὑγρὰ τὰ ἐν τοῖς ἀγγείοις ἐμφερόμενα καὶ κατὰ πᾶν τὸ σῶμα διεσπαρμένα, ἅπερ καλεῖ Ἱπποκράτης χυμοὺς τέσσαρας τοὺς προειρημένους. ἐνορμῶντα δέ ἐστι τὰ

In connection with the last two paragraphs quoted, it should be observed that the term *parenchyma* had by Galen's time become of very wide application, embracing all the above-mentioned tissues. It was used to designate the 'proper flesh' of all organs, the term *flesh* (σάρξ) being applied strictly only to muscles.[1]

Erasistratus' theory of the threefold plait or skein is also treated by Galen at some length in his work *On the natural faculties*, where he discusses his theory that nerves contain both arteries and veins, like a skein woven of three different kinds of thread.[2] He also tells us in the *Ars magna* that Erasistratus believed that arteries were nourished by small veins in their coats, too small to be visible, but seen by the eye of reason.[3] The account given of Erasistratus' doctrine on this point by the Anonymous Londoner agrees almost verbatim with that quoted from the *Introductio*, only there the author takes Erasistratus to task for making assumptions quite beyond the scope of the rules of medicine.[4] What these minimal or 'simple' vessels were supposed to represent is anything but clear, nor is it easy to imagine quite how their interwoven skeins form the organs and the tissues. Some light is thrown on this problem by the admittedly partisan account given by Galen, which seems to suggest that they were of a quasi-atomic character, but different in kind from the atoms postulated by Democritus and Epicurus. Galen is trying to show that Erasistratus' theory of the distribution of nutriment by the filling of a vacuum is not a satisfactory substitute for the 'Hippocratic' theory of ὁλκή or qualitative biological attraction, being in itself logically inconsistent. The crucial instance is that of the nourishment of the

πνεύματα. πνεύματα δὲ κατὰ τοὺς παλαιοὺς δύο ἐστί, τό τε ψυχικὸν καὶ τὸ φυσικόν ... καὶ Ἐρασίστρατος δὲ ὡς ἀρχὰς καὶ στοιχεῖα ὅλου σώματος ὑποτιθέμενος τὴν τριπλοκίαν τῶν ἀγγείων, νεῦρα καὶ φλέβας καὶ ἀρτηρίας παραλείπει τά τε ὑγρὰ καὶ τὰ πνεύματα. δυσὶ γὰρ ὕλαις ταῦτα διοικεῖσθαι λέγει τὸ ζῷον, τῷ μὲν αἵματι ὡς τροφῇ, τῷ δὲ πνεύματι ὡς συνεργῷ εἰς τὰς φυσικὰς ἐνεργείας. οὐ παραλαμβάνει δὲ αὐτὰς ὡς ἀρχάς. πολλὰ δὲ καὶ ἄλλα τῶν σωμάτων εἴδη εὑρίσκεται, οὐκ ἐκ τῆς τριπλοκίας συγκείμενα, οἷον εὐθὺς ὁ ἐγκέφαλος καὶ ὁ μυελὸς καὶ πάντα τὰ ὀστᾶ. τὸν μὲν οὖν ἐγκέφαλον ἢ τὸν μυελὸν παρέγχυμα τροφῆς τολμᾷ λέγειν, ὡς τὴν πιμελήν, καὶ τοῦ ἥπατος καὶ σπληνὸς καὶ πνεύμονος τὴν σύστασιν. τὰ δὲ ὀστέα οὐδὲ παρέγχυμα τροφῆς δύναιτ᾽ ἂν λέγειν, οὐδ᾽ ἐκ τῶν προειρημένων τριγενῶν ἀγγείων πεπλέχθαι.

[1] Galen, *De methodo medendi*, x. 10, K. 730–1 : καλεῖν γοῦν αὐτὴν οὐδὲν κωλύει διδασκαλίας ἕνεκα σαρκοειδῆ φύσιν, ἢ καὶ νὴ Δία τὴν τοῦδέ τινος τοῦ μορίου σάρκα, κατὰ γαστέρα μὲν ἑτέραν ὑπάρχουσαν καθ᾽ ἧπαρ δ᾽ ἑτέραν, ὥσπερ γε καὶ κατὰ ἀρτηρίαν καὶ μῦν. ὠνόμασται δὲ μόνη σάρξ ἡ ἐν μυσί. τῶν ἄλλων οὐδεμίαν ὀνομάζουσι σάρκα πλὴν ὀλίγοι δή τινες.

[2] Galen, *De nat. fac.* ii. 6, K. ii. 96: φλέβας ἔχειν ἐν ἑαυτῷ καὶ ἀρτηρίας τὸ νεῦρον, ὥσπερ τινὰ σειρὰν ἐκ τριῶν ἱμάντων διαφερόντων τῇ φύσει πεπλεγμένην.

[3] Galen, *De usu partium*, vii. 8, K. iii. 537–8: ὅτι καὶ τῶν ἀρτηριῶν αὐτῶν τὸν χιτῶνα καὶ πάντων ἁπλῶς τοῦ ζῴου τῶν μορίων ἐκ φλεβὸς καὶ ἀρτηρίας καὶ νεύρου πεπλέχθαι φησί, καὶ τρέφεσθαί γε πρὸς τῆς ἐν αὐτῷ φλεβὸς ἕκαστον τῆς ἁπλῆς ἐκείνης καὶ λόγῳ θεωρητῆς, οὐδὲν τῆς μεγάλης φλεβὸς ταύτης καὶ συνθέτου δεόμενον.

[4] *Anonymus Londinensis*, xxi. J. 82 : ὁ μὲν γὰρ Ἐρασίστρατος καὶ πόρρω τοῦ ἰατρικοῦ κανόνος προῆλθε. ὑπέλαβεν γὰρ τὰ πρῶτα σώματα λόγῳ θεωρητὰ εἶναι, ὥστε τὴν αἰσθητὴν φλέβα συνεστάναι ἐκ λόγῳ θεωρητῶν σωμάτων, φλεβός, ἀρτηρίας, νεύρου.

nerves. Instead of admitting that they attract nutriment from the visible veins, he postulates his threefold skein of nerve, vein, and artery ending up in invisible 'simple' veins, and endows the nerves themselves with their own invisible veinlets. But this will not really help him, for the nerve, or rather his 'simple' nervelet, must draw its nutriment from the veinlet. It cannot do this by the vacuum principle, because this can only come into operation in the case of visible or perceptible empty spaces. It is true that nerves do contain, according to Erasistratus, cavities of a sort, but these are filled not with blood, but with psychic *pneuma*. Moreover the 'simple' nerve, vein, or artery is so small that if you prick it with the sharpest pin you would tear to pieces all three. The only empty space which could be conceived to exist in the simple nerve would be the purely theoretical one, corresponding presumably to Strato's internal vacuoles, and an empty space which existed only in theory could not compel the adjacent fluid to come and fill it.[1]

On the question of these 'simple' vessels the followers of Erasistratus are not agreed. Are they made up of 'atoms' like those postulated by Democritus and Epicurus? Or are they definitely continuous bodies?[2] The latter hypothesis strikes Galen as being more in accordance with Erasistratus' theory,[3] and of course with that of Strato, as far as our limited knowledge of his actual teaching would seem to permit us to conjecture. If we regard them as compound, then we are reduced to postulating some such jointless particles like those assumed by Asclepiades, and the atomic hypothesis of physiological explanation has come in by the back door.[4] And for the atomic theory as an explanation of the

---

[1] Galen, *De nat. fac.* ii. 6, K. ii. 96–7: αἱ μὲν δὴ φλέβες ἡμῖν οὕτω θρέψονται τοῦ περιεχομένου κατ' αὐτὰς αἵματος ἀπολαύουσαι· τὰ δὲ νεῦρα πῶς; οὐ γὰρ δὴ κἀν τούτοις ἐστὶν αἷμα. πρόχειρον μὲν γὰρ ἦν εἰπεῖν, ἕλκοντα παρὰ τῶν φλεβῶν· ἀλλ' οὐ βούλεται. τί ποτ' οὖν κἀνταῦθα ἐπιτεχνᾶται; φλέβας ἔχειν ἐν ἑαυτῷ καὶ ἀρτηρίας τὸ νεῦρον, ὥσπερ τινὰ σειρὰν ἐκ τριῶν ἱμάντων διαφερόντων τῇ φύσει πεπλεγμένην. ᾠήθη γὰρ ἐκ ταύτης τῆς ὑποθέσεως ἐκφεύξεσθαι τῷ λόγῳ τὴν ὁλκήν . . . ἀλλὰ κἀνταῦθα πάλιν αὐτὸν ὁμοία τις ἀπορία διεδέξατο . . . τῇ μὲν γὰρ πρὸς τὸ κενούμενον ἀκολουθίᾳ πῶς ἂν ἔτι δύναιτο τὴν τροφὴν ἐπισπάσασθαι τὸ ἁπλοῦν νεῦρον, ὥσπερ αἱ φλέβες αἱ σύνθετοι; κοιλότης μὲν γάρ τίς ἐστιν ἐν αὐτῷ κατ' αὐτόν, ἀλλ' οὐχ αἵματος αὕτη γ' ἀλλὰ πνεύματος ψυχικοῦ μεστή. δεόμεθα δ' ἡμεῖς οὐκ εἰς τὴν κοιλότητα ταύτην εἰσάγειν τῷ λόγῳ τὴν τροφὴν ἀλλ' εἰς τὸ περιέχον αὐτὴν ἀγγεῖον . . . πῶς οὖν εἰσάξομεν; οὕτω γάρ ἐστι μικρὸν ἐκεῖνο τὸ ἁπλοῦν ἀγγεῖον, καὶ μέντοι καὶ τῶν ἄλλων ἑκάτερον, ὥστ' εἰ τῇ λεπτοτάτῃ βελόνῃ νύξειάς τι μέρος, ἅμα διαιρήσεις τὰ τρία. τόπος οὖν αἰσθητὸς ἀθρόος κενὸς οὐκ ἄν ποτ' ἐν αὐτῷ γένοιτο· λόγῳ δὲ θεωρητὸς τόπος κενούμενος οὐκ ἦν ἀναγκαστικὸς τῆς τοῦ συνεχοῦς ἀκολουθίας.

[2] Ibid., 97–8: ἐβουλόμην δ' αὖ πάλιν μοι κἀνταῦθα τὸν Ἐρασίστρατον αὐτὸν ἀποκρίνεσθαι περὶ τοῦ στοιχειώδους ἐκείνου νεύρου τοῦ σμικροῦ, πότερον ἕν τι καὶ συνεχές ἐστιν ἀκριβῶς ἢ ἐκ πολλῶν καὶ μικρῶν σωμάτων, ὧν Ἐπίκουρος καὶ Λεύκιππος καὶ Δημόκριτος ὑπετίθεντο, σύγκειται. καὶ γὰρ καὶ περὶ τούτου τοὺς Ἐρασιστρατείους ὁρῶ διαφερομένους. οἱ μὲν γὰρ ἕν τι καὶ συνεχὲς αὐτὸ νομίζουσιν, ἢ οὐκ ἂν ἁπλοῦν εἰρῆσθαι πρὸς αὐτοῦ φασι· τινὲς δὲ καὶ τοῦτο διαλύειν εἰς ἕτερα στοιχειώδη τολμῶσιν.

[3] Ibid., 98: διὸ δή μοι δοκοῦσιν ἀμαθῶς πάνυ τὴν εἰς τὰ τοιαῦτα στοιχεῖα τῶν ἁπλῶν ἀγγείων εἰσάγειν διάλυσιν ἔνιοι τῶν Ἐρασιστρατείων.

[4] Ibid.: εἰ δ' ἐκ πολλῶν σύγκειται, τῇ κηπαίᾳ κατὰ τὴν παροιμίαν πρὸς Ἀσκληπιάδην ἀπεχωρήσαμεν ἄναρμά τινα στοιχεῖα τιθέμενοι. Ibid., 99–100: κάλλιον οὖν μοι δοκεῖ τι καὶ πρὸς

phenomenon of nutrition Galen has no use at all. But even if we do admit that these simple nerves, of which the visible nerves are composed, are continuous bodies we are no further towards explaining their absorption of nutrition by the vacuum principle. For if they are continuous, then any diminution in their volume by wear and tear will leave no empty space, just as the removal of a portion of liquid also fails to do, since the parts, like drops of water, come together again, without creating any vacuum.[1] This analogy of the coalescing drops of water, incidentally, seems much more Stratonian than that of the heap of sand, which we have quoted above.[2] Erasistratus' quasi-atomic particles would, it appears, coalesce like water-drops to form the visible vessels, but that would not prevent them from having internal vacuoles, which in another passage Galen tells us that Erasistratus postulated.[3] This insistence on the vacuum theory only applying to visible empty spaces is quite inconsistent with Erasistratus' theory that in the ultimate 'simple' vessels, which are thin and narrow, nutriment is attracted through the sides of the vessels and deposited in the empty spaces left by the matter which has been carried away.[4] It is, of course, true that nutriment is conveyed through the sides of the veins to the surrounding tissues, but not by the process of the power of the vacuum to cause emptied matter to be replaced.[5]

These passages seem to me to show quite conclusively, Wellmann notwithstanding, that Erasistratus' theory was derived from Strato. They also help to draw attention to one of the more puzzling features of ancient Greek medicine, the baffling ambiguity of the term *neuron*. In this threefold skein of which the tissues were composed, what did the 'nerves' really represent? Were they after all only sinews in disguise, or rather,

---

ἡμᾶς συνεισενέγκασθαι τοῖς Ἐρασιστρατείοις, ἐπειδὴ κατὰ τοῦτο γεγόναμεν, καὶ συμβουλεῦσαι τοῖς τὸ πρῶτον ἐκεῖνο καὶ ἁπλοῦν ὑπὸ Ἐρασιστράτου καλούμενον ἀγγεῖον εἰς ἕτερ' ἄττα σώματα στοιχειώδη διαλύουσιν, ἀποστῆναι τῆς ὑπολήψεως.

[1] Galen, De nat. fac. ii. 6, K. ii. 98–9: καθ' ἑκατέρους γὰρ ἄτοπος ὁ τῆς θρέψεως ἔσται λόγος, ἐκείνοις τοῖς ἁπλοῖς ἀγγείοις τοῖς μικροῖς, τοῖς συντιθεῖσι τὰ μεγάλα τε καὶ αἰσθητὰ νεῦρα, κατὰ μὲν τοὺς συνεχῆ φυλάττοντας αὐτά, μὴ δυναμένης γενέσθαι τῆς πρὸς τὸ κενούμενον ἀκολουθίας, ὅτι μηδὲν ἐν τῷ συνεχεῖ γίνεται κενόν, κἂν ἀπορρέῃ τι· συνέρχεταί γε πρὸς ἄλληλα τὰ καταλειπόμενα μόρια, καθάπερ ἐπὶ τοῦ ὕδατος ὁρᾶται, καὶ πάλιν ἓν γίγνεται πάντῃ, τὴν χώραν τοῦ διαφορηθέντος αὐτῷ καταλαμβάνοντα.

[2] See passage quoted above, p. 202, n. 2.

[3] De nat. fac. ii. 6, K. ii. 99: ἐπὶ γὰρ τῶν αἰσθητῶν μόνων, οὐκ ἐπὶ τῶν λόγῳ θεωρητῶν ἔχει τὴν δύναμιν, ὡς αὐτὸς ὁ Ἐρασίστρατος ὁμολογεῖ διαρρήδην, οὐ περὶ τοιούτου κενοῦ φάσκων ἑκάστοτε ποιεῖσθαι τὸν λόγον, κατὰ βραχὺ παρέσπαρται τοῖς σώμασιν.

[4] Ibid., 105: τοῖς ἐσχάτοις τε καὶ ἁπλοῖς, λεπτοῖς τε καὶ στενοῖς οὖσιν, ἐκ τῶν παρακειμένων ἀγγείων ἡ πρόσθεσις συμβαίνει εἰς τὰ κενώματα τῶν ἀπενεχθέντων κατὰ τὰ πλάγια τῶν ἀγγείων ἑλκομένης τῆς τροφῆς καὶ καταχωριζομένης.

[5] Ibid., 105–6: δεύτερον δ' ἀποδέχομαι τῶν ἐκ τῆς Ἐρασιστράτου λέξεως ὀνομάτων τὸ γεγραμμένον ἐφεξῆς τῷ κατὰ τὰ πλάγια. τί γὰρ φησί; κατὰ τὰ πλάγια τῶν ἀγγείων ἑλκομένης τῆς τροφῆς. ὅτι μὲν οὖν ἕλκεται, καὶ ἡμεῖς ὁμολογοῦμεν, ὅτι δ' οὐ τῇ πρὸς τὸ κενούμενον ἀκολουθίᾳ, δέδεικται πρόσθεν.

in confusion? Some light is thrown on this ambiguity by a passage in the pseudo-Aristotelian treatise *De spiritu*, where we find a theory that the skin is made up of this threefold composition of vein, 'nerve', and artery. The word *nerve* here plainly seems to indicate a sinew-like tissue, for we are expressly told that the artery contains *pneuma* while the 'nerve' does not. Moreover it is capable of tension (τάσις), and is not easily broken, like a blood vessel.[1]

How clearly did Erasistratus recognize the distinction? Jones in his translation of the passage from the Anonymous Londoner, which we have quoted above describing the 'primary bodies', translates νεῦρον by the word sinew. The passage quoted above from the *Introductio* suggests that he regarded all the tissues of the body as made up of the three kinds of vessels plus deposits of nutriment transformed into blood, which might seem to suggest that he thought of the 'nerves' as including sinews, at any rate to supply some 'solidist' elements—elements like ligaments and tendons. The picture given in Galen's *Natural faculties* is rather different, and Brock quite rightly translates νεῦρον by 'nerve' not 'sinew', the nerves being described, as we have just seen, as having cavities which contain psychic *pneuma*. But they are not explicitly said to be hollow tubes, and unlike the veins which contain their nutriment in the form of blood, they need nourishment drawn from without. Moreover their cavities are of a special kind (κοιλότης τις). May not Erasistratus have looked upon them as a special kind of 'sling' or 'bowstring', both words which according to Liddell and Scott are correct translations of the word, which we translate as sinew for want of a better word, concerned with the motion of the limbs as well as with the transmission of perceptions from the sense organs? That Erasistratus knew they were different from ordinary sinews was, as we shall see presently, clear enough, since he may be regarded rightly as the discoverer of what we today call the nervous system, and he knew that their operations were focused in or controlled by the brain. But of the exact nature of these minimal 'elementary' vessels we can obtain no clear idea. They seem to have been a sort of atom, minimal existent particles of a specific character, very different from the atoms of Epicurus or Democritus since they were neither impenetrably solid—they contained internal vacuoles—nor were they provided with hooks for attachment like those conceived by Democritus. They were probably, as Diels pointed out, more like the ἄναρμοι ὄγκοι of Asclepiades. But we are told nothing about their shape. Presumably the 'atomic' vein was different in shape from the 'atomic' artery and the 'atomic' nerve. Nor can we have any precise notion of the way in which

---

[1] Op. cit. 483ᵇ15: τὸ δὲ δέρμα ἐκ φλεβὸς καὶ νεύρου καὶ ἀρτηρίας, ἐκ φλεβὸς μὲν ὅτι κεντηθὲν αἷμα ἀποδίδωσιν, ἐκ νεύρου δὲ ὅτι τάσιν ἔχει, ἐξ ἀρτηρίας δὲ ὅτι διαπνοὴν ἔχει.

they were put together to form the visible veins, arteries, and nerves which were made up of them. For a large vein is quite obviously not an aggregate or bundle of small veins, though a nerve might more easily be considered as such an aggregate. Unfortunately our knowledge of Strato's theories is too small to enable us to judge what Erasistratus really thought about this. He may have thought that when two atomic vein particles combined, they just formed one vein-particle double the size, thus preserving their continuity.

We have, however, seen sufficient evidence to show that the theory which regards Erasistratus' physiological teaching as based on atomism is open to serious qualification. And to regard him as an exponent of the Epicurean philosophy, as we find stated in Singer and Underwood,[1] is, to say the least of it, quite misleading. Nor can we be entirely certain that Galen's reproaches, that though paying lip-service to the teleological conception of the formative wisdom of nature he entirely ruled it out in his theories, are wholly justified. But he certainly made the first systematic attempt of which we have any knowledge in Greek thought to interpret physiological events in mechanical terms. A further example of his 'materialist' (as opposed to 'vitalist') temperament is his denial of another of the main theses of the 'Hippocratic' system, the existence of the innate heat in the living body, which he as well as Praxagoras and Asclepiades regarded as coming to the body from an external source,[2] not to mention his denial of the theory of 'coction' by this innate principle in the stomach. It is time, therefore, to examine a little more closely how this machine of the body consisting of the three kinds of elementary vessels and its various organs and tissues is 'managed' by the two external factors, nourishment and *pneuma*.

Of the four Hippocratic humours, Galen implies that Erasistratus in his theory of digestion only recognizes two—blood and yellow bile. Black bile he entirely omitted.[3] Concerning yellow bile, he took the view that it was entirely useless to the organism,[4] adhering, no doubt, to the

---

[1] Singer and Underwood, *A Short History of Medicine*, 2nd edn. (Oxford University Press, London, 1962), p. 49. 'At the time of the institution of the Medical School at Alexandria, and for long after, there flourished that view of the structure of matter known as "atomic", propounded by the philosopher Democritus. The chief exponent of the theory was Epicurus, whose philosophy was of the order we should now call materialistic. For it the only ultimate realities were atoms and "the void", and everything was ultimately expressible in these terms. Epicurean philosophy was not without its reactions on medicine at Alexandria, where its leading exponent was Erasistratus of Chios.'

[2] Galen, *De tremore, palpitatione, etc.* 6, K. vii. 614: ἐγὼ μὲν γὰρ εἶπον τοῦ κατὰ φύσιν θερμοῦ πάθος εἶναι τὸ ῥῖγος, ἵνα μή τις τοῦ ἔξωθεν νομίσας εἰρῆσθαι, καταψεύδεσθαί με δόξειεν Ἐρασιστράτου καὶ Πραξαγόρου καὶ Φιλοτίμου καὶ Ἀσκληπιάδου καὶ μυρίων ἄλλων, ὅσοι τὸ θερμὸν οὐκ ἔμφυτον ἀλλ' ἐπίκτητον εἶναι νομίζουσι.

[3] Galen, *De atra bile*, 4, K. v. 104: . . . ὥσπερ αὖ πάλιν Ἐρασίστρατος ὅλον παραλιπεῖν.

[4] Galen, *De nat. fac.* ii. 2, K. ii. 78: ἀλλὰ καὶ τὸ χολῶδες ὑγρὸν ἄχρηστον εἶναι παντάπασι τοῖς ζῴοις ἔφασκεν.

doctrine of the Cnidian school which regarded it, if not as a morbid product in itself, as one of the causes of disease, the other being phlegm. He seems to have written very little about it, though he admitted that it was the cause of jaundice and of inflammation of the liver, and agreed that it must be evacuated. He regarded the question of whether it was a by-product of food produced in the stomach, or whether it was a sub-stance mixed up in the actual foodstuffs ingested and so introduced from without, to be a problem the examination of which was quite useless to the physician and the art of medicine.[1] In this connection we may note that Erasistratus, or rather his school, attempted to provide a mechanistic explanation of the secretion of bile into the gall-bladder on iatro-physical lines. He rejected outright the 'vitalistic' theory of 'attraction' (ὁλκή), and tried to explain it on good Stratonian principles. When the blood runs past the mouth of the bile-duct, the bile, being thinner and lighter than blood, passes through the narrower mouth of the bile-duct which the blood is too thick to pass—a doctrine that is criticized by Galen on the ground that the serous constituents of the blood are lighter than bile.[2] Of his theory of the generation of phlegm, Galen can tell us little or nothing, but we know from the Anonymous Parisian that he regarded the obstruction of the internal passages of the nerves by phlegm as responsible for various diseases, such as stroke ('apoplexy').[3] And Galen reports that he thought that the thick and sticky humours—produced by food—were the cause of paralysis, which is due to the infiltration of these into the cavities of the nerves, the channels for the *pneuma* by which voluntary action is brought about. This account is also confirmed by a fragment (No. 20) of the Anonymous Parisian.[4]

[1] Galen, *De atra bile*, 5, K. v. 123: περὶ μὲν οὖν τῆς μελαίνης χολῆς οὐδὲν ὅλως ὁ Ἐρασίστρατος ἔγραψε, περὶ δὲ τῆς ξανθῆς ὀλίγα τε ἅμα καὶ οὐδὲ ταῦθ᾽ ἅπαντ᾽ ἀληθῆ. λέγει μὲν γὰρ οὕτω περὶ αὐτῆς. ἡ δὲ χολώδης ὑγρασία ὅτι μὲν ἀναγκαία ἐστὶν ἀποκρίνεσθαι, πολλὰ τῶν ἐπιγινομένων παθῶν μάρτυρες. οἱ ἴκτεροι γὰρ καὶ αἱ περὶ τὸ ἧπαρ γινόμεναι φλεγμοναὶ καὶ ἄλλα πλείω. πότερον δὲ ἐν τῇ περὶ τὴν κοιλίαν κατεργασίᾳ τῆς τροφῆς γεννᾶται ἡ τοιαύτη ἢ μεμιγμένη ἐν τοῖς προσφερομένοις ἔξωθεν παραγίνεται, οὐδὲν χρήσιμον πρὸς ἰατρικὴν ἐπεσκέφθαι.

[2] Galen, *De nat. fac.* ii. 2, K. ii. 78–9: ἐν μὲν δὴ τοῦτο σφάλμα τῶν ἀποστάντων τῆς ὁλκῆς· ἕτερον δὲ τὸ περὶ τῆς κατὰ τὴν ξανθὴν χολὴν διακρίσεως· οὐδὲ γὰρ οὐδ᾽ ἐκεῖ παραρρέοντος τοῦ αἵματος κατὰ τὰ στόματα τῶν χοληδόχων ἀγγείων, ἀκριβῶς διακριθήσεται τὸ χολῶδες περίττωμα . . . τὸ δὲ μέγιστον καὶ σαφέστατον πάλιν ἐνταῦθ᾽ ἁμάρτημα καὶ δὴ φράσω· εἴπερ γὰρ δι᾽ οὐδὲν ἄλλο, ἢ ὅτι παχύτερον μέν ἐστι τὸ αἷμα, λεπτοτέρα δ᾽ ἡ ξανθὴ χολὴ καὶ τὰ μὲν τῶν φλεβῶν εὐρύτερα στόματα, τὰ δὲ τῶν χοληδόχων ἀγγείων στενότερα, διὰ τοῦθ᾽ ἡ μὲν χολὴ τοῖς στενοτέροις ἀγγείοις τε καὶ στόμασιν ἐναρμόττει, τὸ δὲ αἷμα τοῖς εὐρυτέροις, δῆλον ὡς καὶ τὸ ὑδατῶδες τοῦτο καὶ ὀρρῶδες περίττωμα τοσούτῳ πρότερον εἰσρυήσεται τοῖς χοληδόχοις ἀγγείοις, ὅσῳ λεπτότερόν ἐστι τῆς χολῆς.

[3] AMG (1894), fr. 4: ἀποπληξίας αἰτία. Ἱπποκράτης δὲ καὶ Ἐρασίστρατός φασι περὶ τὸν ἐγκέφαλον φλέγματος ψυχροῦ καὶ παγετώδους γίνεσθαι σύστασιν ὑφ᾽ οὗ καὶ τὰ ἀπὸ τούτου πεφυκότα νεῦρα πληρούμενα μὴ παραδέχεσθαι τὸ ψυχικὸν πνεῦμα, ἀλλ᾽ ἐγκαταπνιγόμενον τοῦτο κινδυνεύειν ἀποσβεσθῆναι.

[4] Galen, *De atra bile*, 5, K. v. 125: ἀλλὰ τούς γε γλίσχρους καὶ παχεῖς αὐτὸς ἀπεφήνατο παραλύσεως αἰτίους γενέσθαι γράψας οὕτως· τὸ μὲν οὖν πάθος συμβαίνει παρεμπτώσεως ὑγρῶν γινομένης εἰς τὰ τοῦ πνεύμονος ἀγγεῖα τὰ ἐν τοῖς νεύροις, δι᾽ ὧν αἱ κατὰ προαίρεσιν κινήσεις

The doctrine that a knowledge of the manner in which these humours are generated is useless to the physician arouses Galen's particular indignation, and it may well indeed appear to us to be a strange view for a pioneer of anatomy to take. But it is possible to find a rather interesting parallel in the history of British medicine, as late as the seventeenth century. The English Hippocrates, the great clinician Thomas Sydenham, adopted a rather similar attitude, disparaging the use of the microscope and expressing the view that physiological processes would always be unknowable. Their detailed study was useless to the clinician, and he advised Sir Hans Sloane against the study of anatomy and botany.[1] Sydenham, it must be remembered, was living in the age of acute controversy between iatro-physicists and iatro-chemists. Perhaps Erasistratus was protesting against the teaching of the iatro-chemists of his day. However that may be, we are entitled to look upon him as the first iatro-physicist. For he performed the first experiment on record to establish the measurement of a physiological process, in order, no doubt, to find confirmatory evidence for his theory of nutrition as the replacement of parts of the body lost through wear and tear. The experiment is recorded in a passage by the Anonymous Londoner. Erasistratus placed a bird, or some other small animal, in a vessel after weighing it, and kept it there for a considerable period without giving it either food or drink. He then weighed it again, together with the total visible excretions passed during the period. He found that the animal and its excreta together weighed a lot less than the animal had weighed before it was put into the vessel, which proved that the body had given off a lot of invisible matter, by way of 'wear and tear'.[2] A rather similar experiment on a human being, to wit himself, was performed by the iatro-physicist Santorio of Capo d'Istria, who was professor at Padua at the beginning of the seventeenth century.

συντελοῦνται . . . ἡ δὲ παρέμπτωσις, φησί, γίνεται τῆς τροφῆς ἀφ' ἧς τὰ νεῦρα τρέφεται. Cf. AMG (1894), fr. 20: Ἐρασίστρατος μέν φησι κατὰ τὸ ἀκόλουθον τῶν ἐν ταῖς φλεψὶν ὑγρῶν εἰς τὰ τῶν νεύρων κοιλώματα δι' ὧν αἱ κατὰ προαίρεσιν κινήσεις γίνονται, παρεμπιπτόντων καὶ τὴν καταφερομένην δύναμιν ἀπὸ τῆς ἀρχῆς εἰς τὸ σῶμα κωλυόντων.

[1] Sydenham's famous remark to Sloane, 'Anatomy and botany, nonsense', must not be taken too seriously, since he was very well aware that the physician, no less than the surgeon, must be thoroughly acquainted at any rate with the gross anatomy of the human body. But his scepticism with regard to the value of post-mortem examinations and the use of the microscope, as well as his distrust of physiological research, read rather strangely today. See Kenneth Dewhurst, *Dr. Sydenham, His Life and Original Writings* (The Wellcome Historical Medical Library, 1966), especially pp. 50, 64, 74, and particularly the essay on 'Anatomy', written by Sydenham in 1668, reproduced on pp. 85–8.

[2] *Anonymus Londinensis*, xxxiii, J. 126: καὶ Ἐρασίστρατος πειρᾶται παρασκευάζειν τὸ προτεθέν. εἰ γὰρ λάβοι τις ζῷον οἷον ὄρνιθα ἤ τι τῶν παραπλησίων, καταθοῖτο δὲ τοῦτο ἐν λέβητι ἐπί τινας χρόνους μὴ δοὺς τροφήν, ἔπειτα σταθμήσαιτο σὺν τοῖς σκυβάλοις τοῖς αἰσθητῶς κεκενωμένοις, εὑρήσει παρὰ πολὺ ἔλασσον τοῦτο τῷ σταθμῷ τῷ δηλονότι πολλὴν ἀποφορὰν γεγενῆσθαι κατὰ τὸ λόγῳ θεωρητόν.

While nourishment maintains the physical framework of the body, *pneuma* has the twofold function of energizing its physiological activities, e.g. digestion, movement, excretion, etc., and also the psychical functions of sensation, intelligence, and voluntary action. *Pneuma*, as we have seen, is taken in from the outer atmosphere, through the nose, mouth, trachea, and bronchi, and the smooth arteries of the lung, the pulmonary veins, into the left ventricle of the heart. All the air taken in by nose and mouth goes to the lungs and the heart, and only from there does it reach the meninges of the brain, where it becomes the 'psychic' or 'animal' spirit, having been transformed from air into 'vital' spirit in the heart. No air goes, as Hippocrates taught, directly from the nose to the cerebral ventricles.[1] What Erasistratus believed to happen to the air on its passage through the lungs via the double system of bronchi and pulmonary veins is not at all clear. Galen criticizes him on account of his inability to explain how the air breathed in becomes the food of the psychic spirit. This is, of course, by a kind of 'digestion' ($\pi \acute{\epsilon} \psi \iota s$), the proper organ of which is the lung.[2] Instead of assuming some qualitative change to be responsible, he seems to have attributed the change in some unintelligible manner to its density, its thickness or thinness, presumably assuming that only the thinnest *pneuma* could penetrate to the brain, once more an iatro-physical explanation.[3] In the same way, Galen continues, he believed that deaths due to suffocation in 'Charon's pits' or in newly-limed houses or through the inhalation of charcoal vapour were brought about by the fact that the *pneuma* inhaled from these sources is so thin that it cannot be contained by the arteries, but easily escapes from the body with the result that the animal perishes from lack of *pneuma*.[4]

Erasistratus' theories concerning the process of respiration are described by Galen as follows. The lungs, we are told in another passage, have no motion of their own. They are moved by the thorax expanding quite mechanically. They draw in air as it expands, in accordance with

---

[1] Galen, *De usu resp.* 5, K. iv. 502: ὁμοίως οἱ περὶ τὸν Ἐρασίστρατον τοῖς περὶ τὸν Ἱπποκράτην τρέφεσθαί φασι τὸ ψυχικὸν πνεῦμα. τοῖς μὲν γὰρ ἐκ τῆς καρδίας διὰ τῶν ἀρτηριῶν εἰς τὰς μήνιγγας, τοῖς δὲ εὐθὺς διὰ τῶν ῥινῶν εἰς τὰς κατὰ τὸν ἐγκέφαλον κοιλίας.

[2] Galen, *De usu partium*, vii. 8, K. iii. 539: ἥ τε σὰρξ τοῦ πνεύμονος ἀερώδης ὁρᾶται καὶ πνεύματος μεστή, σαφῶς εἰς πέψιν ἀέρος ἐνδεικνυμένη, καθάπερ ἡ τοῦ ἥπατος εἰς τὴν τῆς τροφῆς.

[3] Ibid., 540: Ἐρασίστρατον δὲ κἀνταῦθα δέον αἰτιᾶσθαι ποιότητος οἰκειότητά τε καὶ ἀλλοτριότητα, λεπτότητα καὶ παχύτητα, οὐκ οἶδ' ὅπως, αἰτιᾶται τοῦ πνεύματος.

[4] Ibid.: λεπτότητα καὶ παχύτητα, οὐκ οἶδ' ὅπως αἰτιᾶται τοῦ πνεύματος, οἰόμενον ἀπόλλυσθαι διὰ τοῦτο τούς τ' ἐν τοῖς Χαρωνείοις βαράθροις καὶ τοὺς ἐν τῇ νεωστὶ κεχρισμένῃ οἰκίᾳ τιτάνῳ, καί τινος ἐξ ἀνθράκων ὀσμῆς καὶ τῶν ἄλλων τῶν τοιούτων, ἀδυνατοῦντος ἐν τῷ σώματι στέγεσθαι τοῦ πνεύματος ὑπὸ λεπτότητος. Cf. Galen, *De usu resp.* 4, K. iv. 496: πῶς οὖν, φασίν, ἔν τε τοῖς βαρυόδμοις βαράθροις καὶ τοῖς νεωστὶ κεχρισμένοις οἴκοις τιτάνῳ καὶ πρὸς τῆς τοῦ ἐσβεσμένων ἀνθράκων ὀσμῆς πνιγόμεθα; κατὰ μὲν τὸν Ἐρασίστρατον ὅτι λεπτὸς ὢν ἐν ταῖς τοιαύταις καταστάσεσιν ὁ ἀὴρ οὐ στέγεται πρὸς τῶν ἀρτηριῶν, ἀλλ' ἐκκενοῦται ῥᾳδίως καὶ ἐνδείᾳ πνεύματος ἀπόλλυται τὸ ζῷον.

the principle of *horror vacui*, so too contracting as it contracts, like a squeezed sponge from which the water is pressed out.[1] The purpose of respiration is to fill the arteries.[2] This implies a very close connection between respiration, heart-beat, and pulse, the exact nature of which is far from clear. *Pneuma* is drawn into the heart at diastole via the pulmonary veins, in accordance with the *horror vacui*.[3] In accordance with the same principle, when the breath is held or respiration is impeded, animals are asphyxiated, owing to the inability of the heart to attract any *pneuma* from the lung. The reason given for this was that when the breath is held, neither the chest nor the lungs can undergo any change in volume. If therefore the heart draws any air from them a vacuum would be formed, but this is impossible, because if there is to be an attraction of air or *pneuma* by the heart, there must be some part of the vascular system in the thorax which gives it up. But when the breath is held, the volume of the thorax remains unchanged. Therefore the heart cannot receive it.[4] Galen has not much difficulty in pointing out the errors in fact and logic of Erasistratus' rather peculiar argument, for the visible fact is that the heart does go on beating when we hold our breath. It continues its diastole and systole and must therefore on Erasistratus' own principles draw in air, for an expanded heart with a vacuum inside it is impossible.[5] The Erasistratans, if not Erasistratus himself, attempted to overcome the difficulty by assuming that the heart somehow managed to draw *pneuma* from the aorta, notwithstanding its tightly closed valve, under certain 'unnatural' conditions[6]—a doctrine not easily reconciled with their master's, since he, unlike Galen, insisted that all the valves of the heart closed tightly, and permitted no leaking backwards of matter, whether blood or *pneuma*.[7]

---

[1] Galen, *De locis affectis*, v. 3, K. viii. 324–5: προαποδεδειγμένην ἔχοντα τὴν τῆς ἀναπνοῆς ἐνέργειαν ὑπὸ τοῦ θώρακος γιγνομένην, οὐδεμίαν ἔχοντος ἰδίαν κίνησιν τοῦ πνεύμονος, ἀλλ᾽ ὁπότε μὲν ὁ θώραξ διαστέλλοιτο, τῇ πρὸς τὸ κενούμενον ἀκολουθίᾳ συνδιαστελλομένου, κατὰ δὲ τὰς συστολὰς αὐτοῦ συνιζάνοντος εἰς αὐτὸν ὁμοίως τοῖς σπόγγοις οὓς ταῖς χερσὶν περιλαμβάνοντες θλίβομεν.

[2] Galen, *De usu resp.* 1, K. iv. 471: ἐπιπληρώσεως δὲ ἕνεκεν ἀρτηριῶν ἀναπνέομεν, ὡς Ἐρασίστρατος οἴεται. Cf. Galen, *Comment. in Hipp. epidem.* vi, par. vi, K. xviiB. 320: περὶ τῆς εἴσω τε καὶ ἔξω φορᾶς τοῦ πνεύματος . . . τινῶν μὲν ἕνεκα γενέσεως πνεύματος ψυχικοῦ, καθάπερ Ἀσκληπιάδης, ἐνίων δέ, ὡς Ἐρασίστρατος, οὐ τούτου μόνου ἀλλὰ καὶ ζωτικοῦ.

[3] Galen, *De puls. diff.* iv. 2, K. viii. 703: βούλεται γὰρ ἔμπαλιν τῇ καρδίᾳ τὰς ἀρτηρίας σφύζειν, ἐκείνης μὲν ὅτε διαστέλλεται πληρουμένης τῇ πρὸς τὸ κενούμενον ἀκολουθίᾳ.

[4] Galen, *De usu resp.* 2, K. iv. 473, quoted above, p. 211, n. 2.

[5] Ibid., 474–5: τοῖς ἐναργέσιν ὁ λόγος αὐτοῦ μάχεται. βλέπομεν γὰρ ὡς ἕλκει κατὰ τὰς ἐπισχέσεις τῆς ἀναπνοῆς ἡ καρδία τὸν ἐκ τοῦ πνεύμονος ἀέρα. τοῦτο δ᾽ ἕπεται τῷ διαστέλλεσθαι τὴν καρδίαν. οὐδὲ γὰρ ἐνδέχεται κατ᾽ αὐτὸν διαστέλλεσθαι μέν, μηδὲν δ᾽ ἕλκειν, κενὸς γὰρ ἂν οὕτω γένοιτο τόπος. εἰ δ᾽ οὐ διαστέλλεται, δῆλον ὡς οὐδὲ κινεῖται· ἀλλὰ μὴν φαίνεται κινουμένη.

[6] Ibid., 476: πρὸς δὲ τὸ μὴ δύνασθαι παρὰ τῆς μεγάλης ἀρτηρίας ἑλκύσαι τι τὴν καρδίαν διὰ τὴν τῶν ὑμένων ἐπίφυσιν ἀπολογούμενοί φασι περὶ τῆς κατὰ φύσιν οἰκονομίας ταῦτα εἰρηκέναι τὸν Ἐρασίστρατον, οὐ περὶ τῆς βιαίου καὶ παρὰ φύσιν.

[7] Galen, *De usu pulsuum*, 4, K. v. 166: ἀλλ᾽ ἐκεῖνος μὲν ἔοικεν ὑπολαμβάνειν μηδὲν ὅλως εἰς τὴν καρδίαν ἐκ τῶν ἀρτηριῶν μεταλαμβάνεσθαι, πλήν γε διὰ τῶν ἐν πνεύμονι· τὸ δὲ οὐχ οὕτως ἔχει.

However anxious Erasistratus may have been to give mechanical explanations of physiological processes, the knowledge of mechanics current in his day was much too meagre to make this even remotely plausible. Some sort of 'vital' principle had to be assumed by almost every other school of Greek medicine to account for both involuntary and voluntary bodily actions. For in the last resort the behaviour of living things is to all appearance different from that of non-living. And the heart was by tradition the organ in which this principle was supposed to be embodied. Its motions were therefore due to some 'vital' force. They were therefore unable to agree with Erasistratus that the arterial tubes expanded purely mechanically because of the pressure of the *pneuma* expelled from the heart at each systole of the left ventricle.[1] This force was supplied by the inhaled air, which ultimately was responsible for putting into action all the bodily processes. Though he seems to have considered their distinction purely mechanically, Erasistratus believed in the existence of two of the three kinds of 'spirits' which were to play so large a part in the history of European medicine. According to his doctrine, the *pneuma* distributed by the heart through the arterial system was the 'vital' spirit, that which was further elaborated in the brain and distributed from there by the nerves as the 'psychic' or 'animal' spirit.

As to the pulse, Erasistratus was quite certain that it was a quasi-mechanical phenomenon. He was the first to recognize with perfect clarity its direct dependence on the beating of the heart. The expansion of the arteries is caused solely by the pressure of the *pneuma* propelled by the heart in its systole,[2] and their contraction is equally mechanical.[3] He seems at one time to have used the term σφυγμός, as we have already had occasion to note, in the restricted sense of perceptible throbbing in inflammation, following the practice of the older physicians.[4] In another passage, however, Galen implies that he too used the term in its modern sense. Erasistratus, he says, will tell you that the pulse is the movement of the arteries in a process of systole and diastole, which takes place under the influence of the vital and animal faculty for the purpose of

---

[1] Cf. the passage from Galen, *De locis affectis*, quoted above, p. 226, n. 1.

[2] Galen, *Synopsis lib. de puls.* 22, K. ix. 507–8: ὡς δὲ Ἐρασίστρατος ἔλεγε, ὁ σφυγμὸς γίνεται φορᾷ τοῦ παρὰ καρδίας ἐπιπεμπομένου πνεύματος διὰ τῶν ἐν ταῖς ἀρτηρίαις κοιλοτήτων.

[3] Galen, *De usu puls.* 4, K. v. 167 f.: ὡς δ' Ἐρασίστρατος ὑπελάμβανεν, ὀχετῶν ἀψύχων ἔργον, οὐκ ὀργάνων ζωτικῶν αἱ ἀρτηρίαι τοῖς ζῴοις ὑπηρετοῦσιν.

[4] Galen, *De diff. puls.* iv. 17, K. viii. 761: ὅ γε μὴν Ἐρασίστρατος ἔοικεν οὐ τὴν κατὰ φύσιν ἐν ἀρτηρίαις κίνησιν ὀνομάζειν σφυγμὸν ἀλλὰ μόνην τὴν ἐπὶ φλεγμονῇ. δῆλον δὲ ἐκ τῶν ῥήσεων αὐτοῦ τῶν ἐν τῷ πρώτῳ περὶ πυρετῶν, ἐν αἷς κίνησιν μὲν ἀρτηριῶν ὀνομάζει τὸν κατὰ φύσιν ὑφ' ἡμῶν καλούμενον σφυγμόν, ὃν δ' αὐτὸς ἐπὶ φλεγμονῇ τὴν μεταβολὴν ἔχειν φησί, σφυγμὸν φαίνεται καλῶν, ὡς οὐ κατὰ πάσης κινήσεως ἀρτηριῶν ἐπιφέρειν ἡγούμενος χρῆναι τὴν τοῦ σφυγμοῦ προσηγορίαν, ἀλλ' ἐπ' ἐκείνης μόνης, ἥτις ἐξίσταται τοῦ κατὰ φύσιν ὑπὸ τῆς κατὰ τὴν φλεγμονὴν διαθέσεως.

filling the arteries which contain the vital spirit.[1] For Erasistratus in his book on fevers insists that the heart has an 'animal' as well as a 'vital' faculty.[2] The mention of the 'animal' faculty in this connection sounds rather strange, since the arteries are filled with 'vital' not with 'animal' spirit, which exists or comes into being only in the ventricles of the brain, and is carried only in the nervous system. It looks therefore as if the 'animal' power or faculty of the heart may be a vestigial appendix of the Cnidian–Sicilian doctrine of the heart as the seat of consciousness. In this connection it may be appropriate to remember that Chrysippus, according to Galen, thought, in contrast to Erasistratus, that the left ventricle was full of animal spirit,[3] though it is not plain which Chrysippus; it may well have been the physician not the philosopher, though the doctrine agrees perfectly with the Stoic teaching on the primacy of the heart. Galen also tells us that Erasistratus, like Hippocrates, did not devote much attention to the pulse.[4] But from the passage just quoted in a footnote,[5] it is clear that he regarded it as an important symptom in fevers and inflammation. Markellinos reports him as teaching that in fever the pulse in all patients becomes more frequent, and also stronger in most, and that it was a reliable indication of the condition of the fevered patient, which showed the increase or decrease of inflammation, and generally the condition of the whole body.[6] Another reference to his doctrine of the pulse is found in Caelius Aurelianus(?),[7] in which he is also credited with the view that a preternaturally fast pulse is a sign of fever. Erasistratus, as might be expected, appears to have regarded the strength of the pulse as due principally to the strength of the heart-beat, a view in which he was supported later by Asclepiades. But Galen tells us that he

---

[1] Galen, De diff. puls. iv. 2, K. viii. 714: ὁ μὲν γὰρ Ἐρασίστρατος ἐρεῖ τὸν σφυγμὸν εἶναι κίνησιν ἀρτηριῶν κατὰ διαστολὴν καὶ συστολὴν ὑπὸ ζωτικῆς τε καὶ ψυχικῆς δυνάμεως γινομένην, ἐπιπληρώσεως ἕνεκεν ἀρτηριῶν, ἐχουσῶν ἐν αὑταῖς πνεῦμα ζωτικόν.

[2] Ibid., iv. 16, K. viii. 760: αὐτὸς γὰρ ὁ Ἐρασίστρατος ἐν τοῖς περὶ πυρετῶν ἀπεφήνατο σαφῶς, οὐ μόνον ζωτικὴν δύναμιν εἶναι κατὰ τὴν καρδίαν, ἀλλὰ καὶ ψυχικήν.

[3] Galen, De plac. Hipp. et Plat. i. 6, K. v. 185: Ἐρασίστρατος μὲν γὰρ ζωτικοῦ πνεύματος, Χρύσιππος δὲ τοῦ ψυχικοῦ πνεύματος πλήρη φασὶν εἶναι τὴν κοιλίαν ταύτην.

[4] Galen, De diff. puls. i. 2, K. viii. 497: Ἱπποκράτης τό τε ὄνομα τοῦ σφυγμοῦ γράφει καὶ τὴν ἐν αὐτῷ τέχνην οὐκ ἀγνοεῖν ἔοικεν, οὐ μὴν οὔτ' ἐπὶ πλέον ἐξειργάσατο τοῦτο μέρος τῆς τέχνης οὔτ' ἐπὶ πάσης ἀρτηριῶν κινήσεως τοὔνομα φέρει. παραπλήσιον δέ τι φαίνεται ποιεῖν αὐτῷ καὶ ὁ Ἐρασίστρατος.

[5] See n. 2, above.

[6] Markellinos, De pulsibus, 10: τοῖς πυρέσσουσιν ἡ κίνησις πυκνοτέρα μὲν γίνεται πᾶσι, σφοδροτέρα δὲ τοῖς πλείστοις . . . μόνη δ' ἡ περὶ τῇ κινήσει διάθεσις τῶν πυρεσσόντων εὐσύνοπτος καὶ ἀκριβὴς τῷ γε ἕξιν ἔχοντι καὶ οὐ διαψευδομένῳ, ἀλλ' αὐτήν τε τὴν τῆς φλεγμονῆς ἐπίτασιν καὶ ἄνεσιν καὶ τὴν περὶ ὅλον τὸ σῶμα διάθεσιν ἱκανῶς διασημαίνει.

[7] See the treatise De speciali significatione diaeticarum passionum, printed in Valentin Rose, Anecdota Graeca et Graecolatina (Berlin, 1870), ii. 226: 'Alii enim contra naturam effectam mutationem sine externae causae adventu signum febrium vocaverunt . . . alii crebritatem pulsus ultra naturam ut Cleophantes, Chrysippus, et Erasistratus.'

also reckoned the quantity and density of the *pneuma* as contributing to the strength of the pulse.

For Erasistratus does not endow the tunics of the arteries themselves with their own independent power of tension, but he says that the strike of the pulse-beat is generated by the propulsion through the arteries of the *pneuma* forcibly expelled from the heart.[1]

Unlike Herophilus, whom Galen unfortunately followed, Erasistratus has come remarkably close to the facts. He refuses to attribute to the arteries any expansive powers of their own, either independent or heart-derived, other than physical elasticity. They expand only because *pneuma* is forced into them by the contraction of the left ventricle, expanding, as we have seen, at the moment when the ventricle contracts, not at the moment of diastole. But he is far from correct in many of his assumptions. His explanation of the movement of the heart itself is far from satisfactory, and his resort to the principle of the *horror vacui* to explain the attraction of *pneuma* into the left ventricle is anything but 'progressive'. Moreover, he is reported by Galen as having taught that the expansion of different portions of the same artery was successive, not simultaneous. Though modern doctrines of the pulse-wave do not, of course, imply absolute simultaneity, Ewart informs us that 'hardly more than a sixth to an eighth of a second lapses between the beat of any two arteries, however distant from each other'.[2] It is therefore difficult to believe that Erasistratus could have discerned by his naked eye the travel of a pulse-wave at the rate of 20 to 30 feet per second.

Our account of Erasistratus' physiology, though it has led us far from our field, would not be complete even as a sketch without some mention of his doctrine of the nervous system and the working of the brain. From the left ventricle of the heart the vital spirit is propelled via the carotid arteries to the brain, in the description of which Erasistratus showed a great improvement on Herophilus, though, if we may believe Galen, his accurate knowledge of this organ was only acquired late in life. Of the process by which the 'vital' spirit becomes 'animal' we know nothing, since Erasistratus' very numerous discussions on the seats of the *pneumas*, if indeed they touched on it at all, have not been preserved in any

---

[1] Galen, *De diff. puls.* iii. 2, K. viii. 646: Ἀσκληπιάδης . . . τὴν δ' αἰτίαν τῆς σφοδρότητος εἰς πλῆθος καὶ λεπτότητα πνεύματος ἀνοίσει, καθάπερ, οἶμαι, καὶ Ἐρασίστρατος· οὐδὲ γὰρ οὗτος τοῖς χιτῶσιν αὐτοῖς τῶν ἀρτηριῶν μεταδίδωσι τῆς τονικῆς δυνάμεως, ἀλλὰ τῆς καρδίας ἰσχυρῶς ἐκθλιβούσης τὸ πνεῦμα τῇ τούτου διὰ τῶν ἀρτηριῶν φορᾷ τὸ ἀντιβατικὸν ἐν τῇ πληγῇ φησι γεννᾶσθαι.

[2] Ewart, op. cit., p. 37.

quotations by Galen.[1] Indeed it remains a mystery.[2] We are told in the *History of philosophy* that he regarded the membrane of the brain which is called the epicranis (*sic*) as the seat of the soul, in contrast to Strato, who placed it between the eyebrows, and Herophilus, who placed it in the ventricles of the brain, and Democritus and Plato, who placed it in the head as a whole.[3] Galen tells us, in a passage in his treatise on the doctrines of Hippocrates and Plato, that until late in life he thought that all the nerves issued (via the spinal cord?) from the dura mater itself, since he only saw those parts of the nerve which issue from it. But when he became an old man, he retired from practice and devoted himself to anatomy, and changed his opinions. He now recognized that the core of the nerves, as it were, proceeded from the brain itself.[4] That his studies were performed on human not on animal brains seems clear from Galen's account, and the passage cited contains a rather detailed description of the brain and its ventricles which is worth quoting in full, since it contains one of the most surprisingly accurate guesses in the history of comparative anatomy.

I also examined the nature of the brain. It is certainly divided into two parts, like that of other animals, and it has a hollow or ventricle placed longitudinally on each side. These two ventricles are connected with each other, and come together near the place where the two halves of the brain are joined. From here they lead into the so-called 'epencranis', and there is another small ventricle. And each of the two parts of the brain is covered with the membranes, for the epencranis has its own separate covering. The brain is like the small intestine in that it has many folds, and the epencranis itself has even more, and more complicated convolutions. Reflecting on these facts, one learns that, just as the deer, the hare, or any other animal that greatly

---

[1] Herophilus was, for example, the inventor of the notorious rete mirabile, a network of blood vessels lying at the base of the brain, which though something like it may be found in certain domestic animals has no counterpart in the human brain. This network, as we shall see below, was to play a most important role in the physiology of Galen. See below, p. 354.

[2] Galen, *De plac. Hipp. et Plat.* ii. 8, K. v. 281 : Ἐρασίστρατος οὖν οὐχ ἁπλῶς, ὥσπερ οὗτοι, τὸ ζητούμενον λαμβάνων, ἀλλὰ μετὰ κατασκευῆς λόγων οὐκ ὀλίγων ἐκ μὲν τῆς κεφαλῆς φησι τὸ ψυχικόν, ἐκ δὲ τῆς καρδίας τὸ ζωτικὸν ὁρμᾶσθαι πνεῦμα.

[3] Galen (?), *De phil. hist.* 28, K. xix. 315: Δημόκριτος καὶ Πλάτων τὸ ἡγεμονικὸν ἐν ὅλῃ τῇ κεφαλῇ καθίζουσι. Στράτων ἐν τῷ μεσοφρύῳ. Ἐρασίστρατος περὶ τὴν μήνιγγα τοῦ ἐγκεφάλου ἦν ἐπικρανίδα λέγει. Ἡρόφιλος ἐν ταῖς τοῦ ἐγκεφάλου κοιλίαις. This is a suspect source, the accuracy of which may perhaps be gauged by the fact that the author makes Erasistratus call the membrane of the brain the ἐπικρανίς, which sounds suspiciously like the term ἐπεγκρανίς, which, Galen informs us, Erasistratus applied to the cerebellum. Cf. Galen, *De usu part.* viii. 13, K. iii. 673: Ἐρασίστρατος δέ, ὅτι μὲν ἐγκεφάλου σύγκειται ποικιλώτερος ἡ ἐπεγκρανίς— οὕτω γὰρ αὐτὴν ὀνομάζει—καλῶς ἀποφαίνεται· πολύπλοκον δὲ εἶναι φάσκων ἐπ᾽ ἀνθρώπων μᾶλλον ἢ τῶν ἄλλων ζῴων, αὐτήν τε ταύτην καὶ σὺν αὐτῇ τὸν ἐγκέφαλον ὅτι οὐ περίεστιν αὐτοῖς ὁμοίως ἀνθρώπῳ τὸ νοεῖν, οὐκέτ᾽ ὀρθῶς μοι δοκεῖ γινώσκειν.

[4] Galen, *De plac. Hipp. et Plat.* vii. 3, K. v. 602: Ἐρασίστρατος δὲ ἄχρι πολλοῦ τὴν ἔξωθεν μοῖραν ὁρῶν μόνην τοῦ νεύρου, τὴν ἀπὸ τῆς παχείας μήνιγγος ὁρμωμένην ἀπ᾽ ἐκείνης ᾤετο πεφυκέναι σύμπαν τὸ νεῦρον, καὶ μεστά τε τὰ πλεῖστα τούτου τῶν συγγραμμάτων ἐστὶν ἀπὸ τῆς περιεχούσης τὸν ἐγκέφαλον μήνιγγος πεφυκέναι φάσκοντος τὰ νεῦρα. ἀλλ᾽ ὅτε πρεσβύτης ὢν ἤδη καὶ σχολὴν ἄγων μόνοις τοῖς τῆς τέχνης θεωρήμασιν ἀκριβεστέρας ἐποιεῖτο τὰς ἀνατομάς, ἔγνω καὶ τὴν οἷον ἐντεριώνην τῶν νεύρων ἀπ᾽ ἐγκεφάλου πεφυκυῖαν.

excels others in running is well provided with muscles, tendons, and nerves, so man, since he is superior to all other animals in intelligence, has a very convoluted brain. And all the nerves grow out of the brain, and, speaking generally, the brain seems to be the determinant or starting-point of the happenings in the body. For the sensory channel from the nostrils opens on to it, and also those from the ears, and the channels which lead to the tongue and the eyes also grow out of the brain.[1]

Whatever the change in his views about the origin of the nerves, Erasistratus no less than Herophilus believed that the ventricles of the brain were filled with what he called the 'psychic' or 'animal' *pneuma*. It would appear however that he also changed his views on the nature of the nerves themselves. To begin with, at any rate, he seems to have regarded them as hollow vessels, tubes which were the channels of the psychic *pneuma*,[2] provided with minute invisible veins to feed them, in accordance with his theory of the threefold skein.[3] But Wellmann comes to the conclusion that later he regarded them as filled with marrow.[4] The evidence for the nature of this change is far from conclusive. Galen, in the passage which we have just cited, says that he recognized that the pith or core of the nerves all proceeded from the brain in his latest years, but how he conceived this pith or core is quite uncertain. The word ἐντεριώνη, which Galen uses, does, it is true, suggest some kind of solid substance,[5] but Verbecke has pointed out that solid nerves would make

---

[1] Ibid., 602–4: ἐθεωροῦμεν δὲ καὶ τὴν φύσιν τοῦ ἐγκεφάλου, καὶ ἦν ὁ μὲν ἐγκέφαλος διμερής, καθάπερ καὶ τῶν λοιπῶν ζῴων, καὶ κοιλίαν παρὰ τῷ μήκει τῷ εἴδει κειμένην. συντέτρηντο δ' αὗται εἰς μίαν κατὰ τὴν συναφὴν τῶν μερῶν. ἐκ δὲ ταύτης ἔφερεν εἰς τὴν ἐπεγκρανίδα καλουμένην, καὶ ἐκεῖ ἑτέρα ἦν μικρὰ κοιλία, διαπέφρακτο δὲ ταῖς μήνιγξιν ἕκαστον τῶν μερῶν. ἥ τε γὰρ ἐπεγκρανὶς διαπέφρακτο αὐτὴ καθ' ἑαυτὴν καὶ ὁ ἐγκέφαλος παραπλήσιος ὢν νήστει καὶ πολύπλοκος, πολὺ δ' ἔτι μᾶλλον τούτου ἡ ἐπεγκρανὶς πολλοῖς εἰλιγμοῖς καὶ ποικίλοις κατεσκεύαστο. ὥστε μαθεῖν τούτων τὸν θεωροῦντα, ὅτι, ὥσπερ ἐπὶ τῶν λοιπῶν ζῴων, ἐλάφου τε καὶ λαγωοῦ, καὶ εἴ τι ἄλλο κατὰ τὸ τρέχειν πολύ τι τῶν λοιπῶν ζῴων ὑπεραίρει τοῖς πρὸς ταῦτα χρησίμοις, εὖ κατεσκευασμένοις μυσί τε καὶ νεύροις, οὕτω καὶ ἄνθρωπος, ἐπειδὴ τῶν λοιπῶν ζῴων πολὺ τῷ διανοεῖσθαι περίεστι, πολὺ τοῦτ' ἐστὶ πολύπλοκον. ἦσαν δὲ καὶ ἀποφύσεις τῶν νεύρων πᾶσαι ἀπὸ τοῦ ἐγκεφάλου, καὶ καθ' ὅλον εἰπεῖν ἀρχὴ φαίνεται εἶναι τῶν κατὰ τὸ σῶμα ὁ ἐγκέφαλος. ἥ τε γὰρ ἀπὸ τῶν ῥινῶν γιγνομένη αἴσθησις συντέτρητο ἐπὶ τοῦτον, καὶ ἀπὸ τῶν ὤτων. ἐφέροντο δὲ καὶ ἐπὶ γλώσσαν καὶ ἐπὶ τοὺς ὀφθαλμοὺς ἀποφύσεις ἀπὸ τοῦ ἐγκεφάλου. Cf. Galen's somewhat similar account and criticism in De usu partium, viii. 13, quoted above, p. 230, n. 3.

[2] Galen, De nat. fac. ii. 6, quoted above, p. 220, n. 1. Cf. AMG (1894), fr. 20 (quoted above, p. 223, n. 4), where paralysis is attributed by Erasistratus to the infiltration of liquid from the veins into the hollows of the nerves.

[3] Galen, De nat. fac. ii. 6, K. ii. 102: ἀλλ' ἡ μὲν ἁπλῆ φλὲψ ἐξ αὑτῆς τραφήσεται, τὸ νεῦρον δὲ καὶ ἡ ἀρτηρία παρὰ τῆς φλεβός.

[4] Wellmann, in RE. Wellmann's authority for this statement is, of course, Galen, De plac. Hipp. et Plat. vii. 3, K. v. 602, quoted above.

[5] According to Liddell and Scott s.v., the word is used by Theophrastus to describe the pith or heartwood : καλοῦσι δέ τινες τοῦτο (τὸ μεταξὺ τοῦ ξύλου) καρδίαν οἱ δ' ἐντεριώνην· ἔνιοι δὲ τὸ ἐντὸς τῆς μήτρας αὐτῆς καρδίαν, οἱ δὲ μυελόν. Apart from this I have not been able to find any actual quotation from Erasistratus which definitely states that he regarded the interior substance of the nerves as being marrow. Hippocrates uses the word ἐντεριώνη to describe just the interior of a gourd. Cf. the passage referred to in Liddell and Scott, taken from par. 78 of Diseases of women, Book i.

nonsense of his theory of muscular movement.[1] This does not, however, in my opinion, necessarily follow. There does not seem to be any reason why the pith of the nerves should not contain passages sufficient to enable the passing down them of that lightest of all substances, the psychic *pneuma*.

Erasistratus would appear to be the first of the ancient Greeks to make the extremely important distinction between sensory and motor nerves. Herophilus would seem to some extent to have pointed the way, by distinguishing between nerves which have to do with voluntary action and have their origin in the brain and/or the spinal marrow, as distinct from those which connect bones and bind together muscle to muscle and tie the joints together. The distinction of nerves from sinews has begun to make its appearance, but Herophilus has not arrived at the distinction between sensory and motor nerves, as such would both be included in his former category.

The unfortunate ambiguity of the word *neuron* was to persist to the end of the classical period. Herophilus is by tradition the discoverer of the nerves as a separate physiological system, but so little of him has survived that it is far from clear to what extent he really distinguished them absolutely from ligaments and tendons. Nor can we, as we have seen, with any degree of certainty altogether eliminate this confusion, which still exists to some extent in Galen, from Erasistratus, whose theory of the functioning of motor nerves is historically of great interest. Muscles, he taught, are formed of the threefold skein of nerves, arteries, and veins. Each strand has therefore a nerve entwined in it, and it shortens when its central portion is blown out by *pneuma*, for the expansion of the middle portion approximates the two ends.[2] A precisely similar idea is to be found, *mutatis mutandis*, in Borelli, the chief of the

---

[1] Verbecke, *L'Évolution de la doctrine du stoïcisme à S. Augustin* (Paris, 1945), pp. 184 ff.: 'En ce qui concerne les nerfs, la doctrine d'Érasistrate n'est pas constante. Au début de sa carrière, il les considérait comme des vaisseaux remplis du pneuma psychique: cette conception est très notable puisque les nerfs partent tous du cerveau et que le siège du pneuma psychique y est établi. Quant au nerf lui-même, Érasistrate a cru longtemps, nous rapporte Galien, qu'il était de la même substance que la membrane qui entoure le cerveau. Plus tard cependant des dissections plus minutieuses ont renversé ses conceptions: il a découvert que les nerfs ne sont pas des conduites du pneuma, mais que l'intérieur en est rempli de la même substance que le cerveau. Cette découverte a dû renverser de fond en comble les conceptions pneumatologiques d'Érasistrate: en effet quel rôle fait-il désormais attribuer au pneuma contenu dans le cerveau, s'il ne pénètre plus les nerfs pour commander toute l'activité de connaissance et de mouvement de l'homme?'

After quoting the well known passage from Galen's *Isagoge* concerning the two principles which manage the animal economy, he continues: 'Il n'est plus question dans ce texte d'un pneuma psychique ou d'une activité supérieure qui serait exercée par lui: ce silence est assez significatif. Quant au rôle qui est attribué au pneuma, il nous fait penser au πρῶτον ὄργανον d'Aristote et de Galien.'

[2] Galen, *De locis affectis*, vi. 5, K. viii. 429: καὶ γὰρ οὖν καὶ τοὺς μῦς ὁ Ἐρασίστρατος ἐκ τοῦ πληροῦσθαι πνεύματος εἰς εὖρος ἐπιδιδόντας ἀφαιρεῖν φησι τοῦ μήκους, καὶ διὰ τοῦτ' ἀνεσπάσθαι.

iatro-physicists, in his work *De motu animalium*, which was published in
Rome in 1680; only for Borelli the substance that made the middle of
the muscle fibre expand was not 'spirit' but the nervous juice.[1] This
theory was held for a number of years by many physicians. The absence
of any such swelling was only demonstrated experimentally by Swammerdam in 1700.[2]

[1] Borelli, *De motu animalium*, ii. 3, prop. xxii: 'Succus nerveus a voluntate instillari potest
intra musculos.' Borelli compares this nervous juice in prop. xxii with the ebullition caused
by pouring vitriol on *oleum Tartari*, or acids on salts. 'Igitur pariter in musculis non dis-
similis mistura fieri potest ex qua fermentatio et ebullitio subitanea subsequatur, a cujus
mole porositates musculorum repleantur et amplientur, et consequitur turgentia et inflatio.'

[2] For a description of the experiments by which Swammerdam disposed of Borelli's
theory of muscular movement, see Singer and Underwood, op. cit., pp. 133 f., where figures
are reproduced taken from his work.

AFTER the anatomical discoveries of Herophilus and Erasistratus little further progress was made in the knowledge of the heart and the vascular system. The followers of these two great masters contributed nothing, as far as we can judge, to the development of knowledge in this field, and the chief source of potential advance, the ability to dissect human bodies systematically as a part of medical training, came to an end, it would appear, after the expulsion of the physicians from Alexandria by Ptolemy Physkon who reigned from 146 to 117 B.C. Edelstein, indeed, in an early work maintained that this practice continued at Alexandria until the time of Galen,[1] but the only positive evidence which he produces is Galen's statement in the Prologue to his *Anatomical procedures* where he tells us that in the medical school at Alexandria human skeletons were available for the acquisition of first-hand knowledge of the human frame,[2] but in this as well as in other passages he makes it plain that human bodies were not. And the importance of knowledge of the human skeleton is accentuated precisely because our knowledge of the human organs must depend on dissection of monkeys and other creatures like the human animal, and it is only through an accurate knowledge of the human skeleton that we can make the proper morphological analogies.[3] The

---

[1] Edelstein, op. cit., Bd. 3, Heft 2.

[2] Galen, *De anatomicis administrationibus*, i. 2, K. ii. 226: ἔργον δέ σοι γενέσθω καὶ σπούδασμα, μὴ μόνον ἐκ τοῦ βιβλίου τὴν ἰδέαν ἑκάστου τῶν ὀστῶν ἀκριβῶς ἐκμαθεῖν, ἀλλὰ καὶ διὰ τῶν ὀμμάτων σύντονον αὐτόπτην αὐτὸν ἐργάσασθαι τῶν ἀνθρωπείων ὀστῶν. ἔστι δ' ἐν Ἀλεξανδρείᾳ μὲν τοῦτο πάνυ ῥᾴδιον, ὥστε καὶ τὴν διδασκαλίαν αὐτῶν τοῖς φοιτηταῖς οἱ κατ' ἐκεῖνο τὸ χωρίον ἰατροὶ μετὰ τῆς αὐτοψίας πορίζονται.

[3] Ibid., 218–20: ὁποῖόν τι ταῖς σκηναῖς οἱ καλούμενοι κάμακές εἰσιν, καὶ ταῖς οἰκίαις οἱ τοῖχοι, τοιοῦτον ἐν τοῖς ζῴοις ἥ γε τῶν ὀστῶν οὐσία. συνεξομοιοῦσθαι γὰρ αὐτῇ τἆλλα καὶ συμμεταβάλλεσθαι πέφυκεν. οἷον εἰ τῷ ζῴῳ τὸ κράνιον ἢ στρογγύλον, ἀνάγκη καὶ τὸν ἐγκέφαλον τοιοῦτον εἶναι, ὥσπερ γε καί, εἰ πρόμηκες, προμήκης τούτῳ τῷ ζῴῳ καὶ ὁ ἐγκέφαλος. εἰ δὲ γένυες σμικραί, καὶ τὸ πρόσωπον ὅλον στρογγυλώτερον, ἀνάγκη καὶ τοὺς μῦς αὐτῶν εἶναι σμικρούς... διὰ τοῦτο γοῦν καὶ ὁ πίθηκος ἁπάντων τῶν ζῴων ὁμοιότατος ἀνθρώπῳ καὶ σπλάγχνοις καὶ μυσὶ καὶ ἀρτηρίαις καὶ φλεψὶ καὶ νεύροις, ὅτι καὶ τῇ τῶν ὀστῶν ἰδέᾳ. διὰ γὰρ τὴν τούτων φύσιν ἐπί τε δυοῖν βαδίζει σκελοῖν, καὶ τοῖς προσθίοις κώλοις ὥσπερ χερσὶ χρῆται, καὶ στέρνον πλατύτατον ἁπάντων τῶν τετραπόδων ἔχει, καὶ κλεῖς ὡσαύτως ἀνθρώπῳ, καὶ πρόσωπον στρογγύλον καὶ τράχηλον μικρόν. τούτων δ' ὁμοίων ὑπαρχόντων, οὐκ ἐνδέχεται τοὺς μῦς ἑτεροίως ἔχειν. ἐπιτέτανται γὰρ οὗτοι τοῖς ὀστοῖς ἔξωθεν. ὥστε καὶ τὸ μέγεθος αὐτῶν καὶ τὸ σχῆμα μιμοῦνται. τούτοις δ'

prohibition of human dissection did not, of course, imply that the practice of dissecting and vivisecting animal bodies also ceased. There do,
however, seem to have been considerable differences in the attitude
taken up with regard to this practice by the various medical schools
transplanted from Alexandria to Rome. The Empirics were inclined, as
Sir Clifford Allbutt put it,[1] to scoff at the study of anatomy as otiose,
while the Methodists, whose remote ancestor was undoubtedly Erasistratus, with certain exceptions (notably Soranus) were also, it seems,
inclined to look upon it as a matter for idle curiosity. Only the Dogmatists seem to have practised it regularly. Not that it died out even so
in the great medical schools of the Empire, Alexandria, Pergamum,
Laodicea, or Smyrna, to mention only a few. Indeed, before the end of the
first century A.D., if not earlier, the study of anatomy had been established in Rome, as the work of Celsus would clearly appear to imply,
but little or nothing new in the field in which we are interested can be
traced to the period between Erasistratus and Galen. The pseudo-
Galenic work *Medical definitions*, which is considered to be a product
of the Pneumatic school, mentions the Dogmatists, the school which was
founded on the *Hippocratic corpus* and tradition, as practising anatomy
systematically, as opposed to the Empirics, whose knowledge of anatomical facts was gained only incidentally, from the observation of wounds
and other injuries.[2]

There was, however, one department of studies, concerned with the
vascular system more than with the heart, to which a great deal of attention was devoted, namely the examination and analysis of the arterial
pulse. In this field several works have survived, though their attributions
are in some cases doubtful. The more important developments after
Herophilus were chiefly made by the Pneumatic school, founded by
Athenaeus of Attalia, a pupil of the Stoic philosopher Poseidonius[3] (one
of Cicero's masters), who died in Rome at the age of 84 in 51 B.C. They
culminated in the work of Archigenes of Apamea, the Eclectic, who
practised in Rome during the reign of Trajan (A.D. 98–117). None of the
writings of the earlier members of this school has survived, though some
of the therapeutic works of the most influential later physicians of the
school, e.g. Aretaeus of Cappadocia who may have lived in the reign of

---

ἀκολουθοῦσιν ἀρτηρίαι καὶ φλέβες καὶ νεῦρα. καὶ ταῦτ' οὖν ὅμοια τοῖς ὁμοίοις ὀστοῖς. ἐπεὶ τοίνυν
ἥ τε μορφὴ τοῦ σώματος ὁμοιοῦται τοῖς ὀστοῖς, ἥ τε τῶν ἄλλων μορίων φύσις ἕπεται τοῖσδε.

[1] Allbutt, *Greek Medicine in Rome* (London, 1921), pp. 196–7, 317.

[2] Galen (?), *Definitiones medicae*, def. xxxiv, K. xix. 357: ἀνατομή ἐστι θεωρία τῶν ἐν κατακαλύψει σπλάγχνων· εἰσὶ τῆς ἀνατομῆς εἴδη δύο, τὸ μὲν κατ' ἐπιτήδευσιν, τὸ δὲ κατὰ περίπτωσιν. κατ'
ἐπιτήδευσιν μὲν οὖν ἐστιν ἡ ἀπὸ τῶν δογματικῶν παραλαμβανομένη θέα ἕνεκα τῆς ἐν κατακαλύψει
ἤτοι ἐπὶ τῶν ζώντων, ἢ ἐπὶ τῶν τετελευτηκότων, ἢ καὶ ἤτοι ὅλων ἢ μερῶν· κατὰ δὲ περίπτωσιν ἐκ
συντυχίας ἢ ὑπὸ μεγάλης τρώσεως γινομένη· προσχρῶνται δὲ αὐτῇ μόνοι οἱ ἐμπειρικοί.

[3] See F. Kudlien, 'Poseidonius und die Aertzteschule der Pneumatiker', *Hermes*, 90
(1962).

Vespasian, have been preserved. Of Archigenes himself only fragments handed down in quotations, etc., have survived. But we are fairly well acquainted with his doctrines.[1] There are also two smaller works in the *Galenic corpus* which are generally considered, e.g. by Wellmann,[2] to have been written by members of this school, namely the *Medical definitions* and the essay *On the pulse to Antonius*.

The teachings of the Pneumatic school form, as Wellmann has pointed out, a rather curious conflation of the Stoic philosophy with the main doctrines of the so-called Dogmatic school,[3] based on the teachings drawn from the *Hippocratic corpus*, e.g. of the four-humour theory of disease and the four elements which have been transformed into qualities, hot, cold, wet, and dry,[4] together with certain legacies of the Cnidian–Sicilian schools, such as the primacy of the heart as opposed to that of the brain, though this doctrine was not held by all members of the school. One might perhaps have expected that the Alexandrian work on the brain and the nervous system with its insistence on the brain as the seat of consciousness would have disposed once and for all of the conception of the primacy of the heart. But old errors in the field of science even today sometimes die hard, and the science of the two centuries divided by the beginning of the Christian era was not sufficiently coherent or well founded to administer the death-blow to this error. The Stoic philosophy from Zeno onwards, though it adopted Plato's conception of the world-soul, of which it made the human soul as it were a spark, or fragment, refused to follow his location of the reason in the head. Moreover, it tended with its doctrine of *pneuma* to interpret the soul wherever it could, in materialistic terms.[5] For *pneuma* is for the Stoics a rather confusing mixture—a combination of the luminiferous ether, a field of force, and a sort of mind-stuff.[6]

---

[1] Extracts of Archigenes were published by E. Rhode in *Rhein. Mus.* 28, and Archigenes' work is frequently quoted by Antyllus, Soranus, Alexander of Tralles, Oribasius, and Paul of Aegina, as well as by Galen and Aetius.

[2] Wellmann, *Die pneumatische Schule* (Berlin, 1895), pp. 65 ff.

[3] Ibid., part 2, pp. 131–53.

[4] Cf. Galen (?), *Definitiones medicae*, def. xxxi, K. xix. 356: στοιχεῖόν ἐστιν ἐξ οὗ πρώτου καὶ ἁπλουστάτου τὰ πάντα γέγονε καὶ εἰς ὃ ἁπλούστατον τὰ πάντα ἀναλυθήσεται ὂν ἔσχατον. καὶ Ἀθηναῖος ὁ Ἀτταλεὺς ἐν τῷ τρίτῳ βιβλίῳ φησὶν οὕτως· στοιχεῖα τῆς ἰατρικῆς ἐστι καθάπερ τινὲς τῶν ἀρχαίων ὑπέλαβον, τὸ θερμὸν καὶ τὸ ψυχρὸν καὶ τὸ ὑγρὸν καὶ τὸ ξηρόν, ἐξ ὧν πρώτων φαινομένων καὶ ἁπλουστάτων καὶ ἐλαχίστων ὁ ἄνθρωπος συνέστηκε. But these abstract elements would appear to have only a conceptual existence: the material body is composed of the four ὑλικὰ στοιχεῖα, namely earth, air, fire, and water as laid down in def. xxxiii, K. xix. 357: ἐκ τίνων συνέστηκεν ἡμῶν τὰ ὑλικὰ σώματα; ἐκ τεσσάρων· πυρός, ἀέρος, γῆς καὶ ὕδατος· ἅτινα καὶ ὑλικὰ στοιχεῖα καλοῦνται.

[5] Zeno seems to have regarded it, following Anaximenes, as Verbecke points out, op. cit., pp. 21 f., as hot air. See Diogenes Laertius, *Hist. phil.* vii. 157: Ζήνων δὲ ὁ Κιτιεὺς ... πνεῦμα ἔνθερμον εἶναι τὴν ψυχήν. τούτῳ γὰρ ἡμᾶς εἶναι ἐμπνόους καὶ ὑπὸ τούτου κινεῖσθαι. Cf. Rufus, *De nomine partium*, D–R 166: θερμασίαν δὲ καὶ πνεῦμα Ζήνων τὸ αὐτὸ εἶναί φησιν.

[6] Galen (?), *Def. med.*, def. xxix, K. xix. 355: ψυχή ἐστιν οὐσία ἀσώματος αὐτοκίνητος κατὰ

On the vascular system, the Pneumatic school followed Herophilus much more closely than Erasistratus, whose theory of *pneuma* might have been expected to fit their general teaching very conveniently. They accepted the presence of blood in the arteries, and though they regarded the heart as the principal organ, this belief did not inspire them to make any new discoveries about it, in respect either of the manner in which it works or of its physiological significance. They came no nearer to discovering the truth of the circulation. Indeed their theory of *pneuma* rather led them away from it. But they paid great attention to the pulse, the relation of which to the beating of the heart they did not interpret in the simple mechanistic fashion of Erasistratus, but elaborated into an over-complicated series of differentiations the foundations of which had already been laid by Herophilus.

None of the works of the founder of the school, Athenaeus, has survived, but as the writer of the pseudo-Galenic *Medical definitions* informs us, he did write a work with this title,[1] though it is not to be identified with the *Definitions* included in the Galenic canon, which is also regarded both by Diels[2] and by Valentin Rose[3] as proceeding from the Pneumatic school, in spite of the fact that on one point of particular importance it differs from Stoic doctrine in teaching that the brain not the heart is the seat of the governing principle.[4] Athenaeus followed closely the teaching of his master Poseidonius on this point, who like Aristotle, Galen tells us, did not distinguish different parts of the soul or locate these, like Plato, in different parts of the body, but regarded these 'parts' as powers or faculties of a single substance resident in the heart.[5] The date of the *Definitions* cannot be determined with any certainty, but it was probably written some time before Galen, who receives no mention in it, and after Agathinus, who flourished in the first century A.D. and was the master of

Πλάτωνα. κατὰ δὲ τοὺς Στωϊκοὺς σῶμα λεπτομερὲς ἐξ ἑαυτοῦ κινούμενον κατὰ σπερματικοὺς λόγους . . . ἄλλως· ψυχή ἐστι πνεῦμα παρεσπαρμένον ἐν ὅλῳ τῷ σώματι δι' οὗ ζῶμεν καὶ λογιζόμεθα καὶ ταῖς λοιπαῖς αἰσθήσεσιν ἐνεργοῦμεν ὑπηρετοῦντος τοῦ σώματος.

[1] Ibid., Introd., K. xix. 347: μετὰ δὲ τοὺς τούτου χρόνους Ἱπποκράτους οἱ γενόμενοί τινες συνέγραψαν ὅρους, καὶ οὗτοι δὲ οὐ πάντας· δοκοῦσι δὲ ἐπιμελεῖς γεγονέναι ἐν τῇ τοιαύτῃ θεωρίᾳ οἵ τε ἀπὸ τῆς Ἡροφίλου αἱρέσεως καὶ Ἀπολλώνιος ὁ Μεμφίτης, ἔτι δὲ καὶ Ἀθηναῖος ὁ Ἀτταλεύς, ἀλλὰ καὶ οὗτοι οὔτε τῇ τάξει τῇ δεούσῃ ἐχρήσαντο.

[2] H. Diels, 'Ueber das physikalische System des Straton', *Sitzber. d. K. Preuss. Akad. d. Wisschft.* (1893), p. 102, n. 2.

[3] Valentin Rose, *Anecdota Latina et Graeca*, ii (Berlin, 1870), p. 170.

[4] Galen (?), *Def. med.*, def. cxiii, K. xix. 378: ἡγεμονικόν ἐστι ψυχῆς τὸ ἄρχον τῶν μερῶν τῆς ψυχῆς τὸ βασιλεῦον καὶ ἐπιτάσσον, καθιδρυμένον δὲ ἐν τῇ βάσει τοῦ ἐγκεφάλου. οἱ δὲ οὕτως. ἡγεμονικὸν ψυχῆς ἐστι τὸ κατάρχον τῆς ὅλης τοῦ ζῴου διοικήσεως, τεταγμένον δὲ ἐν τῇ καρδίᾳ τοῦ ἐγκεφάλου. The last sentence has a rather curious expression using the word καρδία to describe the ventricle of the brain. May we assume this to be a scribal substitution for the word κοιλία?

[5] Galen, *De plac. Hipp. et Plat.* vi. 2, K. v. 515: ὁ μὲν οὖν Πλάτων καὶ τοῖς τόποις τοῦ σώματος κεχωρίσθαι νομίζων αὐτὰ καὶ ταῖς οὐσίαις πάμπολυ διαλλάττειν, εὐλόγως εἴδη τε καὶ μέρη προσαγορεύει· ὁ δ' Ἀριστοτέλης τε καὶ ὁ Ποσειδώνιος εἴδη μὲν ἢ μέρη ψυχῆς οὐκ ὀνομάζουσιν, δυνάμεις δ' εἶναί φασι μιᾶς οὐσίας ἐκ τῆς καρδίας ὁρμωμένης.

Archigenes, since it mentions four sects, Dogmatists, Empirics, Methodists, and Eclectics, the school of which Agathinus was the founder.[1]

The Stoic teachings of Athenaeus are described in the Galenic(?) treatise, *Introduction or the doctor*. Athenaeus, we are told, regarded the ultimate constituents of the human body as being, not the four elements or first bodies (earth, air, fire, and water), but their qualities, heat, cold, dryness, and wetness, which he practically substantialized. Of these, he regarded two as active (ποιητικά), namely heat and cold, and two as passive (ὑλικά), namely dryness and wetness. And, good Stoic as he was, he brought in a fifth element in the form of *pneuma*, which interpenetrates everything, by which everything is held together and made to function. Instead of attributing disease to the wrong mixture of the four elements and the forces resulting from this, like Hippocrates, Athenaeus, and Archigenes, he attributed both health and disease to the all-pervading *pneuma*—diseases being caused in the first instance by affections of this substance—hence the name of *Pneumatic* as applied to the school.[2] The combination of cosmological and physiological functions allotted to *pneuma* by this school is not always easy to follow, but much light has been thrown on some of the underlying basic conceptions not only by Sambursky,[3] but also in connection with their physiological ideas by Rüsche.[4]

The Pneumatic school linked very closely the *pneuma* and the innate heat, but so little of their writings has survived—of their original founders, Athenaeus and Archigenes, nothing at all—that it is not easy to obtain any exact idea of the manner in which they believed the two to be related to each other. Rufus of Ephesus informs us that Zeno the philosopher identified the two, but that the physicians kept them distinct. For in the animal, *pneuma* and heat are both 'native': the two expressions πνεῦμα σύμφυτον and ἔμφυτον θερμόν are practically equivalent, but, as we have noted, the inborn *pneuma* of the embryo is different

---

[1] Galen (?), *Def. med.*, def. xiv, K. xix. 353: ἰατρικῆς αἱρέσεις αἱ πρῶται δύο ἐμπειρικὴ καὶ λογικὴ καὶ τρίτη μεθοδική. δοκεῖ δὲ τετάρτην αἵρεσιν ἐξευρεῖν Ἀγαθῖνος ὁ Λακεδαιμόνιος, ἣν ὠνόμασεν ἐπισυνθετικήν, ἔνιοι δὲ ἐκλεκτικήν. ἕτεροι τὴν ἑκτικήν.

[2] Galen, *Introductio*, 9, K. xiv. 698 f.: κατὰ δὲ τὸν Ἀθηναῖον στοιχεῖα ἀνθρώπου οὐ τὰ τέσσαρα πρῶτα σώματα, πῦρ καὶ ἀὴρ καὶ ὕδωρ καὶ γῆ, ἀλλ' αἱ ποιότητες αὐτῶν, τὸ θερμὸν καὶ τὸ ψυχρόν, καὶ τὸ ξηρὸν καὶ τὸ ὑγρόν, ὧν δύο μὲν τὰ ποιητικὰ αἴτια ὑποτίθεται, τὸ θερμὸν καὶ τὸ ψυχρόν, δύο δὲ τὰ ὑλικά, τὸ ξηρὸν καὶ τὸ ὑγρόν, καὶ πέμπτον παρεισάγει κατὰ τοὺς Στωϊκούς, τὸ διῆκον διὰ πάντων πνεῦμα, ὑφ' οὗ τὰ πάντα συνέχεσθαι καὶ διοικεῖσθαι. Ἱπποκράτης μὲν οὖν διὰ τριῶν κεχώρηκεν, εἰπὼν στοιχεῖα ἀνθρώπου ἴσχοντα, ἰσχόμενα, ἐνορμῶντα, δι' ὧν τὰ πάντα τῶν μετ' αὐτὸν περιείληφε στοιχεῖα καὶ τὴν κατὰ στοιχείων φυσιολογίαν τε καὶ αἰτιολογίαν τῶν παρὰ φύσιν ... οἱ δὲ περὶ Ἀθηναῖον καὶ Ἀρχιγένην, μόνῳ τῷ διήκοντι δι' αὐτῶν πνεύματι καὶ τὰ φυσικὰ συνεστάναι τε καὶ διοικεῖσθαι, καὶ τὰ νοσήματα πάντα τούτου πρωτοπαθοῦντος γίνεσθαι ἀπεφήναντο, ὅθεν καὶ πνευματικοὶ χρηματίζουσι. Cf. Hippocrates, *De flatibus*, 4: διότι μὲν οὖν ἐν τοῖς ὅλοις ὁ ἀὴρ ἔρρωται, εἴρηται· τοῖς δ' αὖ θνητοῖσιν οὗτος αἴτιος τοῦ τε βίου καὶ τῶν νούσεων τοῖσι νοσέουσι.

[3] Sambursky, *Physics of the Stoics* (London, 1959), especially chs. 1 and 2.

[4] Rüsche, op. cit., pp. 259–75.

from that of the living animal after birth. The infant when it draws its first cold breath changes its character and becomes a living thing or animal. Indeed, Plutarch tells us the Stoics derived the word *psyche* from the verb *psychein*, which means to cool. Wellmann[1] cites as an example of their relation the theory of one of the later Pneumatists. He believes that though for the Pneumatists innate *pneuma* and innate heat are two distinct forces, they believed that the latter was generated by the former owing to the friction engendered in its incessant movement through the body, presumably even in the embryo, and that the cold *pneuma* taken into the heart in respiration was assimilated to the innate *pneuma* and thus became the vehicle of the innate heat, and could therefore be identified with it. The theory of the generation of the innate heat by pneumatic friction is vouched for by a passage taken from the great surgeon Antyllus, which has been preserved in Oribasius. Antyllus appears to have held the view that the heat generated by the friction of the innate *pneuma* was so great that it would be enough to kill one with fever, unless it was cooled by the inspiration of air from the outside.[2]

The process of respiration has, according to the Pneumatists, a double function, that of cooling the innate heat and that of nourishing the vital spirit, a double function which had been inherited from the medical tradition of the age of Aristotle, and even earlier, in accordance with 'Hippocratic' teaching.[3] It also provides material for the generation of the 'animal' or 'psychic' spirit. This theory of the double function of the process of respiration, which we shall find again in Galen, has a fairly long history. The idea that respiration provides nourishment or increase for the *pneuma* is, of course, very old—probably as old as any physiological theory we know of. We have found it, for instance, worked out by the Sicilian school of the fifth century B.C., where the connection between the *pneuma* and the heart is emphasized.[4] The theory of the heart as the centre or seat of the innate heat is also old—quite how old the fragmentary nature of our earlier authorities does not permit us to determine—and the theory of the cooling of this heat must also be of great antiquity. We

---

[1] Wellmann, *Die pneumatische Schule*, p. 137: 'Pneuma und innere Wärme sind ihnen im Grunde verschiedene Kräfte. Das Pneuma ist das Eingeatmete, das sich dem σύμφυτον πνεῦμα assimiliert, während sich die innere Wärme erst aus dem innerem Pneuma in Folge einer durch Reibung verursachten mannigfachen Bewegung entwickelt. Dadurch wird allerdings das Pneuma wesentlich Träger desselben, und kann deshalb mit dem ἔμφυτον θερμόν identificiert werden.'

[2] See the quotation from Antyllus in Oribasius, *C.M.G.* vi. 1. i. 163: τὸ γὰρ πνεῦμα τὴν ἐν ἡμῖν θερμασίαν τῷ πολυκινήτῳ τῆς φορᾶς κατὰ τὴν παράτριψιν ἐγείρει καὶ ζωπυρεῖ, τοσαύτην ἀποτελοῦν διὰ τὸ τῆς ἐνεργείας ἀδιάλειπτον ἐν τῷ σώματι πύρωσιν, ὥστε εἰ μὴ παρ' ἕκαστον ἀναψύχομεν ἑαυτοὺς διὰ τῆς ἀναπνοῆς καταψύξει, λαθεῖν ἂν ὅμοια παθόντας τοῖς εἰς πολλὴν ἐμπεσοῦσιν ἔγκαυσιν.

[3] See above, pp. 79–80, 90–1, 164.

[4] See above, pp. 7–8, 104, 106–7.

found it, as we have already noticed, in Aristotle's treatise *On respiration*,[1] but it is much older than Aristotle.

The account given in the *Definitions* of the heart and the blood vessels is of some interest, since it furnishes a clue to the general ideas of the Pneumatist school on the relations between the vascular and the respiratory systems, as well as introducing a distinction between three kinds of *pneuma*.

The heart is sinew-, muscle-, and vein-like; it also has arteries, and it is shaped like a cone and rather fatty. Out of it grow arteries and veins, through which blood and *pneuma* are set forth. Or else, the heart is like a muscle, and has the shape of a cone, with two ventricles in which are generated the innate heat and the vital *pneuma*. Arteries and veins grow out of it, through which the vital seed and the innate heat are supplied to the whole body.[2]

Blood is defined as wet and hot, the stuff of which the organism is nourished, and there is more of it in the veins than in the arteries.[3] The contents and functions of the two kinds of blood vessel are described as follows:

A vein is a vessel for blood and the natural *pneuma* which is mixed with it, sinew-like, containing perception and the wet and hot substance. It has more blood [than the artery] and less of the vital *pneuma*.[4]

An artery is a vessel containing less but purer blood and more of the natural *pneuma* mixed with it and in a more refined form. It is hotter and drier and more perceiving than the vein, and it moves in a movement of pulsation. [Or else] An artery is a hollow body with two coats, arising out of the heart and supplying vital *pneuma*. It receives or takes in pure air in systole and expels in diastole smoky and sooty superfluities. Bringing in clean air it cools the heart and the innate heat. Now the function of respiration is to cool by means of air. This substance of air also serves to generate and to increase our *pneuma* in generating and adding to the psychic *pneuma*.[5]

---

[1] See above, p. 169.

[2] Galen (?), *Def. med.*, def. xlix, K. xix. 360: καρδία ἐστὶ νευρώδης καὶ μυώδης καὶ φλεβώδης, ἔχουσα καὶ ἀρτηρίας. κωνοειδὴς τῷ σχήματι, ὑποπίμελος, ἐξ ἧς ἐκπεφύκασιν ἀρτηρίαι καὶ φλέβες, δι' ὧν ἐπιπέμπεται αἷμα καὶ πνεῦμα. ἄλλως. καρδία ἐστὶ μυώδης, ἔχουσα σχῆμα κωνοειδὲς καὶ δύο κοιλίας ἐν αἷς γεννᾶται τὸ ἔμφυτον θερμὸν καὶ τὸ ζωτικὸν πνεῦμα, ἐξ ἧς ἐκπεφύκασιν ἀρτηρίαι καὶ φλέβες ἐκφύονται, δι' ὧν χορηγεῖται τῷ παντὶ σώματι ὅ τε ζωτικὸς γόνος καὶ ἡ ἔμφυτος θερμασία.

[3] Ibid., def. lxvi, K. xix. 364: αἷμά ἐστι θερμὸν καὶ ὑγρὸν ἐν ταῖς φλεψὶ πλεῖον, ἐν ἀρτηρίαις ὀλιγώτερον ἐξ οὗ τὸ ζῷον τρέφεται.

[4] Ibid., def. lxxiii, K. xix. 365: φλέψ ἐστιν ἀγγεῖον αἵματος καὶ τοῦ συγκεκραμένου τῷ αἵματι φυσικοῦ πνεύματος, νευρώδης, τὴν αἴσθησιν καὶ τὴν ὑγρὰν καὶ θερμὴν οὐσίαν ἔχουσα. ἔχει δὲ πλεῖον τὸ αἷμα, ὀλιγώτερον δὲ τὸ ζωτικὸν πνεῦμα.

[5] Ibid., def. lxxiv: ἀρτηρία ἐστὶν ἀγγεῖον αἵματος ἐλάττονος καὶ καθαρωτέρου καὶ τοῦ συγκεκραμένου φυσικοῦ πνεύματος πλείονος καὶ λεπτομερεστέρου, θερμοτέρα καὶ ξηροτέρα καὶ αἰσθητικωτέρα τῆς φλεβὸς σφυγμωδῶς κινουμένη. ἄλλως. ἀρτηρία ἐστὶ σῶμα κοῖλον διχίτωνον, ἐκ καρδίας ὁρμώμενον πνεύματος ζωτικοῦ χορηγόν. δέχεται δὲ καθαρὸν ἀέρα ἐν τῇ συστολῇ καὶ ἐκκρίνει ἐν τῇ διαστολῇ τὰ καπνώδη καὶ λιγνυώδη περιττώματα. εἰσφέρουσα οὖν καθαρὸν ἀέρα ψύχει τὴν

This account is of some interest in several points. First, the notion that the blood vessels perceive, a doctrine which it would appear derives ultimately from Empedocles, who located consciousness in the blood surrounding the heart.[1] Secondly, the distinction between the different kinds of *pneuma* also merits attention. The distinction between 'natural' and 'vital' *pneuma* is not easy to grasp. They seem to be two different names given to the same thing. Both arteries and veins contain 'vital' *pneuma*, but that in the arteries is more refined. There can be little doubt that here we have the foundation for the theory developed by the later Galenists, if not by Galen himself, of the three 'spirits', natural, vital, and animal. A rather similar theory of *pneuma* in the veins is also to be found in Apollonius of Pergamum,[2] Galen's native city, a physician of the first century A.D.

It will be remembered also that in the *De corde* of the *Hippocratic corpus* the right ventricle is made to draw, through a leaky pulmonary valve, a certain amount of *pneuma* from the lung, which, no doubt, was to be mixed with the venous blood which fed the tissues.

Definitions cviii and cix define the distinction between respiration and transpiration. The first is performed by the movement of the thorax and the lungs. It consists of two parts, inspiration and expiration. In inspiration air is drawn through the nostrils and the mouth into the brain, and through the pharynx and the lung into the heart. Some of it also passes into the belly. Of the amount taken in, only a small portion is returned into the surrounding air.[3] The second is defined as the involuntary drawing in of air by the natural heat through the surface of the body and the parts lying between the surface and the heart, or in other words, a drawing in of air from all over the body by a process of natural (i.e. unconscious) attraction, and the return of the same through the channels of exit, i.e. the pores.[4]

The picture which emerges from these definitions is anything but clear and consistent—perhaps the most puzzling feature is the notion of the

καρδίαν καὶ τὸ ἔμφυτον θερμόν. ἡ χρεία γοῦν τοῦ σφυγμοῦ αὕτη ἐστί, τὸ ἐμψύχεσθαι διὰ τοῦ ἀέρος. ἔστι δὲ καὶ αὕτη οὐσία τοῦ ἀέρος τὸ προστίθεσθαι τῷ ἡμετέρῳ πνεύματι γέννησις καὶ προσθήκη τοῦ ψυχικοῦ πνεύματος.

[1] See above, p. 18.

[2] See Oribasius, *C.M.G.* vi. 1. i. 218 (quoted by Verbecke, op. cit., p. 198): τὸ μὲν οὖν φλέβας διαιρεῖν πολλάκις τοῦ ἔτους οὐκ ἐπιτήδειον ἡγούμην ἐννοῶν ὅτι ἅμα τῷ αἵματι πολὺ συνεκκρίνεται τὸ ζωτικὸν πνεῦμα.

[3] Galen (?), *Def. med.*, def. cvii, K. xix. 375: ἀναπνοή ἐστι κίνησις θώρακος καὶ πνεύμονος. μέρη δὲ αὐτῆς εἰσι δύο, εἰσπνοὴ καὶ ἐκπνοή. ἢ οὕτως· ἀναπνοή ἐστιν ὁλκὴ ἀέρος διὰ στόματος καὶ μυκτήρων εἰς ἐγκέφαλον καὶ διὰ φάρυγγος καὶ πνεύμονος εἰς καρδίαν. πάρεισι δέ τοι καὶ εἰς τὴν κοιλίαν. καὶ ἐκ τοῦ ληφθέντος πάλιν ὀλίγη τις ἀνταπόδοσις εἰς τὸ περιέχον γίνεται.

[4] Ibid., def. cix: διαπνοή ἐστιν ὁλκὴ ἀέρος ἀπροαίρετος ὑπὸ τοῦ φυσικοῦ θερμοῦ διὰ τῆς ἐπιφανείας ἅμα τοῖς συναπερχομένοις αὐτοῦ σώματος γινομένη. ἑτέρως· διαπνοή ἐστιν ἐκ τοῦ σώματος ὁλκὴ ἀέρος μετ' ὀρέξεως φυσικῆς δι' ὅλου τοῦ σώματος καὶ πάλιν δι' ἐξόδων ἀπόκρισις.

arteries receiving air at systole and expelling it at diastole. If this referred
to the systole and diastole of the heart on Erasistratan principles it
would make sense. But it looks as if this is not what the Pneumatists
believed. The theory that the arteries draw in air at systole, however
contrary it must appear to the most elementary laws of pneumatics,
was, it would seem, held by more than one eminent physician. Thus
Galen tells us that it was held by Archigenes and also by some of his
predecessors, perhaps by Athenaeus, though he is not specifically mentioned.[1] The reason for this preposterous theory alleged to have been
given by its supporters was that they observed that both mouth and
nose narrowed their openings in inspiration and widened them on expiration, a phenomenon seen in sick persons. Galen admits that this phenomenon may indeed sometimes be observed in sick persons, but only
in the cartilaginous endings of the nostrils, and in persons engaged in
running or other forms of violent exercise. But this does not prove anything about the movement of the arteries, even if we were to admit that
their endings were analogous to the lips and the nostrils. Thorax and
lungs expand when they draw in air and contract when they expel it,
and the same process must apply to the arteries also. Moreover the analogy
between pulsation and respiration is confirmed by the fact that the
interval of quiet after systole is much longer than that which occurs
between diastole and systole, just as the interval of quiet which occurs
before inspiration is longer than that occurring after it, i.e. between
inspiration and expiration.[2]

In spite of the fact that they knew that the arteries contained blood,
the Pneumatists reached no further. They realized, as Herophilus had
done, that the pulse was somehow connected with the beat of the heart;
indeed, like Galen after them, they regarded both as a single movement,
but this movement was not connected at all with the transmission of
blood from the ventricles, but with the absorption of air or *pneuma* from
outside the body through the pores of the skin as well as through the
mouth and nose. It should be noted that in the definition of transpiration

---

[1] Galen, *De usu puls.* 4, K. v. 162: καίτοι γιγνώσκω τοὺς περὶ τὸν Ἀρχιγένην καί τινας ἔτι
πρότερον ἐν μὲν ταῖς συστολαῖς πληροῦσθαι τὰς ἀρτηρίας οἰομένους, ἐν δὲ ταῖς διαστολαῖς κενοῦσθαι.

[2] Ibid., 162–3: πρὸς γὰρ τὴν ἕλξιν ἐπιτηδειοτάτην εἶναι νομίζουσι τὴν συστολήν, τεκμαιρό-
μενοι μάλιστα τῷ τε στόματι καὶ ταῖς ῥισὶν κατὰ μὲν τὰς εἰσπνοάς, ὡς ἐκεῖνοί φασι, συστελλομένοις,
κατὰ δὲ τὰς ἐκπνοὰς διαστελλομένοις. ὅπερ ἐπὶ τῶν ἀρρώστων μὲν τὴν δύναμιν ὁρᾶται γιγνόμενον.
οὐδ᾽ οὖν οὐδ᾽ ἐπὶ τούτων, κἂν ἄλλο τι μόριον ᾖ ἐν τοῖς ὑστάτοις καὶ χονδρώδεσι τῶν ῥινῶν. ὁρᾶται
δέ ποτε κἀπὶ τῶν δραμόντων ὠκέως ἢ ἄλλως πως συντόνως γυμναζομένων ... οὐ γὰρ δὴ ἀνάλογον
φήσουσιν ἔχειν ταῖς ἀρτηρίαις τὰ χείλη καὶ τὰς ῥίνας. ἀλλὰ τούτοις μὲν ἀνάλογον τὰ πέρατα
τῶν ἀρτηριῶν, αὐταῖς δὲ ταῖς ἀρτηρίαις αἱ ἀπὸ τούτων ἐπὶ τὴν καρδίαν οἷον ὁδοὶ τοῦ πνεύματός
εἰσιν ... ὥσπερ ἡ φάρυγξ καὶ ὁ πνεύμων, καὶ σύμπας ὁ θώραξ ἐν ταῖς εἰσπνοαῖς διαστέλλεται, καὶ
τὰς ἀρτηρίας οὕτω χρῆναι διίστασθαι, καθ᾽ ὃν ἕλκουσι καιρὸν οὐ καθ᾽ ὃν ἐκπέμπουσι τὸ πνεῦμα.
ἀλλὰ καὶ ἡ μετὰ τὴν συστολὴν αὐτῶν ἡσυχία πολλῷ μακροτέρα γιγνομένη τῆς μετὰ τὴν διαστολήν,
ὥσπερ καὶ ἡ πρὸ τῆς εἰσπνοῆς τῆς μετ᾽ αὐτήν, ἐνδείκνυταί τινα καὶ κατὰ τοῦτο ἀναλογίαν εἶναι
τοῖς σφυγμοῖς πρὸς τὴν ἀναπνοήν.

just cited, no mention is made of the heart, and the channels of exit for the air absorbed through the skin are not specified as arteries, and bear a strong resemblance to the 'pores' of Empedocles. Nor does the description of the later Pneumatist Antyllus make it plain that the 'pores' through which the air is drawn in by the surface of the body are arterioles. His explanation of respiration and transpiration proceeds on the strictly mechanical Erasistratan principle of the *horror vacui*. In both cases the entry of the air from the outside atmosphere is governed by physical law.[1] The principal function of the arteries is to distribute *pneuma* by their pulsation, along with a little of the most refined and lightest blood. But this blood has only one function, to nourish, that is to replace the lighter constituents of worn tissues. It has no need to circulate at all. We have no surviving treatises which give us any consecutive account of the Pneumatists' doctrine of nutrition.

An interesting theory about the medical applications of the Stoic theory of *pneuma* has been put forward by Verbecke, who considers that they represent a 'despiritualization' of the Stoic notion of *pneuma*, as an emphasis on its material aspects as opposed to the 'spiritual' interpretation of *pneuma* as a spark of the world-soul.[2] However that may be, the development of the physiological functions of this somewhat mysterious substance show it to be a sort of conflation of oxygen and the world-spirit. In the light of modern scientific conceptions of metabolism, it is tempting to envisage it in this double role. The Greek theory of respiration and transpiration, as it developed, attempted to combine what in the modern conceptions of physics and chemistry can only be locked upon as contradictory elements. For while both these functions had as their primary purpose the cooling of the innate heat, they also served to maintain and to keep it alive, a conception founded on an analogy based on a complete ignorance of the process of combustion. They knew that a fire could only be maintained by a draught of air,

[1] Antyllus, quoted in Oribasius, *C.M.G.* vi. 1. i. 161: ἐπεὶ τοίνυν ἡ εἰς ἡμᾶς ὁλκὴ τοῦ πνεύματος διαστελλομένου τοῦ θώρακος καὶ τῆς κοιλίας καὶ τῶν καθ' ὅλην τὴν σάρκα πόρων γίνεται. βίᾳ γὰρ ὁ ἀὴρ εἴσω ὠθεῖται πρὸς τὴν ὑπὸ τῆς διαστάσεως γεννηθεῖσαν εὐρυχωρίαν κατὰ τὴν φυσικὴν τοῦ πληροῦσθαι τὸ κενούμενον ἀνάγκην, ἀθροῦν μὲν εἰσερχόμενον διὰ ῥινῶν καὶ στόματος, πολὺ δὲ καὶ διὰ τῶν καθ' ὅλην τὴν ἐπιφανείαν πόρων. Quoted by Verbecke, op. cit., p. 196, n. 53.

[2] Verbecke, op. cit., p. 220: 'Au point de vue de la spiritualisation du pneuma, la pneumatologie médicale marque plutôt une régression. Ceci résulte encore une fois de ce que nous venons de dire. Puisque ce souffle est devenu un élément nécessaire dans le fonctionnement normal de notre organisme, ayant une température et une densité déterminées, il a perdu sa pureté intime avec les corps célestes, et il a été ramené sur terre. Érasistrate insiste même sur le fait que le pneuma ne peut pas être trop subtil, parce qu'il s'échapperait des artères : nous sommes bien loin ici des épithètes stoïciennes par lesquelles les philosophes du Portique affirmaient la subtilité et la pureté incomparables de ce souffle éthéré. Pendant toute la période que nous avons examinée et qui s'étend sur plusieurs siècles, le pneuma médical a donc gardé sa signification purement matérielle : il ne désigne rien d'autre qu'un souffle tiède, élément indispensable de notre vie physiologique.'

hence air was needed to keep alive the innate heat. But this air was not the material of combustion, it had the dual function both of maintaining and of cooling this innate fire. Indeed it acted as a sort of thermostat, keeping the innate heat alive but preventing it from burning up the body. To the Greeks this dual function did not imply any contradiction, because they were completely ignorant of the chemistry of heat production, but they had noticed that flames need air for their maintenance, and that they gave off smoke containing sooty substances. They therefore attributed to respiration and transpiration the further function of eliminating sooty residues, which we should, perhaps not altogether accurately, translate as 'waste products'.

The Pneumatists developed the theory of the pulse on the lines first laid down by Herophilus. The treatise on *Medical definitions* devotes quite a lot of space to pulse-lore. In definition cx the pulse is defined as a 'natural' (unconscious) contraction and expansion of the heart and arteries, and of the brain and its membranes;[1] alternatively, as a movement of the heart and arteries inwards and outwards, for the cooling of the innate heat and the increase of the 'vital tone or tension' and the production of the psychic spirit. This definition is followed by a clinically oriented semi-mystical alternative. The pulse is a truthful messenger of things hidden in the depth of the body and a foreteller of things imperceptible and a proof of things unclear, in harmonic motion and prophetic beat foretelling an unseen condition.[2] In this definition an allusion to the Stoic cultivation of prophecy[3] or divination is clearly indicated. The movement of expansion in diastole and contraction in systole is in three dimensions. Diastole is an expansion, raising up, or upstanding perceptible to the touch, but systole is a contraction or drawing together of the cardiac and arterial walls which is not perceptible as such—here

---

[1] The words 'the brain and its membranes' were added, according to Galen, by the 'corrector' Moschion who revised the writings of Asclepiades, to the traditional definition of the pulse which had come down from Herophilus. See Galen, *De diff. puls.* i. 16, K. viii. 758: ἔνιοι δὲ καὶ αὐτοῖς τούτοις προσέθεσάν τινα, καθάπερ καὶ Μοσχίων ὁ διορθώτης ἐπικληθείς, ἐπειδή τινα τῶν ὑπ' Ἀσκληπιάδου λελεγμένων ἐπανωρθοῦτο, μὴ πάντη πειθόμενος τἀνδρὶ καθάπερ οὐδ' ὁ Ἀλέξανδρος Ἡροφίλῳ. τίς οὖν ὁ τοῦ Μοσχίωνος ὅρος εἰπόντες ἀπαλλαγῶμεν ἤδη καὶ τῶν Ἀσκληπιάδου· σφυγμός ἐστι κίνησις ἴδιος καρδίας καὶ ἀρτηριῶν καὶ φλεβῶν καὶ ἐγκεφάλου καὶ τῆς περὶ αὐτὸν μήνιγγος. Note that the 'corrector' believes in the pulsation of veins.

[2] Galen (?), *Def. med.*, def. cx, K. xix. 375–6: σφυγμός ἐστι διαστολὴ καὶ συστολὴ καρδίας καὶ ἀρτηριῶν φυσική. μέρη δὲ τοῦ σφυγμοῦ εἰσι δύο, διαστολὴ καὶ συστολή. ἢ οὕτως· σφυγμός ἐστι κίνησις κατὰ διαστολὴν καὶ συστολὴν καρδίας καὶ ἀρτηριῶν καὶ ἐγκεφάλου καὶ μηνίγγων φυσικὴ καὶ ἀπροαίρετος. δυνατὸν καὶ οὕτως ὁρίσασθαι· σφυγμός ἐστι κίνησις φυσικὴ καὶ ἀπροαίρετος τοῦ ἐν καρδίᾳ καὶ ἀρτηρίαις θερμοῦ εἰς ἑαυτὸ καὶ ἀφ' ἑαυτοῦ συγκινοῦσα ὁμοίως τήν τε καρδίαν καὶ τὰς ἀρτηρίας. ἄλλως· σφυγμός ἐστι κατὰ διαστολὴν καὶ συστολὴν πρὸς ἔμψυξιν τοῦ ἐμφύτου θερμοῦ καὶ αὔξησιν τοῦ ζωτικοῦ τόνου καὶ γέννησιν τοῦ ψυχικοῦ πνεύματος. ἄλλως· σφυγμός ἐστιν ἄγγελος ἀψευδὴς τῶν ἐν βάθει κεκρυμμένων καὶ ἀφανῶν προφήτης καὶ τῶν ἀδήλων ἔλεγχος ἐν ἁρμονικῇ κινήσει καὶ μαντικῇ πληγῇ διάθεσιν ἀόρατον προαγορεύων.

[3] See Sambursky, op. cit., pp. 66 ff.; also *The Physical World of the Greeks* (London, 1956), pp. 174 f.

the author differs both from Herophilus and Galen—but only inferred logically as taking place.[1] The source (ἀρχή) of the movement is in the heart and the arteries, and the author is at some trouble to explain the three-dimensional expansion of a cylindrical tube about its axis lengthways and in the other two planes. He uses in this connection the simile of the circular waves produced by throwing a stone into a pool of water. Imagine them spreading wider and wider up to a point, and then beginning to become smaller and smaller again.[2] In definitions ccviii to ccxxxiii, the various types of pulse are described. They are divided into three main classes according to various *differentiae*. The first of these is size, measured in three dimensions, and the three classes are big, middling, and small.[3] The next *differentia* is fullness. The full pulse is one which gives the impression to the touch that the coat of the artery has become more perceptible and that the tube itself is fuller and has more body. The empty pulse is one in which the whole circumference of the artery is slender and bubble-like and the liquid in it is scarcely perceptible and has almost vanished, so that when you press it with your fingers you feel that you are in contact with an empty tube. The pulse half-way between these two, i.e. the moderately full one, is the natural pulse.[4] The next *differentia* is that of hardness and softness or what we might call texture. The hard pulse is one in which the artery appears like a sinew or tendon

---

[1] Galen (?), *Def. med.*, defs. ccv and ccvi, K. xix. 402–3: διαστολή ἐστιν ἄρσις καὶ οἷον ἐπανάστασις καρδίας καὶ ἀρτηριῶν καὶ ἐγκεφάλου καὶ μηνίγγων κατὰ μῆκος καὶ πλάτος καὶ βάθος αἰσθητὴ πρὸς τὴν ἔπαρσιν τῆς ἀφῆς, οἱ δὲ οὕτως· διαστολή ἐστι διαίρεσις καὶ οἷον ἐπανάστασις καρδίας καὶ ἀρτηριῶν κατὰ μῆκος καὶ κατὰ πλάτος αἰσθητὴ πρὸς τὴν ἄρσιν τῆς ἀφῆς. συστολή ἐστι συναγωγὴ καὶ σύμπτωσις τούτων κατὰ μὲν αἴσθησιν οὐ κινοῦσα τῷ δὲ εὐλόγῳ καὶ ἀκολούθῳ καταλαμβανομένη.

[2] Ibid., defs. cxi and cxii, K. xix. 377–8: φαμὲν τοίνυν μικτὴν ποιῆσαι τὴν κίνησιν ἔν τε κύκλῳ καὶ ἐπ᾿ εὐθείας. εἰ δὲ μικτή ἐστιν ἡ ταύτης, ὡς εἴρηται, κίνησις εὔλογος ἀπόδειξις τὸ κέντρον. κέντρον δὲ λέγω τὸ μὲν μέσον σημεῖον κατὰ τὴν σύμπτωσιν τῆς ἀρτηρίας διαστελλομένης οὑτωσοῦν ἐπὶ τὰ ἔξω ῥεῖν καὶ πάλιν ἀπὸ τῶν ἔξω ἐπὶ τὸ κέντρον πίπτειν, δόξειν ἐπ᾿ εὐθείας κινεῖσθαι. εἰ δὲ θέλεις αὐτοῖς τοῖς πράγμασι τὴν τῆς ἀρτηρίας θεάσασθαι κίνησιν, ἔστω σοι εἰκὼν σαφὴς τοῦ λεγομένου. ἀναλαβὼν λίθον τις ἀκοντίσει ἐν ὕδατι, εἶτα ἐκ τοῦ λίθου πληγὴν νοήσεις τὴν ἀρτηρίαν, ὁ γενόμενος ἐκ ταύτης κύκλος σαφῆ σοι τὴν διαστολὴν ἀπεργάζεται. εἰ δὲ αὖ πάλιν μὴ ἐπ᾿ ἄπειρον ἰόντα τούτου τὸν κύκλον νοήσεις, ἀλλὰ στάντα καὶ ἀρξάμενον μετ᾿ ὀλίγον ἐλαττοῦσθαι, ἕως ἂν εἰς ἐκεῖνον καταντήσει τὸν τόπον ὅθεν τὴν ἀρχὴν τῆς γενέσεως ἔλαβεν.

[3] Ibid., def. ccviii, K. xix. 404: μέγας ἐστὶ σφυγμὸς ὁ κατὰ μῆκος καὶ βάθος καὶ πλάτος τῆς ἀρτηρίας ἐπὶ πολὺ διϊσταμένης γενόμενος. μικρὸς σφυγμός ἐστιν ὁ τοὐναντίον ἐπ᾿ ἐλάχιστον . . . μέσος ἐστὶν ὁ μεταξὺ τούτων ἀμφοτέρων κατά τε τὸ μῆκος καὶ κατὰ τὸν κύκλον ἀνάλογόν τε καὶ τῆς περιφερείας ὑποπιπτούσης.

[4] Ibid., def. ccix: πλήρης ἐστὶ σφυγμὸς ὁ διάμεσος πρὸς τὴν ἀφὴν ὑποπίπτων, ὥστε καὶ αὐτὸν μὲν τὸν χιτῶνα τῆς ἀρτηρίας ἐπισημότερον δοκεῖν γεγονέναι. μάλιστα δὲ τὸ ἐντὸς αὐτῆς μεστότερόν τε καὶ σωματωδέστερον καταλαμβάνεσθαι. κενός ἐστι σφυγμὸς καθ᾿ ὃν αὐτῆς τε τῆς ἀρτηρίας ἡ περιοχὴ παντάπασιν ἰσχνὴ καὶ πομφολυγώδης ἐστὶν καὶ τὸ ἔγχυμα ἀμαυρὸν καὶ ἐξίτηλον, ὥστε καὶ ἐάν τις πιέσῃ τοῖς δακτύλοις κενεμβατήσεως ἀντίληψιν ὑποπίπτειν. μέσος ἐστὶ σφυγμὸς ὁ σύμμετρος μεταξὺ πλήρους τε καὶ κενοῦ μέσος, καὶ ὃς κατὰ φύσιν ἐστί. This definition of the 'full' pulse is very similar to that of Archigenes quoted by Galen, *De dignosc. puls.* iv. 2, K. viii. 931: ἔστι δὲ πλήρης σφυγμὸς ὁ ναστοτέραν ἐπιδεικνὺς τὴν ἀρτηρίαν καὶ τὴν ὑπόπτωσιν αὐτῆς διασεσαγμένην ἐγχύλως, κενὸς δὲ ὁ πομφολυγώδη τὴν ἔγερσιν τῆς ἀρτηρίας ποιούμενος, ὥστε κατὰ τὸν ἐπιπιεσμὸν τῶν δακτύλων κενεμβάτησιν ὑποπίπτειν.

(νευρώδης), as it were, and beaten hard (ἀπόκροτος). The *pneuma* in it is in a state of tension, so that its beat has something 'apoplectic' about it, that is, it is a hard stroke. In the soft pulse, on the other hand, the artery is soft and relaxed and the *pneuma* inside it is as it were exhausted and its beat very gentle.[1] Here too the middling pulse is the natural one. The next *differentia*, that of wetness and dryness, is perceptible by feeling.[2] Then follows the *differentia* of what we should call temperature, with its two extremes of hot and cold, and its 'natural' mean.[3] The next *differentia* is that of strength—or force. The strong (σφοδρός) pulse is one which has a tense movement and gives a violent or forceful beat, the weak pulse being exactly the opposite.[4] The next *differentia* considered is speed. Here, as in Herophilus, speed is distinguished from frequency. Our author believes he can distinguish the speed of the single motion of dilation, though he has already told us that the actual motion of contraction is imperceptible. He seems to imply that the speed of contraction must be the same as that of dilation, or at any rate, that a quick diastole is always followed by a quick systole.[5] The *differentia* of frequency, which is what we should call the pulse-rate, measures the time interval between two or more beats. The frequent beat is that in which the interval of quiescence between the expansion of the artery and its contraction is small, the infrequent or slow pulse, as we should call it, one in which the intervals of quiescence are long.[6]

The two *differentiae* which follow, orderliness and evenness, do not divide the pulse into three but into two classes. It must either be regular or irregular, even or uneven. By regularity is meant a uniform maintenance of the qualities of the pulse, size, strength, rhythm, or any other *differentia*, and a regular pulse is also one which preserves a certain order in its temporal sequence. This does not mean that the interval between

---

[1] *Def. med.*, def. ccx, K. xix. 405: σκληρός ἐστι σφυγμὸς ἐφ' οὗ νευρώδης, ὡς ἂν εἴποι τις, καὶ ἀπόκροτος ἡ ἀρτηρία φαίνεται καὶ τὸ ἐνὸν πνεῦμα τεταμένον. ὥστε καὶ τὴν πληγὴν ἔχειν τι ἀποπληκτικόν. μαλακὸς σφυγμός ἐστιν ὁ ὑπεναντίος τῷ σκληρῷ ἀνειμένην καὶ ἀπαλὴν ἔχων τὴν ἀρτηρίαν. καὶ τὸ ἐνὸν πνεῦμα ἐκλελυμένον τε καὶ τὴν πληγὴν προσηνεστέραν.

[2] Ibid., def. ccxi: ὑγρὸς σφυγμός ἐστιν ὁ ἁπαλὸς οὔσης καὶ τῆς ἐν αὐτῷ οὐσίας προσηνοῦς τῇ ἁφῇ ὑγρασίαν καί τινα προσβάλλων. αὐχμηρός ἐστι σφυγμός, ὥστε ἐκδεδαπανῆσθαι μὲν τὴν ὑποτεταγμένην ὑγρότητα, ξηρᾷ δὲ καὶ ἀερώδει ἀναθυμιάσει ἀναμιχθῆναι.

[3] Ibid., def. ccxii: θερμὸς σφυγμός ἐστιν ὅταν ἡ ἀρτηρία τῶν πλησίων μερῶν θερμοτέρα ἅπτεται ὥσπερ ἐν ἐκτικῷ πυρετῷ. ψυχρὸς σφυγμός ἐστιν ἐν ᾧ ἡ ἀρτηρία ψυχροτέρα καταλαμβάνεται.

[4] Ibid., def. ccxiii, K. xix. 406: σφοδρός ἐστι σφυγμὸς ὁ τὴν κίνησιν εὔτονον ἔχων καὶ βιαίαν ποιούμενος τὴν πληγήν. ἀμυδρός ἐστιν ὁ ἔκλυτον ἔχων τὸν τόνον καὶ τὴν πληγὴν ποιούμενος ἀσθενῆ.

[5] Ibid., def. ccxiv: ταχύς ἐστι σφυγμὸς ὁ σύντονον ἔχων τὴν διαστολὴν καὶ συστολήν. ἢ ταχὺς σφυγμός ἐστιν ὁ μὲν ἐν ὀλίγῳ χρόνῳ κινουμένης τῆς ἀρτηρίας γινόμενος. βραδύς ἐστι σφυγμὸς ὁ βραδεῖαν ἔχων τὴν διαστολήν τε καὶ τὴν συστολήν. ἢ ὁ ἐν πολλῷ χρόνῳ κινουμένης τῆς ἀρτηρίας γινόμενος.

[6] Ibid., def. ccxv, 407: πυκνὸς σφυγμός ἐστιν ὁ δι' ὀλίγου χρόνου τῆς ἀρτηρίας διαστελλομένης γενόμενος. ἤ, ὅτε βραχύς ἐστιν ὁ χρόνος μεταξὺ τῆς διαστολῆς καὶ συστολῆς. ἀραιός ἐστιν ὁ διὰ πολλοῦ χρόνου τῆς ἀρτηρίας διαστελλομένης γινόμενος. ἢ οὕτως· ἀραιός ἐστι σφυγμός, ὅταν ὁ ἡσυχίας χρόνος τῆς μεταξὺ διαστολῆς καὶ συστολῆς μέσης χρονίζει μακρός.

each beat must be always the same, but that the lengths of beats where they are unequal preserve a certain order or repetitive pattern.[1] By disorder is meant the opposite, e.g. it is now fast, now slow.[2] By evenness is meant something rather different. Evenness of pulse is equality in respect to certain differing qualities of the pulse. An even pulse is one in which the various qualities in each different beat and the time intervals between them remain equal. Inequality can be defined in various ways. Unevenness of pulse is an inequality in respect of certain different qualities, or, in other words, an uneven pulse is one in which some of the beats become stronger or some fainter, or again, an uneven pulse is one in which in respect of one part of the artery it rises higher or lower, and is more blown out or widened, whereas in another it is, as it were, narrowed down. A pulse is uneven in regard to strength when in one part of the artery it makes a more forceful elevation, and in another a rather abbreviated and weak one.[3]

Finally, differences of rhythm are also mentioned. The Pneumatist author adopts the notion of Herophilus that differing rhythms are proper to differing ages, and his distinction of the well-rhythmed, the badly-rhythmed, the wrong-rhythmed, the differently-rhythmed, and the completely rhythmless pulses.[4] He is also acquainted with a number of special abnormal pulse patterns, e.g. the trembling pulse,[5] the crooked pulse which does not follow the axis of the artery,[6] the mouse-tailed or tapering pulse which according to our author appears to be a term covering a

[1] Ibid., def. ccxvi: τάξις σφυγμοῦ ἐστιν σχέσις κατὰ μέγεθος ἢ σφοδρότητα ἢ ῥυθμὸν ἢ ἄλλην τινὰ διαφοράν. τεταγμένος σφυγμός ἐστιν ἐν ᾧ ἡ κατὰ τὰς περιόδους ἀναλογία φυλάττει τινὰ τάξιν. ἢ ἄλλως· τεταγμένος ὁ κατὰ περίοδον ἴσος.

[2] Ibid., def. ccxvii: ἀταξία σφυγμοῦ ἐστιν ἀκαταστασία τῆς κατὰ τοὺς σφυγμοὺς διαφορᾶς. οἱ δὲ οὕτως· ἄτακτος σφυγμός ἐστιν ὁ ποτὲ μὲν πυκνότερος γινόμενος κατά τινας πληγὰς ποτὲ δὲ ἀραιότερος. ἢ ἄτακτός ἐστιν ὁ μηδεμίαν κατὰ τὰς περιόδους τάξιν σῴζων.

[3] Ibid., defs. ccxviii and ccxix, 408: ὁμαλότης σφυγμοῦ ἐστιν ἰσότης κατά τινας τῶν διαφοράς. ὁμαλὸς σφυγμός ἐστιν ὁ ἐφεξῆς ἴσος ὑπάρχων, ἢ ἐν ᾧ πᾶσαι τῶν σφυγμῶν διαφοραὶ ἴσαι μένουσι. ἀνωμαλία σφυγμοῦ ἐστιν ἀνισότης σφυγμῶν κατά τινας τῶν παρεπομένων αὐτοῖς διαφορῶν. οἱ δὲ οὕτως· ἀνώμαλος σφυγμός ἐστιν ἐφ' οὗ ποτὲ μὲν σφοδρότεραι αἱ πληγαὶ γίνονται, ποτὲ δὲ ἀμυδρότεραι. οἱ δὲ πάλιν οὕτως· ἀνώμαλός ἐστι σφυγμὸς ὁ κατὰ μέν τι μέρος ὑψηλότερος ταπεινότερος ὑποπίπτων καὶ ἐπὶ πλεῖον διαφυσωμένης τῆς ἀρτηρίας καὶ ἀνευρυνομένης, κατὰ δέ τι ἐπὶ ποσὸν καὶ ὥσπερ ἀποστενοχωρουμένης. κατὰ σφοδρότητα ἀνώμαλος, ὥσπερ κατὰ μέν τι μέρος τῆς ἀρτηρίας βιαιοτέραν τὴν ἐξαίρεσιν ποιούμενος, κατὰ δὲ ὑποσυμβεβηκυῖαν καὶ ἀσθενεστέραν.

[4] See above, p. 194. Cf. defs. ccxxi and ccxxii, 409: εὔρυθμός ἐστι σφυγμὸς ὁ σῴζων ῥυθμὸν τὸν ἴδιον τῇ ἡλικίᾳ καὶ φύσει καὶ κράσει καὶ τῇ ἑκάστῃ ὥρᾳ καὶ ταῖς ἄλλαις περιστάσεσι. ἄρρυθμός ἐστιν ὁ τὸν ῥυθμὸν οὐδένα τῷ ἑκάστῳ ἴδιον σῴζων· κακόρυθμος σφυγμός ἐστιν ὁ κακῶς τὸν ῥυθμὸν σῴζων, εὐρύθμῳ ἐναντίος. παράρυθμόν φαμεν τὸν ποσῶς προσεγγίζοντα τῇ ἡλικίᾳ ἐφ' ἧς θεωρεῖται ῥυθμὸν μὲν ἔχοντα, μὴ παντάπασι δὲ ὄντα κατ' ἐκεῖνον. ἑτερόρυθμον λέγομεν τὸν ἑτέρας ἡλικίας ῥυθμὸν ἔχοντα. ἔκρυθμος σφυγμός ἐστιν ὁ μηδεμιᾶς ἡλικίας ἤ τινος ἄλλης περιστάσεως παντάπασι ῥυθμὸν ἐκβεβηκώς.

[5] Ibid., def. ccxxiii, 410: τρομώδης ἐστὶ σφυγμὸς ὁ μὴ ὁμαλὴν μηδὲ ἀσάλευτον τὴν πληγὴν ἀναφέρων, ἀλλ' οἷον κινούμενός τις.

[6] Ibid., def. ccxxiv: ἐσκολιωμένος ἐστιν ὁ μὴ ἐπ' εὐθείας τεταγμένης τῆς ἀρτηρίας ἐπιτελούμενος παρὰ τὴν θέσιν.

number of different phenomena. The first-mentioned refers to an uneven movement in different parts of the artery itself. The top or upper parts of the artery, i.e. those nearer to the heart, are contracting, while those lower down are moving in an opposite direction: they are widening themselves while the upper parts are contracting. But the majority of physicians call a pulse mouse-tailed, when its successive beats taper off, each becoming smaller than the one before it. Pulses are also called mouse-tailed when the intervals between the beats grow progressively longer, so that a pulse which has started as frequent becomes rare. Similarly a pulse which starts by being 'quick' (in the Greek sense) and ends up by being slow is also called mouse-tailed.[1]

He also mentions the 'capering' or 'gazelling' pulse whose name was given to it by Herophilus, as well as the 'anting' pulse and the 'spider's web' pulse, though not the 'worming' pulse. The first of these is defined as a pulse in which the movement of expansion seems to have begun, but is not completed, and it then leaps to a big second movement of expansion before the phase of contraction sets in, and the second beat is stronger than the first.[2] This 'capering' pulse is clearly distinguished from the 'double-hammer' pulse, of which more below. The 'anting' pulse is described as small, empty, frequent, and faint, all of these in extreme degree.[3] It seems rather difficult to distinguish from the 'spider's web', which is perhaps best distinguished from it by its irregularity.[4] Among irregular pulses, the 'repetitive' or reversive pulse is defined as one which increases progressively to a certain degree of size or force, and then de-decreases progressively to its initial condition.[5] The 'double-hammer' pulse is also described in terms which differ very considerably from those defined by Galen.[6] This picturesque name appears to have been invented by Archigenes, but the description given by our Pneumatist author is far from adequate to picture the nature of the celebrated *pulsus bis feriens*. The 'double-hammer' is due to an interruption of the systole.

[1] *Def. med.*, def. ccxxv: μύουρός ἐστιν ὁ παρὰ τὴν θέσιν, ὅταν τὰ μὲν ἐπ' ἄνω μέρη τῆς ἀρτηρίας συνάγηται, τὰ δὲ κάτω τοὐναντίον. ἐνταῦθα μὲν ἐπὶ πλέον ἀνευρύνεται, ἐν δὲ τοῖς ἐπ' ἄνω μέρεσι συναιρεῖται. οἱ δὲ πλείους μυουρίζοντα καλοῦσιν, ὅταν ἀπὸ μείζονος τῆς προσαγούσης πληγῆς αἱ ἑξῆς καθ' ὑφαίρεσιν ἀεὶ καὶ μᾶλλον μικρότεραι συντελοῦνται. ὀνομάζονται δὲ καὶ μύουροι οὕτως, ὅταν ἀπὸ τοῦ πυκνοῦ σφυγμοῦ ἀραιότεροι σφυγμοὶ ἀποτελοῦνται. καλεῖται δὲ μύουρος καὶ ὅταν ἀπὸ τοῦ ταχέος (παχέος—K.) βραδύτερος ὁ σφυγμὸς μέγα γίνεται.

[2] *Ibid.*, def. ccxxxi, 412: δορκαδίζων ἐστὶ σφυγμὸς ὅταν ἡ ἀρτηρία δόξασα διεστάλθαι μὴ παντελῶς διεσταλμένη ἐφ' ἑτέραν ἐπεπήδησεν ἀθροώτερον, πρὶν ἔμφασιν συστολῆς παρέχειν, βιαιοτέρα δὲ ἡ δευτέρα γένηται πληγή.

[3] *Ibid.*, def. ccxxxii: μυρμηκίζων σφυγμός ἐστιν ὁ μικρός, κενός, πυκνός, ἀμυδρὸς πάντων ἐπὶ τὸ ἔσχατον κατηγμένος. ἢ οὕτως· μυρμηκίζων ἐστὶν ἀφ' οὗ γίνεται ἡ φαντασία περὶ τοὺς ἐπερειδομένους τῇ ἀρτηρίᾳ δακτύλους οἰονεὶ μύρμηκος περιπατοῦντος.

[4] *Ibid.*, def. ccxxvii, 411: ἀραχνοειδής ἐστι σφυγμὸς ὁ μικρὸς μὴ ἐδρασμένος, ἀλλὰ τρόπον ἀράχνης ὑπὸ βραχείας αὔρας σαλευομένης κινούμενος.

[5] *Ibid.*, def. ccxxxii, 412: παλινδρομῶν σφυγμός ἐστιν ὁ ἐπὶ ποσὸν ἐκβαίνων τὸ μέγεθος ἢ τὴν σφοδρότητα καὶ ἐπὶ τῶν ἄλλων, ἔπειτα εἰς τοσοῦτο πάλιν ἀποκαθιστάμενος.

[6] See below, pp. 411 f.

The retreat of the artery is not completed. A certain halting is observed, depending on the withdrawal of a certain quantity of *pneuma* and its reintroduction, which presumably causes the second beat, after which the full accomplishment of the required systole is completed.[1]

Our Pneumatist, finally, is also acquainted with the 'dropped beat' pulses to which the terms 'intermittent' (διαλείπων) and 'failing' (ἐκλείπων) were applied. The distinction between these terms is not always very clear. It seems to be determined in the first instance by the number of beats dropped, that is by the beat-equivalent of the gap in the series of beats. The 'intermittent' pulse seems originally to have been defined as one in which the pulse omits a single beat. But it came also to be applied to circumstances in which the gap was equivalent to two, three, or even more beats.[2] The 'failing' pulse is defined in the first meaning assigned to it, in almost the same terms but we are then told that the term is also applied to a tapering pulse very like the 'mouse-tailed', in fact the two seem to be identified.[3] The 'dropped beat' pulse was offset by a pulse inserting an extra beat from time to time in its regular succession.[4]

The other treatise which has survived under Galen's name, that dedicated to Antonius, is devoted exclusively to the pulse, after a curiously inaccurate sketch of the main arterial system which, the author tells us, arises from the left 'ear' of the heart, as the so-called aorta, and has the function of distributing air and the vital spirit; it is called 'artery' because it keeps the vital air.[5] He now goes on to inform us that his purpose in this treatise is to distinguish the different kinds of pulses, as indication, almost as causes as it were, of natural, unnatural, and other conditions of the body, such as its elementary mixtures, differences of age and sex, and other circumstances.[6] The author then mentions the

---

[1] Ibid., def. ccxxvi, 410–11 : δίκροτός ἐστι σφυγμὸς ὅταν ἡ δοκοῦσα ἀποχώρησις τῆς ἀρτηρίας μὴ τελεία γίνεται. ἀλλὰ μέλλησμὸς καὶ ἐπὶ ποσὸν ὑπαγωγῆς ἢ τοῦ ἀνακοπέντος πνεύματος, εἶτα ἀπόθεσις τελεία τῆς ὀφειλομένης συστολῆς.

[2] Ibid., def. ccxxviii, 411 : διαλείπων σφυγμός ἐστιν ὅταν τῶν συστολῶν τε καὶ τῶν διαστολῶν ἐπιτελουμένων ἑνὸς σφυγμοῦ χρόνου ἡ ἀρτηρία διαλείπει. οἱ δὲ οὕτως· διαλείπων ἐστὶ σφυγμὸς ἐφ' οὗ οὐκ ἐπὶ δύο μόνον ἀλλ' ἐπὶ τρεῖς ἢ καὶ ἐπὶ πλείους πληγὰς ἡ ἀρτηρία ἐλλείπει διαστολὴν μίαν ἢ καὶ δύο ἢ καὶ πλείους.

[3] Ibid., def. ccxxx: ἐκλείπων σφυγμὸς λέγεται ἐφ' οὗ οὐκ ἐπὶ δύο μόνον, ἀλλ' ἐπὶ τρεῖς καὶ ἐπὶ πλείους πληγὰς ἀκίνητος ἡ ἀρτηρία διαμένει. οἱ δὲ οὕτως· ἐκλείπων ἐστὶν ὁ ἀπὸ μεγέθους ἀρχόμενος καὶ σφοδρότητος ἀεὶ καὶ μᾶλλον ὑφιῶν, καὶ μέχρι μὲν ἔχει τι μέγεθος καλεῖται μυουσίζων ὁ τοιοῦτος, ὅταν δὲ ὑφιῇ μικρότερος, ἐπὶ τὸ μικρότερον ῥέπῃ, ἐκλείπων καλεῖται.

[4] Ibid., def. ccxxix: παρεμπίπτων σφυγμός ἐστιν ὅταν μεταξὺ δυοῖν πληγῶν κατὰ τὴν ἰδίαν τάξιν κινουμένων ἐκ τούτου τις μέση παρεμπίπτῃ πληγή.

[5] Galen (?), De pulsibus ad Antonium, K. xix. 630: ἀρτηρία ἐστὶ σώματος ἐπίμηκες κυκλικὸν δίκην σωλῆνος διχῆ διαιρούντων ἀπὸ καρδίας ἐχόμενον καὶ ἐπὶ τὸ πᾶν σῶμα καταμεριζόμενον ἀέρα καὶ πνεῦμα ζωτικὸν περιέχον. ἀρτηρία δὲ εἴρηται παρὰ τὸ τηρεῖν τὸν ζωτικὸν ἀέρα. αὕτη δὲ ἐκ τοῦ ἀριστεροῦ ὠτίου τῆς καρδίας ἐκ τῆς λεγομένης ἀορτῆς ἐκφύεται.

[6] Ibid., 630–1 : σκόπον ἔχει τὸ παρὸν σύγγραμμα διαγνώσεις εἰπεῖν, καὶ οἱονεὶ αἰτίας ἀπὸ τῆς τῶν σφυγμῶν κινήσεως ποιήσωμεν τῶν κατὰ φύσιν καὶ παρὰ φύσιν καὶ τῶν οὐ φύσει, οἷον κράσεων, ἀνδρῶν τε καὶ γυναικῶν καὶ ἡλικιῶν καὶ ἄλλων συστοίχων.

effects on the pulse of non-natural, as opposed to natural and unnatural, conditions, such as exercise, baths, large meals, wine-drinking, etc. But he does not discuss them, and proceeds immediately to give advice to the physician called to the bed-side of a patient whom he has never seen before. The first thing to consider is whether the patient is a man or a woman, then the patient's nature (fat or thin), then his age, the season of the year, and the climate. From a consideration of these factors the physician will be able to form a guess at what the patient's pulse would be like were he healthy, and from the mental picture so formed he will, on taking the patient's pulse, know accurately the extent to which, deviating from this norm, it shows a diseased condition.[1]

The author now proceeds to divide the variations of the pulse into ten categories: (a) size, (b) speed, (c) strength, (d) texture (hard or soft), (e) frequency, (f) evenness, (g) regularity, (h) fullness, (i) pattern, and (j) temperature. These categories differ somewhat from those laid down in the *Definitions*, and some of them call for passing notice: *strength* is defined as the tone or tension of the pulsative power, and it is noted that an increase in size and frequency makes the pulse strong;[2] with regard to *frequency*, the author has some comments to make on the effects of heat and cold on frequency and also on the speed of the pulse, noting especially the effects of climate—a warm climate makes the pulse large and thick (is this an equivalent to fullness?) and cold the reverse.[3] He now proceeds to reproduce, with certain variations and additions, the well known theory of Herophilus on the characteristic pulses of the different ages. With regard to *evenness*, the author is at pains to point out that evenness and unevenness can be applied to a single beat as well as to a series of beats. In the latter case it is called 'systematic', a term we shall meet also in Galen. Among uneven pulses in a single beat, he mentions the 'capering' or 'gazelling', and the 'double-hammer' pulse. Unevenness, he tells us, is nearly always combined with irregularity, both being due to the weighing down by some cause of the pulsative power or faculty. Among irregularities he classes the 'dropped' beat and the 'inserted'

---

[1] 'Galen', *De pulsibus ad Antonium*, K. xix. 633: ὅταν οὖν ἐπ' ἄρρωστον κληθείς, ὃν οὕπω τεθέασαι, ἐπισκόπει πρῶτον μὲν ἢ ἄρρεν ἢ θῆλύ ἐστι ... εἶτα τὴν φύσιν τοῦ κάμνοντος καὶ τὴν ἡλικίαν αὐτοῦ· καὶ μετὰ ταῦτα τὴν ὥραν τοῦ ἔτους καὶ τὴν χώραν, καὶ συγκρίνας ἅπαντα καὶ στοχασάμενος ὁποῖον ἔδει σφυγμὸν ἔχειν τὸν κάμνοντα, ὁπότε ἦν ὑγίης, τότε γνώσεις ἀκριβῶς τὸ μέγεθος τῆς παρὰ φύσιν γινομένης παρατροπῆς τοῦ σφυγμοῦ.

[2] Ibid., 634: τρίτον γένος τῶν σφυγμῶν τὸ περὶ τὸν τόνον τῆς δυνάμεως ἐν ᾧ θεωρεῖται σφοδρὸς καὶ ἀμυδρὸς καὶ ὁ σύμμετρος. ἡ γὰρ πυκνότης προλαβοῦσα τὸ μέγεθος ποιεῖ τὸν σφυγμὸν σφοδρόν.

[3] Ibid., 635: ἀραιότεροι καὶ βραδύτεροι σφυγμοὶ γίνονται διὰ τὴν τοῦ περιέχοντος ψῦξιν ἤγουν πίλησιν. ὁμοίως δὲ καὶ ἐπὶ τῆς ἑκάστης χώρας κατὰ τὴν ἐκείνης κρᾶσιν καὶ οἱ σφυγμοὶ μεταβάλλονται. εἰ μὲν γὰρ θερμοτέρα ἐστὶ μεγάλους τε καὶ παχεῖς ποιεῖ τοὺς σφυγμούς· εἰ δὲ καὶ ψυχροτέρα, ποιεῖ τὸ ἀνάπαλιν.

beat.[1] Indeed, his description makes it somewhat difficult to distinguish unevenness and irregularity. With regard to (*i*), which I have translated *pattern*, it appears that this is intended to cover the 'dropped' beat and 'inserted' beat, which he seems also to have included under unevenness and irregularity.[2] The last category is supposed to yield much more information than mere temperature. The amount of heat transmitted through the body of the artery informs us by the touch about the condition of the underlying organs and tissues, and reveals faulty mixture of the elements and also 'mordant' conditions (δακνώδεις).[3] The author also gives his account of the 'double-hammer' pulse, obviously derived, unlike that of the *Definitions*, from Archigenes, and attributes its special character to the hardness of the coat of the artery.[4]

So much for our Pneumatists. Unfortunately the dates of the two treatises which we have just been examining are quite uncertain, but it would appear reasonable to suppose that they were composed before Galen wrote his voluminous works on the pulse, since he is never mentioned. Of his predecessors in earlier Imperial days, the most important, and the one from whom he quotes most freely, mostly, it is true, to dissent from him, was Archigenes, the pupil of Agathinus and the founder of the Eclectic school, which seems to have been an offshoot of the Pneumatic. None of his works, as we have already noted, has survived except in quotation and in doxographical excerpts. But Galen tells us that he wrote a great work on the pulse, and instructs us fairly fully as to his doctrines on this subject, which have been sedulously reconstructed by Wellmann in his book on the Pneumatic school. His master Agathinus had written a book on the pulse, of which not very much is known, but it is mentioned in several places by Galen in his treatise *On the differences of pulses*, who gives us some information about a few of the opinions expressed in it, one of which is concerned with a criticism of Philonides 'the Sikel' for his statement that the pulse is confined to the arteries.[5] The significance of Philonides'

---

[1] Ibid., 636: ἕκτον γένος σφυγμῶν τὸ παρὰ τὴν ὁμαλότητα καὶ τὴν ἀνωμαλίαν, ἥτις θεωρεῖται καὶ ἐν ἑνὶ σφυγμῷ καὶ ἐν πλείοσιν. ἐν ἑνὶ μὲν ὡς ἐπὶ δορκαδίζοντος καὶ τοῦ δικρότου. ἡ δὲ ἐν πλείοσι γινομένη λέγεται συστηματικὴ ἀνωμαλία. ὅπου δέ ἐστιν ἀνωμαλία, ἐκεῖ καὶ ἀταξία ὡς ἐπίπαν. εἰ γὰρ διαπίπτει ἡ μία πληγὴ ἢ παρεμπίπτει, καὶ τοῦτο γίνεται βαρυνομένης τῆς δυνάμεως καὶ θλιβομένης ὑπό τινος αἰτίας.

[2] Ibid.: ἕβδομον γένος σφυγμῶν ἐστι τὸ παρὰ τὴν τάξιν καὶ ἀταξίαν. τμηθέντος γὰρ τοῦ ἀνωμάλου σφυγμοῦ εἰς τὸ κατὰ περιόδους ἴσον τε καὶ ἄνισον, ὁ ἄτακτος γίνεται, καὶ οὕτως θεωρεῖται πάλιν κατὰ μίαν πληγὴν καὶ κατὰ τὰς ἀνταποδόσεις. Ibid., 637: ἔννατον γένος σφυγμῶν τὸ παρὰ τὸν ἀριθμὸν ἐν ᾧ μετρεῖται ἀναλογία χρόνου πρὸς χρόνον, ὅθεν οἱ παρεμπίπτοντες, οἱ διαλείποντες.

[3] Ibid.: δέκατον γένος σφυγμῶν ἐστι τὸ παρὰ τὴν θερμασίαν τὴν ἀναδιδομένην διὰ τοῦ σώματος τῆς ἀρτηρίας ἐν ᾧ θεωρεῖται τὸ ποιὸν τῆς ὑποκειμένης ὕλης τοῦ σώματος διὰ τῆς ἁφῆς, οἷον τὸ δύσκρατον καὶ τὸ δακνῶδες.

[4] Ibid., 640: ὁ δὲ δικροτίζων δὶς ἐν τῷ αὐτῷ κρούει τὴν πληγήν. τοῦτο δὲ γίνεται διὰ σκληρότητα τοῦ σώματος τῆς ἀρτηρίας, ἀνακρούοντος γὰρ καὶ παλινδρομοῦντος καὶ βίᾳ φερομένου τοῦ πνεύματος ἐπὶ δευτέραν ἔρχεται πληγὴν ὡς ἐπὶ ἀγκῶνα σφαῖρα.

[5] Galen, *De diff. puls.* iv. 10, K. viii. 748: ἐνταῦθα πολλῶν λόγων ὑπόθεσιν ἑαυτῷ τις πορίσασθαι δύναται . . . ἐὰν τὰ γεγραμμένα Φιλωνίδῃ τῷ Σικέλῳ κατὰ τὸ περὶ τῆς ἰατρικῆς ὄκτω καὶ δέκατον

opinion is not clear. Did he exclude only the veins, or was he excluding the heart from the origination of the arterial pulse? Agathinus apparently regarded the term σφυγμός as having two different meanings, being applied homonymously to two different phenomena, namely (a) the motion of the heart and arteries, and (b) the perception of the throbbing experienced by the patient himself in inflammation,[1] which, as we have seen, appears to have been the more ancient meaning of the word, and was apparently adopted by Archigenes.[2] Galen's full-scale commentary on Archigenes' work on the pulse has been lost,[3] but his numerous criticisms of Archigenes' theories give us a fairly clear picture of his teaching. His definition of the pulse adds the term φυσική to Agathinus' enumeration of διαστολή and συστολή, a term which is intended to imply the absence of voluntary control. 'The pulse is the involuntary expansion or diastole and contraction or systole of the heart and the arteries.' Archigenes, like the Pneumatists, regarded both movements as active processes (ἐνέργειαι), unlike Herophilus and the followers of Asclepiades. Herophilus' doctrine, according to Galen, was, as we have noted, far from clear, for sometimes he seems to regard both movements as active, but for the most part he looks upon contraction alone as active, diastole being a mere reversion to the artery's natural condition.[4] Archigenes classified the pulse according to eight different 'qualities', namely (a) size, (b) strength, (c) speed, (d) fullness, all these being 'classes' or varieties of the single movement of diastole and/or systole; his other four categories were (e) frequency, (f) orderliness, (g) evenness, and (h) rhythm,[5] which are applicable not to the single beat but to a series. The quality of hardness was not included, and for this he is criticized rather unfairly by Galen, since Galen, as we shall see,[6] himself regarded this quality as

προχειρίζηταί τις· ὧν ἐπὶ βραχὺ καὶ Ἀγαθῖνος ἐμνημόνευσε μεμφόμενος αὐτῷ πρῶτον μὲν ὡς μοχθηρῶς ἀποφηναμένῳ τὸν σφυγμὸν ἐν ἀρτηρίαις μόναις γίγνεσθαι.

[1] Galen, De diff. puls. iv. 11, 750: οἰόμενος ὁμωνύμως λέγεσθαι τὸν σφυγμόν· ἄλλως μὲν γάρ, φησί, τὴν τῆς καρδίας καὶ τῶν ἀρτηριῶν κίνησιν λέγομεν σφυγμόν, ἄλλως δὲ τὴν ἐν ταῖς φλεγμοναῖς γινομένην αὐτῷ τῷ κάμνοντι συναίσθησιν. καὶ γὰρ καὶ ταύτην ὁμωνύμως φησὶ καλεῖσθαι σφυγμόν.

[2] Ibid., 752: φαίνεται γὰρ καὶ ὁ Ἀρχιγένης ἠκολουθηκέναι κατὰ τοῦτο τῷ διδασκάλῳ, πολλαχῶς οἰόμενος λέγεσθαι τὸν σφυγμόν.

[3] Cf. ibid., 753: εἴρηται μὲν οὖν μοι περὶ τούτων ἐπ' ὀλίγον κἂν τῷ πρώτῳ τῶν ἐξηγητικῶν ὧν εἰς τὸ περὶ σφυγμῶν Ἀρχιγένους πεποίημαι, τὸν ἀριθμὸν ὀκτώ.

[4] Ibid., 12, 754: ὁ γοῦν Ἀρχιγένης ἐξειργάσθαι δοκῶν τὸν περὶ τῶν σφυγμῶν λόγον ἐν ἑνὶ μεγάλῳ βιβλίῳ, κατὰ τὴν ἀρχὴν αὐτοῦ τόνδε τὸν ὅρον ἔγραψε. σφυγμός ἐστι καρδίας καὶ ἀρτηρίων διαστολὴ φυσική τε καὶ συστολὴ φυσική, προσθεὶς δηλονότι τὸ φυσικὴ τῷ τοῦ Ἀγαθίνου λόγῳ... ἐκ διαστολῆς τε καὶ συστολῆς ὡς μερῶν συγκεῖσθαι νομίζουσι τὸν σφυγμὸν οἱ πνευματικοὶ πάντες, ἐνεργείας ἡγούμενοι τὰς κινήσεις ἀμφοτέρας εἶναι, τῶν περὶ τὸν Ἡρόφιλόν τε καὶ Ἀσκλη-πιάδην οὐχ ὁμοίως δοκούντων φέρεσθαι. τὸν μὲν οὖν Ἡρόφιλον περὶ διαστολῆς τε καὶ συστολῆς ἀρτηριῶν ζήτησιν ἰδίαν ἔχειν μακροτέραν, ἐνίοτε μὲν γάρ σοι δόξει καὶ τὴν διαστολὴν καὶ τὴν συστολὴν ἐνέργειαν νομίζειν, ὡς τὸ πολὺ δὲ μόνην τὴν συστολήν.

[5] Ibid., ii. 4, K. viii. 576–7: ὀκτὼ λέγει ποιότητας παρέπεσθαι τοῖς σφυγμοῖς, μέγεθος, σφο-δρότητα, τάχος, πυκνότητα, πληρότητα, τάξιν ἢ ἀταξίαν, ὁμαλότητα ἢ ἀνωμαλίαν, ῥυθμόν.

[6] See below, p. 401.

not belonging to the pulse as such, but to the coats of the arteries. Without the text of Archigenes' work before us, it is not possible to evaluate the significance of much of Galen's criticism, nor, indeed, is it possible in many instances to make out exactly whom he is criticizing. Thus, for example, the opinions criticized at the end of the third book of *On the differences of pulses* to the effect that a pulse is called hard because of the peculiar quality of the *pneuma* which it contains, or the peculiar properties of its heat, which Wellmann attributed to Archigenes,[1] may not have been his at all, since it seems to me to be more natural to interpret the last sentence of the passage quoted in the footnote[2] as expressly excluding Archigenes. Thus, while agreeing with Wellmann that Archigenes did in fact attribute, like Galen, the quality of hardness in the pulse to the condition of the arterial coat, we should be cautious in attributing to his teaching the definitions of the warm or hot and wet.[3] Archigenes, incidentally, is also criticized for regarding a hard pulse as an invariable accompaniment of fever, in a paragraph which refers to his errors of conception and diagnosis of this kind of pulse, without specifying them.[4]

Most of Galen's criticisms of Archigenes' classification of the different kinds of pulse seem to depend on logical technicalities, rather than on physiology. These considerations take up practically the whole of the second and third books of the treatise *On the differences of the pulses*, and show Galen at his pettifogging worst.

[1] Wellmann, *Die pneumatische Schule*, p. 185.

[2] Galen, *De diff. puls.* iii, *ad fin.*, K. viii. 693 f.: ἐκεῖνο δὲ μόνον, οὐκ ἄλλῳ τινὶ παρονομάζοντες οὔτε κατὰ συμβεβηκὸς οὔτε μεταφέροντες ἢ καταχρώμενοι, προσαγορεύομεν σκληρόν, ἀλλὰ κυρίως τε καὶ πρώτως. ὅταν οὖν τις σκληρὸν σφυγμὸν ἢ κατὰ τὴν τοῦ πνεύματος λέγῃ ποιότητα φαίνεσθαι τοιοῦτον, ἢ καὶ κατὰ τὴν ἰδιότητα τῆς θερμότητος, ἢ κατὰ ἄλλο τι τῶν λαληθέντος μὲν δυναμένων διδαχθῆναι δὲ ἀδυνάτως, οὐκ ἀνεξόμεθα τοῦ τὰ τοιαῦτα δηλονότι ληροῦντός τε καὶ περιλαλοῦντος, ὥσπερ οὐδ' Ἀρχιγένης ἔν τε τῷ περὶ σφυγμῶν αὐτοῦ γράμματι κἂν τῷ δευτέρῳ τῆς τοῦ πυρετοῦ σημειώσεως.

If Archigenes is the person aimed at, surely the word Ἀρχιγένης should read Ἀρχιγένους. The text as it stands in Kühn can surely mean only that Archigenes also would not tolerate such opinions. Moreover the beginning of the chapter refers to persons, no doubt the Pneumatics in the plural. Cf. K. viii. 685: ἐπιδείξαι πειράσομαι κἀνταῦθα τὴν περὶ τὰ ὀνόματα πλημμέλειαν τῶν ἀνδρῶν. Presumably these are the same persons criticized in the previous chapter for their pernicious doctrine of the full pulse, namely, Agathinus, Magnus, Athenaeus, and any other of the Pneumatists. It is true that Archigenes is there included among them, but in this chapter it would appear that he is specifically excepted.

[3] Wellmann, *loc. cit.*: 'Daß er bei der Erklärung des Begriffs der σκληρότης auch die Beschaffenheit der Wärme der Arterie berücksichtigt hat, so glaube ich schließen zu dürfen, daß er den warmen und kalten Puls zu dieser Klasse gerechnet hat ... Vermutlich auch die vom Ps. Galen xix. 211 erhaltenen Definitionen des feuchten und trockenen Pulses hierher.'

[4] Galen, *De febrium differentiis*, 9, K. vii. 311: ὁ σκληρὸς σφυγμὸς οὐκ ἔστιν οὔτ' ἴδιος οὔτ' ἀχώριστος οὐδενὸς γένους πυρετῶν. Ibid., 310: Ἀρχιγένης γὰρ ὅσα πλημμελεῖ περί τε τὴν ἔννοιαν καὶ τὴν διάγνωσιν τοῦ σκληροῦ σφυγμοῦ, διὰ τῆς περὶ σφυγμῶν πραγματείας αὐτάρκως ἐπιδέδεικται. Cf. Galen, *De marcore*, 5, K. vii. 685–6: τὴν σκληρότητα δηλονότι λέγων, ἣν ἀχώριστον ἔθετο σημεῖον ἁπάντων πυρετῶν Ἀρχιγένης. ἀλλ' εἰ μὲν τὸν ὄντως λέγει σκληρὸν (Φίλιππος) ὑπάρχει μὲν τοῖς μαραινομένοις ἅπασι διὰ τὴν ξηρότητα τῶν ἀρτηριῶν, οὐ μὴν σημεῖόν ἐστι πυρετῶν.

When we examine these different categories in rather more detail, the following observations suggest themselves. With regard to size, Archigenes appears to have defined it as the size or volume (ὄγκος) of the uprising (ἐπανάστασις) of the artery, distinguishing the three dimensions of length, breadth, and height.[1] As to speed, Archigenes adopts the traditional notion first put forward by Herophilus. With regard to strength or force, Archigenes rejected the notion of the Pneumatist Magnus that σφοδρότης was a combination of bigness, fullness, and speed.[2] He regarded it as equivalent to the tone or tension of the movement of the artery.[3] He is therefore accused by Galen of confusing cause with effect, though Galen admits that Archigenes is perfectly aware of the peculiar character of the feel of the strong beat.[4] Archigenes seems to have distinguished different kinds of remissness and force in the pulse, and detected through the touch an element of wetness, particularly after meals, as well as a kind of hardness which was, as it were, a jostling of the elbow, a phenomenon occurring in excessively fat persons.[5]

As to the category of frequency, Archigenes accepted the traditional distinction of speed from frequency. Speed describes the quality of the artery's motion, and frequency the duration of the quiescent intervals. This distinction is connected, as Wellmann points out, with the question we have already discussed in connection with Herophilus of the perceptibility of the movement of systole. Agathinus, we noted, denied that the contraction could be felt by the fingers at all.[6] The Pneumatists seem to have

---

[1] Galen, De diff. puls. ii. 6, K. viii. 598: αὐτὸς γοῦν ὁ Ἀρχιγένης μέγεθος εἶναί φησι σφυγμοῦ τὸν ὄγκον τῆς ἐπαναστάσεως τῶν ἀρτηριῶν. ὄγκος δὲ οὐχ ὑπάρχει γραμμῇ, ἀλλὰ μόνοις τοῖς τριχῶς διεστῶσι.

[2] Ibid., iii. 1, K. viii. 640 (quoted by Wellmann, op. cit., p. 179): τί γὰρ δὴ καί φησιν ὁ Μάγνος αὐτῇ λέξει; χρὴ τοίνυν καὶ μέγεθος ἀξιόλογον εἶναι τοῖς σφυγμοῖς καὶ πληρότητα καὶ μετὰ τάχους προσπίπτειν τοῖς δακτύλοις, εἰ μέλλει τις κυριολογεῖν σφοδρὸν σφυγμὸν ὀνομάζων.

[3] Ibid., 2, K. viii. 647: σφοδρὸς μὲν οὖν σφυγμὸς ὁ μείζονα τόνον ἔχων τῆς κινήσεως καὶ ῥοιζώδης ὤν. Cf. Galen, De dignosc. puls. iv. 2, K. viii. 938: ὁ δ' Ἀρχιγένης . . . ὧδε γράφει. ὥστ' ἐκ τοῦ καθ' ἕνα χωρισμοῦ γίνεσθαι καθ' ἑαυτήν τις οὖσα ἡ σφοδρότης ὁ τόνος, ὡς εἶπον τῆς τῶν ἀρτηριῶν κινήσεως. εἶθ' ἑξῆς· φαίνεται δὲ καθ' ὅλην τὴν διαστολὴν τὸ στεγανὸν (τελανὸν—K.) τῆς ὁρμῆς, καθ' ὃ καὶ εἰ προσπιέσαιμεν τοὺς δακτύλους στερεωτέρα ὑποπίπτει ἡ πληγή.

[4] Galen, De diff. puls. iii. 1, K. viii. 644: δοκεῖ δέ τισι ἐν τῇ τῆς ἁφῆς πληγῇ κεῖσθαι, καθ' ὃ καὶ πληγὴν ἀπ' ἀρτηρίας φασὶν αὐτήν τινες . . . φαίνεται δὲ καθ' ὅλην τὴν διαστολὴν τὸ στεγανὸν τῆς ὁρμῆς. καθ' ὃ καὶ εἰ προσπιέσαιμεν τοὺς δακτύλους στερεωτέρα ὑποπίπτει ἡ πληγή, οὐ κατὰ τὸ πέρας τῆς διαστολῆς, ἀλλὰ κατωτέρω τότε γινομένη; also, ibid., 2, 647: σφοδρὸς μὲν οὖν ἐστι σφυγμὸς ὁ μείζονα τόνον ἔχων τῆς κινήσεως, ἀλλὰ προσέθηκε, καὶ ῥοιζώδης ὤν. Ibid., 3, 650: ἀμυδρὸς δὲ ὁ ἐκλελυμένον τόνον ἔχων καὶ ἀσύστροφον τὴν πληγήν.

[5] Ibid., 3, 651: ἔστι δὲ κατὰ τὴν σφοδρότητα τοιαύταις καὶ ἄλλαις ἐντυγχάνειν διαφοραῖς, ἐν αἷς ἐκλελυμένη ἐμπίπτει ἡ πληγὴ καὶ ἀβαρής, ὃν ἀμαυρὸν σφυγμὸν ἤδη τινὲς ἐκάλεσαν. ἄλλη δὲ βαρεῖα μὲν ἔκλυτος ταύτην ἀμυδροῦ σφυγμοῦ διαφορὰν θείη τις ἄν, ἢ δ' οὐκ ἔκλυτος μέν, ἀλλ' οἷον παραπεποδισμένη καὶ εἴσω ῥέπον τὸ βάρος ἔχουσα, πεπιεσμένη καὶ δεδυκυῖα. διαφορὰ κατὰ σφοδρότητα εἴη ἂν σφυγμοῦ καὶ κατὰ τὸν σφοδρόν, ἡ μέν τις πληγὴ εἴη ἂν ἐξεριστική, ὑγρότερος ἐξωθοῦσα τὴν ἁφήν, οἷα ἀπὸ τροφῆς μάλιστα νεαρᾶς ἐγγίνεται. ἡ δὲ δύσθραυστος ἔστι μᾶλλον, οἷον διηγκωνισμένου τοῦ κινοῦντος. ἡ δ' ἐν πείσεσί τισι καὶ ἐπὶ τοῖς ἐν σαρκὶ πλεονασμοῖς φαίνεται.

[6] Galen, De dignosc. puls. i. 3, K. viii. 786: Ἀγαθίνου τοίνυν λέγοντος ἀναίσθητον εἶναι τὴν συστολὴν τῆς ἀρτηρίας, Ἡροφίλου δὲ διὰ παντὸς ὡς ὑπὲρ αἰσθητῆς διαλεγομένου.

varied in their opinions on this subject, like the followers of Erasistratus,[1] while the Empirics maintained that only the 'blow' (πληγή) of the pulse could be felt.[2] Archigenes followed Herophilus in this matter, and maintained, indeed, that in lean persons both the expansion and the contraction of certain arteries could actually be seen.[3] A large number of physicians, however, denied that systole could be felt, at any rate for more than part of the time of the duration of its movement, which, as we shall see, raised many difficulties in the measurement of the rhythm of the pulse, no longer accurately divisible into its four phases of expansion, rest, contraction, rest, a problem which was to exercise the ingenuity of Galen.[4]

Regularity and evenness are both involved in the distinction between the single beat and the series of beats. The attempt to confine them to the latter could not be made to work, since even the single beat could be at least even or uneven. Archigenes seems to differentiate unevenness (ἀνωμαλία) from irregularity (ἀταξία) rather obscurely, if we can credit Galen's account. Galen quotes a number of Archigenes' remarks without their full context, remarks which do not, and were perhaps not intended to, give us a very clear picture. We need not follow Galen in his quibbling objections to Archigenes' formulae. Their meaning would certainly be a good deal plainer if Archigenes' text had survived. Galen's chief objection to Archigenes is that he does not stick logically to the notion of *differentia* as denoting a 'class' of pulse, i.e. the specific qualities of the single beat, because of his introduction of the notions of rhythm and order, regularity, evenness, etc.[5]

With regard to fullness, the characteristic the perception of which as a property of the pulse Galen so strenuously denies,[6] Archigenes appears to have accepted the description of it given in the *Medical definitions*, which we have already quoted. The supposed perception of fullness is a typical feature of post-Herophilian sphygmology from which only the Empirics apparently dissented. The perception was derived from the notion that the arteries were filled with a lot of *pneuma* and a little blood

---

[1] Ibid., 787: εὑρίσκοντες οὖν τοὺς μὲν Ἡροφιλείους σχεδὸν ἅπαντας αἰσθητὴν εἶναι λέγοντας, τοῦ δὲ περὶ τὸν Ἐρασίστρατον χοροῦ τοὺς μὲν ὁμολογοῦντας, τοὺς δ' ἀρνουμένους, καὶ τρίτους ἀπ' Ἀθηναίου τοῦ Ἀτταλέως, ὧν εἷς ἦν Ἀγαθῖνος, ὡσαύτως πρὸς ἀλλήλους διαφερομένους.

[2] Ibid., 776: ὅπερ ἔφαμεν ἐρίζοντας μᾶλλον ἢ ἀληθεύοντας λέγειν τοὺς ἐμπειρικούς, ὡς πληγῆς μόνης αἰσθάνονται, διαστολὴν δ' ἀρτηρίας οὐ γνωρίζουσι.

[3] Ibid., 779: τὸ δ' ὑπὸ τοῦ Ἀρχιγένους λεγόμενον, ὅτι καὶ τῶν ἰσχνῶν ἀνθρώπων αἱ ἐν τοῖς ἀσάρκοις μέρεσιν ἀρτηρίαι φαίνονται τῇ ὄψει διαστελλόμεναι καὶ συστελλόμεναι.

[4] See below, Ch. 7, p. 406.

[5] Galen, *De diff. puls.* ii. 10, K. viii. 629: καὶ πολλὰς παρεγράψαμεν ῥήσεις, οὐχ οὕτως ὑπὲρ τοῦ τῆς διαφορᾶς ὀνόματος σπουδάσαντες, ἀλλ' ἵν' ἐπιδείξωμεν τὸ σημαινόμενον πολυειδὲς ὄν. καὶ γὰρ τὰ γένη πολλάκις διαφορὰς κέκληκε, τά τε πρῶτα καὶ τὰ δεύτερα, καὶ τὰ εἴδη τῶν γενῶν οὐδὲν ἧττον. καὶ ὅσα δὲ μήτε γένη μήτ' εἴδη τέταχεν ὄντα, διαφοραὶ δ' αὐτὸ τοῦτο μόνον καὶ ταύτας διαφορὰς κέκληκεν, ἐν ᾧ καὶ ἡ παρακοὴ τῶν ψευδοδιαλεκτικῶν ἐστι.

[6] See below, Ch. 7, p. 402.

and other humours, the varying proportions of these contents being supposedly perceptible by the touch of the fingers. With regard to rhythm, Archigenes seems to have accepted in general terms the theory propounded by Herophilus[1] concerning the characteristic rhythms of the different ages. He differed from him, however, in one particular, in that he classified the pulse of infants as small, whereas Herophilus thought that it was rather large. He also regarded the 'anting' pulse as fast, whereas Herophilus denied this.[2]

Among Archigenes' descriptions of the different patterns of abnormal pulses, the most interesting to us is that of the 'double-hammer' pulse which, as we have noted, Galen considered that Archigenes was the first to name.[3] Galen accords him some credit for his naming of this pulse and for his simile of the hammer-blow,[4] but criticizes him for the inadequate treatment of its origins or consequences, and of course misses the point of this picturesque description.[5] Archigenes would appear also to have invented another rather picturesque name for a particular kind of pulse pattern. This he called the 'nodding' or 'oscillating' pulse, which, Galen informs us in his *Treatise for beginners*, is found in the wasting condition occurring when certain inflammations have not been dispersed. This pulse is faint and quick and very frequent, and tapers in size in the single beat. Archigenes meant by this term to indicate clearly the short character of the arterial expansion, which has a sort of nodding at each end, not as if its whole volume had been completely curtailed, but as if the parts at both ends had been foreshortened, so that it tapers like a mouse-tail at both ends.[6] What the beginner is to make of this description we must leave to the imagination, nor are we helped by the alternative description given by Galen in his treatise *On the causes of the pulse*,[7] which simply repeats Archigenes word for word. He does, however, suggest in the work *On prognoses from the pulse* that a pulse which 'nods' or 'oscillates' at both ends may not be a symptom of disease, but a

---

[1] See above, pp. 187 f.

[2] Galen, *Synopsis de puls.* 8, K. ix. 453: τὸν γοῦν τοῦ παιδὸς σφυγμὸν ὁ μὲν Ἡρόφιλος ἱκανὸν τῷ μεγέθει φησὶν ὑπάρχειν ὁ δ' Ἀρχιγένης μικρόν. οὕτω δὴ καὶ τὸν μυρμηκίζοντα ταχὺν εἶναί φησιν ὁ Ἀρχιγένης, Ἡρόφιλος δὲ οὐ ταχύν.

[3] See below, the passage quoted, p. 411, n. 4.

[4] Galen, *De praesag. ex puls.* 8, K. ix. 306: ἐξαπατώμενος ὑφ' ὧν ἔλεγεν Ἀρχιγένης, εἰκάζων αὐτὸν ταῖς τῆς σφυρᾶς διπλαῖς πρὸς τὸν ἄκμονα πληγαῖς.

[5] Ibid., 306-7: φαίνεται δέ μοι καὶ ὁ Ἀρχιγένης ἐπιμελῶς παραπεφυλακέναι τοὺς δὶς παίοντας σφυγμούς, οὔτε δ' ἑρμηνεύειν αὐτοὺς ὀρθῶς, οὔτε τὰς διαθέσεις αἷς ἕπονται διαγιγνώσκειν, ἢ οὐκ ἂν ἁπλῶς οὕτως οὔτε ταῖς τῆς σφυρᾶς διπλαῖς πρὸς τὸν ἄκμονα πληγαῖς εἴκασεν αὐτούς.

[6] Galen, *De pulsibus ad tirones*, 12, K. viii. 479-80: οἱ μὲν δὴ ταῖς μὴ λυθείσαις φλεγμοναῖς κατὰ βραχὺ συναπομαρανθέντες ἀμυδροὺς καὶ θάττονας καὶ πυκνοὺς ἄγαν καὶ μυούρους κατὰ μέγεθος ἐν μιᾷ πληγῇ τοὺς σφυγμοὺς ἴσχουσιν. οὓς Ἀρχιγένης ἐπινενευκότας τε καὶ περινενευκότας καλεῖ, σαφῶς δηλοῦν βουλόμενος τὸ κατὰ τὴν διαστολὴν βραχύ, μετὰ τῆς τῶν ἑκατέρωθεν περάτων οἷον ἐπινεύσεως, οὐ γὰρ ὡς κεκομμένων ἀθρόως, ἀλλ' ὡς ἐπικεκομμένων τῶν ἑκατέρωθεν μερῶν εἰς βραχὺ συνεσταλμένων, μύουρος ὢν τῷ μεγέθει καθ' ἑκάτερα τὰ μέρη.

[7] Galen, *De causis pulsuum*, 10, K. ix. 177.

natural developmental idiosyncrasy.¹ The tapering pulse, too, may be a natural condition, but it is mostly a sign of lack of power when the artery is unable to lift itself against the forces which are weighing it down. When this pathological condition becomes very marked, the artery looks as if the pulse has a dent in its upper surface, not extending to its whole circumference, which dent has been called by Archigenes, not inappropriately, γωνίωσις, a word which as far as I know does not occur elsewhere.² Archigenes is, of course, acquainted with the 'dropped-beat' and 'inserted-beat' pulses. He regarded the 'frequent' pulse as more dangerous than the 'rare', and the 'inserted beat' more dangerous than the 'dropped beat', the former because a very quick pulse precedes and accompanies fainting fits and collapse (συγκοπή), the latter because an inserted-beat pulse sometimes occurs in fatal cases of pneumonia and in fevers in which there is obstruction or compression of the most important arteries.³ Galen criticizes this view.

Three other treatises on the pulse of Imperial times before Galen have survived. One of these we have already noted in connection with Herophilus, namely the essay *On the pulse* by Markellinos, which has been edited for the first time in this century (1907) by H. Schoene. The author seems to have been 'an Eclectic with Dogmatist tendencies'. He quotes Archigenes, but he does not mention Galen. Schoene therefore concludes that he must have lived before his time. The treatise, in spite of some rhetorical embellishments, is probably the work of a practising physician. It contains instructions on the proper way of feeling the pulse, and on the danger of doing so brusquely on immediate arrival at the patient's bedside, since the failure first to elicit the confidence of the patient may cause disturbances in the pulse itself. It also contains descriptions of the pulse varieties characteristic of specific diseases. The causes of the pulse are summarily dismissed in a few sentences, outlining three alternative hypotheses which are worth recording. The first of these assigns the role of motive force to the innate heat and the movements of the walls of the arteries. 'The cause of the pulse is a vaporization of the

---

¹ *De praesag. ex puls.* 11, K. ix. 323–4: ἑτέρων δέ γε φύσει περινενευκώς τε καὶ ἐπινενευκὼς ἑκατέρωσε πλέον ἢ κατὰ τὴν κοινὴν φύσιν, οὐ νοσήματος ἤ τινος ὅλως αἰτίας παρὰ φύσιν, ἀλλὰ φυσικῆς διαπλάσεως ἐργασαμένης αὐτόν.

² Ibid., 324: γίγνεται μὲν γάρ, ὡς εἴρηται, μύουρος ὁ σφυγμὸς ἔν τισι παρὰ φύσιν αἰτίοις. εὑρίσκεται μέντοι τισὶ καὶ κατὰ τὴν τῆς διαπλάσεως ἰδιότητα . . . γίνεται δὲ καὶ δι' ἀρρωστίαν δυνάμεως, ἀδυνατούσης ἐπαίρειν τὰ βαρύνοντα· καὶ ὅταν γε τὸ τοιοῦτον πάθος ἰσχυρότερον αὐτῇ γένηται, καμπήν τινα φαίνεται κατὰ τὸ ὕψος ἔχειν ὁ σφυγμός, οὐ κύκλῳ περιφέρειαν, ἥντινα καμπὴν οὐ κακῶς ὁ Ἀρχιγένης ὀνομάζει γωνίωσιν.

³ Ibid., 5, K. ix. 289: ἐναντίοι δ' εἰσὶ τοῖς εἰρημένοις σφυγμοῖς ἕτεροι δύο, τῷ μὲν ἀραιῷ πυκνός, τῷ διαλείποντι δὲ ὁ παρεμπίπτων, οὓς Ἀρχιγένης ἔοικεν οἴεσθαι χαλεπωτέρους εἶναι τῶν προειρημένων, ἐξαπατώμενος ὑπὸ τῶν πυκνῶν, ὅτι καὶ προηγοῦνται καὶ συνεδρεύουσι συγκοπαῖς. ἐπὶ δὲ τῶν παρεμπιπτόντων ὅτι περιπνευμονικοῖς ἐνίοτε προσπίπτουσιν ὀλεθρίως ἔχουσι καὶ πυρετοῖς ἔστιν ὅτε, καθ' οὓς ἔμφραξις ἢ θλῖψίς ἐστιν ἀρτηριῶν κυρίων.

innate heat condensing under the force of attraction in systole and expanding under that of transpiration in diastole, the arteries moving their bodies
in accordance with each of these movements.'[1] The second is clearly of
Erasistratan origin. 'The cause of the pulse is the flowing of *pneuma*
dancing in the arteries in a rhythmic course in obedience to the thrust
of the heart and the force of attraction along the sides of the arteries.'[2]
The third description is much more difficult to follow. 'The cause of
the pulse is the necessary passage of air in accordance with the movement of light substances, since *pneuma* has altogether a tendency to move
outwards by being drawn through the surface and through the mouths
of the arteries in thousands of passages.'[3] These causal considerations
are promptly dismissed; what matters for his purposes, Markellinos
tells us, is the definition of the pulse.[4]

With regard to these he quotes quite a number starting with the
pupil of Herophilus, Baccheius, whose formula runs thus: 'The pulse is
the simultaneous diastole and systole which takes place in all the arteries.[5]
No mention of the heart here but the definition is also quoted by Galen
with the disastrous implication that diastole of heart and arteries, like
systole, was simultaneous.[6] He deliberately rejects Moschion's addition
to the definition of Archigenes which added the brain and its membrane
to the list of pulsating organs, adding that the appearance of pulsation
is derived from that of the arteries they contain.[7] Of all the definitions,
the one he prefers is Archigenes' 'The pulse is the "natural", that is
automatic or quasi-mechanical, expansion and contraction of the heart
and arteries.' He notices, however, incidentally that in conditions arising
out of some diseases, veins may also pulsate, but this is not 'in accordance with nature'.[8] He also accepts Archigenes' eight categories of
the different kinds of pulses, according to size, force, speed, frequency,

[1] Markellinos, *De pulsibus*, ii: τί μὲν οὖν ἐστι κατὰ τὴν γένεσιν ὁ σφυγμός; εἶτ' ἐκθυμίασις
ἐμφύτου θερμοῦ κατὰ τὴν ὁλκὴν συστρεφομένου καὶ κατὰ τὴν διαπνοὴν πρὸς διαστολὴν ἁπλου-
μένου, πρὸς ἀμφοτέρας τὰς κινήσεις τῶν ἀρτηριῶν ἐπαγομένων τὰ σώματα...

[2] Ibid.: εἴτε ῥεῦμα πνεύματος χορεύοντος ἐν ἀρτηρίαις ἐναρμόνιον δρόμον τῇ παρὰ καρδίας
πειθόμενον βολῇ τε καὶ κατὰ τὰ πλάγια τῶν ἀρτηριῶν ὁλκῇ...

[3] Ibid.: εἴτε ὁδὸς ἀέρος ἀναγκαία πρὸς λεπτομέρειαν, ἐπεὶ τὰ πάντα τὸ πνεῦμά ἐστιν ἐξώφορον
ἀεὶ καὶ δι' ἐπιφανείας κατὰ τὸ στόμα τῶν ἀρτηριῶν ταῖς μυρίαις ὁδοῖς ἕλκεται.

[4] Ibid.: εἰς γὰρ τὴν προκειμένην πραγματείαν τί ποτέ ἐστιν ὁ σφυγμὸς ὁρικῶς εἰδέναι χρή,
τὸ δ' ὑφ' οὗ γίνεται ἢ πῶς ἢ δι' ὅτι μὴ ῥηθὲν οὐ λείπει.

[5] Ibid., iii: Βακχεῖος δὲ ὁ Ἡροφίλειος σφυγμὸν εἶπεν εἶναι διαστολὴν καὶ συστολὴν ἐν πάσαις
ταῖς ἀρτηρίαις ἅμα γιγνομένην.

[6] Galen, *De diff. puls.* iv. 6, K. viii. 732: ὁ μὲν οὖν Βακχεῖος ἐν ταῖς ἄλλαις ἀκροάσεσι
τὸν σφυγμὸν εἶναί φησι συστολὴν καὶ διαστολὴν ἅμα ἐν ἁπάσαις ταῖς ἀρτηρίαις γιγνομένην. πρὸς
ὃν ὅρον ἐπηρεαστικῶς μὲν ἀντεῖπον οἱ Ἐρασιστράτειοι... δοκεῖ γὰρ αὐτοῖς ἡ μὲν καρδία πρώτη
διαστέλλεσθαί τε καὶ συστέλλεσθαι τῶν ἀρτηριῶν ἁπασῶν.

[7] Markellinos, *De pulsibus*, iii: ἡ γὰρ μῆνιγξ ἡ περὶ τὸν ἐγκέφαλον εἴπερ καὶ σφύζει, ἀπὸ τῶν
ἀρτηριῶν ἡ καταρχὴ γίγνεται αὐτῇ.

[8] Ibid.: ἡμῖν δὲ ἄριστος εἶναι δοκεῖ ὅρος σφυγμοῦ ὁ καὶ παρὰ Ἀρχιγένει κείμενος· ἔστι δὲ
διαστολὴ καὶ συστολὴ καρδίας καὶ ἀρτηριῶν φυσική.

fullness, order, evenness, and rhythm, to which all other differences can be reduced.[1] The first five of these are divided into three grades, small, large, and medium or moderate, while two of the others only furnish two alternatives, since a pulse must be either even or uneven, regular or irregular. Of the first five of these 'most general characters' (κοινόταται ποιότητες) of the pulse Markellinos has little new to say,[2] but his definition of the strength or force of the beat is interesting in so much as it attempts to interpret this purely mechanically; the strength of the beat is determined by the force exerted on the arterial wall.[3]

Markellinos' chief interest is obviously clinical. What are the various abnormal types of pulse which are signs of danger, and what are the types of pulse characteristic of various diseases? It is perhaps worth while reproducing his account of these different types of abnormal pulse in some detail, since with the loss of the works both of Herophilus and Archigenes, they may give us a slightly clearer insight into their teaching than the mere fragments of quotation which have come down to us. Of the 'gazelling' pulse he tells us that it is dicrotic, inasmuch as it gives two beats in a single motion of diastole. The artery expands, and while it is still in a state of expansion it seems to undergo an apparent but not real contraction though it still remains lifted. It then proceeds to a further expansion and only then embarks on the normal motion of contraction. The two beats are felt as stimuli by the touch, and the second is the stronger. And just as gazelles when they run first take a small step and then suddenly make a big jump which carries them high up off the ground as they leap forward, so the 'gazelling' pulse makes a first faint expansion and then a much larger one. It remains in the expanded state and effects its second expansion before falling back. Herophilus, who was the first to describe this pulse, said that he had only met with one instance of it in the case of a certain eunuch, but Markellinos says that he has constantly come across it in persons suffering from

[1] Ibid., iv: τῷ δὲ σφυγμῷ αἳ λέγονται παρέπεσθαι ποιότητες αἱ κοινόταται ἐπὶ πάντων θεωρούμεναι αἵδε· μέγεθος, σφοδρότης, ἀμυδρότης, τάχος, πυκνότης, πληρότης, τάξις, ὁμαλότης, ῥυθμός. ἅπασαι γὰρ αἱ τοιαῦται διαφοραὶ εἰς ταύτας ὑπαχθήσονται.

[2] Ibid., vi: τὸ δὲ πᾶν οὕτω σαφηνισθήσεται. τοῦ σφυγμοῦ τὰ πρῶτα μέρη λέγομεν εἶναι δύο, διαστολὴν καὶ συστολήν, καὶ τούτων ἑκάτερον διανέμεται διχῇ· ἡ μὲν διαστολὴ εἰς τὸ διαστέλλεσθαί τε καὶ διεστάλθαι. διαστέλλεσθαι μὲν οὖν εἶναι λέγομεν τὸ πρὸς τὸ ἐκτὸς χωρεῖν τὴν ἀρτηρίαν, διεστάλθαι δὲ τὸ πρὸς τὸ ἐκτὸς ἀφικνουμένην τὴν ἀρτηρίαν ἐπιμένειν χρόνον τινὰ ἀκίνητον· καλοῦμεν δὲ τοῦτο ἐπηρέμησιν. συστέλλεσθαι δὲ εἶναί φαμεν τὸ πρὸς ἔνδον ἀναχωρεῖν τὴν ἀρτηρίαν, συνεστάλθαι δὲ τὸ ἀφικνουμένην εἰς τὸ ἔνδον ἐπιμένειν χρόνον τινά. καλεῖται δὲ καὶ τοῦτο ἐπηρέμησις. τεσσάρων οὖν μερῶν τοῦ σφυγμοῦ θεωρουμένων, τὰ μὲν δύο κινήσεις εἰσί, τὰ δὲ δύο ἐπηρεμήσεις. γίνονται τοίνυν ἡ μὲν ταχυτὴς καὶ ἡ βραδυτὴς τῶν κινήσεων ὀνόματα, ἡ δὲ πυκνότης καὶ ἀραιότης τῶν ἐπηρεμήσεων·

[3] Ibid., iv: ἡ δὲ σφοδρότης ἡ ἐν τῷ σφυγμῷ τάττεται μὲν ἐπὶ τῆς κατὰ τὴν ἔξωσιν βίας, ὁπόταν τύχῃ τοιαύτη τις οὖσα. ὥσπερ οὖν κἂν τοῖς ἄλλοις κινουμένοις ἡ σφοδρότης ἐπὶ τῆς ἑκάστου βίας τίθεται, οὕτως ἔχει καὶ ἐπὶ κινήσεως τῶν ἀρτηριῶν.

brain-fever and in heart cases.[1] It is interesting to note that Markellinos makes no mention of Archigenes' 'double-hammer' pulse.

The 'failing' pulse (ἐκλείπων) is described very simply, as one which grows lesser and lesser in size and strength, and also correspondingly in speed and frequency, until it finally becomes imperceptible. This is therefore one of the most serious symptoms, and foreshadows death.[2] The 'intermittent' pulse, on the other hand, does not entail the complete disappearance of arterial motion, but merely its temporary interruption, a period of quiet following on systole. There seems to be a lacuna in the text, but as far as one can reconstruct it by guesswork, Markellinos seems to be distinguishing two factors, the length of the intermission as measured in dropped beats, and the intervals of normal series of beats following each intermission. The seriousness of the condition is increased by the number of beats dropped with each intermission and also by the shortness of the normal intervals between each intermission. In respect of both these factors the 'intermittent' pulse may be either regular or irregular.[3]

Markellinos' account of the intermittent pulse is closely connected with his description of the 'relapsing' or 'reversing' pulse (παλινδρομῶν σφυγμός), which immediately follows. Indeed it is impossible to imagine one without the other. The 'relapsing' pulse is one which remains for a considerable time in systole and gives the impression that the pulse has altogether ceased. It then starts to work again and strikes. The longer the interval of intermittence the more dangerous, since it implies a proportionate loss of vital tone, just as a smaller flame is most easily

[1] Markellinos, De pulsibus, xxxi: ὁ δορκαδίζων σφυγμὸς καλεῖται καὶ διπλασιάζων, ἁπλοῦς δέ ἐστιν ἐν μιᾷ διαστάσει δὶς πλήσσων, εἶτα διαστελλόμενος. διαστᾶσα γὰρ ἡ ἀρτηρία καὶ παρασχοῦσα φαντασίαν συστολῆς, ἔτι μετέωρος τυγχάνουσα, πάλιν προσεπιδιίσταται καὶ τότε τὴν ὀφειλομένην ἀπολαβοῦσα συστολήν, ὁμοίως ἐξερεθίζει τὴν ἁφὴν διπλῆν ἐν τῇ μιᾷ διαστολῇ ποιουμένη τὴν ὁρμήν. ὅθεν καὶ δορκαδίζων ὁ τοιοῦτος ἐκλήθη σφυγμὸς οὐκ ἀτόπως, ὥσπερ γὰρ αἱ δορκάδες ἐν τοῖς δρόμοις τὰ μὲν πρῶτα μικρὰ διαβαίνουσιν εἶτα αἰφνίδιον ἐπὶ τὸ μεῖζον ἐξάλλονται καὶ πρὸς τὸν ἀέρα μετεωρισθεῖσαι πάλιν προσάλλονται πρὶν ἐπιβῆναι τῆς γῆς, οὕτω καὶ ὁ δορκαδίζων σφυγμὸς μικρὰς καὶ ἀμυδρὰς ποιησάμενος τὰς πρώτας διαστολάς, ἐπὶ πλέον διαστέλλεται καὶ μένων ἐν τῇ αὐτῇ διαστολῇ πρὸ τοῦ πεσεῖν πάλιν προσεπιδιιστάμενος πλήσσει τὴν ἁφήν. Ἡρόφιλος μὲν οὖν ὁ πρῶτος ὀνομάσας δορκαδίζοντα σφυγμόν φησι ἅπαξ ἑωρακέναι ἐπί τινος εὐνούχου, ἡμῖν δὲ συνεχῶς ἐπὶ τῶν ἔργων ἐπέπεσεν ἔν τε φρενετικαῖς καὶ καρδιακαῖς διαθέσεσι.

[2] Ibid., xxviii: ὁ ἐκλείπων καλούμενος σφυγμὸς καὶ ἀπ᾽ αὐτοῦ τοῦ ὀνόματος ἐμφαίνει τὸ περὶ αὐτὸν ἰδίωμα. ἐλαττούμενος γὰρ ἀεὶ μᾶλλον κατά τε τὸ μέγεθος καὶ τὴν σφοδρότητα καὶ κατὰ συμμετρίαν τοῦ τάχους καὶ τῆς πυκνότητος, τὸ τέλεον ἐκλείπων οὐκέτι φαίνεται· διὸ καὶ ἐν τοῖς πάνυ χαλέποις καὶ ὀλεθρίοις τοῦτον τίθεμεν ὡς προσημαίνοντα τὸν ὄλεθρον.

[3] Ibid., xxix: ὁ διαλείπων καλούμενος σφυγμὸς παντελῆ μὲν ἀφανισμὸν οὐ ποιεῖ τῆς κατὰ τὴν ἀρτηρίαν κινήσεως, ἀθρόως δὲ ἀποκοπεὶς καὶ ἐφησυχάσας κατὰ τὴν συστολὴν χρόνον τινὰ ἐπανέρχεται πάλιν. καὶ ἔστιν ἐν αὐτῷ ἡ διαφορὰ τοιαύτη τις. διαλείπει γὰρ ἤτοι παρ᾽ ὀλιγωτέρας . . . καὶ τοῦτο γίνεται τεταγμένως ἢ ἀτάκτως· ποτὲ μὲν γὰρ μετὰ πλείονας σφυγμοὺς οἷον τέσσαρας ἢ πέντε διαλείπων, αὖθις μὴ φυλάξας τὴν τάξιν, μετὰ δύο ἢ τρεῖς πληγὰς διαλείπει . . . ἢ τὸ ἔντακτον φυλάσσει, τὴν αὐτὴν ἰσότητα ποιούμενος τῶν κατὰ τὰ διαλείμματα χρόνων. τὸν μὲν οὖν παρ᾽ ὀλιγωτέρας ἀνταποδώσεις σφυγμὸν διαλείποντα μᾶλλον ὀλέθριον νομιστέον, τὸν δὲ παρὰ πλείονας ἧττον, οἷον τὸν παρὰ μίαν κίνησιν τοῦ παρὰ δύο, καὶ τὸν παρὰ δύο τοῦ παρὰ τρεῖς καὶ τὸν παρὰ τρεῖς τοῦ παρὰ τέσσαρας.

extinguished. The distinction between the 'intermittent' and the 're-lapsing' pulse is not very intelligible. The former entails a change from motion to rest, and the latter one from rest to motion.[1] This conception of the relapsing pulse is, as we have seen, quite different from that of the recurrent pulse under the same name described in the *Medical definitions*.[2]

Markellinos' rather picturesque descriptions of the 'anting' and the 'worming' pulse add little to those we have already noted, and it is almost impossible to visualize the significance of the distinction between them.

The last type of pulse to be described is the 'trembling'. This is the most dangerous and most variable of the uneven and irregular pulses. In some parts of the body it feels slow to the fingers, in other parts quiet. Its speed is never constant, it quivers and its motion seems to be a simultaneous combination of both systole and diastole as the artery jumps. Its motion has been compared by the followers of Herophilus to that of a spider's web stretched across the holes of a flute. When the musician blows down it, it vibrates with no uniform motion, but rises higher above this hole than above that, according to the differences in pressure. In the same way the artery expands more freely in this part than in that, in one part more forcibly and in another more feebly.[3]

Another treatise on the pulse which has survived from early Imperial times is the one which has been attributed without any real justification to Soranus. It has survived only in a Latin translation, and was first published by Valentin Rose in his *Anecdota Graeca et Graecolatina*, together with some *Quaestiones medicinales* attributed (also falsely?) to the same source which contain some items also dealing with the pulse. These are

---

[1] Ibid., xxx: ὁ δὲ παλινδρομῶν σφυγμός ἐστιν ὁ πλείονα χρόνον ἐν τῇ συστολῇ μένων καὶ φαντασίαν ἀποτελῶν παντελοῦς ἀσφυξίας. εἶτα πάλιν ἐπανιστάμενος καὶ πλήσσων. ὅσῳ δ' ἂν διὰ πλείονος παλινδρομήσῃ χρόνου, τοσούτῳ μᾶλλόν ἐστιν ὀλεθριώτατος διὰ τὸ τὸν ζωτικὸν τόνον μελετᾶν ἐκ τοῦ κατὰ λόγον ἀπόλλυσθαι. ὅπερ γὰρ τρόπον αἱ λυχνιαῖαι φλόγες μειωθεῖσαι τὸ πῦρ αἰφνίδιον ἐκλείπουσιν, εἶθ' ὅσον οὐ σβέννυται τέλεον, τὸν αὐτὸν τρόπον καὶ ἡ ζωτικὴ δύναμις ἐκ τοῦ κατ' ὀλίγον σβεννυμένη καὶ πρὸς ἐλάχιστον συμπληξαμένη ἀθρόως ἀποκόπτεται. σχέσιν δὲ ὁ παλιν-δρομῶν πρὸς τὸν διαλείποντα ἔχει τοιαύτην συνυπάρχουσαν ἀλλήλοις. οὔτε γὰρ ὁ διαλείπων δύναται νοηθῆναι δίχα τοῦ παλινδρομοῦντος, οὔτε χωρὶς τοῦ διαλείποντος ὁ παλινδρομῶν ... δεῖ γὰρ τὸν μὲν διαλείποντα σφυγμὸν μεταβάλλειν ἐκ κινήσεως εἰς ἀκινησίαν, τὸν δὲ παλινδρομοῦντα τοὐναντίον εἰς κίνησιν ἐξ ἀκινησίας. [2] See above, p. 248, n. 5.

[3] Ibid., xxxv: ὁ δὲ τρομώδης καλούμενος σφυγμὸς ποικιλώτατος καὶ κινδυνωδέστατός ἐστιν ἐκ τῶν ἀνωμάλων καὶ ἀτάκτων τὴν ἐπιπλοκὴν ἔχων. ὅταν γὰρ κατ' ἄλλα μὲν μέρη τάχιον, κατ' ἄλλα δὲ βράδιον ἡ ἀρτηρία προσπίπτῃ τῇ ἁφῇ, καὶ μηδέποτε ἐν αὐτῷ τῷ χρόνῳ, ἀλλὰ καθάπερ κινουμένη τε καὶ κραδαινομένη καταλαμβάνεται καὶ οἷον ἐπιπλοκὴν τῶν κινήσεων ἑκατέρων, τῆς τε κατὰ τὴν διαστολὴν καὶ τῆς κατὰ τὴν συστολὴν ἔχουσα, τηνικαῦτα κέχυται τὸ τάχος καὶ ὁ ῥυθμὸς ἐπὶ τοῦ τοιούτου κινήματος ... καὶ παραδείγμά τι παρὰ τοῖς Ἡροφιλείοις τιθέμενον τοιοῦτον· ὥσπερ γάρ, φασί, τρυπήμασιν αὐλῶν περιτεθέντων λεπτοτάτων ἀραχνίων, ἔπειτα ἐμπνευ-σθέντων ὑπὸ τοῦ μουσουργοῦ τῶν αὐλῶν, πρὸς τὴν διαδρομὴν δὲ καὶ τὴν ἔμπτωσιν τρομώδης αὐτῶν ὁρᾶται κίνησις ἐπὶ τοῖς τρυπήμασιν, οὐκ ἴσης οὐδὲ ὁμαλῆς γινομένης αὐτῶν τῆς διασαλεύσεως ὅλων ἀλλὰ μετεωριζομένων κατ' ἄλλα μὲν μέρη μᾶλλον, κατ' ἄλλα δ' ἧττον καὶ καθ' ἃ μὲν εὐτονώ-τερον ἐπανισταμένων, καθ' ἃ δὲ ἀσθενέστερον, οὕτω δὴ καὶ τὴν ἀρτηρίαν κινεῖσθαι λέγουσιν ἀνωμάλως κατὰ μέν τι διαστελλομένην μέρος. ἐπὶ πλέον, κατὰ δέ τι ἔλαττον καὶ πῇ μὲν βιαιότερον πῇ δὲ ἀσθενέστερον.

written in the form of question and answer, the answer being in the form
of a definition in much the same form as those given in the *Medical definitions*
of Pneumatist origin which we have been examining. That given in the
answer to question 147—'What is the pulse?'—reproduces certain features
of Archigenes' definition, e.g. the insistence on the 'natural' involuntary
motion of the pulse, with the addition made by Moschion of the brain
and the meninges.[1] The pulsation of the brain also seems to be implied
in the treatise *On the pulse*,[2] where the appearance of pulsation in the
veins is also regarded as possible in acute fevers, 'though most authorities
think that a pulsation of the veins is impossible, because they contain
a large amount of blood and only a moderate quantity of *pneuma*.[3]
While accepting the traditional doctrine of the three-dimensional character of the expansion of the arteries, our author does not admit the
distinction between speed and frequency, but he does accept the characteristic differences of speed-frequency proper to the different ages. He
seems to have adopted the Empiric view that only the beat ($\pi\lambda\eta\gamma\acute{\eta}$) of
the pulse can be felt, for he expressly states that in his opinion the terms
fast and slow do not differ in meaning from 'frequent' and 'rare'. But
his description of fast and slow pulses is anything but clear.[4] He also
gives us a description of the 'full' pulse, and its opposite the 'empty'
one, adding that different plenitudes, like different speeds, were regarded
as natural characteristics of the different ages.[5] He also distinguishes
'wet' and 'dry' pulses in a manner which differentiates them from the
'full' and 'empty' kinds.[6]

The third of these treatises on the pulse is that ascribed to Rufus of
Ephesus, like Archigenes and Soranus also a contemporary of Trajan.

[1] *Anecdota Graeca et Graecolatina*, ii. 263: 'Aliter, quid est pulsus? Allevatio et contractio
arteriae procedens de corde et de cerebro per meningem naturaliter sine nostra voluntate.'

[2] Ibid., 276: 'Pulsus est motus arteriarum vel earum partium quae similiter arteriis
moventur.'

[3] Ibid.: 'Plerisque enim visum est venas pulsum habere non posse, quae quidem plurimum
sanguinem continentes et spiritum modicum, in acutis febribus ipso accessionis impetu
quandam imaginem pulsus habere videntur.'

[4] Ibid., 278: 'Veloces sunt qui modico momento quantum velocitas affestinare videtur,
ita diastolen simul et systolen perficere possunt. Proprie enim veloces dicuntur qui ab adsignato singulis aetatibus secundum naturam pulsu, in isdem iterum actatibus veloces in-
veniuntur. Tardi sunt qui longi temporis spatio collecti tardius digitis nostris ceciderunt.
Hos ab spissis et raris multi existimant differre, nos autem unam vim significationis habere
dicimus.'

[5] Ibid.: 'Pleni sunt qui tangentium digitos quadam soliditate ad plenitudinem pulsant.
Proprie autem plenus dictus qui ab adsignato singulis aetatibus secundum naturam pulsu
plenior invenitur. E contra autem inanis est qui tangentium aliquantum digitos oppressus
sustinere non valet, sed citius subcumbit, faciliusque pressura concavatus inferius discedit.
Proprie autem inanis est qui ab adsignato singulis aetatibus secundum naturam in isdem
iterum aetatibus inanior invenitur.'

[6] Ibid.: 'Humidus vero pulsus qui sic digitis occurrit ut non spiritu sed humore quodam
occurrere videatur, e contra siccus ita spiritu inflatur ut humecti pulsus suspicionem habere
non possit.'

Daremberg appears to have had considerable doubts as to its authenticity but his co-editor Ruelle accepted it as genuine, nor, as far as I know, has any conclusive evidence been adduced to show that it could not have been Rufus' work. However, a French critic, Menétrier, thinks that it is much earlier than Rufus, 'probablement même d'un élève d'Hérophile', a judgement which seems to me pure guesswork.[1] The author dissents from Moschion, who as Galen tells us corrected Asclepiades' definition of the pulse by adding the brain and the meninges to the heart and the arteries, and expressly confines the pulse to the latter two. The other portions of the body which appear to pulsate, such as the membranes which surround the brain which in the infant before the skull has properly closed can be seen to 'beat', really derive their movement from the arteries inside them.[2] The process of the pulse is explained as follows: 'The heart, when it draws in breath or *pneuma* from the lungs, first receives it in its left ventricle, then as this contracts immediately afterwards, it furnishes and supplies the *pneuma* to the arteries themselves. The arteries of the body, when they are filled with *pneuma* by the contraction of the heart, give rise to the pulse . . . but when they are emptied they contract . . . The heart produces the pulse when it is being emptied [i.e. at systole] but the arteries when they receive the *pneuma* and are filled.'[3] This is a description, which at first sight looks as if it might have been taken straight out of Erasistratus, so close is it to the facts. For *pneuma* read *blood*, and Rufus would perhaps have discovered the circulation, for he avoided Baccheius' fatal error of the simultaneous expansion and contraction of the heart and the arteries. 'Because heart and arteries', he continues, 'perform their double motion in the same time interval, nearly all the authorities assume that they are both filled simultaneously: I want to establish their error. Those who hold it', he concludes, 'had better learn the facts by going to see a vivisection' (ἀνατομή).[4] He now gives a very vivid description of the actual movement of the living heart.

[1] H. Menétrier, 'A propos du traité du pouls attribué à Rufus, et de la sphygmologie ancienne', *Bull. Soc. Fr. Hist. Med.* 18 (1924), 97–8.

[2] Rufus, *Synopsis de pulsibus*, D–R, 219–20: σφυγμὸς τοίνυν ἐστὶ διαστολὴ καὶ συστολὴ καρδίας καὶ ἀρτηριῶν. μόνα γὰρ ταῦτα τῶν ἐν ἡμῖν τὴν σφυγμικὴν κίνησιν κινεῖται, τὰ δὲ ἄλλα ὅσα δοκεῖ καὶ αὐτὰ σφυγμικῶς κινεῖσθαι, ὡς αἱ περὶ τὸν ἐγκέφαλον μήνιγγες ἐπὶ τῶν παίδων βλεπόμεναι κατὰ μετοχὴν τῶν ἀρτηριῶν κινεῖται.

[3] Ibid., 221: γίνεται δὲ σφυγμὸς οὕτως· ἡ καρδία, ὅταν ἐπισπάσηται ἐκ τοῦ πνεύμονος τὸ πνεῦμα, πρώτη αὐτὸ δέχεται εἰς τὴν ἀριστερὰν αὐτῆς κοιλίαν, εἶτα ἐπισυμπεσοῦσα ἐφεξῆς αὐταῖς ταῖς ἀρτηρίαις ἐπιχορηγεῖ. συμβαίνει οὖν ἐπὶ μὲν τῆς συμπτώσεως πληρουμένων τῶν ἐν τῷ σώματι ἀρτηριῶν τὸν σφυγμὸν ἀποτελεῖσθαι, κενουμένων δὲ συστολήν. αἱ μὲν οὖν ἀρτηρίαι, καθὼς εἶπον, τὸν σφυγμὸν ἀποτελοῦσι πληρούμεναι καὶ δεχόμεναι τὸ πνεῦμα, ἡ δὲ καρδία κενουμένη.

[4] Ibid., 222: ἐπεὶ δὲ ἰσοχρόνως καρδία τε καὶ ἀρτηρίαι τὸν σφυγμὸν ἀποτελοῦσι, καὶ διὰ τοῦτο ὑπολαμβάνουσι σχεδὸν ἅπαντες ὅτι πληρουμένων ἀμφοτέρων ὁμοίως γίγνεται. βούλομαι παραστῆναι τὴν πλάνην αὐτῶν. ὅτι μὲν γὰρ ἰσόχρονον ἐκ τῶν ἀρτηριῶν καὶ τῆς καρδίας τὸν σφυγμὸν γιγνόμενον καταλαμβάνομεν, φανερόν, ὅτι δὲ τῶν ἀρτηριῶν πληρουμένων τῆς δὲ καρδίας κενουμένης τοῦτο γίγνεται· ἐβουλόμην ἀναπέμπειν τοὺς βουλομένους μαθεῖν ἐπὶ τὴν ἀνατομήν.

'Moreover, when the heart draws *pneuma* from the lungs, and is filled on all sides, it moves sideways and is pulled a long distance from the sternum, but when it contracts again and empties itself, returning to its natural shape, it leaps towards the sternum and strikes it, and thus on contracting accomplishes the pulse.'[1] His description of the heart runs into some detail. 'It is shaped like a cone, and its broad part, in which there are also the mouths of its ventricles, adjoins or rests upon the lung, and lies between its four lobes, but its point in the direction of its length stretches upwards towards the sternum, not that it is actually attached to it, any more than its base is to the lung, but it is separated from it. And the heart is enclosed on all sides in a membrane which is called the *pericardium*. And this adjoins the lung at its broader portion and also the breast-bone, near which we said that its point lies, but it is separated from it.'[2]

In all this description there is no mention of the blood, but, as we have seen, blood is not mentioned in the Pneumatist treatises either in connection with the working of the pulse, for the blood in the arterial system was considered to be quite small in quantity, and its role purely passive. The insistence on the practice of and acquaintance with anatomy recalls at once certain passages in the treatise *On the names of human parts*,[3] the genuine authorship of which by Rufus has not been questioned. The description of the heart given in the latter work is not inconsistent with the description we have just quoted, but here the author is more widely concerned with its physiological functions. We are told that the heart is shaped like a pine-cone, it terminates in a peak, that it is like a muscle and 'sinew-like' (not nerve-like, if you please), beating continuously in a pulse-like motion. It has two ventricles that can be seen. The one on the right is called the haematic because it contains more blood, and the one on the left the pneumatic because it contains more *pneuma*. The heart is moved by the storing up of *pneuma*. He also mentions the auricles, and states that many vessels, veins and arteries, flow out from the heart, by which the whole body is provided with vessels.[4] In his treatise *On the*

---

[1] Rufus, *Synopsis de pulsibus*, D–R, 223 : συμβαίνει τοιγαροῦν ὅταν ἐκ τοῦ πνεύμονος ἐπισπάσηται τὸ πνεῦμα, πληρουμένην πανταχόθεν αὐτὴν εἰς τὰ πλάγια χωρεῖν καὶ πολὺ ἀπὸ τοῦ στέρνου ἀφέλ-κεσθαι. ὅταν δὲ πάλιν συμπέσῃ καὶ κενωθεῖσα εἰς τὸ φυσικὸν σχῆμα ἀναδράμῃ, τότε προσάλλεται τῷ στέρνῳ καὶ τὴν πληγὴν ποιεῖ. καὶ οὕτω συμπίπτουσα τὸν σφυγμὸν ἀποτελεῖ.

[2] Ibid., 222 : ἡ καρδία τῷ σχήματι κωνοειδὴς ὑπάρχει, καὶ τὸ μὲν πλατὺ μέρος αὐτῆς, ἐν ᾧ πάρεστι καὶ τὰ στόματα τῶν κοιλιῶν αὐτῆς, τῷ πνεύμονι προσπέφυκε καὶ μεταξὺ τῶν τεσ-σάρων αὐτοῦ λοβῶν κεῖται . . . τὸ δὲ ὀξὺ καὶ παράμηκες ἄνω πρὸς τῷ στέρνῳ οὐχ ὥστε συνδεδέσθαι, ὥσπερ καὶ ἡ βάσις τῷ πνεύμονι, ἀλλά ἐστιν ἀπόλυτον. περιέχεται δὲ πανταχόθεν ἡ καρδία ὑμένι τῷ καλουμένῳ περικαρδίῳ. οὗτος δὲ οὐ μόνον τῷ πνεύμονι προσπέφυκεν ἀρχόμενος ἀπὸ τῶν πλατυτέρων, ἀλλὰ καὶ τῷ στέρνῳ, ἐν οἷς μέρεσιν ἔφαμεν τὸ τῆς καρδίας ὀξὺ ἀπολύτως κεῖσθαι.

[3] Rufus, *De nom. corp. hum. part.*, D–R, 149–50 : τὰ μὲν οὖν ἐπιφανῆ, ὦ παῖ, σὺν τοῖς ὑποκει-μένοις ὀστοῖς οὕτω χρὴ καλεῖν. τὰ δ' ἔνδον τούτονι τὸν πιθηκὸν ἀνατέμνοντες ὀνομάζειν πειρα-σόμεθα.

[4] Rufus, *De anat. corp. hum. part.*, D–R, 177 : τῷ σχήματι στροβιλοειδὴς καὶ ἀπὸ πλατείας βάσεως εἰς κορυφὴν συννεύουσα κωνοειδῶς, τὴν δὲ σύγκρισιν μυώδης τε καὶ νευρώδης παλλομένη

names of human parts, Rufus describes the heart rather differently, as the source (ἀρχή) of heat and of life as well as of the pulse. Its top part is called the head, and its sharp point the bottom, its hollow parts the ventricles. Of these the one on the left, the artery-like one, is thicker, while the one on the right is more vein-like, is thinner, and has a larger cubic capacity than the left ventricle. On each side of the head of the heart are things like wings. They are hollow and soft and pulsate with the rest of the heart and are called its ears.[1]

In the treatise *On the anatomy of human parts*, a description of the blood vessels is found which distinguishes arteries from veins in the way with which we are familiar. Though the arteries contain some blood, they contain much more *pneuma*, and the chief function of the pulse is to distribute *pneuma* to the whole body.[2] In the treatise *On the names*, Rufus tells us of some of the names of the principal vessels, such as the vena cava, and something of the history of these terms, reciting some of the errors of the old anatomists with their description of the splenetic and hepatic veins, which we described in an earlier chapter. He also points out that the ancient physicians of the pre-Hippocratic and Hippocratic ages made no distinction between arteries and veins.[3] He is also one of our principal sources for the statement that Herophilus named the arterial vein and the veinous artery, which we have already examined.

The details of Rufus' description of the various kinds of pulse given in the *De pulsibus* need not concern us, but his comments on one or two of them are perhaps worth mentioning. He is acquainted with the double-beat pulse of which he gives us a definition, and he describes one modification of it without reproducing Archigenes' vivid description of the 'double-hammer'. This kind of pulse is characterized, he tells us, by an interrupted expansion of the artery: first comes an expansion of

συνεχῶς σφυγμικῷ κινήματι, μεσόκοιλος ἔχουσα κοιλίας δύο αἰσθητὰς ἐν αὐτῇ, τὴν μὲν ἐν δεξιοῖς λεγομένην αἱματικήν, διὰ τὸ πλείονος αἵματος εἶναι περιεκτικήν, τὴν δὲ ἐν τοῖς εὐωνύμοις καλουμένην πνευματικήν, διὰ τὸ πνεῦμα πλέον ἐμπεριέχειν, ἢ καὶ κινεῖται κατὰ παράθεσιν τοῦ πνεύματος, ὑμέσι παρὰ ἑκάτερα πλάτεσι κεχρημένη ὠτοειδέαι, διὰ τὸ περὶ αὐτὴν ὠτοειδῶς ἐσχηματίσθαι. ἐκφύεται δὲ ἀπὸ αὐτῆς ἀγγεῖα πλείονα, φλέβες τε καὶ ἀρτηρίαι ἀπὸ ὧν τὸ ὅλον καταγγειοῦται σῶμα.

[1] Rufus, *De nom.*, D–R, 155 f.: ἡ δὲ ἀρχὴ τοῦ θερμοῦ καὶ τοῦ ζῆν καὶ τοῦ σφύζειν καρδία. καὶ ταύτης τὸ μὲν ἄνω, κεφαλή, τὸ δὲ ἄκρον καὶ ὀξύ, πυθμήν, καὶ τὰ κοιλώματα, κοιλίαι. ἡ μὲν παχυτέρα καὶ ἐν ἀριστερᾷ ἀρτηριώδης, ἡ δὲ λεπτοτέρα καὶ ἐν δεξιᾷ φλεβώδης. αὕτη δὲ καὶ εὐρυκοιλοτέρα τῆς ἑτέρας. τὰ δὲ ἑκατέρωθεν τῆς κεφαλῆς ὥσπερ πτερύγια κοῖλα, καὶ μαλακά, καὶ κινητά, ἐν ᾧ πᾶσα σφύζει ἡ καρδία, ὦτα καρδίας.

[2] Rufus, *De anat.*, D–R, 183 f.: φλέβες μέν εἰσιν ἀγγεῖα περιεκτικὰ αἵματος διὰ ὧν τὸ αἷμα εἰς πάντας τοὺς τοῦ σώματος τόπους παραπέμπεται. ἀρτηρίαι δέ εἰσιν ἀγγεῖα περιεκτικὰ αἵματος μὲν ποσῶς, πνεύματος δὲ πλέον πολύ, ἐν οἷς ὁ σφυγμὸς γίγνεται. καὶ τὸ ἀπὸ καρδίας ἐκθλιβόμενον πνεῦμα δἰ αὐτῶν εἰς ὅλον τὸν ὄγκον ἀναδίδοται.

[3] Rufus, *De nom.*, D–R, 162: Ἡρόφιλος δὲ ἀρτηριώδη φλέβα τὴν παχυτάτην καὶ μεγίστην τὴν ἀπὸ τῆς καρδίας καλεῖ φερομένην ἐπὶ τὸν πλεύμονα. ἔχει γὰρ ὑπεναντίως τῷ πλεύμονι πρὸς τὰ ἄλλα· αἱ μὲν φλέβες ἐνταῦθα ἐρρωμέναι καὶ ἐγγυτάτω τὴν φύσιν ἀρτηριῶν· αἱ δὲ ἀρτηρίαι ἀσθενεῖς καὶ ἐγγύτατα τὴν φύσιν φλεβῶν.

considerable size, followed by a second shorter one. It is found in healthy
persons after sharp exercise or other violent activity, and in sick people
chiefly at the stage of rising temperatures.[1] The description given is not
altogether easy to distinguish from the one he gives of Herophilus' 'capering' or 'gazelling' pulse, which also manifests a double beat. 'There is also
a kind of pulse called the capering, when a large pulse having struck,
a short one strikes immediately after, so that it seems as if before the
artery has fully contracted, it starts expanding again.' This pulse, he tells
us, is mostly found in diseases of the chest.[2] He also describes the 'anting'
and the 'worming' pulses. The latter is so small and faint and feeble
that it gives the impression that there is neither contraction nor expansion
of the artery, but a mere eddy or 'rolling' of *pneuma*, in contrast with
the former where both these movements are still just perceptible.[3]
Menétrier attributed the discovery of the 'dicrotic' pulse here described
to Herophilus, and remarks that it still goes by the same name, and is
a recognized symptom in serious attacks of typhoid fever.[4] He identifies
the 'capering' pulse with Corrigan's celebrated 'water-hammer' pulse.[5]

[1] Rufus, *Syn. de puls.*, D–R, 230 : λέγεται δέ τις σφυγμὸς καὶ δίκροτος, ὅταν διαστᾶσα ἡ ἀρτηρία
μείζονα διαστολὴν ἑτέραν ἐπενέγκῃ βραχυτέραν. οὗτος ὁ σφυγμὸς γίγνεται ἐπὶ μὲν τῶν ὑγιαινόντων
ἀπὸ δρόμων ἢ γυμνασίων ἢ ἄλλο τι συντόνως ἡμῶν ἀπεργασάντων. ἐπὶ δὲ νοσούντων ἐν ταῖς
ἀναβάσεσι μάλιστα τῶν πυρεσσόντων εὑρίσκεται.

[2] Ibid., 231 : λέγεταί τις σφυγμὸς καὶ δορκαδίζων, ὅταν μέγας προσπεσὼν εὐθὺς βραχὺς
προσπέσῃ, ὡς δοκεῖν πρὸ τοῦ συσταλῆναι τέλεον τὴν ἀρτηρίαν πάλιν ἐπιδιίστασθαι. οὗτος ὁ
σφυγμὸς εὑρίσκεται μάλιστα ἐν τοῖς περὶ θώρακα νοσήμασιν.

[3] Ibid. : ἔσχατος δὲ πάντων καὶ βραχύτατός ἐστιν ὁ καλούμενος σκωληκίζων. οὗτος δὲ οὕτω
σμικρὸς καὶ ἀσθενὴς ὑπάρχει καὶ ἀμυδρός, ὥστε ἐπὶ μὲν τοῦ μυρμηκίζοντος καὶ βραχυτάτου
παντελῶς ὑπάρχοντος νοεῖται ἡ διαστολὴ καὶ συστολή, ἐπὶ δὲ τούτου οὐδὲ ὅλως, ἀλλὰ οἷον εἴλησις
μόνον καὶ κυλισμὸς τοῦ πνεύματος ἐν ταῖς ἀρτηρίαις ἀποτελεῖται.

[4] Menétrier, op. cit., 97 : 'Le pouls dicrote d'Héraphile est celui que nous décrivions encore
à ce nom, et que nos maîtres nous ont appris à reconnaître dans les formes graves de la fièvre
typhoïde. Il y a bien encore deux soulèvements successifs de l'artère, mais moins brusques,
le premier à peine plus élevé que le second, et avec une mollesse d'action qui marque bien
la défaillance du myocarde.'

[5] Ibid. : 'Ce type me paraît correspondre exactement à ce que nous appelons le pouls
bondissant de Corrigan . . . Le pouls correspondant commence par une rapide et haute éléva-
tion de la paroi artérielle, suivie d'une dépression brusque et plus long mais moins élevé
que le premier, complète la pulsation. Et si maintenant nous comparons cette description
avec l'image que nous donnent les traces sphygmographiques, nous retrouvons tous les
détails ci-dessus énumerés parfaitement figurés par l'ascension brusque, le crochet avec
descente incomplète, et le second soulèvement plus long et moins élevé qui caractérisent le
pouls bondissant de l'insuffisance aortique.' This identification must be treated with great
caution, since in one important particular it fails to agree with the 'gazelling' pulse as described, e.g., by Markellinos, who makes the second expansion of the artery not only longer
but higher than the first.

COMING now to Galen, whose acquaintance with the whole corpus of previous medical writings seems unrivalled and whose skill as an anatomist was matched only by his enterprise as an experimenter and had no equal in the ancient world, we might have expected the barrier which had concealed the circulation to be at last broken down. But it was not to be. Though Galen was much more than an epitomizer of existing knowledge, he was for all his gifts essentially a conservative, and if many of his experiments were certainly original, his temperament was that of a synthesizer, an eclectic who tried to reconcile as far as he could the often irreconcilable doctrines of the great masters of the past. Hippocrates was God, and Galen was his prophet. He was therefore temperamentally unsuited to make the great leap forward. For in spite of his insistence on experiment rather than on authority, he was essentially a conciliator, though his argumentative, not to say pettifogging, prolixity often almost conceals this from the reader's perception. He attempted to combine elements taken from almost every school into an integrated system, an Eclectic-pneumatist-dogmatist, to use the language of his age. The foundation of his medical system is the *Hippocratic corpus*, with all its contradictions and achievements, and the task on which he was to pride himself perhaps more than any other was the reconciliation of the post-Hippocratic discoveries with these sacred scriptures, the higher criticism of which is still engaging the attention of medical historians. He was perfectly aware of the enormous growth of anatomical knowledge since the Hippocratic age, and his debt to Herophilus is freely acknowledged, even too, on the heart, his debt to Erasistratus, whom in so many different connections he so loved to correct and to refute.

We have already seen how close Erasistratus, with his knowledge of heart valves and his postulation of the capillaries, must have come to the discovery of the circulation, and how one of the chief factors preventing him was the theory of Praxagoras, or, to be strictly accurate, that of his father Nicarchos,[1] that arteries contained no blood. When we come to

---

[1] *De plenitudine*, 11, K. vii. 573 f.: ἐν μὲν δὴ ταῖς τοιαύταις διαθέσεσιν οὐδὲν ἐναργὲς γνώρισμα τοῦ κατὰ τὰς φλέβας ἠθροισμένου πλήθους ἐκ (δὲ) τῆς τῶν ἀρτηριῶν κινήσεως ἔνεστι λαβεῖν,

examine the theory of Galen, who knew that the arteries contained at any rate some blood, we may well wonder even more how he too failed, since he was not impeded by the *damnosa hereditas* of Praxagoras' teaching. He went out of his way almost to compose a special treatise arguing 'against Erasistratus' that the arteries as well as the left ventricle contained blood under normal circumstances, and undertook an experiment to prove this in the case of the arteries by ligating an artery in two places and dividing it between the two ligatures.[1] Moreover he accepted Erasistratus' explanation of how the valves in the heart work, as well as his assumption of the interconnecting anastomoses between the arterioles and venules. Here too he cites, as we shall see,[2] experimental evidence to prove this demonstrating the passage of blood from one system to the other. And yet he too failed to discover the circulation.

To understand precisely how it was that he failed to do so we must undertake a really detailed, and in places perhaps tedious, examination of his theories concerning the vascular system. For this purpose, the most convenient starting-point is of course the heart, which is described most fully in two different writings, almost the whole of the sixth book of *On the use of the parts* being devoted to it, as well as the second half of the seventh book of the treatise *On anatomical procedures*. But before we proceed to examine all this rather complicated matter, we may perhaps begin by asking the question whether Galen was himself directly acquainted with the human as contrasted with the animal heart. Daremberg[3] showed quite clearly that he was not, and even accuses him of misreading the location of the heart in the body more like a sophist than an observer. For Galen seems to be arguing that the heart is located right in the centre of the thorax in the physiological as opposed to the anatomical work just mentioned. His words merit exact quotation:

Now most people consider that the heart has been placed, not exactly in the middle, but rather to the left, being deceived by the fact that the beat [σφυγμός] is perceived near the left nipple, the ventricle situated on the left being the starting-point of all the arteries. But there is another ventricle, turned towards the hollow vein and the liver, on the right side of the heart, so that the whole of the heart cannot be said to lie on the left side, but it is precisely in the middle, not only in the horizontal but also in the other two planes defining the height and the depth of the thorax. For the vertebrae are at the same distance from the back of the heart as the sternum is from the front, and the distance of the

εἰ καὶ ὅτι μάλιστα τῷ Νικάρχῳ καὶ Πραξαγόρᾳ δοκεῖ, καίτοι μὴ μεταδιδοῦσι ταῖς ἀρτηρίαις αἵματος.

[1] *De sanguine in arteriis*, 6, K. iv. 724: βρόχῳ γὰρ ἡμεῖς ἑκατέρωθεν τὰς γεγυμνωμένας ἀρτηρίας διαλαμβάνοντες εἶτ' ἐκτέμνοντες τὸ ἐν μέσῳ, δείκνυμεν αἵματος μεστάς.

[2] See below, pp. 282 f.

[3] See the long note appended to his translation of Chapter 2 of the sixth book of *On the use of the parts* (*Œuvres . . . de Galien*, transl. Daremberg, Paris, 1854, i. 383 ff.).

collar-bone from it is the same as that of the diaphragm. And just because it lies right in the middle of the thorax, it properly attracts [the *pneuma*] from all the parts of the lung, while at the same time lying in the safest position, being situated as far as possible from all objects that could impinge upon it through the thorax.[1]

Daremberg points out incidentally that Aristotle agreed with the moderns by placing the heart to the left of the median line, and remarks that it is in the situation of the heart that human anatomy differs most markedly from that of most other mammals. Most mammals have the heart more centrally placed than man and, as we shall see below, the heart is less closely related to the diaphragm, there being quite an appreciable distance between the point where the inferior vena cava traverses the diaphragm and the point where it enters the pericardium. Galen applies to the human body the anatomical location of the heart observable in other mammals in both these respects. In the seventh chapter of the seventh book of *On anatomical procedures*, Galen describes rather more accurately the position of the heart, say in a monkey. Once again he tries to explain away its appearance of lying rather to the left:

You will see in this operation, in addition to what I have stated, that the heart is located midway between the two concavities of the thorax. The appearance of its movement as being more to the left is due to two reasons, first because the animal's pneumatic ventricle is located on the left side, and secondly because the whole organ lies rather towards the left, since its tip, unlike its base, does not lie precisely midway between the right and the left of the thorax. It is not stretched from head to tip precisely in the median line, but it bends slightly, as I have mentioned, towards the left.[2]

In this connection Daremberg pointed out that in most mammals the heart lies much nearer the centre of the thorax than in man, but

---

[1] *De usu partium*, vi. 2, K. iii. 415 f.: νομίζουσι δ' οἱ πολλοὶ μὴ μέσην ἀκριβῶς ἀλλ' ἐν τοῖς ἀριστεροῖς μᾶλλόν πως τετάχθαι τὴν καρδίαν, ἀπατώμενοι τῷ διασημαίνοντι κατὰ τὸν ἀριστερὸν τιτθὸν σφυγμῷ, τῆς ἐνταῦθα τεταγμένης κοιλίας οὔσης τῆς τῶν ἀπασῶν τῶν ἀρτηριῶν ἀρχῆς. ἀλλ' ἔστιν ἑτέρα κοιλία πρός τε τὴν κοίλην ἐστραμμένη φλέβα καὶ τὸ ἧπαρ ἐν τοῖς δεξιοῖς μέρεσιν αὐτοῦ, δι' ἣν οὐκ ἐν τοῖς ἀριστεροῖς τὸ σύμπαν ἡ καρδία τετάχθαι λέγεται, μέση δ' ἀκριβῶς ὑπάρχει, οὐ ταύτης μόνης τῆς διαστάσεως τῆς κατὰ τὸ πλάτος, ἀλλὰ καὶ τῶν ἑτέρων δυοῖν τῶν εἰς τὸ βάθος τε καὶ μῆκος τοῦ θώρακος διηκουσῶν. ὅσον γὰρ οἱ σπόνδυλοι τῆς καρδίας ἀφεστήκασιν ὀπίσω, τοσοῦτον ἔμπροσθεν τὰ στέρνα· καὶ μέν γε καὶ ὅσον αἱ κλεῖς ἄνω, τοσοῦτον κάτω τὸ διάφραγμα. καὶ διὰ ταῦτα μέση κατὰ πάσας τὰς διαστάσεις τοῦ θώρακος κειμένη, δικαίαν μὲν ἐξ ἁπάντων τοῦ πνεύμονος τῶν μερῶν ποιεῖται τὴν ὁλκὴν ἀσφαλέστατα δ' αὐτὴ τέτακται, πάντων τῶν διὰ τοῦ θώρακος αὐτῇ προσπεσουμένων ἔξωθεν ἀπαχθεῖσα πορρωτάτω.

[2] *De anatomicis administrat.* vii. 7, K. ii. 605 f.: ὄψει δὲ κατὰ τὴν τοιαύτην ἐγχείρησιν ἔτι καὶ τοῦτο πρὸς τοῖς εἰρημένοις, ὡς ἥ γε καρδία μέση τέτακται τῶν τοῦ θώρακος εὐρυχωριῶν ἑκατέρας. διασημαίνει δ' ἡ κίνησις αὐτῆς ὡς ἐν ἀριστεροῖς μᾶλλον κειμένης διὰ διττὴν αἰτίαν, ὅτι τε κατὰ τοῦτο τέτακται τοῦ ζῴου τὸ μέρος ἡ πνευματικὴ κοιλία, καὶ ὅτι κέκλιταί πως ὅλη πρὸς τοῦτο μᾶλλον. οὐ γὰρ ὥσπερ ἡ βάσις αὐτῆς ἀκριβῶς ἐστι μέση τῶν τοῦ θώρακος ἀριστερῶν τε καὶ δεξιῶν, οὕτω καὶ ἡ κορυφή· διότι μηδὲ ἀκριβῶς κατάντης ἀπο τῆς ἰδίας βάσεως ἐπὶ τὸ κάτω πέρας ἐκτέταται, παρεγκλίνει δέ, ὡς ἔφην, ἐπὶ τὴν ἀριστερὰν χώραν.

that in the orang-outang it slopes markedly towards the left. It is also much more closely attached to the diaphragm, as it is also in man.[1]

In contrast with the author of the 'Hippocratic' *De corde*, Galen denies that the heart is a muscle, a statement which at first sight appears rather startling. When, however, we examine the reasons for this denial, we shall find that it rests in good part on a purely terminological distinction. The term *muscle* is confined by Galen to those fibrous tissues the function of which is to effect *voluntary* motion.[2] But the action of the heart is involuntary, quite independent of our volition. Indeed, it is so autonomous

[1] Daremberg, loc. cit.: 'La situation du cœur des mammifères est peut-être la circonstance par laquelle il s'éloigne le plus souvent de celui de l'homme, ce qui tient à la marche horizontale de la plupart de ces animaux. Sa position est généralement moins oblique et plus directe d'avant en arrière. Dans les orangs il présente encore cette obliquité d'une manière marquée, et il touche au diaphragme par une aussi grand étendue que chez l'homme. Dans les autres singes il ne répond à ce muscle que par sa pointe, qui conserve un peu d'obliquité à gauche ; et, dans la très-grande partie des autres mammifères, cette pointe n'atteint même pas jusqu'à ce muscle ; elle vient se poser, ainsi qu'une portion de la face inférieure du cœur, sur la partie moyenne du sternum. De sorte que chez ces animaux le cœur est placé sur la ligne médiane du corps ... et à une certaine distance du diaphragme. Comme dans l'homme, il n'est assujetti dans la poitrine que par les gros vaissaux et le sac qui le contient ... Suivant Aristote, et en cela il est d'accord avec Cuvier, le cœur, chez l'homme, dévie sensiblement vers la gauche, tandis que chez les autres animaux il est situé au milieu du thorax. Dans le traité *Des parties des animaux* (II, iv) il dit: "Le cœur a, dans le thorax, la place la plus noble ; il est, en effet, situé vers le milieu, mais plutôt en haut qu'en bas, et plutôt en avant qu'en arrière." Dans ces propositions sur la situation du cœur Galien se montre plus sophiste qu'observateur, et l'on voit évidemment, du reste, qu'il veut rapporter à l'homme ce qui est propre aux animaux. L'opinion du vulgaire, qu'il combat et qui est aussi celle d'Aristote, et de tous les modernes, est la seule vraie pour l'homme. Dans le *Manuel des dissections* (VII, vii) il se montre un peu plus exact, surtout pour ce qui regarde les animaux, quand il dit: "Le cœur occupe le milieu entre les cavités droite et gauche du thorax ; s'il paraît situé plutôt à gauche qu'à droite, cela tient à deux causes: c'est que le ventricule pneumatique est situé de ce côté, et qu'il se porte surtout à gauche, *car la pointe du cœur n'est pas comme la base, située exactement entre les parties droites et gauches du thorax.*" Ainsi un plan divisant le thorax en deux moitiés égales, ne couperait pas en même temps le cœur en deux moitiés parfaitement égales, mais laisserait une partie plus considérable à gauche qu'à droite, la base seule serait atteinte sur la ligne médiane ; tel est, si je ne me trompe, le sens de la phrase soulignée de Galien.'
    In this connection Mrs. Tallmadge May, in her translation of Galen's *De usu partium* (*Galen on the usefulness of the parts of the body*, Cornell University Press, Ithaca, 1968), i. 281, footnote 9, remarks: 'This insistence on a central location for the heart is another example of Galen's tendency to distort facts for the sake of his theory ; for none of the animals which he was in the habit of dissecting has its heart so placed.' Dr. Siegel in his book on *Galen's System of Physiology and Medicine* (Karger, Basel and New York, 1968), Chapter i, insists that Galen's description of the heart is based on that of the ox, which for some reason known only to himself he believes 'he exclusively studied' ; but the anatomical reasons given for this statement seem to me to be far from convincing.

[2] *De anat. admin.* vii. 8, K. ii. 610 f.: ὅτι δ' ἡ τοῦ σώματος τῆς καρδίας οὐσία πάμπολλα διαφέρει μυός, αὐτάρκως ἐπιδέδεικται, μαρτυρούσης αὐτῇ καὶ τῆς ἐνεργείας. ἀβούλητος μὲν γάρ ἐστι καὶ ἄπαυστος, ἔστ' ἂν περιῇ τὸ ζῷον, ἡ τῆς καρδίας κίνησις. ἡσυχάζει δὲ πολλάκις, ἐπεγείρεταί τε πάλιν ἡ τῶν μυῶν, ταῖς ὁρμαῖς τοῦ ζῴου δουλεύουσα. Cf. *De motu musculorum*, i. 3, K. iv. 377: εἰ δέ τῳ δοκεῖ καὶ ἡ καρδία παραπλησίως ἔχειν, οὐκ ἀκριβῶς οὗτος κατεσκέψατο σῶμα μυός, ἢ πάντως ἂν ἔγνω πολὺ διαφέρουσαν αὐτὴν καὶ πάχει καὶ διαπλάσει καὶ πλοκῇ καὶ σκληρότητι μυός. καὶ μὲν δὴ καὶ τοῖς ἔργοις οὐδὲν ἐοίκασιν. ἡ μὲν γὰρ ἐν τῇ διπλῇ καὶ συνθέτῳ κινήσει διὰ παντὸς ἐκ διαστολῆς καὶ συστολῆς συγκειμένη, μηδὲν τῆς ὁρμῆς τοῦ ζῴου πρὸς τὸ γενέσθαι δεομένη· τοῖς μυσὶ δ' οὔθ' αἱ κινήσεις ὅμοιαι, καὶ χωρὶς ὁρμῆς οὐκ ἂν γένοιντο.

that it does not depend even upon the action of the brain and the nervous system. It is the only part of the body which, even when removed from it, retains its power of functioning for a considerable period.[1] But Galen is perfectly aware that the heart-walls are made up of fibres.

Its flesh is hard and not easily injured, being composed of fibres of many different kinds, and because of this, even if it would appear to be like muscles, it is clearly different from them. For muscles have their fibres going only in one direction. Either they have them lying in the direction of their length, or lying at right angles across their breadth, but no muscle has fibres in both directions. But the heart has both length-wise and cross fibres, as well as a third kind running diagonally, inclined at an angle. And in hardness, tone, or tension, and general strength and resistance to injury [δυσπάθεια], the fibres of the heart much surpass all other fibres. For no organ functions so continuously, or moves with such force as the heart.[2]

In the treatise *On anatomical procedures*, he tells us that 'the heart' is made up of fibres of various kinds going in different directions each of which is surrounded by simple flesh. This factor is common not only to all muscles, but also to the stomach and the intestines, the bladder, and the womb, but the fibres do not all have the same strength or thickness, or the flesh the same character. For that in the muscles is redder and softer than that of the stomach and the womb and the intestines. That of the heart is at the same time harder and more varied in its fibres. But the careless observer will not see any difference in the substance of the heart and that of a muscle, just as he will fail to distinguish between a nerve, a ligament, and a tendon.[3] In the same work he informs us that when cooked, the heart tastes quite differently from other organs, each of which has it own flavour.[4]

---

[1] *De plac. Hipp. et Plat.* ii. 6, K. v. 264: ἐκ τούτων τῶν φαινομένων ἕτοιμόν ἐστι συλλογίσασθαι μήτε τὴν καρδίαν εἰς τὴν τῶν σφυγμῶν κίνησιν ἐγκεφάλου τι προσδεῖσθαι, μήτε τὸν ἐγκέφαλον καρδίας. Cf. ibid., vi. 2, K. v. 531: μόνη δ᾿ ἡ καρδία πάντων τῶν ἐν τῷ ζῴῳ μορίων ἐξαιρουμένη μέχρι πλείστου διαφυλάττουσα τὴν κατὰ φύσιν ἐνέργειαν, ὡς ἀρχὴ κινήσεως ἑαυτῇ τε καὶ τοῖς ἀφ᾿ ἑαυτῆς.

[2] *De usu partium*, vi. 8, K. iii. 437 f.: σάρξ ἐστιν ἡ καρδία σκληρὰ καὶ δυσπαθὴς ἐξ ἰνῶν πολυειδῶν συγκειμένη, καὶ κατ᾿ ἄμφω ταῦτα, κἂν εἰ παραπλήσιος εἶναι δοκοίη τοῖς μυσίν, ἐναργῶς αὐτῶν διαφέρει. τοῖς μὲν γὰρ μονοειδής ἐστιν ἡ τῶν ἰνῶν φύσις· ἢ γὰρ εὐθείας μόνον ἔχουσι κατὰ τὸ μῆκος ἑαυτῶν, ἢ ἐγκαρσίας κατὰ τὸ πλάτος, ἅμα δὲ ἑκατέρας οὐδείς. ἡ καρδία δὲ καὶ ταύτας ἀμφοτέρας ἔχει, καὶ τρίτας ἐπ᾿ αὐταῖς τὰς λοξάς. ἀλλὰ καὶ σκληρότητι καὶ τόνῳ καὶ τῇ συμπάσῃ ῥώμῃ τε καὶ δυσπαθείᾳ πολὺ δή τι παραλλάττουσιν αἱ τῆς καρδίας ἶνες ἁπασῶν τῶν ἄλλων. οὐδενὸς γὰρ οὕτως ὀργάνου συνεχές ἢ σφοδρόν ἐστι τὸ ἔργον.

[3] *De anat. admin.* vii. 8, K. ii. 609 f.: ποδηγῆσαι μέντοι τινὰ πρὸς τὴν ἀκριβεστέραν αὐτῶν ἐπίσκεψιν οἷόν τε, τὴν μὲν καρδίαν ἐξ ἰνῶν ποικίλων τῇ θέσει συγκεῖσθαι λέγοντα, περιφυομένης αὐτῶν ἑκάστῃ σαρκὸς ἁπλᾶς. κοινὸν γὰρ τοῦτο καὶ τοῖς μυσὶν ἅπασι καὶ τῇ γαστρὶ καὶ τοῖς ἐντέροις, κύστει τε καὶ μήτρᾳ. οὐ μὴν οὔθ᾿ αἱ ἶνες ἴσην ἰσχὺν ἢ πάχος ἔχουσιν ἐν ἅπασιν, οὔτε ἡ σὰρξ τὴν αὐτὴν ἀκριβῶς ἰδέαν. ἀλλ᾿ ἡ μὲν ἐν τοῖς μυσὶν ἐρυθροτέρα τ᾿ ἐστὶ καὶ μαλακωτέρα τῆς κατὰ τὴν γαστέρα καὶ μήτραν καὶ κύστιν, ἁπασάν τε τῶν ἐντέρων οὐσίαν. ἡ δὲ τῆς καρδίας σκληροτέρα ἅμα καὶ ποικιλοτέρα ταῖς ἰσίν.

[4] *Ibid.*, 611: ἀμέλει κἂν ἐψήσας τις ἅμα καρδίαν τε καὶ μῦν ὁντιναοῦν ἑκατέρου γεύσασθαι βουληθῇ, διαφορὰν εὑρήσει κατὰ τὴν γεῦσιν αὐτῶν οὐ σμικράν. ὥσπερ εἰ σπληνὸς ἢ νεφρῶν ἢ

Though he refuses to call the fibres of the heart, the stomach, and the intestines, bladder, etc., muscles, he is perfectly aware that they move the walls of the heart, and he tells us that we can observe their motion in a heart taken out of a living animal and still beating, or within the breast of the animal itself by excision of the sternum.[1]

When the longitudinal fibres of the ventricles contract, while all the others remain loose, it [the ventricle] becomes smaller in length, but its breadth increases in all directions. Then you will see the whole heart expanding in diastole. On the other hand, when the longitudinal fibres relax and the cross-wise ones contract, then you will observe it contracting in systole. And between these two different motions there is a short period of rest, when the heart has fully embraced its contents, all the fibres being in a state of activity or tension, especially the diagonal, for these play a great part. Those fibres contribute most to the systole which are stretched across inside the ventricles themselves, like ligaments, possessing as they do the greatest strength, and being strong enough, when they come together, to draw inwards the tunics of the heart together with them. For there is in the middle of the two ventricles a thing like a diaphragm, in which the stretched ligaments terminate, connecting it with the bodies covering each ventricle from without which they call its tunic. Now when these tunics [the heart-walls] approach the diaphragm [septum], then the heart is stretched lengthwise, but its breadth is contracted into itself. But when the tunics are at their greatest distance from each other, the breadth of the heart is enlarged, but its length is diminished. And if diastole and systole of the heart are simply the increase in the distance of the walls or tunics from each other and their mutual pulling together, we have discovered how each of these movements takes place.[2]

πνεύμονος ἢ κοιλίας ἢ ἥπατός τε καὶ γλώττης ἤ τινος ἄλλου γεύσαιτο μορίων. ἅπαντα γάρ, ὥσπερ ἁπτομένῳ τε καὶ θεωμένῳ καὶ σκληρότητι καὶ μαλακότητι καὶ πυκνότητι καὶ ταῖς κατὰ χρόαν διαφοραῖς, οὕτω δὲ καὶ τῇ γεύσει διαφέρει.

[1] De usu partium, vi. 8, K. iii. 439: καί σοι θεάσασθαι τὴν τοιαύτην αὐτῶν κίνησιν ἐπὶ τῆς καρδίας ἐστὶν ἐν διτταῖς καταστάσεσιν, ἢ ἐξῃρημένην ἄρτι τοῦ ζῴου καὶ σφύζουσαν ἔτι κατασκεψαμένῳ, ἢ τὸ προκείμενον αὐτῆς ὀστοῦν τὸ στέρνον ὀνομαζόμενον ἐκκόψαντι.

[2] Ibid.: ὅταν μὲν γὰρ εἰς αὐτὰς συνιουσῶν τῶν κατὰ τὸ μῆκος ἐκτεταμένων ἰνῶν τῶν δ' ἄλλων ἁπασῶν χαλωμένων τε καὶ διϊσταμένων, ἔλαττον μὲν γένηται τὸ μῆκος, αὐξηθῇ δὲ τὸ σύμπαν αὐτῆς εὖρος, ἐν τούτῳ μὲν διαστελλομένην ὄψει τὴν ὅλην καρδίαν, ἔμπαλιν δὲ χαλωμένων μὲν τῶν κατὰ τὸ μῆκος, εἰς αὐτὰς δὲ συνιουσῶν τῶν κατὰ τὸ πλάτος, ἐν τούτῳ πάλιν συστελλομένην. ἐν δὲ τῷ μεταξὺ χρόνῳ τῶν κινήσεων ἡσυχία τις γίνεται βραχεῖα, περιεσταλμένης μὲν ἀκριβῶς τῆς καρδίας τοῖς ἐνυπάρχουσιν, ἁπασῶν δὲ τῶν ἰνῶν ἐνεργουσῶν τηνικαῦτα, καὶ μάλιστα τῶν λοξῶν. μέγιστον δέ τι συνεπιλαμβάνουσι, μάλιστα δὲ τὸ πλεῖστον αὐτοὶ διαπράττονται τῆς συστολῆς οἱ ἔνδον ἐν αὐταῖς ταῖς κοιλίαις τῆς καρδίας σύνδεσμοι διατεταμένοι, ῥώμης μὲν ἐπὶ πλεῖστον ἥκοντες, ἱκανοὶ δ' ὄντες, ὁπότε συνιζάνοιεν ἔσω συνεπισπᾶσθαι τῆς καρδίας τοὺς χιτῶνας. ἔστι γὰρ δή τι μέσον ἀμφοτέρων αὐτῆς τῶν κοιλιῶν οἷον διάφραγμα πρὸς ὃ περαίνουσιν οἱ διατεταμένοι σύνδεσμοι, συνάπτοντες αὐτὸ τοῖς σκέπουσιν ἔξωθεν ἑκατέρας τῆς κοιλίας σώμασιν, ἃ δὴ χιτῶνας αὐτῆς ὀνομάζουσιν. ὅταν μὲν οὖν ἐγγὺς ἥκωσιν οἱ χιτῶνες οὗτοι τοῦ διαφράγματος, ἐκτείνεται μὲν τηνικαῦτα τὸ μῆκος τῆς καρδίας, συνιζάνει δὲ εἰς ἑαυτὸ τὸ πλάτος. ὅταν δ' ἐπὶ πλεῖστον ἀφιστῶνται, τὸ μὲν εὖρος αὐξάνεται, τὸ δὲ μῆκος ἔλαττον γίγνεται. καὶ μὴν εἴπερ οὐδέν ἐστιν ἄλλο τὸ διαστέλλεσθαι καὶ συστέλλεσθαι τὴν καρδίαν, ἢ τὸ μὲν τῶν κοιλιῶν αὐτῆς εὖρος ἐπὶ πλεῖστον διΐστασθαί τε καὶ συμπίπτειν, εἴη ἂν ἡμῖν ἐξευρημένον ἑκάτερον αὐτῶν ὅπως γίγνεται.

Galen, in common with all the qualified physicians of his age, was acquainted with the four chambers of the heart, but, like Erasistratus, he regarded only the ventricles as forming the heart proper, the auricles being a sort of process or projection (ἀποφύσεις) of the vessels leading into the ventricles. He compares, in one place, the right auricle to a hand.[1] In another he tells outright that the right auricle is an appendix of the vena cava and that this 'hollow vein' has an appendix leading to the heart, it does not grow out of it. It is an offshoot of the hollow vein which leads directly from the liver to the throat.[2] The auricles are in appearance more like sinews or like skin than the ventricles, and darker in colour, and they are attached to each of the two blood vessels bringing materials into the heart.[3]

They are like sinews and hollow, placed in front of the mouths of the ventricles, and at certain periods they are slack, but when the ventricle dilates in diastole, they contract, like the membranes of the valves, and empty themselves, thereby pressing out the matter they contain, and sending it forward into the heart. And the mouths of the adjacent blood vessels, being with great force pulled inwards by the heart, send on the material pushed into it by the auricles. Now the heart itself has every kind of power of attraction that one could imagine, and receives the matter quickly into the hollows of its ventricles, seizing it, and, as it were, sucking in the matter that is pouring into it.[4]

Looking for analogies, he compares the heart with bellows, which dilate when they suck in air, or with the flames of a lamp which sucks up oil—for the heart, being the source of the innate heat, certainly possesses this attractive power—and even with the magnet, which attracts iron, and he regards the existence of the auricles as singular proof of the wisdom of Providence, since if the heart were to attract blood with its full powers of attraction, the blood vessels might burst. The creator therefore invented the auricles as hollow vessels, reservoirs, as it were,

---

[1] *De usu partium*, vi. 4, K. iii. 420: οἷον χεῖρά τινα τῆς καρδίας ὀρεγούσης αὐτῇ νευρώδη καὶ ἰσχυρὰν ἀπόφυσιν.

[2] Cf. *De plac. Hipp. et Plat.* v. 5, K. v. 538: φαίνεται γὰρ ἡ κοίλη φλὲψ ἀπὸ τοῦ ἥπατος εὐθὺ τῶν σφαγῶν ἀναφερομένη, καὶ ταύτης ἀποβλάστημά τι τὸ εἰς τὴν καρδίαν ἐμφυόμενον οὐκ ἐξ ἐκείνης αὐτή.

[3] *De anat. admin.* vii. 9, K. ii. 615 f.: ὡς γὰρ ἐκεῖνα (τὰ ὦτα) παραπέφυκεν ἑκατέρωθεν τῇ κεφαλῇ, κατὰ τὸν αὐτὸν τρόπον καὶ ταῦτα τῇ καρδίᾳ, νευρωδέστερά τε καὶ δερματωδέστερα φαινόμενα σαφῶς αὐτοῦ τοῦ τῆς καρδίας σώματος . . . ἔστι δέ πως ταῦτα τὰ μόρια καὶ τῇ χρόᾳ μελάντερα καὶ σαφῶς ἐπιφύσεσι δερματώδεσιν ἔοικεν . . . δύο δὲ ταῦτά εἰσιν ἓν καθ' ἑκάτερον τῶν εἰσαγόντων ἀγγείων τὰς ὕλας.

[4] *De usu partium*, vi. 15, K. iii. 480–1: τὰ μὲν γὰρ ὦτα, νευρώδεις τε καὶ κοῖλαι πρὸ τῶν στομάτων ἐπιφύσεις ὑπάρχοντα, χαλαρὰ μὲν τέως ἐστὶ καὶ διὰ τοῦτο κοῖλα. διαστελλομένης δὲ τῆς καρδίας ὁμοίως τοῖς ὑμέσι τεινόμενά τε καὶ στενούμενα, καὶ διὰ τοῦτο τὰς ὕλας ἐκθλίβοντα προπέμπει τῇ καρδίᾳ. τὰ δ' ἐφεξῆς αὐτῶν στόματα τῶν ἀγγείων, διὰ τὸ σφοδρῶς ὑπὸ τῆς καρδίας εἴσω τείνεσθαι παραπέμπει τὰς ὑπὸ τῶν ὤτων ἐπωθουμένας ὕλας. αὐτὴ δὲ ἡ καρδία πάσας ὅσας ἄν τις ἐπινοήσῃ δυνάμεις ὁλκῶν ἔχουσα, διὰ ταχέων ὑποδέχεται κόλποις τῶν κοιλιῶν ἀναρπάζουσα καὶ οἷον ἐκροφοῦσα τὰς εἰσρεούσας ὕλας.

of the heart's nourishment. For if there were no auricles and the heart were to pull with all its might, there would not be sufficient room for the whole volume of blood or *pneuma* to pass, and the vena cava and the pulmonary vein (for the right auricle pumps blood and the left auricle *pneuma*) would burst. The auricles therefore, even if they were misnamed, were not created in vain.[1] The blood vessels leading into the ventricles are both soft, and this is in order that they should contract easily, which makes them also easy to burst.[2] That is why the vein-like artery (pulmonary vein) has a venous not an arterial character.[3] The auricles also help the ventricles to fill quickly, for they are both thin and sinew-like, their thinness contributing greatly to their power of contraction, while their sinew-like property gives strength to their walls.[4]

As to the ventricles, the wall of the left one is rather thick and hard, since it is destined to be the cover of the ventricle of the *pneuma*, whereas the wall of the right ventricle is thin and soft. This is a suitable arrangement for ensuring the equilibrium of the heart, since it was better that the *pneuma* should be contained in the thicker ventricle, while the larger volume of blood in the right ventricle balances the thicker fabric of the left.[5] Galen knows that the left ventricle reaches right down to the apex, whereas the right one starts some way up the septum and has a different shape,[6] a fact that had already been noted by the author of the 'Hippocratic' *De corde*, who was aware that the cubic capacity of the left was smaller than that of the right.[7]

[1] *De usu partium*, vi. 15, 481–2: ἐμοὶ μὲν δοκεῖ κἂν διασπάσαι τι τῶν ἀγγείων ἁπάσαις ἅμα χρωμένη τῆς ὁλκῆς ταῖς δυνάμεσιν, εἰ μή τι κἀνταῦθα θαυμαστὸν ἐπικούρημα τοῦ μηδὲν γενέσθαι τοιοῦτον ὁ δημιουργὸς ἡμῶν ἐτεχνήσατο, προσθεὶς ἔξωθεν ἑκατέρου τῶν εἰσαγόντων στομάτων τὰς ὕλας ἰδίαν κοιλότητα καθάπερ τι ταμεῖον τροφῆς, ὡς μὴ κινδυνεύσῃ ποτὲ ῥαγῆναι τὸ ἀγγεῖον, ἑλκούσης μὲν ἀθρόως τε καὶ σφοδρῶς ἐνίοτε τῆς καρδίας, αὐτὸ δ' οὐκ ἔχον ὑπὸ στενότητος ὅσον αἰτεῖ παρασχεῖν ἀφθόνως. ὥσπερ γὰρ εἴ τις ἀγγεῖον ἀέρος πλῆρες ἐκκενώσειε διὰ τῆς ὀπῆς ἐκμυζήσας τῷ στόματι ῥήξειεν ἄν, εἰ ἐπὶ πλέον βιάζοιτο, κατὰ τὸν αὐτόν, οἶμαι, τρόπον ἡ καρδία πολλαπλασίαν ἑκατέρου τῶν ἀγγείων τῆς εὐρότητος ἀθρόως ἐκπληροῦσθαι δεομένη κοιλότητι διέρρηξεν ἄν ποτε καὶ διέσπασεν αὐτὰ βιαίως ἕλκουσα, μηδεμιᾶς ἔξωθεν αὐτῇ προστιθείσης κοιλότητος οἷα νῦν ἐστι καθ' ἑκάτερον τῶν ὤτων. οὔκουν μάτην τὰ τῆς καρδίας ὦτα γέγονεν, ἀλλ' ὠνόμασται μάτην.

[2] *Ibid.*, 483: λεπτὸν δ' ἀγγεῖον καὶ μαλακὸν ὥσπερ εἰς τὸ συστέλλεσθαι ῥᾳδίως ἐπιτηδειότερον, οὕτως εἰς τὸ διασπασθῆναι τεινόμενον ἑτοιμότερον.

[3] *Ibid.*, 482–3: τά τε γὰρ ἄλλα καὶ λεπτὰ τοῖς χιτῶσιν ἄμφω ταῦτά ἐστι τὰ ἀγγεῖα, τὸ μὲν ὅτι φλέψ ἐστιν ἄντικρυς, τὸ δ' ὅτι τὴν ἀρτηρίαν τοῦ πνεύμονος ἄμεινον ἐδείκνυτο φλεβώδη γενέσθαι.

[4] *Ibid.*, 484: διὰ τοῦτο δέ, οἶμαι, καὶ τῶν ὤτων ἑκάτερον ἰσχνὸν ἅμα καὶ νευρῶδες ἐγένετο, πρὸς μὲν γὰρ τὸ συστέλλεσθαι ῥᾳδίως ἡ λεπτότης αὐτῶν μέγιστον συντελεῖ· πρὸς δὲ τὸ μηδὲν πάσχειν ἡ ῥώμη τοῦ σώματος, ἰσχυρότατον γὰρ τὸ νευρῶδες.

[5] *Ibid.*, 16, K. iii. 487: καὶ γὰρ οὖν καὶ τὸ σῶμα αὐτὸ τὸ ἐν ἀριστερᾷ μὲν πᾶν ἱκανῶς παχύ τε καὶ σκληρόν ἐστιν, ὡς ἂν τῆς πνευματικῆς κοιλίας μέλλησον γενήσεσθαι σκέπασμα, τὸ δ' ἐν τοῖς δεξιοῖς λεπτὸν καὶ μαλακόν, ἵν' ἅμα μὲν οἰκείως ἑκάτερον ἔχοι ταῖς ὕλαις, ἅμα δ' ἰσόρροπον ἐργάζοιτο τὴν καρδίαν. τό τε γὰρ πνεῦμα παχυτέρῳ στέγεσθαι χιτῶνι βέλτιον ἦν. τό τε τοῦ κατὰ τὴν δεξιὰν κοιλίαν αἵματος βάρος ἰσόρροπον ἔχειν τὸν ὄγκον τῆς ἀριστερᾶς.

[6] *De anat. admin.* vii. 11, K. ii. 623: ὄψει δὲ δήπου γυμνώσας ὅλην τὴν καρδίαν, τὴν μὲν ἀριστερὰν κοιλίαν αὐτῆς ἀνήκουσαν ἐπ' ἄκραν τὴν κορυφήν, τὴν δεξιὰν δὲ πολὺ κατωτέρω παυομένην καὶ περιγραφὴν δὲ πολλάκις ἰδίαν ἔχουσαν.

[7] See above, p. 86.

The doctrine of the function and structure of the two ventricles is found in two of the more important of Galen's physiological works, the essay on the teachings of Hippocrates and Plato, and also in the treatise *On the use of the parts*.[1] These important treatises make it quite plain that he believed that *pneuma* was drawn into the heart from the lung, though, as we shall see in due course, he expresses, in one of the works dealing with the pulse and its connection with respiration, some apparent doubt as to the quantity of *pneuma* so absorbed into the heart itself.[2] But the attribution of the tougher and thicker nature of the wall of the left ventricle to its function of containing *pneuma* seems to be quite central to his physiological conception of how the heart worked. The arteries did of course contain blood, but in much smaller quantities than the veins—a doctrine which was generally held by most schools of medical thought.

Galen describes the valves of the heart at considerable length in a number of passages which need detailed examination. Each ventricle has two mouths fitted with membranes, one mouth having the membranes turning inwards to let matter into the ventricle, and the other with membranes turned outwards to facilitate its exit. All except one of these 'mouths' have three membranes or 'cusps'. This one has only two. In the outlet valves the membranes are shaped like a sigma. The inlet valve of the right ventricle, which modern anatomy still calls the tricuspid valve, lies at the root of the hollow vein. Galen, as we have seen, regards this hollow vein as including the superior and inferior vena cava in a single vessel with a side channel opening into, or rather constituting, the right auricle. The outlet valve of the right auricle opens into the artery-like vein (pulmonary artery) leading to the lung. Here it divides into a system of many branches. The inlet valve of the left ventricle has only two cusps—it is still sometimes called the bicuspid as well as the mitral valve—and therefore does not close with the speed or with the accuracy of the tricuspid. This idea, as we shall see, plays an important part in determining Galen's notions on the movement of the blood. The bicuspid lies at the base of the left auricle, which forms the terminal process of the 'smooth' or vein-like artery leading out of the lung which we call the pulmonary vein. The outlet of the left ventricle is the sigmoid valve opening into the 'great artery', the aorta, which is the trunk of the arterial system. The inlet and outlet valves close alternately; when the inlet valves are open the outlet valves are closed, and vice versa, the purpose of both kinds of valve being to prevent back-flow. In a detailed study like the present, a full translation of the principal passages dealing with the valves of the

[1] *De usu partium*, vi. 16, from which we have been quoting. Cf. *De plac. Hipp. et Plat.* v. 5.
[2] See below, pp. 342 f.

heart will not be amiss. In the second book of his *On anatomical procedures* Galen says:

But when you cut open [the word he uses is *unfold*] the auricles like this, then the body of the heart itself will be visible, and each of the above-described mouths or valves, and then the membranes which lie at the insertion of the auricles, three on the right ventricle and two on the left. The shape of their construction is like the barbs of darts or arrows. Indeed they have been called three-barbed by some of the anatomists. Now these you will be able to examine accurately in a heart which has been taken out of the thorax, as you will also be able to examine the two remaining valves, those of the vessels that lead matter out of the heart, in the case of the right ventricle into the lung, namely the artery-like vein, and in that of the left ventricle the vessel of the great artery, which carries its contents to the whole body of the animal. On these mouths or valves you will again see on each side three membranes arranged in the form of a sigma, leaning outwards from the heart, as those of the three-barbed lean inwards.[1]

In Chapter 7 of the sixth book of *The use of the parts*, we find the following description of the valves of the left ventricle:

And there are the mouths of the two vessels of the left ventricle, which physicians are accustomed to call the pneumatic. For through these two mouths the heart is put in continuity of communication, through the smaller with arteries of the lung [pulmonary veins] and through the larger with all the arteries of the animal.[2]

In the eleventh chapter of the same book, we are given a description of the pulmonary valve and its functions:

For the more forcibly the thorax presses inwards, squeezing out the blood, by so much the more tightly do the membranes close the valve [of the pulmonary artery]. For they grow outwards from within, and in a circle embrace the whole mouth. And each of them has its form and size accurately fitted, so that when they are all of them drawn so as to stand in their 'upright' position they form a single large lid blocking the whole 'mouth'. They are turned outwards by the contents of the ventricle coming from within it, and point

---

[1] *De anat. admin.* vii. 9, K. ii. 616 f.: ἀναπτύξαντος δέ σου ταυτὶ τὰ ὦτα, τότε τὸ σῶμα τῆς καρδίας αὐτὸ φανεῖται, καὶ τῶν εἰρημένων στομάτων ἑκάτερον, εἶθ' ὑμένες οἱ κατὰ τὴν ἔμφυσιν ἐπικείμενοι, τρεῖς μὲν ἐπὶ τῆς δεξιᾶς κοιλίας, δύο δ' ἐπὶ τῆς ἀριστερᾶς, ὧν τὸ σχῆμα τῆς συνθέσεως ἔοικε ταῖς τῶν βελῶν γλωχῖσι. ταῦτά τοι καὶ τριγλώχινας αὐτὰς ὠνόμασαν ἔνιοι τῶν ἀνατομικῶν. ἀλλὰ ταῦτα μὲν ἔνεστί σοι κἀπὶ τῆς ἐξῃρημένης τοῦ θώρακος καρδίας ἀκριβῶς ἐπισκέψασθαι, καθάπερ γε καὶ τὰ λοιπὰ δύο στόματα τῶν ἐξαγόντων τὰς ὕλας ἀγγείων, ἐκ μὲν τῆς δεξιᾶς κοιλίας εἰς τὸν πνεύμονα τὸ τῆς ἀρτηριώδους φλεβός, ἐκ δὲ τῆς ἀριστερᾶς εἰς ὅλον τοῦ ζῴου τὸ σῶμα τὸ τῆς μεγάλης ἀρτηρίας. ἐφ' ὧν αὖ πάλιν ἑκατέρωθεν θεάσῃ τρεῖς ὑμένας σιγμοειδεῖς τὸ σχῆμα νεύοντας ἔξω τῆς καρδίας ὥσπερ οἱ τριγλώχινες εἴσω.

[2] *De usu partium*, vi. 7, K. iii. 436: ἔστι δὲ δὴ ταῦτα δυοῖν ἀγγείων στόματα κατὰ τὴν ἀριστερὰν αὐτῆς κοιλίαν, ἣν τοῖς ἰατροῖς ἔθος ὀνομάζειν ἐστὶ πνευματικήν. διὰ γὰρ δὴ τούτων τῶν στομάτων ἡ καρδία διὰ μὲν τοῦ μικροτέρου ταῖς κατὰ τὸν πνεύμονα, διὰ δὲ τοῦ μείζονος ἁπάσαις ταῖς κατὰ τὸ ζῷόν ἐστιν ἀρτηρίαις συνεχής.

outwards, folding upon the actual tunic of the vein, so as to allow the contents easily to pass outwards, since they open and unbar the mouth to its greatest extent. But if something were to be carried from outside the ventricle inwards, that would automatically close the membranes together into one piece, so that they fold upon one another and make of themselves as it were a tightly closed door . . .

And the purpose of all of them is the same, to prevent matter from flowing backwards, each of them in its own fashion, two of them to prevent any of the contents of the heart which are going outwards from returning back into it, and two, those in the mouths of the vessels bringing matter in, to prevent any matter from flowing back out of it.[1]

In Chapter 14, he gives a general description of the valves.

There are four mouths in the heart. Three of them are closed by three membranes, but there are only two membranes in the mouth of the vein-like artery. The membranes of all of them grow out of the mouths themselves. Starting from there, some extend inwards into the ventricles of the heart, so as to fit into them with secure fastenings, and some bend outwards at the place where each of the two vessels first emerges from the heart. Now there are on the artery-like vein, which, as we have said, feeds the lung, three membranes which bend outwards, membranes which from their shape are called sigma-shaped or sigmoid by those who have an accurate knowledge of anatomy. And on the vein which brings blood into the heart [the vena cava] there are on this too three membranes leaning from the outside inwards, and they are larger, thicker, and stronger than the former [the sigmoid]. And there is no third mouth on the right ventricle.

Now the vein which feeds the lower part of the thorax, and which forms a crown round the heart, for they call it the coronary, has the beginning of its projection beyond or outside the membranes. But on the other ventricle of the heart [the left] there is one mouth, the largest of them all, the mouth of the great artery, out of which all the arteries in the animal grow. And on this there are also attachments of three membranes like a sigma, pointing from within outwards. The other mouth is that of the vein-like artery, which subdivides into the lung [the pulmonary vein]. It has the attachments of two membranes, the shape of which none of the experts in anatomy has ventured to compare with any known object, unlike the sigmoid. For they have not called them three-barbed from their shape, but they gave them a name from

---

[1] Ibid., 11, K. iii. 459–60: ὅσον γὰρ ἂν ἔσω ἐπωθῇ σφοδρότερον ὁ θώραξ ἐκθλίβων τὸ αἷμα, τοσούτῳ μᾶλλον ἀκριβῶς ἀποκλείουσι τὸ στόμα οἱ ὑμένες. ἔσωθεν γὰρ ἔξω πεφυκότες ἐν κύκλῳ τε περιειληφότες ἅπαν τὸ στόμα, καὶ σχῆμα καὶ μέγεθος ἀκριβὲς ἕκαστος οὕτως ἔχων, ὡς εἰ ταθεῖεν καὶ σταῖεν ὀρθοὶ σύμπαντες, εἰς γίνεσθαι μέγας ἅπαν ἐπιφράττων τὸ στόμα, πρὸς μὲν τῶν ἔσωθεν ἔξω φερομένων ἀνατρεπόμενοί τε καὶ καταπίπτοντες εἰς τὸ ἐκτὸς ἐπ' αὐτὸν τῆς φλεβὸς τὸν χιτῶνα διεξέρχεσθαι ῥᾳδίως αὐτοῖς ἐπιτρέπουσι, ἀνοιγνυμένου τε καὶ διοιγομένου τοῦ στόματος ἐπὶ πλεῖστον. εἰ δ' ἔξωθεν εἴσω τι φέροιτο, τοῦτ' αὐτὸ συνάγει τοὺς ὑμένας εἰς ταὐτόν, ὡς ἐπιβαίνειν ἀλλήλοις καί τινα οἷον πύλην ἀκριβῶς κεκλεισμένην ἐξ αὐτῶν συνίστησι . . . χρεία δ' αὐτῶν ἐστιν ἁπάντων μὲν κοινή, κωλῦσαι παλινδρομεῖν εἰς τοὐπίσω τὰς ὕλας. ἰδία δ' ἑκατέρων τῶν μὲν ἐξαγόντων αὐτὰς ἐκ τῆς καρδίας, ὥστε μηκέτ' εἰς ἐκείνην ἐπανέρχεσθαι .τῶν δ' εἰσαγόντων, ὡς μηκέτ' ἀντεκρεῖν ἐξ αὐτῆς.

their closing in on each other. But the accuracy of their fitting does resemble the barbs of darts. Now it is the membranes on the mouth of the hollow vein which are properly called three-barbed, but these, since they are not three, but only two, we could not rightly call tricuspid. Why on this mouth only there are two membranes, for nature has not been negligent, I will tell you a little later.

It is only reasonable to expect that the membranes growing on the vessels which carry matter into the heart should be large and strong, and on those which carry matter out of it weaker.

I shall now try to explain also nature's preparations for the attraction and expulsion of matter. Now even given an actual inspection of the parts, it is difficult to explain these matters clearly, but without such inspection almost impossible. We must however try to give as clear an explanation as possible of these processes. The ends of the membranes leaning inwards from the outside, which we said were strong and large, all have their outside edges fixed into the heart itself, attached to it by very strong bonds or fastenings. Now when the heart expands, each of these bonds is stretched by the heart's distension and pulls itself, bending back the membranes, as it were, towards the body of the heart itself. When all three membranes have been bent backwards towards the heart, the mouths of the vessels are opened, and the heart easily draws in the matter in them through a broad passage. Besides which the vessel, i.e. the ventricle itself, in these circumstances stretches and attracts and conducts the matter through or past the membranes into itself. For it is not possible for the membranes to be pulled open by the heart, and for the vessel that is contiguous to them to be unaware of this attraction. So as the result of one action which the heart performs in diastole, the membranes are pulled by their fastenings and bent inwards into the ventricle of the heart, and being folded back in a circle, they open the mouth inwards. Meanwhile the vessels are pulled in through the membranes towards the heart, and their contents flow into the ventricles without hindrance, since they no longer meet with any resistance, all the factors through which a very quick transit of matter can be brought about, combining to contribute to this effect. For matter to be moved from one place to another must either be attracted or hit or propelled by something or transmitted. And all these things happen to the matter at the diastole of the heart. For the heart itself pulls, and the cavities of the auricles which lie in front of it, propel, and the vessels transmit it. And in this movement, of all of these motions the actual diastole of the heart is the source [ἀρχή].[1]

---

[1] De usu partium, vi. 14, K. iii. 476 ff. : τεττάρων ὄντων ἐν τῇ καρδίᾳ στομάτων, τρεῖς μὲν ἐφ' ἑκάστῳ τῶν ἄλλων ὑμένες εἰσί, δύο δ' ἐπὶ τῆς ἀρτηρίας τῆς φλεβώδους μόνης. ἐκφύονται μὲν οὖν ἅπαντες ἐξ αὐτῶν τῶν στομάτων, ἐντεῦθεν δ' ὁρμηθέντες, οἱ μὲν εἴσω προίασιν εἰς τὰς τῆς καρδίας κοιλίας, ὥστε καὶ συνάπτονται πρὸς αὐτὰς ἰσχυροῖς δεσμοῖς, οἱ δ' ἐκτὸς ἀποκλίνουσιν ἵνα πρῶτον ἀνίσχει τῆς καρδίας ἑκάτερον τῶν ἀγγείων. εἰσὶ δ' ἐπὶ μὲν τῆς φλεβὸς τῆς ἀρτηριώδους, ἣν τὸν πνεύμονα τρέφειν ἐλέγομεν, ἔσωθεν ἔξω νεύοντες ὑμένες τρεῖς ἀπὸ τοῦ σχήματος ὑπὸ τῶν ἀκριβεστέρως τὰς ἀνατομὰς ἐχόντων ὀνομαζόμενοι σιγμοειδεῖς. ἐπὶ δὲ τῆς εἰσαγούσης τὸ αἷμα φλεβός, τρεῖς μὲν κἀπὶ ταύτης ἔξωθεν εἴσω νεύοντές εἰσιν, ἀλλὰ πολὺ καὶ πάχει καὶ ῥώμῃ καὶ μεγέθει διαφέρουσιν ἐκείνων. ἄλλο δὲ τρίτον οὐκ ἔστι κατὰ τὴν δεξιὰν κοιλίαν στόμα. καὶ γὰρ ἡ τὰ κάτω τοῦ θώρακος τρέφουσα καὶ ἡ περιστεφανοῦσα τὴν καρδίαν, οὕτω γὰρ αὐτὴν καὶ ὀνομάζουσιν, ἔξω τῶν ὑμένων τὴν ἀρχὴν τῆς ἐκφύσεως ἔχουσι. καὶ μέν γε καὶ κατὰ τὴν ἑτέραν κοιλίαν τῆς καρδίας ἐν μὲν στόμα

From these descriptions it is clear that Galen had a fairly accurate idea of the way in which the heart works.[1]

Another point worth noting is that Galen was evidently acquainted with the coronary system of vessels providing the blood-supply to the heart itself,[2] though his interpretation of it is topsy-turvy because he thought that it was the coronary veins not the coronary arteries that were responsible for conveying blood to the body of the heart.[3] In another matter too he made a more fatal error, which has become historically

τὸ μέγιστον ἁπάντων ἐστὶ τὸ τῆς ἀρτηρίας τῆς μεγάλης, ἀφ' ἧς ἅπασαι πεφύκασιν αἱ κατὰ τὸ ζῷον ἀρτηρίαι, τρεῖς δὲ καὶ τούτῳ σιγμοειδῶν ὑμένων ἐπιφύσεις ἔσωθεν ἔξω φερομένων εἰσίν. ἕτερον δὲ τὸ στόμα τὸ τῆς φλεβώδους ἀρτηρίας, τῆς εἰς τὸν πνεύμονα κατασχιζομένης, ἔξωθεν ἔσω πεφυκότων ὑμένων δυοῖν ἐπίφυσιν ἔχει, ὧν τὸ σχῆμα τῶν γιγνωσκομένων οὐδενὶ προσεικάσαι τῶν ἀνατομικῶν ἀνδρῶν ἐπεχείρησεν οὐδεὶς ὥσπερ καὶ τῶν σιγμοειδῶν. οὐδὲ γὰρ οἱ τριγλώχινας αὐτοὺς ὀνομάσαντες ἀπὸ τοῦ καθ' ἕκαστον σχήματος, ἀλλ' ἀπὸ τῆς πρὸς ἀλλήλους συντάξεως ἐποίησαν τοὔνομα. καὶ γὰρ ἀκριβῶς ἡ σύνθεσις αὐτῶν ἔοικεν ἀκίδων γλωχῖσιν· ἀλλὰ τοὺς μὲν ἐπὶ τῷ τῆς κοίλης φλεβὸς στόματι, τρεῖς ὄντας, οὕτως ὀνομάζειν ἐγχωρεῖ. τοὺς δ' ἐπὶ τῷ τῆς φλεβώδους ἀρτηρίας, οὐκέτ' ἂν ὀρθῶς τις ὀνομάζοι οὕτως δύο ὄντας. διὰ τί μὲν οὖν ἐπὶ τούτῳ μόνῳ τῷ στόματι δύο γεγόνασιν ὑμένες (οὐδὲ γὰρ οὐδὲ τοῦτ' ἠμέληται τῇ φύσει) μικρὸν ὕστερον ἐρῶ. ὅτι δ' εὐλόγως ἐπὶ μὲν τοῖς εἰσάγουσι τὰς ὕλας ἀγγείοις ἰσχυροὶ καὶ μεγάλοι πεφύκασιν ὑμένες, ἐπὶ δὲ τοῖς ἐξάγουσιν ἀσθενέστεροι, τά τ' ἄλλα τὰ περὶ τὴν ὁλκὴν καὶ τὴν ἔκπεμψιν τῶν ὑλῶν τῇ φύσει παρεσκευασμένα λέγειν ἤδη πειράσομαι. ἔστι μὲν οὖν καὶ μετ' αὐτῆς τῶν μορίων τῆς θέας ἑρμηνεύεσθαι σαφῶς διὰ τοιαῦτα χαλεπόν, ἀπούσης δ' ἐκείνης ἐγγὺς ἀδύνατον. πειρατέον δ' ὅμως, εἰς ὅσον οἷόν τε σαφέστατα διεξελθεῖν αὐτά. τῶν ἔξωθεν ἔσω φερομένων ὑμένων, οὓς ἰσχυροὺς καὶ μεγάλους ὑπάρχειν ἔφαμεν, ἁπάντων εἰς αὐτὴν τὴν καρδίαν ἀνῆπται τὰ πέρατα, δεσμοῖς εὐρώστοις συνεχόμενα. διαστελλομένης οὖν αὐτῆς, ἕκαστος τῶν δεσμῶν τούτων τεινόμενος ὑπὸ τῆς κατὰ τὴν καρδίαν διαστάσεως, ἐφ' ἑαυτὸν ἕλκει καὶ οἷον ἀνακλᾷ τὸν ὑμένα πρὸς τὸ σῶμα τῆς καρδίας αὐτό· πάντων οὖν ἀνακλωμένων ἐκ κύκλῳ τῶν τρίων ἐπὶ καρδίαν, ἀνοίγνυνταί τε τῶν ἀγγείων τὰ στόματα, τὰς θ' ὕλας τὰς ἐν αὐτοῖς ἡ καρδία ῥᾳδίως ἐπισπᾶται δι' εὐρείας ὁδοῦ. τά τε γὰρ ἄλλα καὶ αὐτὸ τὸ ἀγγεῖον νῦν ἐν τούτῳ πρὸς ἑαυτὸ ἐπισπᾶται τείνουσα καὶ προσαγομένη διὰ τῶν ὑμένων. οὐ γὰρ ἐνδέχεται τούτου μὲν ἕλκεσθαι πρὸς ἐκείνης, τὸ συνεχὲς δὲ αὐτοῖς ἀγγεῖον ἀναίσθητον εἶναι τῆς ὁλκῆς ὥσθ' ὑπὸ μιᾶς ἐνεργείας, ἣν ἡ καρδία ποιεῖται διαστελλομένη, τοὺς μὲν ὑμένας ἑλκομένους ὑπὸ τῶν δεσμῶν εἰς αὐτὴν τὴν κοιλίαν ἀνακλίνεσθαι τῆς καρδίας, ἐν κύκλῳ δὲ τούτων ἀναπτυσσομένων εἰς τοὐπίσω διοίγεσθαι τὸ στόμα, κἂν τούτῳ τά τε ἀγγεῖα διὰ τῶν ὑμένων ἕλκεσθαι πρὸς τὴν καρδίαν, τὰς δ' ἐν αὐτοῖς ὕλας εἰς τὰς κοιλίας αὐτῆς ἀκωλύτως εἰσρεῖν, ὡς ἂν μήτ' ἀντιπράττοντος ἔτι μηδενός, ἁπάντων τε τῶν αἰτίων, ὑφ' ὧν ἂν γένοιτο ταχίστη μετάστασις ὑλῶν εἰς ταὐτὸ συντελούντων. ἢ γὰρ ἕλκεσθαι χρὴ τὸ μεθιστάμενον, ἢ βάλλεσθαι πρός τινος, ἢ παραπέμπεσθαι. καὶ ταῦτα σύμπαντα ταῖς ὕλαις ὑπάρχει, διαστελλομένης τῆς καρδίας. ἕλκει μὲν γὰρ αὐτή, πέμπουσι δ' αἱ προκείμεναι κοιλότητες αἱ κατὰ τὰ ὦτα, παραπέμπει δὲ τὰ ἀγγεῖα. καὶ τούτων ἁπάντων τῆς κινήσεως ἀρχὴ μία τῆς καρδίας αὐτῆς ἡ διαστολή.

[1] See R. Siegel, 'Galen's ideas on the heartbeat', *Proceedings of the Sixth International Congress of the History of Medicine* (1949), pp. 209–13; and his remarks on p. 32 of his book on *Galen's System of Physiology and Medicine.*

[2] *De usu partium*, vi. 17, K. iii. 498–9: ἐπεὶ δ' ἕκαστον, οἷόν ἐστι, τοιαύτης χρῄζει καὶ τροφῆς, εὐλόγως ἡ μὲν καρδία παχέος, ὁ πνεύμων δ' ἀτμώδους αἵματος ἐδεήθη· καὶ τοῦτ' αἴτιον τοῦ μὴ τρέφεσθαι τὴν καρδίαν ἐξ ἑαυτῆς, ἀλλὰ καὶ πρὶν ἐμφῦναι τῇ δεξιᾷ κοιλίᾳ τὴν κοίλην φλέβα, μέρος αὐτῆς τηλικοῦτον ἡλίκον μάλιστα τρέφειν ἱκανόν ἐστι τὴν καρδίαν, ἀποσχισθὲν ἐλίττεσθαί περὶ τὴν κεφαλὴν αὐτῆς ἔξωθεν, καὶ εἰς ἅπαντα τὰ μέρη διασπείρεσθαι. τούτῳ δ' εὐλόγως ἀρτηρία συμπεριφέρεταί καὶ συγκατασχίζεται τῆς μεγάλης αὖ καὶ ἥδε τηλικοῦτον ἀποβλάστημα γενόμενον, ἡλίκον ἔμελλε μάλιστα τήν τε προειρημένην ἀναψύχειν φλέβα καὶ τοῖς ἔξω μέρεσι τῆς καρδίας τὴν εὐκρασίαν τῆς ἐμφύτου φυλάξειν θερμασίας.

[3] Ibid., 496: οἱ τοίνυν ἐν τῇ καρδίᾳ φαινόμενοι βόθυνοι κατὰ τὸ μέσον αὐτῆς μάλιστα διάφραγμα τῆς εἰρημένης ἕνεκα κοινωνίας ἐγένοντο· τά τε γὰρ ἄλλα καὶ προκατειργασμένον ἐν ταῖς φλεψὶ τὸ αἷμα μεταλαμβάνειν ταῖς ἀρτηρίαις ἦν ἄμεινον.

For more modern views of the permeability of the septum, see below, p. 334, n. 2.

notorious, namely his assumption of the permeability of the interventricular septum—an error which, as we shall see in due course, was
not such an anatomical blunder as has generally been supposed, however
mistaken the physiological consequences deduced from it. But his reasonings from comparative anatomy were by no means always inaccurate.
He notes that all animals do not have the same number of ventricles in
their hearts. Only those that breathe through lungs have two. Fishes,
for example, have only one, and Aristotle was quite wrong in supposing
that the larger warm-blooded animals have three.[1] Before leaving Galen's
account of the heart's anatomical structure, we should note his description of the rather mysterious feature which was also postulated by
Aristotle,[1] the bone in the heart. This is more clearly visible in large
animals:

A sort of bone is found at the head of the heart in large animals, the use
of which has perhaps been correctly described by Aristotle, who says that
it is a sort of fixture or seat for the heart, and that it is found in large animals.
For it is clear that a heart suspended in a large thorax probably needs some
part of this kind. A more proper description than bone would be the following. Everywhere nature fits the beginnings [we should say ends] of ligaments
either to a cartilage or to a cartilage-like bone. She was not destined to forget
either the ligaments in the heart, for of this kind are the membranes at the
mouths of the blood vessels, or the coats of the arteries, which are of the same
texture as a ligament, but she fitted, as we have shown in our works on anatomy, the ends of all these structures into the cartilage-like bone. Now in
large animals, it is cartilage-like bone, but in very small ones, it is a kind of
cartilaginous sinew-like body. Every heart has in the same place a hard kind
of substance to fulfil this same need in every animal.[3]

Galen rather prided himself on having demonstrated this bone in the
heart of an elephant, which, so he tells us, he was able to persuade one

---

[1] *De usu partium*, vi. 9, K. iii. 441 : πλῆθος μὲν δὴ τῶν κοιλιῶν τῆς καρδίας . . . οὐκ ἴσον ἐν ἅπασι
τοῖς ζῴοις ἐστίν, ἀλλ᾽ ὅσα μὲν ἐξ ἀέρος εἰσπνεῖ διὰ φάρυγγος καὶ ῥινῶν καὶ στόματος, εὐθὺς μὲν καὶ
πνεύμων τούτοις ἐστίν, εὐθὺς δὲ καὶ τῆς καρδίας ἡ δεξιὰ κοιλία, τοῖς δ᾽ ἄλλοις ἅπασιν οὔτε πνεύμων
ἐστίν, οὔτ᾽ ἐν τοῖς δεξιοῖς τῆς καρδίας εὐρύτης οὐδεμία . . . οὔκουν ὀρθῶς Ἀριστοτέλης διῃρεῖτο περὶ
τοῦ πλήθους τῶν ἐν τῇ καρδίᾳ κοιλιῶν, εἰς μέγεθος καὶ μικρότητα τοῦ σώματος ἀνάγων αὐτῶν
τὸν ἀριθμόν. οὔτε γὰρ τοῖς μεγίστοις ζῴοις ἅπασι τρεῖς, οὔτε τοῖς ἐλαχίστοις ἐστὶ μία.

[2] *De part. an.* 3. 4, 666ᵇ17–21. *De hist. an.* 2. 15, 506ᵃ8–10.

[3] *De usu partium*, vi. 19, K. iii. 501–3: ἐπεὶ δὲ καὶ ὀστοῦν εὑρίσκεταί τι κατὰ τὴν κεφαλὴν
τῆς καρδίας ἐν τοῖς μεγάλοις ζῴοις, εὔλογον ἂν εἴη καὶ τὴν ἐκείνου χρείαν μὴ παρελθεῖν. ἔστι μὲν
οὖν ἴσως καὶ ἡ Ἀριστοτέλους εἰρημένη λόγον ἔχουσα. στήριγμα γάρ τι καὶ οἷον ἕδραν εἶναί φησι τῆς
καρδίας αὐτό, καὶ διὰ τοῦτο ἐν τοῖς μεγάλοις ζῴοις εὑρίσκεσθαι. δῆλον γὰρ ὡς ἐν μεγάλῳ θώρακι
μεγάλην καρδίαν αἰωρουμένην εὔλογον ἦν δήπου καὶ τοιούτου μορίου. κάλλιον δ᾽ ἂν ὧδε
λέγοιτο· πανταχοῦ τῶν συνδέσμων τὰς ἀρχὰς ἡ φύσις ἢ εἰς χόνδρον ἢ εἰς ὀστοῦν ἀνάπτει χονδρῶδες.
οὔκουν οὐδὲ τῶν κατὰ τὴν καρδίαν συνδέσμων, (ἐκ τούτου γὰρ τοῦ γένους εἰσὶν οἱ ἐπὶ τοῖς στόμασι
τῶν ἀγγείων ὑμένες,) ἀλλ᾽ οὐδὲ τοῦ χιτῶνος τῶν ἀρτηριῶν ὁμοίου συνδέσμῳ τὴν τοῦ σώματος
οὐσίαν ὄντος ἔμελλεν ἀμελήσειν, ἀλλὰ καὶ τούτων ἁπάντων εἰς τουτὶ τὸ χονδρῶδες ὀστοῦν ἀνῆψε
τὰς ἀρχάς, ὡς ἐν ταῖς ἀνατομικαῖς ἐγχειρήσεσιν ἐδείκνυμεν. ἐν μὲν οὖν τοῖς μεγάλοις ζῴοις
ὀστοῦν ἐστι χονδρῶδες, ἐν δὲ τοῖς μικροῖς νευροχονδρῶδές τι σῶμα. πᾶσά γ᾽ οὖν ἔχει καρδία κατὰ
τὸν αὐτὸν τόπον οὐσίαν τινὰ σκληρὰν ἕνεκα τῶν αὐτῶν χρειῶν ἐν ἅπασι τοῖς ζῴοις γεγενημένην.

of Caesar's cooks to let one of his colleagues remove[1] and send him. The larger the animal the more bone-like the structure, and he insists that in very large animals, it should be called not a bone-like cartilage but a cartilage-like bone.[2]

With regard to the distinction between the two kinds of blood vessels, veins and arteries, Galen accepts the nomenclature which was derived from Herophilus, under which all vessels connected with the right side of the heart were called vein, and all those with the left side arteries, which gave rise to the rather paradoxical appellations of the vein-like artery for the pulmonary vein, and the artery-like vein for the pulmonary artery.

If possible, it would be preferable to distinguish the blood vessels in the lungs by the pulse, but as this cannot be done with any clarity, it is best to retain the classification of the blood vessels according to the ventricle with which they are connected, with the additional qualification describing the nature of their structure. We must therefore call the vessel that carries *pneuma* (the pulmonary vein) an artery, even if it has the structure of a vein, and the vessel that carries blood to the lungs a vein— for its function is to convey nourishment—although it has the structure of an artery.[3]

Galen is quite clear on the anatomical difference between arteries and veins and also on their different behaviour. Starting out from the fact, first noted by Herophilus, that arteries are tubes with walls six times as thick as veins,[4] he goes on to describe their different anatomical characteristics. Veins have only one coat or tunic, arteries two,[5] an outer and

---

[1] De anat. admin. vii. 10, K. ii. 620: ἀρθείσης μέντοι τῆς καρδίας, ὑπὸ τῶν τοῦ Καίσαρος μαγείρων, ἔπεμψά τινα τῶν γεγυμνασμένων ἑταίρων περὶ τὰ τοιαῦτα παρακαλέσοντα τοὺς μαγείρους ἐπιτρέψαι τὸ κατ' αὐτὴν ὀστοῦν ἐξελεῖν. καὶ οὕτως ἐγένετο.

[2] Ibid., 619: ὅσῳ γ' ἂν ᾖ τὸ τοῦ ζῴου γένος, ἀξιολογώτερον τῷ μεγέθει τοσούτῳ πλέον ὀστώδους οὐσίας ὁ χόνδρος ἐπικέκτηται. καὶ κατά γε τὰ μέγιστα ... προσήκει καλεῖν αὐτὸν τηνικαῦτα χονδρῶδες ὀστοῦν, οὐ χόνδρον ὀστώδη. In this connection, Ogle, in a note in his translation of *The parts of animals* in the Oxford Aristotle states: 'It is not uncommon to find, in large mammalia, especially in pachyderms and ruminants, a cruciform ossification in the heart below the origin of the aorta. In the ox this is a normal formation, as also in the stag. But in pachyderms, or at any rate in the horse, it is only found in old individuals and appears to be the result of a pathological degeneration.'

[3] De anat. admin. vii. 4, K. ii. 600: ἠκολουθήσαμεν δ' ἡμεῖς, ὡς ἄμεινον τιθεμένοις ὅσοι τὸ μὲν ἐκ τῆς ἀριστερᾶς κοιλίας τῆς καρδίας ἐκφυόμενον ἀγγεῖον ὠνόμασαν ἀρτηρίαν φλεβώδη, τὸ δ' ἐκ τῆς δεξιᾶς ἀρτηριώδη φλέβα, βέλτιον εἶναι νομίζοντες ἐπειδὴ τῷ σφύζειν οὐκ ἐναργῶς αὐτὰ διαγιγνώσκομεν, ὡς ἀρτηρίαν μὲν ὀνομάσαι τὸ πνευματικὸν ἀγγεῖον, ἀλλ' ἐπεὶ φλεβὸς ἔχει χιτῶνα, προσθεῖναι τὸ φλεβῶδες, φλέβα δ' αὖ πάλιν θάτερον ἀπὸ τῆς χρείας προσαγορεύσαντες, ἐπειδὴ δὲ καὶ τοῦτο τὸ σῶμά ἐστιν ἀρτηρίας, ἀρτηριώδη προσθέντες. ἄριστον μὲν γάρ, ὡς ἔφην, τῷ σφύζειν τε καὶ μὴ σφύζειν αὐτὰ διακρίνεσθαι. τούτου δ' οὐ πάνυ τι ταῖς αἰσθήσεσι διαγιγνωσκομένου σαφῶς, ἀπὸ μὲν τῆς πρὸς τὰς κοιλίας τῆς καρδίας ἑκατέρας κοινωνίας θέσθαι τοὔνομα, προσθήκην δ' ἀπὸ τῆς σωματικῆς οὐσίας ποιήσασθαι.

[4] De usu partium. vi. 10, K. iii. 445: ἐν μὲν γὰρ τοῖς ἄλλοις ἅπασι μορίοις, τῆς ἴσης ἀρτηρίας τῇ φλεβὶ τὸ πάχος τῶν χιτώνων οὐκ ἴσον, ἀλλ' εἰς τοσοῦτον ἄρα διενήνοχεν, ὡς Ἡρόφιλος ὀρθῶς ἐστοχάσθαι δοκεῖ, τὴν ἀρτηρίαν τῆς φλεβὸς ἑξαπλασίαν ἀποφηνάμενος εἶναι τῷ πάχει.

[5] De nat. fac. iii. 11, K. ii. 181: ταῦτ' ἄρα καὶ ὁ τῆς φλεβὸς χιτὼν εἷς ὢν ἐκ πολυειδῶν ἰνῶν ἐγένετο, καὶ τῶν τῆς ἀρτηρίας, ὁ μὲν ἔξωθεν ἐκ τῶν στρογγύλων, ὁ δ' ἔσωθεν ἐκ μὲν τῶν εὐθειῶν πλείστων, ὀλίγων δέ τινων σὺν αὐταῖς καὶ τῶν λοξῶν.

an inner one with fibres going different ways, indeed they may even have three, each with its own special character. The outer coat of the arteries is about as thick as that of the veins, but the inner coat is about five times as thick, and much harder, being made up of crosswise as opposed to lengthwise fibres, whereas the outer coat is like that of the veins, with fibres going lengthwise, some rather slanted, but with no cross-fibres. The inner coat has on its inward surface a sort of skin, almost like a spider's web to look at, which can be seen in the big arteries. Some people regard this as a third coat.[1] The arteries must be porous, since they take part in the process of respiration and pulsation. At their diastole they take in air, and at their systole they expel sooty matter.[2] Their coats have a power or faculty of expanding, by which they attract matter from the environment from all directions.[3] The hardness of their inner coats contributes greatly to the force of the arterial beat, and so to the power of distinguishing the systole.[4] Galen thus conceives the coats of the arteries as being full of porous openings, which are connected not only like mouths opening into intestines and the stomach, but also into the outer skin.[5] These porous openings are quite distinct from the anastomoses of the capillary system, which he inherited from Erasistratus. They are, of course, on a microscopic scale, too small to enable even thin fluids like the arterial blood to pass. They serve only to let what we should call gaseous substances to pass through them. Yet this is not quite correct, for they also permit those light elements contained in the blood, which are proper to each particular type of tissue, to be absorbed through them.

While accepting the capillary system, Galen was not prepared to do so without some experimental evidence in its favour. These anastomoses between veins and arteries could, in his opinion, be proved by the fact that if you kill an animal by severing many large arteries, all the blood in its body will run out, and you will find the veins as well as the arteries

---

[1] *De anat. admin.* vii. 5, K. ii. 601 : δύο δ' εἰσὶν οἱ τῆς ἀρτηρίας ἴδιοι χιτῶνες, ὁ μὲν ἔξωθεν οἷός περ ὁ τῆς φλεβός, ὁ δ' ἔνδον πενταπλάσιός που τῷ πάχει τοῦδε καὶ μέντοι καὶ σκληρότερος εἰς ἐγκαρσίας ἴνας διαλυόμενος· ὅ γε μὴν ἔξωθεν, ὁ καὶ ταῖς φλεψὶν ὑπάρχων, εὐθείας τε καὶ ἐνίας μετρίως λοξὰς ἔχει τῶν ἰνῶν, ἐγκαρσίαν δ' οὐδεμίαν. ὁ δ' ἔνδον χιτὼν τῆς ἀρτηρίας, ὁ πάχυς καὶ σκληρός, οἷον δέρμα τι κατὰ τὴν ἐντὸς ἐπιφάνειαν ἔχει παραπλήσιον ἀραχνίῳ σαφῶς, φαινόμενον μὲν ἐπὶ τῶν μεγάλων ἀρτηριῶν, ὃν ἔνιοι τρίτον ἀρτηρίας τίθενται χιτῶνα.

[2] *De pulsuum causis*, 4, K. ix. 6 f. : οὕτως ἡ τοὺς σφυγμοὺς ἐργαζομένη δύναμις δι' ὀργάνων τῶν ἀρτηριῶν τὸ ἑαυτῆς ἔργον, τὴν φυλακὴν τῆς ἐμφύτου θερμασίας ἀποτελεῖ . . . καὶ τοίνυν ἐπειδὰν μὲν τὴν ψύχουσαν οὐσίαν ἕλκη διαστέλλεται τὸ σῶμα τῶν ἀρτηριῶν, ἐπειδὰν δὲ τὸ αἰθαλῶδες ἐκκρίνῃ συστέλλεται.

[3] *De sanguine in arteriis*, 7, K. iv. 730 : ἆρα τὸ δεύτερον, τῷ εἶναί τινα δύναμιν ἐν τοῖς χιτῶσιν αὐτῶν, ὑφ' ἧς διαστέλλονται, πᾶν ἕλκεται τὸ συνεχὲς ἐκ παντὸς μέρους αὐτῶν, ὅθεν ἂν ἐγχωρῇ.

[4] *De dignosc. puls.* i. 6, K. viii. 801 : ἐλέχθη δ' ὅτι καὶ ἡ σκληρότης συντελεῖ τι πρὸς τὴν τῆς συστολῆς διάγνωσιν . . . τῷ γὰρ πληγῆς βιαίῳ μέγα συμβάλλεται καὶ ἡ τοῦ χιτῶνος τῆς ἀρτηρίας σκληρότης.

[5] *De usu pulsuum*, 4, K. v. 164 : πάμπολλοι πόροι ταῖς ἀρτηρίαις, οἱ μὲν ἐν αὐτοῖς τοῖς χιτῶσιν, οἷον ὀπαί τινες, ἄλλοι δὲ δίκην στομάτων εἰς ἔντερα καὶ γαστέρα, καὶ τοῦτο δὴ τὸ ἐκτὸς δέρμα περαίνονται.

are emptied.[1] Moreover, almost everywhere each artery is accompanied by a vein, though some veins are without accompanying arteries.[2] The function of these anastomoses between the capillary arteries and veins all over the body is to facilitate the exchange of blood and *pneuma* between the two systems.[3] It is here that we come up against one of the greater obstacles to the true understanding of the circulation—an obstacle which Galen, in spite of the knowledge of the capillaries, failed to surmount, owing, in the last resort, to the fatal residual legacy of the teaching of Praxagoras' pneumatism.

To realize the true nature of this obstacle, we must examine in some detail Galen's theories of the relations between the heart and the lungs, between breathing and blood movement. The principal anatomical basis of his teaching is the supposed connection between the tracheo-bronchial system and the pulmonary veins.

There grows out of the left ventricle of the heart an artery whose structure is like a vein. First, it is split up into as many branches as the lung has lobes. After that, in each of these lobes the branches divide into smaller and smaller branches, until they are finally exhausted. And the innumerable ends of these last branches, which are like the twigs of a tree, coincide with the ends of those of the 'rough artery' [trachea], the windpipe, which also distributes itself in branches all over the whole lung, just like the vein-like artery.[4]

In this case Galen does not in fact use the term *synanastomoses*, but elsewhere he does tell us that the artery-like vein, or rather its capillary branches, have synanastomoses with those of the vein-like artery.[5] It

---

[1] *De nat. fac.* iii. 15, K. ii. 207: τοῦ δ' ἐκ τῶν φλεβῶν εἰς τὰς ἀρτηρίας μεταλαμβάνεσθαί τι πρὸς τοῖς εἰρημένοις ἱκανὸν καὶ τό γε τεκμήριον. εἰ πολλὰς καὶ μεγάλας ἀρτηρίας διατεμὼν ἀποκτεῖναι δι' ἐκείνων βουληθεὶς τὸ ζῷον, εὑρήσεις αὐτοῦ τὰς φλέβας ὁμοίως ταῖς ἀρτηρίαις ἐκκενουμένας, οὐκ ἂν τούτου ποτὲ γενομένου χωρὶς τῶν πρὸς ἀλλήλας αὐταῖς ἀναστομώσεων.

[2] *De usu partium,* xvi. 13, K. iv. 338: εὑρήσεις οὖν φλέβας μέν τινας ἀρτηριῶν χωρίς, ἀρτηρίαν δ' οὐδεμίαν ἄνευ τῆς συζύγου αὐτῇ φλεβός. This general statement is somewhat modified in the treatise On anatomy of arteries and veins, 10, where Galen names the aorta and the pulmonary artery and one going to the shoulder-blades and the left armpit—quite apart from certain arrangements in the foetal blood vessels. See K. ii. 828–9: αἱ δὲ ἄλλαι ἀρτηρίαι χωρὶς φλεβῶν εἰσιν, οὐκ ἐπὶ τῶν κυουμένων μόνον, ἀλλὰ καὶ ἤδη τῶν τελείων ζῴων, αἵ γε ἐκ τῆς καρδίας, αἱ μεγάλαι, μία μὲν ἡ ἐπὶ τὸν πέμπτον τοῦ θώρακος καθήκουσα σπόνδυλον, ἑτέρα δὲ ἡ ἐπὶ τὰς σφαγὰς ἀναφερομένη, καὶ τρίτη πρὸς ταύταις, ἣν ἔφην ἐπ' ὠμοπλάτην τε καὶ μασχάλην ἀριστέραν ἰέναι.

[3] *De usu partium,* vi. 10, quoted below.

[4] *De plac. Hipp. et Plat.* ii. 4, K. v. 228–9: κατὰ γὰρ τὴν ἀριστερὰν κοιλίαν τῆς καρδίας ἐκφύεταί τις ἀρτηρία φλεβώδης τὸ σῶμα, τὸ μὲν πρῶτον εἰς τοσαῦτα μόρια σχιζομένη ὅσοι περ ἂν ὦσιν οἱ τοῦ πνεύμονος λοβοί. μετὰ ταῦτα δὲ ἤδη καθ' ἕκαστον αὐτῶν ἑκάστη διανέμεται εἰς πολλὰ γιγνομένη μόρια, μέχρι περ ἂν ἀναλωθῇ σύμπασα. τοῖς δὲ ἐσχάτοις αὐτῆς πέρασι, παμπόλλοις οὖσιν οἷόν περ δένδρου βλάσταις, εἰς ταὐτὸν ἥκει τὰ τῆς τραχείας ἀρτηρίας πέρατα, τὸν αὐτὸν τρόπον εἰς ὅλον τὸ σπλάγχνον μερισθείσης ὄν περ ἡ φλεβώδης ἀρτηρία.

[5] *De usu partium,* vi. 10, K. iii. 455: συνανεστόμωνται μὲν αἱ ἀρτηρίαι ταῖς φλεψὶ καθ' ὅλον τὸ σῶμα, καὶ μεταλαμβάνουσιν ἐξ ἀλλήλων αἷμα καὶ πνεῦμα διά τινων ἀοράτων τε καὶ στενῶν ἀκριβῶς ὁδῶν ... συστελλομένου δὲ τοῦ θώρακος, ὠθούμεναί τε καὶ ἔσω πιλούμεναι πανταχόθεν ἰσχυρῶς, αἱ ἐν τῷ πνεύμονι φλεβώδεις ἀρτηρίαι ἐκθλίβουσι μὲν αὐτίκα δὴ μάλα τὸ ἐν αὐταῖς πνεῦμα, μεταλαμβάνουσι δέ τι διὰ τῶν λεπτῶν ἐκείνων στομάτων τοῦ αἵματος.

seems quite clear, however, that Galen thought that the pulmonary veins, besides being connected with the pulmonary arteries, were also connected with the bronchial system, for, as we shall see later, these connections must be responsible for the leakage into it of a small quantity of blood in certain cases of wounds or disease.[1] The pulmonary vein is slender, as compared with the vena cava and the aorta, and has only one coat.[2] Its function is to assist respiration by conveying air or *pneuma* to the heart,[3] for just as trees draw all their nourishment through their roots, so does the heart draw air from the lungs, through this system of arteries;[4] though in a passage which we shall examine later, Galen seems rather uncertain whether in fact the heart does actually take up any air from the lungs.[5]

The other vessel leading direct from the heart to the lungs is the pulmonary (vein-like) artery, the function of which is to provide nourishment for the lungs from the right ventricle. It has two tunics of the same character as an artery,[6] and it is very large,[7] since the lung needs a great deal of nourishment, as it is soft, very hot, and in continuous movement, while the hard parts of the body, particularly the bones, need very little.[8] Galen is, moreover, sufficiently acquainted with the dispensations of providence to tell us why it has two coats like the arteries, and not just one like the veins. The lung and the heart stand in reciprocal contributory relations of barter, the lungs supplying *pneuma* to the heart, and the heart nourishment to the lungs, nourishment which has originated from the liver.[9] It was better that the blood providing this nourishment should not come directly from the vena cava. All-wise nature therefore invented the pulmonary valve and changed the coats of the veins and arteries in the lungs, making the veins like arteries and the arteries like veins.[10]

---

[1] See below, p. 309.

[2] De ven. et art. anat. 9, K. ii. 816: ἀρχὴ μὲν τούτων (τῶν ἀρτηριῶν) ἐστὶν ἡ ἀριστερὰ κοιλία τῆς καρδίας. ἐντεῦθεν δὲ μία μὲν εἰς τὸν πνεύμονα κατασχίζεται, λεπτὴ καὶ μονοχίτων καθάπερ αἱ φλέβες.

[3] Ibid., 817: ὡσαύτως γάρ τοι καὶ ἥδε διὰ τῆς εἰσπνοῆς ὠφέλειαν εἰς τὸν πνεύμονα κατασχίζεται.

[4] De plac. Hipp. et Plat. vi. 3, K. v. 525: ἑτέραν δ' ἀρτηρίαν ἐκ τῆς αὐτῆς κοιλίας τῆς καρδίας ἐκφερομένην, τὴν εἰς τὸν πνεύμονα κατασχιζομένην ἀνάλογον τῷ καθήκοντι μέρει τῆς ῥιζώσεως εἰς τὴν γῆν. ὥσπερ γὰρ ἐκ τῆς γῆς τὰ φυτὰ διὰ τῶν ῥιζῶν ἅπασαν ἐπισπᾶται τὴν τροφήν, οὕτως ἐκ τοῦ πνεύμονος ἡ καρδία τὸν ἀέρα διὰ τῶν εἰρημένων ἀρτηριῶν.

[5] But see below, p. 343.

[6] De ven. et art. anat. 2, K. ii. 786: κἀκ ταύτης εἰς τὸν πνεύμονα τὸν αὐτὸν ἔχουσα χιτῶνα τῷ τῶν ἀρτηριῶν.

[7] De usu partium, xvi. 14, K. iv. 341: πνεύμονι δὴ μεγίστη φλὲψ ἐκ καρδίας ἐμπέφυκεν.

[8] Ibid., 340: πνεύμονι μὲν οὖν ἅπανθ' ὑπάρχει τὰ πρὸς τὴν κένωσιν ἔτοιμα, μαλακώτατός τε γάρ ἐστι καὶ θερμότατος, ἐν κινήσει τὲ διηνεκεῖ, τοῖς δ' ὀστοῖς ὥσπερ ἐκ διαμέτρου τἀναντία, καὶ γὰρ σκληρὰ καὶ ψυχρὰ καὶ τὸν πλείω τοῦ βίου χρόνον ἡσυχάζοντα.

[9] Ibid. vi. 10, K. iii. 444: ἀμοιβὴν γάρ τινα τῷ πνεύμονι τὴν ἐκ τοῦ ἥπατος θρέψιν ἔοικεν ἀντιπαρέχειν ἡ καρδία, καὶ τοῦτον ἀντεισφέρειν αὐτῷ τὸν ἔρανον ἀνθ' οὗ λαμβάνει παρ' ἐκείνου πνεύματος.

[10] Ibid., 445: οὐ γὰρ δὴ μάτην οὐδ' ὡς ἔτυχεν ἡ πάντα σοφὴ φύσις, ὥσπερ οὐδ' ἄλλο οὐδὲν ἐποίησεν ἐν ἅπασι τοῖς ζῴοις, οὕτως οὐδ' ἐπὶ πνεύμονος. ἐνήλλαξε γὰρ τῶν ἀγγείων τοὺς χιτῶνας, ἀρτηριώδη μὲν ἐργασαμένη τὴν φλέβα, φλεβώδη δὲ τὴν ἀρτηρίαν.

For owing to the continual expansion and contraction of the thorax and the lung, its blood vessels are subject to great pressure. As the 'arteries' carry *pneuma*, their soft coats can easily contract and expand with their venous tunics, but the 'veins' carrying nourishment would be greatly inconvenienced by this pressure due to respiration and their coats must therefore be thick in order to enable them to perform their function.[1] Moreover each part of the body is nourished by those elements in the blood which are most like its own substance. Now the lung is of all organs the lightest and rarest. Its body is, as it were, made of a sort of bloody foam, and therefore it needs thin, vaporous, and clean or pure blood, which the arteries were designed to carry, not the thick and 'muddy' blood which nourishes the liver. Hence the vessels which carry it must be of the opposite kind to the veins which convey the blood from the liver, whose thin and loose coats allow thick blood to be supplied to the tissues which surround them. So the vessel feedings the lungs only permits the thinnest elements of the blood to percolate. Now the arteries with their thick and closely-knit coats only let a little vaporous blood percolate into the tissues which surround them in the other parts of the body, but to the lungs alone they permit this kind of blood to percolate in large quantities being unable to contain it owing to their rareness and thinness.[2] But this theory is developed in a far from consistent argument. Galen now proceeds to tell us that owing to the thickness of their tunics, the 'veins' in the lungs—the artery-like veins—only let through very little nourishment to the lungs; the function of providing the bulk of the nourishment is therefore assumed by the lung's vein-like arteries, which on account of their single thin tunics supply the lungs with a lavish quantity of thin, clean, vaporous blood.[3] The nourishment

[1] Ibid., 449: ἀλλ' οὔτε εἰσπνεόντων οὔτ' ἐκπνεόντων ἐχρῆν ὡσαύτως διαστέλλεσθαι ταῖς ἀρτηρίαις τὰς φλέβας, ὅτι μηδὲ τὴν αὐτὴν ὑπηρεσίαν πεπίστευνται. τὰς μὲν γὰρ ὑποδοχὰς τοῦ πνεύματος ἡ φύσις ἐτέμετο ῥᾳδίως μὲν πληροῦσθαι δεομένας εἰσπνεόντων, ἑτοίμως δ' ἐκπνεόντων τε καὶ φωνούντων ἐκκενοῦσθαι. τὰς δ' αὖ φλέβας οἷον ταμιεῖα τῆς τροφῆς ἐδημιούργησεν, οὔτε διαστέλλεσθαι δεομένας εἰσπνεόντων, οὔτ' ἐκπνεόντων συστέλλεσθαι. καλῶς οὖν εἶχε ταῖς μὲν μαλακὸν ἀπεργάσασθαι τὸ σῶμα, ταῖς δὲ σκληρόν.
[2] Ibid., 450 f.: τρέφεται μὲν γὰρ ἕκαστον ἐκ τῆς ὁμοίας ἑαυτῷ τροφῆς, ὡς καὶ τοῦτο ἀποδέδεικται· κοῦφον δ' ἐστὶ καὶ μανὸν καὶ οἷον ἐξ ἀφροῦ τινος αἱματώδους πεπηγότος τὸ τοῦ πνεύμονος σῶμα, καὶ διὰ τοῦτο δεόμενον ἀτμώδους καὶ λεπτοῦ καὶ καθαροῦ τοῦ αἵματος, οὐχ ὥσπερ τὸ ἧπαρ, ἰλυώδους τε καὶ παχέος, ὅθεν ἔμπαλιν αὐτῷ τὰ τῶν ἀγγείων ἔχει μάλιστα μὲν τοῖς καθ' ἧπαρ, ἤδη δὲ καὶ τοῖς ἄλλοις τοῦ ζῴου μορίοις. τοῖς μὲν γὰρ ἀραιός τε καὶ λεπτὸς ὁ χιτὼν ὑπάρχων τοῦ χορηγοῦντος ἀγγείου τὸ αἷμα πλεῖστον τοῦ παχέος ἑτοίμως τοῖς περιέχουσι διαδίδωσι. τῷ δὲ πνεύμονι παχὺς καὶ πυκνὸς γενόμενος οὐδὲν ὅτι μὴ τὸ λεπτότατον ἐπιτρέπει διεξέρχεσθαι· καὶ τοῖς μὲν ἄλλοις αἱ ἀρτηρίαι παχεῖαι καὶ πυκναὶ γεννηθεῖσαι παντάπασιν ὀλίγον ἀτμώδους αἵματος τοῖς περικειμένοις μορίοις ἕλκειν ἐπιτρέπουσι. τῷ δὲ πνεύμονι μόνῳ πάμπολυ τὸ τοσοῦτον μεθιᾶσιν, ὑπὸ μανότητός τε καὶ λεπτότητος ἀδυνατοῦσαι στέγειν. This passage is reproduced almost word for word in Galen's *Commentary IV to Hippocrates' Treatise on nourishment*. See K. xv. 382 ff.
[3] *De usu partium*, vi. 10, 451-2: ὅσον οὖν ἔλαττον αἱ φλέβες αὐτῷ μεταδιδόασι τροφῆς, πυκναὶ καὶ παχεῖαι γενόμεναι, τοῦτο πᾶν πληροῦσιν αἱ ἀρτηρίαι, λεπτὸν καὶ καθαρὸν καὶ ἀτμῶδες αἷμα δαψιλῶς αὐτῷ διαπέμπουσαι.

of the lungs thus takes place in an opposite manner from that of the other parts of the body. For the lung the principal source of nourishment is the arteries, not the veins.[1] Pretty as it sounds, this account is quite illogical. We have been told that the reason for the arterial character of the vein conveying blood from the heart is that it prevents the muddier elements in the blood from percolating into the lungs, for which they are a wholly improper food. Now we are informed that, after all, the nourishment of the lungs does in fact take place through vessels with vein-like coats, which easily let through these inappropriate nutritive elements. We shall revert to this dilemma presently, in our account of Galen's theories of what happens in the heart.[2] He was evidently not satisfied with the explanation here given, for elsewhere he produces quite a different theory. In a parallel passage in the fourth commentary on 'Hippocrates' *De alimento* we find quite a different explanation of the matter. The small amount of matter that is able to percolate through the thick arterial coats of the artery-like veins (pulmonary arteries) is compensated for by the size and number of these vessels.[3]

To return to the account given in the *Use of the parts*, of which we have been giving such a full précis. In a passage in the sixth book Galen explains nature's arrangements for the feeding of the lungs as follows. In order to provide for their nourishment, she invented the pulmonary valve, so that the pressure of the thorax on the pulmonary artery in the continual process of breathing in and breathing out should not result in a futile process of backward and forward movement of the blood in this vessel, to and fro between the lung and the heart. Were this valve not there, with each contraction of the lung the blood in the pulmonary artery would be squeezed back into the right ventricle,[4] and the purpose of this artery-like vein and its branches of carrying nutriment to the lung would be frustrated.[5] But the existence of this valve, which shuts after the expulsion of its contents by the right ventricle into the pulmonary artery,[6] enables the systole of the left ventricle and the pressure of the thorax and the lung to propel the blood to the end of its smallest branches, where they open into those of the vein-like artery (pulmonary vein). The pulmonary veins with their soft thin coats yield much more readily

---

[1] *De usu partium*, vi. 10, K. iii. 451 : ὥστε πάντῃ τῷ πνεύμονι τὰ περὶ τὴν τροφὴν ὑπεναντίως ἔχει τοῖς ἄλλοις ἅπασι τοῦ ζῴου μορίοις.

[2] See below, pp. 305 ff.

[3] *Comment. IV in Hipp. de alimento*, iv, K. xv. 384 : ἔτι δὲ μεγίστας ἐν αὐτῷ φλέβας, ἵνα ὅσον ἀπολείπεται τοῦ τρέφειν ἱκανῶς, διὰ τὴν τοῦ χιτῶνος πυκνότητα τοῦτ' ἐκ τοῦ μεγέθους αὐτῶν ἀναπληροῦται.

[4] *De usu partium*, vi. 10, K. iii. 453–4, quoted below, p. 313, n. 1.

[5] Ibid. : εὔδηλον ἤδη πηλίκον τι βλάψει τὴν ὅλην ἀναπνοὴν εἰ διαστέλλοιτο καὶ συστέλλοιτο τὰ τῆς τροφῆς ὄργανα. χρὴ γὰρ ἡσυχάζειν ἀκριβῶς αὐτά.

[6] Ibid., 11, 459 : θλίβεσθαι μέν τι καὶ συστέλλεσθαι τὰς φλέβας ἀναγκαῖον, οὐ μὴν ἐκκενοῦσθαί γε αὖθις εἰς τοὐπίσω διὰ τοῦ στόματος ὑπὸ τῶν ὑμένων κλείεσθαι φθάνοντος.

to the pressure of the thorax—the lung has no power of movement in itself—and expel all the *pneuma* they contain into the left ventricle of the heart, thus drawing into themselves blood from the capillary branches of the pulmonary artery, the artery-like vein, which drips drops of blood into the capillaries of the pulmonary veins, the vein-like arteries, for the purpose of feeding the lung. How great a good this is for the lung, will be quite clear to those who remember his discussion on nutrition.[1] But the resources of nature were not exhausted by the mere invention of the pulmonary artery and the pulmonary valve. The nutrition of an organ as hot and as constantly in motion as the lung required not only a large number of big artery-like veins to make up for the small amount of blood which could escape through their coats, it also required three other devices to assist it. One of these is heat. It is the nearness of the lungs to the heart, the source of the innate heat, which breaks up the nourishment provided by the blood into small particles and diffuses it in a form ready to become vaporized. The second is the expansion of the lung on breathing in, which seizes by force certain elements even from the densest organs. And the third is the action of the heart itself. For the blood which goes to the lungs comes straight from it, and goes only to them, after having been worked over by it carefully and rendered thinner.[2] For the right ventricle, in the last resort, exists only for the sake of the lungs.[3] As we have noted, Galen knew that fishes and other creatures which have no lungs only have one ventricle. He was also aware that consequently the vascular arrangements of the foetus *in utero* were different from those existing after birth, and he understood in some respects why this is so.

The development of the embryo is divided by Galen into four stages. The first is one in which the form of seed predominates, the second, which results from the proliferation of the blood vessels in the umbilical cord, shows the embryo as a flesh-like conglomeration, but neither heart, nor liver, nor brain has yet been differentiated. In the third stage all three primary organs are plainly visible, and a sketch-work of all the other members, though the organs of the belly are still rather vague, still more so the limbs. Finally, in the fourth or final stage, when all the limbs have been articulated, Hippocrates no longer calls the foetus an embryo, but

---

[1] Ibid., 10, 456–7: συστελλομένου δὲ τοῦ θώρακος, ὠθούμεναί τε καὶ ἔσω πιλούμεναι πανταχόθεν ἰσχυρῶς αἱ ἐν τῷ πνεύμονι φλεβώδεις ἀρτηρίαι ἐκθλίβουσι μὲν αὐτίκα δὴ μάλα τὸ ἐν αὐταῖς πνεῦμα, μεταλαμβάνουσι δέ τι διὰ τῶν λεπτῶν ἐκείνων στομάτων τοῦ αἵματος, ὅπερ οὐκ ἂν μετειλήφθη ποτὲ παλινδρομεῖν, εἴπερ οἷόν τ' ἦν εἰς τοὐπίσω διὰ τοῦ μεγίστου στόματος ἡλίκον τῆς φλεβὸς ταύτης ἐστὶ τὸ πρὸς τῇ καρδίᾳ. νυνὶ δ' ἐν τῷ θλίβεσθαι μὲν πανταχόθεν ἀποκεκλεῖσθαι δὲ τῆς διὰ τοῦ μεγάλου στόματος ἐπανόδου, στάζει τι διὰ τῶν λεπτῶν ἐκείνων στομάτων εἰς τὰς ἀρτηρίας. πηλίκον δὲ τοῦτ' ἐστὶν ἀγαθὸν τῷ πνεύμονι, ταχὰ μὲν ἤδη φαίνεται τῷ γε μεμνημένῳ τῶν ὑπὲρ τῆς θρέψεως αὐτοῦ λόγων.

[2] Ibid., 452, quoted below, p. 305, and n. 1.

[3] Ibid., 9, 442: ἡ μὲν γὰρ δεξιὰ κοιλία τοῦ πνεύμονος ἕνεκα γέγονεν.

already a child.[1] During the whole of this process of development it is the seed which acts as the craftsman (δημιουργός) or organizing principle. It is the bearer, as we might say, of genetic information, and the course of the development is determined at each stage by biological needs. At the beginning its only biological need is growth, and the organ which is in charge of the growing process is the liver. The embryo in its very early stages has grown a skin, and the umbilical veins which have united at the navel of the foetus almost immediately after penetrating this skin divide again; just as the seed of a plant—and the embryo at this stage is a plant —throws out two shoots from one of which the roots develop and from the other the stem and branches, so the umbilical veins, united at the navel, as soon as they penetrate the skin of the embryo divide into two big branches. Each of these proliferates near the point of junction into two sets of progressively smaller divisions between which the flesh of the liver with its two gates is deposited like a sort of stuffing.[2] From the lower gate on the underside of the liver the veins grow out which supply the materials for the intestines, etc. The upper gate exists for the sake of the great vein which stretches along the whole of the body, the so-called vena cava, but which Hippocrates called the hepatic because he saw it growing out of the liver.[3] This throws off branches to the thoracic membranes, the diaphragm, and the pericardium as well as to the right ventricle of the heart.[4]

[1] Galen, De semine, i. 9, K. iv. 542–3: διελώμεθα τέσσαρσι χρόνοις τὴν σύμπασαν τῶν κυουμένων δημιουργίαν. πρῶτος μέν, ἐν ᾧ κατὰ τὰς ἀμβλώσεις τε καὶ κατὰ τὰς ἀνατομὰς ἡ τοῦ σπέρματος ἰδέα κρατεῖ . . . ἐπειδὰν δὲ πληρωθῇ μὲν τοῦ αἵματος, ἡ καρδία δὲ καὶ ὁ ἐγκέφαλος καὶ τὸ ἧπαρ, ἀδιάρθρωτα μὲν ἔτι καὶ ἄμορφα, πῆξιν δ' ἤδη τινὰ καὶ μέγεθος ἀξιόλογον ἔχῃ, δεύτερος μὲν οὗτος ὁ χρόνος ἐστί, σαρκοειδὴς δὲ καὶ οὐκέτι γονοειδής ἐστιν ἡ οὐσία τοῦ κυήματος . . . τρίτος ἐπὶ τῷδε χρόνος, ἡνίκα, ὡς εἴρηται, τὰς μὲν τρεῖς ἀρχὰς ἔστιν ἰδεῖν ἐναργῶς, ὑπογραφὴν δέ τινα καὶ οἷον σκιαγραφίαν, ἁπάντων τῶν ἄλλων μορίων. ἐναργεστέραν μὲν γὰρ ὄψει τὴν περὶ τὰς τρεῖς ἀρχὰς διάπλασιν, ἀμυδροτέραν δὲ τὴν τῶν κατὰ τὴν γαστέρα μορίων, καὶ πολὺ δὴ τούτων ἔτι ἀμυδροτέραν τὴν κατὰ τὰ κῶλα . . . τέταρτος δ' οὗτός ἐστι καὶ τελευταῖος χρόνος, ἡνίκα ἤδη τά τ' ἐν τοῖς κώλοις ἅπαντα διήρθρωται, καὶ οὐδ' ἔμβρυον ἔτι μόνον, ἀλλ' ἤδη καὶ παιδίον ὀνομάζει τὸ κυούμενον ὁ θαυμάσιος Ἱπποκράτης, ὅτε καὶ ἀσκαρίζειν καὶ κινεῖσθαί φησιν, ὡς ζῷον ἤδη τέλειον.

[2] Galen, De foetuum formatione, 3, K. iv. 667–8: ἡ γὰρ ἐξ ὀμφαλοῦ φλὲψ ἅμα τῷ πρώτως εἰς τὴν ἐντὸς χώραν ἀφικέσθαι τοῦ περὶ τὸ κυούμενον δέρματος εὐθέως σχίζεται δίχα, καθάπερ εἰς δύο μόρια μέγιστα κατὰ τὰ πολλὰ τῶν δένδρων ὁρᾶται τὸ πρέμνον διαιρούμενον, εἶθ' ἑκατέρας τῶν φλεβῶν τῶνδε δίκην κλάδου ἀποφυούσης ἑτέρας φλέβας, ἐκείνων τε πάλιν ἑτέρας, εἶτα τούτων γεννωμένων ἄλλας, ἄχρι περ εἴς τινα πέρατα τελευτήσωσιν ἑκάτεραι τῶν κατασχίσεων, ἡ τοῦ ἥπατος ἴδιος οὐσία . . . ἐν κύκλῳ τε περιφέρεται καὶ τὰ μεταξὺ τῶν σχίσεων ἀναπληροῖ, καθάπερ τις στοιβή . . . καὶ διὰ ταύτην γε τὴν αἰτίαν αἱ δύο πύλαι τοῦ ἥπατος ἐγένοντο τοῖς ἐμβρύοις.

[3] Ibid., 668–9: τῆς μὲν ὑψηλοτέρας πύλης γενομένης ἕνεκα τοῦ γεννηθῆναι τὰς κατὰ τὸ ἧπαρ ἁπάσας, τῆς ταπεινοτέρας δὲ ἕνεκα τοῦ τὰς εἰς τὴν γαστέρα καὶ σπλῆνα, καὶ τὸ ὑπόλοιπον, ἔντερά τε πάντα. συμπληρωθέντος δὲ τοῦ ἥπατος, ἐκ μὲν τῶν κατὰ τὰ κυρτὰ μέρη φλεβῶν αὐτοῦ καθάπερ ἔκ τινων ῥιζῶν ἀθροίζεται στέλεχος ἡ μεγίστη τῶν ἐν τῷ σώματι φλεβῶν, ἣν διὰ τοῦτο κοίλην ὀνομάζουσι κατ' ἐξοχὴν δή τινα πρὸς τὰς ἄλλας φλέβας, ἐνδεικνύμενοι τὸ μέγεθος αὐτῆς· Ἱπποκράτης δ' ἀπὸ τοῦ ἥπατος, ὅθεν ἑώρα τὴν ἔκφυσιν ἔχουσαν, ἡπατῖτιν ἐκάλεσεν.

[4] Ibid., 669: τὸ μέν τι κάτω φέρεται κατὰ μέσης τῆς ῥάχεως ἐστηριγμένον, τὸ δ' ἄνω διὰ μέσου τοῦ θώρακος ἐπὶ τὸν τράχηλον ἀναφέρεται, πρώτας μὲν ἀποφύσεις εἰς τὸ διάφραγμα

While this development has been proceeding, the arteries have been forming from the materials provided from the umbilical arteries, which have carried it, one on each side of the bladder, and have developed the arterial system past the point where the two branches of the abdominal aorta unite, to the vicinity of the heart. From this hotter blood the ventricles of the heart appear to be formed, but it is not quite clear whether Galen thought that venous blood contributed to the formation of the right ventricle, which is less hot than the left,[1] the seat of the innate heat. Simultaneously with the formation of the heart, the upper portions of the two main blood vessels must be developed, since once the ventricles have been formed and the two main blood vessels, the vena cava and the aorta, connected up with them, the hotter blood pouring in from the aorta and the cooler from the vena cava, the heart begins to beat, and the arteries to pulsate. The embryo has now become an animal; up to this stage it has only been a plant.[2] The third principal system, that of the nerves, is not required until the foetus has been fully formed, but its starting-point (ἀρχή) the brain comes early into being, though at this stage it is much smaller than the liver. Both the arterial and the nervous systems need blood for their development. Hence the preponderant size of the liver in the early stages of development, indeed until the time of birth.[3]

With the details of Galen's views on the development of the foetus,

---

ποιούμενον οὐ σμικράς, ἐπ᾽ αὐταῖς δ᾽ ἑτέρας πάντως λεπτὰς εἴς τε τοὺς διαφράττοντας ὑμένας τὸν θώρακα καὶ τὸν περικάρδιον χιτῶνα, μετὰ δὲ ταῦτα εἰς τὴν δεξιὰν κοιλίαν τῆς καρδίας καὶ τὸν θώρακα.

[1] Compare the two following passages, both from the third chapter of the treatise *On the formation of foetuses*. In the first (K. iv. 662), Galen compares the formation of the heart with that of the lung; he suggests two alternatives: οὐ μήν, ὥσπερ ἐπὶ τῆς τοῦ ἥπατος γενέσεως οὐδὲν ὑπολείπεται ζήτημα, κατὰ τὸν αὐτὸν τρόπον ἐπὶ τῆς καρδίας φαίνεται . . . τῇ καρδίᾳ δὲ τὴν ὕλην, ἐξ ἧς τὴν γένεσιν ἕξει, παρὰ τῆς κυούσης ἤτοι διὰ τῶν ἀρτηριῶν ἀναγκαῖόν ἐστιν ἢ διὰ μέσου τοῦ ἥπατος χορηγεῖσθαι κατὰ τὴν ἐξ αὐτοῦ φερομένην φλέβα μετέωρον εἰς τὴν τῶν ἄνω τοῦδε τοῦ σπλάγχνου μορίων γένεσιν.

In the latter (K. iv. 670) he appears to think that the matter for the heart is derived from the arterial blood of the mother: ἐκ ταύτης οὖν τὴν καρδίαν πιθανόν ἐστιν ἀρυομένην αἷμα θερμοτέραν πολλῷ τοῦ κατὰ τὰς φλέβας εἰς τοσοῦτον καὶ αὐτὴν θερμοτέραν γίνεσθαι τοῦ ἥπατος, εἰς ὅσον καὶ τὸ αἷμα τοῦ αἵματός ἐστι θερμότερον. οὐσῶν δὲ δυοῖν αὐτῆς κοιλιῶν, εἰς μὲν τὴν δεξιὰν τὸ ἐκ τοῦ ἥπατος παραγίνεται, μετρίως θερμὸν ὑπάρχον, εἰς δὲ τὴν ἀριστερὰν πολλῷ θερμότερον τοῦδε τὸ διὰ τῶν ἀρτηριῶν.

[2] Ibid., 670: ὅταν δὲ τὰς κοιλίας σχῇ καὶ τὰς ὕλας ἀμφοτέρας, ὡς ἂν ἤδη πεπληρωμένης αὐτῶν τῆς οὐσίας, αὐτή τε σφύζει καὶ τὰς ἀρτηρίας ἅμα ἑαυτῇ κινεῖ τὴν αὐτὴν ἑαυτῇ κίνησιν, ὥστε τὸ κυούμενον οὐ μόνον ὡς φυτὸν ἔτι τὴν διοίκησιν ἔχειν, ἀλλὰ καὶ ὡς ζῷον.

[3] *De usu partium*, xv. 6, K. iv. 241 f.: πλέονι μὲν οὖν μέτρῳ τῆς τῶν ἄλλων ἀναλογίας ὑπερέχει τὸ ἧπαρ ἐν τοῖς πρώτοις χρόνοις, ὑπερέχει δ᾽ οὐκ ὀλίγῳ καὶ μέχρι τῆς ἀποκυήσεως . . . πλέονος δ᾽ οὔσης τῷ κυουμένῳ ζῴῳ τῆς ἐκ τῶν φλεβῶν χρείας, ὡς ἂν ἄχρι πλείστου διοικουμένῳ δίκην φυτοῦ, τὴν ἀρχὴν τούτων εὐθέως ἀπὸ τῆς πρώτης γενέσεως ἰσχυροτάτην εἰργάσατο. ἐν μὲν γὰρ ἐγκεφάλῳ καὶ τῇ καρδίᾳ καὶ τοῖς ἀπ᾽ αὐτῶν ἐκπεφυκόσιν ὀργάνοις ἢ παρὰ τῶν φλεβῶν ἀναγκαία χρεία, χωρὶς αἵματος μήτε γεννηθῆναι μήτ᾽ αὐξηθῆναι δυναμένοις· ἥπατι δὲ καὶ φλεβὶν ἀρτηριῶν μὲν ὀλίγη χρεία, νεύρων δ᾽ οὐδεμία, πρὶν τελειωθῆναι. διὰ τοῦτ᾽ οὖν ἰσχυρὸν μὲν καὶ μέγα τὸ φλεβῶδες γένος εὐθὺς ἐξ ἀρχῆς ἡ φύσις ἀπειργάσατο, τῶν δ᾽ ἄλλων ἑκάτερον ἐπὶ τούτοις αὖθις αὐξάνειν ἤρξατο.

interesting as they are, we cannot here concern ourselves. But his conception of the movement of the blood, once the vascular system has been fully developed, calls for examination. His description of the placenta shows that he was, as one might expect, fairly accurately informed as to its general structure, except for the one cardinal mistake of supposing the continuity of the maternal with the foetal blood vessels, though in default of any knowledge of the circulation of the blood, he is quite ignorant of its true function. He has observed the villi, though whether he regards these—the so-called κοτυληδόνες (a word of somewhat variegated meaning, including the suckers of an octopus as well as any cup-shaped hollow or cavity, even the socket of the hip-joint)—as belonging to the uterus rather than the chorion, as 'Hippocrates' seems to have done,[1] is not quite clear. These 'suckers', Galen tells us, though their name is derived from the plant of that name, not from the squid, form a secure bond attaching the chorion to the womb. Though their existence in the human womb has been denied, they are found in cows, goats, and suchlike animals.[2] He distinguishes the blood vessels, it would seem, from the surrounding 'fat-like fleshy processes' of the villi, and it is the vessels alone which actually form the connections between the chorion and the womb.[3] These vessels which, both veins and arteries, are small and many, form a network in the chorion and join together like the roots of a tree to form a tree-trunk or stalk, though this is a double one. It contains two veins and two arteries, forming the umbilical cord, which enters the body of the foetus at the navel.[4] At each of the mouths of the vessels which

[1] *Comment. in Hipp. aphorism.* xlv, K. xviiB. 837 f. The aphorism quoted deals with abortions at two or three months pregnancy and reads as follows: ὁκόσαι δὲ μετρίως τὸ σῶμα ἔχουσαι ἐκτιτρώσκουσι δίμηνα καὶ τρίμηνα ἄτερ προφάσιος φανερῆς, ταύτησιν αἱ κοτυληδόνες μύξης μεσταί εἰσι καὶ οὐ δύνανται γοῦν κρατέειν ὑπὸ τοῦ βάρεος τὸ ἔμβρυον, ἀλλ' ἀπορρήγνυνται. Galen comments thus: εἰκὸς γὰρ ταῖς τοιαύταις μυξώδη τὰ στόματα τῶν εἰς τὴν μήτραν καθηκόντων ἀγγείων ὑπάρχειν, ἐξ ὧν ἤρτηται τὸ χορίον (χωρίον K.)—ἃ δὴ καὶ κοτυληδόνας ὠνόμασεν.

[2] *De uteri dissectione,* 10, K. ii. 905–6: κατὰ ταῦτα καὶ αἱ κοτυληδόνες εἰσί, δεσμὸς ἀσφαλὴς τῷ χορίῳ πρὸς τὴν μήτραν γεγενημέναι καίτοι τὴν τῆς ἀνθρώπου μήτραν οὔ φασιν ἔχειν κοτυληδόνας. γίγνεσθαι γὰρ αὐτὰς ἐπί τε βοῶν καὶ αἰγῶν καὶ ἐλάφων καὶ τοιούτων ἑτέρων ζῴων, σώματα πλαδαρὰ ὑπόμυξα τῷ σχήματι ἐοικότα κοτυληδόνι, τῇ πόᾳ τῇ κυμβαλίτιδι, ὅθεν περ καὶ τοὔνομα αὐταῖς . . . ὥστε ἔχοι ἂν ἡ γυναικεία μήτρα κοτυληδόνας.

[3] *Comment. in Hipp. aphorism.* xlv, 838: ἃ δὴ καὶ κοτυληδόνας ὠνόμασεν, οὐχ ὡς ἔνιοι νομίζουσι τὰς ἐπιτρεφομένας ἀδενώδεις σάρκας αὐταῖς. ἔν τε γὰρ τῷ πρώτῳ τῶν γυναικείων αὐτός φησιν, ἦν δὲ αἱ κοτυληδόνες φλέγματος περίπλεες ἔωσι, τὰ καταμήνια γίνεται ἐλάσσονα.

[4] *De uteri dissectione,* 10, 906: ἀρχόμενα οὖν τὰ τοῦ χορίου ἀγγεῖα ἐντεῦθεν, ὅθεν περ εἴρηται, διαπλέκει τε τὸ χορίον, ἀλλήλοις τε μίγνυνται καὶ συμφύεται. ὁ δὲ τρόπος αὐτῆς τῆς συνόδου τοιόσδε τίς ἐστιν. ἐννόησον ῥίζας δένδρου πολλάς τε καὶ λεπτὰς κατὰ δύο καὶ τρεῖς ἀλλήλαις ἑνουμένας, ὥστε ἐξ αὐτῶν ἑτέρας ῥίζας γίνεσθαι μείζους μὲν τῷ μεγέθει ἐλάττους δὲ τῷ ἀριθμῷ, κἀκείνας πάλιν συνιούσας ἀλλήλαις ἑτέρας ὡσαύτως ποιεῖν . . . καὶ τοῦτο ἀεὶ γινόμενον, ἕως εἰς ταὐτὸ ἐλθοῦσαι σύμπασαι τελευτήσωσιν ὑπ' ἀκρὰν τῆς γῆς τὴν ἐπιφάνειαν εἰς τὸ τοῦ δένδρου μέρος ἐκεῖνο ὃ καλεῖται στέλεχος. καὶ γάρ τοι τὰ ἀγγεῖα ταῦτα, οἷον ῥίζαι τινὲς οὖσαι, πολλαὶ καὶ μικραὶ συμφύονται καὶ συμφύονται γίνεται μείζονα τῶν προτέρων. εἶτα ἐφεξῆς μείζονα γινόμενα περατοῦνται σύμπαντα εἰς δύο οἷον στελέχη, φλέβας μὲν τὰ φλεβώδη, ἀρτηρίας δὲ τὰ ἀρτηριώδη, ἑκάτερον ἐξ ἑκατέρου μέρους, δεξιοῦ τε καὶ ἀριστεροῦ, ἐμβαλλούσας εἰς τὸ ἔμβρυον κατὰ τὸν ὀμφαλόν.

penetrate the wall of the uterus (through which the menstrual blood passes, the matter from which in conjunction with the male seed the embryo is formed) a new vessel grows at the time of pregnancy, an artery at the mouth of each artery, and a vein at the mouth of each vein, so that the number of new vessels is the same as that of those which have their terminal mouths in the wall of the uterus.[1] The fact that in the chorion and its very complicated network of blood vessels vein only joins to vein, and artery to artery, to form the umbilical cord, is cited by Galen as a proof of the marvellous artistic skill of nature.[2]

The function of the umbilical cord he conceives to be the supplying of blood and *pneuma* to the growing embryo.[3] The fact that the circulation of the foetal blood system is entirely independent and separate from that of the mother was quite unknown to him, though, as we have already noted, he was aware of the fact that the heart and arteries of the foetus have their own independent beat and pulse. If his anatomical conceptions of the development of the foetus seem strange to us today, we should remember that the anatomy of the chorion and the placenta was only worked out in gross detail by the Hunter brothers in the second half of the eighteenth century. Galen's mistake in assuming a direct connection between the foetal and the maternal blood supply was therefore quite natural, since he was able to follow the course of both the arteries and the vein of the umbilical cord as they were continued in the body of the foetus. He traced quite correctly the continuation of the umbilical vein to the liver, though, *pace* Siegel,[4] I am unable to find any evidence that

---

[1] *De usu partium*, xv. 4, K. iv. 224–5: ἐφ' ἑκάστῳ δὴ στόματι τῶν εἰς τοὐντὸς τῆς μήτρας ἀφηκόντων ἀγγείων, δι' ὧνπερ καὶ τὸ καταμήνιον εἰς αὐτὴν ἐφέρετο, γεννᾶται παρὰ τὸν τοῦ κύειν καιρὸν ἕτερον ἀγγεῖον, ἀρτηρία μὲν ἐπὶ τῷ τῆς ἀρτηρίας στόματι, φλὲψ δ' ἐπὶ τῷ τῆς φλεβός, ὥστ' εἶναι τὸν ἀριθμὸν ἴσα τὰ γεννώμενα τοῖς εἴσω τῆς μήτρας περαίνουσι στόμασι.

[2] Ibid., 226: τὸ γὰρ ἐν τοσαύτῃ φορᾷ τῇ μεταξὺ παμπόλλων ἀγγείων ἀλλήλοις ἀναμιγνυμένων μηδεπώποτε φλέβα μὲν ἀρτηρίᾳ εὑρίσκεσθαι, ἀρτηρίαν δὲ φλεβὶ ἐμφῦσαι, ἀλλ' ἀεὶ γνωρίζειν τὸ οἰκεῖον καὶ ἐνοῦσθαι, τοῦτο μόνον τέχνης θαυμαστῆς, οὐ τύχης ἀλόγου τεκμήριον.

[3] Ibid., 231: εὐθὺς οὖν ἑκάτερον τὸ ζεῦγος τῶν ἀγγείων ἡ φύσις ἐν ἐπιτηδείῳ χωρίῳ κατέθετο, καὶ διὰ τούτων οἷον πρέμνων τινῶν ἐκ τῆς μήτρας ἕλκει τὸ ἔμβρυον αἷμα καὶ πνεῦμα.

[4] See his article entitled 'Galen's experiments and observations on the pulmonary blood-flow', *Am. J. Cardiol.* 10 (1962), 738–45, where he remarks: 'Galen described how blood flows from the placenta through the umbilical vein into the portal vein of the foetus near the liver; how a short shunt diverts the blood from passage through this organ and connects the portal vein directly with the inferior vena cava. Today, this shunt is called the ductus Arantii. Thus blood can flow from the placenta directly into the right atrium.'
So too in his book (op. cit., p. 59) he repeats this erroneous statement. It is interesting to compare Galen's actual words in the passage cited by Siegel in this connection, from the thirteenth book of *Anatomical procedures* in Duckworth's translation from the Arabic. (*Galen on Anatomical Procedures; the later books* (Cambridge, 1962).) 'As for the animal which is on the point of being born you will see in it two arteries which go from the placenta to the foetus, travelling in the umbilical cord, and those are the two of which we spoke earlier (*umbilical arteries*), likewise the artery (*umbilical vein*) which runs to the liver near to that part of it which is called the porta hepatis. This place is rightly named "porta", since through it enters the blood which comes from the pregnant mother to the foetus in the same way as

he was acquainted with the ductus venosus Arantii. He simply tells us that the single vein derived from the two in the cord travels directly to the underside or hollow side of the liver. He was also correct in assuming that the two arteries of the cord pass one on each side of the bladder (in the form of the right and left hypogastric arteries) into the two internal iliac arteries, branches of the iliac fork of the abdominal aorta.[1] But his passion for symmetry misled him rather badly in the anatomy of the cord itself. It plainly had two arteries, therefore it must also have two veins, though these, he tells us, are united immediately after passing the umbilicus of the foetus.[2] He was also aware that since *in utero* the lungs were not working nature had to make certain special provisions to supply the embryo with blood and *pneuma*. He knew that the vascular arrangements of the foetus differ from those of the animal after birth, but his failure to grasp the notion of the circulation of the blood led him badly astray in his interpretation of their meaning. He deals with them at great length in two books of *On the use of the parts*, from which I shall have to make rather extensive quotations in the next few paragraphs. In the twentieth and twenty-first chapters of the sixth book he describes nature's methods of supplying *pneuma* to the embryo when the lungs are not yet functioning, and he explains a vivisectional experiment from which he draws his conclusions. He also returns to the same subject in the sixth chapter of the fifteenth book.

The essential feature of these arrangements is to relieve the foetal heart of the responsibility of furnishing the foetal body with either blood or *pneuma*. This purpose is accomplished by means of a direct connection

provisions for nourishment reach the interior of the body through its portals. From this spot the blood which the mother transfers to the offspring arrives at the convexity of the liver and the hollow surface of the liver of the offspring. From here the blood which reaches the hepatic convexity passes to the vena cava, and this vein delivers it and distributes it in the whole of the body of the foetus, just as will be delivered subsequently in fully formed bodies. But the blood which comes to the hollow aspect of the liver travels further in the portal vein until it reaches to the intestines, the stomach, the omentum, and the spleen.'

The idea that Galen was acquainted with the ductus venosus seems to have been shared by other modern historians. Thus, as D. M. Franklin pointed out in his article 'A survey of the growth of knowledge about certain parts of the foetal cardio-vascular apparatus', *Ann. Sci.* 5 (1941), 57–89, even the great Needham in the first edition of his *History of Embryology* slipped up on this point, observing that he has not succeeded in discovering a passage in Galen in which such knowledge was exhibited. I have been no more successful.

[1] *De plac. Hipp. et Plat.* vi. 6, K. v. 559: οὔτ᾽ ἐπὶ τὴν μεγάλην ἀρτηρίαν ἡ φορά. περιλαβοῦσαι γὰρ ἑκατέρωθεν τὴν κύστιν εἰς τὸ κάταντες ἔρχονται μέχρι περ ἂν ἐντύχωσι ταῖς ἐπὶ τὰ σκέλη τοῦ κυουμένου φερομέναις ἀρτηρίαις.

[2] *De usu partium*, xv. 4, K. iv. 226–7: τέτταρα γὰρ οὖν ἐνταῦθα τὰ πάντ᾽ ἐστὶν ἀγγεῖα, δύο μὲν ἀρτηρίαι, δύο δὲ φλέβες ... τὸ δὲ μήτε τὰς φλέβας εἰς ἄλλο τι καταφύεσθαι σπλάγχνον ὑπερβαινούσας τὸ ἧπαρ, μήτε τὰς ἀρτηρίας ἀλλαχόσε ποι φέρεσθαι πλὴν ἐπὶ τὴν μεγάλην ἀρτηρίαν ... πῶς οὐ θαυμαστόν; ... ἀλλὰ τὰς μὲν φλέβας εἰς τὰ τοῦ ἥπατος σιμά, τὰς δ᾽ ἀρτηρίας εἰς τὴν ἐπ᾽ ὀσφύϊ μοῖραν τῆς μεγάλης ἀρτηρίας ... τὰς μὲν γὰρ φλέβας ἔστιν ἰδεῖν εὐθέως μετὰ τὸν ὀμφαλὸν εἰς ταὐτὸν ἀλλήλαις ἰούσας καὶ μίαν γενομένας.

of the vena cava with the vein-like artery or pulmonary vein, through a
common opening between them, and the existence of a vessel joining the
aorta to the pulmonary artery.[1] The foetal heart, that is its two ventricles,
is thus bypassed; the maternal blood which has been distributed through
the umbilical veins into the liver and thence into the vena cava passes
via the opening straight into the pulmonary veins and into the quiescent
foetal lung, while the arterial blood from the mother, passing into the
aorta abdominalis, has no need to enter the left foetal ventricle. Once
having entered the aorta, it can find a direct passage via the ascending
aorta into the upper, and via the iliac arteries to the lower portions of the
foetal body. The only organ it could not so reach would be the lungs.
Nature therefore provided a foetal connection between the aorta and the
pulmonary artery, enabling it to do so. This connection, the ductus
arteriosus, wastes away soon after birth. Galen describes these arrangements as follows, in the sixth book of the treatise under discussion:

For nature, by opening up the thick solid-coated vessel of the lung [pulmo-
nary artery] into the great artery [aorta], and the vena cava into the thin and
loose-textured vessel [pulmonary vein], gave the lungs a fair share of both blood
and *pneuma*, while at the same time relieving the heart of service with respect
to them. So that it is not surprising that the heart, sending neither blood nor
pneuma to the lungs, nor furnishing a supply of them to the arteries that go all
over the animal's body, as it does in animals after birth, only needs in the foetal
condition an extremely small quantity to ensure its own living existence.[2]

These arrangements are also described in the fifteenth book, where
Galen puts the position in the following paragraph:

Now it is right to admire nature also in this matter. When the lungs merely
had to grow [i.e. in their foetal condition], she simply supplied them
with blood,[3] but when their function changes into movement she made

---

[1] Ibid. vi. 20, K. iii. 507: ἡ μὲν γὰρ (φύσις) οὔτ' ἀργῶς οὔτ' ἀπρονοήτως, ἀλλ' (ἅπερ οὗτοι
λέγουσι) προτέρα λελογισμένη καὶ γιγνώσκουσα, μὴ τῆς αὐτῆς δεῖσθαι διοικήσεως τὸν ἔτι κυούμενον
καὶ διαπλαττόμενον καὶ ἀκίνητον πνεύμονα τῷ τετελειωμένῳ καὶ ἤδη κινουμένῳ, τὸ μὲν ἰσχυρὸν
καὶ παχὺ καὶ στεγανὸν ἀγγεῖον ἀνεστόμωσε πρὸς τὴν μεγάλην ἀρτηρίαν, τὸ δ' ἀσθενὲς καὶ
μανὸν καὶ λεπτὸν εἰς τὴν κοίλην φλέβα.

[2] Ibid., 509: ἀναστομώσασα γὰρ εἰς μὲν τὸ παχὺ καὶ στεγανὸν ἀγγεῖον τοῦ πνεύμονος τὴν
μεγάλην ἀρτηρίαν, εἰς δὲ τὸ λεπτὸν καὶ μανὸν τὴν κοίλην φλέβα, καὶ τῷ πνεύμονι μέν, ὡς εἴρηται,
μετέδωκεν ἀμφοτέρων τῶν ὑλῶν δικαίως, καὶ τὴν καρδίαν δ' οὐδὲν ἧττον ἠλευθέρωσε τῆς περὶ
αὐτὸν ὑπηρεσίας. ὥστ' οὐδὲν ἔτι θαυμαστόν, εἰ μήθ' αἷμα μήτε πνεῦμα τῷ πνεύμονι πέμπουσα,
μήτε ταῖς καθ' ὅλον τὸ ζῷον ἀρτηρίαις αὐτὴ χορηγοῦσα, καθάπερ ἐπὶ τῶν τελείων, εἰς μόνην τὴν
ἰδίαν ζωὴν ἐδεήθη πνεύματος ὀλιγίστου παντάπασιν.

[3] I have here translated the word ἀκριβές as *simply*, though Kühn in his Latin translation
renders it by the word *purum* and Mrs. Tallmadge May (op. cit. ii. 670) by the word 'pure'.
The important point to remember is that here 'pure' cannot mean 'refined' in the sense that
arterial blood in the adult is 'refined'. Nor is the blood that passes through the foramen ovale
mixed with *pneuma*, except for the very small amount of *pneuma* contained in the maternal
venous blood which is the ultimate source of the foetal blood.

their flesh light, giving it feathers as it were, so that it could easily be distended and contracted by the thorax. The connection between the vena cava and the vein-like artery [pulmonary vein] in the foetus also came into being for the same reason. Since, I think, this vessel [the pulmonary vein] serves as a vein for the organ, it was necessary for the other [sc. the artery-like vein] to change its function by fulfilling the function of an artery. For this reason nature also connected this vessel with the great artery [aorta]. But here there was some interval between the two vessels, so she fashioned a third small vessel to join them both together. In the case of the other two vessels [sc. the vena cava and the pulmonary vein], since these two vessels touched one another, she made as it were a common hole between them, and devised a membrane to act as a cover to this hole, which readily inclined towards the vessel leading to the lung, so that it would yield to the pressure of blood pushed in a stream from the vena cava, but would prevent any of this blood from flowing back into it.[1]

The meaning of this rather obscure passage can perhaps best be interpreted by reference to a sentence in the *De venarum et arteriarum dissectione*, where Galen states that this foetal duct is an artery, not only in its structure (i.e. it has a thick coat), but also in its function, that is to say, it conveys both blood and *pneuma*,[2] the latter being derived from the maternal arterial system. This passage just quoted shows quite clearly that Galen was acquainted with both the foramen ovale and the ductus arteriosus now called after Botallo, as Daremberg did not fail to point out.[3] The opening to which Galen refers was a 'hole' in what we call the auricular septum, which he describes with great accuracy. He knows that

___

[1] *De usu partium*, xv. 6, K. iv. 243–4 : ἄξιον οὖν ἐστι κἀν τῷδε θαυμάζειν τὴν φύσιν, ἡνίκα μὲν ἐχρῆν αὐξάνεσθαι μόνον τὸ σπλάγχνον, ἀκριβὲς αἷμα χορηγοῦσαν αὐτῷ, μεταπεσόντος δ' εἰς τὸ κινεῖσθαι, κούφην τὴν σάρκα καθάπερ τι πτέρωμα ποιήσασαν, ὅπως ἑτοίμως ἀπὸ τοῦ θώρακος διαστέλλοιτό τε καὶ συστέλλοιτο. διὰ ταῦτα τοιγαροῦν ἐγένετο καὶ ἡ τῆς κοίλης φλεβὸς πρὸς τὴν ἀρτηρίαν τὴν φλεβώδη σύντρησις, ἐπὶ τῶν ἔτι κυουμένων, ἅτε δ', οἶμαι, τοῦ ἀγγείου τούτου τῆς φλεβὸς ὑπηρετοῦντος τῷ σπλάγχνῳ, θάτερον ἀναγκαῖον ἦν εἰς ἀρτηρίας χρείαν μεταπεσεῖν, καὶ διὰ τοῦτο συνέτρησε καὶ τοῦτο ἡ φύσις εἰς τὴν μεγάλην ἀρτηρίαν. ἀλλ' ἐνταῦθα μέν, ἐπειδὴ διάστημά τι μεταξὺ τῶν ἀγγείων ἦν, ἕτερον τρίτον μικρὸν ἀγγεῖον, ἄμφω συνάπτον ἐδημιούργησεν. ἐπὶ δὲ τῶν ὑπολοίπων τῶν δυοῖν, ἐπειδὴ καὶ ταῦτ' ἔψαυεν ἀλλήλων, οἷον ὀπήν τινα κοινὴν ἀμφοῖν ἐποιήσατο, καί τινα κατ' αὐτῆς ὑμένα δίκην ἐπιθήματος ἐτεχνήσατο, πρὸς τὸ τοῦ πνεύμονος ἀγγεῖον ἑτοίμως ἀνακλινόμενον, ὅπως εἴκῃ μὲν τῇ ῥύμῃ τῆς φορᾶς τοῦ αἵματος ἐκ τῆς κοίλης ἐπιρρέοντος, ἀποκωλύοι δ' αὖθις εἰς αὐτὴν ἀπανέρχεσθαι τὸ αἷμα. The term *small*, as applied to the ductus, is anatomically incorrect (see Franklin, op. cit.), but Galen may after all only be referring to its length.

[2] *De ven. et art. dissect.* 10, K. ii. 828 : καὶ μέντοι καὶ ἡ ἐκ τῆς μεγάλης ἀρτηρίας εἰς τὴν ἀρτηριώδη φλέβα, κυουμένων ἔτι τῶν ζῴων, ἀπόφυσίς ἐστι καὶ κατάφυσις, οὐ κατὰ τὸ σῶμα μόνον ἀλλὰ κατὰ τὴν χρείαν ἐπὶ τῶν κυουμένων ἐστὶν ἀρτηρία.

[3] See his translation of the *De usu partium* in his first volume, p. 252. Mrs. May in her translation (op. cit. i. 331, footnote 102) raises the question whether Galen was the first to discover these structures. She observes that H. F. Killian in his work, *Über den Kreislauf im Kinde das noch nicht geatmet hat* (Karlsruhe, 1826), says that they were known to Herophilus, but fails to give any evidence for this assertion, and wisely adds that if Galen had been the first to distinguish anything so striking, he might have been expected to say so.

the septum secundum opens into the left atrium, that it is pushed open by the pressure of the blood from the right atrium, whereas blood coming in the opposite direction would close it, and that it closes itself very soon after birth. The process of sealing up usually takes place, he tells us, in animals in one or two days, but may in certain cases require three or four days or even longer. Even after this interval you may see the membrane in the process of growing over the hole, but not yet completely united with the edges of the septum. But when this process is completed and the animal begins to attain its full growth, you would not believe that such a hole had ever existed when you look at the completely continuous structure.[1] In a similar manner, the ductus joining the aorta to the pulmonary artery not only ceases to grow after birth, when all the other parts of the animal are growing, but it can be seen to become thinner and thinner, until as time progresses, it dries up completely and wears away.[2]

The supply of *pneuma* to the lungs, which after birth obtain it through the trachea in respiration, also requires special arrangements in the foetus. During the whole of their intra-uterine existence they are, of course, inactive. Not yet being filled with air, they are red, not as after birth whitish. This is because they obtain their nourishment from a vessel with a thin coat, the pulmonary vein, which lets through the thicker kind of blood which has come from the liver via the vena cava and the foramen ovale. When the foramen closes up after birth, the lungs are fed by a thick-coated vessel, namely the artery-like vein or pulmonary artery, which only permits a very small quantity of blood, and that only of the thinnest and lightest kind, to pass into their tissues. Much *pneuma* comes into them and very little blood. Since animals' lungs move continuously so long as they remain alive and continue to breathe, the blood in the lungs is cut down by the *pneuma* in accordance with its double motion, the one which it acquires from the arteries, and the one which it acquires from the whole lung. So the flesh of the lungs becomes thinner and softer than before and like foam. The result is that it changes from its intra-uterine condition, when it was red, heavy, and dense, into that of the breathing animal, which is light, pale, and of a loose texture.[3]

---

[1] *De usu partium*, xv. 6, K. iv. 244–5: παντὸς δ' ἐπέκεινα θαύματος ἡ μετὰ ταῦτα σύμφυσις τοῦ προειρημένου τρήματος. καὶ γὰρ τῶν ἄρτι γεγενημένων ζῴων, ἢ πρὸ μιᾶς ἢ δυοῖν ἡμερῶν, ἐπ' ἐνίων δὲ καὶ τεττάρων καὶ πέντε καὶ πλεόνων, ἔστιν ὅτε συμφυόμενόν ἐστιν εὑρεῖν τὸν ἐπὶ τοῦ τρήματος ὑμένα, συμπεφυκότα δ' οὐδέπω. τελειωθέντος δὲ καὶ τὴν οἰκείαν ἀκμὴν ἀπολαβόντος τοῦ ζῴου θεασάμενος τὸ χορίον ἅπαν ἀκριβῶς στεγανόν, ἀπιστήσεις γεγονέναι ποτὲ τὸν χρόνον ἡνίκα διετέτρητο.

[2] Ibid., 245–6: οὕτω δὲ καὶ τὸ συνάπτον ἀγγεῖον τὴν μεγάλην ἀρτηρίαν τῇ κατὰ τὸν πνεύμονα φλεβί, τῶν ἄλλων ἁπάντων τοῦ ζῴου μορίων αὐξανομένων, οὐ μόνον ἀναυξές, ἀλλὰ καὶ λεπτότερον ἀεὶ φαίνεται γινόμενον, ὡς ἐν χρόνῳ προϊόντι παντάπασιν ἀπομαραίνεσθαί τε καὶ ξηραίνεσθαι.

[3] Ibid., 242: διὰ τί δὲ καὶ ὁ πνεύμων ἐπὶ τῶν ἔτι κυουμένων ἐρυθρός ἐστιν, οὐχ ὥσπερ ἐπὶ τῶν τελέων ζῴων ὑπόλευκος; ὅτι τρέφεται τηνικαῦτα καθάπερ τἆλλα σπλάγχνα δι' ἀγγείων ἕνα χιτῶνα

The provision of these two elementary necessities to the lungs would appear to be plain sailing. Their provision to the foetal heart raises a number of difficulties. These arrangements are almost impossible to decipher, because of the difficulty of reconciling the statement we have just quoted, that the foetal heart is relieved of all responsibility for providing either blood or *pneuma* to the foetal vascular system, with the discovery which Galen was probably the first to make, that both the heart and the arteries of the foetus 'pulsate', and with the findings or rather the conclusions drawn from an experiment which he devised and carried out.

The provision of the *pneuma* required by the heart of the foetus presents a problem. Its needs are minimal, only just the small amount needed to keep it alive and working as it were *in vacuo*. Whence and how does it procure this? Galen answers this question very ambiguously, to say the least of it.

In the first place [or 'certainly', μάλιστα μέν] it is able, I think, to obtain it even from the great artery itself, since the membranes forming the valves were not, as we have already shown above, invented by nature for the purpose of ensuring that absolutely nothing could get past them, but rather in order to prevent any large and compact body of matter entering the heart. The heart could moreover also attract blood mixed with *pneuma* from the lungs, through the valve which has only two membranes, [sc. the mitral or bicuspid], for this vessel [sc. pulmonary vein] receives blood from the vena cava in the embryo through a certain opening of considerable size. Now it has been demonstrated

λεπτὸν ἐχόντων· εἰς ταῦτα γὰρ ἐκ τῆς κοίλης φλεβὸς ἀφικνεῖται τὸ αἷμα κατὰ τὸν τῆς κυήσεως καιρόν. ἀποκυηθέντων δὲ τυφλοῦται μὲν ἡ τῶν ἀγγείων σύντρησις, ἐμπίπτει δ᾿ εἰς αὐτὰ πνεῦμα πλεῖστον, ὀλίγιστον δ᾿ αἷμα, καὶ τοῦτο ἀκριβῶς λεπτόν. ἀλλὰ καὶ κινεῖται τηνικαῦτα διηνεκῆ κίνησιν ὁ πνεύμων, ἀναπνέοντος τοῦ ζῴου. κοπτόμενον μὲν οὖν ἀπὸ τοῦ πνεύματος τὸ αἷμα κατὰ διττὴν κίνησιν, ἥν τε ἐκ τῶν ἀρτηριῶν ἔχει, καὶ ἣν ἐξ ὅλου τοῦ πνεύμονος ἐπικτᾶται, λεπτότερον ἔτι καὶ μαλακώτερον ἑαυτοῦ καὶ οἷον ἀφρῶδες γίνεται. καὶ διὰ τοῦτο μεταπίπτει τῆς σαρκὸς τοῦ πνεύμονος ἡ φύσις ἐξ ἐρυθρᾶς καὶ βαρείας καὶ πυκνῆς εἰς λευκὴν καὶ κούφην καὶ ἀραιάν.

This passage is not altogether clear since the use of the term artery is ambiguous. Is Galen here referring to the tracheal system or to the system of the pulmonary veins? Perhaps in referring to arteries he may be including in that term both systems, the rough as well as the smooth. For according to his teaching there was some connection between the two systems the exact nature of which, as we shall see presently, is anything but clear. Nor is it at all easy to reconcile the statement that after birth very little blood passes into the lung with statements made elsewhere, when he is dealing with the quantity of nutrition needed by that organ owing to its intense respiratory activity. On the whole I am inclined to think that he means the windpipes here. The lung is a sort of bag inflated by the bronchial system which blows air not only into the tubes leading to the heart, but also into the interstices between the three sets of pipes which constitute the flesh of the lung. In the post-natal condition the pulmonary artery conveys only the refined, or at any rate partially refined, blood to the lung, to feed its foam-like tissues, but in the foetal condition, there does not seem to be any reason why it should convey blood to the lung at all. If it does so, it must be blood mixed with *pneuma*, which has been derived from the maternal system via the umbilical arteries and the foetal aorta. The important point is that both blood and *pneuma* supplied to the foetal lungs short-circuit the foetal heart.

above that it [sc. the pulmonary vein] receives its share of blood in the fully formed animal [i.e. after birth] from the haematic (which in the case of the embryo are the pneumatic) organs through many fine orifices too small to be seen, so that in the foetal condition it receives its share of *pneuma* even more readily. We must add, too, that what happens in the embryo is no small additional testimony to the fact that the two classes of blood vessels anastomose with each other, and also to the existence of some *pneuma* in the veins.

For, if you take a female animal with the embryo still attached to the mother, and open up the abdominal cavity and the uterus, after the manner described in *Anatomical procedures*, and tie a ligature round the (foetal) arteries at the umbilicus, all the arteries in the placenta will cease to pulsate while those of the embryo itself will continue pulsating. If now you tie the ligature round the veins at the umbilicus, the arteries in the embryo will also stop pulsating. This makes it plain that the power which makes the arteries in the placenta move starts out from the heart of the embryo. It also shows that it is through the openings or anastomoses with the veins that the arteries obtain their supplies of *pneuma*, by means of which the innate heat can be preserved up to a certain time at least. It is not therefore impossible in the heart itself for some assistance also to be furnished by the vessel which contains blood [the pulmonary vein] to the innate heat in its left ventricle, for the sake of which animals have need both of respiration and the pulse.[1]

It also proves, incidentally, that Erasistratus' statements that blood and *pneuma* can never mix were neither self-consistent nor in accordance with the facts.[2]

The argument of these two paragraphs is rather difficult to follow. As Mrs. May has pointed out (in a footnote to her translation of the passage

[1] *De usu partium*, vi. 21, K. iii. 509–11 : ὁ μάλιστα μέν, οἶμαι, κἀξ αὐτῆς τῆς μεγάλης ἀρτηρίας οἷόν τ᾽ ἦν αὐτῇ λαμβάνειν. ἡ γὰρ τῶν ὑμένων ἐπίφυσις, ὡς ἔμπροσθεν ἐδείξαμεν, οὐκ εἰς τὸ μηδὲν ὅλως, ἀλλ᾽ εἰς τὸ μήτε πολὺ μήτ᾽ ἀθρόως εἰς αὐτὴν παραγίγνεσθαί τι, πρὸς φύσεως ἐξευρέθη. καὶ μέντοι κἀκ τοῦ πνεύμονος αἷμα καὶ πνεῦμα μεμιγμένον οἷόν τέ ἐστιν ἕλκειν αὐτῇ διὰ τοῦ στόματος, ἐφ᾽ ᾧ μόνῳ δύο χιτῶνας ἐλέγομεν ἔξωθεν ἔσω πεφυκότας ἐπικεῖσθαι. τοῦτο γὰρ δὴ τὸ ἀγγεῖον ἐπὶ τῶν κυουμένων ἐκ μὲν τῆς κοίλης φλεβὸς αἷμα δέχεται διά τινος ἀναστομώσεως ἀξιολόγου τὸ μέγεθος· ἐκ δὲ τῶν ἐν μὲν τοῖς τελείοις αἱματικῶν, ἐν δὲ τοῖς ἔτι κυουμένοις πνευματικῶν ὀργάνων, ἐδείχθη μὲν ἔμπροσθεν αἷμα μεταλαμβάνον ἐπὶ τῶν τελείων ζῴων κατὰ πολλὰς καὶ λεπτὰς ἀναστομώσεις ἐκφευγούσας τὴν ὄψιν ἑτοιμότερον δ᾽ αὖ ἐπὶ τῶν ἔτι κυουμένων τὸ πνεῦμα μεταλαμβάνει. καὶ γὰρ δὴ καὶ τοῦτο ἔτι προσθεῖναι χρὴ φαινόμενον ἐπὶ τῶν ἐμβρύων οὐ σμικρὸν τεκμήριον αὐτοῦ τε τοῦ συνανεστομῶσθαι πρὸς ἄλληλα τὰ δύο γένη τῶν ἀγγείων καὶ τοῦ μετεῖναί τι καὶ ταῖς φλεψὶ πνεύματος. εἰ γάρ, ἔτι προσεχομένου τοῦ κυουμένου τῇ μητρί, διελὼν τὸ ἐπιγάστριον αὐτῆς καὶ τὰς ὑστέρας, καθ᾽ ὃν εἴρηται τρόπον ἐν ταῖς ἀνατομικαῖς ἐγχειρήσεσι, βρόχους ταῖς κατὰ τὸν ὀμφαλὸν ἀρτηρίαις περιβάλοις, αἱ κατὰ τὸ χόριον ἄσφυκτοι πᾶσαι γενήσονται, τῶν κατ᾽ αὐτὸ τὸ ἔμβρυον ἔτι σφυζουσῶν· εἰ δὲ δὴ καὶ ταῖς φλεψὶ ταῖς κατὰ τὸν ὀμφαλὸν ἐπιβάλοις τοὺς βρόχους, οὐκ ἂν οὐδὲ αἱ κατὰ τὸ ἔμβρυον ἀρτηρίαι σφύζοιεν ἂν ἔτι. κἂν τῷδε δῆλον ἅμα μέν, ὡς ἡ κινοῦσα τὰς κατὰ τὸ χόριον ἀρτηρίας δύναμις ἀπὸ τῆς τοῦ κυομένου καρδίας ὅρμαται, ἅμα δὲ καὶ ὡς διὰ τῶν φλεβῶν κατὰ τὰς ἀναστομώσεις εὐποροῦσιν αἱ ἀρτηρίαι πνεύματος, ὑφ᾽ οὗ διασώζεσθαι δύναται τὸ ἔμφυτον θερμὸν ἄχρι γοῦν τινος. οὔκουν οὐδὲ κατὰ τὴν καρδίαν αὐτὴν ἀδύνατον ἐκ τοῦ αἷμα περιέχοντος ἀγγείου γενέσθαι τινὰ ὠφέλειαν τῆς κατὰ τὴν ἀριστερὰν αὐτῆς κοιλίαν ἐμφύτου θερμεσίας, δι᾽ ἣν καὶ τῆς ἀναπνοῆς καὶ τῶν σφυγμῶν ἐδείχθη τὰ ζῷα δεόμενα.
[2] Ibid., 511: τὰ δ᾽ ὑπὸ Ἐρασιστράτου λεγόμενα περὶ τοῦ μηδ᾽ ὅλως ἐπιμίγνυσθαι τὰς ὕλας οὔτε τοῖς φαινομένοις οὔτ᾽ ἀλλήλοις ὁμολογεῖ.

quoted),[1] it is the pulmonary artery [artery-like vein] and its branches
which carry blood to the lung in the adult and *pneuma* in the foetus. In
the adult, this vessel carries blood from the right ventricle which has
come direct from the liver to the lung. This, owing to the inosculations
of its terminal branches with those of the pulmonary vein, drips in
small quantities into the vein-like artery [pulmonary vein], which
carries *pneuma* to the heart. In the foetus the *pneuma* follows the
same route. Venous or unrefined blood derived from the maternal
system through the umbilical veins from the vena cava goes through the
foramen ovale into the lungs via the pulmonary vein, passing through the
inosculations into the branches of the pulmonary artery, the artery-
like vein. Blood mixed with *pneuma* derived from the maternal arterial
system via the arteries of the umbilical cord, the aorta of the foetus,
and the ductus arteriosus reaches the foetal lung through the pulmonary
artery. The heart therefore to get this *pneuma* has to draw it through
the inosculations of the branches of the pulmonary artery with those
of the pulmonary vein, via the mitral valve. But this does not appear to be
the source of *pneuma* for the foetal heart indicated by the experiment
just described. The ligation of the arteries in the umbilical cord does not
stop the foetal heart and arteries from beating. This proves that they do
not derive this power from the maternal heart and arteries, but they must
obtain the *pneuma* this power implies somehow from the maternal blood.
This is shown by the fact that when the umbilical veins are ligated, the
beating of the foetal heart and arteries ceases. The blood derived from the
maternal veins must therefore contain some *pneuma*. Where this *pneuma*
comes from we are not told, but as far as I can judge, its most likely
source would seem to be the air contained in food or drink ingested. At
any rate its amount is very small, just sufficient to animate the foetal
heart and arteries. After a refutation of Erasistratus' theory of the
complete separation of blood and *pneuma*, Galen proceeds to make
obscurity more obscure in the following paragraph.

For it has been demonstrated in the paragraphs immediately above, first,
that the arteries are not dilated because they are filled with *pneuma* coming
from the heart, and secondly that with each dilation they attract some matter
from the veins, and, thirdly, that in the embryo it is necessary when the pulmonary vein receives blood from the vena cava, that when the heart is at diastole
not a little of this blood passes into the left ventricle, since the membranes
of the mitral valve, being turned from outside inwards, place no obstacle in
its way. So that the heart appears to be plainly the source of the power which
moves the arteries, not only in the creature after birth, but also in the embryo.[2]

[1] May, op. cit. i. 331, n. 102.
[2] *De usu partium*, vi. 21, K. iii. 511–12 : δείκνυται γὰρ ἐκ τῶν εἰρημένων ἀρτίως ἅμα μέν, ὡς οὐ
διότι πληροῦνται τοῦ παρὰ καρδίας πνεύματος αἱ ἀρτηρίαι, διὰ τοῦτο διαστέλλονται, ἅμα δ' ὡς ἕλκουσί
τι κἀκ τῶν φλεβῶν καθ' ἑκάστην διάστασιν, ἅμα δὲ καὶ ὡς ἀναγκαῖόν ἐστιν ἐπὶ τῶν ἐμβρύων αἷμα

Galen never tells us what happens to this blood which has entered the left ventricle. It is therefore not easy to conjecture exactly of how it is disposed. For at the systole of the foetal heart it should surely be expelled through the valve closing the aorta. But we have just been told that the foetal heart is relieved of all responsibility of supplying blood or *pneuma* either to the lungs or to the arteries throughout the body. This way there is no escape from our dilemma. The foetal heart and arteries beat, but there is no indication that Galen thought they propelled blood. It seems to me quite possible that he thought that the maternal blood which reached the foetal right ventricle via the liver, the vena cava, and the tricuspid valve, and the left ventricle via the bicuspid valve, remained there oscillating between the two ventricles. Since it is quite clear that the pulmonary valve remained closed, no blood passing through it to the lung. The aortal valve therefore might also have remained shut in the foetal condition. The blood in the heart, i.e. the ventricles, could be no doubt engaged in providing the material for its growth. Nor, as it seems to me, is any better way provided by the hypotheses of Siegel,[1] who in his articles on Galen gives the following explanation of his conception of the foetal blood-movement.[2]

Thus in the first of these he tells us:

Galen clearly stated that the purpose of the close contact between the maternal and foetal arterial blood vessels is the exchange of air between the maternal and foetal blood. He wrote that the maternal vessels supply the foetus sufficiently with air to keep it alive, and that a small amount of blood may pass directly from the mother through the placenta into the foetal blood vessels. Galen did realize that the blood in the umbilical vessels was aerated. He thought that the aerated blood passed from the placenta through the umbilical vein through the right heart into the aorta of the foetus and from there into the periphery of the body. In addition he (Galen) incorrectly assumed that some of the blood went directly from the placenta upwards through the aorta of the foetus to the left ventricle. Thus Galen contradicted the result of his own observations that the pulsation of the umbilical arteries is directly away from the heart.

παρὰ τῆς κοίλης φλεβὸς δεχομένης τῆς ἀρτηρίας τῆς φλεβώδους ἕλκεσθαι, δηλονότι διαστελλομένης τῆς καρδίας, ἐξ αὐτῆς οὐκ ὀλίγον εἰς τὴν ἀριστερὰν κοιλίαν, τῆς γε τῶν ὑμένων ἐπιφύσεως οὐδὲν κωλυούσης, ἔξωθεν γὰρ ἔσω φαίνονται πεφυκότες. ὥστε τῆς μὲν δυνάμεως ἡ καρδία ταῖς ἀρτηρίαις ἐναργῶς φαίνεται χορηγοῦσα τῆς κινούσης αὐτάς, οὐ μόνον ἐπὶ τῶν τελείων ἤδη ζῴων, ἀλλὰ καὶ ἐπὶ τῶν ἔτι κυουμένων.

[1] See his three articles: 'Historical Milestones. Galen's experiments and observations on pulmonary blood-flow and respiration', *Am. J. Cardiol.* 10 (Nov. 1962) ; 'Why Galen and Harvey did not compare the heart to a pump', *Am. J. Cardiol.* 15 (July 1967) ; 'The influence of Galen's doctrine of the pulmonary blood-flow on the development of modern conceptions of the circulation', *Arch. f. Gesch. d. Med.* xlvi (1962) ; and his paper, 'Galen's ideas on the heartbeat', delivered at the XIXth International Congress on the History of Medicine, held at Basel in 1964.

[2] The author's view of Galen's conception of blood-flow is shown in Fig. 5. See also the note at the end of the chapter.

In his article in *Sudhoffs Archiv*, Siegel says:

Galen described correctly how in the unborn foetus the venous blood flows from the placenta through the umbilical veins into the vena cava and the right atrium bypassing the liver through another shunt. He recognized that the open foramen only prevents the blood from entering through the pulmonary artery into the lungs of the foetus which remain collapsed until after birth. He further observed correctly that a small amount of blood still passes into the right chamber of the heart. He discovered that this blood was short-circuited from the pulmonary artery into the aorta by using an extra-cardial shunt, which is now called the ductus Botalli. Galen further observed that shortly after birth the ductus Botalli and the bypass around the liver close up, and that now the entire blood flows from the right heart into the lungs.

The idea of an exchange of air between the maternal and the foetal blood seems to me to be quite misleading. The whole of the blood in the foetus is supplied by the mother, not, as seems to be here stated, a small amount. The arterial type of blood needed by the foetus was supplied by its mother through the umbilical arteries. The whole point of the experiment of ligating the umbilical vessels was to show that venous blood, or to speak more accurately the blood coming from the mother's veins through the umbilical cord into the vena cava of the foetus, does in fact contain some *pneuma*. For the blood coming to the foetal arteries from the mother through the arterial vessels of the cord did not reach the foetal heart at all.

With regard to the second passage, I can find no evidence that Galen was acquainted with the ductus Arantii venosus. On the contrary, he expressly tells us that the umbilical vein leads into the 'concave' ($\tau \grave{\alpha}$ $\sigma\iota\mu\acute{\alpha}$) not the 'convex' ($\tau \grave{\alpha}$ $\kappa\upsilon\rho\tau\acute{\alpha}$) side of the liver, because that is where the gall-bladder is, and it was better for the maternal blood to be purified of its excess of bile before being distributed to all the tissues of the foetal body.[1] There could therefore be no question of a liver-avoiding shunt. Nor can I find any passage in which Galen tells us that a small amount of the blood entering the right atrium passes into the right ventricle. Finally, it was quite foreign to Galen's teaching that all the blood after birth flows from the right heart into the lungs. Not only does a large proportion of it not enter the right side of the heart at all, but even of the amount which does enter the right ventricle a large proportion goes not to the lungs but through the septum to the left ventricle. It cannot be emphasized too strongly that for Galen blood production does not start until after birth in the newborn infant. For blood is essentially the product of nutrition. The animal starts its extra-uterine life with a full

---

[1] *De usu partium*, xv. 4, K. iv. 230: διὰ τί δ' ἡ φλὲψ οὐκ εἰς τὰ κυρτὰ τοῦ ἥπατος, ἀλλ' εἰς τὰ σιμὰ καταφέρεται; διότι τὸ τῆς χολῆς ἀγγεῖον ἐνταῦθα ἐτέτακτο, καὶ βέλτιον ἦν καθαρθῆναι τὸ αἷμα πρὶν εἰς ὅλον τὸ ζῷον διανέμεσθαι.

complement of blood all furnished by its mother. It is only when it begins feeding that it starts producing its own blood.

In the account of the foetal circulation given in his book on Galen's physiological system, Siegel continues to attribute to Galen the modern notion of the placental function. Thus he tells us:

Galen recognized that the foetal blood takes up air from the mother's blood in the placenta and that the aerated blood, circumventing the right heart and the lungs, proceeds directly to the left heart and further to the arterial tree of the foetus. He was most fascinated by the discovery that at the time of birth the circulation of the blood changes from the foetal to the adult type. He observed that only *after* birth does the blood, coming from the vena cava, flow through the right chamber and the lungs before arriving at the left heart. He devoted much space to the description of the minute details of the foetal circulation and its changeover after birth. His discoveries were not fully appreciated, at least not in recent times.[1]

Galen also recognized that the flow of blood in both mother and foetus was controlled by two entirely separate mechanisms.

Siegel then quotes a passage from the account of the experiment we have just examined, adding:

This proved to Galen that the heart of the foetus was beating, a fact denied by some medieval writers. For Galen, the heart was always the leading force of the blood flow. His observation of the different rates of the foetal and the maternal heart served as additional evidence of a complete separation of both circulations.[2]

This assumption is quite unacceptable, as the passages which we have reviewed make abundantly plain. The whole idea of a foetal circulation was quite foreign to Galen's ideas. The blood of the foetus, derived entirely from the mother, had an inseparably connected double function, that of nutrition *plus* growth in the exercise of which it was entirely consumed, an exclusively one-way traffic. I therefore find it impossible to agree with Siegel's diagrammatic representation of Galen's notions (See the note at the end of this chapter).

Here we seem to have come upon another missed clue, which might have put him on the track of the circulation. For to us the most obvious conclusion to be drawn from the experiment is the independence of the foetal from the maternal circulation. As it is, the discovery of the beating of the foetal heart was only potentially important, a noteworthy contribution to physiological knowledge which he never seems to have attempted to think out. Hence he never appears to have asked himself the question what happens to the contents of the pulsating foetal heart.

Siegel, if I understand him correctly, postulates the reception by the right foetal ventricle of a certain amount of blood from the right auricle

[1] Siegel, *Sudhoffs Archiv* (1962), p. 59.   [2] Ibid., p. 62.

through the bicuspid valve, not all the blood entering the right auricle being transmitted through the foramen ovale into the left auricle and the venous artery (pulmonary vein). This blood from the right ventricle is propelled through the pulmonary artery, but not to the lung; it passes via the ductus arteriosus to the aorta and, if Galen's statement that the foetal heart distributes no blood to the arteries of its body be accepted, it must be presumed, though Siegel does not state this, that it must somehow pass through the valve opening from the foetal left ventricle into its aorta in reverse direction into the heart. Indeed Siegel's diagram indicates a double arrow in the portion of the aorta between its junction with the ductus arteriosus and the left ventricle, which must be supposed to indicate a two-way traffic.

Galen also discovered that in the foetus a certain amount of blood flows from the right atrium into the right ventricle and is expelled by the contraction of the right heart into the pulmonary artery. Galen described accurately how another shunt sends this blood from the pulmonary artery directly into the aorta, thus again bypassing the lungs.[1]

The conception of this intra-cardial minimal circulation is certainly fascinating, but I can find no passage in Galen which would justify its assumption. This way madness lies. It seems to me much safer to assume that Galen's thinking was like that of many of his predecessors and successors, lacking in consistency. It is interesting to note, in this connection, that it was Leonardo da Vinci who was the first, as far as we know, to observe that the blood systems of mother and offspring were completely separate, a fact noted by Needham in his *History of Embryology*.[2]

Finally, we may perhaps be more ready to understand the paradox of the foetal heart which beats but does not expel its contents when we remember that Galen's physiological mechanics were hardly his strong point. Before we can deal conclusively with this topic, there are some

[1] Siegel in his first article (*Am. J. Cardiol.* 1962), p. 743. This statement is repeated in almost identical words in his book on Galen's physiological system, p. 60, opposite to which appears as Fig. 5 the identical diagram as Fig. 4 in the article referred to.

[2] Needham, op. cit. (2nd edn. 1959), p. 97 quoted by Franklin in the article cited above: 'Da Vinci . . . was ahead of his time in stating that the veins of the child do not ramify in the substance of the uterus of its mother, i.e. he recognized the separateness of the foetal and the maternal vascular systems.'

Cf. Leonardo's note (Q. III. 7, v), reproduced in K. D. Keele's *Leonardo da Vinci on Movement of the Heart and Blood* (London, 1952): 'The veins and arteries of the uterus of woman have such a mixture of contacts with the extreme veins of the navel-string of her child . . . as the mesenteric veins ramifying in the liver have with the ramification of the veins which descend from the heart into the same liver . . . But the veins of the child do not ramify in the substance of the uterus of its mother, but in the placenta which takes the place of a shirt in the interior of the uterus which it coats, and is connected (but not united) with this by means of cotyledons.'

This passage seems to show that Leonardo had grasped the essential principle involved, but the first person to have drawn the explicit conclusion actually from Galen's experiment, would appear to have been the Dutchman Adrian Spigel or Spieghel (1578–1625).

features concerning the physiological processes which Galen imagined in the lung which need to be examined a little more closely. As we have already noted, he thought that the function of the right ventricle was to supply nutriment to the lungs, since only animals that breathe have a right ventricle—fishes have only one.[1] But the blood which enters the right ventricle from the liver is thick and muddy—quite unsuitable to nourish such a delicate organ. Hence the thick arterial coat of the artery-like vein (pulmonary artery), which is required to prevent the thicker elements of the blood from penetrating into the pulmonary flesh.[2] What then happens to these elements? At systole they must pass into the pulmonary artery. How then do they pass out of it and how are they disposed of? No consistent theory of their disposal seems to have been formulated by Galen, who was evidently hesitating between two quite inconsistent explanations. For we are told in another account that the crude muddy blood from the liver is transformed in the right ventricle into the light and vaporous kind which is suitable food for the lung, through the agency of the innate heat, which, though primarily resident in the left ventricle, appears to be sufficiently present in the right ventricle to effect this operation.[3]

Now it is true that according to Galen, the special type of blood which is conveyed by the arterial system receives its final elaboration under

[1] *De plac. Hipp. et Plat.* viii. 1, K. v. 658 f.: ἐναντίως ἔσται τῷ φαινομένῳ καὶ ἐν ταῖς τῶν ἰχθύων ἀνατομαῖς εὑρισκομένῳ. οὐδενὸς οὖν αὐτῶν ἡ καρδία δεξιὰν ἔχει κοιλίαν, ὅτι μηδὲ πνεύμων ἐστὶ τοῖς ζῴοις ἐκείνοις. Cf. *De usu partium*, vi. 9, K. iii. 441 f.: ἀλλ᾽ ὅσα μὲν ἐξ ἀέρος εἰσπνεῖ διὰ φάρυγγος καὶ ῥινῶν καὶ στόματος, εὐθὺς μὲν καὶ πνεύμων τούτοις ἐστίν, εὐθὺς δὲ καὶ τῆς καρδίας ἡ δεξιὰ κοιλία, τοῖς δ᾽ ἄλλοις ἅπασιν οὔτε πνεύμων ἐστὶν οὔτ᾽ ἐν τοῖς δεξιοῖς τῆς καρδίας εὐρύτης οὐδεμία.

[2] *Comment. IV in Hipp. de alimento,* 4, K. xv. 382–3: δεῖται γοῦν ἀτμώδους καὶ λεπτοῦ καὶ καθαροῦ τοῦ αἵματος, οὐχ ὥσπερ τὸ ἧπαρ ἰλυώδους καὶ παχέος. ὅθεν ἔμπαλιν αὐτῷ τὰ τῶν ἀγγείων ἔχει, μάλιστα μὲν τοῖς καθ᾽ ἧπαρ· ἤδη δὲ καὶ τοῖς ἄλλοις τοῦ ζῴου μορίοις. ἐκείνων μὲν γὰρ ἀραιός τε καὶ λεπτός ὁ χιτών ἐστι τοῦ ἀγγείου τοῦ τὸ αἷμα χορηγοῦντος. διὸ πλεῖστον τοῦ παχέος ἑτοίμως τοῖς περιέχουσι διαδίδωσιν. ὁ δὲ τοῦ πνεύμονος παχὺς καὶ πυκνὸς καὶ διὰ τοῦτο οὐδὲν πλὴν τὸ λεπτότατον ἐᾷ διεξέρχεσθαι.

[3] See Siegel, *Galen's System of Physiology and Medicine,* pp. 38 f. Siegel seems to be aware of the contradiction involved in these two accounts, but it does not appear to me that his explanation, or rather circumvention of the problem, given in his book, carries much conviction: 'Galen wrote briefly that the blood was prepared and thinned in the right chamber before entering the lungs. He assumed that thus the blood is prepared to serve as nourishment for the lungs. It cannot be decided if the line concerning the preparation of the blood in the right ventricle was later added to the original text. In view of the obvious contradiction of this passage to Galen's concept of respiration, one is inclined to regard the idea of a preparation of the blood in the right chamber as a falsification of the original text. Galen already complained of many falsifications of his books. This cannot be proved. But one becomes reluctant to accept such an apparent contradiction as Galen's own error. Galen was usually logical and pointed often at unsolved problems. In the autobiographical treatise which he published during his life he complained bitterly of such distortions of his treatises by scribes and imitators. Therefore it appears acceptable to discard the idea of a preparation of the blood in the right heart as unimportant for our understanding of Galen's system of blood-flow, although it was extensively discussed in medieval literature.'

the influence of the innate heat resident chiefly in the left ventricle, but that does not exclude a preliminary elaboration, under the same influence, in the right ventricle, in order to prepare the particular nutrition required by the lungs. Indeed, to reject this theory would be to make nonsense of the very carefully argued discussion of the lung's nutrition, which can hardly be regarded as a foreign interpolation. The most probable explanation seems to me to be that in his search for a teleological reason for the arterial nature of the artery-like vein (pulmonary artery) and the vein-like nature of the venous artery (pulmonary vein), Galen was at first content with the notion that the arterial coat of the pulmonary artery could be explained by the need for excluding from the lungs the thicker 'muddier' elements, and that he thought that the nutrition of the lungs took place through the pulmonary artery. It was only when he had worked out the notion of the capillary connections of the pulmonary arteries with the pulmonary veins that he realized the necessity of the processing in the right ventricle, since the blood which feeds the lungs through the venous coats of the vein-like arteries must already have been separated from its thicker elements. He found no difficulty in finding a function for the arterial coats of the vessel conveying blood from the right ventricle to the lung, since in order to fulfil its function of conveying nutriment it had to be protected from thoracic pressure.

Siegel, with his theory of Galen's discovery of the pulmonary transit, is able to dispose of this problem. Galen, he tells us, thought that

[the blood] is rendered more fluid by mechanical agitation in the right ventricle to become fit for passing through the invisible anastomoses in the lungs and the equally small pores of the interventricular septum. Such transit appeared unlikely when the blood would have remained sluggish after leaving the liver. This assumed mechanical elaboration of the blood by the right heart does not contradict the other tenets of Galen's doctrine of respiration and blood-flow.[1]

That may very well be true, but in fact Galen nowhere mentions such mechanical agitation. In every passage, even the one that Siegel cites, the influence which is responsible for separating the thicker from the more volatile constituents of the blood is heat, the innate heat, whose principal residence is the left ventricle, but which is present not only in the right ventricle but also in the lungs themselves, though of course in a lesser degree. Thus we are told, in the passage in question, that

nature has realized that three other means of assistance would be necessary to ensure the plentiful supply of nutriment to the lung; one, the plenty of local heat, to break down and liquefy all the nutriment, so as to make more ready to vaporize; another is the expansion of the lung in inspiration, which

___

[1] Siegel, *Galen's System of Physiology*, p. 82.

forcibly snatches something even from the most thick-textured organ; and thirdly, the greatest of all, the fact that the blood sent out from the heart only to the lung is accurately processed and thinned out in it [the heart].[1]

That the 'processing' is done by the innate heat is clearly indicated. What is not so clear is quite what this process in the right ventricle consists of. What happens to the thicker muddier elements which are no proper food for the foam-like tissue of the lung? Siegel seems to imagine that they are just melted down, without the production of smoky or sooty superfluities. Are these produced in the left ventricle only, being the product of the processing of the crude blood together with *pneuma* by the innate heat? But, as Siegel himself admits, the right ventricle does contain some *pneuma*, for the veins contain a little misty air, as Hippocrates taught.[2] It seems to me, therefore, that the problem of the residues still remains. If they are produced in the right ventricle, and/or in the pulmonary artery itself, what becomes of them? Do they pass on with the rarefied blood into the pulmonary veins? This would not appear at all possible, since the venous coats of the vein-like artery (pulmonary vein) would let them pass into the flesh of the lung. We must assume therefore that they pass into the tracheal system of the rough arteries which are connected with the vein-like arteries. But Galen never tells us, and the misty *pneuma* contained in the veins would not appear to be either sufficient or of the right character to transform these residues into particles small enough to pass through the extremely fine orifices of the terminal bronchi, which are too fine to admit any blood. Nor presumably can they pass through the interventricular septum, which Galen tells us has pores too small to admit any but the finer elements of the blood.[3] It does not appear to me to be possible to extract a completely consistent story out of Galen's account. Meanwhile it is important to note that the question of the evacuation of 'waste products' through the valve from the right heart into the pulmonary artery has been assumed by some authorities to have been taught by Galen.

Two of the German historians of medicine, namely Haeser[4] and

[1] *De usu partium*, vi. 10, K. iii. 452: καὶ μέν γε καὶ ἄλλας τρεῖς ἐπικουρίας τῷ πνεύμονι πρὸς εὐπορίαν τροφῆς ἡ φύσις ἐγίνωσκεν ἐξ ἀνάγκης ἐσομένας· μίαν μὲν τὸ πλῆθος τῆς ἐγχωρίου θερμότητος εἰς λεπτὰ καταθραυούσης καὶ διαχεούσης ἅπασαν τὴν τροφήν, ὡς ἀτμίζειν ἑτοιμότερον, ἑτέραν δὲ τὴν ἐν ταῖς εἰσπνοαῖς τοῦ πνεύμονος διάστασιν, ἐξαρπάζουσάν τι βιαίως κἀκ τῶν πυκνοτάτων ὀργάνων, καὶ τρίτην, ἣ μεγίστη πασῶν, ἀπὸ καρδίας ἐπιπεμπομένου μόνῳ τῷ πνεύμονι τοῦ αἵματος, ἀκριβῶς ἐν ἐκείνῃ κατειργασμένου τε καὶ λελεπτυσμένου.

[2] Ibid., 16, K. iii. 491: ἐδείχθη γὰρ οὖν ἡμῖν δι' ἑτέρων ὡς ἐν ἅπασι πάντ' ἐστί, καθάπερ Ἱπποκράτης ἔλεγε, καὶ μετέχουσιν αἱ μὲν ἀρτηρίαι λεπτοῦ καὶ καθαροῦ καὶ ἀτμώδους αἵματος, αἱ δὲ φλέβες ὀλίγου καὶ ὀμιχλώδους ἀέρος.

[3] *De nat. fac.* iii. 15, K. ii. 207 f.: ὡσαύτως δὲ καὶ κατ' αὐτὴν τὴν καρδίαν ἐκ τῆς δεξιᾶς κοιλίας εἰς τὴν ἀριστερὰν ἕλκεται τὸ λεπτότατον, ἔχοντός τινα τρήματα τοῦ μέσου διαφράγματος αὐτῶν.

[4] H. Haeser, *Lehrbuch der Geschichte der Medizin und der epidemischen Krankheiten* (3d edn., Jena, 1875), i. 359: 'Das in der Leber gebildete Blut gelangt durch die Venae hepaticae

Pagel,[1] to the somewhat exaggerated indignation of Fleming,[2] have indeed assumed that Galen believed these 'waste products' to be evacuated from the right ventricle through the pulmonary artery into the lungs and the tracheal system. Nor is this at all an improbable suggestion, even if it is not expressly stated by Galen. For the three systems of vessels which occupy the lungs all have their terminal ramifications leading to adjacent minute orifices, and we are told that those of the tracheal system are so small that they will not permit the passage of blood from either of the other two. Galen may very well therefore have thought that at the synanastomoses of the terminal branches of the artery-like vein (the pulmonary artery) with those of the vein-like artery (the pulmonary vein), the 'sooty gases' escaped into the final ramifications of the 'rough arteries' (the bronchial tubes). For we shall see that it is by no means certain that Galen regarded these anastomoses as anything more than a juxtaposition of orifices.

The relation between the three sets of vessels in the lungs needs perhaps rather more detailed consideration. The fullest description of that organ, which Galen, like other Greek doctors, regards as being a single structure divided at the top into two parts, is given in the seventh book of *On the use of the parts*, where he explains that the lung, like the liver, is a sort of 'tissue' ($\pi\lambda\acute{\epsilon}\gamma\mu\alpha$) of a very large number of vessels, the spaces between being filled up by a kind of stuffing of soft flesh. There are three sets of vessels, each with a single origin. Their respective starting-points are the left ventricle of the heart, the right ventricle, and the pharynx. Proceeding from these starting-points, they all divide up in similar fashion, since the lung is divided into a right and a left portion. The windpipe divides at the bottom of the neck, while both the vein-like artery (pulmonary vein) and the artery-like vein (pulmonary artery) divide immediately after leaving the heart into their right and left branches. He then goes on to describe their successive divisions in the formation of the four lobes and the little fifth one in the right cavity of the thorax, which forms a cushion for the vena cava. The outside of the lobes is enveloped in a thin membrane.[3]

und die aufsteigende Hohlvene zum rechten Herzen, in welchem, vermöge der demselben eingepflantzten Wärme, die unbrauchbaren Bestandtheile der "Ruß" ($\lambda\iota\gamma\nu\acute{\upsilon}s$) von den brauchbaren geschieden werden wo bei der Expiration durch die als dann sich öffnenden halb-mondformigen Klappen der Arteria pulmonalis in die Lungen, und von da nach außen geführt werden.'

    [1] Fleming also quotes an almost identical passage from Julius Pagel, *Einführung in die Geschichte der Medizin* (Berlin, 1898), i. 124: 'Das in der Leber bereitete Blut geht durch die Venae hepaticae und Vena cava ascendens zum rechten Herzen, in welchem sich die unbrauchbaren Stoffe als $\lambda\iota\gamma\nu\acute{\upsilon}s$ (Ruß, Fumus) ausscheiden, um bei der Ausatmung durch die zu diesem Zwecke öffnenden halb-mondformigen Klappen der Arteria pulmonalis aus dem Körper geführt zu werden.'

    [2] Fleming, op. cit.

    [3] *De usu partium*, vii. 2, K. iii. 517–18: $\pi\lambda\acute{\epsilon}\gamma\mu\alpha$ δή τι καὶ τοῦτό ἐστι τὸ σπλάγχνον, ὥσπερ καὶ τὸ ἧπαρ, ἀγγείων παμπόλλων μαλακῇ σαρκὶ καθαπερεὶ στοιβῇ τινι τὰς μεταξὺ χώρας ἀναπεπληρω-

Of the three sets of tubes, the two kinds of artery, the rough and the smooth, and the artery-like vein, only the first, which is also called the bronchus by some authorities, contains no blood. But even though it never carries any blood in its interior, its coat is provided with small veins which furnish it nourishment.

The functions of the three types of tubes in the lung are carefully distinguished. That of the trachea or bronchus is to afford a passage for the outside air required for the voice and for respiration. The lung has no power of movement of its own. It is moved by the muscles of the thorax and the diaphragm. When these expand the thoracic cavity, air passes into the trachea in accordance with the principle of the *horror vacui*,[1] and when they contract it, the air is pushed out in expiration. The artery-like veins or pulmonary arteries also have a single function, that of conveying nutriment in the form of light and *pneuma*-like blood to the lungs. The smooth arteries (pulmonary veins) on the other hand perform a triple function. They connect with the ramifications of the bronchus and so convey *pneuma* to the heart, they convey nutrition to the lung, and they also evacuate from the left ventricle the 'waste products' engendered by the innate heat during the mixture (or combination?) of blood with *pneuma* in the preparation of arterial blood, besides providing a continual cooling[2] to the innate heat, and food for the generation of the psychic spirit, the first stage of its preparation taking place in the light airy flesh of the lungs.[3] They, like the bronchus, carry a two-way traffic of gaseous materials. They also carry a one-way traffic of light, clean vaporous blood, going in the direction

μένον. ὁρμᾶται δὲ τῶν ἀγγείων τὸ μὲν ἐκ τῆς ἀριστερᾶς κοιλίας τῆς καρδίας, τὸ δὲ ἐκ τῆς δεξιᾶς, τὸ δὲ ἐκ τῆς φάρυγγος. ἔπειτ' ἐντεῦθεν προιόντα κατασχίζεται τρόπον ὁμοιότατον ἅπαντα, δίχα μὲν τὸ πρῶτον, ὅτι καὶ τοῦ πνεύμονος αὐτοῦ τὸ μὲν ἐν τοῖς δεξιοῖς ἐστι, τὸ δ' ἐν τοῖς ἀριστεροῖς τοῦ ζῴου μέρεσιν, ὑμέσιν ἰσχυροῖς διειργόμενον· ἔπειτα δ' ἑκάτερον αὐτῶν αὖθις εἰς ἕτερα τμήματα δύο τέμνεται, διότι καὶ τοῦ πνεύμονος ἐν ἑκατέρῳ μέρει δύο ἐστὸν λοβοί· καὶ οὕτως ἤδη τέτταρα τὰ πάντα μόρια τῶν εἰρημένων ἀγγείων ἑκάστου γενόμενα κατασχίζεται πολυειδῶς εἰς τοὺς τέτταρας λοβοὺς τοῦ πνεύμονος. πέμπτου δ' ὄντος λοβοῦ μικροῦ κατὰ τὴν δεξιὰν εὐρυχωρίαν τοῦ θώρακος, ὃν ἕδραν τέ τινα καὶ οἷον ὑποστόρεσμα τῆς κοίλης φλεβὸς ἔφαμεν ὑπάρχειν, ἀπὸ τῶν εἰς τὸν παρακείμενον αὐτῷ λοβὸν τὸν μέγαν ἀγγείων νενεμημένων ἀποβλαστήματα μικρὰ φερόμενα παντὶ κατασχίζεται. περιέχει δέ τις ἔξωθεν ὑμὴν λεπτὸς ἅπαντας τοὺς λοβούς, τῶν παρὰ τὸν στόμαχον εἰς τὴν γαστέρα καταφερομένων νεύρων μόρια ἄττα δεχόμενος.

[1] Ibid., 4, 523: διαστελλομένου γὰρ ἐν ταῖς εἰσπνοαῖς ἅπαντος τοῦ θώρακος, ὡς ἐν τοῖς περὶ κινήσεως αὐτοῦ δέδεικται λόγοις, εἶτα τῇ πρὸς τὸ κενούμενον (κινούμενον Κ.) ἀκολουθίᾳ πάντῃ τὸν πνεύμονα διαστέλλοντος.

[2] Ibid., 9, K. iii. 545: ὅτι μὲν οὖν τὰς λείας ἀρτηρίας ἁπάσας εἰς μίαν ἀρχὴν ἀνεστόμωσε τὴν ἀριστερὰν κοιλίαν τῆς καρδίας, ἵνα περ ἡ τῆς ἐμφύτου θερμασίας ἐστὶν ἀρχή, κατὰ τοῦτο μὲν ὡς ἀνάψυξιν συνεχῆ τῇ καρδίᾳ παρασκευάσασαν αὐτήν, ἐπαινεῖσθαι δίκαιον. ὅτι δὲ διά τε τῶν αὐτῶν τούτων ἐν ταῖς τῆς καρδίας συστολαῖς, ὅσον αἰθαλῶδες ἐν αὐτῇ καὶ λιγνυῶδες ἀποχεῖται, καὶ πολὺ μᾶλλον ἔτι διὰ τῆς μεγάλης ἀρτηρίας εἰς τὰς ἄλλας ... ὑμνεῖσθαι προσήκει.

[3] Ibid.: τὸ δὲ καὶ τὴν τοῦ πνεύμονος σάρκα μαλακὴν καὶ μανὴν καὶ ἀφρώδη ποιῆσαι χάριν τοῦ τὸν ἔξωθεν ἀέρα προσπίπτειν, ὡς τροφὴν οἰκείαν προνοησαμένην αὐτὴν τῷ πνεύματι τῷ ψυχικῷ, αυμάζεσθαι δίκαιον.

of the heart.[1] The permanent insufficiency of the mitral valve, which this implies, is required to permit the two-way passage of gaseous material to and from the left ventricle, and there can be no question that the valve *could* admit blood as well as *pneuma* into the left ventricle, since its membranes turn inwards. But if it does, why has nature to provide the alternative route for blood from the right to the left ventricle directly through the pores in the septum? There can be very little doubt that Galen thought that the whole of the blood entering the left ventricle reached it through the septum in this way. He seems to have believed that the quantity of matter passing into the left ventricle was in any case not large. The arteries branching from the aorta contained much less blood than the veins, and the amount of *pneuma* passing into the smooth arteries from the trachea was very small.[2]

The arrangements here described would certainly appear to imply that the smooth arteries were joined at their capillary extremities both to the tracheal system and to the pulmonary arteries as we call them today, though the exact nature of these joints is not altogether clear. Galen may have implied some difference between 'synanastomosis' and 'anasto-mosis' without the particle? This I believe to be possible, since in the passage quoted above, p. 283, n. 4, he simply tells us that the ends of the trachea come to the same place or coincide with those of the pulmonary venules. He makes no mention of their 'mouths' joining in this passage from the treatise *On the opinions of Hippocrates and Plato*. In the treatise *On the use of the parts*, he makes the arteries and the veins all over the body 'synanastomose'. Did he then think that the terminal venules of the pulmonary veins were as it were forked, one prong joining up with the bronchiole and the other with the pulmonary arteriole? Or did he agree with Aristotle that the bronchioles just ended in the tiny interstices of the flesh of the lung? That there could be some connection or rather passage of blood from the pulmonary venules into the bronchioles was, of course, a matter well known to all physicians from very early times, and Galen tries to explain this by assuming that in normal health the ends of the air-tubes are too small in diameter to admit even the refined blood which feeds the lung.[3] But in another passage he seems to imply that

---

[1] *De usu partium*, vii. 8, K. iii. 537 : ἀλλ' αἵ γε πρὸς τὴν καρδίαν τὰς τραχείας μέλλουσι συνάπτειν αἱ λεῖαι, πολλάκις μὲν ἐδείχθησαν ἤδη λεπτὸν καὶ καθαρὸν καὶ ἀτμῶδες αἷμα περιέχειν, καὶ μὴ μόνον πνεύματος ὑπάρχειν ὄργανον.

[2] Ibid., 539 : ἀλλ' ἕν γε τῷ κατὰ φύσιν ἔχειν αὐτό τε τὸ μεταλαμβανόμενον ἐκ τῶν τραχειῶν εἰς τὰς λείας πνεῦμα παντελῶς ὀλίγον, ἥ τε σὰρξ τοῦ πνεύμονος ἀερώδης ὁρᾶται καὶ πνεύματος μεστή.

[3] *De usu partium*, vii. 8, 539 : ἐπειδὴ γὰρ αἱ μὲν ἄλλαι πᾶσαι καθ' ὅλον τὸ ζῷον ἀρτηρίαι μετέχουσιν αἵματος, ὥσπερ καὶ ἡ ἀριστερὰ κοιλία τῆς καρδίας, αἱ τραχεῖαι δὲ μόναι καθαραὶ τυγχάνουσιν οὖσαι, διὰ μέσων τῶν λείων συνήφθησαν τῇ καρδίᾳ, πάντως που καὶ τὰ τούτων στόματα πρὸς τῆς μηδὲν ἀλόγως ἐργαζομένης φύσεως εἰς τοῦθ' ἥκει συμμετρίας, ὡς ἀτμῷ μὲν καὶ πνεύματι δίοδον ἔχειν, αἵματι δὲ καὶ ταῖς οὕτω παχείαις οὐσίαις ὑπάρχειν ἄβατον.

any actual opening of the venule into the tracheole is caused only by wounds or by disease.

The trachea is completely void of blood in the state of health [κατὰ φύσιν ἔχειν] of the animal. But when some breakage occurs or some opening of a passage [ἀναστόμωσις] or erosion of one of the vessels of the lung, some blood may also pass into this artery, which obstructs the *pneuma* by occupying its proper channel. The animal then starts coughing and the blood is brought up through the pharynx into the mouth.[1]

The meaning of the word anastomosis used here is not altogether clear. Does Galen only mean by it 'an opening-wide of the mouth'? Or does he use it in the sense of 'opening a passage' into 'the trachea'? This he apparently regards as a morbid phenomenon. Some light on this problem is perhaps thrown by another passage in the same book, where he says that if the terminal orifices of the bronchioles alter their normal size proportionately to those of the terminal branches of the pulmonary artery by opening wider (ἀναστομωθέντα), blood passes from the smooth artery into the trachea and causes coughing, etc.[2] This would seem to suggest that the bronchiole opens into the pulmonary venule. On the other hand, I am inclined to think that Galen may have believed that a large portion of the air drawn in through the trachea did not go into the smooth artery at all, but went directly into the flesh of the lung, where its transformation into psychic spirit was begun.[3] But whatever the actual nature of the connection between the two sets of vessels, there is no doubt that Galen believed, when he wrote the most important of his physiological works,[4] that air passed from the lung to the left ventricle of the heart by the pulmonary veins, being drawn in from the trachea. He also believed that the pulmonary veins contained a considerable quantity of what we should call 'arterial' blood.[5] For in an earlier passage in the treatise from which we have been quoting, he states that the other organs of the body only attract a very small quantity of blood through the arteries. Only the lungs absorb this fine blood in any quantity, for there is no other organ the flesh of which is so light, rare, and aerated (πνευματῶδες).[6] The need of the lung for its special food in large quantities is

---

[1] Ibid., 3, 521: ταύτῃ μὲν γὰρ ἀτμώδους αἵματος καὶ λεπτοῦ καὶ καθαροῦ μέτεστιν οὐκ ὀλίγον· ἡ δὲ τραχεῖα τελέως ἐστὶν αἵματος ἄμοιρος, ἔν γε τῷ κατὰ φύσιν ἔχειν τὸ ζῷον. ἐπειδὰν δέ τις ἢ ῥῆξις, ἢ ἀναστόμωσις, ἢ διάβρωσις ἀγγείου κατὰ τὸν πνεύμονα γένηται, τότ' ἐκχεῖται μέν τι καὶ εἰς τήνδε τὴν ἀρτηρίαν αἵματος, ἐνοχλεῖ δὲ τῷ πνεύματι καταλαμβάνον αὐτοῦ τὰς ὁδούς, καὶ οὕτως ἤδη βήττει μὲν τὸ ζῷον, ἀναφέρεται δὲ τὸ αἷμα διὰ τῆς φάρυγγος εἰς τὸ στόμα.

[2] Ibid., 8, 539: καὶ εἴποτ' ἄρα τὴν κατὰ φύσιν ἀπολέσειε συμμετρίαν ἀναστομωθέντα, διαδίδοταί τι ταῖς τραχείαις ἀρτηρίαις ἐκ τῶν λείων αἷμα, καὶ βῆχά τε παραχρῆμα ποιεῖ καὶ ἀναγωγὴν αἵματος.

[3] Ibid., 9, 545, quoted above, pp. 307, n. 2. [4] But see below, pp. 339–43.

[5] De usu partium, vii. 8, 544: καὶ μέν γε καὶ τῶν ἀρτηριῶν ὁ χιτὼν ἀπεδείχθη λεπτὸς γεγονέναι πρὸς τὸ τρέφεσθαι τὸν πνεύμονα πλείστῳ τῷ παρ' αὐτῶν αἵματι, καθαρῷ καὶ λεπτῷ καὶ ἀτμώδει τὴν φύσιν ὑπάρχοντι, καὶ πρὸς τὸ ῥᾳδίως ἑλκούσῃ τῇ καρδίᾳ μεθιέναι τὸ πνεῦμα.

[6] Ibid., vi. 10, K. iii. 451–2: καὶ τοῖς μὲν ἄλλοις αἱ ἀρτηρίαι παχεῖαι καὶ πυκναὶ γεννηθεῖσαι παντάπασιν ὀλίγον ἀτμώδους αἵματος τοῖς παρακειμένοις μορίοις ἕλκειν ἐπιτρέπουσι· τῷ δὲ

particularly emphasized, and on Galen's physiological principles it is difficult to see how the passage of any leftover nutriment from the pulmonary veins into the left ventricle could serve any useful biological purpose, since the requirements of the other organs of the body for this aerated type of blood have already been amply met by the direct passage of blood from the right ventricle through the septum. I can find no passage in which Galen actually speaks of any blood—in the adult, as opposed to the foetus—passing from the pulmonary vein through the mitral valve into the left ventricle, though as Siegel points out there are no passages which deny this.

Galen could not have conceived that more than a few drops of blood entered the left ventricle through the mitral valve, and in fact he nowhere says that this actually happens, though as a good disciple of Hippocrates he might perhaps have believed it did, since Hippocrates, he tells us, in connection with the presence of a little *pneuma* in the veins, taught that none of the constituents of the body is absolutely pure.[1] We shall therefore be in good company when we maintain that Galen thought that only *pneuma* passed inwards through the mitral valve. Granjel, whose summary of Galen's doctrines on the movement of the blood is in many ways the best short account I have come across, insists that all the blood which is carried outward from the heart and liver to the organs is consumed by them,[2] including, of course, the lungs. The blood transmitted by the vein-like artery has the exclusive mission of nourishing the lung's tissues,[3] and the pulmonary vein, when it enters the heart, carries exclusively air or *pneuma*.[4]

Nevertheless the notion that Galen really discovered the circulation of the blood has fascinated, not to say hypnotized, quite a number of the modern historians of Greek medicine. Thus, for example, Bañuelos,

πνεύμονι μόνῳ πάμπολυ τὸ τοιοῦτον μεθιᾶσιν, ὑπὸ μανότητός τε καὶ λεπτότητος ἀδυνατοῦσαι στέγειν. ὥστε πάντη τῷ πνεύμονι τὰ περὶ τὴν τροφὴν ὑπεναντίως ἔχει τοῖς ἄλλοις ἅπασι τοῦ ζῴου μορίοις, ὥσπερ καὶ τὰ τῆς τοῦ σώματος ἰδέας. οὔτε γὰρ οὕτω μανὸν καὶ κοῦφον καὶ πνευματῶδες εὕροις ἂν ἕτερόν τι μόριον, ἀλλ᾽ οὐδὲ ἐγγὺς οὕτως αἵματι καθαρῷ καὶ λεπτῷ καὶ ἀτμώδει τρεφόμενον. ὅσον οὖν ἔλαττον αἱ φλέβες αὐτῷ μεταδιδόασι τροφῆς, πυκναὶ καὶ παχεῖαι γενόμεναι, τοῦτο πᾶν πληροῦσιν αἱ ἀρτηρίαι, λεπτὸν καὶ καθαρὸν καὶ ἀτμῶδες αἷμα δαψιλῶς αὐτῷ διαπέμπουσαι. ἀλλ᾽ οὐδέπω τοῦθ᾽ ἱκανὸν οὕτω θερμῷ καὶ πολυκινήτῳ σπλάγχνῳ.

[1] *De usu partium*, vi. 16, K. iii. 491 f.: ἐδείχθη γὰρ οὖν ἡμῖν δι᾽ ἑτέρων, ὡς ἐν ἅπασι πάντ᾽ ἐστί, καθάπερ Ἱπποκράτης ἔλεγε, ... καὶ ὅλως μηδὲν εἶναι τῶν ἐν τῷ σώματι καθαρὸν ἀκριβῶς, ἀλλὰ πάντα πάντων μετέχειν.

[2] Granjel, *Bol. Soc. esp. Hist. méd.* 1 (1961) loc. cit.: 'Para Galeno, y es ella opinión reiteradamente formulada en sus escritos, la sangre marcha del hígado del corazón a la periferia, a las distintas regiones orgánicas, y en ellas agotado se consume nutriendo las estructuras morfológicas.'

[3] Ibid.: 'Lo que occurre en todo el organismo ... acontecería, como queda apuntado, en el propio pulmón, donde la sangre a él enviada por el ventrículo derecho tendría como exclusiva misión nutrir al pulmón.'

[4] Ibid.: 'Arteria venosa, vaso según Galeno que únicamente trasportaría aire o pneumo.'

whose admiration of Galen as an anatomist could hardly be described as being 'this side of idolatry',[1] in a number of articles published in the *Gaceta médica española*,[2] and in a book published in Barcelona in 1946,[3] maintained quite unequivocally that he was acquainted not only with the pulmonary, but also with the systemic circulation. His conclusions are summed up in an article (quoted and refuted by Entralgo).[4] Bañuelos's theories were quickly demolished in his own country, with respect to the pulmonary circulation by De la Granda,[5] as well as by Granjel, while Entralgo dealt chiefly with the systemic. But Bañuelos is not the only modern interpreter of Galen to assume that he was acquainted with both the greater and the lesser circulation. Pezopoulos and Lamera make the same claim on his behalf, a claim which they would appear to maintain by implication rather than by rational evidence. With the intention of proving that the circulation was known to the ancient Greek physicians in general,[6] they have assembled a fairly extensive collection of quotations, chiefly from the *Hippocratic corpus* and Galen, but with additional citations from Plato and Aristotle, and one or two modern historians; but unfortunately I have so often found their references unreliable that quite apart from any conclusions which they draw from them, they are often grossly misleading. Moreover in one case at least, the text appears to have been tampered with. Thus in quoting the passage from Galen's

[1] See his article, 'Opiniones de Galeno sobre el tratamiento de las enfermedades febriles', *Gac. méd. esp.* 21 (1947), which contains the following statement: 'Vemos que Galeno no es solamente el gran naturalista, y acaso el más grande disector de todos los tiempos, y fundador de la fisiológica, experimental, sino también uno de los más grandes clínicos que ha tenido la humanidad, en el sentido de hacer estudiado profondamente los mas graves problemas patológicos y clínicos de la medicina en qualquier aspecto.'

[2] Bañuelos, 'Los grandes errores en el estudio de la circulación': 'De nuevo sobre Galeno y la circulación': 'Conoció Galeno la circulación de la sangre?' *Gac. méd. esp.* 20, 21, 22 (1946-8).

[3] Bañuelos, *El problema de la circulación de la sangre. Nuevos hechos y nuevas ideas* (Barcelona, 1946).

[4] Lain Entralgo, 'Conoció Galeno la circulación de la sangre?', *Méd. clín.* (1946): Bañuelos's conclusions read textually as follows: 'Tenemos que concluir con las siguientes afirmaciones: *Primera.* Galeno conoció con exactitud la sangre en sus círculos mayor y menor. *Segunda.* Harvey expuso en su famoso libro la doctrina de Galeno, solamente en parte y de modo incompleto, limitándose apracticar algunas vivisecciones de las que Galeno realizó, no añadiendo ecos transcendientes a lo dicho por Galeno, y incorriendo, por el contrario, en errores importantes. Tiene el enorme mérito de que su descripción es más claro y comprensible... *Tercera.* Servet expusó solamente en unos frases resumiendolas, algunas ideas de Galeno sobre la circulación menor. Esto puede verse en el libro de Harvey traducido recientemente por Izquierdo.'

[5] See his article, 'Galeno y Servet', *Gac. méd. esp.* 22 (1948); and his book, *Sistema metadialéctico de la Medicina* (Madrid, 1942), p. 204.

[6] S. N. Pezopoulos and I. K. Lamera, op. cit., prologue, p. 1: 'Ἡ τοιαύτη τοῦ ἐπιμάχου τούτου ζητήματος ἀνακίνησις ἐπιβάλλει ἡμῖν τοῖς Ἕλλησιν ἰατροῖς τὸ καθῆκον τῆς μετὰ προσόχης ἐρεύνης τῶν ἀρχαίων κειμένων, πρὸς ὁριστικὴν λύσιν τοῦ προβλήματος, καὶ ἀποκατάστασιν τῆς ἱστορικῆς ταύτης ἀληθείας. Ἔχοντες ἀπόλυτον πεποίθησιν ὅτι οἱ ἀρχαῖοι ἐγίνωσκον ἄριστα τὴν κυκλοφορίαν προβαίνομεν εἰς τὴν ἔκθεσιν τῶν ἀποδείξεων, κτλ. Cf. ibid., p. 37: ἐκ τῶν μέχρι τοῦδε ἐκτεθέντων φρονοῦμεν ὅτι σαφῶς ἐξάγεται ὅτι οἱ ἀρχαῖοι εἶχον τελείαν γνῶσιν τῆς κυκλοφορίας καὶ τοῦ ἔργου αὐτῆς.

Anatomical procedures (vi. 9, K. ii. 616) quoted by me, p. 273, n. 3, in which he describes the auricle as the terminal processes of the vessels leading matter into the heart through the inlet valves, they substitute the word αἷμα for the word ὕλας which actually appears in the text.[1] It is, to put it mildly, a little difficult to take seriously a work which asserts that Hippocrates was acquainted with the valves in the veins many centuries before their discovery by Fabricius.[2]

To return to works in the English tongue. Even so careful a scholar as Prendergast through his failure to appreciate the alimentary function of the blood in the lungs made Galen outline the idea of the pulmonary circulation. Thus he says :[3]

The idea of the pulmonary circulation is clearly outlined by Galen. And to this teaching Harvey found it convenient to turn when dealing with the re-actionaries of his day, those who would admit nothing unless upon authority . . . Galen points out that a transfer of blood from the branches of the pulmonary artery to those of the pulmonary veins takes place, and that this blood reaches the heart. But this doctrine is deduced from an indefensible hypothesis about the action of the pulmonary valve. This valve was supposed to remain closed during the contraction of the thorax, during which some of the blood is pressed out from the arteries into the veins through the anastomoses of these vessels in the lung, and the propulsive power of the heart is completely underrated.

It is a brilliant speculation, but Galen fails to grasp its real or relative value. It would be unwise to stress too much the importance of it in his physical system. It is enough to admit that he outlined the path by which the pulmonary circulation could be effected.

With the cautious conclusions contained in the last paragraph we can thoroughly agree, but the argument about the pulmonary valve seems to me to be based on a misunderstanding. Galen was quite aware that the heartbeat was completely independent of the respiratory motion of the thorax and that pulmonary diastole and systole in respiration were normally less frequent than those of the heart and arteries. Moreover, one of the reasons given for the hard arterial coat of the artery-like vein is precisely to ensure its incompressibility, in order to enable this vessel to ensure a steady uninterrupted flow of nutriment to the lungs. But the movements of the thorax are so powerful, especially when we breathe very hard or shout very loud, that the pulmonary artery is unable wholly to resist their pressure, especially on its smaller branches, with the result that unless the barrier of the pulmonary valve existed, the blood would flow back into the heart when the thorax compressed the lungs, thus

---

[1] Pezopoulos and Lamera, op. cit., p. 37, quotation no. 205.

[2] Ibid., p. 4: καὶ μὴ δὲν φέρεται εἰς πάντα τὰ συγγράμματα Fabricio d'Aquapendente (1574) ὡς ὁ πρῶτος παρατηρήσας τὰς ἐν ταῖς φλεψὶ βαλβίδας; Καὶ ὅμως τὰς βαλβίδας ταύτας περιγράφει σαφῶς ὁ Ἱπποκράτης ὑποδεικνύων καὶ τὸ ἔργον αὐτῶν.

[3] Prendergast, op. cit.

giving rise to a most unsuitable movement of purposeless backward and forward motion of the blood destined to feed the lungs.[1] But thanks to the existence of the valve, this does not occur. All that the pressure of the thorax does in respect of the blood in the pulmonary artery is to squeeze a little blood from the mouth of each of its arterioles into the pulmonary venules with which it is connected, while at the same time pressing out the *pneuma* which it contains back into the trachea. This transfer of blood from arteriole to venule could not take place if the pulmonary valve did not exist.[2] This process need not, as Prendergast appears to imply, entail the permanent closure of the pulmonary valve during the period of thoracic contraction, since the systole of the right ventricle opening the valve would automatically prevent any backflow. Prendergast is, however, quite right when he insists that Galen enormously underrated the propulsive force of the heart's action, which he thought was only sufficient to propel the blood from the right ventricle as far as the extremities of the ramifications of the pulmonary artery, but I am not convinced that he therefore handed over to the thoracic contraction the task of moving it forward in the pulmonary veins.

Peller, too, seems to me to underestimate the nutritional function of the blood passing through the lung. Its relative abundance in the lung need not imply that it produces a surplus which trickles back into the heart. For the lung is a very large organ in continuous motion, and in the last resort blood has only one function, that of feeding, that is, replacing spare parts or supplying additional ones in the case of growth. He describes the double source of the blood in the left ventricle as follows:

Of blood in the right heart, a part was supposed to pass through the aforementioned invisible intra-ventricular channels to the left heart, while another

---

[1] *De usu partium*, vi. 10, K. iii. 453–4: εἰ γὰρ καὶ ὅτι μάλιστα παχὺ καὶ σκληρὸν ἐδημιουργήθη τὸ ἀγγεῖον, ὡς μήτε διαστέλλεσθαι ῥᾳδίως μήτε συστέλλεσθαι, ἀλλ' οὐκ εἰς τοσοῦτόν γε σκληρόν ἐστιν, ὡς μηδ' ὅλως νικᾶσθαι πρὸς οὕτως ἰσχυροῦ καὶ μεγάλου καὶ σφοδρῶς ἐνεργοῦντος ὀργάνου, τοῦ θώρακος, καὶ μάλισθ' ὅταν ἀθρόως ἐκπνέομεν ἢ μέγα φωνῶμεν, ἤ πως ἄλλως ἔσω προσάγωμεν ἐκ παντὸς μέρους αὐτόν, ἅπαντας ἰσχυρῶς ἐκτείνοντες τοὺς μῦς. οὐδὲ γὰρ οὐδὲ καθ' ἕνα τῶν τοιούτων καιρῶν ἐγχωρεῖ παντάπασιν ἄθλιπτα καὶ ἀσύμπτωτα φυλάττεσθαι τὰ τῆς φλεβὸς ταύτης ἀποβλαστήματα. καὶ μὴν εἰ θλίβοιτο καὶ συστέλλοιτο, παλινδρομήσει ῥᾳδίως ἐξ ἁπάντων αὐτῶν ἐπὶ τὸ πρῶτον στόμα τὸ αἷμα καὶ μεταληφθήσεται πάλιν εἰς τοὐπίσω. κἂν τούτῳ τρίτον ἤδη τὸ ἄτοπον, αὐτό τε τὸ αἷμα μάτην κινεῖσθαι δίαυλόν τινα τοῦτον ἀκατάπαυστον, ἐν μὲν ταῖς διαστολαῖς τοῦ πνεύμονος ἐπιρρέον τε καὶ πληροῦν ἁπάσας τὰς κατ' αὐτὸν φλέβας, ἐν δὲ ταῖς συστολαῖς οἷον ἄμπωτίν τινα κινούμενον εὐρίπου δίκην, ἀεὶ τῇδε κἀκεῖσε μεταβαλλόμενον οὐδαμῶς αἵματι πρέπουσαν φοράν.

[2] Ibid., 455–6: εἰ δ' ἦν τὸ στόμα τὸ μέγα τῆς ἀρτηριώδους φλεβὸς ἀναπεπταμένον ὡσαύτως ἀεί, μηδὲν τῆς φύσεως ἐξευρούσης μηχάνημα, κλείειν αὐτὸ καὶ αὖθις ἀνοιγνύναι δυνάμενον ἐν τοῖς προσήκουσι καιροῖς, οὐκ ἄν ποτε διὰ τῶν ἀοράτων καὶ μικρῶν στομάτων εἰς τὰς ἀρτηρίας μετειλήφθη τὸ αἷμα συστελλομένου τοῦ θώρακος ... συστελλομένου δὲ τοῦ θώρακος, ὠθούμεναί τε καὶ ἔσω πιλούμεναι πανταχόθεν ἰσχυρῶς αἱ ἐν τῷ πνεύμονι φλεβώδεις ἀρτηρίαι ἐκθλίβουσι μὲν αὐτίκα δὴ μάλα τὸ ἐν αὐταῖς πνεῦμα, μεταλαμβάνουσι δέ τι διὰ τῶν λεπτῶν ἐκείνων στομάτων τοῦ αἵματος, ὅπερ οὐκ ἂν μετειλήφθη ποτέ, παλινδρομεῖν εἴπερ οἷόν τ' ἦν εἰς τοὐπίσω διὰ τοῦ μεγίστου στόματος, ἡλίκον τῆς φλεβὸς ταύτης ἐστὶ τὸ πρὸς τῇ καρδίᾳ.

portion was thrown into the pulmonary artery, in order to provide the lung with the required nutritional elements. The function of the valves at the root of the pulmonary artery was known : they had to prevent regurgitation. In this artery the blood could not remain for long : it was pushed forward by two periodical forces. First, with each systole some new blood entered the artery, and space had to be made for it. Second, with each expirium the inter-thoracic space was reduced, and therefore the pulmonary artery squeezed. Prevented from reflux, the blood was forced through the anastomoses into the pulmonary veins, and further to the left heart, where it joined the blood which had passed the septum.[1]

This account, though in the main following pretty closely Galen's description of these processes, misses one of the important points. The pressure of the thorax, according to him, makes itself felt only in the peripheral branches of the pulmonary artery, and as we have already noted, he nowhere speaks of the blood entering the left ventricle. The views of both Prendergast and Peller have been criticized by Fleming,[2] whose verdict on this point, however much we may disagree with him on others, seems to sum up the position very justly. 'Drs. Peller and Prendergast seem overly [sic] confident of Galen's having postulated a pulmonary circulation with passage of blood as well as air through the venous artery.' The motion of the *pneuma* through the pulmonary veins was indeed, Galen insists, due to thoracic pressure, but I am less confident that we can assume it to have also been the prime mover of the blood, since this would leave out of account the attractive force of the tissues of the lung itself, which plays such an important part in the metabolism, and indeed the motion, of the venous blood into the various tissues.[3]

But the most persistent of the modern upholders of the idea that Galen discovered the pulmonary circulation—or shall we call it more accurately the pulmonary transit?—is Siegel, the author of four essays to which we have already referred. Thus in the first of these,[4] he maintains that Galen 'outlined the mechanism of the pulmonary circulation, but his discovery was misunderstood during the entire middle ages'. The principal passages on which he bases this hypothesis have all been quoted in the preceding paragraphs. The one on which he lays the greatest stress is that dealing with the foetal circulation, which we have just been discussing, in which Galen tells us that the heart of the foetus could draw blood mixed with *pneuma* from the lungs. Siegel simply takes this statement as being applicable to the animal after birth, without making any reference to the fact that in the passage in question, Galen is dealing with the peculiar conditions of the intra-uterine existence. Thus Siegel simply tells us :

The adult heart can draw from the lungs the blood mixed with air (*pneuma*) through the opening which has only two valves (i.e. mitral or bicuspid) and

[1] Peller, op. cit.   [2] Fleming, op. cit.
[3] See below, pp. 329 f.   [4] Siegel, *Am. J. Cardiol.* (1962).

which *leads into the left chamber of the heart*. But in the foetus this chamber actually receives blood from the vena cava through a certain anastomosis (i.e. the foramen ovale of the atrial septum), which is remarkably wide.[1]

Now apart from the somewhat arbitrary assumption that this peculiarity of the foetal condition persists after birth, even as a potentiality, there is little to object to in this statement. It is when he attempts to find evidence for the fact that this actually *does* happen that we must part company. Siegel, on grounds that I have not been able to understand, concludes from the account of certain experiments described in the treatise *On anatomical procedures* that Galen was convinced that the blood-flow into the left side of the heart could not be maintained only through the ventricular septum, but that some passed by way of the pulmonary vein. Thus Siegel tells us:

In order to study what would happen when the communication between lungs and heart were interrupted [*sic*], Galen tried to ligate the pulmonary veins before their entry into the left atrium. He carefully avoided collapse of the lungs by preventing any injury to the pleura or tearing the fragile blood vessels themselves. Although he did not succeed in ligating the veins as they passed through the hilus of the lungs, he did tie the vessels close to the heart. He wrote:

'All the arteries became motionless since they were, of course, deprived of the supply from the lungs that fills them. The animal died at once.'

The experimental interruption of blood in the warm-blooded organism after ligation of the pulmonary veins demonstrated to Galen that the blood-flow into the left side of the heart could not be maintained only through the pores of the interventricular septum. Galen recognized that the left heart depended on the blood arriving from the vena cava and the right heart after passing through the lungs.[2]

A similar statement is also made in Siegel's book.[3]

If we compare these pronouncements with Galen's actual words, we can only be astonished, to say the least of it, at the conclusions drawn. In the first place, it is a little curious to find that the experiment attributed by Siegel to Galen was never performed by him at all, and that the conclusions drawn from it were not Galen's at all, but those of another doctor who had claimed to have performed it—a claim which Galen himself indignantly repudiates on the ground that it was impossible to perform. In order that the reader may draw his own conclusions from the evidence, I quote the passage in full.

. . . and, moreover, to expose the error of those who say that such and such symptoms seize on the animal if one ligates the large artery, or as some say,

---

[1] Ibid., p. 743 (italics Siegel's). The same statement occurs also in his book, *Galen's System of Physiology and Medicine*, p. 52.

[2] Siegel, *Am. J. Cardiol.* (1962), p. 740.   [3] Siegel, *Galen's System*, pp. 55 f.

the venous artery [pulmonary vein] running into the lungs. For on this they do not all say the same. For no such ligation can be made without the thorax being perforated, nor, if it were, could it bind the root of the artery so exactly as to block its aperture.

I found by experience that this was always said by those who could not expose the heart without perforation but who, under pressure, immediately perforated the thorax, saying that the operation was difficult; and that it was for this reason that they had postponed it, for, they said, had they exposed it, they would have put the ligature round it and demonstrated clearly what they promised.

In contrast to them, what I promise I perform. For I expose the heart easily without damage to the membranes partitioning the cavity of the thorax. Then I ask them to put the ligature round the vessels springing from the heart. Under compulsion, without effecting anything, they get so far as to tear apart some of the membranes and make a perforation. At that point they say they ought not to make any further attempt. But again I speedily expose the heart in another animal for them, and present this to them, and force them to make another attempt, until they are put to shame over their impudent pretences.

It is not possible to ligature the course of the vessel. It can be done round the base of the heart, but the animal dies at once. One who said that if the venous artery [pulmonary vein] be ligated when the heart is exposed without perforating the thorax, the lungs remain expanded, had a like experience when he was refuted before many witnesses by one of my colleagues.

Such a combination of pretentious humbug and rash confidence is shown by some in their behaviour to the ignorant, particularly when they come to speak of the venous artery which divides [almost] within the auricle. Others say they have ligatured it, for, they say, it comes forth single and that then these two things happen: firstly, that all the arteries in the body become motionless, being, of course deprived of the supply from the lungs which fills them; secondly, that the lungs remain at an equal distance apart, for obviously the heart is drawing nothing from them. Yet others profess to show the lungs moving after a ligation of the arteria tracheia [trachea]—and some have actually recorded this in writing without adding how they observed the lungs, whether without a perforation of the thorax, or with one. Either is unbelievable. For with this perforation the whole process of respiration is destroyed, while if it be not perforated you cannot see within the thorax at all, except by excising a rib and leaving the pleura unharmed.[1]   (trs. Singer.)

[1] De anat. admin. vii. 14, K. ii. 636–8: ἔτι τε πρὸς τούτῳ τοῖς φάσκουσιν, εἰ διαλάβοι τις βρόχῳ τὴν ἔκφυσιν τῆς μεγάλης ἀρτηρίας, ἢ ὡς ἕτεροί τινες, τῆς εἰς τὸν πνεύμονα φερομένης τῆς φλεβώδους, τάδε τινὰ καταλαμβάνει τὸ ζῷον τὰ συμπτώματα, λέγουσι δ' οὐ τὰ αὐτὰ πάντες, ὡς ἂν ψευδομένους δείξωμεν, ὅτι μήτε περιβληθῆναί τις δύναται βρόχος ἄνευ τοῦ συντρηθῆναι τὸν θώρακα, μήτ' εἰ περιβληθῇ, σφίγγειν ἀκριβῶς οὕτως τὴν ῥίζαν τῆς ἀρτηρίας, ὡς ἀποφράξαι τὸ στόμιον αὐτῆς. λεγόντων δ' ἐπειράθην ἀεὶ ταῦτα τῶν μηδὲ γυμνῶσαι καρδίαν δυναμένων ἄνευ συντρήσεως, ἀλλ' εἰ καὶ βιάσαιτό τις αὐτούς, εὐθέως συντρησάντων τὸν θώρακα, φασκόντων χαλεπὸν τυχεῖν τούτου, καὶ διὰ τοῦτο ἀναβαλλομένων τὴν χειρουργίαν εἰς αὖθις, ὡς, εἴ γ' εὐτυχηθείη γυμνωθῆναι, περιβάλλοντες ἂν τὸν βρόχον ἀπέδειξαν σαφῶς, ἅπερ ἐπηγγείλαντο. τούτοις οὖν ἡμεῖς ἔμπαλιν ἀπαγγελλόμεθά τε καὶ πράττομεν. γυμνώσαντες γὰρ τὴν καρδίαν ῥᾳδίως ἄνευ τοῦ τρῶσαί τινα τῶν διαφραττόντων ὑμένων τὸ κύτος τοῦ θώρακος, ἀξιοῦμεν αὐτοὺς περιβαλεῖν τὸν βρόχον τοῖς τῆς καρδίας ἐκφυομένοις

The conclusions which I am able to hazard on the implication of Galen's experiments are very different from Siegel's—they are those of missed clues.[1] To us, since Harvey's discovery of the circulation, it is more than a little tempting to ask whether here, too, another clue has been missed. Is Galen's allegation of the absolute impossibility of ligating the pulmonary vein at its point of emergence from the heart in all animals a watertight affirmation? Is it possible to suppose that some skilful and/or lucky operator may have succeeded in tying ligatures round all four branches of the pulmonary veins? And, if so, might he not have observed that before the animal actually died and the heart stopped beating entirely, the pulse in the arteries had become imperceptible? As to the behaviour of the lungs, is it necessary to suppose that the animal would immediately stop breathing? The critical point involves, of course, Galen's conception of the auricles as not belonging to the heart proper but to the two blood vessels, the vena cava and the pulmonary vein.

In his second article,[2] Siegel presents a picture of Galen's doctrines on the movement of the blood, which while bringing out some important points not generally emphasized by commentators yet seems to me to be seriously misleading. Thus he tells us correctly that

Galen never suggested that the heartbeat accounted entirely for the motion of the blood. In the first place he thought that the right heart did not impel blood through the veins to the periphery of the body, and secondly he thought that the inferior vena cava carried only a small part of the blood to the right atrium.

ἀγγείοις. οἱ δ' ἄχρι τοσούτου βιάζονται μέν, ἀνύουσι δ' οὐδέν, ἄχρι τοῦ διασπάσαι τινὰ τῶν ὑμένων σύντρησίν τ' ἐργάσασθαι· τηνικαῦτα γὰρ οὐδ' ἐπιχειρεῖν ἔτι χρῆναί φασιν. ἀλλ' ἡμεῖς τε ἐν τάχει πάλιν ἐφ' ἑτέρου ζῴου γυμνώσαντες αὐτοῖς τὴν καρδίαν παρέχομεν, ἀναγκάζομέν τε πάλιν ἐγχειρεῖν, ἄχρι περ ἂν ἀσχημονήσωσιν ἐφ' οἷς ἠλαζονεύσαντο. τῇ μὲν γὰρ ἐκφύσει τῶν ἀγγείων περιβάλλειν τὸν βρόχον οὐχ οἷόν τε· τῇ βάσει δὲ τῆς καρδίας ἐγχωρεῖ μέν, ἀλλ' εὐθέως ἀποθνήσκει τὸ ζῷον. τοιοῦτον γάρ τι καὶ τῷ φάσκοντι, τῆς φλεβώδους ἀρτηρίας βρόχῳ διαληφθείσης, ὅταν καρδία γυμνωθῇ χωρὶς τοῦ συντρῆσαι τὸν θώρακα, διεσταλμένον ἀεὶ διαμένειν τὸν πνεύμονα, συνέβη παθεῖν ἐπὶ πολλῶν μαρτύρων ὑπό τινος τῶν ἡμετέρων ἑταίρων ἐλεγχθέντι. τοσαύτη τινὲς ἀλαζονείᾳ τε ἅμα καὶ τόλμῃ περὶ ὧν οὐκ ἴσασι πρὸς τοὺς οὐκ εἰδότας χρῶνται, καὶ μάλιστα ὅταν ἐπὶ τῆς φλεβώδους ἀρτηρίας ὁ λόγος αὐτοῖς γίγνηται, τῆς ἔνδον ἔτι τοῦ τῆς καρδίας ὠτὸς σχιζομένης. οὐ δέ γ', ὡς μονοφυοῦς ἀνισχούσης αὐτῆς, βρόχον ἐπιβεβληκέναι φασί, καὶ συμβῆναι τὸ ζῷον ἐκεῖνο παθεῖν ἄμφω ταῦτα, τὰς μὲν ἐν ὅλῳ τῷ σώματι πάσας ἀρτηρίας ἀκινήτους ἔχειν, ὡς ἂν δηλονότι τὴν χορηγίαν τοῦ πληροῦντος αὐτὰς πνεύματος ἀφῃρημένας, μένειν δ' ἐν ἴσῃ διαστάσει τὸν πνεύμονα, μηδὲν δηλαδὴ μηδ' ἐκ τούτου τῆς καρδίας ἑλκούσης. ἕτεροι δὲ τῇ τραχείᾳ φασὶν ἀρτηρίᾳ βρόχον περιβάλλοντες ἐπιδεικνύναι κινούμενον τὸν πνεύμονα, μηκέτι λέγουσιν ἢ διαγράφουσι, καὶ γὰρ γέγραπται πρὸς τινῶν ταῦτα, πῶς ἐθεάσαντο συστελλόμενον τὸν πνεύμονα, πότερον ἄνευ τοῦ συντρηθῆναι κατὰ τὸν θώρακα τὸ ζῷον, ἢ συντρηθέντος· ἑκάτερον γὰρ ἄτοπον. συντρηθέντος μὲν διαφθείρεται τὰ κατὰ τὴν ἀναπνοὴν ἅπαντα· πρὶν δὲ συντρηθῆναι, τὴν ἀρχὴν οὐδ' ἰδεῖν ἐστιν αὐτόν, εἰ μή τις ἄρα βούλοιτο πλευρὰν ἐκκόψας ἀπαθῆ φυλάξαι τὸν ὑπεζωκότα.

[1] Siegel, Am. J. Cardiol. (1962), pp. 740 f.; Galen's System of Physiology, pp. 56 f.
[2] Siegel, Am. J. Cardiol. 15 (1967), 117 sqq.

This last statement, though correct, does not appear to be consistent with the proposition quoted above[1] that after birth Galen believed that the entire blood flows from the right heart into the lungs. Siegel nevertheless concludes that

The increase of blood volume in the vena cava, due to the blood formation in the liver, and the rhythmically increased pressure of the thorax during respiration, appeared to Galen to be the main mechanical factors responsible for the entry of the blood into the right auricle.

Another factor which he omits to mention is the attractive force of the expansion of the right ventricle itself, which, working on the principle of the *horror vacui* so dear to Erasistratus, was admitted by Galen to be a factor, though not the principal factor, effecting the entry of blood from the main stream of the vena cava, arising out of the liver, to the right chamber of the heart.[2]

The main points of Siegel's description are contained in the following paragraphs:

Galen described the subsequent contraction of the right auricle driving blood into the right chamber, and wrote that this blood is expelled by the right heart through the pores of the inter-ventricular septum, as well as through the pulmonary artery and its anastomoses to the left heart. But he believed that even this flow depended more upon the respiratory movements of the thorax than upon the contraction of the heart. Galen thought that the sturdy walls and valves of the pulmonary artery prevented a backward motion of the blood during the expiratory contraction of the thorax, but that the thin walls of the pulmonary vein yielded to the compression of the contracting thorax during expiration. By this mechanism the blood was squeezed into the left atrium. Obviously Galen regarded the pumping force of the right chamber of the heart as insufficient to propel the blood through the anastomoses in the lungs as well as through the inter-ventricular septum into the left heart. Thus the forward flow of blood from the right to the left heart seemed to depend less upon the pumping action of the heart than upon the action of the thoracic muscles. It is difficult to imagine that Galen would have believed the heart to be a pump that depends upon a force acting on the pipes leading into and from the pump.

Galen thought that during systole only the transverse fibres of the ventricular walls contracted; whereas the other muscle layers actually dilated. This assumed mechanism of the heart muscle could not remind Galen of any type of pump. The pressure and suction pumps of antiquity were either the rigid piston-type or the bellows type without valves. The heart certainly does not resemble the piston-operated pump with rigid walls. The bellows pump has elastic walls that fold during compression and stretch during the extension of the pump. But in Galen's time the latter was obviously operated without valves. Also Galen and his contemporaries probably could not have conceived of a pump in which one part contracted, while the other part dilated during

_____
[1] See above, p. 300.   [2] See below, p. 369.

each phase of motion. Thus the heart did not lend itself to comparison with either type of mechanical pump.

This question of the failure of Galen to compare the heart to a pump seems to me to be rather unimportant. The comparison of the arterial system, including the left ventricle to bellows, is common enough in Galen's writings. But Siegel is certainly right to draw attention to the comparatively secondary function assigned by Galen to the contraction of the ventricles in the distribution of the blood, either to the lungs or to the organs and peripheral portions of the body and the limbs. And though he is in my opinion wrong in assuming that blood was believed by Galen to make an actual transit from right to left heart via the lungs, he is correct in assuming that Galen thought 'that the peripheral utilization of the blood was very slow, *since it never seemed to return to the heart*' (my italics), and that he 'underestimated both the quantity of the peripherically directed venous blood-flow and the amount of arterial blood driven by the left heart into the arteries'. Siegel concludes that Galen believed that the contraction and expansion of the arteries in pulsation could exert sufficient force to propel the blood to the peripheral organs, 'consequently it was unnecessary to postulate a strong pumping action of the cardiac chambers', and that the arterial flow 'was the result both of the left ventricular systole and the rhythmic dilation and contraction of the arteries, which together performed the double action of drawing blood from the heart and propelling it forward'. This, as we shall have reason to see, constitutes one of the rather puzzling riddles of his haemodynamics. In this connection it is important to remember a factor which Siegel does not mention in his analysis, the notion that the most powerful action of both heart and arteries was dilation, not contraction.[1] The heart and the arteries were conceived by him as a very powerful form of what we today would call a suction pump.

Siegel is correct, too, when he maintains that Galen thought that 'the peripheral utilization of both arterial and venous blood created an additional suction promoting the flow of both . . . towards the peripheral organs'. But I am unable to understand the reason for this arrangement which Siegel postulates, when he tells us that Galen 'pointed out that otherwise a vacuum would be created, an idea unthinkable to the scientists of his time'. That surely was the theory of Erasistratus, which Galen spent so much time in refuting.[2] Nor can I assent to Siegel's conclusion:

Far from being considered a pump, the heart was believed to serve as the organ of heat production, by which the inhaled air was thought to convey

---

[1] *De usu partium*, vi. 15, K. iii. 484: καὶ ἡ τῆς ἐν τῷ διαστέλλεσθαι κινήσεως ἰσχὺς ὑπερεῖχε τῆς ἐν τῷ συστέλλεσθαι. βιαιότερον γὰρ ἕλκειν ἀνάγκη τὴν καρδίαν διαστελλομένην, ἥπερ ἐκθλίβειν συστελλομένην.

[2] A large portion of his treatise *On the natural faculties* is devoted to this refutation. See below, pp. 329 f.

heat to the blood. Galen actually suggested a similarity between the left chamber of the heart and a coal furnace, since like his predecessors he believed that the main function of the left ventricle was to furnish heat for the entire body. In disproving older erroneous concepts, Galen had demonstrated, *first*, that the arteries and therefore the left heart contain only blood, and, *secondly*, that air or the heat derived from the inhaled air must be absorbed by the blood. Therefore Galen assumed it was most likely that the motion of heat from the left heart supported the other forces that drive the blood into the arteries. Galen compared the arteries to the pipes of a hot-air furnace, in which the air had no other propelling force than its own spontaneous motion. Thus Galen's faulty doctrine of respiration based on the assumption of heat production by 'combustion' of blood in the left heart, suggested this additional mechanical explanation of the forward flow of the blood.

Siegel here seems to me to have been rather seriously misled by his knowledge of biochemical processes first discovered by Lavoisier. The idea that body-heat was produced by the interaction of the blood with the inhaled air was wholly contrary to Galen's ideas. Everywhere he insists that the function of the inspired air is to *cool* the innate heat in the left ventricle. This was the traditional theory inherited from 'Hippocratic' times and shared, incidentally, by Aristotle. Without such cooling, the innate heat would burn the body up, and the result would be the death of the organism. Indeed this burning-up is the cause of the natural death of old age which results when the cooling process of respiration is no longer functioning, and the greatly diminished innate heat is still sufficient to cause a mortal desiccation or withering ($\mu\acute{\alpha}\rho\alpha\nu\sigma\iota\varsigma$).[1]

Thus, while we may accept Siegel's description of the forces propelling the blood from the right ventricle through the lungs as correct, we cannot accept the notion that they amount to what we moderns call the pulmonary transit. Siegel seems to have ignored the reasons given by Galen for the venous nature of the vein-like artery, namely its truly venous function of nutrition.

Nor is Siegel justified in claiming that Galen made a great discovery, that he was able to prove that blood vessels, by which he presumably means both veins and arteries, 'never contain any free air'.[2] Indeed Siegel ventures the statement that 'All other physicians of antiquity assumed that the pulmonary veins contained only air',[3] which can hardly be defended historically. The doctrine that both veins and arteries contained both blood and *pneuma* in differing proportions goes back, as we have seen, to the *Hippocratic corpus*. We must therefore, I think, abandon the attempt to attribute to Galen this discovery, even if we accept as correct Siegel's statement that 'Galen never wrote that the entire blood flowing

---

[1] See below, p. 441.
[2] Siegel, *Arch. f. Gesch. d. Med.* xlvi (1962), 312.
[3] Siegel, *Am. J. Cardiol.* 10 (1962).

into the lungs is utilized by this organ'. In his latest book,[1] which only came into my hands after I had finished writing, Siegel adopts a distinction between *circulation* and *transit* which brings his version of Galen's doctrine much nearer what I conceive to be the truth. He tells us that

Galen assumed that only a few drops of blood entered the left heart from the pulmonary vein with each respiratory cycle. We, therefore, should not speak of a blood-flow through the pulmonary vessels or lesser circulation, but of a slow transit of blood through assumed anastomoses of these vessels. The use of the term circulation presumes a co-ordination between the amounts passing through both pulmonary and peripheral vessels and also indicates a return flow.

Again Siegel fails to mention the chief function of this slow transit, namely the nutrition of the continually expanding and contracting lung. There can be no doubt that no Renaissance commentators before Servetus and Colombo believed that he taught that some blood passed from the right ventricle to the left via the lungs.[2] Harvey however did, as well as his contemporary Hofman. Prendergast may very well be correct in supposing that Harvey was to some extent trying to find shelter from the storms aroused by his discovery under the authority of Galen. For he quotes extensively from the *De usu partium* to show that Galen had believed in a pulmonary transit in the seventh chapter of the *De motu cordis*.[3] Realdo Colombo also, as Siegel points out,[4] cites Galen as his authority for the transport of aerated blood from the lungs to the left ventricle, as the primary function of the lungs, in a passage which is perhaps a trifle ambiguous. But Fernel seems to have maintained that Galen taught that all the blood passing into the pulmonary veins was

[1] Siegel, *Galen on Sense Perception* (Karger, Basel and New York, 1970), p. 4.
[2] See J. J. Bylebyl and W. Pagel, 'The chequered career of Galen's doctrine on the pulmonary veins', in *Medical History*, xv (1971), 218.
[3] Cf. *De motu cordis*, ch. vii, English text of 1653, ed. G. Keynes (London, 1928), p. 51: 'But seeing there are some such persons which admit of nothing, unless there be an authority alleged for it, let them know, that the very same truth may be proved from *Galen's* own words, that is to say, not only that the blood may be transfused out of the *vena arteriosa* into the *arteria venosa* and thence into the left ventricle of the heart, and afterwards transmitted into the arteries, but also that this is done by a continued pulse of the heart, and motion of the lung while we breathe.' p. 54: 'That argument which *Galen* brings for the passages of the blood through the right ventricle out of the *vena cava* into the lungs, we may more rightly use for the passages of the blood out of the veins through the heart into the arteries, changing only the terms. It does therefore clearly appear from the words and places of *Galen*, a divine man, father of Physicians, both that the blood doth pass from the *vena arteriosa* into the little branches of the *arteria venosa*, both by reason of the pulse of the heart and also because of the motion of the lungs and thorax. (See the commentarie of the most learned *Hofmannus* upon the sixth book of *Galen*, *De usu partium*, which book I saw after I had written these things.)'
[4] Siegel, *Arch. f. Gesch. d. Med.* (1962). The passage quoted from Colombo is taken from *De re anatomica libri XV* (Venice, 1559), p. 224, translated as follows: 'It is unlikely that Galen, the great philosopher and only comparable to Hippocrates, should not have recognized this function of the lungs.'

used up in the process of nutrition.[1] The relation of the discovery of the pulmonary circulation to Galen's teaching has been admirably summed up by Wilson.[2] Speaking of all three 'discoverers', namely Ibn-an Nafis, Servetus, and Colombo, he remarks:

Their discoveries were almost certainly independent in each case, but all three seem to begin their reasoning from the same literary source, namely the passage at the end of the tenth chapter of the sixth book of Galen's *De usu partium*, where Galen shows that blood which has passed into the pulmonary artery, from the right ventricle of the heart, must pass through the anastomoses between arteries and veins into the pulmonary vein when the lungs collapse in expiration.

Wilson then quotes the passage in question and comes to the conclusion that Galen considered these arrangements to serve principally for the nourishment of the lung, but he points out:

Although in the passage quoted Galen mentions all the elements of the pulmonary pathway and the mechanism by which blood might pass at least part of the way along it, his own interpretation of the pulmonary pathway is that it is purely nutritional. In his system of physiology Galen had to provide for the passage of blood from the right ventricle, but he did this by means of his postulated pores in the inter-ventricular septum. Yet if the existence of these pores is once questioned, then the way is open for the reinterpretation of the pulmonary pathway which Galen has described.

It would, I think, be difficult to find a better summing up of this controversy. So we must leave the matter there.[3]

But in order to discover how it was that Galen who came so near to it yet failed to reach it, we must follow a little more closely his teaching on the mutual relations of the two substances which Erasistratus first declared to be responsible for managing the economy of the organism, namely blood and *pneuma*. The first point to notice is that Galen, though by and large a very accurate observer, did make two important mistakes. He failed to discover the valves in the veins and he assumed the transit of blood through the pores in the interventricular septum. But he postulated the capillaries and he understood the function of the heart's valves as

---

[1] Siegel, ibid.

[2] Leonard Wilson, 'The problem of the discovery of the pulmonary circulation', *J. Hist. Med.* 17 (1962), 229–44.

[3] This chapter had already been written before May's admirable translation of the *De usu partium* came into my hands. She too would appear to believe that Galen taught a rudimentary kind of transit via the lungs of blood from the right to the left ventricle. In a footnote (op. cit., i. 301, n. 43) she remarks: 'The blood coming through the pulmonary artery to the lungs also has in his view two fates, as he will shortly explain. The larger part is used for nutrition of the lung, which needs a great deal, since it is such a porous highly active viscus, but some of it is forced by the compression of the thorax in expiration through the minute inosculations into the pulmonary veins. Thus it will be seen that Galen had a very rudimentary conception of a pulmonary circulation.'

closing inlets and outlets. He even, as we have just seen, had discovered
the path for a possible pulmonary circulation. It was his physiology rather
than his anatomy that led him astray. For it was physiology that led him
to regard the source of the veins as being not the heart but the liver,
a doctrine which, as we have noted, is to be found in several of the pre-
Aristotelian physicians. And it was this doctrine which blinded his eyes
to any inkling of a circulatory process. And the doctrine was essentially
physiological rather than anatomical. Galen's topographical scheme of
the vascular system was reasonably correct; it was his physiological
interpretation of the facts which was at fault.

The implications of this conception of two roots for the vascular
system needs to be worked out rather carefully. It was 'Hippocrates' who,
according to Galen, founded the doctrine that all arteries are rooted in
the heart and all veins in the liver.[1] The vascular system is, or rather its
two parts each are, compared to a tree, an analogy which Galen works
out with great care. As 'Hippocrates' had observed long before him, all
arteries are rooted in the heart.[2] The aorta is the trunk from which all the
arteries of the body diverge, like the branches of a tree. Those entering
and spreading themselves through the lung, i.e. the pulmonary veins, are
the roots. So too in the case of the veins, all the veins branching forth into
every part of the body grow out of the vena cava, and those that go to the
belly and the intestines are analogous to the roots. Immediately on
emerging from the convex surface of the liver, the vena cava goes in
a straight line to both the halves of the body, the upper and the lower.[3]
The liver is the only place in the body out of which all the veins in the
body grow, though there are some who say they all grow out of the right
ventricle of the heart[4]—the theory of Erasistratus which Galen so

---

[1] Galen, De plac. Hipp. et Plat. i. 7, K. v. 199: οὕτως γὰρ οἶμαι καὶ τὸν Ἱπποκράτην προσ-
εικάσαντα ῥίζωσιν ἀρτηριῶν ἀποφαίνεσθαι, τὴν καρδίαν, ὥσπερ ἀμέλει τῶν φλεβῶν τὸ ἧπαρ.

[2] See above, p. 36, n. 3.

[3] Ibid., vi. 3, K. v. 531 f.: καί μοι δοκεῖ καὶ ὁ Ἱπποκράτης ἐντεῦθεν ἐπὶ τὰ ζῷα μεταφέρων
τοὔνομα ῥίζωσιν εἰρηκέναι τῶν μὲν ἀρτηριῶν τὴν καρδίαν τῶν δὲ φλεβῶν τὸ ἧπαρ. ὡς γὰρ ἀπὸ
τῆς ῥιζώσεως τῶν φυτῶν αἱ ῥίζαι μὲν κάτω, τὸ δὲ στέλεχος ἄνω φύεται, κατὰ τὸν αὐτὸν τρόπον
ἐκ μὲν τῆς καρδίας ἥ τε εἰς τὸν πνεύμονα καὶ ἡ εἰς ὅλον τὸ ζῷον, ἐκ δὲ τοῦ ἥπατος ἥ τ' εἰς τὴν κατὰ
τὴν γαστέρα καὶ εἰς τὸ σύμπαν σῶμα. ῥίζαις μὲν οὖν ἐοίκασιν αἱ εἰς τὴν γαστέρα καθήκουσαι
φλέβες, ὡς καὶ τοῦτ' αὐτὸς Ἱπποκράτης ἔδειξε φάμενος· ὡς γὰρ τοῖς δένδροις ἡ γῆ, οὕτω τοῖς
ζῴοις ἡ γαστήρ, τὸ δ' οἷον πρέμνον ἡ κοίλη φλέψ ἐστιν, ἐκ μὲν τῶν κυρτῶν τοῦ ἥπατος ἐκπεφυκυῖα,
φερομένη δ' ἐκ τοῦ ἥπατος εὐθεῖα πρὸς ἑκάτερα τοῦ ζῴου τὰ μέρη, τὰ ἄνω καὶ τὸ κάτω. Cf.
Comment. IV in Hipp. de aliment. 6, K. xv. 388 f.: καὶ ταῖς μὲν κατὰ τὴν καρδίαν ἀρτηρίαις αἱ
κατὰ τὸ ἧπαρ φλέβες ἀνάλογον ἔχουσιν. καὶ ὥσπερ ἡ ἐκ τῆς ἀριστερᾶς κοιλίας τῆς καρδίας ἀρτηρία
φυομένη πρέμνον τῶν καθ' ὅλον τὸ ζῷόν ἐστι τῶν ἀρτηριῶν, τὸν αὐτὸν τρόπον ἀπὸ τῆς κοίλης
φλεβὸς αἱ καθ' ὅλον τὸ ζῷον ἀποπεφύκασι φλέβες οἷον κλάδοι τινὲς ὡς ἀπὸ στελέχων. ταῖς δ'
οἷον ῥίζαις τῶν ἀρτηριῶν, ταῖς εἰς τὸν πνεύμονα κατασχιζομέναις, ἐκ τῆς καρδίας ἀνάλογον αὖ
πάλιν αἱ κατὰ τὴν γαστέρα τε καὶ τὸν σπλῆνα καὶ τὸ μεσεντέριον ἔχουσι φλέβες.

[4] De plac. Hipp. et Plat. viii. i, K. v. 657: ἑτέρα (ἀπόδειξις) ἐκ τοῦ μηδὲν ἄλλο μόριον εὑρίσκεσθαι κατὰ τὸ ζῷον, ᾧ συμφυεῖς εἰσιν αἱ φλέβες ἅπασαι, λαμβανομένη. τὴν γὰρ ἐκ τῶν κυρτῶν
τοῦ ἥπατος ἐκφυομένην φλέβα τὴν κοίλην, ἔνιοί φασι τῆς δεξιᾶς ἐν τῇ καρδίᾳ κοιλίας ἐκπεφυκέναι.

wrong-headedly combated. The veins, he tells us, which connect the
stomach, the large intestines, the spleen, the rectum, and the omentum,
do not grow out of the vena cava at all, but out of a vein whose starting-
point is not the convex but the concave side of the liver, the so-called
door, the focal point of the portal system, and the portal vein is quite
separate from the vena cava. But this, he continues, will not help those
who regard the heart as the starting-point (ἀρχή) of the veins, for the
heart too is not connected with the portal system. The liver is connected
both with the portal system and the vena cava.'Hippocrates', indeed, called
the vena cava the liver vein, for the liver is the origin of all the veins, and
therefore of the nutritive faculty.[1] The passage from the vena cava leading
to the right ventricle of the heart Galen regards as a sort of side channel
or backwater. The vena cava is at its broadest below the liver, the part
that stretches up through the diaphragm is less broad, and still less broad
than either of these is the right auricle, the part of the vena cava that
grows into the heart.[2] In this connection Daremberg pointed out that
this notion, as well as his description of the mediastinum, shows that he
had no direct knowledge of the human heart. In man the vena cava
penetrates the pericardium immediately after crossing the diaphragm,
whereas in most other mammals there is an interval of some length
between the point where it traverses the diaphragm and the point where
it enters the heart.[3] According to Galen, the vena cava goes up right past

---

[1] *De plac. Hipp. et Plat.* viii. 1, 657–8: ἀλλ' αἵ γ' ἐκ τῶν σιμῶν τῆς ἥπατος ἀνάλογον ῥίζαις
εἰς τὴν γαστέρα, τήν τε νῆστιν καὶ τὸ λεπτὸν ἔντερον καὶ τὸ τυφλὸν καὶ τὸ κῶλον εἴς τε τὸ ἀπευθυ-
σμένον ὀνομαζόμενον, καὶ τὸν σπλῆνα καὶ τὸ ἐπίπλοον ἤκουσαι φλέβες, οὐκ ἀπὸ ταύτης πεφύκασιν,
ἀλλ' ἔστιν ἑτέρα φλέψ, ἀπασῶν τούτων ἀρχὴ κατὰ τὰς πύλας τοῦ ἥπατος τεταγμένη. πῶς οὖν
ἔτι ἀρχὴ τῶν φλεβῶν ἡ δεξιὰ τῆς καρδίας ἔσται κοιλία μήτε τῶν εἰρημένων φλεβῶν μήτε πρὸς
αὐταῖς τῶν ἐν τοῖς σιμοῖς τοῦ ἥπατος συναπτομένων τῇ καρδίᾳ; ἧπαρ δὲ καὶ ταύταις ἁπάσαις
συνῆπται ταῖς φλεψὶν καὶ ταῖς καθ' ὅλον τὸ σῶμα διὰ τῆς ἐκ τῶν κυρτῶν αὐτοῦ μερῶν
ἐκπεφυκυίας, ἣν οἱ μὲν πλεῖστοι τῶν ἰατρῶν κοίλην ὀνομάζουσι διὰ τὸ μέγεθος. Ἱπποκράτης
δὲ καὶ ὅσοι τὰ τούτου πρεσβεύουσιν, ἡπατῖτιν ἀπὸ τοῦ σπλάγχνου προσονομάζουσιν, ὅθεν ἐκπέφυκεν
αὕτη. τοιγαροῦν ἤδη σοι δευτέρα περὶ ἥπατος ἀπόδειξις, ὡς ἁπασῶν ἐστι φλεβῶν ἀρχή, διὰ
τοῦτο δὲ καὶ τῆς θρεπτικῆς δυνάμεως.

[2] *Ibid.*, vi. 3, K. v. 532: εὐρύτατον μὲν οὖν αὐτῆς ἐστι τὸ κάτω τοῦ ἥπατος, ἧττον δ' εὐρὺ τὸ
διὰ τῶν φρενῶν ἀνατεταμένον, ἔλαττον δὲ ἀμφοτέρων τὸ τῇ καρδίᾳ ἐμφυόμενον.

[3] Daremberg, op. cit. 387, n. 1: 'Maintenant quelles sont ces tuniques communes qui ser-
vent à fixer la veine cave? Galien l'indique lui-même: ce sont les plèvres. En effet, la portion
de la veine cave qui représente pour nous la *veine cave supérieure* dans la partie libre, c'est
à dire celle qui n'est pas renfermée dans le péricarde, est recouverte à droite et en arrière
par le feuillet séreux droit du médiastin. Quant à la portion de la *veine cave inférieure* contenue
dans la cavité thoracique, chez l'homme elle pénètre immédiatement dans le péricarde
après avoir traversé le diaphragme; mais chez la plupart des mammifères la *veine cave inférieure* a un véritable trajet *intra-thoracique* avant de pénétrer dans le péricarde, à cause
de la situation même de ce sac qui est plus ou moins distant du diaphragme.'

Cf. i. 438 n. 1: 'Galien ne mentionne pas les adhérences de cette tunique (le péricarde)
au diaphragme: mais cela n'a rien d'étonnant, car chez les singes . . . comme je l'ai moi-
même vérifié sur le magot, l'adhérence du péricarde au diaphragme est nulle ou presque
nulle. Cuvier dit encore que les prolongements du médiastin qui s'avancent à partir du

the heart and ascends to the throat.[1] In the treatise *On the dissection of veins and arteries*, he seems to treat the pulmonary arteries, the vein-like ones, as if they were a pair of branches of the vena cava, remarking that its branches mostly go in pairs. He treats the diaphragm as marking the division between the upper and the lower 'hollow vein', and lists the following branches for the upper portion. Above the diaphragm the first pair which goes off is the one into the diaphragm itself. Then there are a number of hair-like vessels which go into the membranes forming the partition of the thorax and the pericardium. After that comes the rather large opening into the right auricle, and that from the auricle into the right ventricle of the heart, the big one, and the branches from the right auricle to the lungs, which have arterial coats, and he mentions also the coronary vein, which he calls a very small vessel.[2] But to pursue these branches in further detail is unnecessary. The important point to note is that, in accordance with the arrangements just described, the majority of the blood created in the liver does not go into the heart at all.[3]

The flesh of the liver, besides being the starting-point of the veins, is also the chief instrument of sanguinification. That is why the veins coming from the stomach and the intestines, which have united in the portal vein, are again divided into many branches in the liver itself. Why could not nature have kept them united in a single large cavity or ventricle in the liver? Erasistratus' theory was that this division was necessary in order to separate the blood from the yellow bile, but on closer examination this notion would appear to be untenable. Nature could easily have separated the superfluity of the bile without such a complicated network of veins, as is clearly shown in the case of the kidneys, which do not have such a network, and yet all the blood which is fed into the hollow vein is quickly relieved of the urine it contains by these organs, which are not even in contact with it.[4] The real reason is that the nourishment conveyed

diaphragme sur les côtés du péricarde suppléent aux adhérences de cette enveloppe avec le muscle.'

[1] Galen, *De ven. et art. dissect.* 2, K. ii. 787: παρελθοῦσα γὰρ ἡ κοίλη τὴν καρδίαν ἐπὶ τὰς σφαγὰς ἀναφέρεται.

[2] Ibid., 786: ἀποφύονται δὲ φλέβες, ἀπὸ μὲν τῆς ἄνω φερομένης αἵδε· πρώτη μὲν συζυγία κατ' αὐτὰς τὰς φρένας, εἶθ' ἑξῆς τριχοειδεῖς τινες πλείους, εἴς τε τοὺς διαφράττοντας ὑμένας τὸν θώρακα καὶ τὸν περικάρδιον χιτῶνα. μετ' αὐτὰς δ' ἱκανῶς ἀξιόλογος εἰς τὸ τῆς καρδίας οὖς τὸ δεξιόν. ἐκ δὲ τοῦ ὠτὸς εἴς τε τὴν δεξιὰν κοιλίαν τῆς καρδίας τὴν μεγάλην, κἀκ ταύτης εἰς τὸν πνεύμονα, τὸν αὐτὸν ἔχουσα χιτῶνα τῷ τῶν ἀρτηριῶν, καί τις ἄλλη μικροτάτη κατὰ τὴν ἐκτὸς ἐπιφάνειαν τῆς καρδίας, εἰς ὅλον τὸ σπλάγχνον διασπειρομένη.

[3] See above, p. 273, n. 2.

[4] *De usu partium*, iv. 13, K. iii. 303 f.: τί δήποτε γὰρ . . . τὰς πολλὰς φλέβας ἐκείνας τὰς ἐκ τῆς κοιλίας τε καὶ τῶν ἐντέρων ἁπάντων ἀναφερούσας τὴν τροφὴν εἰς τὸ ἧπαρ ἑνώσασα κατὰ τὰς πύλας ἡ φύσις, αὖθις εἰς παμπόλλας κατέτεμεν; ἥνωσε μὲν γὰρ αὐτάς, ὡς μιᾶς δεομένη, ἔσχισε δ' εὐθὺς ὡς μάτην ἑνώσασα, ἐνόν γ' αὐτῇ, μίαν ἐργασαμένη μεγάλην ἐν τῷ σπλάγχνῳ κοιλίαν αἱματικήν, ἐμφῦσαι ταύτῃ κάτωθεν μὲν τὴν ἀναφέρουσαν τὸ αἷμα φλέβα τὴν ἐκ τῶν πυλῶν, ἄνωθεν δὲ τὴν διαδεξομένην τε καὶ παντὶ τῷ σώματι διακομίσουσαν. τὰ μὲν οὖν ὑπὸ Ἐρασιστράτου λεγόμενα

to the liver must remain in it for some time, in order to be perfectly turned into blood. If the liver were made hollow, like a single-ventricled heart, this would mean that the humour or liquid supplied to it from the belly would pass straight through it. The narrow veins into which the portal vein divides thus serve the same purpose as the pylorus and the coils of the small intestine.[1] The veins in the liver are the thinnest in the whole body, and they are placed in the flesh of the organ, so as to keep them safe from injury. Part of the function of the network of veins in the liver is to separate the (excess of) yellow bile from the nutritional contents. The passages which draw off the yellow bile are therefore placed in front of the veins which distribute the blood to the hollow vein, in order that it may receive its blood in a purified condition.[2]

The liver is the seat of the faculty of nutrition. The three principal activities of an animal are: (a) those connected with will or choice, centred in the brain, (b) those called vital, centred in the heart, and (c) those connected with nourishment, called natural.[3] Hence, as we shall presently see, the division of *pneuma* or 'spirits' into the three categories, animal-psychic, vital, and natural. The liver is the common place of digestion for the whole organism,[4] the process of 'cooking' (πέψις), which takes place in the stomach being only a preliminary operation. The veins of the portal system, which convey the nourishment from the stomach (and the intestines) to the liver do so by a power of attraction,

διακρίσεως ἕνεκα τῆς ξανθῆς χολῆς ἐνδείκνυται τὴν σχίσιν τῶν ἐν ἥπατι φλεβῶν γεγονέναι. φανείη δ' ἄν, εἴ τις ἀκριβέστερον αὐτὰ διασκέπτοιτο, κακῶς εἰρημένα, δυναμένης γε τῆς φύσεως, καὶ χωρὶς τοσαύτης τε καὶ τοιαύτης πλοκῆς διακρίνειν τὰ περιττώματα, καθότι σαφῶς ἐπὶ τῶν νεφρῶν ἐνεδείξατο. πάμπολλοι γοῦν τῶν κωθωνιζομένων ἀμφορέας ὅλους ἐκπίνοντες ἀνάλογόν τε τῷ πλήθει τοῦ πόματος οὐροῦντες, οὐκ ἐμποδίζονται περὶ τὴν διάκρισιν, ἀλλ' ἑτοιμότατα καὶ ῥᾷστα τὸ παραγενόμενον εἰς τὴν κοίλην αἷμα καθαίρεται πρὸς τῶν νεφρῶν ἅπαν, οὐδὲ ψαυόντων τῆς φλεβός.

[1] *De usu partium*, iv. 13, K. iii. 305: οὔκουν διακρίσεως ἕνεκεν ἡ φύσις ἐποίησε τὴν τοσαύτην πλοκὴν τῶν κατὰ τὸ ἧπαρ ἀγγείων ἀλλ' ὑπὲρ τοῦ χρονίζουσαν ἐν τῷ σπλάγχνῳ τὴν τροφὴν αἱματοῦσθια τελέως. εἰ γὰρ ὡς ἐπὶ τῆς καρδίας μίαν εἰργάσατο μεγάλην κοιλίαν, οἷον δεξαμένην τινά, κᾆπειτ' εἰς αὐτὴν διὰ μιᾶς μὲν φλεβὸς εἰσῆγε τὸ αἷμα, δι' ἑτέρας δ' ἐξῆγεν, οὐκ ἀκαρῆ χρόνον κατὰ τὸ ἧπαρ ἔμενεν ὁ ἐκ τῆς γαστρὸς ἀναφερόμενος χυμός, ἀλλὰ διεξήρχετ' ἂν ἑτοίμως δι' ὅλου τοῦ σπλάγχνου τῇ τῆς ἀποδόσεως ῥύμῃ φερόμενος, ἕνεκα δὲ τοῦ μένειν ἐπὶ πλέον καὶ ἀλλοιοῦσθαι τὴν τροφὴν τελέως αἱ τῶν διεξόδων στενότητες ἐγένοντο, ὥσπερ ἐπὶ μὲν τῆς γαστρὸς ὁ πυλωρός, ἐπὶ δὲ τῶν ἐντέρων αἱ ἕλικες.

[2] Ibid., 306 f.: ταῦτ' ἄρα καὶ αὐτὰς τὰς φλέβας τὰς κατὰ τὸ ἧπαρ ἁπασῶν ἰσχνοτάτας τῶν καθ' ὅλον τὸ σῶμα φλεβῶν ἐδημιούργησεν· ἐκείνας μὲν γὰρ ὡς ἂν μήτε γειτνιώσας τῇ τῆς αἱματώσεως ἀρχῇ καὶ δυσπαθείας δεομένας εὐλόγως ἰσχυρὰς ἀπειργάσατο . . . τὰς δὲ κατὰ τὸ ἧπαρ ἰσχνοτάτας, ὡς ἂν μήτε παθεῖν τι κινδυνευσούσας (ἥδρασμέναι γὰρ ἀκριβῶς εἰσιν ἐν τῷ σπλάγχνῳ) καὶ κάλλιον ἂν οὕτω τὴν αἱμάτωσιν ἐργασομένας, ὅτι δὲ βέλτιον ἦν ἐπὶ ταῖς ἀναφερούσαις τὴν ἐκ τῆς κοιλίας τροφὴν φλεψὶ προτέρους τῶν διαδεξαμένων φλεβῶν τοὺς ἕλκοντας τὴν ξανθὴν χολὴν τετάχθαι πόρους . . . κεκαθαρμένον γὰρ ἤδη καλῶς τὸ αἷμα τῇ τῶν ἀγγείων τούτων ἐπικαίρῳ θέσει διαδέχοιτ' ἂν ἡ κοίλη φλέψ.

[3] *Comment. III in Hipp. de aliment.* xxv, K. xv. 362: τριῶν μὲν οὖν οὐσῶν, ἔμαθες ὅτι ὁ ἐγκέφαλός ἐστιν ἀρχὴ τῶν προαιρετικῶν ἐνεργειῶν, ἡ καρδία δὲ τῶν ζωτικῶν ὀνομαζομένων, τὸ δὲ ἧπαρ τῶν περὶ τροφῆς, ἃς δὴ καὶ φυσικὰς ὀνομάζουσι.

[4] *De usu partium*, iv. 2, K. iii. 268: οὕτω καὶ αὗται τὴν ἐν τῇ γαστρὶ κατειργασμένην τροφὴν ἀναφέρουσιν εἴς τι κοινὸν ὅλου τοῦ ζώου πέψεως χωρίον, ὃ καλοῦμεν ἧπαρ.

that mysterious power which Galen makes responsible for most, if not for every, movements of the blood. They also play a part in preparing in a suitable manner for the operation of that organ.[1] By the time that it reaches the liver, the nutriment has already become, as it were, an imperfect rough sketch of blood, with a confused resemblance to it.[2] Indigestible, hard, and insoluble elements have already been purged from it in the stomach, but other elements which require further digestion are still present. In this semi-digested condition it arrives in the liver in the form of a liquid—this character being supplied by what we drink— to receive a further digestion under the influence of the innate heat, the process being compared to the fermentation of certain kinds of wine, which takes place with effervescence that produces the so-called 'flower' and the deposit of lees. In the process of sanguinification there are two by-products, one a thick and muddy one,[3] the other a light thin one. The thick and muddy 'lees' represent the black bile, to be deposited in the spleen, but the light and thin yellow bile is poured along with the blood into the hollow vein, and goes to all portions of the body,[4] the bile that is separated off into the gall-bladder being, presumably, only a superfluity or excess. The blood, which has thus been diluted with drink, does not, however, retain all its liquid. The superfluity is strained off by the kidneys.[5]

The process of sanguinification is the work of the flesh of the liver, which is the essence or substance of the organ and has its own special character, though it was regarded by Erasistratus as a mere deposit of

[1] Ibid., 269: καὶ τὰς μὲν φλέβας οὐ παραγούσας μόνον τὴν τροφὴν ἐκ τῆς γαστρός, ἀλλ' ἑλκούσας ἅμα καὶ προπαρασκευαζούσας τῷ ἥπατι τὸν ὁμοιότατον ἐκείνῳ τρόπον.

[2] Ibid., 3, 269: αὐτὸ δὲ τὸ ἧπαρ ἐπειδὰν αὐτὴν παραλάβῃ, πρὸς τῶν ὑπηρετῶν ἤδη παρεσκευασμένην, καὶ οἷον ὑπογραφήν τινα καὶ ἀμυδρὸν εἶδος αἵματος ἔχουσαν, ἐπάγει τέλεον αὐτῇ τὸν κόσμον εἰς αἵματος ἀκριβῶς γένεσιν.

[3] Ibid., 269–70: ἀλλ' ἐπεὶ τῶν κατὰ τὴν γαστέρα τὰ μὲν οὕτω μοχθηρά, καθάπερ ἐν τῷ σίτῳ γῆ καὶ λίθοι καὶ τὰ τῶν ἀγρίων σπέρματα ὀσπρίων, διεκέκριτο, τὸ δ' οἷον ἄχνη καὶ πίτυρον, ἑτέρας καθάρσεως ἐδεῖτο ... ἄμεινον δ' ἂν εἴη εἰς εἰκόνος ἐνεργείαν, μὴ ξηροῖς σιτίοις, ἀλλ' ὑγρῷ χυμῷ προπεπεμμένῳ μὲν ἤδη καὶ προκατειργασμένῳ, δεομένῳ δὲ τελειωτέρας πέψεως, ὁμοιῶσαι τὸν ἐκ τῆς κοιλίας διὰ τῶν φλεβῶν εἰς τὸ ἧπαρ ἀναφερόμενον χυλόν. ἔστω δή τις οἶνος, ἄρτι μὲν τῶν βοτρύων ἐκτεθλιμμένος, ἐγκεχυμένος δ' ἐν πιθάκναις, ὑπὸ δὲ τῆς ἐμφύτου θερμότητος ἔτι κατεργαζόμενός τε καὶ διακρινόμενος καὶ πεττόμενος καὶ ξέων, καὶ αὐτῶν τῶν περιττωμάτων τὸ μὲν βαρὺ καὶ γεῶδες, ὅπερ, οἶμαι, τρύγα καλοῦσιν, ἐν τοῖς πυθμέσι τῶν ἀγγείων ὑφιστάσθω, τὸ δ' ἕτερον, τὸ κοῦφόν τε καὶ ἀερῶδες, ἐποχείσθω· καλεῖται δ' ἄνθος τοῦτο ... νόει μοι τὸν ἐκ τῆς κοιλίας εἰς τὸ ἧπαρ ἀναδοθέντα χυλὸν ὑπὸ τῆς ἐν τῷ σπλάγχνῳ θερμασίας, ὥσπερ τὸν οἶνον τὸν γλεύκινον ζέοντα τε καὶ πεττόμενον καὶ ἀλλοιούμενον εἰς αἵματος χρηστοῦ γένεσιν· ἐν δὲ τῇ ζέσει ταύτῃ τὸ μὲν ὑφιστάμενον αὐτῷ τῶν περιττωμάτων, ὅσον ἰλυῶδές τε καὶ παχύ, τὸ δ' ἐπιπολάζον, ὃ δὴ λεπτόν τε καὶ κοῦφον οἷον ἀφρός τις ἐποχεῖται τῷ αἵματι.

[4] De atra bile, 6, K. v. 127: διὰ τούτων μὲν οὖν ὑπαχθέντες οἱ ἄριστοι τῶν παλαιῶν ἰατρῶν τε καὶ φιλοσόφων ἀπεφήναντο καθαιρέσθαι τὸ ἧπαρ ὑπὸ τοῦ σπληνὸς ἕλκοντος εἰς ἑαυτὸν ὅσον ἰλυῶδες ἐν αἵματι.

[5] De usu partium, iv. 6, K. iii. 273: ταύτας οὖν τὰς λεπτὰς ὑγρότητας, ὅταν τὸ σφέτερον ἔργον πληρώσωσιν, οὐκέτ' ἐν τῷ σώματι χρὴ μένειν ἄχθος ἀλλότριον ἐσομένας ταῖς φλεψί. καὶ ταύτης ἕνεκα τῆς χρείας οἱ νεφροὶ γεγόνασιν.

nutriment or parenchyma. If you examine it, you will see that it is very like blood. Imagine blood turned vaporous by heat and then condensed, and you have just the flesh of the liver.[1] The purpose or aim of each part of the body which changes nutriment is to make the matter changed like itself. So the chyle from the stomach taken in by the liver is changed bit by bit by the flesh of that organ into its own nature, and so becomes thicker and redder, until it is finally assimilated to it.[2] But the whole of the blood cannot become liver-flesh. Blood is therefore something that is not completely assimilated; it is, as it were, halfway between food and flesh, being as far removed qualitatively from flesh as it is from the liquid product of digestion in the stomach.[3] With a more detailed examination of the functions of the liver we need not concern ourselves, but it is worth while noting that Galen regards the liver as the source of the living functions which are common to vegetables and animals, and he accepts the Platonic hypothesis that the liver is the seat of the appetitive part of the soul, as well as that of the faculty of nutrition which had been assigned to it by Aristotle. Indeed, for Galen it is the seat or starting-point ($\dot{a}\rho\chi\dot{\eta}$) of many powers or faculties ($\delta v\nu\dot{a}\mu\epsilon\iota\varsigma$), or more properly of an essence ($o\dot{v}\sigma\dot{\iota}a$) of the soul.[4] Now the physiological implications of the doctrine that the liver is the starting-point of the veins are for Galen all-important. The liver is in charge of the 'vegetative' function of nutrition, and just as a plant draws nourishment from its roots, and propels it to its leaves through its stalk, so the liver, not the heart, is responsible for distributing the blood. The liver is not a mere ancillary organ preparing a necessary material, but is itself in charge of the distribution of nutriment.[5] What this rather mysterious power of distribution amounted to, Galen never properly explains, but he does tell us quite a lot about the way in which the blood is actually distributed. And here we must make a distinction between venous and arterial blood: the latter is distributed if not by, at

---

[1] *De usu partium*, iv. 12, K. iii. 298: ἀπολείπεται τοίνυν ἡ οἷον σὰρξ τοῦ ἥπατος, ἥπερ δὴ καὶ ἴδιός ἐστιν οὐσία τοῦ σπλάγχνου ... καὶ μέντοι καὶ σαφῶς εἴ τις αὐτῆς κατασκέψαιτο τὴν φύσιν, ἐγγυτάτω φανεῖται τοῦ αἵματος· εἰ γὰρ ἐννοήσεις ὑπὸ θερμότητος ἐξατμιζόμενον αἷμα καὶ παχυνόμενον, οὐδὲν ἄλλο εὑρήσεις γιγνόμενον ἢ τὴν τοῦ ἥπατος σάρκα.

[2] *Ibid.*, 298–9: ἕκαστον τῶν ἀλλοιούντων μορίων τὴν τροφὴν οἷον σκοπόν τινα ἔχει καὶ τέλος ἑαυτῷ συνεξομοιῶσαι τὸ ἀλλοιούμενον. εἰ δὲ ἐννοήσεις τὸν ἐκ τῆς κοιλίας ἀναλαμβανόμενον χυλὸν ἀλλοιούμενον ὑπὸ τῆς σαρκὸς τοῦ ἥπατος καὶ κατὰ βραχὺ μεθιστάμενον εἰς τὴν ἐκείνου φύσιν, παχύτερος ἑαυτοῦ καὶ ἐρυθρότερος ἐξ ἀνάγκης ἔσται πρὶν ὁμοιωθῆναι τελέως ἐκείνῃ.

[3] *Ibid.*, 299: ὥστ' εἴπερ τέλος μέν ἐστι τῇ σαρκὶ τοῦ ἥπατος ὁμοιῶσαι τὴν τροφὴν ἑαυτῇ, τοῦτο δ' ἀθρόως οὐκ ἐνδέχεται γενέσθαι, τὸ μέσον ἀμφοῖν ἔσται τὸ αἷμα, τοσούτῳ τῆς σαρκὸς τοῦ ἥπατος ἀπολειπόμενος, ὅσῳ πλεονεκτεῖ τοῦ κατὰ τὴν γαστέρα πεπεμμένου χυμοῦ.

[4] *De plac. Hipp. et Plat.* vi. 3, K. v. 521: τοιαύτης γὰρ δυνάμεως ἀρχὴ τὸ ἧπαρ, οἷα καὶ τοῖς φυτοῖς ὑπάρχει ... ὕστερον ἐπιδειξόντων ἡμῶν ἀκριβέστερον, ὡς πολλῶν ἐστι δυνάμεων ἀρχὴ τὸ ἧπαρ, καὶ κάλλιον οὐσίαν ψυχῆς ὀνομάζειν, οὐ δύναμιν ἐν ἑκάστῳ τῶν τριῶν σπλάγχνων περιεχομένην, ἐν ἐγκεφάλῳ μὲν λογιστικήν, ἐν καρδίᾳ δὲ θυμοειδῆ, κατὰ δὲ τὸ ἧπαρ ἐπιθυμητικήν, ἢ φυτικήν, ἢ γενετικήν, ἢ ὡς οἱ περὶ τὸν Ἀριστοτέλην θρεπτικήν.

[5] *Ibid.*, vi. 4, K. v. 534: φαίνεται γὰρ οὐχ ὡς ὑπηρέτης ἡγουμένῳ προπαρασκευάζων ἐπιτήδειον ὕλην τὸ ἧπαρ, ἀλλ' ὡς αὐτὸς ὁ ἡγούμενος ἐξουσίαν ἔχων τοῦ διανέμειν αὐτήν.

any rate through, the heart; of the former, only the amount necessary to feed the flesh of the lung, and to provide the blood-content of the arterial system, which contains very much less blood than the venous. Every part of the body below the diaphragm obtains its blood straight from the liver, and so also do the parts above. The diaphragm itself, the pericardium and the mediastinum all obtain their nourishment from the vena cava before it actually reaches the heart, and the upper parts of the body also obtain their nourishment from the vena cava, that is from the liver.[1] How then is the quantity needed to give nourishment to the upper parts of the body made to reach them? For the lower parts of the body, gravity no doubt helps, but the real force distributing the blood-supply is something quite different. The thing which really moves it is the power of attraction (ὁλκή) which every organ or tissue possesses. This quasi-magnetic power is strongest in the liver and the heart. The power of attraction is visualized by Galen as something nearly automatic. It does not involve the psychic or even the vital spirit. It can pull against gravity and its nature resembles the pull of the magnet or loadstone.[2]

In the treatise *On the natural faculties* Galen explains that there are two kinds of attraction: one of these is the power of the *horror vacui* of which Erasistratus made so many applications; the other is based on a kind of qualitative affinity or appropriateness of qualities. Air is attracted into bellows when they open by the former, iron by the magnet in accordance with the latter. Moreover the attraction which results from creating a vacuum acts primarily on what is light, whereas that resulting from appropriateness of qualities frequently acts on heavy bodies if they should be more appropriately related.[3] Now, just as the heart attracts blood and the liver the chylified nutriment contained in the veins coming from the stomach and the intestines, so every organ or tissue attracts from the blood the elements appropriate to its character. These elements are all derived from what has been eaten and drunk. What is left over after the stomach and the intestines have eliminated what we today would call

---

[1] Ibid., 535: πάντα γὰρ ὅσα κάτω τοῦ διαφράγματός ἐστι τοῦ ζῴου μόρια παρ' ἥπατος ἀναμφισβητήτως ἔχει τὸ αἷμα, καίτοι πλείω τῶν ἡμίσεών ἐστι. μᾶλλον δ' ὅτι καὶ αὐτὸ τὸ διάφραγμα καὶ ὁ περικάρδιος ὑμὴν ἅμα τοῖς ἄλλοις ὑμέσι τοῖς πλησίον, ὅσοι τε διαφράττουσι τὸν θώρακα, καὶ ὅσοι περιαλείφουσι τὸν πνεύμονα, τὴν τροφὴν ἐκ τῆς κοίλης ἔχει, πρὶν ἐπὶ τὴν καρδίαν ἀφικέσθαι, διδαχθῶμεν, ὑπὸ τῆς ἀνατομῆς εἰσόμεθα τὰ πλείω τῶν τοῦ ζῴου μορίων ἐξ ἥπατος τρεφόμενα προφανῶς τε καὶ ἀναμφισβητήτως. ἐπιδειχθήσεται μὲν γὰρ ... ὅτι καὶ τὸ ἄνω τῆς καρδίας ἅπαν ἐξ ἥπατος ἔχει τὴν τροφήν.

[2] No law of inverse squares for him; the scalp and the brain 'attract' their nutriment quite as powerfully and efficiently as any other part of the body.

[3] De nat. fac. iii. 15, K. ii. 206: δύο εἰσὶν ὁλκῆς εἴδη, τὸ μὲν τῇ πρὸς τὸ κενούμενον ἀκολουθίᾳ, τὸ δ' οἰκειότητι ποιότητος γιγνόμενον. ἑτέρως μὲν γὰρ εἰς τὰς φύσας ὁ ἀήρ, ἑτέρως δὲ ὁ σίδηρος ὑπὸ τῆς Ἡρακλείας ἐπισπᾶται λίθου καὶ ὡς ἡ μὲν πρὸς τὸ κενούμενον ἀκολουθία τὸ κουφότερον ἕλκει πρότερον, ἡ δὲ κατὰ τὴν τῆς ποιότητος οἰκειότητα πολλάκις, εἰ οὕτως ἔτυχε, τὸ βαρύτερον, ἂν τῇ φύσει συγγενέστερον ὑπάρχῃ.

waste products, the superfluities, is needed by the liver, and in the same
way the other parts of the body which are served by the venous system
receive in suitable form the blood that is left over when the liver has
nourished itself. For the liver changes the material it attracts from stomach
and intestines into something which is more suited to the parts to which
the blood is distributed after it leaves the liver. These attract into themselves the blood so prepared through the veins, namely those branching
off from the hollow vein, and render it more suitable for the parts which
are further away, by a kind of pre-digestion, and this process goes on
until the nutriment has reached every part of the body.[1] For each of the
organs of an animal is compounded of simpler parts, but they all have an
essence or substance (οὐσία) of their own, unlike that of any other of the
parts of the animal body; for example, the stomach, spleen, brain, kidney,
tongue, eyes, bladder, and womb, each have their own special character.[2]
So too arteries, veins, bones, and 'nerves', cartilages, ligaments, and fat,
each have their special pattern of being (εἶδος) and special function
(ἐνεργεία).[3]

How this rather complicated process works is far from clear, but the
movements of substances in the veins that it must entail are far from
constituting a one-way traffic. For the blood, before it can become a
suitable *Nährstoff* for all the other parts of the body, has to be purged of
certain superfluities, and there are three organs, and only three, which
nature has designed to do this, namely the gall-bladder, the kidneys, and
the spleen. The gall-bladder, being placed immediately adjacent to the
liver, provides no difficulties; it is able to draw off the excess of yellow
bile by its own special ducts. The way the spleen works is rather more
complicated. It is connected with the liver, not by a branch of the vena
cava but by a branch of the portal vein.[4] But it draws off from the blood
already manufactured in the liver the thick and earthy elements, or

[1] *De plac. Hipp. et Plat.* vi. 8, K. v. 567–8: ὥσπερ οὖν τὸ τῆς γαστρὸς λείψανον ἐπιτήδειον
γίνεται τῷ ἥπατι, κατὰ τὸν αὐτὸν τρόπον τοῖς μεθ' ἧπαρ ἅπασι τὸ τούτου πάλιν αὐτοῦ περιττόν. οὐδ'
οὖν αὐτοῦ τοῦ ἥπατος ἐκείνων ἕνεκεν ἀλλοιώσαντος τὴν τροφήν, ἀλλὰ καθ' ὃν εἴρηκα τρόπον,
ἡνίκα μεταβάλλοντός τε καὶ ἀλλοιοῦντος ἐπιτηδειότερα ἐν τῷδε γίγνεται τοῖς μεθ' ἧπαρ μορίοις. ὡς
γὰρ αὐτὸ διὰ τῶν φλεβῶν εἵλκυσεν ἐκ γαστρός τε καὶ τῶν ἐντέρων τὴν τροφήν, οὕτως, ὅσα μετ'
ἐκεῖνο τέτακται δι' ἄλλων ἕλκει φλεβῶν εἰς ἑαυτά, κἄπειτ' αὖθις ἕτερα, καὶ τοῦτο ὑπάρχει γιγνόμενον, ἄχρι περ ἂν εἰς ἅπαν ἀφίκηται τοῦ ζῴου μόριον ἡ τροφή, παρασκευάζει δ' ἕκαστον ἀεὶ καὶ
προπέττει τὸ μεθ' αὑτὸ κατὰ τὸ συνεχὲς τῆς διαδόσεως.

[2] Ibid., 568: οὕτως οὖν καὶ τὸ ἧπαρ παρομοιοῖ τὸν ἐκ τῆς κοιλίας ἀναδοθέντα χυλὸν ἑαυτῷ,
τοῦτ' ἔστι τῇ σαρκί τε καὶ τῇ οὐσίᾳ τῇ ἑαυτοῦ τῷ καλουμένῳ πρὸς ἐνίων ἰατρῶν παρεγχύματι.
ἕκαστον γὰρ τῶν ὀργανικῶν τοῦ ζῴου μορίων, σύνθετον ὑπάρχον ἐξ ἑτέρων μορίων, πάντως ἴδιόν
τι τοιοῦτον ὑπάρχει κατὰ τὴν οὐσίαν, οἷον οὐκ ἄλλο καθ' ὅλου τοῦ ζῴου τὸ σῶμα. τὸ γοῦν τῆς
γαστρὸς σῶμα τὸ ἴδιον, οἷον οὐκ ἄλλο τῶν πάντων ἐστίν. ὡσαύτως δὲ καὶ τὸ τοῦ σπληνός, ἐγκεφάλου
τε καὶ νεφρῶν, καὶ γλώττης, καὶ ὀφθαλμῶν, καὶ κύστεως καὶ μητρῶν.

[3] Ibid., 569: ὡσαύτως δὲ καὶ νεύρῳ καὶ φλεβὶ καὶ ὀστῷ καὶ χόνδρῳ καὶ ὑμένι καὶ συνδέσμῳ
καὶ πιμελῇ. κατὰ δὲ τὸ ἴδιον εἶδος ἑκάστης οὐσίας ἰδίαν ἀναγκαῖον εἶναι τὴν ἐνεργείαν.

[4] *De ven. et art. dissect.* 25, K. ii. 781: τῶν δὲ ἀξιολόγων ἀποφύσεων τῆς ἐπὶ πύλας φλεβός,
πρώτη μέν ἐστιν ἡ εἰς τὸ σιμὸν τῆς γαστρὸς φερομένη, δευτέρα δὲ ἡ εἰς τὸν σπλῆνα.

rather their superfluities, which the body does not require.[1] These waste products are therefore, according to Galen, not drawn off before they have reached the liver by the portal vein, but this vein draws them off after the blood has been formed in the liver. The portal vein for a portion of its course must therefore contain a two-way traffic, since the splenetic vein is one of its branches. In the matter of the kidneys also a two-way traffic in a part of the venous system seems to be implied. For if the urine is a superfluity or waste product of the blood, the blood must go into the kidneys by the renal vein, and out again by the same route. But this is not the end of the story. For the kidneys seem to perform a double function. Besides eliminating excess liquid from venous blood, they also purge the arterial blood of its excess of serous fluid. Here again, two-way traffic must be implied, and Erasistratus is chidden because he failed to realize the significance of the anatomical fact that the arteries leading into the small kidneys are as large as the very big veins leading into them. This would not have been the case if the arteries contained only *pneuma*.[2] In fact if we try to work out the route of the blood created by the liver in the various portions of the venous—and to a lesser degree, perhaps, the arterial—systems, the movements seem to become quite hopelessly complicated, that is, if the logic of Galen's physiological premisses is to be followed out to its paradoxical conclusions. For, on his principles, it would appear that *all* the blood created in the liver has to be purged by passing through the kidneys, as well as the arterial blood prepared in the left ventricle of the heart. Hence the large size of both kinds of blood vessels going into the kidney. Or can this task be left to the quasi-magnetic qualitative attraction? I rather think not. And even if this rather desperate way out is attempted, we still have a great deal of two-way traffic of materials, *pace* Fleming,[3] from the upper parts of the body, for example to the renal arteries and veins. Not that this raised any difficulties for Galen, for he regarded two-way traffic in the portal system as normal, indeed as essential. For the portal system, as well as drawing nutrition from the intestines and the stomach, has also to feed these organs. The same double function would seem to belong to the corresponding arteries. During long fasts a certain amount of nutriment drawn back from the liver into the stomach through the same veins by which it was presented to the liver during the absorptive process. The

---

[1] *De nat. fac.* ii. 9, K. ii. 138: τὸ γὰρ ἱκανῶς παχὺ καὶ γεῶδες καὶ τελέως διαπεφευγὸς τὴν ἐν ἥπατι μεταβολὴν ὁ σπλὴν εἰς ἑαυτὸν ἕλκει.

[2] *De usu partium*, v. 5, K. iii. 364: οὐκ ἂν ἔχοι λέγειν οὔτ' Ἐρασίστρατος οὔτ' ἄλλος τις, ὃς ἂν ἡγῆται πνεῦμα μόνον ἐν ἀρτηρίαις περιέχεσθαι, τὴν χρείαν τοῦ μεγέθους τῶν εἰς τοὺς νεφροὺς ἐμφυομένων ἀρτηριῶν, εἰ γὰρ δὴ τὰς φλέβας μόνον ἐκκαθαίρουσιν οἱ νεφροί, καὶ διὰ τοῦτο εἰς αὐτοὺς καίτοι σμικροὺς ὄντας μέγισται καταφύονται, τὰς ἀρτηρίας οὐκ ἐχρῆν ὁμοίως εἶναι ταῖς φλεψὶ μεγάλας.

[3] Fleming, op. cit.

veins situated between the liver and the stomach thus fulfil a double purpose. When the alimentary canal contains a lot of food, this is drawn up into the liver; when it is empty and in need of nutriment, the nutriment is again attracted away from the liver by the same veins. The mouths of the arteries supplying the intestines also take up a little food, but most is taken by the veins.[1] And if the arteries can take up food, presumably they can also return it, though it is not at all certain that Galen believed this, since the food elements carried by the arteries were probably too refined to satisfy any of the gross needs of the belly. It is therefore not at all surprising that Galen tells us that the blood in the veins does not move with great force, unlike that in the arteries. The reason which he gives for this fact is that the blood in the veins contains little or no *pneuma*, and that the veins which carry it do not pulsate.[2] Hydrodynamics was not exactly his strong suit.

Two points in connection with Galen's theory just described are perhaps worth noting. First, in this process of 'purging' of the blood, what takes place is not strictly speaking an elimination of 'waste products' but the extrusion of an excess of some humour which is a normal constituent of the healthy body. It is only the excess of yellow or of black bile that is accumulated in the gall-bladder and the spleen, and finally eliminated through the digestive tract. In the same way, it is only the excess of serous fluid in the blood that is eliminated through the kidneys. For the blood needs a certain amount of the thick and muddy substances composing the black bile just as it does the light, bitter elements composing the yellow bile,[3] and the watery elements providing the blood serum.[4] Galen's physiology is built up on the basis of the four 'Hippocratic' (or must we say Polybian?) humours. He does not adopt the Cnidian theory

[1] *De nat. fac.* iii. 13, K. ii. 188 f.: τούτου δ' ἔτι μᾶλλον οὐ χρὴ θαυμάζειν, εἰ δι' ὧν εἰς ἧπαρ ἀνεδόθη τι φλεβῶν ἐκ γαστρός, αὖθις εἰς αὐτὴν ἐξ ἥπατος ἐν ταῖς μακροτέραις ἀσιτίαις δύναται ἕλκεσθαι ἡ τροφή ... τί θαυμαστόν ἐστι διττὴν ὑπηρεσίαν τε καὶ χρείαν εἶναι ταῖς φλεψὶ ταῖς ἐν μέσῳ τεταγμέναις ἥπατός τε καὶ τῶν κατὰ τὴν κοιλίαν, ὥσθ' ὅποτε μὲν ἐν τούτοις ἄφθονος εἴη περιεχομένη τροφή, διὰ τῶν εἰρημένων εἰς ἧπαρ ἀναφέρεσθαι φλεβῶν, ὅποτε δ' εἴη κενὰ καὶ δεόμενα τρέφεσθαι διὰ τῶν αὐτῶν αὖθις ἐξ ἥπατος ἕλκεσθαι; Cf. *De usu partium*, iv. 17, K. iii. 329: τὰ καθήκοντα ἀρτηριῶν εἰς ἔντερα στόματα βραχύ τι τῆς τροφῆς ἀναλαμβάνει, τὸ δὲ πλεῖστον αἱ φλέβες.

[2] *De plac. Hipp. et Plat.* vi. 8, K. v. 573: τὸ μὲν γὰρ ἐξ ἥπατος ὁρμώμενον οὐ περιφέρεται σφοδρῶς, ὅτι μήτε πνευματῶδές ἐστι, μήθ' ὅλως σφύζουσιν αἱ περιέχουσαι φλέβες αὐτό.

[3] *De nat. fac.* 9, K. ii. 138: τῶν δ' εἰρημένων (χυμῶν) ἐστί τις χρεία τῇ φύσει, καὶ τοῦ παχέος καὶ τοῦ λεπτοῦ, καὶ καθαίρεται πρός τε τοῦ σπληνὸς καὶ τῆς ἐπὶ τῷ ἥπατι κύστεως τὸ αἷμα καὶ ἀποτίθεται τοσοῦτόν τε καὶ τοιοῦτον ἑκατέρου μέρους, ὅσον καὶ οἷον, εἴπερ εἰς ὅλον ἠνέχθη τοῦ ζῴου τὸ σῶμα, βλάβην ἡντιναοῦν εἰργάσατο. τὸ γὰρ ἱκανῶς παχὺ καὶ γεῶδες καὶ τελέως διαπεφευγὸς τὴν ἐν τῷ ἥπατι μεταβολὴν ὁ σπλὴν εἰς ἑαυτὸν ἕλκει. τὸ δ' ἄλλο τὸ μετρίως παχὺ σὺν τῷ κατειργάσθαι πάντῃ φέρεται. δεῖται γὰρ ἐν πολλοῖς τοῦ ζῴου μορίοις παχύτητός τινος τὸ αἷμα.

[4] *De usu partium*, iv. 6, K. iii. 273: ταύτας οὖν τὰς λεπτὰς ὑγρότητας, ὅταν τὸ σφέτερον ἔργον πληρώσωσιν, οὐκέτ' ἐν τῷ σώματι χρὴ μένειν ... καὶ ταύτης ἕνεκα τῆς χρείας οἱ νεφροὶ γεγόνασιν, ὄργανα κοῖλα στομάχοις τοῖς μὲν ἕλκοντα, τοῖς δ' ἐκπέμποντα τὸ λεπτὸν τοῦτο καὶ ὑδατῶδες περίττωμα. Cf. ibid. v. 6, K. iii. 371: καὶ μὴν εἴπερ αὐτάρκως μὲν οἱ ἀμφότεροι καθαίρουσι τὸν ὀρρὸν τοῦ αἵματος, ἔστι δὲ πολλαπλάσιον τὸ περίττωμα τοῦτο τῶν ἄλλων περιττωμάτων.

that bile and phlegm are as such the causes of disease. Both black and yellow bile are distributed by the veins normally, mixed with phlegm and blood in all healthy persons. All the four humours in the mother partake in the processes of reproduction and growth.[1]

Secondly, his acceptance of the idea, shared by the Pneumatists, that the arteries contain blood, does not, in default of any idea of circulation, enable him to give any more plausible account than Erasistratus did of the distribution of blood to the tissues throughout the body. The substitution of 'attraction' for the *horror vacui* does not really carry us any nearer to the truth. It is a kind of teleosmosis which can hardly be interpreted as an anticipation of any biochemical verities. For the *main* direction of the blood moving in the veins is for Galen, as for Erasistratus, away from not towards the heart. Blood flows out from the liver to the extremities both upwards and downwards, only a small proportion of it passing through the heart at all. The surprising thing is that Galen, master-dissector and expert in comparative anatomy, never discovered the valves in the veins. But even had he done so would he have recognized their significance? One cannot help suspecting from his general ignorance of elementary physics that he very well might have failed to do so.

We must now follow up the destiny of that portion of the blood which is drawn from the vena cava into the right ventricle. Part of it, as we have seen, goes through the artery-like vein, the pulmonary artery, to feed the lung. The rest passes through the invisible perforations in the interventricular septum into the left ventricle,[2] where it undergoes a profound change. The blood which enters the right ventricle is exactly the same in quality as that which has been produced in the liver and is distributed throughout the body by the veins.[3] That which comes out of the left ventricle and passes through the sigmoid valve into the aorta is very different, both in colour and in consistency. The arterial blood is much lighter and 'yellower', which we can translate best as 'brighter'.[4] Galen, with his long and copious practice of vivisection, had observed, as

---

[1] *De elementis ex Hippocrate*, ii. 5, K. i. 506: διὸ καὶ ὅσοι τῶν ἰατρῶν τε καὶ φυσικῶν ἐξ αἵματος μόνου γίνεσθαι καὶ τρέφεσθαι τὸ ζῷον ἀπεφήναντο, ... ἀλλ' Ἱπποκράτης φυσικώτερον ἔτι καὶ τούτων ἐκ τῶν τεττάρων χυμῶν καὶ τὴν γένεσιν, καὶ τὴν αὔξησιν, καὶ τὴν θρέψιν εἶναί φησι τοῖς σώμασιν ἡμῶν ... Cf. *De simp. men. temp. et fac.* x. 13, K. xii. 275: ἔμαθες γὰρ εἶναι τοὺς πάντας ἐν ἑκάστῳ τῶν ἐναίμων ζώων χυμοὺς τέτταρας, αἷμα καὶ φλέγμα καὶ χολὴν ξανθήν τε καὶ μέλαιναν.

[2] *De nat. fac.* iii. 15, K. ii. 207–8: ὡσαύτως δὲ καὶ κατ' αὐτὴν τὴν καρδίαν ἐκ τῆς δεξιᾶς κοιλίας εἰς τὴν ἀριστερὰν ἕλκεται τὸ λεπτότατον ἔχοντός τινα τρήματα τοῦ μέσου διαφράγματος αὐτῶν.

[3] *De plac. Hipp. et Plat.* vi. 4, K. v. 537: ὅμοιον γὰρ τό τ' ἐν τῇ δεξιᾷ κοιλίᾳ τῆς καρδίας αἷμα καὶ τὸ κατὰ πάσας τὰς φλέβας ὅλῳ τῷ ζῴῳ καθάπερ γε καὶ τὸ κατὰ τὰς ἀρτηρίας ἁπάσας ὅμοιόν ἐστι τῷ κατὰ τὴν ἀριστερὰν κοιλίαν.

[4] Galen, *De locis affectis*, i. 1, K. viii. 5: τὸ δ' ἐξακοντιζόμενον αἷμα σφυγμωδῶς ἀρτηρίαν (τετρῶσθαι σημαίνει)· εὐθὺς δὲ τοῦτο καὶ θερμότερόν ἐστι καὶ λεπτομερέστερον καὶ ξανθότερον τοῦ κατὰ τὰς φλέβας.

Aristotle had before him, the difference in colour between arterial and venous blood. He had also noticed that blood spurts out of a cut artery, whereas the flow from a cut vein is steady and slower. Nor was he inaccurate in observing the pits (βόθυνοι) in the interventricular septum. His historic error, as recent examinations of a minute nature have shown, lay not so much in assuming that these pits ended in perforations or small channels (τρήματα),[1] as in supposing that a large quantity of blood could pass by these channels from the right to the left ventricle. The traditional legend taught to every schoolboy of these non-existent passages, whose non-existence was first pointed out by Vesalius, is in fact far from accurate. For since the time of Vieussens and Thebesius, their existence has been known and in recent times been investigated by several physiologists interested in the minutiae of the cardiacal circulation.[2] Blood vessels forming a continuous passage larger than capillaries do exist in the septum of the human heart, but their haemodynamic significance is minimal. It was perhaps an inevitable result of the revolution caused in physiological thought by Harvey's discovery that they should have been, with certain exceptions,[3] overlooked for nearly three centuries. To Galen the existence of these passages seemed to be proved, or at any rate confirmed, by the fact that the vena cava, whose termination is the right auricle, is much larger than the 'vein' which leads out of the right ventricle, the pulmonary artery, a fact which he interpreted to mean that not all the blood which enters the right ventricle from the vena cava is expelled into the lungs. Some of it must therefore be supposed to pass directly into the left ventricle.[4] In the absence of any

---

[1] De nat. fac. iii. 15, K. ii. 208: τρήματα ... ἃ μέχρι μὲν πλείστου δυνατὸν ἰδεῖν, οἷον βοθύνους τινὰς ἐξ εὐρυτάτου στόματος ἀεὶ καὶ μᾶλλον εἰς στενώτερον προϊόντας. οὐ μὴν αὐτά γε τὰ ἔσχατα πέρατα δυνατὸν ἔτι θεάσασθαι διά τε σμικρότητα, καὶ ὅτι τεθνεῶτος ἤδη τοῦ ζῴου κατέψυκταί τε καὶ πεπύκνωται πάντα.

[2] For a recent description of these 'anastomoses', see an article (to which my attention was drawn by Walter Pagel) by Gerhard Richter, entitled 'Morphologische Besonderheiten der Herzscheidewand und ihre historische Bewertung', Arch. f. Gesch. d. Med. xlix (1965), 391–400. These peculiarities of the septum, though not universally present, would appear to be relatively common. Thus Richter writes (op. cit., p. 392): 'An 5 von 28 normalen Erwachsenherzen, ... ließen sich durch Tuscheinjektion sog. transeptale Anastomosen zwischen dem rechten und dem linken Ventrikel nachweisen. Ihre Existenz verdanken sie der Kommunikation der vasa minima profunda untereinander. Diese Anastomosen haben keineswegs — wie man annehmen könnte — nur den Durchmesser von Kapillaren. Neben histologischen Untersuchungen läßt sich auch die Tatsache belegen, daß bereits bei einem geringerem Injektionsdrucke, der etwa den physiologischen Verhältnissen entspricht, eine beträchtliche Menge der Injektionsflüssigkeit vom rechten in den linken Ventrikel gelangt.'

[3] Notably, inter alios, Gassendi, Swedenborg, and von Haller in the seventeenth and eighteenth centuries and Abernethy, who wrote a paper on them entitled 'Observations on the foramina in the basin of the heart', Phil. Trans. Soc., 1798.

[4] De nat. fac. iii. 15, K. ii. 208–9: δεύτερον δὲ κἀκ τοῦ, δυοῖν ὄντοιν στομάτοιν ἐν τῇ δεξιᾷ τῆς καρδίας κοιλίᾳ, τοῦ μὲν εἰσάγοντος τὸ αἷμα πολλῷ μείζονος, τοῦ δ' ἐξάγοντος ἥττονος, πολλῷ μεῖζον εἶναι τὸ τοῦ εἰσάγοντος. ὡς γὰρ οὐ παντὸς τοῦ αἵματος, ὅσον ἡ κοίλη φλὲψ δίδωσι τῇ

quantitative indication, it is not possible to know how much blood passed this way, but I am inclined to believe that it was the whole of the arterial blood, for reasons that I have already indicated. The blood passing into the lungs was all used up as food for that vigorous and therefore hungry organ. Moreover the amount of blood in the arterial system was universally regarded as small compared with that contained in the venous. It would appear that Galen was therefore not quite as wrong as has been supposed.

Galen's account of what happens to the blood which enters the right ventricle was, as we have already seen, far from consistent. The innate heat, he told us, breaks up, dissolves, and disperses the thick or earthy elements in the blood already in the right ventricle, for it is only the lighter type of blood which can pass through the interstices of the porous septum.¹ These combustion products of the thicker and earthier elements seem to be the source of the sooty superfluities (περιττώματα) which are generated by the excess of vital heat in the heart and evacuated to the lungs by the insufficient mitral valve, the one with only two membranes.² If so, it is clear that they must also pass through the interventricular septum with the purified blood into the left ventricle. But these superfluities are mostly produced in the left ventricle.

The doctrine of Galen on these matters is not always easy to follow. In the treatise *On the opinions of Hippocrates and Plato* we have rather a different picture. Galen here tells us, in a passage we have already quoted,³ that the blood in the right ventricle is the same as that in all the veins, while that in the arteries all over the body is the same as that in the left ventricle. After telling us the well-known traditional difference between the two types of blood—that that in the veins is thicker and darker—he adds rather a curious footnote that sometimes it is not. The arterial blood may sometimes be thicker than the venous, but it is always hotter. The blood in the right ventricle receives nothing special in

καρδίᾳ, πάλιν ἐξ ἐκείνης ἐκπεμπομένου τῷ πνεύμονι, μείζων ἐστὶν ἡ ἀπὸ τῆς κοίλης εἰς αὐτὴν ἔμφυσις, τῆς ἐμφυομένης εἰς τὸν πνεύμονα φλεβός. οὐδὲ γὰρ τοῦτ᾽ ἐστιν εἰπεῖν, ὡς ἐδαπανήθη τι τοῦ αἵματος εἰς τὴν αὐτοῦ τοῦ σώματος τῆς καρδίας θρέψιν ... εἰ δὲ καὶ δαπανᾶταί τι, ἀλλ᾽ οὐ τοσοῦτόν γε μείων ἐστὶν ἡ εἰς τὸν πνεύμονα φλὲψ ἄγουσα τῆς εἰς τὴν καρδίαν ἐμφυομένης, ὅσον εἰκὸς εἰς τροφὴν ἀνηλῶσθαι τῆς καρδίας, ἀλλὰ πλέονι πολλῷ. δῆλον οὖν ὡς εἰς τὴν ἀριστερὰν μεταλαμβάνεται κοιλίαν.

¹ *De usu partium*, vi. 17, K. iii. 496: οἱ τοίνυν ἐν τῇ καρδίᾳ φαινόμενοι βόθυνοι κατὰ τὸ μέσον αὐτῆς μάλιστα διάφραγμα τῆς εἰρημένης ἕνεκα κοινωνίας ἐγένοντο. τά τε γὰρ ἄλλα καὶ προκατειργασμένον ἐν ταῖς φλεψὶ τὸ αἷμα μεταλαμβάνειν ταῖς ἀρτηρίαις ἦν ἄμεινον, ἵν᾽ ὅπερ ἡ γαστὴρ πρὸς τὰς φλέβας, τοῦτ᾽ ἐκεῖνα πρὸς τὰς ἀρτηρίας ὦσιν.

² Ibid., 15, 485–6: εὐλόγως οὖν ἐφ᾽ ἑνὸς μόνου τοῦ στόματος τοῦ τῆς φλεβώδους ἀρτηρίας δυοῖν ἐμφύσεις ὑμένων ἐγένοντο, μόνῳ γὰρ τούτῳ βέλτιον ἦν οὐκ ἀκριβῶς κλείεσθαι, διότι καὶ μόνῳ συγχωρεῖν ἦν ἄμεινον εἰς τὸν πνεύμονα φέρεσθαι τοῖς ἐκ τῆς καρδίας λιγνυώδεσι περιττώμασιν, ἃ διὰ μὲν τὸ πλῆθος τῆς ἐμφύτου θερμασίας ἀναγκαῖον ἴσχειν αὐτῇ, συντομωτέραν δ᾽ ἑτέραν οὐκ εἶχεν ἐκροήν.

³ See above, p. 333, n. 3.

addition from the ventricle itself.[1] This would not, however, exclude a different kind of change involving abstraction rather than addition. Where then does the change from 'venous' to 'arterial' blood take place? In the right or in the left ventricle? The answer would appear to be in both. The liver-blood has some of its 'impurities' removed by the innate heat in the right ventricle, and the blood which passes to the left ventricle through the septum already possesses some of the arterial blood's characteristics. It contains only the lighter elements—but the main process of transformation takes place in the left ventricle, which is the principal source of the innate heat.

What happens to it, then, when it passes to the left ventricle? Here, it would appear, it meets with the *pneuma* which has been drawn into the left ventricle through the respiratory passages. This brings us up against one of the most difficult problems in Galen's physiology. What is the relation between the blood and the *pneuma* in the left ventricle, and how has the *pneuma* reached the heart? To obtain a consistent account of these matters seems to be impossible. The theory found in the main treatises is, however, quite clear. The left ventricle contains a mixture of blood and *pneuma*, or some other form of coexistence of these two substances. This is indicated by the fact that the vein-like artery, the pulmonary vein, is much smaller than the aorta. For the pulmonary vein only conveys *pneuma* to the heart, while the aorta conveys both *pneuma* and blood out of it. 'And in the same way the artery which carries the *pneuma* from the lung to the heart is also much smaller than the great artery [just as the pulmonary artery is much smaller than the vena cava] out of which all the arteries of the body grow, since it receives some addition of blood from the right ventricle';[2] a passage which seems to imply that no blood passes into the heart through the pulmonary vein. But in what form the combination or coexistence of these two substances in the heart and arteries consisted is anything but clear. *Pneuma*, which is simply air when it is drawn into the nostrils, is taken into the body in respiration, some of it goes straight to the brain, but most of it to the lungs and from there to the left ventricle of the heart. *Pneuma* also enters the body by quite a different

---

[1] *De plac. Hipp. et Plat.* vi. 4, K. v. 537: τὸ δὲ κατὰ τὴν δεξιὰν κοιλίαν αἷμα τὴν αὐτὴν ἰδέαν ἔχει τῷ τ' ἄλλῳ παντὶ καὶ τῷ κατὰ τὸ ἧπαρ, ὡς ἂν οὐδὲν ἐξαίρετον ἐπικτώμενον ἐν τῇ δεξιᾷ κοιλίᾳ.

[2] *De usu partium*, vi. 17, K. iii. 497 f.: ταῦτ' οὖν ἅπαντα καθ' ὅλον τε τοῦ ζῴου τὸ σῶμα καὶ πρὸ τούτων ἐν αὐτῇ τῇ καρδίᾳ καλῶς ἡ φύσις ἅπαντα παρεσκευάσατο, τὴν κοινωνίαν ἐξευροῦσα ταῖς φλεψὶ πρὸς τὰς ἀρτηρίας διὰ τῶν λεπτῶν ἐκείνων στομάτων. καὶ διὰ τοῦτο μείζων ἐστὶν ἡ εἰς αὐτὴν ἐμφυομένη φλὲψ τῆς ἐκφυομένης, καίτοι κεχυμένον γε τὸ αἷμα διὰ τὴν ἐν αὐτῇ θερμασίαν ὑποδεχομένης· ἀλλ' ἐπεὶ πολὺ κατὰ τὸ μέσον διάφραγμα καὶ τὰς ἐν αὐτῷ διατρήσεις εἰς τὴν ἀριστερὰν μεταλαμβάνεται κοιλίαν, εὐλόγως ἡ εἰς τὸν πνεύμονα φλὲψ ἐμφυομένη τῆς εἰσαγούσης εἰς τὴν καρδίαν τὸ αἷμα μείων ἐστί. ὡσαύτως δὲ καὶ ἡ ἐκ τοῦ πνεύμονος εἰς τὴν καρδίαν ἀρτηρία παράγουσα τὸ πνεῦμα καὶ αὐτὴ πολὺ μείων ἐστὶ τῆς μεγάλης ἀρτηρίας, ἀφ' ἧς αἱ κατὰ τὸ σῶμα πεφύκασιν ἅπασαι, διότι τε προσλαμβάνει τι τοῦ παρὰ τῆς δεξιᾶς κοιλίας αἵματος ἡ μεγάλη ἀρτηρία, καὶ διότι πασῶν ἔμελλεν ἀρχὴ γενήσεσθαι τῶν καθ' ὅλον τὸ ζῷον ἀρτηριῶν.

route, via the skin into the arteries when they expand.[1] The arteries
therefore also contain both blood and air or *pneuma*, but here the difficulty
begins to arise. Do the arteries contain a double source of *pneuma*, the
heart and the skin? For when the left ventricle contracts and expels its
contents into the aorta, we should expect the mixture of blood and *pneuma*
contained in it to pass into the arteries. But this does not appear to
happen. For though the blood passes into the arteries through the aortal
valve—how it can do so is a bit of a mystery, since when it opens at
systole the arteries are also contracted—the *pneuma*, together with the
combustion-products produced by the operation of the innate heat on the
venous blood, passes up to the lungs again through the insufficient
mitral valve and, owing to the pressure of the thorax, passes through the
windpipe and the mouth and out again into the air on expiration.

Both the heart and the arteries pulsate, and, as we have already noted,
the power of pulsation comes to the arteries from the heart. The process of
pulsation is twofold. When the heart and the arteries dilate at diastole,
they draw in air from the lungs and the skin for three purposes, namely
(a) the cooling of the innate heat in the heart, (b) ventilation, the supply
of air or *pneuma* to maintain this innate fire, and (c) the generation of
the psychic or animal spirit.[2] When heart and arteries contract simultaneously at systole, they expel waste products generated in them from
the blood and the humours.

We have demonstrated that the sooty superfluity is generated in the blood
by the innate heat, and in greatest quantity when it is hotter. There is then
clearly a need for its elimination, and nature has provided a technique for
supplying this need, superfluities from the heart being eliminated by expiration, and those generated throughout the body by the contraction of the arteries.
The superfluities from the arteries as well as those from the veins—for the
veins were demonstrated to have synanastomoses with the arteries—are straightway excreted through the skin, being pressed out by the systole of the arteries.[3]

One of the points to be noticed in connection with this theory is the
apparent identification of *pneuma* with air, which should never be lost

[1] De nat. fac. iii. 14, K. ii. 204: θαυμαστὸν οὐδέν σοι φανεῖται τὰς ἀρτηρίας, ὅσαι μὲν εἰς τὸ δέρμα
περαίνουσιν αὐτῶν, ἐπισπᾶσθαι τὸν ἔξωθεν ἀέρα διαστελλομένας.
[2] De plac. Hipp. et Plat. viii. 8, K. v. 708–9: τὸ δὲ ἕτερον ὃ καλεῖται σφυγμός, ὑπό τε τῆς καρδίας
καὶ τῶν ἀρτηριῶν γίγνεται, τῇ μὲν διαστολῇ διὰ τῶν εἰς τὸ δέρμα καθηκόντων στομάτων ἑλκουσῶν
τῶν ἀρτηριῶν εἰς τὸ σῶμα τὸν ἔξωθεν ἀέρα τριῶν ἕνεκα χρειῶν, ἐμψύξεως, ῥιπίσεως, γενέσεως
πνεύματος ψυχικοῦ, τῇ συστολῇ δ' ἐκθλιβουσῶν ὅσον αἰθαλῶδες ἢ καπνῶδες ἐγεννήθη κατ' αὐτὰς
τῶν χυμῶν.
[3] Comment. VI in Hipp. epidem. VI, sect. 6, K. xviiB. 317: διὰ τὴν ἔμφυτον θερμασίαν ἐδείξαμεν
γεννᾶσθαι τὸ λιγνυῶδες περίττωμα κατὰ τὸ αἷμα, καὶ μάλισθ' ὅταν ᾖ θερμότερον· ἀποκρίσεως
οὖν αὐτῷ χρεία δηλονότι, καὶ ταύτην ἡ φύσις ἐτεχνήσατο τοῖς μὲν ἐκ τῆς καρδίας ἐκκριθησομένοις
διὰ τῆς ἐκπνοῆς τοῖς δὲ καθ' ὅλον τὸ σῶμα διὰ τῆς τῶν ἀρτηριῶν συστολῆς. τὰ μὲν ἐκ τούτων τε
καὶ τῶν φλεβῶν, ἐδείχθησαν γὰρ αὐταῖς συνανεστομωμέναι, διὰ τοῦ δέρματος εὐθέως ἐκκρίνεται
τῇ συστολῇ τῶν ἀρτηριῶν ἐκθλιβόμενα.

sight of. *Pneuma* has, even according to the schoolboy's Liddell and Scott, a number of different though related meanings, such as 'a blowing', 'a wind', 'a blast', 'breeze, odour, scent, breathed air, breath', besides the later or less classical meanings of 'spirit', 'ghost', and 'inspiration'; why therefore not just 'oxygen'? But however tempting it may be to interpret Galen's *pneuma* in the light of Lavoisier's discoveries, this would be highly misleading. For all that, the ancient Greek theories of respiration some-times appear to be almost uncannily anticipative.

That the arteries contain both blood and *pneuma* is sufficiently authenti-cated, but how are these combined? Here difficulties of interpretation at once arise. What exactly is it that the arteries contain? Blood certainly, and *pneuma*, but is this *pneuma* just air, or is it a different though related substance derived from air? And what is its relation to the blood? It is, I think, impossible, as some commentators of recent date, notably Hall,[1] have pointed out, to find any single consistent answer to these questions in the very large number of different writings. The best we can do, then, is to follow up certain, by no means always consistent lines of argument which Galen uses.

Let us begin by examining his views on the relation between blood and *pneuma* in the arteries. Do they just exist side by side, and if so, in what form? As separate layers, as it were, or is there a more intimate mixture, or is the *pneuma* entirely absorbed by the blood? That blood and *pneuma* simply exist side by side would seem to be natural enough, but Galen may have to look for a more intimate connection. For he denies that any *pneuma* can be seen to escape from a cut artery when arguing against Erasistratus' theory of the escape of *pneuma* previous to the emergence of blood. I am not at all convinced, however, that he might not have ad-mitted that some *pneuma* escapes from a cut artery *with* the blood. Siegel seems to me to be claiming too much when he says: 'It was one of his great discoveries that blood vessels never contain any free air.'[2] For in one passage, Galen actually speaks of blood and *pneuma* being in the arteries without fighting with each other.[3] We find quite frequent allusions to a mixture of blood and *pneuma* in the arteries, but it would, I think, be rather misleading to interpret this as a 'solution' of *pneuma* in the blood, since, as Hall points out, it is inconsistent with his theory of the inter-change of blood and *pneuma* through the capillary system.[1] Moreover, it is also difficult to reconcile with the theory of arterial respiration just described. Did Galen really believe that all the *pneuma* absorbed by the arteries was immediately dissolved or taken up by the blood in the arterial system? And what about the *pneuma* absorbed by the left ventricle

---

[1] Hall, op. cit.

[2] In the article published in *Arch. f. Gesch. d. Med.* (1962).

[3] *De sanguine in arteriis*, 6, K. iv. 723: ... καὶ πῶς ἀμάχει δύναται συνεῖναι τὸ αἷμα τῷ πνεύματι.

at each diastole? Hall, while maintaining that Galen's denial of the Erasistratan theory of the escape of *pneuma* could be accounted for by the belief
that the *pneuma* was dissolved in the blood, which would thus be the
vehicle of the *pneuma* taken up by the blood in the left ventricle, nevertheless concludes that 'There is no evidence that Galen entertained this
conception and much (particularly in his account of the anastomoses
between veins and arteries) to indicate that he did not'. For the chief
function of these anastomoses, as we have seen,[1] was to effect the inter-
change between blood and *pneuma*, which could hardly be conceived if
the *pneuma* was dissolved in the blood.

The question indeed of the taking up of air or *pneuma* by the heart
points to a fundamental ambiguity in Galen's teaching, which no logical
juggle can turn into a consistent structure. In several passages, both in the
important physiological treatise *On the use of the parts* and in the essay *On
the opinions of Hippocrates and Plato*, he appears to have no doubt at all that
air is actually drawn into the left ventricle of the heart from the atmosphere through the lungs, but in others he seems to imply that little or
none of the inspired air actually reaches the heart. Some of these passages
must now be examined in detail.

In the sixth book of *On the opinions of Hippocrates and Plato*, Chapter three,
after describing the aorta, he speaks of 'another artery coming out of the
same ventricle of the heart, the one that divides up into branches in the
lung, just as the roots of a plant do in the earth'. For as plants draw all
their nourishment from the earth through their roots, so the heart draws
air from the lungs through the said arteries.[2] Nothing could very well be
plainer than this statement. So too in the treatise *On the use of the parts*,
there are several statements equally uncompromising. 'The need for
respiration in animals has been shown to arise from the heart, since the
heart somehow needs some of the substance of the air, but mostly because
it wants to be cooled because of the boiling heat.'[3] 'The heart draws
pneuma not immediately from the outside, but through the lungs and
expels it back into them.'[4] 'Indeed, nature made the heart one of the

---

[1] See above, p. 283.

[2] *De plac. Hipp. et Plat.* vi. 3, K. v. 524–5: καὶ πρῶτον μὲν ἐπίσκεψαι τὴν μεγίστην ἀρτηρίαν,
ἥτις ὥσπερ πρέμνον ἐκφύουσα τῆς καρδίας διασχίζεται, τῷ μὲν ἑτέρῳ μέρει τῷ μικροτέρῳ πρὸς
τὴν κεφαλὴν ἀναφερομένη, θατέρῳ δὲ τῷ μείζονι κατὰ τῆς ῥάχεως ἐκτεταμένη. θέασαι δ' ἐξῆς ἅπαντ'
αὐτῆς τὰ βλαστήματα πάντοσε τοῦ σώματος φερόμενα, καθ' ὃν ἐν τῷ πρώτῳ γράμματι λέλεκται
τρόπον, ἑτέραν δ' ἀρτηρίαν ἐκ τῆς αὐτῆς κοιλίας τῆς καρδίας ἐκφερομένην, τὴν εἰς τὸν πνεύμονα
κατασχιζομένην ἀνάλογον τῷ καθήκοντι μέρει τῆς ῥιζώσεως εἰς τὴν γῆν. ὥσπερ γὰρ ἐκ τῆς γῆς
τὰ φυτὰ διὰ τῶν ῥιζῶν ἅπασαν ἐπισπᾶται τὴν τροφήν, οὕτως ἐκ τοῦ πνεύμονος ἡ καρδία τὸν ἀέρα
διὰ τῶν εἰρημένων ἀρτηριῶν.

[3] *De usu partium*, vi. 2, K. iii. 412: ἡ χρεία τῆς ἀναπνοῆς τοῖς ζῴοις ἐδείχθη διὰ τὴν καρδίαν
γίγνεσθαι, τὸ μέν πού τι δεομένην καὶ αὐτὴν τοῦ ἀέρος τῆς οὐσίας, τὸ δέ τι πλεῖστον ὑπὸ θερμότητος
ζεούσης ἀναψύχεσθαι ποθοῦσαν.

[4] Ibid., 414: οὔτ' ἔξωθεν εὐθύς, ἀλλ' ἐκ τοῦ πνεύμονός τε καὶ εἰς τὸν πνεύμονα τήν θ' ὁλκὴν
τοῦ πνεύματος ἡ καρδία καὶ αὖθις τὴν ἔκπεμψιν ποιεῖται.

respiratory organs, though not the only one. She clothed the heart with the lung.'[1] 'Respiration supplies the cold quality to the heart and breathing out enables it to discharge the boiling and as it were smoky products of combustion.'[2] Moreover, as we have already noted,[3] the whole structure of the heart with the thicker wall of the left ventricle was designed because it was to contain *pneuma*; and the intimate connection of the trachea and the bronchial system with the pulmonary veins, that is of the 'rough' with the 'smooth' arteries, is explained by the fact that the rough arteries provide for the respiratory needs of the heart through the smooth arteries (the pulmonary veins).[4] The smooth arteries all converge into a single channel opening into the left ventricle, the source of the innate heat, in order to provide a continuous cooling to the heart.[5] When the lung expands, only air is drawn in through the throat into the hard arteries, and from the right ventricle only blood goes into the veins, but from the left comes something that is a mixture of both. Before describing the mechanics of respiration, he recalls, in words almost identical with those presented in the third book of *On the natural faculties*, which we shall quote later in this chapter,[6] the application of the 'law' of the *horror vacui* to the expansion of the lungs as the result of the movement of the thorax. This 'law' states that when a vacuum is created, the lighter elements are first drawn in to fill it before the heavier ones, and more readily through a wide than through a narrow opening.[7] Applied to pulmonary expansion this means that the contents drawn into the lung from the heart and blood vessels will be as just indicated, first air through the hard arteries, then air mixed with blood from the left ventricle, and, finally, (heavy) blood from the right ventricle and the veins.[8]

---

[1] *De usu partium*, vi. 2, K. iii. 414: διὰ ταῦτα μὲν οὖν ἡ φύσις οὐκ αὐτὴν μόνην τὴν καρδίαν ἀναπνευστικὸν ἐποίησεν ὄργανον, ἀλλ᾽ ἔξωθεν αὐτῇ περιέθηκε πνεύμονα.

[2] *Ibid.*, 412: ἀναψύχει δ᾽ αὐτὴν (τὴν καρδίαν) ἡ μὲν εἰσπνοὴ χορηγίᾳ ποιότητος ψυχρᾶς, ἡ δ᾽ ἐκπνοὴ τοῦ ζέοντος ἐν αὐτῇ καὶ οἷον συγκεκαυμένου καὶ λιγνυώδους ἀποχύσει.

[3] See above, p. 274.

[4] *De usu partium*, vii. 8, K. iii. 543: ἑκατέραις γὰρ αὐταῖς ἔδει πλησιάζειν, τῇ μὲν λείᾳ διότι τὴν χρείαν τῆς ἐκπνοῆς τῇ καρδίᾳ διὰ μέσης ἐκείνης ἡ τραχεῖα παρέχει.

[5] *Ibid.*, 545: ὅτι μὲν οὖν τὰς λείας ἀρτηρίας ἁπάσας εἰς μίαν ἀρχὴν ἀνεστόμωσε τὴν ἀριστερὰν κοιλίαν τῆς καρδίας ἵνα περ ἡ τῆς ἐμφύτου θερμασίας ἐστὶν ἀρχή, κατὰ τοῦτο μὲν ὡς ἀνάψυξιν συνεχῆ τῇ καρδίᾳ παρασκευάσασαν αὐτὴν (τὴν φύσιν) ἐπαινεῖσθαι δίκαιον.

[6] *De nat. fac.* iii. 15, K. ii. 207: see below, p. 368, n. 1.

[7] *De usu partium*, vii. 9, K. iii. 546: ὅτι μὲν οὖν ὁ πνεύμων ἅπασαν ἐκπεπλήρωκε τὴν εὐρυχωρίαν τοῦ θώρακος, καὶ ὡς, εἴτε διαστέλλοιτο, συνδιαστέλλεται κατὰ πᾶν καὶ αὐτός, εἴτε συστέλλοιτο συστέλλεται, ἐν τοῖς περὶ κινήσεως αὐτῶν ἔμαθες ὑπομνήμασιν. ἀλλὰ καὶ ὡς τοῖς ἕλκουσιν ἅπασιν ὀργάνοις τῇ πρὸς τὸ κενούμενον ἀκολουθίᾳ πρότερον ἕπεται τοῦ βαρυτέρου τὸ κουφότερον, καὶ ὡς διὰ τῶν εὐρυτέρων στομάτων ἑτοιμότερον αὐτοῖς πληροῦσθαι, καὶ ταῦτα ἐν ἐκείνοις ἔμαθες.

[8] *Ibid.*, 546–7: καὶ μέν γε καὶ ὡς τῶν μὲν τραχειῶν ἀρτηριῶν ἓν ἁπασῶν ἂν εἴη στόμα μέγιστον, ἀνέχον εἰς τὴν φάρυγγα, τῶν δὲ λείων ἕτερον ἓν εἰς τὴν ἀριστερὰν κοιλίαν τῆς καρδίας, ὥσπερ γε καὶ τῶν φλεβῶν εἰς τὴν δεξιάν, καὶ ὡς ἐκ μὲν τῆς φάρυγγος ἀὴρ ἕλκεται μόνος εἰς τὰς τραχείας

For when the lung is expanded, the first thing that will follow to fill up the vacuum will be the lightest element, namely the atmospheric air, which will fill the rough arteries. The second to follow will be the contents of the left ventricle of the heart, which will fill the smooth arteries. Third and last the blood will follow. But before the rough arteries are completely filled with *pneuma* it is not possible for any portion of the other two to be taken in. Moreover, since this is so, it would only be possible for anything to pass from the heart into the smooth arteries and the veins, if the thorax was still in process of expanding, and the rough arteries had already reached their maximum expansion. But if the thorax stopped expanding at the exact moment that they had reached their maximum distension, there would no longer be any time left for either the smooth arteries or the veins to expand in. For since the lung would no longer be expanding because the thorax had ceased to expand, none of its parts could make any expansion. It is therefore clear that if we can prove that when the rough arteries alone are expanded, the lung receives its maximum expansion, it would be proved that they alone are filled by the act of breathing in.[1]

The meaning of this passage is anything but clear, and has been interpreted by Renaissance commentators in a way which to me at any rate seems quite fantastic. Thus Riolanus,[2] Spigelius,[3] and Laurentius,[4] among others, assert consistently that the third function of the pulmonary veins is to carry *arterial* blood to the lung, the other two being to carry air to the heart and to remove 'soot' from it via the lungs. Did Galen really think that the movement of the expansion of the thorax pulled blood and *pneuma* out of the heart's ventricles? I find it difficult to believe that he could have entertained such an idea, even in view of his complete misunderstanding of the way in which the mitral valve functions. It seems to me that Galen is merely putting a hypothetical consequence forward,

ἀρτηρίας, ἐκ δὲ τῆς δεξιᾶς κοιλίας αἷμα μόνον εἰς τὰς φλέβας, ἐκ δὲ τῆς ἀριστερᾶς ἐξ ἀμφοῖν τι μικτόν. εἰ δὴ ταῦτα μνημονεύοις ἅπαντα συνθεὶς αὐτά, ῥᾳδίως ἐξευρήσεις τοῦ προκειμένου τὴν ἀπόδειξιν.

[1] Ibid., 547–8: διαστελλομένου γὰρ τοῦ πνεύμονος, πρῶτον μὲν ἀκολουθήσει τὸ κουφότατον, ὅ δή ἐστιν ὁ ἔξωθεν ἀήρ, καὶ πληρώσει τὰς τραχείας ἀρτηρίας· δεύτερον δὲ τὸ ἐκ τῆς ἀριστερᾶς κοιλίας τῆς καρδίας, καὶ πληρώσει τὰς λείας· ἔσχατον δὲ καὶ τρίτον ἐπὶ τούτοις τὸ αἷμα· πρὶν δὲ τὰς τραχείας ἀρτηρίας τελέως πληρωθῆναι πνεύματος, εἰς οὐδέτερον τῶν ἄλλων ἐνδέχεταί τι μεταληφθῆναι, καὶ μήν, εἴπερ τοῦθ' οὕτως ἔχει, μόνως ἂν οὕτως ἐγχωρήσειεν εἴς τε τὰς λείας ἀρτηρίας καὶ τὰς φλέβας εἰσρυῆναί τι παρὰ τῆς καρδίας εἰ διαστέλλοιτο μὲν ὁ θώραξ ἔτι, φθάνοιεν δ' ἔχειν ἤδη τὴν μεγίστην αἱ τραχεῖαι διάστασιν. εἰ δ' ἅμα μὲν ὁ θώραξ παύοιτο διαστελλόμενος, ἅμα δ' ἐκεῖναι τὴν μεγίστην ἔχοιεν διάστασιν, οὐδεὶς ἔτ' ἀπολείπεται χρόνος, οὔτε ταῖς λείαις ἀρτηρίαις, οὔτε ταῖς φλεψὶν ἐν ᾧ διαστήσονται· μηκέτι γὰρ τοῦ πνεύμονος διαστελλομένου, διότι μηδ' ὁ θώραξ, οὐδὲ τῶν μορίων αὐτοῦ δύναιτ' ἂν ἔτι διαστέλλεσθαί τι. δῆλον οὖν, ὡς εἴπερ ἐπιδείξαιμεν, ὅτι τὴν μεγίστην τοῦ πνεύμονος διάστασιν αἱ τραχεῖαι μόναι διαστελλόμεναι καταλαμβάνουσιν, εὐθὺς ἂν ἀποδεδειγμένον εἴη, ὅτι καὶ μόναι κατὰ τὰς εἰσπνοὰς πληροῦνται.

[2] Riolanus, *Anthropographia* (Paris, 1626), p. 367.

[3] Spigelius, *De humani corporis fabrica* (Venice, 1627), p. 302.

[4] Laurentius, *Hist. Anatom.* (ed. Frankfurt, 1602), p. 820. I am indebted to Pagel for drawing my attention to the implications of this passage, and for this and the two preceding references.

in order to refute it by the experiment which he describes in the immediately following sentence, which goes to prove that the distension or expansion of the lung is due entirely to the sucking in of air into the tracheal system. So he goes on to explain that if you blow air down the larynx of a dead animal, the lungs will be fully expanded but the veins and the arteries of the lung will keep their volume unchanged.[1] The heart can therefore only attract *pneuma* by its own diastole, just as it returns it in systole. The smooth arteries, the pulmonary veins, serve the heart, and the rough arteries, the bronchial system, the lungs. And the principles on which they work are quite different, for the movements of the heart are unconscious—they proceed from nature—while those of the thorax take place not automatically, but as the result of the activity of the vital principle, since it was better that respiration should be our conscious action, always subservient to the will of the animal.[2]

In this, the chief of Galen's physiological works, the doctrine is quite clear. Air, breath, or *pneuma* is drawn into the heart at diastole and expelled from it at systole, yet in the treatise *On the usefulness of respiration* we find what appears to be quite a different doctrine. In that treatise he discusses the question whether we need the substance of the air breathed in, or only its quality, or both of them, and comes to the conclusion that nothing at all or very little of the *substance* of the air is taken up into the heart.[3] What the organism needs is its cooling quality. Erasistratus was wrong in supposing that the heart needs the substance of the air. This can be proved by the fact that if we hold our breath with our lungs full of air, we choke,[4] though the heart has plenty of air to draw on. Indeed we choke all the more violently and the more quickly the fuller our lungs are of air. Galen appears to think that you hold your breath by closing or shutting off the trachea, no doubt through the epiglottis.[5] If you do this with your lungs full of air and then compress your thorax, the heart will continue to beat, drawing air into itself, but nevertheless you will choke,

---

[1] *De usu partium*, vii. 9, K. iii. 548 : ἐπὶ τεθνεῶτος ἤδη τοῦ ζῴου διὰ τοῦ λάρυγγος ἐμφυσῶν πνεῦμα πληρώσεις μὲν δή που τὰς τραχείας ἀρτηρίας, διϊσταμένων δ' ἐπὶ πλεῖστον ὄψει τὸν πνεύμονα τὸν ἴσον ὄγκον ἐν αὐτῷ τῶν τε λείων ἀρτηριῶν καὶ τῶν φλεβῶν φυλαττουσῶν.

[2] Ibid., 548–9 : πότ' οὖν εἰς τὴν καρδίαν ἕλκεται τὸ πνεῦμα; κατὰ τὰς διαστολὰς αὐτῆς δηλονότι, καθάπερ γε καὶ κατὰ τὰς συστολὰς αὖθις ἐκκρίνεται. τὰς μὲν γὰρ λείας ἀρτηρίας ὑπηρετεῖν χρὴ ταῖς τῆς καρδίας κινήσεσι, τὰς δὲ τραχείας ταῖς τοῦ πνεύμονος. ὅτι δὲ ἀρχαὶ δύο τούτων τῶν κινήσεών εἰσιν, ὅλῳ τῷ γένει διαφέρουσαι, καὶ ὡς αἱ μὲν τῆς καρδίας ὑπὸ τῆς φύσεως, αἱ δὲ θώρακος ὑπὸ τῆς ψυχῆς γίγνονται, δέδεικται πολλάκις· ἀλλὰ καὶ ὅτι βέλτιον ἦν ἡμέτερον ἔργον εἶναι τὴν ἀναπνοήν, ὑπηρετοῦσαν ἀεὶ τοῦ ζῴου τῇ βουλήσει.

[3] See his précis of his conclusions described in *De sanguine in arteriis*, 6, K. iv. 724–5 : ἀποδέδεικται δ' ἡμῖν ἐν τῷ περὶ χρείας ἀναπνοῆς, ὡς ἤτοι παντελῶς ὀλίγον, ἢ οὐδὲν ὅλως τῆς τοῦ πνεύματος οὐσίας εἰς τὴν καρδίαν μεταλαμβάνεται.

[4] *De usu respirationis*, 2, K. iv. 473 : ἐπεὶ τοίνυν εἰσπνεύσαντες μὲν τῆς μὲν οὐσίας εὐπορeῦμεν, πνιγόμεθα δ' οὐδὲν ἧττον.

[5] Ibid., 478 : πανταχόθεν μὲν γὰρ ἐν ταῖς τοιαύταις ἐνεργείαις θλιβόμεν τε τὸν θώρακα καὶ συστέλλομεν βιαίως κλείσαντες τὸν ἄνω πόρον τῆς τραχείας ἀρτηρίας.

and the more quickly the more you have breathed in.[1] What the heart needs therefore must be a certain quality of the air. One of the reasons why Galen asks this question of substance or quality[2] would appear to be the fact that the air breathed out is of the same volume as the air breathed in, in spite of the fact that some of the *pneuma* has been absorbed by the heart and the arteries.[3] In the treatise *On blood in the arteries*, which is aimed at Erasistratus, he goes so far as to say that most of the physicians and the most accurate have been of the opinion that the heart needs not the substance but the quality of the air.[4]

The apparent contradiction is, I believe, explained in part if we interpret the word μεταλαμβάνεται (which I have translated *taken up* in the passage quoted in note 3 to the previous page) to mean something like absorption, i.e. incorporation into the substance of the heart. The *pneuma* that is drawn into the left ventricle with each heart-beat at diastole is expelled back into the lung together with the sooty super-fluities at each systole. In the same treatise Galen still admits that the heart *does* take in some air at diastole equivalent in volume to the dis-tention of the left ventricle, and that at systole it sends it to the neighbour-ing arteries.[5] What Galen is trying to tell us is that the air taken in by the heart from the lung does not enter into any, what we should call today, chemical combination with it or with the blood it contains. It merely imparts to the ventricle its quality of cold. To maintain that it is the air taken in from the lung which feeds the innate heat or creates heat by its reaction with the blood is, in my opinion, quite foreign to Galen's way of thinking; nor is it the air which acting on the venous blood breaks it up and separates its lighter constituents to form 'arterial' blood. That is the function of the innate heat. But cold is not the only quality which air contributes to the maintenance of life. It also, chiefly in the arteries, combines with vapours of the blood to produce the vital spirit.

[1] Ibid., 479: ἔστι γὰρ ἑκάστῳ τὴν πεῖραν ἀφ' ἑαυτοῦ λαβεῖν, μυριάκις εἰσπνεύσαντα πλεῖστον, θλίβειν πανταχόθεν τὸν θώρακα καὶ μηδὲν ἀντεκπνέοντα· φανήσεται γὰρ σφύζουσα μὲν ἐν τούτῳ ἡ καρδία, πνιγόμενος δ' ὁ ἄνθρωπος, καὶ τοσοῦτόν γε μᾶλλον καὶ θᾶττον πνιγόμενος, ὅσον πλεῖον εἰσέπνευσεν.

[2] Ibid., I, 473: τοῦτ' οὖν πρῶτον διορισόμεθα, πότερον αὐτῆς τῆς οὐσίας χρῄζομεν τοῦ κατὰ τὴν εἰσπνοὴν ἐρχομένου ἀέρος, ἢ τῆς ποιότητος, ἢ ἀμφοτέρων.

[3] Ibid., 5, K. iv. 511: διὰ τί δέ, τῆς καρδίας εἰς ἑαυτήν τι παρὰ τοῦ πνεύμονος ἑλκούσης ἀέρος ἐπιπεμπούσης τε ταῖς πλησίον ἀρτηρίαις, ὅμως γε ὁ ἐκπνεόμενος οὐδὲν ἐλάττων φαίνεται τοῦ κατὰ τὴν εἰσπνοὴν ἑλχθέντος, εἰρήσεται μὲν δι' ἑτέρων ἐπὶ πλέον, ἀποχρήσει δὲ καὶ νῦν εἰπεῖν τόδε μόνον, ὡς ἀτμός τις ἐκπνεῖται τοὐπίπαν ἴσος τῷ πλήθει τῆς μεταληφθείσης μοίρας τοῦ πνεύματος εἴς τε τὴν καρδίαν καὶ τὰς ἀρτηρίας.

[4] *De sanguine in arteriis*, 6, K. iv. 724: καθάπερ τοῖς πλείστοις τε καὶ ἀκριβεστάτοις ἔδοξεν ἰατροῖς τε ἅμα καὶ φιλοσόφοις, οἳ μὴ τῆς οὐσίας ἀλλὰ τῆς ποιότητος αὐτοῦ δεῖσθαί φασι τὴν καρδίαν ἐμψύχεσθαι ποθοῦσαν, καὶ ταύτην εἶναι χρείαν τῆς ἀναπνοῆς.

[5] *De usu respirationis*, 5, K. iv. 510 f.: ὅτι μὲν οὖν εἰς τὴν καρδίαν ἕλκεταί τις ἀέρος μοῖρα κατὰ τὰς διαστολὰς αὐτῆς ἀναπληροῦσα τὴν γενομένην κένωσιν, τὸ μέγεθος αὐτό γε τῆς διαστάσεως ἱκανὸν ἐνδείξασθαι. ὅτι δὲ καὶ εἰς τὸν ἐγκέφαλον εἰσπνεῖται, δι' ἑτέρας ἐπιδέδεικται πραγματείας.

I am unable to follow Siegel when he suggests that this quality to which Galen is referring is 'heat'.[1] Siegel attributes to Galen the doctrine that air is predominantly heat,[2] quoting a phrase from the treatise *On the mixture and powers of simple drugs* without giving any context or, indeed, informing his readers that the passage in question is not stating Galen's own doctrine, but merely stating the different views taken by certain famous philosophers, such as Aristotle and his school, who conceived air as being hot, in contrast to the Stoics who regarded it as being cold.[3] Siegel indeed goes much further. He attributes to Galen, if I understand him correctly, a view which would imply that the heat, the essential 'quality' of the air absorbed by the heart, is the source of the body's heat which is produced by the combustion of the blood by the innate heat continued chiefly in the left ventricle of the heart. Thus in his first article he tells us:

> The ancients assumed, and so did Galen, that most of the body heat was generated in the left ventricle by the interaction of blood and air.[4]

In his book on Galen's physiological system, Siegel gives an elaboration of Galen's doctrine of combustion and its relation to respiration and the blood-flow which I am unable to follow. My random quotations may therefore do less than justice to his interpretation. But if I understand him correctly, he believes that the essence of Galen's doctrine was that the heat of the body is maintained by the absorption of the 'quality' of heat from the inhaled air. Thus he tells us:

> Of all the existent qualities Galen regarded the quality of heat as the most important factor for the understanding of respiration and combustion. Heat

---

[1] See the chapter on 'Respiration and combustion' in his *Galen's System of Physiology*, pp. 135–78.

[2] Ibid., p. 153.

[3] Galen, *De temperamentis simplicium*, ii. 20, K. xi. 509–10: λεγόντων οὖν τῶν φιλοσόφων θερμὸν εἶναι τοὔλαιον καὶ τεκμήριον τιθεμένων οὐ σμικρόν, ὡς οἴονται, τὸ τάχος τῆς εἰς τὴν φλόγα μεταβολῆς ἀντιλέγοντες ἔνιοι τουτὶ μὲν ὑπάρχειν αὐτῷ φασιν, ὅτι λεπτόν τ' ἐστὶ καὶ ἀερῶδες. ἐκ δὲ τοῦ πήγνυσθαι ταχέως ἐν τῷ χειμῶνι σαφῶς ἀναδείκνυσθαι τὴν ψύξιν. οὐ μόνον γὰρ οἴνου καὶ ὄξους, ἀλλὰ καὶ αὐτοῦ τοῦ ὕδατος ἑτοιμότερον ὑπὸ τοῦ ψυχροῦ νικᾶσθαι. πρὸς ταῦτα δὲ ἀντιλέγοντες ἕτεροι, τὸ μὲν ἀερῶδες ὑπάρχειν αὐτὸ συγχωροῦσιν καὶ φαίνεσθαί γε σαφῶς τοῦτό φασιν ἐκ τῆς κουφότητος, οὐ μὴν καὶ ψυχρόν γε εἶναι τὴν δύναμιν ὁμολογοῦσιν. ἀέρα γὰρ ἅπαντα θερμὸν ὑπάρχειν τὴν φύσιν, ὡς δηλοῖ καὶ ἡ γένεσις αὐτοῦ. λεπτυνθὲν οὖν καὶ λυθὲν ὑπὸ θερμότητος ὕδωρ, ἀέρα γίγνεσθαι. καὶ δῆλον ὡς ἐντεῦθεν αὐτοὺς διαδέχεται μέγιστον ζήτημα, τὸ καὶ τοῖς ἐνδοξοτάτοις φιλοσόφοις ἠμφισβητημένον, Ἀριστοτέλους μὲν καὶ τῶν ὑπ' αὐτοῦ θερμὸν ὑπολαμβανόντων εἶναι τὸν ἀέρα, τῶν δ' ἀπὸ τῆς στοᾶς ψυχρόν.

Unfortunately this is not the only example of quotations applied out of context in order to prove a point. Thus Siegel tells us that Galen clearly stated that blood and air enter the pulmonary veins at the same time, quoting a passage from *De nat. fac.* iii. 15: 'The (left) heart does not only get air from the lungs but also blood from the right heart through these anastomoses', without mentioning the fact that the anastomoses here referred to are without any question the pores in the interventricular septum.

[4] Siegel, *Galen's System of Physiology*, p. 744.

seemed to be the predominant constituent of air, the main agent of fire, and essential for life.[1]

Galen tried to establish that, like in the burning flame, only a *quality* of air is being absorbed by respiration.[2]

He described how the addition of air renders the blood 'enriched' and 'thinned' during its passage through the lungs, the absorbed air remaining invisible.

The factor incorporated in the blood was mostly defined as *pneuma zotikon*, the *vital spirit*. This expression corresponded more to the common use in the writings of the scientists and philosophers of his time than the term 'quality of heat'.

[Here follow translations of two quotations describing the vital and the psychic spirits, their seat and generation, one from the *Ars Magna* (see below, p. 351) and the other from the third Commentary on Hippocrates *On nourishment*, identical but for one word with n. 1 on p. 359 taken from *On the opinions of Hippocrates and Plato*.]

The fact that Galen used the terms quality and *pneuma* interchangeably and as synonyms was the reason for many misinterpretations of his writings. We have always to remember that he indicated that only an invisible and not measurable quality of heat was absorbed from the inhaled air, when he spoke of the vital *pneuma* carried by the blood through the arterial system.[3]

Siegel believes that Galen found experimental evidence for the contention that only a quality of the air and not any measurable quantity was absorbed by the lung in respiration in an experiment which is briefly described in the treatise on the use of breathing. Galen, he tells us, tried to measure the amount of air absorbed by the lungs of patients breathing from an inflated bladder tied round the mouth and nose, 'without any leakage' during the duration of the experiment. The volume of the bladder apparently did not change at all. But this was not, in fact, what Galen was trying to prove by his experiment, nor does it describe it accurately. What Galen actually wrote was as follows:

We can learn clearly from the following account what appears to happen concerning the intake of breath from the proper artery of the lung (i.e. the windpipe) into the arteries all over the body, namely that it is certainly very small, if indeed it exists at all. For placing round the mouth and nose of a boy a large ox-bladder, or some other such vessel, in such a way that nothing he breathed in could escape by a side channel, we saw him breathing a whole day long without any impediment. From which it is plain that the arteries of an animal have very little need if any at all of qualities from the outside, and particularly of heat.[4]

---

[1] Ibid., p. 151.   [2] Ibid., pp. 153 f.
[3] Ibid., p. 155.

[4] *De usu resp.* 5, K. iv. 504–5: μαθεῖν δὲ ἐναργῶς ἔστιν ἐξ οὗ μέλλομεν εἰπεῖν φαινομένου περὶ τῆς οἰκείας πνεύμονος εἰς τὰς καθ' ὅλον ἀρτηρίας μεταλήψεως τοῦ πνεύματος, ὡς ἤτοι βραχὺ ἔτι παντελῶς, ἢ οὐδ' ὅλως γίγνεται. περιτιθέντες γὰρ παιδὸς τῷ στόματι καὶ ταῖς ῥισὶ μεγάλην κύστιν βοείαν, ἤ τι τοιοῦτον ἕτερον ἀγγεῖον, ὡς μηδαμῇ παραπνεῖσθαι μηδὲν τῆς ἀναπνοῆς δι'

From this experiment and the statement made at the conclusion of the same treatise that the amount of expired air is not smaller than that of the inspired air and 'that the volume of exhaled vapor remains in all respects equal to the air (*pneuma*) which is taken up into the heart and arteries during inspiration', Siegel concludes that the 'fumes' or 'waste products' produced in the left ventricle of the heart did not occupy any space at all.[1] The evidence for this startling conclusion I can nowhere find in any statement made by Galen, nor can I find any passage in which Galen suggests that the vital spirit is to be identified with the 'not-space-occupying' quality of heat. The idea that the innate heat is reinforced or maintained by heat derived from in-breathed air seems to me to be fundamentally mistaken.

Siegel's contention that Galen did not accept the doctrine of Aristotle that respiration serves mainly to cool the heart[2] seems to me curious, in view of the emphasis he places *passim* on the importance of this function. To select only one instance out of so many, in the ninth chapter of the seventh book *On the use of the parts*, Galen informs us that the first and foremost function of respiration is to preserve the innate heat, since animals deprived of the possibility of refrigeration or cooling die immediately.[3] Siegel appears to have misunderstood the meaning of the phrase the 'preservation (φυλακή, σωτηρία) of the innate heat', as his explanation of the increased rate of respiration in cases of *boulimia* would appear to indicate.

[Galen] agreed with Aristotle that we breathe more rapidly in fever 'when more heat seems to have accumulated around the heart and the thorax'. But he noticed that respiration is equally increased in cold temperature or when patients suffer from *boulimia*, a type of prostration (shock) during which they became very cold. Galen concluded from these clinical observations that the purpose of respiration could not only be to cool the heart, but also to raise the lowered body temperature by increased breathing, thus enhancing the combustion in the left ventricle.[4]

If we examine Galen's actual words in their context, we shall, I am convinced, be faced with a very different picture. Galen, it is true, has to contest the argument that if the prime object of breathing is to cool the

---

ὅλης ἡμέρας εἴδομεν ἀκωλύτως πνέοντα αὐτόν. ἐξ οὗ δῆλον, ὡς ἤτοι μικρὸν παντελῶς ἢ οὐδ᾽ ὅλως αἱ κατὰ τὸ ζῷον ἀρτηρίαι ἔχουσι τῶν ἔξωθεν ποιοτήτων ἀνάγκην, καὶ μάλιστα τῆς θερμότητος.

[1] Siegel, op. cit., p. 157. The passage from Galen quoted by him in this connection reads as follows: ἀποχρήσει δὲ καὶ νῦν εἰπεῖν τόδε μόνον, ὡς ἀτμός τις ἐκπνεῖται τοὐπίπαν ἴσος τῷ πλήθει τῆς μεταληφθείσης μοίρας τοῦ πνεύματος εἴς τε τὴν καρδίαν καὶ τὰς ἀρτηρίας.

[2] Siegel, op. cit., p. 162.

[3] *De usu partium*, vii. 9, K. iii. 544: ἐπειδὴ γὰρ ἡ χρεία τῆς ἀναπνοῆς, ἡ πρώτη μὲν καὶ μεγίστη, φυλακὴ τῆς ἐμφύτου θερμασίας ὑπάρχειν ἐδείκνυτο, δι᾽ ἣν καὶ παραχρῆμα διαφθείρεσθαι τὰ ζῷα στερούμενα τῆς ἀναψύξεως.

[4] Siegel, op. cit., p. 162.

innate heat, we should expect the need for breathing in cases of *boulimia*, which is a complaint characterized not only by cold but also by abnormal hunger, to be reduced to a minimum, yet patients afflicted with it and those who have been exposed to severe frost, who need to be heated not cooled, make great efforts to breathe.[1] But his explanation is quite different from that put forth by Siegel. Galen tries to resolve this difficulty by an appeal to the analogy of combustion. With the details of his theory we need not concern ourselves, but he postulated three requisites for maintaining a fire: fuel, and two movements of heat, one upward, a general dissemination as it were, and the other downward to the source of the kindled flame. If either of these movements is eliminated, the fire will cease to burn, just as it does when all the fuel has been used up. The maintenance of a fire depends on a balance between heat and cold. Every flame needs a moderately cold atmosphere. Too much heat makes the upward movement excessive; all the heat is dispersed, with the result that the inward motion is destroyed, while too much cold extinguishes the upward or outward movement.[2] Flames can be kept alight only by moderately hot or cold draughts of air. It is not improbable that similar or analogous conditions apply to the body-heat of animals. The fuel from which it is kindled is the blood, and the innate heat itself has an innate principle of double movement. If it is deprived of either of these movements, it is of necessity also deprived of the other, so that if you deprive it either of blood or of respiration an animal dies immediately,[3] just as the flame of a lantern can be extinguished by smothering it, i.e. by depriving it either of air or of fuel. Now assume that the heart is analogous to the wick of the lantern, and the blood to the oil, while the bowl corresponds to the lung,[4] which Galen proceeds to compare with a cupping glass in a series of phrases which we need not go into. A more

---

[1] Galen, *De usu resp.* 3, K. iv. 485: ἀλλὰ πάλιν εἰ κατεψυγμένων τῶν αὐτῶν τούτων ὀργάνων, ὡς ἔν τε τοῖς βουλίμοις καλουμένοις, κἀπειδάν τις ἰσχυρῷ ὁμιλήσῃ κρύει, μὴ ὅτι ψύχει τὴν ἐν ἡμῖν θερμασίαν, ἀλλὰ καὶ θερμαίνει, δι' ὀλίγου δεῖν ἅπασαν ἐψυγμένην, ὅμως εἰσπνέειν ὀρεγόμεθα, δόξει ἐναντιοῦσθαι, τὴν ἀναπνοὴν ἐμψύξεως ἕνεκα γίνεσθαι.

[2] Ibid., 490: ταῦτ' ἄρα συμμέτρως ψυχροῦ τοῦ περιέχοντος ἀέρος δεῖται πᾶσα φλόξ. ὁ μὲν γὰρ ὑπερβαλλόντως ἔκθερμος τὴν ἔξω κίνησιν αὐτῆς ἀμέτρως ἐργαζόμενος, ὁ δὲ ψυχρὸς τὴν ἔσωθεν σβέννυσιν. ἀμφότεροι τοίνυν ῥιπιζόμενοι ἀσυμμέτρως ἀναστέλλουσι τὴν φλόγα πρὸς τὴν ὕλην, ὥσπερ καὶ τὸ ψυχρόν· τὸ δὲ ὑπερβαλλόντως κινεῖσθαι σκεδάννυσιν, ὥσπερ καὶ τὸ θερμόν. τῶν δὲ τὴν ἔξω κίνησιν ἄμετρον ἐργαζομένων ἐστὶ καὶ σικύα καὶ πᾶν, ὅ τί περ ἂν τῶν ὑπὸ τῆς ἐντὸς φλογὸς ἀέρα διακεκαυμένων εἴρηται πρὸς τὴν ἔξω τοῦ πυρὸς τῶν ψυχρῶν ὁμιλίαν ἰέναι. ἡ δὲ συμμετρία σωτηρία τῆς πάσης φλογός ἐστιν.

[3] Ibid.: οὕτως οὖν οὐκ ἀπεικὸς ἔχειν κἀπὶ τῆς ἐν τοῖς ζῴοις θερμασίας. ὕλην μὲν ὅθεν ἀνάπτεται τὸ αἷμα, σύμφυτον δὲ ἔχουσα κινήσεως ἀρχὴν ἐφ' ἑκάτερα, τῆς ἑτέρας στερηθεῖσα, καὶ τῆς λοιπῆς ἐξ ἀνάγκης στερίσκεται· καὶ διὰ τοῦτ' αὐτό, ἐάν τε ἀναπνοῆς εἴρξῃς, ἐάν θ' αἵματος, εὐθέως διαφθείρεται.

[4] Ibid., 491: καὶ γὰρ καὶ τὴν τοῦ λύχνου φλόγα ἅμα ἀφαιρήσεις καταπνίξας ἢ παντάπασιν ἐλαίου στερήσας. ἀνάλογον οὖν τίθεσο τῇ μὲν θρυαλλίδι τὴν καρδίαν, τῷ δὲ ἐλαίῳ τὸ αἱματῶδες, τῷ δὲ ὀργάνῳ τὸν πνεύμονα. This analogy must not be taken too literally. The innate heat, as we shall see, does not consume any portion or element of the body.

relevant analogy follows, that of a chimney. A furnace choked with soot does not burn, but if you provide an air vent, the soot will be blown away, and the fuel will spring into flame—a fact from which Galen tells us that he drew the conclusion that the body had a great need of breathing out, in order to eliminate the soot-like element of the blood. For smoke and soot and suchlike residues produced by burning fuel extinguish a fire quite as readily as water.[1] The function of breathing in respect of the innate heat is a double one, to ventilate the seat or origin (ἀρχή) of the innate heat by causing the complete evacuation of the 'smoky' wastes, and to effect a moderate refrigeration; this double function can be embraced under the single term of 'safeguarding' (σωτηρία).[2] Nowhere is there any suggestion that breathing supplies any external element of heat. The innate heat is an independently existing entity. It can be quenched by too much cooling, and also by the accumulation of too great a quantity of 'waste products'. Breathing gives it the moderate cooling it requires, as well as preventing it being choked by sooty or smoky residues.

Galen's theory of respiration and its relation to the heart and arteries is not easy to translate into a coherent system. The supply of *pneuma* to the heart, which is the chief function of respiration, is not so simple as it looks. For the question was to be bedevilled by the philosophical distinction between substance and quality which we have just examined. All authorities who have written about the innate heat, so Galen tells us, are agreed that respiration is concerned with its preservation, but exactly how they were not able to state clearly. Some of them say its function is cooling, others ventilation, and others strengthening, and the analogy which has attracted them most is that of fire or flame. For when deprived of air a flame dies, just as an animal does.[3] The analogy between respiration and combustion is worked out at length in a parallel whose details we need not go into. Just as a fire needs a moderate amount of air, for too much would blow it out, of a suitable temperature, and its sooty residues also need elimination if it is to be kept alight, so the innate heat, whose chief source is the heart, needs to have its temperature kept constant by a 'circulation' of air in the left ventricle and the arteries. It

---

[1] *De usu resp.* 3, K. iv. 491: ἐγὼ δὲ καὶ κάμινον ἰδὼν σβεννυμένην ὑπὸ τοῦ μὴ διαπνεῖσθαι, κἄπειτα αὐτὴν παρανοιχθεῖσαν πολὺ μὲν αἰθαλῶδες ἐκπνεύσασαν, πολὺ δ' ἔξωθεν εἰσπνεύσασαν τὸν ἀέρα καθαρόν, ἐπ' ἀμφοτέροις ἀναλάμψαι, οὐ μικρὰν τῆς ἐκπνοῆς ἐλογισάμην εἶναι τὴν χρείαν εἰς τὸ κενοῦν τὴν οἷον λιγνὺν τοῦ αἵματος. αἴθαλος γὰρ καὶ καπνὸς καὶ λιγνὺς καὶ πᾶν τὸ τοιοῦτον περίττωμα τῆς καιομένης ὕλης οὐδὲν ἧττον ὕδατος ἀποσβέννυσθαι πέφυκε τὸ πῦρ.

[2] *Ibid.*, 4, 493: οὐκοῦν ἔκ τε τοῦ ῥιπίζεσθαι τὴν ἀρχὴν τῆς ἐμφύτου θερμασίας, κἄκ τε τοῦ συμμέτρως ἐμψύχεσθαι, κἄκ τοῦ τὸ οἷον καπνῶδες αὐτῆς ἅπαν ἀπορρεῖν, ἐν ἀθροίζεται κεφάλαιον, ἡ σωτηρία τῆς κατὰ φύσιν θερμασίας.

[3] *Ibid.*, 3, K. iv. 487: κινδυνεύουσι γὰρ ἅπαντες ὅσοι περὶ τῆς ἐμφύτου θερμασίας παρήκασί τι, τὴν μὲν σωτηρίαν αὐτῆς ὀνειρώττειν, οὐ δύνασθαι δὲ ἀκριβῶς καὶ διηρθρημένως ἐξηγήσασθαι τὸ σφέτερον νόημα, καὶ διὰ τοῦτο, οἶμαι, οἱ μὲν ἔμψυξιν, οἱ δὲ ῥίπισιν, οἱ δὲ καὶ ῥῶσιν γράφουσι. μάλιστα δὲ αὐτούς, οἶμαι, προτρέπειν τὰ περὶ τὰς φλόγας φαινόμενα· ταύτας γὰρ ἐναργῶς ὁρῶμεν οὕτως ταχέως ἀπολλυμένας, ὅταν ἀποστερηθῶσιν ἀέρος, ὥσπερ τὰ ζῷα.

would appear then that though none of the air breathed in in respiration is absorbed by the heart, what is taken in goes out again in expiration from the left ventricle, together with the 'waste products' produced by the action of the innate heat upon the blood, and this in and out movement keeps the temperature of the heart steady (within limits) through the medium of its cooling quality. Respiration also 'feeds' the vital and animal spirits, but this takes place only in inspiration.[1] In the same way the air taken in at diastole by the arteries has a similar double function, but this function is exercised independently by the arteries, and no *pneuma* passes into them through the lungs via the heart.[2] Their function is to guard the innate heat and to nourish the psychic *pneuma*.[3]

What exactly then is this pneuma? That there are at least two kinds we have noted, the 'animal' or 'psychic', and the 'vital', and as we shall see, Galen may also have tentatively recognized a third variety, 'natural' spirit. The psychic (and the vital) spirit is derived in part from the air taken in in respiration and transpiration, and in some of the passages which we have quoted from, the air is taken via the lungs into the heart. In others, however, before reaching the heart, it has already undergone a kind of transformation, likened by Galen to digestion. This transformation seems to take place in two stages. In the flesh of the lung it is worked on, it receives a 'processing' (ἐργασία), a first working over, since the qualities necessary for it to become the food of the psychic spirit cannot be conferred upon it instantaneously. It has to undergo changes analogous to those of digestion, the flesh of the lung corresponding to that of the liver.[4]

In the heart and? the arteries it undergoes a further transformation, being changed, presumably into 'vital' spirit, its final and greatest transformation taking place in the brain, in the ventricles of which it is perfected, as fully elaborated 'psychic' spirit.[5] The distinction between the two kinds of 'spirit' is not always easy to maintain with great clarity. But they have different functions and different locations in the body, the

---

[1] Ibid., 5, K. iv. 510: αὕτη μὲν οὖν (ἀνάψυξις καὶ ῥίπησις) ἡ μεγίστη χρεία τῆς ἀναπνοῆς· δευτέρα δὲ θρέψις τοῦ ψυχικοῦ πνεύματος. γίνεται δ' ἡ προτέρα δι' ἀμφοτέρων τῆς ἀναπνοῆς μερῶν, εἰσπνοῆς τε καὶ ἐκπνοῆς, τῆς μὲν οὖν ἀναψυχούσης τε καὶ ῥιπιζούσης, τῆς δὲ τὸ αἰθαλῶδες ἀποχεούσης. ἡ δευτέρα δὲ διὰ τῆς εἰσπνοῆς μόνης.

[2] Ibid., 504, quoted above, p. 345, n. 4.

[3] *De usu partium*, i. 16, K. iii. 45-6: ἀρτηριῶν δὲ φυλάττειν τε τὴν κατὰ φύσιν θερμασίαν καὶ τρέφειν τὸ πνεῦμα τὸ ψυχικόν.

[4] Ibid., vi. 8, K. iii. 540: εὔλογον γὰρ οὐκ ἀθρόον οὐδ' ἐξαίφνης τὸν ἔξωθεν ἀέρα τοῦ κατὰ τὸ ζῷον πνεύματος γίνεσθαι τροφήν, ἀλλὰ κατὰ βραχὺ μὲν ἀλλοιούμενον, ὥσπερ γε καὶ τὰ σιτία, δεχόμενον δὲ τὴν οἰκείαν ποιότητα τῷ συμφύτῳ πνεύματι χρόνῳ πλείονι, καὶ ταύτης τῆς ἀλλοιώσεως τὸ πρῶτον ὄργανον ὑπάρχειν τὴν τοῦ πνεύμονος σάρκα, καθάπερ γε καὶ τῆς εἰς αἷμα μεταβολῆς ἡ σὰρξ τοῦ ἥπατος ἐδείκνυτο τὴν αἰτίαν ἔχειν.

[5] Ibid., 541: τὸ δ' ἐκ τῶν τραχειῶν ἀρτηριῶν πνεῦμα, τὸ ἔξωθεν ἐλχθὲν ἐν μὲν τῇ σαρκὶ τοῦ πνεύμονος τὴν πρώτην ἐργασίαν λαμβάνει, μετὰ ταῦτα δὲ ἐν τῇ καρδίᾳ τε καὶ ταῖς ἀρτηρίαις, καὶ μάλιστα ταῖς κατὰ τὸ δικτυοειδὲς πλέγμα τὴν δευτέραν, ἔπειτα τὴν τελεωτάτην ἐν ταῖς τοῦ ἐγκεφάλου κοιλίαις ἔνθα δὴ καὶ ψυχικὸν ἀκριβῶς γίγνεται.

'home' of the vital spirit being the heart and arteries, that of the psychic the brain.[1] They both come into existence in a rather similar way, as the result of the 'bubbling' or 'vaporization' of the arterial blood caused by the innate heat in conjunction with the breath, the air drawn in from the outer atmosphere.[2] The function of the vital spirit is to be the instrument of the vital processes in the body, i.e. those which make and keep the animal alive and make it something essentially different from a stone or a clod of earth; that of the psychic to be the instrument of the activities concerned with action, will, and choice. With regard to this psychic *pneuma*, Galen is at great pains carefully to distinguish it from the soul, the essence of which he regards as being an unknown.[3] The soul resides, indeed, in the brain, but it is not to be identified with the *pneuma* in its ventricles. The *pneuma* is only an instrument for effecting perception and voluntary action. The vital spirit, composed as we have just described from 'breath' and the vapours given off by the blood and the humours, undergoes a further vaporization in the network of blood vessels in the brain, a sort of redistillation which turns it into the psychic spirit.[4] This doctrine of vaporization (ἀναθυμίασις) seems to be an old one. It may very well derive from Empedocles, and the 'boiling' of the blood is to be found in Plato, in a passage from the *Timaeus* quoted by Galen himself.[5] In the passage we have just quoted, Galen includes the other 'humours' besides the blood as constituents of the *pneuma*, but in most places the vaporization of blood only is referred to.

Of the existence of a vital spirit Galen appears to be less certain than of the existence of the psychic spirit. In a passage in the fifth chapter of the twelfth book of the *Ars magna*, his principal work on the art of healing, he says:

We have shown clearly that the brain is, as it were, the fount of the psychic *pneuma*, which is watered and nourished by breathing in and by the matter

---

[1] *De plac. Hipp. et Plat.* vii. 3, K. v. 608: τὸ μὲν οὖν κατὰ τὰς ἀρτηρίας πνεῦμα ζωτικόν ἐστί τε καὶ προσαγορεύεται, τὸ δὲ κατὰ τὸν ἐγκέφαλον ψυχικόν.

[2] For this process of ἀναθυμίασις, see below, pp. 353 f.

[3] *Comment. V in Hipp. epidem. VI*, sect. 5, K. xviiB. 247 f.: πέπεισμαι καὶ πρός γε τούτῳ τὸ κατὰ τὰς κοιλίας αὐτοῦ πνεῦμα πρῶτόν τι τῶν ὀργάνων εἶναι τῶν ψυχικῶν, ὅπερ ἦν μοι προπετέστερον ἀποφηναμένῳ ψυχῆς οὐσίαν εἰπεῖν. Cf. *De usu resp.*, 5, K. iv. 501: εἴπωμεν δὲ προτέρως πῶς καλοῦμέν τι ψυχικὸν πνεῦμα, ἀγνοεῖν ὁμολογοῦντες οὐσίαν ψυχῆς.

[4] *De plac. Hipp. et Plat.* vii. 3, K. v. 605–6: ἐκ τούτων οὖν τῶν φαινομένων ἴσως ἄν τις ὑπονοήσειε τὸ κατὰ τὰς κοιλίας τοῦ ἐγκεφάλου πνεῦμα δυοῖν θάτερον, εἰ μὲν ἀσώματός ἐστιν ἡ ψυχὴ τὸ πρῶτον αὐτῆς ὑπάρχειν, ὡς ἂν εἴποι τις, οἰκητήριον, εἰ δὲ σῶμα τοῦτ' αὐτὸ πνεῦμα τὴν ψυχὴν εἶναι . . . βέλτιον οὖν ὑπολαβεῖν ἐν αὐτῷ μὲν τῷ σώματι τοῦ ἐγκεφάλου τὴν ψυχὴν οἰκεῖν, ἥτις ποτ' ἂν ᾖ κατὰ τὴν οὐσίαν . . . τὸ πρῶτον δ' αὐτῆς ὄργανον εἰς τε τὰς αἰσθήσεις ἁπάσας τοῦ ζῴου καὶ προσέτι τὰς καθ' ὁρμὴν κινήσεις, τοῦτ' εἶναι τὸ πνεῦμα. Cf. *ibid.*, 608: τὸ δὲ κατὰ τὸν ἐγκέφαλον ψυχικόν, οὐχ ὡς οὐσία ψυχῆς ὑπάρχον, ἀλλ' ὡς ὄργανον πρῶτον αὐτῆς οἰκούσης κατὰ τὸν ἐγκέφαλον, ὁποία τις ἂν ᾖ τὴν οὐσίαν.

[5] *Ibid.*, vi. 8, K. v. 573: ὡς οὖν ἀρτηριῶν, οὕτως καὶ τοῦ πνευματώδους τε καὶ τοῦ ζέοντος αἵματος ἀρχή τε καὶ πηγὴ τοῖς ζῴοις ἐστὶν ἡ καρδία, καὶ διὰ τοῦτο καὶ τὸ θυμοειδὲς ἐνδείκνυται τῆς ψυχῆς ἐν αὐτῇ κατῳκῆσθαι. ταῦτ' ἄρα καὶ ὁ Πλάτων τὴν καρδίαν ἔλεγεν πηγὴν τοῦ περιφερομένου κατὰ πάντα μέλη σφοδρῶς αἵματος.

urnished by the net-like complex of arteries [δικτυοειδὲς πλέγμα, a structure which does not exist in the human brain]. But our proof of the vital *pneuma* was not equally clear. It is, however, not improbable or difficult to believe that it seems to be contained in the heart and the arteries, and like the former (the psychic) nourished principally by breathing in, but also by the blood. And if there is also such a thing as the 'natural' *pneuma*, that would be contained in the liver and the veins.[1]

This qualifying phrase, 'if there is such a thing', also occurs in a slightly different form in connection with the psychic spirit itself. Here, the doubt expressed seems to concern not so much its existence as its character. 'Nor is this definition (λόγος)', we are told, 'impossible, that the psychic *pneuma* is a sort of boiling up or vaporization of good blood, if it [or there] is one.'[2] This has been taken to mean, e.g. by Hall, that Galen was not altogether happy about the division of this *pneuma* into two, and still less into three, kinds. Hall connects these doubts not unreasonably with Galen's agnosticism on the essence of the soul. 'He never makes it clear whether there are three distinct spirits, or whether the *pneuma psychicon* and the *pneuma zootikon* are the same aerial *pneuma* qualified by its location in the brain and in the arteries, or, finally, whether they are modifications of aerial *pneuma*.'[3]

This seems to me to indicate rather too much scepticism on Galen's part. As I hope to show, he certainly believed in two different sorts of *pneuma*, the 'vital' and the 'psychic', each concerned with different functions. Whether he actually believed in three different kinds is much less certain. Hall is inclined to take Sir Michael Foster[4] to task for having found also a 'natural' spirit 'in the Galenic blood', adding, somewhat brusquely, that 'there seems to be no authority for this'. But the 'authority' of the passage just quoted from the *Ars magna* cannot, in my opinion, be set aside quite so arbitrarily. It is, as far as I am aware, the only passage in Galen's genuine works in which a 'natural' spirit is postulated, as a possibility at any rate, and it is quoted also by Temkin in his learned article 'On Galen's pneumatology',[5] who cites it as the unique reference in the whole of Galen's genuine works, since he naturally rejects the *Medical definitions*, in which two other mentions of it occur, as being

---

[1] *De methodo medendi*, xii. 5, K. x. 839: τοῦ μὲν δὴ ψυχικοῦ πνεύματος ἐναργῶς ἐδείξαμεν οἷον πηγήν τινα οὖσαν τὸν ἐγκέφαλον, ἀρδομένου καὶ τρεφομένου διά τε τῆς εἰσπνοῆς καὶ τῆς ἐκ τοῦ δικτυοειδοῦς πλέγματος χορηγίας. τοῦ δὲ ζωτικοῦ πνεύματος οὐχ ὁμοίως μὲν ἐναργῶς ἡ ἀπόδειξις ἦν, οὐ μὴν ἀπίθανόν γε κατά τε τὴν καρδίαν αὐτὸ καὶ τὰς ἀρτηρίας δοκεῖν περιέχεσθαι, τρεφόμενον καὶ τοῦτο μάλιστα μὲν ἐκ τῆς ἀναπνοῆς, ἤδη δὲ καὶ τοῦ αἵματος. εἰ δέ ἐστί τι καὶ φυσικὸν πνεῦμα, περιέχοιτ' ἂν καὶ τοῦτο κατά τε τὸ ἧπαρ καὶ τὰς φλέβας.

[2] *De usu partium*, vi. 17, K. iii. 496: οὐδὲ γὰρ οὐδ' οὗτος ὁ λόγος ἀδύνατος, ὡς ἀναθυμίασίς τις, εἴ γε ἐστίν, αἵματος χρηστοῦ τὸ ψυχικὸν πνεῦμα.

[3] Hall, op. cit.

[4] Foster, *History of Physiology* (Cambridge University Press, London 1924), pp. 12 f.

[5] Temkin, op. cit.

spurious.[1] He also points out, in agreement with Drabkin,[2] that the doctrine of the three kinds of spirit was never incorporated in his physiological works, and that the first formulation of the doctrine of the three spirits as part of Galen's teaching is to be found in the *Isagoge* of Johannitus, the Arabic translator, Hunain ibn Ishaq.[3] But the defenders of the traditional view adopted by Foster have one or two other passages, which though they do not mention a 'natural' spirit could be interpreted as implying its existence. Thus, for example, in this same fifth chapter of the twelfth book of the *Ars magna* we are told that the essence of the powers or faculties, by which our physiological economy is managed, consists of *pneuma* and the mixture of solid bodies,[4] the four elements which make up the organs which these faculties need. These faculties, we are told elsewhere, are three in number, the psychic, the vital, and the natural, whose respective seats are the brain, the heart, and the liver.[5] In the *Synopsis on the pulse*, he mentions all three kinds of powers or faculties. Since the operative power of the psychic faculties is the psychic spirit, and that of the vital faculties the vital spirit, it would seem to be quite logical to assume that the 'natural' faculties are operated by a 'natural' spirit.[6] Moreover, in a passage in the *Introduction* we are told that the ancients divided *pneuma* into two classes, natural and psychic.[7]

Whatever his doubts on the 'natural' spirit, Galen seems to have held firmly enough to the existence of the vital and the psychic spirits as two distinct entities, neither of which was absolutely constant in its character. *Pneuma* varies in accordance with the state of the humours and the

[1] The two passages occur in Deff. lxxiii and lxxiv, K. xix. 365: φλέψ ἐστιν ἀγγεῖον αἵματος καὶ τοῦ συγκεκραμένου τῷ αἵματι φυσικοῦ πνεύματος. ἀρτηρία ἐστὶν ἀγγεῖον αἵματος ἐλάττονος καὶ καθαρωτέρου καὶ τοῦ συγκεκραμένου φυσικοῦ πνεύματος πλείονος καὶ λεπτομερεστέρου.

[2] M. R. Cohen and E. Drabkin, *A Source-Book for Greek Science* (New York, 1948), p. 486.

[3] Temkin quotes the following passage from this treatise (text of the Articella, Venice, 1491): 'Thus there are three spirits: first, the natural, which takes its origin from the liver; second, the vital from the heart; and third, the psychic from the brain. Of these the first is diffused from the liver over the whole body through the veins which have no pulse. The second is directed from the heart into the whole body by the arteries. And the third is directed from the brain into the whole body by the nerves.'

[4] *De methodo medendi*, xii. 5, K. x. 837–8: ἐπεὶ δὲ ἡ οὐσία τῶν διοικουσῶν ἡμᾶς δυνάμεων ἔν τε τῷ πνεύματι καὶ τῇ τῶν στερεῶν σωμάτων ἐστὶ κράσει.

[5] *Comment. III in Hipp. de aliment.* x, K. xv. 292–3: οὐσῶν δὲ τριῶν ἐν ἡμῖν, τῆς ψυχικῆς καὶ ζωτικῆς καὶ φυσικῆς (δυνάμεως), αἵπερ διοικοῦσι τὸ ζῷον καὶ ἑτερογενεῖς ἀλλήλων εἰσίν, ὥσπερ ἐκ πηγῆς τινος ἰδίας ἑκάστη παντὶ τῷ σώματι διανέμεται. ἔστι δ' ἡ μέν τις αὐτῶν εἰς τὸ τρέφεσθαι τὸ ζῷον ἀναγκαία καὶ κοινὴ πρὸς τὰ φυτά. καὶ οἷον πηγὴν ἔχει τὸ ἧπαρ . . . ἑτέρα δὲ οὐ μόνον ὡς φυτοῖς ἡμῖν ἢ ζῷσιν, ἀλλὰ καὶ ὡς ζῴοις ὑπάρχουσα ψυχὴ κατὰ τὴν καρδίαν ἵδρυται . . . τρίτη δὲ ἐν ἐγκεφάλῳ ἐστὶ ψυχὴ λογική, τῶν κατὰ προαίρεσιν ἐνεργειῶν ἅμα ταῖς αἰσθήσεσιν ἐξηγουμένη.

[6] *Synopsis de puls.* 21, K. ix. 492: μεγάλην δὲ ἔφην ἔχειν ἰσχὺν ἐν τοῖς πυρετώδεσι νοσήμασι τὴν ῥώμην τῆς τὰς ἀρτηρίας κινούσης δυνάμεως ἣν καὶ ζωτικὴν ὀνομάζομεν . . . ἀλλ' ἐπισκεπτόμεθα τηνικαῦθ' ὅπως ἔχει ῥώμης ἡ ψυχικὴ δύναμις· ἄμεινον μὲν οὖν ἀμφοτέρας ἐρρῶσθαι καὶ πρὸς αὐταῖς γε τρίτην τὴν φυσικὴν ὀνομαζομένην, ἧς ἀρχὴ τὸ ἧπάρ ἐστιν ὥσπερ τῆς μὲν ζωτικῆς ἡ καρδία, τῆς ψυχικῆς δ' ὁ ἐγκέφαλος.

[7] *Introductio sive Medicus*, cap. 9, K. xiv. 697: ἐνορμῶντα δέ ἐστι τὰ πνεύματα. πνεύματα δὲ κατὰ τοὺς παλαιοὺς δύο ἐστί, τό τε ψυχικὸν καὶ τὸ φυσικόν.

character of the atmospheric air.¹ The business of the physician is to keep
it, as well as the solid constituents of the body, in their natural condition
both of quality and quantity.² About this process of vaporization his conceptions seem rather vague. It arises from air breathed in through the
nose and the mouth, and also from air transpired through the pores of
the skin into the arteries meeting with or acting upon the blood. Various
names can be given to it, anyone who likes can call it aeration or rarefac-
tion or dissolution into vapour, or even diffusion.³ In another passage
he even speaks of it as 'boiling'.⁴ None of these expressions conveys to us
any exact idea of the process, but that perhaps is only to be expected, in
view of the very primitive notions of ancient Greek chemistry.

Galen, though very vague on these points, attempts in a characteristic
way to establish the difference between the vital and the psychic *pneuma*
by an experiment. Erasistratus had thought, as we have seen,⁵ that the
pneuma responsible for working the nervous system was produced in
the brain from the *pneuma* that had come up from the left ventricle of the
heart via the carotid artery, since he did not believe in any direct intake
of *pneuma* into the brain via mouth and nose. Galen, on the other hand,
following the 'Hippocratic' tradition, believed that *pneuma* reaches the
brain directly without passing through the lungs and the heart. In order
to prove this, he ligated the carotid arteries of an animal on both sides.
The animal went on breathing and moving without hindrance for a
whole day. At the end of the day Galen killed it, since it might later have
died from remoter consequences of ligation. What surprised him was
that even when the vascular connections between the two principal
organs of the body, the heart and the brain, had been interrupted, the
rest of the animal functions were so little disturbed.⁶ He does admit,

---

¹ *De methodo medendi*, xii. 5, K. x. 840: ἡ δὲ τοῦ πνεύματος ἀλλοίωσις διά τε μοχθηροὺς γίγνεται
χυμούς, καὶ τὴν τοῦ περιέχοντος ἀέρος κακίαν.

² Ibid., 838: τὴν τοῦ πνεύματος οὐσίαν ἅμα τοῖς στερεοῖς σώμασι φυλακτέον ἡμῖν ἐστιν ἐν ταῖς
νόσοις, ὥστε καὶ τῇ ποιότητι καὶ τῇ ποσότητι καθ' ὅσον ἐνδέχεται κατὰ φύσιν ἔχειν αὐτά.

³ Ibid., xi. 2, K. x. 742: ἐπειδὴ δὲ τῆς δυνάμεως οὐσία συνεπληροῦτο διά τε τοῦ πνεύματος καὶ
τῆς σαρκώδους ἰδέας τῶν στερεῶν, ἐκ τῶν ὁμοίων ἑκάστῳ πορίζεσθαι χρὴ τὴν διαμονήν. τῷ μὲν
πνεύματι διὰ τῆς ἀναπνοῆς τε καὶ διαπνοῆς καὶ τῆς ἐκ τοῦ αἵματος ἀναθυμιάσεως, ἐξέστω δὲ
κἀνταῦθα τῷ βουλομένῳ καλεῖν ἀέρωσιν, ἢ λεπτοποίησιν αἵματος, ἢ εἰς ἀτμοὺς λύσιν, ἢ χύσιν, ἢ
ὅπως ἂν αὐτὸς ἐθέλοι.

⁴ *De plac. Hipp. et Plat.* vi. 8, K. v. 573: ὡς οὖν ἀρτηριῶν, οὕτως καὶ τοῦ πνευματώδους τε καὶ
τοῦ ζέοντος αἵματος ἀρχή τε καὶ πηγὴ τοῖς ζῴοις ἐστίν ἡ καρδία.

⁵ See above, pp. 225 ff.

⁶ *De usu resp.* 5, K. iv. 502: ἐπισκεψώμεθα τουτὶ τὸ φαινόμενον οὗ πολλάκις ἐπειράθημεν. ἐν
γὰρ τῷ βρόχοις διαλαμβάνεσθαι τὰς κατὰ τὸν τράχηλον ἀρτηρίας οὐδὲν πάσχει τὸ ζῷον, οὔτ' εὐθὺς
οὔθ' ὕστερον, ὡς ἡμεῖς ἐνίοτε πειρώμενοι ἐν βρόχοις αὐτὰς διαλαμβάνομεν· ὅλην δὲ ἡμέραν τὸ ζῷον
εἰσπνέον τε καὶ ἐκπνέον καὶ κινούμενον ἀκωλύτως ἰδόντες, νυκτὸς ἤδη βαθείας ἐσφάξαμεν, οὐκέθ'
ἡγούμενοι τὴν ἐπὶ πλέον πεῖραν πίστιν ὑπάρχειν· δύνασθαι γὰρ ἐν τοσούτῳ χρόνῳ διὰ τοὺς περι-
κειμένους βρόχους συμπαθῆσαί τι τῶν κυριωτάτων μορίων. ἐθαυμάζομεν οὖν τὰς ἐκ τῶν κυριωτάτων
τῶν ζωτικῶν ὀργάνων, τῶν τῆς καρδίας, εἰς τὰ κυριώτατα τῶν ψυχικῶν τὸν ἐγκέφαλον τεταμένας
ἀρτηρίας, οὕτως ἄλυπον τῷ παντὶ βίῳ τὴν βλάβην ἐχούσας εὑρίσκοντες ... ἀπολείπεται γοῦν, ἤτοι

however, in another account he gives of the same experiment that though he was able to make the animal run quite well for a long time, it eventually became unable to run any more.[1] This experiment proved, according to Galen, that the brain did not need *pneuma* coming from the heart. We must assume therefore, either that there were sufficient 'exhalations' to maintain it from the existing blood in the brain, or that the brain inhaled sufficient air to maintain it through the nose. The first of these assumptions appears unlikely, since the arteries supplying blood and *pneuma* to the brain were intercepted by the ligature. Therefore the psychic *pneuma* must obtain most of its nourishment through the nose. Galen does, however, appear to believe that it may get a little *pneuma* from the heart as well as blood.[2] The net-like complex, the rete mirabile, as the medieval disciples of Galen called it, which is an arterial network arising out of the carotid artery and lying at the base of the brain, contains a sufficient reserve of psychic *pneuma* to enable an animal with ligatured carotids to carry on for quite some time. This net-like tissue of blood vessels is distinguished by Galen from the choroid plexus, the 'placenta-like' plexus which lines the ventricles of the brain, where the final elaboration of the psychic *pneuma* takes place. Both are conceived as networks of blood vessels containing both veins and arteries. The former lies at the base of the brain, wrapped up in a fold of the dura mater, the 'thick membrane', and from it the arteries go up into the brain to form the various networks of many branches in this organ including the networks lining the ventricles, the choroid plexus in which the psychic *pneuma* is given its final elaboration.[2] This net-like complex is something of a mystery. Herophilus, as we have seen, appears to have been the first to describe it, and Galen gives us two other descriptions, one in the treatise *On the opinions of Hippocrates and Plato*, and the other in the book *On the use of the parts*, besides the one here quoted.[3]

τὴν ἀναθυμίασιν αὐτῷ τὴν ἐκ τοῦ αἵματος ἱκανὴν ὑπάρχειν, ἢ τὴν διὰ τῶν ῥινῶν εἰσπνοήν. ἀλλ᾽ οὐδὲ τὴν ἀναθυμίασιν εἰκὸς γίγνεσθαι δαψιλῆ, βρόχῳ διαληφθεισῶν τῶν ἀρτηριῶν . . . ἀναγκαῖον οὖν ἐκ τῆς διὰ τῶν ῥινῶν ἐστιν ὡς τὴν πλείστην εἶναι τροφὴν τῷ ψυχικῷ πνεύματι.

[1] De usu pulsuum, 2, K. v. 155: ἐπεὶ δὲ μέχρι μὲν πολλοῦ καλῶς ἔτρεχε, μέχρι παντὸς δ᾽ οὐκ ἠδύνατο, ζητεῖν ἐδόκει χρῆναι, διότι μέχρι μὲν πολλοῦ ἔτρεχε, μέχρι παντὸς δ᾽ οὐκ ἠδύνατο, καὶ πάλιν αὐτὸ μέχρι πολλοῦ οὐ διαρκεῖν, ἀλλ᾽ εὐθέως ἐκλύεσθαι δαπανωμένου τοῦ ψυχικοῦ πνεύματος.

[2] Ibid., 154: ὥστ᾽ οὐδὲν θαυμαστόν, ὀλίγης αὐτῷ παρὰ καρδίας χορηγουμένης τῆς ἐπικουρίας ὀλίγην εἶναι καὶ τὴν βλάβην τῶν καρωτίδων λεγομένων ἀρτηριῶν βρόχοις διαληφθεισῶν.

[3] Ibid., K. v. 155–6: ἀλλὰ καὶ αὐτοῦ τούτου τὸ δικτυοειδὲς πλέγμα πρὸς τῶν ἀμφὶ τὸν Ἡρόφιλον κληθέν, ἐδόκει τὴν αἰτίαν ἔχειν. ἐκεῖ γὰρ αἱ ἐπὶ τὸν ἐγκέφαλον ἀνιοῦσαι καρωτίδες ἀρτηρίαι, πρὶν διελθεῖν τὴν σκληρὰν μήνιγγα, σχίζονται πολυειδῶς ὑπ᾽ αὐτῆς, περιπλεκόμεναι κατὰ πολλοὺς στίχους, ὡς εἰ νοήσαις ἀλλήλοις ἐπικείμενα δίκτυα πλείω, καὶ χώραν παμπόλλην, ἣν καλοῦσιν ἐγκεφάλου βάσιν, καταλαμβάνουσιν, ἐνὸν αὐταῖς εὐθὺς μὲν διεκπεσεῖν τὰς μήνιγγας, ἐμφῦναι δὲ εἰς τὸν ἐγκέφαλον, οὗ περ ἐξ ἀρχῆς ἱέναι. τοῦτ᾽ οὖν τὸ θαυμαστὸν πλέγμα πρὸς τῆς μηδὲν εἰκῆ ποιούσης φύσεως ἐν οὕτως ἀσφαλεῖ χώρᾳ ταχθῆναι, μεγάλης τινὸς ἐδόκει χρείας ἐνδεικτικὸν ὑπάρχειν. ἀλλ᾽ ἐπειδὴ τὴν τῶν ἐντέρων ἕλικα καὶ τὴν τῶν εἰς τοὺς ὄρχεις ἐμφυομένων ἀγγείων ἀκριβοῦς τε πέψεως ἕνεκα τῶν περιεχομένων ὑλῶν καὶ προσέτι δαψιλοῦς παρασκευῆς ταῖς

The description of this plexus given in the first-mentioned treatise is the more elaborate, and perhaps a little more precise. After referring to the choroid plexus as first instrument or organ of the soul, he continues with the following description of the retiform:

Now you would even more expect this *pneuma* to come into being through its being breathed by the blood vessels, particularly the arteries, into the ventricles of the brain, when you have examined the retiform plexus which is formed from the arteries which go into the brain, where they first traverse the underside of the skull and reach the inside of it by the so-called base of the brain. For there nature has prepared no small space like a bed-chamber for this retiform plexus surrounded by the dura mater, into which area a large portion of what are called the carotid arteries penetrates. At each end they form a single vessel, but between these single vessels they divide into many branches creating a far from simple network, one with many strands, lying on top of each other, and all of them intertwining with one another and fastened to one another. Moreover from this plexus which I have described, a pair of arteries emerges of the same size as those which originally grew out of the carotids, and is carried up into the brain. This pair of vessels weaves itself with very many branches into all the other parts of the brain including the plexuses formed round the ventricles. Now the *pneuma* in the arteries is, and is called, the vital, but that in the brain the psychic.[1]

The description given in the second treatise mentioned expressly compares the plexus to the nets of fishermen. It is not at all easy to follow:

The feature called by the anatomists the net-like plexus, the most wonderful object in this region, is situated here. It surrounds the gland [hypophysis] completely and reaches a long way to the rear, since practically the whole base of the brain has this plexus extending underneath it. It is a far from simple network, but it is as if you took a number of fisherman's nets and spread them out one on top of the other. It has this additional property, that each layer is continuously attached to the next one, so that you could not just take

ἑξῆς ἐνεργείαις ἑωρῶμεν γεγενημένην, εὔλογον ἐδόκει κἀνταῦθα τοιοῦτόν τι μεμηχανῆσθαι τὴν φύσιν ἅμα τε κατεργαζομένην πολλῷ χρόνῳ τὴν ἐν ταῖς ἀρτηρίαις ὕλην, αἷμα θερμὸν καὶ λεπτὸν καὶ ἀτμῶδες ὑπάρχουσαν, ἅμα τε κατασκευάζουσαν τροφὴν δαψιλῆ τῷ κατὰ τὸν ἐγκέφαλον ψυχικῷ πνεύματι.

[1] De plac. Hipp. et Plat. vii. 3, K. v. 607 : ἔτι δ᾽ ἂν μᾶλλον ἐλπίσαις γίγνεσθαι τὸ πνεῦμα τοῦτο, τῶν ἀγγείων ἀναπνεόντων αὐτό, καὶ μάλιστα τῶν ἀρτηριῶν, εἰς τὰς κοιλίας τοῦ ἐγκεφάλου, τὸ δικτυοειδὲς ἰδὼν πλέγμα γιγνόμενον ἐκ τῶν ἐρχομένων εἰς τὴν κεφαλὴν ἀρτηριῶν, ὅταν πρῶτον ὑπερβᾶσαι τὸ κράνιον ἐντὸς αὐτοῦ γένωνται κατὰ τὴν καλουμένην ἐγκεφάλου βάσιν. ἐνταῦθα γὰρ οὐκ ὀλίγην χώραν ἡ φύσις οἷον θαλάμην τινὰ τῷ δικτυοειδεῖ τῷδε παρεσκεύασε πλέγματι περιεχομένην ὑπὸ τῆς παχείας μήνιγγος, εἰς ἣν χώραν ἀπὸ τῶν καρωτίδων ὀνομαζομένων ἀρτηριῶν οὐ σμικρά τις ἀφικνουμένη μοῖρα, καθ᾽ ἑκάτερον μέρος ἓν ἀγγεῖον, εἶτα κατασχιζόμεναι πολυειδῶς οὐχ ἁπλοῦν ἐργάζονται καὶ τὸ δίκτυον, ἀλλ᾽ ἐπ᾽ ἀλλήλοις κείμενα πολλὰ μετὰ τοῦ συνῆφθαί τε καὶ συμπεφυκέναι πάντα. καὶ πάλιν γε κατὰ τοῦ πλέγματος τοῦδε τηλικούτου ζεύγους ἀρτηριῶν ἐκφυομένου, ἡλίκον ἐξ ἀρχῆς ἦν τὸ παρὰ τῶν καρωτίδων ἧκον, εἰς τὸν ἐγκέφαλον ἀναφέρεται τά τ᾽ ἄλλα μέρη διαπλέκον αὐτοῦ παμπόλλαις ἀπονεμήσεσι καὶ τὰ κατὰ τὰς κοιλίας ἐργαζόμενα πλέγματα. τὸ μὲν οὖν κατὰ τὰς ἀρτηρίας πνεῦμα ζωτικόν ἐστί τε καὶ προσαγορεύεται, τὸ δὲ κατὰ τὸν ἐγκέφαλον ψυχικόν.

hold of one of them. For each would follow the other in series if you pulled one of them, since they are all attached to each other in a row. Nor can you compare it to any man-made network on account of the fineness of its constituent threads and their close packing. Now it is not made of any matter casually thrown together, but of the arteries which run up from the heart to the head, a very large portion of which nature laid down in this network. For some short branches of these arteries go off into the neck and the face and the exterior of the head, and the scalp. But all the rest, which runs straight up from its source, carried up through the thorax and the neck to the head, is gratefully received by this portion of the skull, which lets it through its perforation and sends it on without any trouble into the inside of the head. Now the dura mater, too, might have received it and let it straight through in the direction in which it pointed by means of a perforation. Indeed one might have expected from all these conditions that the carotids would be in a hurry to get into the brain. But this was not the case. Once they had passed through the bottom of the skull, they split up, in the first place into many very small fine arteries in the space between it and the dura mater. And straightway spreading to the front, to the back and to the left and to the right in a network, they create the opposite impression that they have forgotten the way to the brain. But this is not true either. For all these arteries again unite like roots to form a trunk, so that another pair of arteries emerges equal in size to that which first went up through the skull, and this pair goes through perforations in the dura mater into the brain.[1]

The existence of any structure of this type at the base of the human brain must be denied, and it has generally been assumed that Galen was describing a vascular network which does exist at the base of the brain of certain domestic animals, but, as we have seen, the first

[1] De usu partium, ix. 4, K. iii. 696–8 : τὸ δὲ καλούμενον ὑπὸ τῶν ἀνατομικῶν δικτυοειδὲς πλέγμα μέγιστον θαῦμα τῶν ἐνταυθοῖ τέτακται, περιλαμβάνον μὲν ἐν κύκλῳ καὶ αὐτὸν τὸν ἀδένα, παρῆκον δὲ καὶ εἰς τοὐπίσω μέχρι πλείστου. πᾶσα γὰρ ὀλίγου δεῖν ἡ τοῦ ἐγκεφάλου βάσις ὑποτεταγμένον ἔχει τοῦτο τὸ πλέγμα. ἔστι δ' οὐχ ἁπλοῦν τὸ δίκτυον, ἀλλ' ὡς εἰ καὶ ταῦτα τὰ δίκτυα τῶν ἁλιέων πλείω λαβὼν ἐπ' ἀλλήλοις ἐκτείναις. πρόσεστι δὲ τῷ τῆς φύσεως ἐκείνῳ δικτύῳ τὸ τὰς ἐπιβολὰς ἀεὶ θατέρου συνῆφθαι θατέρῳ, καὶ μὴ δύνασθαι μόνον ἐν ὁτιουν λαβεῖν ἐξ αὐτῶν· ἕπεται γὰρ καὶ τὰ ἄλλα τῷ ληφθέντι κατὰ στοῖχον, ἁπάντων ἑξῆς ἀλλήλοις συνημμένων. οὐ μὴν οὐδὲ τῇ λεπτότητι τῶν συντεθέντων οὐδὲ τῇ πυκνότητι τῆς συνθέσεως ἔχοις ἂν αὐτῶν παραβαλεῖν οὐδὲν τῶν ἀνθρωπείων τούτων δικτύων. οὐ μὴν οὐδ' ἐξ ὕλης τῆς ἐπιτυχούσης γέγονεν, ἀλλὰ τῶν ἀπὸ τῆς καρδίας ἐπὶ τὴν κεφαλὴν ἀναφερομένων ἀρτηριῶν τὴν μὲν μεγίστην μοῖραν ἡ φύσις ὑπεβάλετο τῷ θαυμαστῷ τούτῳ πλοκάμῳ. βραχεῖαι γάρ τινες αὐτῶν ἀποβλαστήσεις εἴς τε τὸν τράχηλον καὶ τὸ πρόσωπον καὶ τακτὸς τῆς κεφαλῆς ἀπεχώρησε μόρια. τὸ δ' ἄλλο πᾶν ὃ ὄρθιον ἐξ ἀρχῆς ἐγένετο, διά τε τοῦ θώρακος καὶ τοῦ τραχήλου πρὸς τὴν κεφαλὴν ἀναφερόμενον, ὑπεδέξατο μὲν εὐμενῶς ἡ ταύτῃ μοῖρα τοῦ κρανίου, καὶ διατρηθεῖσα παρέπεμψεν ἀλύπως εἴσω τῆς κεφαλῆς· ὑπεδέδεκτο κἂν ἡ μῆνιγξ ἡ παχεῖα, καὶ κατ' εὐθὺ τῆς ἐκείνων ὁρμῆς ἤδη διετέτρητο· καὶ δόκησις ἦν ἐκ τούτων ἁπάντων ἐπείγεσθαι πρὸς τὸν ἐγκέφαλον αὐτάς. ἀλλ' οὐκ ἄρα τοῦθ' οὕτως εἶχεν. ὑπερβᾶσαι γὰρ τὸ κρανίον, ἐν τῇ μεταξὺ χώρᾳ τούτου τε καὶ τῆς παχείας μήνιγγος, πρῶτα μὲν ἐσχίσθησαν εἰς πολλὰς πάνυ σμικρὰς καὶ λεπτὰς ἀρτηρίας. ἑξῆς δὲ τὸ μέν τι πρόσω τῆς κεφαλῆς, τὸ δ' ὀπίσω, τὸ δ' εἰς ἀριστερὰ τὸ δ' εἰς δεξιὰ δι' ἀλλήλων φερόμεναί τε καὶ περιπλεκόμεναι πάλιν ἑτέραν δόκησιν ἐναντίαν παρέσχον, ὡς ἐπελάθοντο τῆς ἐπὶ τὸν ἐγκέφαλον ὁδοῦ. ἀλλ' οὐκ ἄρ' οὐδὲ τοῦτ' ἀληθὲς ἦν. αὖθις γὰρ ἐκ τῶν πολλῶν ἐκείνων ἀρτηριῶν ὥσπερ ἐκ ῥιζῶν εἰς πρέμνα τῆς συναγωγῆς γενηθείσης, ἐξέφυ ζεῦγος ἀρτηριῶν ἕτερον, ἴσον τῷ κατ' ἀρχὰς ἀνιόντι, καὶ οὕτως ἤδη διὰ τῆς παχείας μήνιγγος ἡμάτιων εἰς τὸν ἐγκέφαλον ἔδυ.

description of this network comes from Herophilus, who was presumably acquainted with the human brain, and Galen himself must have been pretty intimately acquainted with the brains of monkeys, as his very detailed accounts of how to dissect them (the brains) in the eighth and ninth books of the *Anatomical procedures* show.[1] We cannot assume that he is trying to describe the choroid plexus, since he carefully distinguishes this from the retiform, nor can we identify it with the tela choroidea of the third ventricle which he would have regarded as part of the choroid. Goss, who greatly admires the accuracy of Galen's anatomical descriptions,[2] has suggested that by the net-like plexus Galen means the circle of Willis,[3] an interesting suggestion, to a certain extent topographically appropriate, but as Siegel has pointed out,[4] in creatures which have both, the circle lies well above the rete, the latter, as Galen describes it, being below the dura mater. The circle of Willis in man is located above the dura mater surrounding the hypophysis and the infundibulum,[5] the 'stalk' of the pituitary gland. The animal in which this network is perhaps most noticeable is the ox, a species in which, according to Sisson and Grossmann,[6] a rete mirabile, which they define as 'a network intercalated in the course of an artery', is formed, among others, by the middle meningeal artery, which enters the cranial cavity through the foramen ovale and also by branches 'which take the place of the internal carotid artery'. These enter the cranial cavity through the foramen orbito-rotundum.

They concur with the branches of the occipital, vertebral, middle meningeal, and condyloid arteries in the formation of an extensive rete mirabile cerebri on the cranial floor around the sella turcica.[7]

This description seems to fit pretty closely with that of Galen who, we may be all but certain, never dissected a human brain, although he dissected brains of oxen and domestic animals by the score. No doubt confident that Herophilus had derived his knowledge of this structure from the dissection of the human brain, he took it for granted that the

---

[1] The ninth book in the Greek text abruptly ends with the sixth chapter, but the remainder of it has come down to us in an Arabic version of Hunain ibn Ishaq rendered into English by Duckworth (Cambridge University Press, London, 1962).

[2] See his presidential address to the American Association of Anatomists (1965).

[3] C. M. Goss, 'The precision of Galen's anatomical descriptions compared with Galenism', *Anat. Rec.* 152 (1965); and his translation of Galen's treatise *On the anatomy of muscles for beginners*, in the same volume.

[4] Siegel, *Galen's System of Physiology*, pp. 109 f.

[5] Ibid., p. 111; see the note to the diagram to the section on circle of Willis.

[6] S. Sisson and J. D. Grossmann, *The Anatomy of Domestic Animals* (Philadelphia, 1948), p. 626.

[7] Ibid., p. 723. I am indebted for reference to this work to Dr. Siegel.

human brain also contained such a network of arteries. Siegel has found another candidate in the human brain for the rete. He suggests that in man the internal carotid artery after passing through the petrous bone forms such a network below the dura mater, citing as his authority the anatomical atlas of Spalteholz.[1] Another less probable candidate is also suggested by Siegel in a footnote.[2] My anatomical knowledge does not entitle me to form any judgement on this difficult point, except perhaps to raise the question whether structures so comparatively small as the circle of Willis and Spalteholz's rete foraminis ovalis could answer for so conspicuous a complex as Galen would appear to postulate.

Galen's account of the generation of the psychic *pneuma*, which is given in the seventh book of the treatise *On the opinions of Hippocrates and Plato*, is so obscure that we shall be forced to quote it in full. After having described the disturbances of function caused by brain injuries involving the ventricles, he explains that when these are emptied of the *pneuma* by an injury, an animal remains alive, but without sensation or the power of movement until the *pneuma* has again been able to form itself, when the ventricles again close up. If therefore the psychic *pneuma* were the soul, its escape would cause immediate death, which it does not.[3]

Therefore it is reasonable to suppose that this [psychic] *pneuma* is generated in the ventricles of the brain and for that reason no small quantity of arteries and veins terminates there. These form the so-called placenta-like or choroid plexus, and that is the first tool or instrument of the soul.[4]

He now goes on to describe the retiform plexus in the words which we have already quoted, and explains that just as the vital spirit is formed from the vaporization or exhalation of blood and the humours (together with *pneuma*) in the arteries, so the psychic spirit is formed by the further

---

[1] W. Spalteholz, *Handatlas der Anatomie des Menschen*, 3 vols., 7th edn. (Hirzel, Leipzig, 1913–14); i. 5, 2. 400, fig. 445.

[2] Siegel, op. cit., p. 112, n. 33: 'It is conceivable but unlikely that Galen interpreted a venous network as rete. We find in H. G. Gray, *Anatomy of the Human Body*, 27th edn., pp. 740, 742 . . . that a network of *veins*, the rete foraminis ovalis, unites the cavernous sinus with the pterygoid plexus through the foramen ovale. Further, that the sinus intercavernosus ant. and post. form a venous circle with the cavernous sinuses around the hypophysis. This basilar plexus consists of several interlacing venous channels which are located *between* layers of the dura mater, above the occipital bone. They communicate with the anterior venous plexus of the cervical vertebra. Since venous and arterial vessels are intermingled, an error was quite possible.'

[3] *De plac. Hipp. et Plat.* vii. 3, K. v. 606: διὸ καὶ κενωθέν, ἄχρις ἂν αὖθις ἀθροισθῇ, τὴν μὲν ζωὴν οὐκ ἀφαιρεῖσθαι τὸ ζῷον, ἀναίσθητον δὲ καὶ ἀκίνητον ἐργάζεσθαι· καίτοι γε εἴπερ ἦν αὐτὸ ἡ τῆς ψυχῆς οὐσία συνδιεφθείρετ' ἂν αὐτῷ κενουμένῳ παραχρῆμα τὸ ζῷον.

[4] Ibid.: εὔλογον οὖν γεννᾶσθαι τουτὶ τὸ πνεῦμα κατὰ τὰς κοιλίας τοῦ ἐγκεφάλου, καὶ διὰ τοῦτο ἐκεῖσε τελευτᾶν ἀρτηριῶν τε καὶ φλεβῶν οὐκ ὀλίγον πλῆθος, ἐξ οὗ τὰ καλούμενα χοροειδῆ πλέγματα γέγονεν, ὄργανον δ', ὡς ἔφην, εἶναι τὸ πρῶτον αὐτὸ τῆς ψυχῆς. ἔτι δ' ἂν μᾶλλον ἐλπίσαις γίγνεσθαι τὸ πνεῦμα τοῦτο, τῶν ἀγγείων ἀναπνεόντων αὐτό, καὶ μάλιστα τῶν ἀρτηριῶν, εἰς τὰς κοιλίας τοῦ ἐγκεφάλου.

elaboration of the vital spirit.[1] The retiform plexus was formed as a sort of labyrinth—today we might say laboratory?—close to the brain for the elaboration of the psychic spirit,[2] though only the laboratory for the first stage in the production of this rather mysterious entity. Its final elaboration only takes place in the choroid plexus of the ventricles of the brain. This first elaboration is compared and contrasted with the secretion of semen, and of milk, though these are much less powerful products. Nature, wishing to ensure that the material of which they are composed remains a sufficient time in the organs which produce them to ensure their thorough processing, invented a lot of complicated passages for their reception in the breasts and in the testicles. But the psychic *pneuma* needs much more careful and accurate elaboration than even the semen. In an interesting passage he compares the retiform plexus with the 'variciform' plexus of the spermatic cord, and remarks that the former is much more complicated than the latter.[3]

But the physics of the final elaboration of the psychic spirit are anything but easy to translate into modern terms, in spite of Galen's remarkably correct ideas of the vascular anatomy of the brain. Thus he has a general acquaintance with the venous sinuses which he connects with the torcular Herophili,[4] and he has some general idea of the superior cerebral veins,[5] though he regards the former as reservoirs of venous blood to feed the brain. In the brain, in contradistinction to many other parts of the body (e.g. the intestines and the stomach), veins and arteries run very close together and in many cases even touch one

---

[1] Ibid., 608 : ὥσπερ δὲ τὸ ζωτικὸν πνεῦμα κατὰ τὰς ἀρτηρίας τε καὶ τὴν καρδίαν γεννᾶται, τὴν ὕλην ἔχον τῆς γενέσεως ἔκ τε τῆς εἰσπνοῆς καὶ τῆς τῶν χυμῶν ἀναθυμιάσεως, οὕτω τὸ ψυχικὸν ἐκ τοῦ ζωτικοῦ κατεργασθέντος ἐπὶ πλέον ἔχει τὴν γένεσιν.

[2] Ibid., 608–9 : εἰκότως καὶ κατὰ τὸν ἐγκέφαλον ἐκ τοῦ ζωτικοῦ πνεύματος ἐργαζομένη (ἡ φύσις) τὸ ψυχικόν, οἷον λαβύρινθόν τινα ποικίλον ἐδημιούργησε πλησίον ἐγκεφάλου τὸ δικτυοειδὲς πλέγμα.

[3] Ibid., 608 : ἐχρῆν γὰρ δήπου μᾶλλον ἁπάντων αὐτὸ μεταβολῆς ἀκριβοῦς τυχεῖν. εἴπερ οὖν τό τε σπέρμα καὶ τὸ γάλα, καίτοι γ' ἀπολειπόμενα τῇ δυνάμει τοῦ ψυχικοῦ πνεύματος, ὅμως ἡ φύσις ἀκριβῶς κατεργάζεσθαι δεομένη πολυχρόνιον αὐτοῖς ἐμηχανήσατο τὴν ἐν τοῖς πεπτικοῖς ὀργάνοις διατριβήν, καὶ διὰ τοῦτο τῷ μὲν σπέρματι τὴν πρὸς τῶν ὄρχεων ἕλικα παρεσκεύασε, τῷ δὲ γάλακτι τὸ μῆκος τῶν εἰς τοὺς τιτθοὺς ἰόντων ἀγγείων. Cf. *De usu partium*, ix. 4, K. iii. 700, where the retiform plexus is compared with the 'variciform' : ἀλλ' ὅσῳ τὸ κατὰ τὸν ἐγκέφαλον πνεῦμα ψυχικὸν ἀκριβεστέρας ἐδεῖτο κατεργασίας τῆς τοῦ σπέρματος, τοσούτῳ καὶ τὸ δικτυοειδὲς πλέγμα τοῦ κιρσοειδοῦς πολυπλοκώτερον ἐγένετο. καλῶς οὖν ἐν ἐκείνοις ἐπεδείκνυτο τοῖς ὑπομνήμασιν ἡ γένεσις τοῦ κατὰ τὸν ἐγκέφαλον πνεύματος ψυχικοῦ, τὸ διὰ τῶν ἀρτηριῶν ἀναφερόμενον τὸ ζωτικὸν ὕλην οἰκείαν ἔχειν.

[4] *De usu partium*, ix. 6, K. iii. 708 : συμβάλλουσι δὲ κατὰ τὴν κορυφὴν τῆς κεφαλῆς αἱ παράγουσαι τὸ αἷμα διπλώσεις τῆς μήνιγγος εἰς χώραν τινὰ κενήν, οἷον δεξαμένην, ἣν δὴ καὶ δι' αὐτὸ τοῦτο προσαγορεύειν ἔθος ἐστὶν Ἡροφίλῳ ληνόν.

[5] Ibid., 708–9 : ἐντεῦθεν δ' οἷον ἐξ ἀκροπόλεώς τινος ἅπασι τοῖς ὑποκειμένοις μορίοις ὀχετοὺς ἐπιπέμπουσιν· οὐδ' ἔστιν ἔτι τὸν ἀριθμὸν εἰπεῖν τῶν ἐκροῶν, ὅτι μηδὲ τὸ πλῆθος τῶν τρεφομένων ἀριθμῆσαι μορίων. ἐκρέουσι δὲ τινὲς μὲν ἐξ αὐτῆς τῆς μέσης χώρας εἰς τὴν παρακεφαλίδα πᾶσαν, ἐσχισμένοι τε καὶ κατατετμημένοι τρόπον ὁμοιότατον τοῖς κατὰ τὰς πρασιάς, τινὰς δ' ἐκ τοῦ πρόσω φερομένου τοῦ τὸν ληνὸν ἐκδεχομένου φαίης ἂν ἀγωγοῦ τινος αἵματος, ὃν καὶ αὐτὸν ἐκ τῆς παχείας μήνιγγος εὐμηχάνως ἐτεχνήσατο.

another externally. But in the case of the brain nature has made quite different arrangements. Both types of vessel are in many places at a considerable distance from each other,[1] and nature found it better to ensure that veins and arteries should meet in the brain coming in opposite directions. The arteries come up from the heart and pass through the retiform plexus and then continue upwards into the brain; the veins, on the other hand, pass downwards into it from the venous sinuses at the crown.[2] A large number of both veins and arteries have their terminations in the choroid plexus of the ventricles, and both are spread all over the other parts of the brain. Now many veins and arteries reach down to the stomach and the intestines, which secrete bile and phlegm and certain other humours of this kind, while retaining in themselves the blood and the vital spirit. In the same way in the ventricles of the brain the veins secrete their surpluses (presumably of humours other than blood?), while the arteries most of all breathe *pneuma*. Nature made special arrangements that the substances escaping through their mouths should permeate the whole of the brain, while they are still contained in the blood vessels, they go in them all over the body, but once secreted, they become subject to the natural laws, as we should say, of gravitation, the light and thin ones are carried upwards and the heavy and thick ones downwards. Now those of the arteries in the ventricles whose ends point downwards discharge no *pneuma* into the ventricles, except so much as the motion of the artery itself may push out, but from those arteries which point upwards towards the brain, a continual stream of *pneuma* processed in the retiform plexus keeps pouring, as much, in fact, as the arteries in the plexus transmit. Now the *pneuma* is not able to pass quickly through the plexus on account of the complicated structure of its vessels, turning now up, now down, now left, now right. It is therefore processed throughout a long stay in the plexus before being discharged straight into the brain's ventricles.[3] It consequently undergoes extensive alterations.[4]

---

[1] *De usu partium*, ix. 4, 703: ἔπειτα δέ, ὅτι μεγάλα τὰ μεταξὺ τῶν ἀγγείων ἔσχε διαστήματα.

[2] Ibid., 5, 705: οὐκ ἄρα θαυμάσομεν τὴν πρόνοιαν τοῦ δημιουργοῦ, μέχρι μὲν αὐτῆς τῆς κεφαλῆς ἀπὸ τῆς καρδίας διὰ τοῦ θώρακός τε καὶ παντὸς τοῦ τραχήλου τὰς φλέβας ἅμα ταῖς ἀρτηρίαις ἀναγαγόντος, ἐντεῦθεν δὲ τὰς μὲν ἀρτηρίας ἐπὶ τὸ δικτυοειδὲς πλέγμα, τὰς φλέβας δ' ἐπ' ἄκραν τὴν κορυφὴν τῆς κεφαλῆς ἀναγαγόντος. Cf. ibid., 703-4: . . . ἀναμνησθῆναι πασῶν τῶν κατὰ τὸ σῶμα φλεβῶν καὶ ἀρτηριῶν, ὅπως εἰς ἅπαντα τὰ μόρια τὰ δεόμενα τῶν ἀγγείων ἀμφοτέρων ἐμφύονται, ὡς ἐγγὺς ἀλλήλων καὶ πλησίον οὕτω πολλάκις, ὥστε καὶ ψαύειν τὰς εἰς κοιλίαν καὶ νῆστιν καὶ πᾶν τὸ λεπτὸν ἔντερον καὶ τὸ κῶλον . . . κατὰ δέ γε τὸν ἐγκέφαλον ὅτι βέλτιον ἦν ἐκ διαφερόντων χωρίων, μᾶλλον δ' ἐναντίων πάντη τὴν εἰς αὐτὸν ποιήσασθαι κατάφυσιν . . .

[3] Ibid., 4, 700-2: ὅ τε γὰρ ὅλος ἐγκέφαλος ὑπὸ τούτων τῶν ἀρτηριῶν διαπλέκεται, πολυειδῶς σχισθεισῶν, καὶ πολλαὶ τῶν ἀποσχίδων εἰς τὰς κοιλίας αὐτοῦ τελευτῶσιν, ὥσπερ οὖν καὶ τῶν ἐκ τῆς κορυφῆς κατιουσῶν φλεβῶν. ἐξ ἐναντίων μὲν γὰρ τόπων ἐμβάλλουσι ταῖς ἀρτηρίαις, εἰς ἅπαντα δ' ὡσαύτως αὐτοῦ τὰ μόρια διανέμονται, τά τε ἄλλα καὶ κατ' αὐτὰς τὰς κοιλίας. ἀλλ' ὥσπερ εἰς τὴν γαστέρα καὶ τὰ ἔντερα καθήκουσιν ἀρτηρίαι τε καὶ φλέβες πάμπολλαι, χολὴν μὲν καὶ φλέγμα καὶ τινας ἑτέρας τοιαύτας ὑγρότητας εἰς τὴν ἐκτὸς εὐρυχωρίαν ἀποχέουσαι, στέγουσι δ' ἐντὸς αὐτῶν τό θ' αἷμα καὶ τὸ πνεῦμα τὸ ζωτικόν, οὕτως εἰς τὰς κατὰ τὸν ἐγκέφαλον κοιλίας αἱ μὲν φλέβες ὡσαύτως

(For footnote 3 cont. and 4 see page 361 opposite)

It is not easy to make out quite what this double processing of the vital spirit in the retiform plexus and in the ventricles is supposed to consist of. So far as the arteries of the plexuses are concerned, it would appear that they merely breathe in the *pneuma* that has been drawn into the brain through the nose, by the rather complicated passages through the sponge-like bone at the base of the skull.[1] Being arteries they are in a continual state of alternate expansion and contraction. When they arrive at the retiform plexus they contain the light sort of blood and vital spirit which is the 'steam' (ἄτμος) of the arterial blood 'fed' by *pneuma*. A process of further exposure to the *pneuma* in the brain taking place in both plexuses, but principally in the retiform, completes the transformation of the *pneuma* they contain into its final psychic form, and this is breathed out by them into the ventricles from the choroid plexus. The part played by the veins of the choroid plexus, and in the retiform, if they exist there at all which appears to be doubtful—a fact which might be adduced in favour of Goss's identification of it with the circle of Willis—is very far from clear, and Galen's accounts of it appear to differ. What are these 'superfluities' which are excreted by the veins into the ventricles? In a passage in the ninth book of the *Anatomical procedures*, Galen describes the venous sinus of the torcular which he qualifies as 'callous' (not to be confused with the corpus callosum), a sort of depository for the imperfectly processed alimentary products from the adjacent portions of the brain.[2] It is difficult to see what part these can play in the development of

ἐκκρίνουσι μὲν τὰ περιττώματα, τὸ δ' αἷμα κατέχουσιν, αἱ δ' ἀρτηρίαι τὸ πνεῦμα καὶ μάλιστα πάντων ἀναπνέουσιν. αὗται μὲν γὰρ ἐκ τῶν κάτωθεν ἀναφέρονται μερῶν, αἱ φλέβες δ' ἐκ τῆς κορυφῆς εἰς αὐτὸν καθήκουσι, προνοησαμένης καὶ τοῦτο θαυμαστῶς τῆς φύσεως, ἵν' αἱ διεκπίπτουσαι τῶν κατ' αὐτὰς στομάτων οὐσίαι διεξέρχωνται τὸν ὅλον ἐγκέφαλον. ἔστ' ἂν μὲν γὰρ ἐν αὐτοῖς τοῖς ἀγγείοις ὦσι περιεχόμεναι, πάντη τοῦ σώματος ἅμ' ἐκείνοις ἴασιν· ἐπειδὰν δ' ἅπαξ αὐτῶν ἐκπέσωσι, κατὰ τὴν οἰκείαν ἑκατέρα φέρεται ῥοπήν, ἄνω μὲν ἡ κούφη τε καὶ λεπτή, κάτω δὲ ἡ παχεῖά τε καὶ βαρεία. τῶν μὲν οὖν εἰς τὰ κατὰ τὴν κοιλίαν μόρια περαινουσῶν ἀρτηριῶν κατάντη τὴν θέσιν ἐχουσῶν, οὐδὲν εἰς τὴν ὑποδεχομένην εὐρυχωρίαν ἐμπίπτει πνεῦμα, πλὴν ὅσον ἂν ὑπ' αὐτῶν τῶν ἀγγείων τῆς ἐνεργείας προωθῆταί ποτε. τῶν δ' εἰς τὸν ἐγκέφαλον ἀνάντης μὲν ἡ θέσις, ἐκρεῖ δ' ἀεὶ τὸ καλῶς κατειργασμένον ἐν τῷ δικτυοειδεῖ πλέγματι, τοσοῦτον ἑκάστοτε ἐπιφερόμενον, ὅσον ἂν αἱ κατ' αὐτὸ προπέμπωσιν ἀρτηρίαι. οὐ γὰρ δὴ καὶ ταύτας γε δύναται ταχέως διεξελθεῖν, ἀλλ' ἴσχεται κατά τε τὰς ἄνωθεν κάτω καὶ τὰς εἰς τὸ πλάγιον ἐπιστροφάς τε καὶ καμπάς, πολλάς τε καὶ πολυειδεῖς οὔσας, παντοίως ἀλώμενον. ὥστε ἐν ταύταις μὲν χρόνῳ παμπόλλῳ μένον κατεργάζεται, κατεργασθὲν δ' εὐθέως ἐμπίπτει ταῖς κοιλίαις τοῦ ἐγκεφάλου. Cf. *Comment. III in Hipp. de alimento* i, K. xv. 263: ὥσπερ δὲ τὸ ζωτικὸν πνεῦμα κατὰ τὰς ἀρτηρίας τε καὶ καρδίαν γεννᾶται, τὴν γένεσιν ἔκ τε τῆς εἰσπνοῆς ἔχον καὶ τῆς τῶν χυμῶν ἀναθυμιάσεως, οὕτω τὸ ψυχικὸν ἐκ τοῦ ζωτικοῦ κατεργασθέντος ἐπὶ πλέον ἔχει τὴν γένεσιν.

4 Ibid., xvi. 10, K. iv. 323: τρέφουσι γὰρ αὗται τὸ ψυχικὸν ἐν ἐγκεφάλῳ πνεῦμα, πολὺ δή τι παραλλάττον τῇ φύσει πάντων τῶν ἄλλων πνευμάτων, ὥστ' οὐδὲν θαυμαστὸν ἐπὶ πλεῖστον προπεμπομένης καὶ προκατειργασμένης καὶ πάντα τρόπον ἠλλοιωμένης χρῄζειν αὐτὸ τροφῆς.

1 Ibid., viii. 6, K. iii. 651: προστίθησιν αὐτῷ ἡ φύσις ὀστοῦν ποικίλως κατατετρημένον, ὥσπερ σπογγίαν, ὑπὲρ τοῦ μηδ' ἄλλο τι προσπίπτειν ἔξωθεν σκληρὸν σῶμα, μήτ' ἀκραιφνῆ τὴν ψῦξιν, εἰσπνεόντων ἡμῶν, εὐθὺ τῶν κατὰ τὸν ἐγκέφαλον ἰέναι κοιλιῶν.

2 *De anatomicis admin.* ix. 3, K. ii. 718 f.: ἤτοι γ' ἔκκοπτε πᾶσαν μέχρι τῶν κατὰ τὸν ληνὸν χωρίων, ἢ ᾗπερ ἐκπέφυκεν ἀνατείνας ἐπ' αὐτῶν ἐκείνων κατάθες. σὺ δὲ τὴν χώραν, ἣν ἐγύμνωσας, ἐπιμελῶς κατάσκεψαι, τυλώδη πως οὖσαν, ὡς φαίνεσθαί τινα φυσικὴν ἐνταῦθα ὑπάρχειν κοιλότητα,

the psychic spirit. In a passage in the treatise *On the opinions of Hippocrates and Plato*, we are told that this psychic *pneuma*, which is in the ventricles, is produced, a little of it perhaps from the veins which terminate in them, but the most important part of it in the arteries of the retiform plexus.[1]

The reason here expressed seems to be based merely on the fact that the veins contain some *pneuma*, i.e. vital spirit, but the 'superfluities' still need explanation. I can only hazard the guess that perhaps Galen considered that the arterial blood, since it had undergone so much purification, needed some elements of the humours which could only be provided from the venous blood. Whatever the truth of this matter, there can be no doubt that the working over of the vital spirit in the brain produced a fairly large quantity of 'smoky residues'. The evacuation of these what we should call gaseous products appears to have created no difficulties for him. Being gaseous they naturally travel upwards, and their tenuous nature enables them to pass quite easily through the soft matter of the brain which simply closes automatically after they have made their way through it.[2] Nor is the texture of the two membranes enveloping the brain, the pia and the dura mater, or the diploon or marrow of the skull or pericranium any obstacle. The skull however presents a more formidable problem. It has to act as an efficient protection for the brain from all possibilities of external injury, and yet it has also to let through these 'waste products'. Nature solved this problem by making the skull rather spongy in its texture and by inventing the sutures which form an easy passage for these redundancies.[3] The thicker are evacuated only through the sutures, but the thinner find their way through the skull itself.[4]

δεχομένην τῶν ὑπερκειμένων τε καὶ περικειμένων σωμάτων τὰ μὴ κατεργασθέντα τελέως τῆς τροφῆς, ἃ καλοῦσιν ἰδίως περιττώματα.

[1] *De plac. Hipp. et Plat.* iii. 8, K. v. 356: γένεσις δὲ τῷ πνεύματι τῷδε τῷ κατὰ τὰς κοιλίας αὐτοῦ τάχα μέν τις ὀλίγη καὶ ἐκ τῶν εἰς αὐτὰς περαινομένων γίγνεται φλεβῶν, τὴν πλείστην δὲ καὶ κυριωτάτην αἱ κατὰ τὸ δικτυοειδὲς πλέγμα τὸ κατὰ τὴν τοῦ ἐγκεφάλου βάσιν ἀρτηρίαι χορηγοῦσιν, αἵτινες ἀπὸ τῆς καρδίας ἀναφέρονται.

[2] *De usu partium*, ix. 1, K. iii. 686 f.: διττοὺς καὶ τοὺς τῆς ἐκκρίσεως αὐτοῖς ἐτέμετο πόρους, τοὺς μὲν τὰ κοῦφα κενώσοντας ἐπὶ τὸ ὑψηλότερον ἄγουσα, τοὺς δὲ τὰ βαρέα τε καὶ κάτω ῥέποντα κατάντεις ἐργασαμένη ... ἀλλ' ἐν μὲν τοῖς ὑγροῖς τε καὶ μαλακοῖς τοῦ σώματος μέρεσιν οὐδ' ἀποτέτακταί τις ἐξαίρετος ὁδὸς οὐδεμιᾷ τῇ τοιαύτῃ κενώσει, πεφυκότος γε δὴ παντὸς ὑγροῦ καὶ μαλακοῦ σώματος εἴκειν μὲν ἑτοίμως καὶ διίστασθαι τοῖς μεθ' ὁρμῆς ὠκυτέρας δι' αὐτοῦ φερομένοις, ἀπελθόντων δ' αὖθις ἐκείνων, συνέρχεσθαί τε καὶ συμφύεσθαι παραχρῆμα τὴν ἀρχαίαν ἀπολαμβάνον ἕνωσιν.

[3] Ibid., 687–9: ταῦτ' ἄρα κατὰ μὲν αὐτὸν τὸν ἐγκέφαλον καὶ τὰς μήνιγγας καὶ τὸ περὶ τὴν κεφαλὴν δέρμα πόρους ἀφωρισμένους εἰς ἀτμῶν κένωσιν οὔτ' ἀναγκαῖον ὑπάρχειν, οὔτ' εἴπερ ἦσάν τινες οἷόν τ' ἦν αὐτοὺς αἰσθήσει διαγνῶναι, φθάνοντάς γε δὴ συνιζάνειν εὐθὺς ἅμα τῷ κενωθῆναι ... ἀλλ' ἐπεὶ τὸν ἐγκέφαλον ἀναγκαῖον ἦν ἀσφαλεῖ φρουρεῖσθαι περιβόλῳ καὶ διὰ τοῦθ' ἡ φύσις οὐ δέρματι μόνῳ ... τὴν φυλακὴν ἐπίστευσεν, ἀλλ' οἷον κράνος τι πρότερον αὐτῷ περιέβαλε τὸ πρὸ τοῦ δέρματος ὀστοῦν, οὐ μόνον τῆς δαψιλεστέρας παρὰ τὰ λοιπὰ μόρια κενώσεως, ἀλλ' οὐδὲ τῆς μετρίας εὐπορήσειν ἔμελλεν, εἰ μὴ πολλὰς ἀναπνοὰς αὐτῷ παρεσκεύασεν, ἅμα μὲν σηραγγοειδὲς ἐργασαμένη τὸ τῆς κεφαλῆς ὀστοῦν, ἅμα δὲ καὶ συνηρθρωμένον ποικίλως ταῖς ὀνομαζομέναις ῥαφαῖς.

[4] Ibid., 691: τὰ μὲν οὖν παχύτερα τῶν αἰθαλωδῶν περιττωμάτων διὰ τούτων κενοῦται μόνων, τοῖς λεπτοτέροις δὲ καὶ αὐτὸ τὸ κρανίον ἐστὶ βάσιμον.

How the psychic spirit works is only explained in a rather superficial comparison. Just as the heart in systole and diastole alternately draws in and sends out again blood and *pneuma*, so the brain when it wishes to send out any of the psychic spirit in its ventricles to any portion performs a similar motion of transmission.[1] It is a little difficult to reconcile this explanation with the distinction we have already noted between the involuntary character of the heart's action and the voluntary character of respiration.[2]

With the function of the psychic *pneuma* in the operation of the nervous system, both sensory and motor, we cannot concern ourselves further here. To return then to the blood and the arteries. The function of the arteries, with their dual content of blood and *pneuma*, is, as we have seen, to guard or preserve the innate heat and to nourish the psychic (and vital) spirit,[3] as well as to feed all those parts of the body which, like the lungs, need the lighter, purer, and more finished type of blood. This arterial blood, bright red, thin, and like *pneuma*, is generated in the left ventricle whence it is distributed, Galen does not tell us exactly how, to all parts of the body.[4] Its function, like that of the venous blood from which it is derived, is nourishment. All parts of the body do not require the same kind of nourishment; those needing lighter material draw it from the arteries, not only the lungs but tissues all over the body, while thicker parts draw it from the veins.[5] But most parts need both kinds. Thus muscles, for instance, are provided with both arteries and veins.[6] It would appear that the arteries keep their blood and *pneuma* separately, not in a state of combination, since in certain diseases, presumably, they may become over-filled with blood, leaving no space for *pneuma*. This prevents them from pulsating and drawing in air from the atmosphere, thus suffocating and extinguishing the innate heat, so that the patient loses consciousness and power of moving.[7] The blood in the arteries is hotter

---

[1] De plac. Hipp. et Plat. iii. 8, K. v. 355–6: ὥσπερ γὰρ αὐτὸ τὸ σῶμα τῆς καρδίας ἐξ ἑαυτοῦ διαστελλόμενόν τε καὶ συστελλόμενον ἐν μέρει τὰς ὕλας τε ἕλκει καὶ αὖθις ἐκπέμπει, κατὰ τὸν αὐτὸν τρόπον ὁ ἐγκέφαλος, ἐπειδὰν προέληται τοῦ περιεχομένου κατὰ τὰς ἑαυτοῦ κοιλίας πνεύματος, ὃ δὴ καὶ ψυχικὸν ὀνομάζομεν, ἐπιπέμψαι τινὶ μορίῳ, τὴν εἰς τοῦτ᾽ ἐπιτηδείαν κίνησιν κινηθεὶς οὕτως ἐπιπέμπει.

[2] See above, p. 270.

[3] De usu partium, i. 16, K. iii. 45 f.: ἀρτηριῶν δὲ φυλάττειν τε τὴν κατὰ φύσιν θερμασίαν καὶ τρέφειν τὸ πνεῦμα ψυχικόν.

[4] Comment. I in Hipp. de humoribus, K. xvi, 12 f.: αἵματος δὲ ξανθοῦ καὶ λεπτοῦ καὶ πνευματώδους ἡ μὲν πρώτη γένεσις ἐν τῇ καρδίας ἀριστέρᾳ κοιλίᾳ. διανέμουσι δὲ καὶ παράγουσιν εἰς ὅλον τὸ ζῷον αἱ ἀρτηρίαι.

[5] De semine, i. 2, K. iv. 554: πρῶτον μὲν οὖν ἕλκει τὰ μέλλοντα θρέψασθαι τὸν οἰκεῖον ἕκαστον ἐκ τοῦ αἵματος χυμὸν ... καὶ ὡς τὸ μὲν παχυτέρου δεῖται τοῦ αἵματος, τὸ δὲ λεπτοτέρου, καὶ τὸ μὲν θερμοτέρου, τὸ δὲ ψυχροτέρου, καὶ τὸ μὲν φλεγματωδεστέρου, τὸ δὲ μελαγχολικωτέρου· ἀτὰρ οὖν καὶ ἀκριβεστέρου καὶ καθαρωτέρου δεῖταί τινα, καὶ αὖθις ἕτερα μὲν καθαρωτέρου, τὰ δ᾽ ὀρρωδεστέρου, καὶ δὴ καὶ τελεωτάτου κατειργασμένου.

[6] Comment. III in Hipp. de alimento, K. xv. 259: ἅπας δὲ μῦς ἀρτηρίας τε καὶ φλέβας ἔχει καὶ διὰ τούτων τρέφεται.

[7] De causis morborum, 3, K. vii. 14: ἐπειδὰν δὲ ἀποληφθῶσιν αἱ κατὰ τὸ ζῷον ἀρτηρίαι, τοῦτ᾽ ἔστιν οὕτω πληρωθῶσιν αἵματος ὡς μηδεμίαν ἔτι κενὴν ἀπολείπεσθαι χώραν ἐν αὐταῖς, εἰς ἣν ἐν τῷ

than that in the veins, and it moves much faster.[1] The *pneuma* which they carry is also hot, particularly in the large arteries and the thorax.[2] The arteries have need of blood to feed their coats. At each diastole they draw blood from the veins through the capillaries into their coats, taking from this blood the lighter constituents.[3] At each systole they press or squeeze *pneuma* through the capillaries into the veins,[4] whose coats are fed simply by the blood which flows through them.[5] The arteries at systole only press *pneuma* through the capillaries, since it would not appear that the whole contents of the arterioles' blood as well as *pneuma* are pressed into the venules, for this blood would not perform any useful function, as the venous coats do not need nourishment, but they do need *pneuma* to keep them 'alive', even though the action of both types of blood vessel is merely 'natural', i.e. it is not subject to voluntary control. Galen seems to distinguish quite clearly the vital functions conferred by the blood from those conferred by the nerves. This is shown in his account of the movement of muscles. Muscles contain, as Erasistratus was the first to point out, arteries, veins, and nerves. The first two of these irrigate the body of the muscle, and convert it from being a mere three-dimensional non-living solid to a live thing something like a plant. But it is the nerve that makes it more than a plant, and confers upon it the powers of perception, movement, and impulse.[6] But a plant is alive, and a stone is not, and the vein as a part of an animal must be alive too, and so must have a share of the vital *pneuma*. In this account be it noted, there does

διαστέλλεσθαι τὸν ἔξωθεν ἀέρα ἐπισπᾶν δυνήσονται, καταπνίγεται μὲν ἐν τῷδε καὶ ἔμφυτον θερμόν, ἀκίνητοι δὲ καὶ ἀναίσθητοι διὰ ταχέων οἱ οὕτω παθόντες ὅλῳ τῷ σώματι γίγνονται.

[1] De dogm. Hipp. et Plat. vi. 8, K. v. 573–4: τὸ δ' ἐκ τῆς ἀριστερᾶς κοιλίας τῆς καρδίας ὁρμώμενον θερμότερόν τε τοῦδε καὶ πνευματῶδες ἱκανῶς ἐστιν, ὡς ἂν σφυζόντων αὐτοῦ τῶν ἀγγείων.

[2] De semine, ii. 5, K. iv. 633: ἐπεὶ μᾶλλον ἐργάζεσθαί τι τοῦτο πέφυκε πολὺ πνεῦμα θερμόν, ταῦτά τοι καὶ ἀρτηρίας μείζονάς τε καὶ ἰσχυρότερον ἔχει σφύζουσας.

[3] De usu partium, vi. 10, K. iii. 455: συνανεστόμωνται μὲν αἱ ἀρτηρίαι ταῖς φλεψὶ καθ' ὅλον τὸ σῶμα, καὶ μεταλαμβάνουσιν ἐξ ἀλλήλων αἷμα καὶ πνεῦμα διά τινων ἀοράτων τε καὶ στενῶν ἀκριβῶς ὁδῶν.

[4] De nat. fac. iii. 14, K. ii. 204–5: θαυμαστὸν οὐδέν σοι φανεῖται τὰς ἀρτηρίας, ὅσαι μὲν εἰς τὸ δέρμα περαίνουσιν αὐτῶν, ἐπισπᾶσθαι τὸν ἔξωθεν ἀέρα διαστελλομένας· ὅσαι δὲ κατά τι πρὸς τὰς φλέβας ἀνεστόμωνται τὸ λεπτότατον ἐν αὐταῖς καὶ ἀτμωδέστατον ἐπισπᾶσθαι τοῦ αἵματος. Cf. ibid., 207: καὶ τοίνυν καὶ ταῖς ἀρτηρίαις τε καὶ τῇ καρδίᾳ, ὡς μὲν κοίλοις τε καὶ διαστέλλεσθαι δυναμένοις ὀργάνοις, ἀεὶ τὸ κουφότερον ἀκολουθεῖ πρότερον, ὡς δὲ τρέφεσθαι δεομένοις εἰς αὐτοὺς τοὺς χιτῶνας.

[5] De usu pulsuum, 5, K. v. 165: διὰ γοῦν τούτων τῶν ἀναστομώσεων ἐκ τῶν φλεβῶν ἕλκουσι μὲν ἐν ταῖς διαστολαῖς ἀρτηρίαι, ἐκθλίβουσι δὲ εἰς αὐτὰς ἐν ταῖς συστολαῖς. Cf. De nat. fac. ii. 96: αἱ μὲν δὴ φλέβες ἡμῖν οὕτω θρέψονται τοῦ περιεχομένου κατ' αὐτὰς αἵματος ἀπολαύουσαι.

[6] De musculorum motu. i. 1, K. iv. 371–2: ἣν (τοῦ μυὸς σάρκα) ὥσπερ τινὰ χώραν μοι νόει πολλοῖς ὀχετοῖς ἀρδευομένην, ἑνὶ μὲν τῷ πρόσθεν εἰρημένῳ τῷ νεύρῳ, δύο δ' ἄλλοις, τῷ μὲν αἵματος θερμοῦ καὶ λεπτοῦ καὶ ἀτμώδους, τῷ δὲ ψυχροτέρου τε καὶ παχυτέρου, καλεῖται δ' αὐτῶν τὸ μὲν ἀρτηρία, τὸ δὲ φλέψ. οὗτοι μὲν οὖν οἱ ὀχετοὶ τὴν ἀρχὴν ἀπὸ καρδίας καὶ ἥπατος ἔχοντες, τὸ σῶμα τῶν μυῶν ἄρδουσι καὶ διὰ τούτους οὐκέτι χώρα τις ἁπλῶς, ἀλλ' οἶον φυτὸν ὁ μῦς γίνεται, διὰ δὲ τὸν τρίτον ὀχετόν, τὸν ἀπὸ τῆς μεγάλης ἀρχῆς οὐ φυτὸν ἀλλ' ἤδη κρεῖττον φυτοῦ, προσλαβὼν αἴσθησίν τε καὶ κίνησιν τὴν καθ' ὁρμήν, οἷς τὸ ζῷον τοῦ μὴ ζῴου διαφέρει.

not seem to be any place for 'natural' *pneuma*. In order to function at all, the veins then must contain some *pneuma*, and Galen does indeed tell us that they do so. This, at least, seems to be the interpretation of the passage in the sixteenth chapter of the sixth book of the work *On the use of the parts*, where he says that while the arteries are full of thin, clean, and vaporous blood, the veins have a little dewy air.[1]

The question of *pneuma* in the veins has been examined by Temkin,[2] who notes that in one treatise, that *On the opinions of Hippocrates and Plato*, he seems to imply that there is no *pneuma* at all in the veins. 'But', he comments, 'such extreme formulations can be counterbalanced by many references, which, in the aggregate, weaken considerably the difference between the composition and function of the venous blood on the one hand, and the arterial on the other.' Venous blood, according to Temkin, has three sources of *pneuma*: (*a*) the useful and vaporous parts of the winds developed in the abdomen, (*b*) juices of chyle and blood, which exhale some *pneuma* so that even psychic *pneuma* may be engendered from the veins in the cerebral ventricles, and (*c*) the synanastomoses of the capillaries. These sources need a careful examination. As to (*a*), Galen is discussing the useful functions of the peritoneum. Among these is the control of flatulence. If the food ingested is very πνευματώδης, which I can only translate as *windy*, the wind has to be eliminated, since digestion releases it. Some of it comes off in eructations, and some of it in farting, but the part of it which is both vaporous and good or useful is taken up into the veins.[3] Here, I cannot help feeling, we must be a little cautious. The word πνευματώδης, which I have translated as *windy*, can, of course, without doing any violence to the Greek language, be given the rendering of *pneuma*-like; but is this word being used by Galen as a technical physiological term, or merely in a more colloquial sense? I am inclined to think the latter. The part of abdominal wind which is absorbed by the veins is surely that which is steamy, i.e. containing a good deal of liquid and certain nutritious particles. But air, we must remember, is the raw material of *pneuma*, so that it is quite possible that the wind absorbed by the veins might be converted into this mysterious substance, but of this, except in this one sentence, Galen tells us no more. Nor is it easy to suppose that the 'superfluities' excreted by the veins in the ventricles of the brain can really be the venous *pneuma* derived from these sources. However that may be, Galen certainly believed that the veins

---

[1] De usu partium, vi. 16, K. iii. 491 : καὶ μετέχουσιν αἱ μὲν ἀρτηρίαι λεπτοῦ καὶ καθαροῦ καὶ ἀτμώδους αἵματος, αἱ δὲ φλέβες ὀλίγου καὶ ὀμιχλώδους ἀέρος.

[2] O. Temkin, 'On Galen's Pneumatology', *Gesnerus*, viii, pp. 180–9.

[3] De usu partium, iv. 9, K. iii. 292 : καὶ εἰ πάνυ πνευματώδη τὰ ἐδηδεσμένα τύχῃ, καὶ πέπτεται, καὶ ἀναδίδοται ῥᾳδίως. τὸ μὲν γάρ τι τῆς φύσης αἱ ἐρυγαὶ κενοῦσι, τὸ δέ τι κάτω διεξέρχεται, ὅσον δ' ἀτμῶδες ἅμα καὶ χρηστόν, εἰς τὰς φλέβας ἀναλαμβάνεται. καὶ πρὸς ταῦτ' οὖν ἅπαντα χρήσιμόν ἐστι τὸ περιτόναιον.

ending in the choroid plexus do contribute a little *pneuma* to the ventricles.[1] Probably the easiest way to account for its origin would be to suppose that not all the *pneuma* drawn into the venous system through the capillary system is used up in giving life to the veins, and that therefore a surplus remains. But the term surplus is so often applied to the 'waste products' that its use here must give rise to some doubt or questioning. And whatever the source of this venous *pneuma*, there is no question of any circulation of it, or of the blood. The mutual interchange of blood and *pneuma* through the capillaries has nothing to do with any such idea. For the blood in both veins and arteries has no other function than that of feeding. The notion of circulation would be no less incongruous to Galen than it was to Erasistratus.

Galen never gives us a specific list of those organs or tissues that are fed by arterial as opposed to venous blood. The lungs are fed, it is true, with a light kind of blood, but this is not, it would appear, the fully perfected arterial variety, since it comes from the right ventricle, and has not undergone the final elaboration by the innate heat in the left. The blood too that feeds the coats of the arteries themselves is only the lightest portion of the blood which has percolated from the veins; the thick residues presumably never leave the venous system. Here again we come across an apparent inconsistency. The lung is undoubtedly the lightest tissue of the body, and is fed by the lightest blood, yet the actual source of its blood-supply is the right ventricle where the innate heat is smaller than it is in the left, and its elaboration of the blood less thorough than that which takes place in the presence of *pneuma*, for the bulk of the sooty superfluities are certainly produced in the left not the right ventricle. Moreover, it should not be forgotten that the arteries have a double function. Besides being the channels for the lightest nutriment of the cleanest blood, which is quite small in volume, they contain much more *pneuma* than blood, and their function is to distribute and maintain at a suitable temperature the innate heat, which appears to vary in different organs. Thus the liver has only very small arteries. These do not seem to have any feeding to do, nor need they supply the liver with much vital spirit. Their chief business is to maintain the innate heat at a moderate temperature.[2] In the spleen, however, they play a much more important part. The function of the spleen is that of purging the blood produced in the liver of its 'melancholic' thick and earthy elements,[3]

---

[1] See the passage from *The opinions of Hippocrates and Plato* quoted above, p. 355.

[2] *De usu partium*, iv. 13, K. iii. 307: εὐλόγως δὲ καὶ μικραὶ πάνυ γεγόνασιν, ὡς ἂν εἰς ἔμψυξιν μόνον ὑπηρετοῦσαι τῷ σιμῷ τοῦ σπλάγχνου, μήτε δ' αἵματος δεόμεναι μεταλαμβάνειν, οὐδέπω γὰρ ἀποτέθειται τὰ περιττώματα, μήτε τὸ ζωτικὸν πνεῦμα πολὺ παρέχειν τῷ ἥπατι, καθάπερ ἄλλοις τισὶν ὀργάνοις, ἀλλ' οὐδὲ τρέφειν αὐτοῦ τὴν σάρκα λεπτῇ καὶ ἀτμώδει τροφῇ.

[3] Ibid., 15, 316: ὡς ἔστιν ὁ σπλὴν ὄργανόν τι καθαρτικὸν τῶν ἐν ἥπατι γεννωμένων ἰλυωδῶν καὶ παχέων καὶ μελαγχολικῶν χυμῶν.

a process which takes a lot of time. This is brought about chiefly by the arteries, which are large and thick and distributed throughout its volume, where they have to work very hard in their continuous movement reinforcing the strength of the innate heat, which comes from the heart in the process of breaking up and transforming those humours which have been produced in the liver. The lightest elements of this thick hepatic blood are used to feed the actual tissues of the spleen,[1] which is lighter than that of the liver, though not so light as that of the lungs. The part of the blood that cannot be worked up into any form that is at all suitable for alimentary purposes is discharged into the alimentary canal through another mouth.[2] The thick blood that is to be purged is contained in the veins, but the pulsation of the arteries, it would appear, breaks up the earthy elements, and the arteries absorb and discharge the gaseous superfluities produced.[3]

We come now to one of the paradoxes of Galen's physiology. By and large, the blood moves in one direction, outward from the heart, but it is not the heart which supplies the principal motive power. Material passes into the heart, and as we have noted the heart 'sends it out', but it is not the expulsive force of the heart's systole which drives it on its way, at any rate for any large distance. Galen can give us no adequate mechanical explanation of how the blood moves in the arteries any more than in the veins. As we have seen, the majority of the blood in the veins bypasses the heart altogether, and even in the lungs the heart's movement does not do any more than propel the blood through the artery-like vein to the end of its ramifications. From that point it is the movement of the thorax which pushes it through the capillaries of the pulmonary veins. In a similar way the contraction of the left ventricle does not appear to carry the blood any distance up or down the aorta. Other forces very

---

[1] Ibid., 317: ἑλκύσας δ' (ἀπὸ τοῦ ἥπατος) οὐκ εὐθὺς εἰς τὴν κοιλίαν ἀποκρίνει, ἀλλ' αὐτὸς πρότερον κατεργάζεται καὶ μεταβάλλει κατὰ πολλὴν σχολὴν χρώμενος εἰς τὴν ἐνέργειαν ταύτην μάλιστα ταῖς ἀρτηρίαις, αἳ δὴ πολλαὶ καὶ μεγάλαι καθ' ὅλον εἰσὶ τὸ σπλάγχνον οὐκ ἀργῶς οὐδ' ὡς ἔτυχεν ὑπὸ τῆς φύσεως αὐτῷ δοθεῖσαι, ἀλλ' ὅτι γε τῷ διηνεκεῖ τῆς κινήσεως καὶ τῇ τῆς ἐμφύτου θερμασίας ἰσχύϊ τῆς παρὰ τῆς καρδίας αὐταῖς ἐπιρρεούσης κατεργάζεσθαι καὶ καταθραύειν καὶ μεταβάλλειν καὶ ἀλλοιοῦν δύναται τὸ πάχος τῶν ἐξ ἥπατος εἰς σπλῆνα μεταβαλλομένων χυμῶν.
[2] Ibid.: ὁπόσον δ' ἄν τι καὶ τὴν ἐν τούτῳ διαφύγῃ κατεργασίαν καὶ μὴ δυνηθῇ εἰς αἵματος ἰδέαν λεπτοῦ καὶ χρηστοῦ κατεργασθῆναι, καὶ παντάπασιν ἄχρηστον ᾖ πρὸς θρέψιν, εἰς τὴν γαστέρα τοῦτο διά τινος ἑτέρου φλεβώδους ὁ σπλὴν ἐξερεύγεται στομάχου.
[3] Ibid., 319–20: τὸ μὲν γὰρ ἑλκόμενον εἰς τὸν σπλῆνα παχύτερόν ἐστι τοῦ κατὰ τὸ ἧπαρ. ἀλλ' ἐπεὶ κατεργασθὲν ὑπὸ τῶν ἀρτηριῶν τῶν ἐνταῦθα σὺν ἅμα καὶ ταῖς φλεψί, πολλῷ στεγανώτερον ἐχούσαις τὸν χιτῶνα τῶν ἐν τῷ ἥπατι φλεβῶν, οὐχ ὁλοσχερὲς καὶ παχὺ τῇ σαρκὶ τοῦ σπληνός, ἀλλὰ λεπτόν τε καὶ κατὰ βραχὺ διαπέμπεται, διὰ τοῦτο καὶ ἡ σὰρξ τοῦδε τοῦ σπλάγχνου μανωτέρα μέν ἐστι καὶ κουφοτέρα τῆς κατὰ τὸ ἧπαρ ... αὗται μὲν οὖν αἱ προειρημέναι δύο χρεῖαι τοῦ πλήθους τῶν κατὰ τὸν σπλῆνα πεφυκυιῶν ἀρτηριῶν. καί τις ἐπ' αὐταῖς ἄλλη τρίτη κατὰ τὴν ἰδίαν αὐτῶν ἐνέργειάν τε καὶ χρείαν. δέδεικται γάρ, ὡς ἡ κίνησις αὐτῶν ἕνεκα φυλακῆς μάλιστα τῆς ἐν ἑκάστῳ μέρει ἐμφύτου θερμασίας γέγονεν, ἐμψύχουσα μὲν ταῖς διαστολαῖς τῷ ψυχρὰν ἐπισπᾶσθαι ποιότητα, καθαίρουσα δ' ἐξ αὐτῶν ταῖς συστολαῖς τὸ λιγνυῶδες περίττωμα.

soon take over its direction. Two of these are specifically detailed, the systole and diastole of the arteries, for the arteries perform their own systole and, more important, diastole, quite independently of the heart, even if their power of moving is derived from it. This, as we have seen, would result in a perpetually alternating forward and backward movement, were it not for the existence of the aortic (and pulmonary) valves.[1] But there seems to be a two-way traffic in the arteries no less than in the veins, caused by the variable needs of the tissues for nutriment. Nor is this two-way traffic, even so, absolutely ruled out in the case of the three-cusped valves—the bicuspid being bicuspid precisely in order to permit it—for these valves are not hermetically sealed. Even the aortic valve permits a small quantity of regurgitation.[2] None of the valves can therefore prevent a small quantity of backflow taking place. Moreover, the conformation of the aorta, no less than that of the vena cava, is such as to make it possible for blood to bypass the heart in theory, if not in practice. And Galen may have thought that the arterial blood from the top part of the body was passed through the kidneys in this way.

But though the main stream of arterial blood is outwards from the heart to the various organs of the body, that is not the whole story. We have already noted what looks like a periodical reflux of the current of foodstuffs absorbed from the alimentary canal back to the digestive organs, and it does not appear logical to restrict this reflux only to the veins. Galen expressly insists that there is no difficulty in assuming that the same channel may be used to draw nutriment and to discharge it at different times.[3] And since the arteries absorb some foodstuffs, a limited degree of reflux may be postulated in them also. So far as the veins are concerned, this reflex plays a very important part. Not only are waste products discharged into the veins and through the veins into the stomach, but in conditions of long-practised fasting, actual food is also drawn back into the stomach from the liver.[4] Moreover, purgative drugs draw their appropriate humours from all over the body by the same openings

---

[1] De nat. fac. iii. 13, K. ii. 203: κατὰ μὲν γὰρ τὰς ἀρτηρίας ἱκανῶς ἐναργὲς τὸ τοιοῦτο, ὥσπερ καὶ κατὰ τὴν καρδίαν τε καὶ τὸν θώρακα καὶ τὸν πνεύμονα. τούτων γὰρ ἁπάντων διαστελλομένων τε καὶ συστελλομένων ἐναλλάξ, ἀναγκαῖον ἐξ ὧν εἱλκύσθη τι πρότερον, εἰς ταῦθ' ὕστερον ἐκπέμπεσθαι. καὶ ταύτην ἄρα τὴν ἀνάγκην ἡ φύσις προγιγνώσκουσα, τοῖς ἐν τῇ καρδίᾳ στόμασι τῶν ἀγγείων ὑμένας ἐπέφυσε κωλύσοντας εἰς τοὐπίσω φέρεσθαι τὰς ὕλας.

[2] See below, p. 394.

[3] De nat. fac. iii. 13, K. 186 f.: οὐ μὴν οὐδὲ τὸ διὰ τοῦ αὐτοῦ πόρου τὴν ὁλκὴν γίνεσθαι καὶ τὴν ἀπόκρισιν ἐν διαφόροις τοῖς χρόνοις οὐδὲν ἔτι χαλεπὸν ἐξευρεῖν.

[4] Ibid., 188: μηκέτι θαυμάζωμεν, εἰ καὶ διὰ τῶν φλεβῶν ἡ φύσις ἐκκρίνει πολλάκις εἰς τὴν γαστέρα περιττώματα. τούτου δ' ἔτι μᾶλλον οὐ χρὴ θαυμάζειν, εἰ, δι' ὧν εἰς ἧπαρ ἀνεδόθη τι φλεβῶν ἐκ γαστρός, αὖθις εἰς αὐτὴν ἐξ ἥπατος ἐν ταῖς μακροτέραις ἀσιτίαις δύναται ἕλκεσθαι ἡ τροφή. τὸ γὰρ τοῖς τοιούτοις ἀπορεῖν ὅμοιόν ἐστι δήπου τῷ μηκέτι πιστεύειν μηδ' ὅτι τὰ καθαίροντα φάρμακα διὰ τῶν αὐτῶν στομάτων ἐξ ὅλου τοῦ σώματος εἰς τὴν γαστέρα τοὺς οἰκείους ἐπισπᾶται χυμούς, δι' ὧν ἔμπροσθεν ἡ ἀνάδοσις ἐγένετο, ἀλλ' ἕτερα μὲν ζητεῖν ἀναδόσεως, ἕτερα δὲ καθάρσεως στόματα.

through which their absorption originally took place. When the food-canal is empty and in need of nutriment, this is again attracted from the liver by the same veins.[1] The power of attraction of the different organs varies, the heart has greater powers of attraction and rejection than the liver, the liver than the stomach and the intestines, and the arteries than the veins, but the relative power of attraction of each organ may vary. At one time the liver has the greater power, at another the stomach.[2] Each of the parts, when it has attracted its own special humour and made use of it, hastens to discharge all surpluses as quickly as it can, and this discharged surplus obeys the laws of mechanical movement,[3] i.e. heavy products move downwards and light ones move upwards. This means that matter can be attracted from the extreme surfaces of the skin back into the stomach, as 'Hippocrates' pointed out when he maintained that not merely *pneuma* or excess or surplus matter, but actual nutriment is brought down from the outer surface to the original place from which it was taken up.[4] Indeed there is a sort of 'struggle for existence' among the different organs, both for the nutrition to be absorbed and for its excretion, and the 'strongest' part or organ passes on its superfluities to the weaker.

Now just as the parts draw food from each other, so also they sometimes deposit their excess substances in each other, and just as the stronger prevailed when the two were exercising traction, so it is also when they are depositing. This is the cause of the so-called fluxions, for every part has a definite inborn tension, by virtue of which it expels its superfluities, and, therefore, when one of these parts becomes weaker—owing, of course, to some special condition—there will necessarily be a confluence into it of the superfluities from all the other parts. The strongest part deposits its surplus matter in all the parts near it; these again into other parts which are weaker; these next into yet others; and this goes on for a long time, until the superfluity, being driven from one part into another, comes to rest in one of the weakest of all; it cannot flow from this into another part, because none of the stronger ones will receive

---

[1] Ibid., 188–9: τί θαυμαστόν ἐστι διττὴν ὑπηρεσίαν τε καὶ χρείαν εἶναι ταῖς φλεψὶ ταῖς ἐν τῷ μέσῳ τεταγμέναις ἥπατός τε καὶ τῶν κατὰ τὴν κοιλίαν, ὥσθ' ὁπότε μὲν ἐν τούτοις ἄφθονος εἴη περιεχομένη τροφή, διὰ τῶν εἰρημένων εἰς ἧπαρ ἀναφέρεσθαι φλεβῶν, ὁπότε δ' εἴη κενὰ καὶ δεόμενα τρέφεσθαι, διὰ τῶν αὐτῶν αὖθις ἐξ ἥπατος ἕλκεσθαι;

[2] Ibid., 189: φύσει μὲν καὶ κοινῇ πᾶσιν ἀνθρώποις τε ἅμα καὶ ζῴοις ἡ μὲν καρδία τοῦ ἥπατος, τὸ δ' ἧπαρ ἐντέρων τε καὶ γαστρός, αἱ δ' ἀρτηρίαι τῶν φλεβῶν, ἑλκύσαι τε τὸ χρήσιμον ἑαυταῖς ἀποκρῖναί τε τὸ μὴ τοιοῦτον ἰσχυρότεραι. καὶ καθ' ἕκαστον δ' ἡμῶν ἰδίως ἐν μὲν τῷδε τῷ καιρῷ τὸ ἧπαρ ἰσχυρότερον ἕλκειν, ἐν δὲ τῷδε ἡ γαστήρ.

[3] Ibid., 193: ταῖς γὰρ ἐναντίαις δυνάμεσιν ἐναντίας κινήσεις τε καὶ φορὰς τῶν ὑλῶν ἀναγκαῖον ἀκολουθεῖν. ἕκαστον γὰρ τῶν μορίων, ὅταν ἑλκύσῃ τὸν οἰκεῖον χυμὸν ἔπειτα κατάσχῃ καὶ ἀπολαύσῃ, τὸ περιττὸν ἅπαν ἀποθέσθαι σπεύδει, καθότι μάλιστα δύναται τάχιστά τε ἅμα καὶ κάλλιστα, κατὰ τὴν τοῦ περιττοῦ ῥοπήν.

[4] Ibid., 193–4: τί δὴ θαυμαστόν, εἰ κἀκ τῆς ἐσχάτης ἐπιφανείας τῆς κατὰ τὸ δέρμα μέχρι τῶν ἐντέρων τε καὶ τῆς γαστρὸς ἀφικνεῖταί τι μεταλαμβανόμενον· ὡς καὶ τοῦθ' Ἱπποκράτης ἡμᾶς ἐδίδαξεν, οὐ πνεῦμα μόνον ἢ περίττωμα φάσκων, ἀλλὰ καὶ τὴν τροφὴν αὐτὴν ἐκ τῆς ἐσχάτης ἐπιφανείας αὖθις ἐπὶ τὴν ἀρχήν, ὅθεν ἀνηνέχθη καταφέρεσθαι.

it, while the affected part is unable to drive it away.[1] (Transl. Brock, Loeb edition.)

With the interesting clinical implications of this theory we cannot concern ourselves in this essay; suffice it to point out some of its physiological consequences, which make Galen's physiology so difficult to understand. For here as elsewhere Galen is dominated by two principles, to us quite irreconcilable, his conception of the laws of gravity and levity, and his notion of what Brock, in his introduction to the translation of the work *On the natural faculties*, has rendered by the phrase 'specific selection', and I call 'quasi-magnetic or qualitative attraction'. In the passages which I have just been quoting, the contradiction between these two principles is particularly apparent. The movements described, which belong in the first place to the liquids composing the venous blood stream, clearly imply the notion of a periodic ebb and flow, which Fleming[2] has brusquely taken Foster and others to task for attributing to Galen. Fleming, after expressing his surprise 'to find that Galen's view of the motion of the heart in the blood and lungs was misconstrued by some of the leading German historians of medicine', attributes 'a second major error'—we have already examined the first—to Foster, citing a passage from his *Lectures on the history of physiology in seventeenth and eighteenth centuries*[3] which reads as follows:

Thus from the right side of the heart there is sent to the body generally along the great veins, and to the lungs along the artery-like vein (the pulmonary artery) a flow, followed by an ebb, of crude blood, endowed with natural spirits only, blood serving the lower stages of nutrition. Blood flows through the artery-like vein (the pulmonary artery) to the lungs for nourishment of the lungs, just as it flows through the other veins for the nourishment of the rest of the body: in both cases there is an ebb as well as a flow along the same channel.

The notion of ebb and flow, which roused Fleming's indignation, certainly does not appear to be quite accurate so far as the lungs are concerned, but it would be quite wrong therefore to repudiate the notion *in toto*, which, with a single exception, Fleming would have us do, with the admonition that 'Insufficiently qualified statements that Galen believed in an ebb and flow of venous blood are too numerous to mention'.

---

[1] *De nat. fac.* iii. 13, K. ii. 190–1 : ὥσπερ οὖν ἐξ ἀλλήλων ἕλκει τὰ μόρια τροφήν, οὕτω καὶ ἀποτίθεταί ποτ' εἰς ἄλληλα τὸ περιττόν· καὶ ὥσπερ ἑλκόντων ἐπλεονέκτει τὸ ἰσχυρότερον, οὕτω καὶ ἀποτιθεμένων καὶ τῶν γε καλουμένων ῥευμάτων ἤδε ἡ πρόφασις. ἕκαστον γὰρ τῶν μορίων ἔχει τινὰ τόνον σύμφυτον, ᾧ διωθεῖται τὸ περιττόν. ὅταν οὖν ἐν ἐξ αὐτῶν ἀρρωστότερον γένηται κατά τινα διάθεσιν, ἐξ ἁπάντων εἰς ἐκεῖνο συρρεῖν ἀνάγκη τὰ περιττά. τὸ μὲν γὰρ ἰσχυρότατον ἐναποτίθεται τοῖς πλησίον ἅπασιν, ἐκείνων δ' αὖ πάλιν ἕκαστον εἰς ἕτερ' ἄττα τῶν ἀσθενεστέρων, εἶτ' αὖθις ἐκείνων ἕκαστον εἰς ἄλλα καὶ τοῦτ' ἐπὶ πλεῖστον γίγνεται, μέχρι περ ἂν ἐξ ἁπάντων ἐλαυνόμενον τὸ περίττωμα καθ' ἕν τι μείνῃ τῶν ἀσθενεστάτων· ἐντεῦθεν γὰρ οὐκέτ' εἰς ἄλλο δύναται μεταρρεῖν, ὡς ἂν μήτε δεχομένου τινὸς αὐτὸ τῶν ἰσχυροτέρων μήτ' ἀπώσασθαι δυναμένου τοῦ πεπονθότος.

[2] Fleming, op. cit.

[3] Foster, op. cit., p. 12.

Both Foster and Singer[1] were not, in my opinion, entirely correct in the idea that blood was distributed to the body from the right side of the heart to the great veins. As Fleming rightly pointed out, Galen did not believe that more than a comparatively small portion of the blood entered the right ventricle at all, as we have already had occasion to note. And, so far as the lungs were concerned, he expressly excluded such a forward and backward motion as being prevented by the pulmonary valve. But precisely this backward and forward movement was postulated for the portal system in particular, though, of course, the inward or forward motion was of the raw material of semi-processed blood into the liver. But the motion of nutriment drawn by the hungry liver in the fasting state cannot be anything but fully formed blood. Nor are the movements just described confined to the portal system. It would appear that 'waste products' from all over the body are eliminated through the vascular system, which seems to imply that they were carried in the blood-stream. Finely-divided faecal residues flow downwards from the tissues back into the liver and thence back into the stomach and intestines from which they are finally eliminated, and not only faecal residues but surpluses of yellow bile and serum, the latter of which are evacuated as urine.[2] But the state of affairs in the venous system is simplicity itself compared with what goes on in the arterial. For here there are three different principles at work, the law of gravity, the law of the *horror vacui*, and the law, presumably, of qualitative attraction and repulsion as well. The combination of the first two ensures that at systole, when the heart and arteries dilate, matter is drawn into them, both blood and *pneuma*. The right ventricle draws blood through the tricuspid valve from the right auricle, an appendage of the vena cava, while the left ventricle draws *pneuma* through the mitral valve, and the finest parts of the blood through the pores in the septum; and the arteries, on dilating, also attract matter, in virtue of the principle of the *horror vacui*. This principle is combined with the law of gravity, in as much as the attraction works first on the lightest and thinnest substances and then progressively upon the heavier and thicker. Now the lightest of all substances in the body is

---

[1] Fleming, op. cit., quotes from C. Singer, *A Short History of Science to the Nineteenth Century* (Oxford University Press, London, 1941), pp. 91–2: 'For the venous blood that entered this important branch, the right side of the heart, the Galenic scheme reserved two possible fates. The greater part remained a while in the ventricle, parting with its impurities, which were carried off (by the artery-like vein now called the pulmonary artery) to the lung, and there exhaled. These impurities being discharged, the venous blood in the right ventricle ebbed back again into the general venous system.'

[2] Galen, *De nat. fac.* iii. 13, K. ii. 190: καὶ τοῦ γε μὴ πεινῆν ἐνίοτε τὸ ζῷον ἡ περιουσία τῆς ἐν ἥπατι τροφῆς αἰτία· κρείττονα γὰρ ἔχουσα καὶ ἑτοιμοτέραν τροφὴν ἡ γαστὴρ οὐδὲν δεῖται τῆς ἔξωθεν· εἰ δέ γέ ποτε δέοιτο μέν, ἀποροίη δέ, πληροῦται περιττωμάτων. ἰχῶρες δέ τινές εἰσι ταῦτα, χολώδεις τε καὶ φλεγματώδεις καὶ ὀρρώδεις, οὓς μόνους ἑλκούσῃ μεθίησιν αὐτῇ τὸ ἧπαρ, ὅταν ποτὲ καὶ αὐτὸ δέηται τροφῆς.

pneuma in the first place, and vapour in the second; in the third place that portion of the blood which has been carefully elaborated and refined.[1] In accordance with the principle of the *horror vacui*, all hollow organs capable of dilating attract the lighter matter first, but in so far as they require nourishment it is into their coats, which are the real bodies of these organs, that their proper nourishment is drawn.[2] What happens in the arteries would therefore be something like this. The blood which has been properly refined is propelled into the aorta. The aorta itself and the arteries which lie nearest to it, those which pass up from the heart to the neck, and that which lies along the spine, that is the aorta ascendens and the aorta descendens, and their branches draw mostly from the heart itself, while those which go to the stomach and intestines also draw from the heart as well as the numerous veins in its neighbourhood.[3] From the heart itself they draw refined blood, and from the veins the lightest elements; they do not obtain any of the thick, heavy nourishment provided in the portal system, since in accordance with the progressive action of the *horror vacui*, they are full before this can exert itself upon the heavier matter.[4] The arteries which reach the skin draw in, presumably through the pores, atmospheric air into their cavities, while those which anastomose at any point with the veins attract the thinnest and lightest elements of the venous blood.

It is clear from this description that the heart is for Galen not the only, even if it is the principal, source of the motion of the arterial blood. He has no conception of the force exerted upon the blood by the contraction of the heart muscle. He therefore has to supplement his supply of arterial blood from other sources, and to do this he has to rely on the mysterious force of 'qualitative attraction'. This would appear to entail in the arteries as well as in the veins a good deal of two-way traffic. For if the main stream of arterial blood runs outwards from the heart to the periphery, the blood drawn in from the veins through the capillaries would seem to be travelling in the opposite direction. Yet perhaps this conclusion is not justified, since Galen may very well have thought that the blood drawn into the coats of the arteries at their diastole, as well as the small amounts

---

[1] *De nat. fac.* iii. 14, K. ii. 205: ἐν γὰρ τῇ πρὸς τὸ κενούμενον ἀκολουθίᾳ τὸ κουφότατόν τε καὶ λεπτότατον ἔπεται πρότερον τοῦ βαρυτέρου τε καὶ παχυτέρου· κουφότατον δ' ἐστὶ καὶ λεπτότατον ἁπάντων τῶν κατὰ τὸ σῶμα πρῶτον μὲν τὸ πνεῦμα, δεύτερον δ' ὁ ἀτμός, ἐπὶ τούτῳ δὲ τρίτον, ὅσον ἂν ἀκριβῶς ᾖ κατειργασμένον τε καὶ λελεπτυσμένον αἷμα.

[2] *Ibid.*, 15, 207: καὶ τοίνυν καὶ ταῖς ἀρτηρίαις τε καὶ τῇ καρδίᾳ, ὡς μὲν κοίλοις τε καὶ διαστέλλεσθαι δυναμένοις ὀργάνοις, ἀεὶ τὸ κουφότερον ἀκολουθεῖ πρότερον, ὡς δὲ καὶ τρέφεσθαι δεομένοις εἰς αὐτοὺς τοὺς χιτῶνας, οἳ δὴ τὰ σώματα τῶν ὀργάνων εἰσίν, ἕλκεται τὸ οἰκεῖον.

[3] *Ibid.*, 14, 205-6: ὥστε καὶ τῶν εἰς τὴν γαστέρα τε καὶ τὰ ἔντερα καθηκουσῶν ἀρτηριῶν, ἀπὸ τῆς ἐπὶ ῥάχει πεφυκυίας, ἁπασῶν τὴν ὁλκὴν ἐν τῷ διαστέλλεσθαι γίνεσθαι παρά τε τῆς καρδίας αὐτῆς καὶ τῶν παρακειμένων αὐτῇ φλεβῶν παμπόλλων οὐσῶν.

[4] *Ibid.*, 206: οὐ γὰρ δὴ ἔκ γε τῶν ἐντέρων καὶ τῆς κοιλίας τροφὴν οὕτω παχεῖάν τε καὶ βαρεῖαν ἐν ἑαυτοῖς ἐχόντων δύναταί τι μεταλαμβάνειν, ὅ τι καὶ ἄξιον λόγου, φθάνουσαι πληροῦσθαι τοῖς κουφοτέροις.

derived from their anastomoses with the veins, was consumed in the coats of the arteries themselves. But the question of two-way traffic in the arteries cannot be so summarily and easily dismissed. Though Galen does not tell us of any faecal residues carried back by the arteries to the alimentary canal, there was at least one element which had to be evacuated from arterial no less thoroughly than from venous blood, namely excess of water, which is drawn off by the kidneys.[1] The forces at work in the arteries are not at all easy to visualize. Galen's explanation of 'qualitative' attraction seems to be full of contradictions. In some passages which we have quoted it is made responsible for the distribution of blood through the venous system, by a kind of 'quasi-magnetic' attraction, or what I might perhaps call a teleosmosis, yet in another he tells us that the magnet can attract only objects placed very close to it. The principle of the *horror vacui* can, on the other hand, act at a great distance.[2] Water can be sucked up through a tube of any length.[3] Galen attempts to overcome this difficulty by introducing a comparison between the arterial system and that of a scheme of garden irrigation. Moisture cannot be distributed from a distance. A pool or channel of water will not distribute moisture peripherically. To distribute it systematically over a wide area many small conduits are needed, made of such a size and placed at such intervals as will enable the intervening spaces to absorb the moisture they need.[4]

So also is it in the body of animals. Numerous conduits distributed through the various limbs bring them pure blood, much like the garden water-supply, and, further, the intervals between these conduits have been wonderfully arranged by Nature from the outset, so that the intervening parts should be plentifully provided for when absorbing the blood, and that they should never be deluged by a quantity of superfluous fluid running at unsuitable times.[5]　(trs. Brock.)

Not a very convincing essay in hydrodynamics.

[1] See above, p. 331.
[2] *De nat. fac.* iii. 15, K. ii. 210: ἀλλ' ὑπομνήσαντας, ὡς δύο ἐστὶν ὁλκῆς εἴδη, τῶν μὲν εὑρείαις ὁδοῖς ἐν τῷ διαστέλλεσθαι τῇ πρὸς τὸ κενούμενον ἀκολουθίᾳ ποιουμένων τὴν ἕλξιν, τῶν δ' οἰκειότητι ποιότητος, ἐφεξῆς λέγειν, ὡς τὰ μὲν πρότερα καὶ πόρρωθεν ἕλκειν τι δύναται, τὰ δὲ δεύτερα ἐκ τῶν ἐγγυτάτων μόνον.
[3] Ibid.: αὐλίσκον μὲν γὰρ ὅτι μήκιστον εἰς ὕδωρ ἔνεστι καθέντι ῥᾳδίως ἀνασπᾶν εἰς τὸ στόμα δι' αὐτοῦ τὸ ὑγρόν.
[4] Ibid.: σαφέστατα δ' ἂν αὐτὸ μάθοις ἐπὶ τῶν ἐν τοῖς κήποις ὀχετῶν· ἐκ τούτων γὰρ εἰς μὲν τὰ παρακείμενα καὶ πλησίον ἅπαντα διαδίδοταί τις ἰκμάς, εἰς δὲ τὰ πορρωτέρω προσελθεῖν οὐκέτι δύναται, καὶ διὰ τοῦτο ἀναγκάζονται πολλοῖς ὀχετοῖς μικροῖς ἀπὸ τοῦ μεγάλου τετμημένοις εἰς ἕκαστον μέρος τοῦ κήπου τὴν ἐπίρρυσιν τοῦ ὕδατος ἐπιτεχνᾶσθαι· καὶ τηλικαῦτά γε τὰ μεταξὺ διαστήματα τούτων τῶν μικρῶν ὀχετῶν ποιοῦσιν, ἡλίκα μάλιστα νομίζουσιν ἀρκεῖν εἰς τὸ ἱκανῶς ἀπολαύειν ἕλκοντα τῆς ἑκατέρωθεν αὐτοῖς ἐπιρρεούσης ὑγρότητος.
[5] Ibid., 211: οὕτως οὖν ἔχει κἂν τοῖς τῶν ζῴων σώμασιν. ὀχετοὶ πολλοὶ κατὰ πάντα τὰ μέλη διεσπαρμένοι παράγουσιν αὐτοῖς αἷμα καθάπερ ἐν κηπίῳ ὑδρείαν τινά. καὶ τούτων τῶν ὀχετῶν τὰ μεταξὺ διαστήματα θαυμαστῶς ὑπὸ τῆς φύσεως εὐθὺς ἐξ ἀρχῆς διατέτακται πρὸς τὸ μήτ' ἐνδεῶς χορηγεῖσθαι τοῖς μεταξὺ μορίοις ἕλκουσιν εἰς ἑαυτὰ τὸ αἷμα, μήτε κατακλύζεσθαί ποτ' αὐτὰ πλήθει περιττῆς ὑγρότητος ἀκαίρως ἐπιρρεούσης.

The underlying difficulty is surely due to the double purpose which the arteries have to play in Galen's physiological system. For besides being part of the vascular or blood-distributing system, they are also an essential part of the respiratory system. Their diastole and systole are the means by which *pneuma* is distributed to the body, and certain 'waste products' eliminated. The mechanics of this are comparatively simple. In accordance with the principle of the *horror vacui*, *pneuma* is drawn in at diastole and 'waste products' are expelled at systole. This bellows action is difficult to reconcile or to combine with the pumping action of the heart required to propel the arterial blood to the periphery of the body, in spite of the invention of the back-stop of the aortic valve. The principal function of the *pneuma* taken into the arteries is to 'feed' the vital spirit, which confers upon the various tissues the qualities of living matter. That is why a portion of it has to be conveyed through the capillary arterioles to the venules, for the veins, too, are living matter. And in its final form as psychic spirit, it has to work the nervous and muscular systems. We cannot therefore regard it as forming a single compound with or even as a solution in the blood. It maintains always and everywhere its separate identity, even if it does not appear as 'free' air.

We must now pass to the relation of the *pneuma* to the other fundamental principle, condition, or entity, call it what you will, which makes life possible, the innate heat. Babies are born warm to touch and corpses are cold. Unless therefore the innate heat can be preserved in proper condition, neither too hot nor too cold, health, and in the last resort life itself, ceases to exist. The maintenance and distribution of the innate heat are two of the many functions of the blood, no less than the nutrition of the tissues. In one passage, Galen speaks of the blood as if it were the logs by which the fire of life is maintained.[1] The focus of this central-heating system is the left ventricle of the heart, and by means of this innate heat all the main physiological functions connected with nutrition, growth, digestion, the production of all the humours, and the qualitative changes assumed by the surplus products, are carried out, as well as the changes involved in the production of blood. Though its principal source is the heart, there is also a large store of it in the liver.[2] And the functions of the innate heat are not exclusively physical. The natural heat in the

---

[1] *De venae sectione*, 5, K. xi. 262: οὐ μόνον ἡ τροφὴ τοῖς τοῦ ζῴου μέρεσιν ἐξ αἵματός ἐστιν, ἀλλὰ καὶ ἡ κατὰ φύσιν θερμασία τὴν διαμονὴν ἐξ αἵματος ἔχει, καθάπερ ἐκ τῶν ἐπιτηδείων καίεσθαι ξύλων τὸ κατὰ τῆς ἑστίας πῦρ, ὑφ' οὗ καὶ τοὺς οἴκους ὁρῶμεν ὅλους θερμαινομένους.

[2] *De nat. fac.* ii. 4, K. ii. 89: καὶ τὴν πέψιν ἀλλοίωσίν τιν' ὑπάρχειν καὶ μεταβολὴν τοῦ τρέφοντος εἰς τὴν οἰκείαν τοῦ τρεφομένου ποιότητα, τὴν δ' ἐξαιμάτωσιν ἀλλοίωσιν εἶναι καὶ τὴν θρέψιν ὡσαύτως καὶ τὴν αὔξησιν ἐκ τῆς πάντη διαστάσεως καὶ θρέψεως γίνεσθαι, τὴν δ' ἀλλοίωσιν ὑπὸ τοῦ θερμοῦ μάλιστα συντελεῖσθαι, καὶ διὰ τοῦτο καὶ τὴν θρέψιν καὶ τὴν πέψιν καὶ τὴν τῶν χυμῶν ἁπάντων γένεσιν, ἤδη δὲ καὶ τοῖς περιττώμασι τὰς ποιότητας ὑπὸ τῆς ἐμφύτου θερμασίας ἐγγίνεσθαι.

liver generates blood, but the larger quantity in the heart was given us to generate courage and wrath, as both Hippocrates and Plato observed.[1] But the analogy with fire or flame must not be carried too far, since it may be misleading. A theory which was fashionable among the younger doctors was that the innate heat was like a fire, which receives its heat from such combustible material as wet logs. For newly-born animals are all damp, and they grow slowly, just as a fire almost choked by the dampness of the logs with which it is fed grows very slowly, while it is overcoming the dampness. When it has succeeded in doing this, it burns brightly until it has consumed all its fuel. It then dies down through lack of fuel, and quenches itself, this latter process corresponding to old age and death.[2] Galen objects that the analogy here depicted is false, even if it does appeal to nearly all the younger doctors. Flame has its origin from the destruction of combustible material, but the innate heat, which fashions the organism, stands in quite a different relation to living creatures. These are made to grow and are governed by it, and there is no period during which the innate heat with its plastic and many other powers is not extended throughout the body. It attracts nutriment into itself and governs the matter of the body, adding to it and increasing it, quite unlike flame, which merely consumes it.[3] The innate heat does not consume the body—even though in fevers it may do so—and it is true that our bodies grow old and finally die because of it, in so far as they dry up by a purely natural process.[4] Just as a fire, in order to keep itself

---

[1] *Comment. V in Hipp. epidem. vi*, sect. 5, K. xviiB. 252: θερμασία μέν τις ἔμφυτος ἐν ἥπατι περιέχεται καθ' ἣν αἷμα γεννᾶται· θερμασία δὲ ἑτέρα πλείων ἐστὶ κατὰ τὴν καρδίαν εἰς θυμοῦ γένεσιν ἡμῖν δοθεῖσα. Cf. *Comment. III in Hipp. de alimento ix*, K. xv. 289, which contains the self-same words.

[2] *De marcore*, 3, K. vii. 673–4: ὥσπερ αἱ φλόγες, ὅταν ἐμπέσωσιν ὑγροῖς ξύλοις, ἐν ἀρχῇ μὲν ὑποτύφονταί τε καὶ οἷον καταπνίγονται, μικραὶ παντάπασιν οὖσαι, καὶ ἀσθενεῖς, ἐν δὲ τῷ χρόνῳ προήκοντι κατὰ βραχὺ μὲν ἐκλάμπουσί τε καὶ αὔξονται, κατὰ βραχὺ δὲ τῆς ὕλης ἐγκρατεῖς γίνονται καὶ τέλος ἐπὶ μήκιστον αἴρονται μέγεθος, ὅταν ἁπάσης κρατήσωσιν, ὅπερ ἐστὶν αὐταῖς ἀκμή τε καὶ ῥώμη· κᾆπειτα ἐντεῦθεν ἤδη τῆς τροφῆς ἐπιλειπούσης ταύτης, μαραίνονταί τε καὶ σβέννυνται. κατὰ τὸν αὐτὸν τρόπον ἡ ἐν ἡμῖν, φασί, θερμότης ἐνδεδεμένη τῷ τοῦ ζῴου σώματι καθάπερ ὕλῃ τινί, τὸ μὲν πρῶτον ὑγρά τίς ἐστι καὶ ἀσθενής, αὐξανομένη δὲ μέχρι τῆς τῶν ἀκμαζόντων ἡλικίας ἐκλάμπει τε καὶ αὐξάνεται καὶ ἐπὶ πλεῖστον αἴρεται μεγέθους, καὶ μιμεῖται τοῦ πυρὸς τὴν φλόγα. τοὐντεῦθεν δὲ τροφῆς ἀπορίᾳ μαραίνεται κατὰ βραχύ, καὶ τοῦτό ἐστι τὸ γῆρας, ὕστερον δὲ ἤδη καὶ ἀποσβέννυται, ὅπερ ἐστὶν ὁ θάνατος.

[3] Ibid., 674: οὗτος ὁ λόγος εὐδοκιμεῖ παρὰ πᾶσιν ὀλίγου δεῖν τοῖς νεωτέροις ἰατροῖς τε καὶ φιλοσόφοις, οὐκ ὢν ἀληθής, ἐμοὶ γοῦν κριτῇ, παραβάλλων γέ τοι τὴν φλόγα τοῦ πυρὸς τῇ τῶν ζῴων θερμασίᾳ, μηδὲ τοῦτ' αἰσθανόμενος, ὡς ταῖς μὲν φλοξὶν ἡ γένεσις ἐκ τῆς κατὰ τὴν ὕλην ἐστὶ φθορᾶς, ὅθεν περιεξάπτονται, τὰ ζῷα δὲ οὐχ οὕτως ὑπὸ τοῦ διαπλάττοντος αὐτὰ τῆς ἐμφύτου θερμότητος ἔτυχεν ἀλλ' ὡς αὐξηθησόμενα καὶ διοικηθησόμενα παρ' αὐτῆς, οὐδέ ἐστί τις χρόνος ἐν ᾧ διὰ πάσης αὐτῆς οὐκ ἐκτέταται τὸ σύμφυτον ἡμῖν θερμὸν δυνάμεις ἔχον, οὐχ αἷς διαπλάττει μόνον, ἀλλὰ καὶ πολλὰς ἑτέρας. καὶ γὰρ ἕλκει τὴν τροφὴν ἐφ' ἑαυτό, καὶ τὴν ὕλην διοικεῖ καὶ προστίθησι καὶ προσφύει καὶ ὁμοιοῖ, καί, συλλήβδην εἰπεῖν, ἅπαντα τἀναντία ταῖς φλοξὶν ἀπεργάζεται περὶ τὴν σύμφυτον ὕλην ἑαυτῇ.

[4] Ibid., 676: ἀληθὲς μέν ἐστι τὸ διὰ τὴν ἔμφυτον θερμότητα γηράσκειν τε τὰ σώματα καὶ τελευτῶντα διαφθείρεσθαι· ψευδὴς δὲ ὁ τρόπος ὃν οὗτοί φασιν, οὐ γὰρ ὡς ἡ φλὸξ τὰ ξύλα, ταύτῃ καὶ

alive, needs both air and fuel, so the innate heat to maintain itself needs blood and air. If deprived of either, it is immediately extinguished.[1] Hence the need for respiration and for the provision of both blood and air in the pulsating (heart and) artery. How the innate heat can be fed by the blood Galen cannot explain to us, but the analogy with combustion haunts him. And if for *pneuma* we read oxygen, we arrive once more at an astonishing Hellenic intuition of the way the body works.

It is not altogether easy to understand what Galen meant by the phrase σύμφυτος θερμασία. Is it a quality, or is it a thing? Its grammatical formulation certainly suggests the former, nevertheless it often looks as if the latter notion approximates more closely to his conception of it. For he distinguishes between its essence and its quality. In the *Commentary on Hippocrates' aphorisms* he tries to establish what amounts almost to a distinction between temperature and quantity of heat. The temperature corresponding to the 'quality', and the quantity to the 'essence'.[2] Indeed he endows it with qualities as if it were a thing,[3] and to all intents and purposes identifies it, in another passage, with the innate *pneuma*.[4] The heart, he tells us, as Hippocrates pointed out, is the source of the vital functions, indeed, the source of life itself. It is therefore the principle (ἀρχή) and source or fountain (πηγή) of the innate heat, without which an animal cannot remain alive or begin to live, and from it the innate heat proceeds to all parts of the animal continuously and at all seasons, and it runs back to the heart so as to constitute an exchange (ἀμοιβή) or alternation, such as that which, we have told you, is necessary to life.[5]

τὸ σύμφυτον θερμὸν τῶν ζῴων ἀναλίσκει τὰ σώματα . . . τὸ μέν τοι ξηραίνεσθαι τὰ σώματα κατά τινα φυσικὴν ἀκολουθίαν, καὶ γίνεσθαι τοῦτο διὰ τὴν ἔμφυτον θερμότητα παντὸς μᾶλλον ἀληθές ἐστιν.

[1] *De usu resp.* 3, K. iv. 490 f.: οὕτως οὖν οὐκ ἀπεικὸς ἔχειν κἀπὶ τῆς ἐν τοῖς ζῴοις θερμασίας. ὕλην μὲν ὅθεν ἀνάπτεται, τὸ αἷμα, σύμφυτον δὲ ἔχουσα κινήσεως ἀρχήν, ἐφ᾽ ἑκάτερα, τῆς ἑτέρας στερηθεῖσα, καὶ τῆς λοιπῆς ἐξ ἀνάγκης στερίσκεται· καὶ διὰ τοῦτ᾽ αὐτό, ἐάν τε ἀναπνοῆς εἴρξῃς, ἐάν θ᾽ αἵματος, εὐθέως διαφθείρεται. καὶ γὰρ καὶ τὴν τοῦ λύχνου φλόγα ἅμα ἀφαιρήσεις καταπνίξας ἢ παντάπασιν ἐλαίου στερήσας.

[2] *Comm. in Hipp. aph.* 14, K. xviiB. 405–6: ἐπὶ μὲν τῶν ἀμίκτων, ὡς ἂν εἰ καὶ δυοῖν ἐχόντοιν ὕδωρ ὁμοίως θερμὸν ἐν δεξαμέναις ἀνίσοις περιεχόμενον, τὸν μὲν ἕτερον πλέον ἔχειν λέγομεν τὸ θερμόν, ᾧ μείζων ἡ δεξαμένη, τὸν ἕτερον ἔλαττον . . . ἐνίοτε δὲ οὐ πρὸς τὸ πλῆθος ἀναφέροντες τῆς οὐσίας τὸν λόγον, ἀλλὰ πρὸς τὴν ποιότητα μόνην, τῷ μέν τινι πλέον εἶναί φαμεν, τῷ δ᾽ ἧττον τὸ θερμόν.

[3] Ibid., 407: ἡ γὰρ οὐσία τοῦ ἐμφύτου θερμοῦ ἀερώδης καὶ ὑδατώδης ὑπάρχει.

[4] *De simplicibus*, v, K. xi. 730 f.: ἀλλ᾽ ἡμᾶς χρὴ μήτε παρακούειν αὐτοῦ ('Ιπποκράτους) καὶ γιγνώσκειν ἔμφυτον εἰρῆσθαι θερμόν, ὅπερ καὶ πνεῦμα ἑκάστῳ τῶν ζῴων ὀνομάζομεν, ὑπὲρ οὗ καὶ Ἀριστοτέλης ἔγραψεν. οὐδὲν δὲ κωλύει καὶ τὴν αἱματικὴν οὐσίαν καὶ ἀερῶδες θερμὸν ἔμφυτον ἀκούειν ἅμα τῷ πνεύματι.

[5] *Comment. III in Hipp. de aliment.*, sect. 25, K. xv. 362: νῦν δὲ ἐπειδὴ ἐν τῇ καρδίᾳ ἡ ἀρχὴ τῆς ζωῆς συνίσταται καὶ αὕτη ἐστιν ἀρχή τε καὶ πηγὴ τῆς ἐμφύτου θερμασίας, ἧς ἄνευ οὐ δύναται ζῷόν ποτε ζῆν . . . ἐξ αὐτῆς γὰρ ὁρμῶσα ἡ ἔμφυτος θερμότης εἰς πάντα τοῦ ζῴου μόρια, καὶ τὰ ἐγγυτάτω καὶ τὰ πορρωτάτω, ἅπερ αὐτὸς ἔσχατα λέγει, κατὰ πᾶσαν ὥραν καὶ πάντα χρόνον ἀφικνέεται καὶ πάλιν εἰς αὐτὴν παλινδρομεῖ, ὡς τοιαύτην τινὰ γενέσθαι ἀμοιβήν, οἵαν δὴ ἔφαμεν πολλάκις πρὸς τὴν ζωὴν ἀναγκαῖον εἶναι.

The passage quoted from 'Hippocrates' is of course one of those on which the 'circulationists' have relied to prove that the Father of medicine was acquainted with the circulation of the blood. But its meaning would appear to be quite different. The innate heat returns to the heart, but this must not be taken to imply that the blood does so too. 'Hippocrates' realized that there was a proper moderation (συμμετρία) at which the innate heat should be maintained, but the value of this idea was very much diminished by the absence of any clear distinction between temperature and the amount of heat, and the idea, curious to us today, that the 'hotness' of the different parts of the body should vary, and vary too at the different seasons of the year. The heart was, and had to be, much hotter than the rest of the body, for it was the source of the innate or natural heat which was located in the left ventricle. Indeed, if you put your finger into the ventricle of an animal, preferably the left one, which you have vivisected in a cold atmosphere, and which has consequently died through the cooling of the heart, you will find that it still has a lot of heat—much more than the other parts; for a given quantity of heat which is a very small one for the heart is a very large one for the other parts.[1] The proper temperature of the heart needs to be maintained by respiration through the lungs and transpiration through the arteries, and the natural temperature for the body and its different parts varies with age. Babies and young growing animals should be hotter than grown adults, and adults hotter than old men.[2] For, as Hippocrates taught, babies have most innate heat and old men least.[3] The translation of our modern notions of temperature and quantity of heat in terms of the 'essence' and the 'quality' of the innate heat is far from accurate, as may be shown by the following quotation describing the 'Hippocratic' doctrine. 'But the innate heat is of a good mixture (εὔκρατος), being present in respect of its "essence" (οὐσία) chiefly in the blood and the phlegm, and with regard to its "quality" it is mixed (ποιότης εὔκρατος) of hot and cold in the correct proportions.'[4] Let those who will translate this into physics.

[1] De usu resp. 2, K. v. 158 f.: οὐχ ὅμοιον οὖν ἐστι τὸ κατὰ φύσιν τῇ τε καρδίᾳ καὶ τοῖς ἄλλοις μορίοις· τὴν μὲν γὰρ ζεῖν ἀεὶ χρή, τοῖς δ' ἀρκεῖ τὸ μὴ παντάπασι καταψύχεσθαι . . . τάχιστα γὰρ ἀποθνήσκει τὸ ζῷον, εἰ καταψύξεις τὴν καρδίαν . . . ἀλλ' εἰ, κατεψυγμένης ἤδη, καὶ διὰ τοῦτο τοῦ ζῴου τεθνεῶτος ἐθέλοις παραχρῆμα τρώσας ὁποτέραν οὖν τῶν κοιλιῶν, καὶ μᾶλλον τὴν ἀριστερὰν καθεῖναι δάκτυλον εἰς αὐτήν, αἰσθήσῃ πολλῆς τῆς θερμασίας, καὶ πολύ γε πλείονος ἢ ἐν τοῖς ἄλλοις μορίοις τοῖς κατὰ φύσιν διακειμένοις· τὸ γὰρ ἴσον μέρος τῆς θερμασίας ἐλάχιστον μὲν τῇ καρδίᾳ, πάμπολυ δὲ τοῖς ἄλλοις ἐστί.

[2] Comment. II in Hipp. de nat. hom., sect. 12, K. xv. 154: θερμότατος γὰρ ἄν γε ῥηθῇ τῷ ἐμφύτῳ (θερμῷ). τοῦτο γάρ ἐστι πλεῖστον τοῖς παιδίοις.

[3] De plac. Hipp. et Plat. viii. 7, K. v. 704: τὰ αὐξανόμενα πλεῖστον ἔχει τὸ ἔμφυτον θερμόν. Ibid., 703: γέρουσι δ' ὀλίγον τὸ θερμόν . . . ψυχρὸν γὰρ τὸ σῶμα.

[4] Ibid., 703: τὸ δ' ἔμφυτον θερμὸν εὔκρατον εἶναι κατὰ μὲν οὐσίαν ἐν αἵματι καὶ φλέγματι τὴν ὕπαρξιν ἔχον μάλιστα, κατὰ δὲ ποιότητα μικτὸν ὂν εὐκράτως ἐκ θερμότητός τε καὶ ψυχρότητος.

In maintaining the natural heat in its proper condition with regard to both quantity and quality, the chief mechanism is the beat of the heart and the pulsation of the arteries, for both of which the Greeks used the single term σφυγμός. That these two movements were clearly connected with each other had been obvious to all physicians since Herophilus, but on the exact nature of this relation there was no agreement. Erasistratus, in spite of his adoption of Praxagoras' error of the bloodless arteries, had it nearly right. And unbeknown to himself, had discovered yet another clue, namely that if you bind a limb with a tourniquet, the veins are distended and the blood from an opened vein will flow more copiously.[1] But Galen, in spite of the fact that he knew and had proved by experiment that both the left ventricle and the arteries contain blood, and was also acquainted with the phenomenon mentioned by Erasistratus, never managed to grasp this simple problem in hydrodynamics. He even devised a rather ingenious experiment, which again might, to our hindsight, have been expected to yield the answer, but as we shall see presently, either his observation was faulty, or his technique inadequate.

In order to prove that arteries had their own power of pulsation, even if ultimately derived from the heart and they did not dilate, as Erasistratus had assumed, simply because they were elastic tubes, obeying the ordinary laws governing inorganic matter, as we might have said, he performed the experiment which he describes in the treatise *On blood in the arteries*, and in his work *On anatomical procedures*. In the latter he says:

You must expose one of the big arteries near the skin, like the one in the groin, which is the one I use most frequently to perform this experiment. You must tie a ligature round it in its upper part. Then with the fingers of your left hand compress it as far as possible below the ligature, but above the point where it throws off any large branch. In the portion between these two points, you make a straight longitudinal cut, large enough to be able to insert a hollow tube between the ligature and the fingers of your left hand. You must have prepared a thin reed, like those we use for writing, or a bronze tube specifically selected for this purpose, and it is sufficient for it to be of a finger's length. It is clear that while you are performing this operation, there will be no haemorrhage from the artery that is being divided, since the higher portion from which the blood flows has been shut off by a ligature, and the part below the cut no longer pulsates, on account of the ligature and because it is being compressed by your fingers. You can therefore take plenty of time in inserting the hollow tube under the portion of the coat of the artery which has been cut, and you can wrap a thin bandage round the artery and the tube taking care to see that no portion of the tube projects beyond the coat. The diameter of

---

[1] *De venae sectione*, i, K. xi. 148, where Galen quotes the following passage from Erasistratus: ἐν γὰρ τοῖς ἀποδουμένοις μέρεσι τοῦ σώματος πλεῖον αἷμα ἀπολαμβάνεται. δηλοῖ δὲ ἥ τε διάτασις τῶν φλεβῶν καὶ ἡ φλεβοτομία. πολὺ γὰρ πλεῖον ῥεῖ, ὅτε ἀποδεθῇ τὸ φλεβοτομούμενον μέρος τοῦ σώματος.

the tube should be such that, when it is inserted, the coat does not lie loosely upon it, because we want it to remain in its place. It must neither bulge beyond the upper edge of the cut, nor must there be any space left between the cut and the upper surface of the tube. When it has been properly fitted, loosen the ligature, and as an extra precaution you can, if you wish, transfer the fingers you used to compress the artery to that portion of it which contains the tube. Now if the tube is fitted and bound accurately, it will not require any further handling or support from you, and you will then be able quietly to observe that the portion of the artery above the tube continues to pulsate, as it did before you applied the ligature, but that the portion below it is absolutely devoid of any pulse.[1]

The conclusions to be drawn from the experiment are more clearly described in the work *On blood in the arteries*:

It is clear therefore that if the power of pulsating remains inactive, that is because arteries are not moved by the heart, but by the heart sending forth to them the power of movement through their coats or tunics. Hence Erasistratus' statements on the movement of the arteries are altogether false. For before the cessation of movement in the denudated artery in the portions below the ligature—a cessation which could not take place before the ligature was tied—it is possible to see the whole artery moving at the same time, not one part of it first and the other afterwards, as Erasistratus alleges. And that is another of his completely absurd statements. For though one might maintain that while, before the artery is filled with blood, the passage of *pneuma* was so swift that it escapes perception which part of the artery was the first to be dilated, when it has been filled with blood, the *pneuma* is not able to reach the termination of the artery from the heart so quickly as before. This theory would not however explain the movement of the lower part of the artery after the insertion of the hollow tube, but before the tying of the

---

[1] *De anat. admin.* vii. 16, K. ii. 646–8 : ἡ δ' ἐγχείρησίς ἐστι τοιάδε. τῶν ἐγγὺς τοῦ δέρματος ἀρτηριῶν τῶν μεγάλων χρὴ γυμνώσαντα μίαν, οἵα πέρ ἐστιν ἡ κατὰ τὸν βουβῶνα, μάλιστα γὰρ ἐπ' ἐκείνης εἴωθα ποιεῖσθαι τὴν ἀνατομὴν τήνδε, βρόχον περιβάλλειν τοῖς ὑψηλοτέροις αὐτῆς μέρεσιν, εἶτα τοῖς δακτύλοις τῆς ἀριστερᾶς χειρὸς αὐτὴν σφίγγοντα τὴν ἀρτηρίαν, ὅσον οἷόν τε πορρωτάτω μὲν τοῦ βρόχου, πρὶν δ' ἀποβλάστημα ποιήσασθαι μέγα, διατέμνειν αὐτὴν κατὰ τὸ μῆκος εὐθείᾳ τομῇ, τηλικοῦτον ὡς ἐνθεῖναι δύνασθαι κοῖλόν τι σῶμα μεταξὺ τοῦ βρόχου καὶ τῶν δακτύλων. παρεσκευάσθω δή σοι κάλαμος τῶν λεπτῶν, οἷς γράφομεν, ἢ χαλκοῦν τι τοιοῦτον ἐπίτηδες γεγονός· ἀρκεῖ δ' εἶναι τοῦτο τῷ μήκει δακτυλαῖον. εὔδηλον οὖν, ὡς κατὰ τὴν ἐνεργείαν ταύτην οὐδεμία γενήσεται τῆς διῃρημένης ἀρτηρίας αἱμορραγία, τοῦ μὲν ὑψηλοτέρου μέρους, ὅθεν ἐπιρρεῖ τὸ αἷμα, βρόχῳ διειλημμένου, τοῦ ταπεινοτέρου δὲ μήτε σφύζοντος ἔτι διὰ τὸν βρόχον, ὑπό τε τῶν δακτύλων σφιγγομένου. κατὰ πολλὴν οὖν σχολὴν ἔνεστί σοι τὸ καθιέμενον εἰς τὴν ἀρτηρίαν σῶμα κοῖλον ὑποκείμενον ποιῆσαι τῷ διῃρημένῳ μέρει τοῦ χιτῶνος αὐτῆς, εἶτα περιλαμβάνειν ἐν κύκλῳ λίνῳ λεπτῷ τὴν ἀρτηρίαν ἅμα τῷ καλάμῳ, προνοούμενον ὅπως μηδὲν ὑπερεκπίπτῃ τῆς κατὰ τὴν ἀρτηρίαν τομῆς τοῦ καλάμου. τῷ πάχει δὲ ἔστω τηλικοῦτος ὁ κάλαμος, ὡς ἔφην, ὥστε τὸν χιτῶνα τῆς ἀρτηρίας μὴ χαλαρὸν ἐγκεῖσθαι, βουλόμεθα γὰρ αὐτὸν κατὰ χώραν μεῖναι, μήτ' ἀνώτερον τῆς κατὰ τὴν ἀρτηρίαν διαιρέσεως ἐνεχθέντα, μήτε κατώτερον. γενομένου δὲ τούτου, λῦσον μὲν τὸν βρόχον, αὐτὸς δὲ ὑπὲρ ἀσφαλείας, εἰ βούλει, μετάθες τοὺς δακτύλους οἷς ἔσφιγγες τὴν ἀρτηρίαν, ἐπὶ τὴν περὶ τῷ καλάμῳ μοῖραν αὐτῆς, εἴ γε μήν, ὡς εἶπον, ἐσφηνωμένος τ' εἴη καὶ δεδεμένος ἀκριβῶς ὁ κάλαμος, οὐδὲν ἔτι δεήσεταί σου κρατοῦντος, ἀλλ' ἐφ' ἡσυχίας μὲν δὴ οὕτως ὑπάρξει σοι θεάσασθαι τὸ μὲν ἀνώτερον τοῦ καλάμου τῆς ἀρτηρίας ἔτι καὶ νῦν σφύζον, ὡς ἔμπροσθεν, ἄσφυκτον δ' ἀκριβῶς γιγνόμενον αὐτοῦ τὸ κατώτερον.

ligature. The fact that after the ligature has been tied pulsation ceases in
the parts of the artery distal to the tube shows clearly that the power of
dilation of the arteries is communicated to their coats by the heart, and not
by the matter flowing through the tube.[1]

The power of pulsation thus transmitted is compared by Galen to what
we should today call a nervous impulse. When we decide to move our
toes, we do so immediately, though the decision to move them is not
made in the toe itself, but the power of movement is communicated to it
instantaneously.[2]

This experiment, which seems to have fascinated Galen—he demonstrated it repeatedly—is also described in his work *On anatomical procedures* in rather greater detail and with certain added precautions about
seeing that the tube fits the artery properly, that it does not slip, and that
no blood escapes through the cut. In this instance he tells us that he used
a goat and that the artery he operated on for preference was the femoral
artery, that in the groin.

It rather looks as if this experiment was a set exercise of the anatomy
school in Alexandria, for Galen tells us that Erasistratus himself had
performed it.[3] If this is correct, it is curious to find that he still persisted
in maintaining Praxagoras' theory of the bloodless arteries. But the
obvious to posterity is often far from obvious to the present.

It might appear even more curious that Galen failed to observe the
pulsation of the artery after he had loosened the ligature below the
inserted cannula, but the fact is that repeated performances in modern
times of Galen's experiment do not seem to have yielded consistent
results, since the days of the Renaissance. Thus as late as 1965 Malato,
an Italian physiologist, contributed a paper to the twenty-first National
Congress of the History of Medicine held in Perugia, entitled 'On an
experiment of Galen repeated several times and not yet yielding a

---

[1] *De sang. in art.* 8, K. iv. 733–5: δῆλον οὖν, ὡς εἰ μὲν δύναμις ἀτρεμοίη, οὐ κινεῖσθαι παρὰ τῆς
καρδίας αὐτάς, διὰ δὲ τῶν χιτώνων αὐτὴν ἐπιπέμπεσθαι. τὰ δὲ ὑπὸ Ἐρασιστράτου περὶ κινήσεως
τῶν ἀρτηριῶν εἰρημένα ψευδῆ παντελῶς ἐστιν. πρὸ γὰρ τοῦ παύσασθαι τῆς γεγυμνωμένης ἀρτηρίας
τὴν κίνησιν ἐν τοῖς μετὰ τὸν βρόχον μέρεσιν, ὅπερ οὐκ ἐχρῆν γίγνεσθαι πρὸ τοῦ βρόχον αὐτῇ
περιβαλεῖν, ἔνεστι θεάσασθαι πᾶσαν ἐνὶ χρόνῳ κινουμένην, οὐ τὸ μὲν αὐτῶν πρότερον μόριον, τὸ δ'
ὕστερον, ὅπερ Ἐρασίστρατος βούλεται. καίτοι καὶ ταῦτ' αὐτῷ δεινῶς ἄτοπα. πρὶν μὲν γὰρ αἷμα
περιέχειν αὐτήν, ἴσως ἄν τις οὕτως ὠκεῖαν εἶναι τὴν τοῦ πνεύματος φορὰν συνεχώρησεν, ὡς
λανθάνειν τὴν αἴσθησιν, ποιά ποτ' ἐστὶ μόρια τῆς ἀρτηρίας τὰ διαστελλόμενα πρότερα· πεπληρωμένης δὲ αἵματος, οὐκ ἐγχωρεῖ τὸ πνεῦμα τάχα οὕτως ὡς πρόσθεν ἀπὸ τῆς καρδίας ἐπὶ τὰ πέρατα
τῆς ἀρτηρίας διεξέρχεσθαι. ἀλλ' εἰ καὶ τοῦτο οὕτως ἔφην, ἴσως οὐ συγχωρήσειεν ἤ γε μετὰ τὸ
καταστῆναι τὸν κοῖλον κάλαμον εἰς τὴν ἀρτηρίαν τῶν κάτω μερῶν αὐτῆς κίνησις, πρὶν περιβληθῆναι
τὸν βρόχον. ἀκινησία δέ, περιβληθέντων, ἐναργῶς ἐνδείκνυται δύναμιν ἀπὸ καρδίας ἐπιπέμπεσθαι
τοῖς χιτῶσι τῶν ἀρτηριῶν τὴν διαστέλλουσαν αὐτάς, οὐχ ὕλην διὰ τῆς κοιλότητος.

[2] *Ibid.*, 735: ὡς γὰρ καὶ τὸν τοῦ ποδὸς δάκτυλον κινῆσαι προελόμενοι παραχρῆμα κινοῦμεν
αὐτόν, οὐ τὸν λογισμὸν ἔχοντες ἐν αὐτῷ τῷ μορίῳ, διαδοθείσης δέ τινος ἐπ' αὐτὸν ἐν ἀκαρεῖ χρόνῳ
δυνάμεως, οὕτω κἀπὶ τῆς καρδίας καὶ τῶν ἀρτηριῶν γίγνεται.

[3] *De anat. admin.* vii. 16, K. ii. 648: διηγεῖτό γε μὴν ἐναντίως ὁ Ἐρασίστρατος ὑπὲρ αὐτοῦ,
φαίνεσθαι λέγων κινούμενον τὸ κάτω τοῦ καλάμου.

conclusive result'.[1] One of the more famous of these repetitions was that performed by Harvey in 1649.[2] He wrote of it as follows:

For the moment you have thrown your ligature around the artery upon the reed or tube, immediately, by the force of the blood thrown in, it is dilated beyond the circle of the tube, by which the flow is impeded, and the shock is broken; so that the artery which is tied only pulsates obscurely, being now cut off from the full force of the blood which flows through it, the shock being reverberated, as it were, from that part of the vessel which is above the ligature; but if the artery below the ligature be now divided, the contrary of what has been maintained will now be apparent, from the spurting of the blood through the tube . . . I can state, after having made the trial, that the inferior part will continue to pulsate, if the experiment be properly performed; and whilst they say that when you have undone the ligature, the inferior arteries begin to pulsate again, I maintain that the part below beats less forcibly, when the ligature is untied, than it did when the thread was still tight. But the effusion from the wound confuses everything and renders the whole experiment unsatisfactory . . . so that nothing certain can be shown, by reason, I have said, of haemorrhage.[3]

On this description Forrester comments pertinently: 'It is evident that Harvey's tube fitted very loosely in the artery.' He (Harvey) goes on to mention a case he saw himself, where parts of the aorta were turned to bone, and so presumably could not conduct the impulse onwards, yet in this case the impulse did travel past and down the leg vessels. He regarded

[1] Marco T. Malato and G. B. Scarano, 'Su di un esperimento di Galeno più volte ripetuto e non ancora concluso', *Riv. stor. med.* X, fasc. 2 (1966), with full quotation of sources.

[2] J. M. Forrester, 'An experiment of Galen's repeated', *Proc. R. Soc. Med.* 47, 241–4.

[3] Quoted by Forrester, ibid., from Harvey's *Exercitationes anatomicae, etc.* (1649), Exerc. altera (Sydenham Soc. edn., London, 1847, p. 111). It will be remembered that in the preface to the *De motu cordis* Harvey stated that he had not performed Galen's experiment, and expressed the opinion that it could not properly be carried out on a living body, because it would cause too violent an eruption of blood, and also because the reed could not be made to prevent leakage from the wound without a ligature, but he has no doubt that the blood would spurt through and beyond the reed. 'Nec ego feci experimentum Galeni nec recte posse fieri vivo corpore, ob impetuosi sanguinis ex arteria eruptionem puto; nec obturabit sine ligatura vulnus fistula; et per fistulae cavitatem ulterius prosilire sanguinem dubito.' The original of the passage quoted by Forrester reads as follows: 'Hoc experimentum memoratur a Vesalio . . . sed neque Vesalius, neque Galenus dicit experimentum hoc fuisse ab ipsis sicut a me probatum . . . Nam super calamum aut fistulam quamprimum ac vinculo arteriam strinxeris, supra ligaturam arteria, statim ab impulsu sanguinis desuper impacti, dilatatur ultra orbitam fistulae; inde et fluxus inhibetur et impetus refringitur; ita ut arteria vinculo subdita obscure admodum pulset, quia est sine impetu transeuntis sanguinis, eo quod supra ligaturam reverberatur: sin vero infra fistulam abscissa arteria fuerit, videre licebit contrarium, ex saltu sanguinis projecti et per fistulam impulsi, sicut solet evenire (ut in libello de sanguinis motu notavi) in aneurismate ab exesis arteriae tunicis . . . expertus dico subditam partem pulsaturam, si recte fiat experientia, et cum solveris vinculum, ubi asserunt subditas arterias repulsare, aio minus pulsare partem subditam soluto quam stricto vinculo. Verum sanguinis e vulnere prosilientis effusio omnia perturbat, et irritum experimentum et vanum reddit adeo ut nihil certi, ob impetum sanguinis, ut dixi, demonstrari possit.'

this as a natural equivalent of Galen's experiment.[1] Harvey had been anticipated in the repetition of the experiment already by Vesalius,[2] who reported a result which if not perfectly identical with Galen's, seemed nevertheless to confirm his theory that the power of pulsation was communicated to the arteries by the heart through their tunics. For Vesalius reports that if you insert the tube, as Galen did, into the cut made in the artery and bind a ligature over the tube, blood and spirits runs right through the tube, but the portion of the artery below the tube no longer pulsates. If however you untie the ligature over the tube, the part of the artery below it pulsates no less forcibly than that above it.[3] Galen, it would appear, never released the ligature over the inserted reed and found the pulse restored to the parts of the artery below it; he only applied the ligature after he had inserted the tube. He did not undo it and see the pulse restored to the parts distal to the cannula. Another contemporary of Harvey, De Wale, says he repeated the experiment more than once, but he hints that the passage in Galen describing the experiment may be corrupt, since the operation is a very difficult one, and loss of blood may be caused by spurting such as to cause the death of the animal, or at any rate to weaken it sufficiently to prevent any pulsation in the remoter parts.[4] If however Galen's account is genuine,

---

[1] Harvey, loc. cit.: 'Alio quoque viro nobilissimo et fortissimo, aortam partemque magnae arteriae juxta cor in os rotundum conversam novi. Ita Galeni experimentum, vel saltem ejus analogon (quod industria non inventum, casu repertum) satis manifestum facit, impressionem pulsificae facultatis, constrictione vel ligatura tunicarum arteriae, non impediri ut inde arteriae subditae non pulsarent.'

[2] See M. P. Amacher, 'Galen's experiment on the pulse and the experiment repeated', *Arch. f. Gesch. d. Med.* xlviii (1964).

[3] Vesalius, *De corporis humani fabrica*, vii, cap. 19: 'Item in arteriis vivorum sectionem vix requirimus, quanquam licebit alicui arteriam in inguinem procedentem nudare, vinculoque intercipere, ac intueri partem arteriae vinculo subtensam non amplius pulsare. Atque ita levi negotio observatur in arteriis sanguinem natura contineri, si quando arteriam in vivis aperimus. Ut autem certiores fiamus, pulsandi vim non arteriae inesse, aut contentam in arteriis materiam opificem existere, verum a corde eam virtutem pendere, praeterquam quod arteriam vinculo interceptam non amplius sub vinculo pulsare cernimus, licebit inguinis femorisve arteriae longam sectionem inducere, et canaliculum ex arundine tam crassum assumere, quanta arteriae est capacitas: et ita illum sectioni indare, ut superior canalis pars altius in arteriae cavitate pertingat, quam sectionis superior sedes: et ita inferior quoque canalis pars, seorsum magis ipsa inferiori sectionis parte protrudatur: ac dein vinculum arteriae circundetur, quod ipsius corpus super canalem stringat. Quum enim id fit, sanguis quidem et spiritus per arteriam ad pedem usque excurrit, verum tota arteriae pars canali subdita non amplius pulsat. Soluto autem vinculo, arteriae pars canali succedens non minus quam superior pulsum ostendet.'

[4] De Wale, *De motu chyli et sanguinis epistula, etc.*, in *Opera Selecta Nederlandicorum de Arte Medica* (Amsterdam, 1922), pp. 106 f.: 'Equidem verum est in *Galeni* libello, *an sanguis in arteriis contineatur*, verbis ultimis asseri, intrusa arteriis cannula, arteriaque supra cannulam ligata, ultra ligaturam arteriam non pulsare, etiamsi sanguis per cannulam pelli possit. Sed mutilum enim esse locum mihi suspicio est, quod ea ratione qua ibi describitur succedere rarissime et difficillime operatio possit: libera enim arteria praescribitur ibi secanda e qua dissecta, nemo non novit quanta vis sanguinis exileat, adeo ut vel moriatur animal, vel prae languore nullae arteriae vel saltem non remotiores queant pulsare.'

and he succeeded in performing the operation he describes, the fact that
he did not perceive any pulse below the cannula may have been due to the
fact that the lumen of the cannula was too small. He himself had tried the
experiment on a rabbit ligating the aorta in two places, but the animal
had died with the result that no pulse could be felt either above or below
the cannula. And it is not at all easy to find an artery that can be conveniently operated on. He had himself never succeeded in performing it
properly since the animal always died of haemorrhage, or what is more
remarkable, of convulsions. Yet he was convinced that the only cause of
the pulse that need be postulated was the impulsion of the blood in the
arteries.[1]

Another slightly younger contemporary of Harvey, the Italian physician Thomaso Cornelio de Cosenza, described a repetition of the experiment in *Progymnasimenta physica*, a work published in Venice in 1663.[2]
He excuses Galen's failure to perceive any pulsation below the cannula on
the ground that this can be very feeble, and that the reason why he did
not observe it may have been the small diameter of the cannula's lumen,
which may have obstructed the passage of the blood, or the fact of
clotting which it requires great care and observation to avoid.[3]

But the most impressive repetition of this experiment in the generations
fairly close to Harvey's discovery was that made at Montpellier by
Raymond Vieussens, who performed it in the presence of a distinguished company of witnesses, including Chicoyneau, Regis, Chirac,
Rouve, and Marmaduke Whitham, on 13 December 1680. Vieussens

[1] Ibid.: 'Sed locus integer sit, et ubi jam describitur operatio successerit, fieri potuit ut
languente prorsus animali ob sanguinis effluxum, citra cannulam pulsus sentiretur, quod
cannula intrusa arteriam reddens angustiorem ex parte sanguinem sisteret, ut facile sanguis
replere arteriam possit et attollere. Ita non raro vidimus arterias quae vel languidum vel
nullum exhibebant pulsum, manifestum edidisse quando non ita remote a corde compri-
merentur. Ultra vero cannulam a *Galeno* pulsus non fuit animadversus, quod per cannulam
arteria multo angustiorem minus sanguinis arteriae reciperent. Et tale quid facile potuisse
contingere in cuniculo animadvertimus, cujus aortae, ea utrinque ligata ligatura animal
emoreretur, operae pretium non videbatur supra cannulam arteriam ligare, visi tamen nobis
sumus aliquem usque ad cannulam pulsum sentire, nullum vero potuimus supra aut ultra
cannulam. Nec praeterea id experimentum nobis unquam successit, quod haud facile sit
commodam arteriam invenire. Et ea ubi oblata debiteque dissecta sit ocyssime tamen animal
aut haemorraghia, aut, quod mirum est, convulsione morietur, ut non aliud appareat quam
impulsum sanguinem arterias posse permeare, ut ab eo quoque arterias posse distendi. Nec
aliam videri ad arteriarum pulsum causam arcessendam, cum ab his peragi pulsus possit.'

[2] I am indebted for the reference and the quotation to Malato and Scarano, op. cit.

[3] Ibid., pp. 104 ff.: 'Atqui ego non omnem Galeno fidem in hac re derogandam velim:
quippe mihi haec aliquando licuit experiri, ligata utrinque hic et illinc arteria, spatioque
inter vincula diffisso, fistulam per vulnus in arteriam inserui, ac discissam arteriae partem
praetenui filo fistulae alligavi: tum disruptis confestim prioribus vinculis, sanguis per fistulam
permanabat in ulteriorem arteriae partem. At interea videre erat arteriam ultra vinculum,
sed paulo obscurius, pulsantem. Quod autem ejusmodi motum Galenus non animadverterit
causam fuisse suspicor calami crassitudinem, quia quoniam exiguo pertusus erat foramine,
trajectioni sanguinis officere potuit. Ad haec accidit quod sanguis intra fistulam facile coit
atque densatur, quapropter tale experimentum navum industriumque postulat observatorem.'

describes his performance of the operation in the following terms. He prepared, in the first place, a number of little tubes varying in diameter and length. The animal he chose was a dog, and the artery chosen the aorta descendens, the two ligatures being placed immediately below the diaphragm and above the division of the iliac branches. The longitudinal cut was made between the two ligatures, and the whole of the blood contained by the artery between them was pressed out and the piece of the artery between the ligatures wiped with a sponge which had been placed in warm water. The tubes had also been placed in warm water, and one was inserted into the cut artery which exactly fitted its cavity without any undue distention. Two tight ligatures were then placed over the portion of the artery enveloping the tube and precautions were taken to avoid coagulation of blood which was to enter the tube. When the two ligatures above and below the tube were removed, all the audience were able to convince themselves both by sight and by touch that the artery pulsated both above and below the tube, the pulsation below the tube being of almost equal force as that above it.[1]

But Vieussens did not content himself with a single experiment. He now embarked upon a significant variation. This time, he blocked the tube to be inserted in the artery with a piece of sponge, taking care to keep it at least at blood heat to prevent coagulation, while at the same time he refrained from tying any ligatures over the inserted tube. Yet not a drop of blood escaped through the aperture of the incision. After the ligature above and below the tube had been loosened, no pulsation below the tube was observed.

The conclusions drawn from this result by Vieussens were the following: Neither Galen's theory that the power of pulsation was transmitted

---

[1] Reported in Le Clerc and Manget, *Bibliotheca Anatomica* (2nd edn., Geneva, 1699), ii. 129: 'Istam vero opinionem sequentibus confirmamus experimentis, quae multis adhibitis cautionibus, die decima tertia mensis Decembris anni 1680 fecimus in Theatro Anatomico Montpeliensis Academiae, Medicinae Studiis celeberrimae, coram Illustrissimo Viro supra laudato, D. Chicoyneau et coram Viris Clarissimis, Dom. D. Regis, Chirac, Rovve, et Marmaduco Witham, Doctoribus Medicis Meritissimis. Primum itaque tubulos plures quorum alii aliis longiores, et alii aliis crassiores erant, in aquam calidam immisimus. Secundo, canis tabulae affixi abdomine aperto, et arteriis tum mammariis, tum epigastricis ligatis, renem sinistrum, lienem, stomachum et intestina supra dextrum latus reclinavimus, et arteria musculari superiore, una cum vena quae alias adiposa dici solebat, ligata, descendentem aortae truncum paulo infra diaphragma et paulo supra iliacos ejus ramos vinculo strinximus: partem illius utrique vinculo intermediam, cultro anatomico aperuimus: ex ipsa totum quem continebat sanguinem per compressionem extraximus: ac subinde postquam arteriam ipsam bina inter vincula, spongia aqua tepefacta imbuta, fovimus: e tubulis in aqua calefactis unum in cavitatem illius intrusimus, qui eam penitus replebat, nec praeter modum distendebat. Praeterea arteriam eandem super tubulo vinculis duobus arctissimis obligavimus: adeo ut aperta ejus pars inter posteriora haec vincula reperiretur. His diligenter quantum potuimus peractis, praedictis cautionibus servatis, ne sanguis tubuli cavitatem subiturus in ipsa concresceret, et prioribus solutis vinculis, aeque valide fere infra ac supra tubulum arteriam pulsare, clarissimi viri supra nominati visus et ipsius tactus ministerio perceperunt.'

to the artery by the heart through the arterial coats, nor that of Willis that it was transmitted by animal spirits permeating the annular fibres of the arterial coats, can any longer be maintained. The only possible theory which fits the facts is that the pulse is due to the expansive force of the blood transmitted or propelled by the heart.

In order to demonstrate quite conclusively the falsity of Galen's theory, accepted in a somewhat modified form by Willis, that the power of pulsation was transmitted to the arteries from the heart through their tunics by a quasi-nervous impulse, he repeated the experiment just described with certain variations. This time he inserted a tube which had been blocked with a piece of sponge. When the ligatures were removed after the tube had been inserted, no pulsation was observed below the tube. This fact he believed to show that the pulsation of the arteries was caused entirely by the pressure of the blood propelled through them by the ventricular contraction of the heart.[1]

One might have thought that after so convincing a demonstration, the falsity of Galen's observation would have been accepted as no longer open to dispute, but three repetitions of the experiment during the present century appear to have yielded divergent results. Two of these yielded results inconsistent with Galen's observations, but the third

---

[1] Ibid.: 'Supra allato peracto experimento, arteriam iterum paulo infra diaphragma et paulo supra iliacos ejus ramos circumligavimus, binisque vinculis, quibus ipsa super tubulo stringebatur solutis, tubulum e cavitate illius extraximus, ipsiusque tubuli cavitatem pauca spongia obturavimus, eumque calentem in aquam immisimus, et dum calefiebat, arteriam spongia, aqua tepefacta imbuta, ut antea fovimus, quo pristinum illi calorem redderemus. Quod cum peractum esset, obturatum et non nihil calefactum tubulum in cavitatem illius denuo indidimus: nec ipsam ligavimus; et tamen, ne una quidem sanguinis gutta per apertionem illius incisione factam effluxit. Quia totam eius cavitatem replebat tubulus. Iis peractis, bina solvimus vincula quibus arteriam strinxeramus. Iisque solutis, haec licet identidem aqua paululum calida foveretur; infra tubulum minime pulsavit. Quae cum verissima sint, neque Galeni neque Willisii opinio stare potest: nam si arteriae vel pulsificam quandam facultatem e corde manantem, earumque tunicas subeuntem (uti vult Galenus), vel per spiritum animalem annulares mediae ipsarum tunicae fibras permeantem, ut Willisio placet, dilatarentur et contraherentur: dum arteria strictissime super tubulum stringitur: quod fit per primum experimentum, infra tubulum minime pulsare deberet: etenim tunc facultas pulsifica, si quae sit, et spiritus animalis intercipiuntur, ipsam tamen pulsare certissimum esse pronuntiamus. Quod si arteriarum dilatatio a fluente intra cavitates ipsarum sanguine non penderet, uti secundum fit experimentum, arteria infra tubulum prius obturatum, pulsare deberet cum per illum neque pulsificae facultatis, neque spiritus animalis praepediatur influxus: eam tamen dum secundum tentatur experimentum, nequaquam pulsare sensibus patet. Neque oggerat aliquis, arteriam infra vincula pulsare non tantum quod effervescentem e ventriculis cordis depulsum, propriam inter cavitatem sanguinem admittat, sed etiam quod eadem infra vincula nerveis instructa sit propaginibus per quas spiritum animalem, praecipuam dilatationis et contractionis suae causam recipit, siquidem eam a nervis et a vicinis quibusvis partibus, quantum fieri potuit, liberavimus ac separavimus, dum praedictis in experimentis conficiendis nostram posuimus operam. Quae cum ita sint, arteriarum dilatationem a sola sanguinis vi expansiva praedicti impulsus pendere existimabimus: donec spiritum animalem per tunicas quibus ipsae constant diffusum, ipsarum motui peragendo conducere, solido quodam experimento clare evicantur.' I am indebted for these quotations to the article of Malato and Scarano, to which I have referred.

seems to have confirmed Galen's report that after the insertion of the tube and the release of the original ligatures, no pulse distal to the tube could be observed. The explanation of these apparently contradictory results lies wholly beyond a layman's competence, even if common sense seems so strongly to support the negation of Galen's findings. To dismiss their confirmation as the result of incompetence would be presumptuous. I therefore decided to include an account of Malato's experiment, though I found it expedient to omit some of his technical explanations.

The first of the experiments in question, that of Forrester, was performed on the carotid artery of a dog anaesthetized with ether. Forrester described his results as follows:

The right common carotid artery was exposed and dissected free of the vaso-sympathetic trunk and internal jugular vein. The pulse was found to be readily palpable but not visible. The blood flow was controlled by proximal and distal retractors, and the arterial wall was incised longitudinally for a distance just sufficient to allow the insertion of a glass tube about one inch long, and of thin wall. The tube was wide enough to fit snugly and slightly to dilate the arterial wall.

The blood loss at this stage was negligible, and the pulse in the distal part of the artery beyond the tube was found to be still clearly palpable and expansile, but of diminished force and volume. A ligature of linen thread which was probably Galen's material (Kühn, ii. 647; J. S. Milne, *Surgical Instruments in Greek and Roman Times*) was then applied round the artery at the segment containing the tube, and just proximal to the incision. This produced no change in the pulse in the distal part of the artery; in a further attempt to elicit arterial spasm, a second ligature was applied over the tube just distal to the incision, but without result.

At this point an interval of ten minutes was allowed to elapse, to see whether clotting would occur in the tube, but no change in the distal pulse was found. No anti-coagulants had been employed. At this stage, too, a further possibility was raised, that Galen had inadvertently included the vagus nerve in his ligature and caused cardiac inhibition by tying it, similar to the well-known inhibition seen on electrical stimulation of the vagus . . . However, to test the possibility, a femoral cannula was inserted and the blood-pressure recorded by kymograph for the remainder of the experiment. The original ligatures were removed and the distal pulse again observed, in view of Harvey's observation that this step diminished the pulse; but no change was found, although some slight haemorrhage followed the removal of the ligatures. Another ligature was then applied as before, but including the right vago-sympathetic trunk. No cardiac inhibition resulted; there was a transient rise in blood-pressure, without alteration of the pulse-rate or character of distal pulse. Finally the left vagosympathetic trunk was also ligated, without including the common carotid, and a repetition of the same events observed. At the conclusion of the experiment the distal pulse was observed ninety minutes after the start of the experiment, to find whether evidence of clotting had appeared, but it was still unchanged.

Thus it has not been possible to demonstrate the reason for Galen's observation. No arterial spasm was produced by manœuvres resembling his. No sign of clotting was observed within a reasonable time. The hypothesis that he crushed his tube is only a matter for speculation. And in our experiment the result of including the vagus in the ligature was rather that of section of the vagus than that of stimulation.

A similar clearly anti-Galenic result was also obtained by Amacher, who operated on the femoral artery of a dog and used as cannula a copper tube 0·625 in. long with an interior diameter of 0·125 in. The dog was anaesthetized with phenobarbitol, which has little effect on the peripheral blood-pressure. He describes his results as follows:

The pulse was at all times plainly visible distal to the tube, both before and after the ligature was tightened. Tightening the ligature did not change the magnitude of the pulse observed distal to the tube. The artery was considerably distended proximal to the cannula, so that the pulse was very noticeable there. The pulse appeared of lower magnitude in the portion of the artery distal to the cannula, especially when compared with that in the distended portion proximal to the tube. The tube was removed from the artery after ten minutes. No clotting of blood was observed within the tube.

In view of these two very careful experiments yielding positive results disproving Galen's findings, it is interesting to read of Malato's opposite conclusions. Malato used a reed (canna de campo) with one end of it cut into the shape of the mouthpiece of a flute. His reed was 25 mm long, with a diameter of about 4 mm, and the animal operated on was a lamb, one and a half years old and weighing 7 kg. Malato found that immediately after the insertion of the tube the pulse below it ceased, and that the application of the ligature round the cannula made no difference. Why therefore, asks Malato, did Galen maintain that before the application of the ligature round the cannula the pulse below the tube was still beating? Malato hints that Galen's 'observations' were clearly predetermined by his own particular physiological theories, namely his belief that the power of pulsation was transmitted by the heart via the coat of the artery, while at the same time paying a tribute to his skill in devising and his technical ability in carrying out the experiment. He therefore rejects as grossly inaccurate the results reported by Vieussens. He insists that no pulse will be observed, as Galen maintained, even if he did so for the wrong reasons.[1]

---

[1] Malato and Scarano, op. cit.: 'Perchè allora Galeno afferma che l'arteria continuava a pulsare dopo l'introduzione del tubo, e cessava di pulsare solo dopo la ligatura? Abbiamo qui uno dei chiari esempi di esperimenti addatti a dimostrazione de un credo preconcetto. Galeno

To the common sense of the layman it seems very difficult to suppose that Galen's observation of the absence of the pulse could have been accurate in view of the negative result obtained by several careful repetitions of his experiment. But the question is evidently far from simple, seeing that Amacher points out that from the standpoint of modern theory it cannot readily be judged *a priori* what the results of such an experiment would be.

The cross-sectional areas through which the blood flows differ greatly along the sections of the artery concerned and the tube. The distensibility of the artery is affected by the surgery on the surrounding structures. When the experiment was described to two physiologists now engaged on research on the circulation, they did not agree as to whether or not the pulse would be visible distal to the copper pipe and constricted tunic of the artery.

It is perhaps a little difficult for us to understand how, in view of all his experiments and his extensive experience as surgeon to the gladiators at Pergamum, such an intelligent practitioner as Galen could have missed discovering the circulation. In his great work *On the method of Medicine*, he devotes practically the whole of the fifth book to the consideration of the treatment of divided, wounded, and injured blood vessels. The details of the various techniques described lie outside the scope of this essay, but in general he recognizes two main methods of arresting haemorrhage from injured vessels, namely, tamping and the application of clot-forming drugs, and the application of ligatures. Thus, in the case of a wound, the instruction given is to place the fingers round the 'mouth' or aperture of the vessel, gently pressing its edges together and holding it thus until a clot is formed, which will stop the flow of blood. In the case of the deeper-lying vessels the size and position of the injury and the nature of the vessel itself, whether artery or vein, can best be discovered by manipulation with a hook to raise the vessel and twist it slightly. If meanwhile the flow of blood continues, one must try, if the vessel be a vein, to arrest bleeding by the application of ischaemic drugs, such as resin, gypsum, etc., without tying a ligature. If the vessel be an artery a ligature must be used, and we are sometimes compelled to use this also in the case of large veins. The safest way is to tie this ligature, and then to divide the vessel on the further side of the knot, which should be tied at the 'root' of the vessel, that is the side nearer the heart, in the case of an artery, and nearer the liver, in the case of a vein, for all veins, according to Galen, arise, as we have seen, out of the liver.[1]

voleva dimostrare che la pulsazione era dovuta alla trasmissione attraverso le tuniche della arteria di una certa virtù pulsifica proveniente del cuore, e a tale scopo adattò il risultato.

Ciò nonostante è doveroso riconoscere la genialità dell'impostazione dell'esperimento, e la capacità tecnica della sua esecuzione.

[1] Galen, *De methodo medendi*, v. 3, K. x. 318–19: αὐτίκα μὲν ἐπιβαλλέτω τὸν δάκτυλον ἐπὶ τὸ

Having seen quite clearly the correct direction of the arterial blood-flow, he somehow missed, in spite of his occasional application of the technique of ligation to the larger veins, discovering the direction of the venous flow. But we must remember that if he had observed it, or thought he had observed it, he might very well have distrusted his own observation, since to accept it as a fact would have exploded the whole foundations on which ancient Greeks had built their physiological constructions. We may guess too, perhaps, that the real reason for this failure may be summed up in a single word, haemorrhage, as the last sentence in the passage just quoted from Harvey would appear to suggest.

Galen evidently spent a great deal of time in investigating experimentally both by dissection and by vivisection the actual working of the heart. Thus he describes in some detail a vivisectional technique by which a live heart can be exposed and its actual working observed, the important condition being not to perforate—or tear—any of the membranes lining and dividing the cavities of the thorax, since once this happens the whole breathing function is destroyed, the lung collapses, and the animal dies immediately.[1] He also describes an actual case in which he was able to observe the living heart of one of his patients, who was still alive at the time of writing. The patient was the slave of Marullus the mimographer. He had been hit on the sternum in the palaestra. The injury had been neglected and he was also given the wrong treatment. After about four months pus appeared in the injured part. The physician who was treating him wished to evacuate this, and made an incision which he thought he had caused to heal quickly and to form a scar. The place again became inflamed and produced an abscess. Another incision was

στόμιον τοῦ κατὰ τὸ ἀγγεῖον ἕλκους, ἐρείδων πρᾳέως καὶ πιέζων ἀνωδύνως, ἅμα τε γὰρ ἐφέξει τὸ αἷμα καὶ θρόμβον ἐπιπήξει τῇ τρώσει. καὶ μέντοι κἂν εἰ διὰ συχνοῦ βάθους εἴη τὸ αἱμορραγοῦν ἀγγεῖον, ἀκριβέστερον ἂν καταμάθοις τήν τε θέσιν αὐτοῦ καὶ τὸ μέγεθος καὶ πότερα φλὲψ ἢ ἀρτηρία ἐστί· μετὰ δὲ ταῦτα διαπείρας ἀγκίστρῳ ἀνατεινέτω τε καὶ περιστρεφέτω μετρίως. μὴ ἐπισχεθέντος δ' ἐν τῷδε τοῦ αἵματος, εἰ μὲν φλὲψ εἴη, πειράσθω χωρὶς βρόχου στέλλειν τὸ αἷμα, τῶν ἰσχαίμων τινὶ φαρμάκων. ἄριστα δ' αὐτῶν ἐστι τὰ ἐμπλαστικά, συντιθέμενα διά τε τῆς φρυκτῆς ῥητίνης καὶ ἀλεύρου πυρίνου χνοῦ καὶ γύψου καὶ ὅσα τοιαῦτα. εἰ δὲ ἀρτηρία ἐστί, δυοῖν θάτερον, ἢ βρόχον περιθείς, ἢ ὅλον διακόψας τὸ ἀγγεῖον, ἐφέξεις τὸ αἷμα. βρόχον δ' ἀναγκαζό-μεθά ποτε καὶ ταῖς μεγάλαις φλεψίν, ὥσπερ γε καὶ διατέμνειν ποτ' αὐτὰς ὅλας, ἐγκαρσίας δηλονότι. καταστα ίη δ' ἄν τις εἰς ἀνάγκην τοῦδε κατὰ τὰς ἐκ πολλοῦ βάθους ὀρθίας ἀναφερομένας, καὶ μάλιστα διὰ στενοχωρίας τινὸς ἢ μερῶν κυρίων. ἀνασπᾶται γὰρ οὕτως ἑκάτερον τὸ μέρος ἑκατέρω-θεν, καὶ κρύπτεται καὶ σκέπεται πρὸς τῶν ἐπικειμένων σωμάτων ἡ τρῶσις. ἀσφαλέστερον δ' ἄμφω ποιεῖν, βρόχον μὲν τῇ ῥίζῃ περιτιθέναι τοῦ ἀγγείου τέμνειν δὲ τοὐντεῦθεν. ῥίζαν δ' ἀγγείου καλῶ τὸ πρότερον αὐτοῦ μέρος, ἤτοι τῷ ἥπατι συνάπτον ἢ τῇ καρδίᾳ.

[1] De anat. admin. vii. 12, K. ii. 631: καὶ μὴ τρῶσαι τοὺς διαφράττοντας ὑμένας τὸν θώρακα· τρωθέντος γὰρ οὑτινοσοῦν ἀναγκαῖόν ἐστι περιπεσεῖν τὸ ζῷον ἐκείνοις τοῖς συμπτώμασι, ἃ κατὰ τὸν ἑξῆς λόγον εἰρήσεται γίγνεσθαι συντετρημένου τοῦ θώρακος. Ibid., cap. 15, 639: εὔδηλον δ' ὅτι διὰ ταχέων ἀποθνήσκει τὸ ζῷον ἐπὶ τῇ τοιαύτῃ χειρουργίᾳ πνιγόμενον ὡς ἂν ἀπολλυμένης αὐτῷ τῆς ἀναπνοῆς.

made, but this time the wound could not be made to heal.[1] At this point Galen was called in, among a number of other physicians.

All agreed that the trouble was that the slave's sternum had rotted away, and the movement of his heart was plainly visible on the left side. But no one had the courage to cut away the diseased bone, for they thought the result of such an operation would inevitably involve the perforation of the thoracic membrane, with fatal consequences. I said that I would cut it away without making any perforation such as that mentioned by my colleagues. But I refused to make any promises about effecting a real cure, for it could not be seen whether, or to what extent, the parts underneath the sternum had been affected. When the place was exposed, it was found that no more of the sternum had been affected than had at first been visible, wherefore I was the more encouraged to proceed with the operation, since the ends of the sternum to which the arteries and veins are attached were both seen to be uninjured. I removed the diseased part of the bone, which was just that place where the peak of the pericardium is attached, and the bare heart was visible since the pericardium at that place had also rotted. The immediate outlook for the slave was anything but hopeful, but he was completely cured in no great length of time.[2]

Galen goes out of his way to demonstrate the utility of vivisections exposing the living heart. He describes three surgical operations to be performed on the living animal, which have some common and some individual features: (a) in order to inspect the arteries of the lung, one incision made at the bend of the ribs is sufficient; (b) in addition to this, another incision may be made through the other part of the thorax; (c) this is an operation in which the heart is exposed, but the thorax is not perforated. There is nothing miraculous in this. For, he says, it is possible for some wounding of the thorax to occur without actual perforation taking place. What they call perforation is an incision which penetrates into the thoracic cavity in which the lung is situated. All other cuts which wound the membrane but do not perforate it are just called

[1] *De anat. admin.* vii. 12–13, 631–2: ὅπου γε ὁ Μαρύλλου τοῦ μιμογράφου παῖς ἐθεραπεύθη καὶ ζῇ νῦν ἔτι, καίτοι γυμνωθείσης αὐτῷ ποτε τῆς καρδίας . . .

πληγεὶς ἐκεῖνος ὁ παῖς ἐν παλαίστρᾳ κατὰ τὸ στέρνον ἠμελήθη μὲν τὸ πρῶτον, ὕστερον δ᾽ οὐ καλῶς προυνοήθη. καὶ μετὰ τέσσαρας που μῆνας ἐφάνη πῦον ἐν τῷ πληγέντι μορίῳ. τοῦτο κομίσασθαι βουλόμενος ὁ θεραπεύων, ἔτεμε τὸν παῖδα, καί, ὡς ᾤετο, διὰ ταχέων εἰς οὐλὴν ἤγαγεν. εἶτ᾽ αὖθις ἐφλέγμηνε, καὶ αὖθις ἀπέστη καὶ αὖθις ἐτμήθη, καὶ οὐκέθ᾽ οἷόν τε εἰς οὐλὴν ἀχθῆναι.

[2] Ibid., 632–3: ὡς δὲ πᾶσιν ἐδόκει σφάκελος εἶναι τοῦ στέρνου τὸ πάθος, ἐφαίνετο δὲ καὶ ἡ τῆς καρδίας κίνησις, ἐκ τῶν ἀριστερῶν αὐτοῦ μερῶν, οὐδεὶς ἐκκόπτειν ἐτόλμα τὸ πεπονθὸς ὀστοῦν· ᾤοντο γὰρ ἐξ ἀνάγκης ἐπ᾽ αὐτῷ σύντρησιν ἔσεσθαι τοῦ θώρακος. ἐγὼ δ᾽ ἐκκόψειν μὲν ἔφην αὐτὸ χωρὶς τοῦ τὴν καλουμένην ἰδίως ὑπὸ τῶν ἰατρῶν σύντρησιν ἐργάσασθαι· περὶ μέντοι τῆς παντελοῦς ἰάσεως οὐδὲν ἐπηγγελλόμην, ἀδήλου ὄντος εἰ πέπονθε καὶ μέχρι πόσου πέπονθε τῶν ὑποκειμένων τι τῷ στέρνῳ. γυμνωθέντος οὖν τοῦ χωρίου πλέον οὐδὲν ἐφάνη τοῦ στέρνου πεπονθότος, ἢ ὅπερ ἐξ ἀρχῆς εὐθὺς ἐφαίνετο, διὸ καὶ μᾶλλον ἐθάρρησα πρὸς τὴν χειρουργίαν ἐλθεῖν, ἀπαθῶν γε τῶν ἑκατέρωθεν ὀφθέντων περάτων οἷς ὑποπεφύκασιν αἵ τ᾽ ἀρτηρίαι καὶ φλέβες. ἐκκοπέντος δὲ τοῦ πεπονθότος ὀστοῦ, κατ᾽ ἐκεῖνον μάλιστα τὸν τόπον ἐν ᾧ ἐμπέφυκεν ἡ τοιαύτη κορύφη τοῦ περικαρδίου, καὶ φανείσης γυμνῆς τῆς καρδίας, ἐσέσηπτο γὰρ ὁ περικάρδιος κατὰ τοῦτο, παραχρῆμα μὲν οὐκ ἀγαθὴν ἐλπίδα περὶ τοῦ παιδὸς εἴχομεν, ὑγιάσθη δὲ εἰς τὸ παντελὲς οὐκ ἐν πολλῷ χρόνῳ.

woundings, not perforations. The reason why perforation must at all cost be avoided is, as we have seen, because it results in the death of the animal, thus defeating the purpose of the operation, which is to see how the living heart works. What, Galen now asks, is the use of exposing the heart? The answer given is : (a) in order that we may observe accurately the way in which it pulsates; is it at diastole or at systole that it comes up to the region of the sternum and hits the thorax?—a question to which we are not given the answer; (b) in order that when we have exposed the great artery in an animal, we can perceive accurately whether the artery contracts at the moment when the heart expands, and expands at the moment when the heart contracts, or whether both heart and arteries contract and expand simultaneously; (c) in order that we may take hold of the heart between our fingers, or with a pair of forceps, 'as I am in the habit of doing, because it so easily jumps out of our fingers', and that we may observe with what symptoms the animal is seized when the heart is so grasped. In order, too, to establish what actually does happen if one tries to tie off in a noose the great artery where it emerges from the heart (the aorta), or the vein-like artery, the pulmonary vein;[1] operations which Galen does not consider possible in the living creature, as we have already noted.[2]

As to the first two of these questions, neither of which is here answered, we may perhaps be entitled to suppose that like Rufus, he was aware that the heart approaches nearest to the sternum at systole, but we cannot be at all certain, since for him diastole was the most important and powerful motion of the heart,[3] and the answer that he gives to the second, in so many other contexts, is palpably wrong. As Prendergast has remarked: 'Unfortunately he came to the conclusion that the diastole of the heart

---

[1] Ibid., 14, 634–6: τρεῖς ἔλεγον εἶναι χειρουργίας ἐπὶ ζῶντος τοῦ ζῴου γιγνομένας, τὸ μέν τι κοινὸν ἐχούσας ἀλλήλαις, τὸ δ᾽ ἑκάστῃ ἴδιον. ἤτοι γὰρ ἕνεκα τοῦ θεάσασθαι τὰς ἀρτηρίας τοῦ πνεύμονος, ἀρκεῖ μία τομὴ γιγνομένη κατὰ τὰς καμπὰς τῶν πλευρῶν, ἢ καὶ πρὸς ταύτῃ τις ἑτέρα, κατὰ τὸ λοιπὸν μέρος τοῦ θώρακος, ἧς τὴν χρείαν ὀλίγως ὕστερον ἐρῶ. τρίτη δὲ ἐπ᾽ αὐταῖς ἐγχείρησις, καθ᾽ ἣν ἡ μὲν καρδία γυμνοῦται, σύντρησις δ᾽ οὐ γίγνεται τοῦ θώρακος. οὐδὲν δήπου θαυμαστόν ἐστι, τρῶσιν μὲν τοῦ θώρακός τινα γενέσθαι, σύντρησιν δὲ μή. τὴν γὰρ εἰς τὰς εὐρυχωρίας αὐτοῦ, καθ᾽ ἃς ὁ πνεύμων τέτακται, διἴσχουσαν τομὴν ὀνομάζουσι σύντρησιν, ἡ δ᾽ ἄλλη πᾶσα διαίρεσις αὐτοῦ τρῶσις μὲν λέγεται, σύντρησις δ᾽ οὐ καλεῖται. τίς οὖν ἡ χρεία τοῦ γυμνοῦν οὕτω τὴν καρδίαν ἐστίν; ἵνα πρῶτον μὲν ἐν ὁποίῳ τρόπῳ σφύζει θεασώμεθα σαφῶς, καὶ πότερον ἐν τῷ διαστέλλεσθαι πλήττει τὸν θώρακα, προσερχομένη τοῖς κατὰ τὸ στέρνον χωρίοις, ἢ καθ᾽ ὃν χρόνον συστέλλεται· δεύτερον δ᾽ ἵνα γυμνώσαντες ἀρτηρίαν μεγάλην ἐν τῷ ζῴῳ, καθάπερ ὁρᾶτέ με τὴν ἐν τῷ βουβῶνι γυμνοῦντα, κατανοήσωμεν ἀκριβῶς, εἴτε καθ᾽ ὃν ἡ καρδία διαστέλλεται χρόνον, ἡ ἀρτηρία συστέλλεται, διαστελλομένη, καθ᾽ ὃν ἡ καρδία συστέλλεται, ἢ καὶ διαστέλλονται καὶ συστέλλονται κατὰ τοὺς αὐτοὺς χρόνους ἀμφότερα· τρίτον, ἵνα τοῖς δακτύλοις διαλαμβάνοντες ἢ καὶ πυράγρᾳ τὴν καρδίαν, ὡς ἐγὼ ποιεῖν εἴωθα, διὰ τὸ ῥᾳδίως αὐτὴν ἐκπηδᾶν τῶν δακτύλων, ἴδωμεν, ὁποῖόν τι σύμπτωμα καταλαμβάνει τὸ ζῷον· ἔτι τε πρὸς τούτῳ τοῖς φάσκουσιν εἰ διαλάβοι τις βρόχῳ τὴν ἔκφυσιν τῆς μεγάλης ἀρτηρίας, ἤ, ὡς ἕτεροί τινες, τῆς εἰς τὸν πνεύμονα φερομένης, τῆς φλεβώδους, τάδε τίνα καταλαμβάνει τὸ ζῷον συμπτώματα.

[2] See above, pp. 315 f.

[3] De usu partium, vi. 15, K. iii. 484: εἰς ὅσον καὶ ἡ τῆς ἐν τῷ διαστέλλεσθαι κινήσεως ἰσχὺς ὑπερεῖχε τῆς ἐν τῷ συστέλλεσθαι.

and the arteries took place simultaneously. Perhaps it is some justification to plead Harvey's early difficulties with this problem, when he "found the task so truly arduous" and almost concluded with Fracastorius that the motion of the heart was only comprehensible to God.'[1] Nor is his description of the living heart actually working as clear as might be desired. He has seen both auricles and ventricles expand and contract, he knows that the contraction of the auricles precedes that of the ventricles, and he has a general idea of the auricles as reservoirs for holding and transmitting blood and *pneuma* into the ventricles. He knows too that both ventricles contract simultaneously, not as some of his contemporaries maintained only the left. He also 'knew' that all the arteries contract at the same time,[2] which is of course not strictly true, but for all practical purposes known to him a sufficient approximation to the truth.

He does, too, give us an interesting though not entirely accurate account of the dying heart as the result of a vivisection in which the heart was exposed. Progressively the movements of both ventricles become smaller and separated by long intervals of quiescence. The diastole of the right ventricle now is seen to effect its expansion in a manner peculiar to its own nature. You will observe this more particularly when the ventricles approach the point when they cease to move altogether. First the parts nearest to the apex of both ventricles stop moving, and then those progressively higher up, until finally only the bases of the ventricles, i.e. the top parts, are left in motion. And when these too have ceased to move, a small, not very perceptible, motion of the auricles is still seen to take place at long intervals. This phenomenon puzzles Galen, and must be left to be examined at further leisure, for it is not in accordance with reason that when the body of the heart itself has stopped moving, its appendages should continue to move for some time.[3] What Galen did not observe is that it is the right auricle which is the *ultimum moriens*, causing, before it dies, the evacuation of the blood from the main arteries, a condition which may have been noted, as we have seen, by physicians before the days of Hippocrates.[4] This insistence on the idea that the auricles are

---

[1] Prendergast, op. cit., p. 1842.

[2] *De anat. admin.* vii. 15, K. ii. 640 : πρόκειται γάρ σοι κατὰ τὴν τοιαύτην ἀνατομὴν θεάσασθαι τῆς καρδίας ἀμφοτέρας τὰς κοιλίας σφυζούσας ὁμοίως, οὐχ, ὥς τινές φασι, μονὴν τὴν ἀριστεράν. ἐκ περιουσίας δ' ἐναργέστερον ἔτι ὄψει νῦν ἢ πρόσθεν, εἴτε ἐναλλὰξ ἢ κατὰ τὸν αὐτὸν χρόνον τε καὶ ῥυθμὸν αἱ καθ' ὅλον τὸ ζῷον ἀρτηρίαι διαστέλλονται καὶ συστέλλονται.

[3] Ibid., 640–1 : ἐπὶ προσήκοντι δὲ χρόνῳ, βραχεῖαι μὲν ἑκατέρας τῆς κοιλίας αἱ κινήσεις, ἡσυχίαις μακραῖς διαλαμβανόμεναι, σαφὴς δὲ καὶ τῆς δεξιᾶς κοιλίας διαστολὴ κατὰ τὴν ἰδίαν αὐτῆς φύσιν ἐπιτελουμένη, καὶ μάλισθ' ὅσα περ ἂν ἐγγὺς ἀκινησίας ἥκωσι, κατόψει τὰ τοιαῦτα. πρῶτον μὲν γὰρ αὐτῶν ἑκάτερα παύεται κινούμενα τὰ πρὸς τῇ κορυφῇ· δεύτερον δὲ τὰ τούτων ἐφεξῆς· καὶ ταῦτ' ἀεὶ γίγνεται, μέχρις ἂν αἱ βάσεις μόναι ἀπολειφθῶσι κινούμεναι. καὶ τούτων αὖθις παυσαμένων, ἀμυδρὰ καὶ βραχεῖα κίνησις ἐκ μακρῶν διαλειμμάτων ἐν τοῖς ὠσὶ τῆς καρδίας φαίνεται. τούτου μὲν οὖν τοῦ φαινομένου τίς ποτ' ἐστὶν ἡ αἰτία ζητητέον ἐπὶ σχολῆς· οὐ γάρ ἐστιν εὔλογον αὐτοῦ τοῦ σώματος τῆς καρδίας ἐπὶ πλείονα χρόνον φαίνεσθαι κινουμένας τὰς ἐπιψύσεις.

[4] e.g. Alcmaeon and Diogenes of Apollonia. See above, pp. 8, 27.

appendages of the blood vessels and not part of the heart itself provides Galen with another puzzle. The right auricle is a budding off or appendix of the 'hollow vein', but if you perform the appropriate operation, you will see it pulsating like the arteries. Does it like them receive its power of pulsation from the heart, so that it shakes violently as the blood rushes into the heart, or is there a two-way traffic of blood in the auricle itself, or does the 'hollow vein' receive this power of pulsating in some other way? Galen puts the question and then avoids answering it by saying that this is superfluous for his present purposes to inquire.[1] The left auricle, of course, provides him with no such difficulty, for it is the termination of an artery, and the business of arteries, except, of course, the pulmonary, is to pulsate.

Finally, before we leave Galen's account of the functioning of the heart and the blood vessels, there is one rather curious point which calls for comment, his doctrine of permanent and normal 'mitral insufficiency'. He has a generally correct view of the valves and their functions of preventing back-flow into the ventricles, but he is badly misled by his teleological misinterpretation of the anatomical structure of the bicuspid valve, which he regards as a supremely clever device of nature to permit a two-way traffic of what we should call gaseous matter in and out of the left ventricle, *pneuma* coming in from the lungs, and sooty vapours, the 'waste products' of combustion by the vital or innate heat going out, via the pulmonary veins, into the bronchial system, and so into the atmosphere. This doctrine of mitral insufficiency, which looks today like a desperate expedient to preserve the traditional orthodoxy of the pneumatic content of the arteries, and its corollary, the function of the heart as one of the respiratory organs, was combined by Galen with a still more extraordinary theory. For him, not even the aortal sigmoid valve nor the sigmoid pulmonary valve—to say nothing of the tricuspid—was completely blood-, or even *pneuma*-tight. Similarly the epiglottis, which according to the 'Hippocratic' theory, we have already noted,[2] permitted a small quantity of the drink swallowed to go down the windpipe, with a final destination of the heart, was also regarded by Galen as not completely water-tight,[3] in contrast to Erasistratus, who ridiculed this

---

[1] *De plac. Hipp. et Plat.* vii. 7, K. v. 563: ἐὰν οὖν ἅμα τε τοῦτο ποιήσῃς καὶ τέμῃς ὄρθιον, ὡς εἴρηται, τὸν δεξιὸν θώρακα, τῆς δεξιᾶς κοιλίας τῆς καρδίας ἐναργῶς ὄψει τὸν σφυγμόν. οὐ λήσεταί σε οὐδὲ τὸ καταφυόμενον εἰς αὐτὴν ἀγγεῖον, ὅπερ ἐστὶν ἀποβλάστημα τῆς κοίλης ὁμοίως ταῖς ἀρτηρίαις σφύζον. εἴτε δὲ τῷ δέχεσθαι δύναμιν ἐκ τῆς καρδίας ἄχρι τοῦ βράττεσθαι ἐπιρρέουσαν, εἴτε τοῦ αἵματος τῆς ἐπὶ τἀναντία φορᾶς τῇ κατὰ τὸ δεξιὸν οὖς, εἴτε ἄλλῳ τινὶ τρόπῳ τὴν κίνησιν ταύτην ἡ κοίλη φλὲψ λαμβάνει, περιττὸν ἐν τῷ παρόντι σκοπεῖν.

[2] See above, pp. 85 f.

[3] See the passage quoted above, p. 83, n. 3, as well as *De usu partium*, iv. 8, K. iii. 282, where the epiglottis is stated to have the function of preventing liquid in any considerable quantity from going into the lungs. καὶ γὰρ καὶ τοῦτ' ἄμεινον ἦν εἴς τε τὴν τῶν περιεχομένων ἐν τῷ στόματι σιτίων ὁλκήν, καὶ ὅπως ἡ γλῶττα κατασπῷτο σὺν τοῖς κατὰ τὰ παρίσθμια μυσίν, ὑφ'

theory, but accepted by the Anonymous Londoner.[1] Galen's theory of valvular insufficiency is explained in his great physiological work *On the use of the parts*, where, after describing the 'insufficient' bicuspid valve, he continues:

Perhaps someone would imagine that nothing at all goes back past the mouths of the other three vessels. But this is not true. For during the time taken by the actual closing of the membranes, of necessity some blood and *pneuma* must go past and be attracted into the heart. And when the heart is contracting, before the valves are completely shut, something must be sent back, during the time in which they are shutting. Moreover, even when the membranes are completely closed, it is possible occasionally, when the heart moves rather violently, that some matter may flow past them, not only *pneuma* and vapour, but also blood itself. For as we demonstrated in the case of the rough artery, it is not possible that no fraction of the liquids drunk should get past [the epiglottis]; we must suppose the same thing to happen here. Nature has discovered a method of preventing matter going past the valves in any quantity, but she was unable to invent a fortification strong enough to ensure that absolutely nothing at all, not even a very small portion, should do so. For it has been demonstrated to us by other authorities that everything is in all things, as Hippocrates remarked, and the arteries contain thin, clean, and vaporous blood, and the veins a little moist air. . . . So too it was demonstrated that *pneuma* goes past into the stomach through drinking and through respiration, and that there is nothing in the whole body that is absolutely pure. But all things partake of all things, though not in equal proportions . . . So when the thorax is opened up, both ventricles are seen to pulsate, but they do not contain blood and *pneuma* in equal quantities. For there is a far greater quantity of blood in the right ventricle, and a far greater quantity of *pneuma* in the left.[2]

ὧν τῆς τάσεως ἁπάντων ἀνατεινομένου τοῦ λάρυγγος καὶ προσανατρέχοντος τῇ ἐπιγλωττίδι κα πωμαζομένου πρὸς αὐτῆς, ἀθρόον ὑγρὸν ἐμπίπτειν κωλύεται τῷ πνεύμονι.

[1] *Anonymus Londinensis*, xxiii, J. 89: διηθεῖται δὲ εἰς κοιλίαν ὀλίγον διὰ τοῦ στομάχου καθ' ἡμᾶς, οὐ μὴν κατὰ τὸν Ἐρασίστρατον.

[2] *De usu partium*, vi. 16, K. iii. 490–2: ἐκ τούτων οὖν ἴσως ἄν τις ὑπονοήσειε μηδὲν ὅλως εἰς τοὐπίσω φέρεσθαι κατὰ τὰ λοιπὰ τρία στόματα τῶν ἀγγείων, ἀλλ' οὐχ ὧδ' ἔχει τἀληθές. ἐν ᾧ γὰρ χρόνῳ συμβαίνει κλείεσθαι τοὺς ὑμένας, ἀναγκαῖον ἐν τούτῳ φθάνειν ἑλκόμενον εἰς τὴν καρδίαν αἷμα καὶ πνεῦμα, καὶ μέν γε κἂν τῷ συστέλλεσθαι, πρὸ τοῦ κλεισθῆναι πάλιν ἀντιπέμπεσθαι κατὰ τὸν τοῦ συγκλείεσθαι χρόνον. ἀλλὰ καὶ κεκλεισμένων ἤδη τῶν ὑμένων ἐνδέχεταί ποτε, τῆς καρδίας σφο-δρότερον κινουμένης, παραρρυῆναί τι μὴ μόνον ἀτμοῦ καὶ πνεύματος, ἀλλὰ καὶ αὐτοῦ τοῦ αἵματος. ὡς γὰρ ἐπὶ τῆς τραχείας ἀρτηρίας ἐπεδείκνυμεν, ἀδύνατον ἦν μηδὲν παρηθεῖσθαί τι τῶν κατα-πινόντων ὑγρῶν, οὕτως ἔχειν χρὴ νομίζειν κἀνταῦθα· τοῦ πλήθους αὐτῶν ἐξευρῆσθαι τῇ φύσει κώλυμα, τοῦ δ' ὅλως μηδὲν παραρρεῖν μηδὲ τοὐλάχιστον ἀδύνατον εὑρεθῆναί τι φυλακτήριον. ἐδείχθη γὰρ οὖν ἡμῖν δι' ἑτέρων ὡς ἐν ἅπασι πάντ' ἐστί, καθάπερ Ἱπποκράτης ἔλεγε, καὶ μετ-έχουσιν αἱ μὲν ἀρτηρίαι λεπτοῦ καὶ καθαροῦ καὶ ἀτμώδους αἵματος, αἱ δὲ φλέβες ὀλίγου καὶ ὁμιχλώ-δους ἀέρος. οὕτω δὲ καὶ διὰ τοῦ στομάχου παραρρεῖν εἰς τὴν γαστέρα τὸ πνεῦμα καταπινόντων τε καὶ εἰσπνεόντων ἐδείκνυτο, καὶ ὅλως μηδὲν εἶναι τῶν ἐν τῷ σώματι καθαρὸν ἀκριβῶς, ἀλλὰ πάντα πάντων μετέχειν· οὐ μὴν ἐξ ἴσου γε, κἂν τούτῳ τὸ μὲν αἵματος ἤ τινος ἄλλης τροφῆς εἶναι, τὸ δὲ πνεύματος ὄργανον. οὕτω τοίνυν καὶ αἱ τῆς καρδίας αὐτῆς κοιλίαι σφύζουσαι μὲν ἀμφότεραι φαίνονται διοιγομένου τοῦ θώρακος, οὐ μὴν ὡσαύτως γε ἐν ἀμφοῖν αἷμα καὶ πνεῦμα περιέχεται· πλεονεκτεῖ γὰρ οὐκ ὀλίγῳ κατὰ μὲν τὴν δεξιὰν ἡ τοῦ αἵματος οὐσία, κατὰ δὲ τὴν ἀριστερὰν ἡ τοῦ πνεύματος.

This doctrine of the leaky valves and leaky epiglottis, which had already been rejected by Erasistratus, is not easy for us to understand. It seems to be based on metaphysical rather than scientific reasoning, and it is tempting to see in it a residue of the doctrine of Anaxagoras who pointed out that from bread and water arose hair, veins, arteries, flesh, muscles, and bones, yet how can hair be made of what is not hair, and flesh of what is not flesh? His solution to this problem was to postulate a great plurality of 'seeds', and an original plurality in a state of the universe in which all things were together, infinite both in quantity and in smallness. Thus he is reported as teaching that 'everything is called that of which it has most in it, though as a matter of fact it has everything in it'.[1] There is of course no difficulty in accounting for the fact that Galen accepted it, since it was one of the most characteristic of the doctrines attributed to Hippocrates, who must have been right. But Galen had to discover some philosophical reasons for adopting it. He therefore looks out for some reasons of a quasi-physiological kind to justify, for example, the minimum degree of aortic insufficiency. The arteries receive much from the heart, but they also give it something, though of course much less than they receive, on account of the aortic valve. Erasistratus thought that the heart received nothing at all from the arteries, except from those in the lungs, the pulmonary veins, but he was wrong. The membranes of this valve are not absolutely tight, since in certain conditions when the animal is subjected to violent extremities, some back-flow is necessary. The heart must be able to attract both blood and *pneuma* from all directions. If the arteries give anything to the heart, they must also be able to return it. It would be quite unreasonable, therefore, to suppose that they could draw matter from all directions, including the heart, but could only return it in all directions but one, i.e. the heart. Moreover, Galen

---

[1] Burnet, *Greek Philosophy*, pp. 79 f. The relevant passages from Anaxagoras are as follows:

Fr. 1 (D–K, vol. 2, 32): ὁμοῦ πάντα χρήματα ἦν ἄπειρα καὶ πλῆθος καὶ σμικρότητα· καὶ γὰρ τὸ σμικρὸν ἄπειρον ἦν. καὶ πάντων ὁμοῦ ἐόντων οὐδὲν ἔνδηλον ἦν ὑπὸ σμικρότητος. πάντα γὰρ ἀήρ τε καὶ αἰθὴρ κατεῖχεν, ἀμφότερα ἄπειρα ἐόντα· ταῦτα γὰρ μέγιστα ἔνεστιν ἐν τοῖς σύμπασι καὶ πλήθει καὶ μεγέθει.

Fr. 10 (D–K, 36 f.): ὁ δὲ Ἀναξαγόρας παλαιὸν εὑρὼν δόγμα, ὅτι οὐδὲν ἐκ τοῦ μηδαμῇ γίνεται, γένεσιν μὲν ἀνῄρει, διάκρισιν δ' εἰσῆγεν ἀντὶ γενέσεως. ἐλήρει γὰρ ἀλλήλοις μὲν μεμίχθαι πάντα, διακρίνεσθαι δ' αὐξανόμενα· καὶ γὰρ ἐν τῇ αὐτῇ γονῇ καὶ τρίχας εἶναι καὶ ὄνυχας καὶ φλέβας καὶ ἀρτηρίας καὶ νεῦρα καὶ ὀστᾶ, καὶ τυγχάνειν μὲν ἀφανῆ διὰ μικρομερείαν, αὐξανόμενα δὲ κατὰ μικρὸν διακρίνεσθαι. πῶς γὰρ ἄν, φησίν, ἐκ μὴ τριχὸς γένοιτο θρίξ, καὶ σὰρξ ἐκ μὴ σαρκός; οὐ μόνον δὲ τῶν σωμάτων, ἀλλὰ καὶ τῶν χρωμάτων ταῦτα κατηγόρει· καὶ γὰρ ἐνεῖναι τῷ λευκῷ τὸ μέλαν καὶ τὸ λευκὸν τῷ μέλανι. τὸ αὐτὸ δὲ ἐπὶ τῶν ῥοπῶν ἐτίθει, τῷ βάρει τὸ κοῦφον σύμμικτον εἶναι δοξάζων καὶ τοῦτο αὖθις ἐκείνῳ.

Cf. the passage quoted from Theophrastus in Simplicius, *In phys.* 27 (D–K, 15): πάντα γὰρ τὰ ὁμοιομερῆ οἷον ὕδωρ ἢ πῦρ ἢ χρυσὸν ἀγένητα μὲν εἶναι καὶ ἄφθαρτα, φαίνεσθαι δὲ γινόμενα καὶ ἀπολλύμενα, συγκρίσει καὶ διακρίσει μόνον, πάντων μὲν ἐν πᾶσιν ἐνόντων, ἑκάστου δὲ κατὰ τὸ ἐπικρατοῦν ἐν αὐτῷ χαρακτηριζομένου. χρυσὸς γὰρ φαίνεται ἐκεῖνο, ἐν ᾧ πολὺ χρύσιον ἐστί, καίτοι πάντων ἐνόντων. λέγει γοῦν Ἀναξαγόρας ὅτι ἐν παντὶ παντὸς μοῖρα ἔνεστι· καὶ ὅτων πλεῖστα ἔνι, ταῦτα ἐνδηλότατα ἓν ἕκαστον ἔστι καὶ ἦν.

adds, this theory is a great improvement on that of Erasistratus, since through that we simply cannot account for the whole body breathing together and all the body fluids running into one another (in the famous words of Hippocrates already quoted above).[1] This can only be explained if we assume that the arteries draw matter from all directions and also return it in all directions. For only in this way can every part be cooled and purged through the different motions of the arteries, and the benefits of their activities be communicated to the whole organism.[2]

[1] See above, p. 80, n. 3.

[2] *De usu pulsuum*, 5, K. v. 166 f. : παρὰ δὲ τῆς καρδίας λαμβάνουσι μὲν πλεῖον, διδόασι δ᾽ ἔλαττον. αἰτία δ᾽ αἱ τῶν ὑμένων ἐπιφύσεις, ὑπὲρ ὧν αὐτάρκως Ἐρασιστράτου διειλεγμένου, περιττὸν ἡμᾶς νῦν γράφειν. ἀλλ᾽ ἐκεῖνος μὲν ἔοικεν ὑπολαμβάνειν, μηδὲν ὅλως εἰς τὴν καρδίαν ἐκ τῶν ἀρτηριῶν μεταλαμβάνεσθαι, πλήν γε διὰ τῶν ἐν πνεύμονι· τὸ δὲ οὐχ οὕτως ἔχει. τάχα μὲν γὰρ καὶ τὰ κατ᾽ αὐτὸν τὸν τῆς φύσεως νόμον διοικουμένου τοῦ ζῴου μεταλαμβάνεταί τι μικρόν. οὐχ οὕτως γάρ μοι δοκοῦσιν ἀκριβῶς ἀποφράττειν τὸ στόμα τῆς μεγάλης ἀρτηρίας οἱ ὑμένες, ὡς μηδὲν ἐξ αὐτῆς εἰς τὴν καρδίαν παλινδρομεῖν· εἰ δὲ μή, ἀλλά τοί γε, βιαίας τινὸς περιστάσεως καταλαβούσης τὸ ζῷον, ἀναγκαῖον οὕτως γίνεσθαι . . . εἰ μὲν γάρ τι καὶ τῇ καρδίᾳ μεταδιδόασιν αἱ ἀρτηρίαι παντα-χόθεν ἂν οὕτως ἕλκοιέν τε καὶ αὖθις ἀντιπέμποιεν· εἰ δὲ μή, πανταχόθεν μὲν ἕλξουσιν, ἐπιπέμψουσιν δὲ καί, πλὴν εἰς τὴν καρδίαν, πανταχόσε. καί μοι δοκεῖ πολλῷ βέλτιον εἶναι τοῦτο τὸ δόγμα τῶν Ἐρασιστρατείων ὑποθέσεων· οὐδὲ γὰρ συμπνοῦν οὐδὲ σύρρουν εἶναι τὸ σῶμα δυνατὸν ἑαυτῷ, τῶν ἀρτηριῶν ἑλκουσῶν μὲν πανταχόθεν, μὴ ἐκπεμπουσῶν δὲ πανταχόσε. καὶ μὲν δὴ τὸ τῆς ἐνερ-γείας αὐτῶν χρηστὸν ὧδ᾽ ἂν μᾶλλον εἰς ἅπαν ἐκταθείη τὸ ζῷον. οὕτω γὰρ ἅπαν μόνον ἀναψύχεσθαί τε καὶ καθαίρεσθαι δυνήσεται, ταῖς τῶν ἀρτηριῶν διαφόροις κινήσεσι ἐπιστατούμενον.

Note added in Proof

Readers may perhaps find it difficult to follow the account given in this chapter of Dr. R. E. Siegel's view on Galen's conception of the blood-movements in the foetus *in utero*. I had hoped to avoid this obscurity, to say nothing of the danger of misrepresenting them, by the inclusion of his own diagram contained in his book *Galen's System of Physiology and Medicine* (Karger, Basle and New York 1968). I therefore applied for permission to repro-duce it. But the conditions laid down by Dr. Siegel for this reproduction included an assurance that it 'will not be attached to a text which supports the opposite opinion' to those expressed by himself on Galen's assumption of the pulmonary transit, and were of course impossible to accept.

7 · GALEN'S PULSE-LORE

Two fundamental assumptions which underlie all Galen's thinking on the pulse must constantly be remembered. The first of these is that, unlike Erasistratus and Rufus, he insists that the expansion and contraction of both heart and arteries is simultaneous. At the moment of the ventricles' systole, the arteries too are contracted, and at the moment of diastole expanded. And the second is the logical consequence of the first, namely that when the arteries are contracting the aortic valve is open, and that when they are expanding it is closed. This rather paradoxical situation accounts for the slight degree of aortic regurgitation that he postulates, but it leaves him with the paradoxical situation that the heart is compelled to force what blood there is in the left ventricle through the aorta when it is at its narrowest, and this blood is only prevented at the immediately following diastole from being forced back into the heart by the closure of that valve. No wonder, then, that he was compelled as we saw in the last chapter, to postulate other forces than the left ventricle's contraction to supply the peripheral tissues with the *pneuma*-like or pneumaticized type of blood. The chief function of the arteries was to act as a kind of bellows, drawing in air at diastole and expelling it, together with the 'waste products' of 'combustion' at systole, moreover, the arteries, unlike the veins, were essentially elastic. Both movements, systole as well as diastole, were variable quantities determined ultimately by physiological needs. Arterial elasticity as conceived by Galen must not, however, be interpreted in modern terms. It was something rather different implying a double process. For diastole and systole are two separate and independent movements; systole, unlike expiration, which is a remission or relaxation of the thorax, a cessation of its active contraction, corresponds rather to the process of blowing, which is an active expulsion of air, as opposed to the merely passive process of expiration. It is not just the return of the artery to its normal condition after the activity of expansion.[1] For

---

[1] *De usu pulsuum*, 7, K. v. 172 f.: ἐφεξῆς ἂν εἴη σκεπτέον, εἰ, ὥσπερ ἡ ἐκπνοὴ ἄνεσίς ἐστι καὶ οἷον ἀνάπαυσις τῆς ἐνεργείας τοῦ θώρακος, ἡ ἐκφύσησις δὲ ἐνέργεια, καὶ διὰ τοῦτο τὸ μᾶλλόν τε καὶ ἧττον ἔχει, τῆς ἐκπνοῆς οὐκ ἐχούσης, οὕτως καὶ ἡ συστολὴ μὲν ἐν τοῖς σφυγμοῖς ἔκλυσις τῆς ἐνεργείας ἐστὶ τῶν ἀρτηριῶν, ἕτερον δέ τι ταύτῃ παρακείμενον ἀνάλογος ταῖς ἐκφυσήσεσιν ἡ ἐνέργεια. καί μοι δοκεῖ καὶ τοῦτο παντὸς μᾶλλον ἀληθὲς εἶναι.

though the artery after the distention of diastole does return to its natural or neutral size, after a momentary pause it contracts to smaller than its 'natural' size, returning then back again to normal before starting once more to expand. And the size and speed of the two movements of expansion and contraction have no direct relation to one another. These are determined by two different physiological needs, namely the need for cooling, which determines the character of the motion of diastole, and the need for the expulsion of sooty waste products, which determines the character of systole. These two needs vary considerably under different conditions: for example, when a person is sleeping after a heavy meal, diastole is smaller and slower—terms the exact meaning of which we shall examine further presently—while systole is both faster and its contraction greater, the coats of the arteries approaching more closely to each other.[1]

In studying the pulse and the causes of its variations or varieties, there are three main factors which have to be considered, namely the physiological need, the pulsative power, due ultimately to the vital spirit, and the state of the organs of pulsation, the heart and the arteries.[2] The physiological need is double, corresponding to the two movements of diastole and systole. The need for diastole is determined by the necessity of taking in air from the atmosphere, which, as we have seen, performs the double function of cooling and maintaining at its proper temperature the innate heat, and generating, in conjunction with the arterial blood, the vital and the psychic spirit or *pneuma*. The need for systole is the immediate evacuation of sooty superfluities, by-products or 'waste products' resulting from the 'combustion' of the humours by the innate heat.[3] The need for diastole is determined by two main factors, the increase of the bodily heat and the expenditure of the psychic spirit, that of systole by the quantity of 'waste products' generated. The pulsative power or faculty may be either strong or weak in varying degrees. The third factor, the state of the organs, namely the arteries, though they derive their power of pulsation from the heart, is determined by the hardness or softness of their coats.[4] Other things being equal, a soft coat

---

[1] De usu pulsuum, 7, K. v. 173 f.: ἐναργῶς δὲ μαρτύρια πάμπολλα τῶν ἐν τοῖς σφυγμοῖς φαινομένων, οἷον εὐθέως τὰ κατὰ τοὺς ὕπνους ἐπὶ τῶν ἐδηδοκότων δαψιλῶς. ἐν τούτοις γὰρ ἐκλύεται μὲν ἡ διαστολὴ μικροτέρα τε ἅμα καὶ βραδυτέρα γινομένη, ἐπιτείνεται δὲ κατ' ἄμφω ἡ συστολή, καὶ γὰρ ὠκυτέρα ἢ πρόσθεν καὶ ἐπὶ πλέον εἴσω κατιοῦσα φαίνεται.

[2] De causis pulsuum, i. 1, K. ix. 1: τῶν τοὺς σφυγμοὺς τρεπόντων αἰτίων, τὰ μὲν τῆς γενέσεως αὐτῶν ἐστιν αἴτια, τὰ δὲ τῆς ἀλλοιώσεως μόνον· τῆς γενέσεως μὲν ἥ τε χρεία δι' ἣν γίγνονται, καὶ ἡ δύναμις ὑφ' ἧς, καὶ τὰ ὄργανα δι' ὧν διατείνονται.

[3] Ibid., 3, K. ix. 5: περὶ δὲ τῆς χρείας αὐτῶν ἀναμνησθῆναι χρὴ τῶν ἐν ἑτέροις ἀποδεδειγμένων, ὅτι φυλακῆς ἕνεκα τῆς καθ' ὅλον τὸ σῶμα θερμασίας γεγόνασιν ἐμψύχοντές τε ταύτην καὶ εἴ τι λιγνυῶδες ἐκ τῆς τῶν χυμῶν συγκαύσεως ὑποτρέφοιτο, τοῦτ' εὐθέως ἀποκρίνοντες. εἴρηται δ' ἐν ἐκείνοις ὡς καὶ τῇ γεννήσει τοῦ ψυχικοῦ πνεύματος συντελοῦσι.

[4] Ibid., 4, K. 7: τῆς μὲν δὴ δυνάμεως αἱ διαφοραὶ ῥώμη τε καὶ ἀρρωστία ἐστί, τῆς δ' ἐμφύτου θερμασίας ἐκπύρωσίς τε καὶ κατάψυξις, τοῦ δὲ τῶν ἀρτηριῶν χιτῶνος σκληρότης τε καὶ μαλακότης.

makes for a 'large' pulse, because a soft coat is more easily dilated than a hard one.

Variations arising in the need for the pulse are met by changes in its size, speed, and frequency. The size of the pulse is measured by the quantity of dilation and contraction, the speed by the time taken by each of the two movements of the single beat, and the frequency by the time interval between successive beats, which is determined largely by the length of the intervals between the time of quiescence and their variations. Thus, should the biological need of the organism be increased by excess of heat or of 'waste products',[1] the natural reaction will be for the pulse to become larger, stronger, and more frequent, provided that a sufficient margin of pulsative power is available, and that the coats of the arteries are not hard. For if there be a lack of power, or if the arteries be hard, the pulse can become neither large nor quick, since under these conditions the artery cannot expand as far as it should, nor can it, through lack of power, make its diastole quick.[2] The first reaction on an increase in heat is to enlarge the diastole of the arteries to its maximum. If this is not sufficient to meet the need for cooling, an increase in the pace of diastole helps to fulfil the need, but if it is even greater, as it may well become in acute fever, an increase in frequency occurs through the shortening of the intervals of quiescence, which indeed may seem to disappear altogether, leaving the two movements apparently continuous with one another.[3] A reverse process takes place when the innate heat diminishes. This makes the pulse small, slow, and rare or infrequent.[4] The terms large, small, quick, slow, frequent, and rare are all relative terms. The standard with reference to which they are defined is the

---

[1] Ibid., K. 6–7: καὶ τοίνυν ἐπειδὰν μὲν τὴν ψύχουσαν οὐσίαν ἕλκῃ διαστέλλεται τὸ σῶμα τῶν ἀρτηριῶν, ἐπειδὰν δὲ τὸ αἰθαλῶδες ἐκκρίνῃ, συστέλλεται. πλεονεκτεῖ δὲ ποτὲ μὲν ἡ τοῦ διαστέλλεσθαι, ποτὲ δὲ ἡ τοῦ συστέλλεσθαι χρεία.

[2] Ibid., 5, K. 9: πλείονος θερμασίας ἠθροισμένης ἐν τῷ σώματι μείζονος μὲν χρῄζειν ἀνάγκη τὸ ζῷον τῆς ἀναπνοῆς μειζόνων δὲ καὶ σφυγμῶν. ᾧ δὲ λόγῳ μειζόνων τούτῳ καὶ θαττόνων τε καὶ πυκνοτέρων . . . χρῄζει γάρ, ἵνα τοιοῦτοι γενηθῶσι, δυνάμεως μὲν ἐρρωμένης, ὀργάνων δὲ μαλακῶν· εἰ γὰρ ἀσθενὴς ἡ δύναμις ἢ σκληρὸν ᾖ τὸ ὄργανον, οὔτε μεγάλους αὐτοὺς οὔτε ταχεῖς ἐνδέχεται γενέσθαι, τοῦ μὲν ὀργάνου διὰ σκληρότητα δυσπειθοῦς γινομένου τῇ κινούσῃ δυνάμει, τῆς δυνάμεως δ' αὐτῆς δι' ἀρρωστίαν ἀδυνατούσης ἐξαίρειν τὰς ἀρτηρίας εἰς ὅσον προσήκει.

[3] Ibid., 5, 11–12: ἂν γοῦν αὐξηθῇ μὲν ἡ θερμασία μόνη, φυλάττοιντο δ' ἥ τε δύναμις καὶ οἱ χιτῶνες τῶν ἀρτηριῶν ἄτρεπτοι, μείζους τε καὶ θάττους ἐξ ἀνάγκης οἱ σφυγμοὶ γενήσονται. καὶ συναυξηθήσονταί γε τῷ πλήθει τῆς θερμασίας ἄχρι περ ἂν ἐπὶ τὴν μεγίστην ἀφίκωνται διαστολήν. τάχιστοι δὲ οὐδὲ νῦν οὐδέ ποτε φανοῦνται πρὶν τὴν θερμασίαν ὑπὲρ τὴν μεγίστην αὐξηθῆναι διαστολήν. τότε δ' ὑπὲρ τὴν μεγίστην αὔξεται διαστολήν, ὅταν ἐνδεῶς ὑπ' αὐτῆς ἀναψύχηται. τὸ τοίνυν λεῖπον ἐπανισοῖ τηνικαῦτα τῷ τάχει τῆς κινήσεως, καὶ οὕτως οἱ σφυγμοὶ τάχιστοι γίνονται. ἀρκεῖ δ' οὐδὲ ταῦτα τῇ μεγάλως ἐκπυρωθείσῃ, ἀλλ' ὃν ἡσύχασε πρότερον χρόνον μεταξὺ τῶν κινήσεων, ἤδη καὶ τοῦτον συντέμνει. πολλάκις δ' οὕτως βραχὺν ἀπέφηνεν, ὡς συνεχεῖς ἀλλήλαις δοκεῖν τὰς κινήσεις μηδαμῇ σχιζομένας ἡσυχία . . . τριῶν γὰρ ὄντων τρόπων ἐπικουρίας ἐν ἁπάσαις ὑπερβολαῖς, πᾶσιν ὁμοῦ χρῆται . . . τούτων δὲ τὸ μὲν πρῶτον μεγίστους ποιεῖ τοὺς σφυγμούς, τὸ δὲ δεύτερον ταχίστους, τὸ δὲ τρίτον πυκνοτάτους.

[4] Ibid., 6, 12: εἴη δ' ἄν, οἶμαι, δῆλον ἤδη καὶ περὶ τῶν ἐν ταῖς ἐνδείαις τῆς ἐμφύτου θερμασίας ἑπομένων σφυγμῶν . . . οἰκεῖοι δ' εἰσὶν μάλιστα μὲν ὅ τε μικρὸς καὶ βραδὺς ἤδη δὲ καὶ ὁ ἀραιός.

moderate pulse of the man with the most perfect constitution in his most normal undisturbed condition.[1] If, for any reason, he became cold, the first visible change in his pulse to appear would be rareness: it would become less frequent, the next symptom to make its appearance would be slowness, and the third, smallness. But so long as the power remained strong, the pulse could not become either very slow or very small, but it could become very infrequent, and would of course be both slower and smaller than the normal.[2]

Galen now proceeds in a characteristic manner to work out the permutations and combinations of excess or deficiency of these three factors, need, pulsative power, and arterial elasticity, in the details of which we are not compelled to follow him; but there is one point which deserves notice. A large deficiency in power, combined with a large increase in biological need, as for example in the heat generated in a high fever, produces a very characteristic pulse, small and slow, but very frequent,[3] which we shall meet again in the terminal stages of many diseases.[4]

Galen tells us that he was deeply fascinated by the phenomenon of the pulse. Certainly, he devoted to this rather narrow subject quite a disproportionate volume of his writings—four treatises of four books each, a synopsis of his own works on the pulse, an essay on the use of the pulse, as well as a short introductory treatise for beginners.[5] He defines the pulse as an expansion and contraction of the arteries, the power of effecting which is communicated to their coats by the heart. The artery being a three-dimensional vessel, its expansion must also take place in three dimensions, each contraction also being measured in the dimensions of length, breadth, and height, and each of these dimensions has three degrees, large, small, and medium or moderate, only the medium degree being strictly speaking according to nature, whereas the others are contrary to nature in respect of their excess or deficiency.[6] A single beat or

---

[1] De causis pulsuum, i. 7, K. ix. 23: οἱ ἂν ἄριστα τῆς κατασκευῆς τοῦ σώματος ἔχωσιν, οὔτε βραδεῖς οὔτ' ὠκεῖς ἀλλὰ συμμέτρους ὑπάρχειν φύσει τοὺς σφυγμούς. τοῖς δ' αὐτοῖς τούτοις οὐδὲ μεγάλους οὐδὲ μικροὺς ἀλλὰ τοὺς μέσους ἀμφοῖν, τοὺς συμμέτρους, οὐδὲ πυκνοὺς ἢ ἀραιοὺς ἀλλὰ καὶ τοὺς ἐν τούτῳ γένει συμμέτρους.

[2] Ibid., 24–5: εἰ μέντοι ψυχρότερος ἑαυτοῦ ὁ τοιοῦτος ἄνθρωπος γένοιτο, πρώτη μὲν ἡ ἀραιότης ἐναργῶς φαίνεται, δεύτερα δ' ἡ βραδυτής, τρίτη δ' ἡ μικρότης . . . ἂν μέντοι πλείων ἡ ψῦξις γένηται, καὶ διὰ τοῦτο τὰ τῆς χρείας ἱκανῶς ἐκλυθῇ, συνεκλυθήσεται μὲν οὕτως καὶ τὸ τάχος τῆς κινήσεως, μικροτέρα δ' εὐθὺς ἔσται καὶ ἡ διαστολή, ἐπὶ πλεῖστον δὲ προϊούσης τῆς ψύξεως, ἀραιοτάτους μέν, οὐ μὴν καὶ βραδυτάτους τε καὶ μικροτάτους ἀνάγκη γενέσθαι τοὺς σφυγμούς, ἀλλ' ἀρκεῖ βραδυτέρους ἀεὶ καὶ μικροτέρους τῶν κατὰ φύσιν γίνεσθαι· τελέως γὰρ βραδεῖς ἢ μικροὶ τῆς δυνάμεως ἐρρωμένης οὐκ ἄν ποτε γένοιντο.

[3] Ibid., 8, 26: εἰ μὲν ἐπὶ πλέον ὑπ' ἀμφοτέρων τῶν αἰτίων δυναστεύοιτο ἥ τε δύναμις ἱκανῶς ἄρρωστος εἴη καὶ τὸ θερμὸν πυρῶδες, μικροὶ καὶ βραδεῖς οἱ σφυγμοὶ καὶ πυκνότατοι γίνονται.

[4] See below, p. 414.

[5] De dignoscendis pulsibus, i. 1, K. viii. 770: ἐγὼ μέν γε ἀφ' οὗ τὸ πρῶτον εἰς ἰατροὺς φοιτᾶν ἠρξάμην παῖς ἔτι ὤν, θαυμαστήν τινα ἐπιθυμίαν ἔσχον τῆς περὶ τοὺς σφυγμοὺς τέχνης.

[6] De pulsibus ad tirones, 2, K. viii. 455: ἀπτομένῳ δέ σοι, φανεῖται διαστελλομένη κατὰ πᾶσαν διάστασιν ἡ ἀρτηρία. τρεῖς δ' εἰσὶ διαστάσεις παντὸς τοῦ σώματος, εἰς μῆκος, βάθος καὶ πλάτος.

movement, be it of contraction or expansion, must therefore be of one of these three degrees in each of the three dimensions, it must be either long, medium, or short, and either broad, medium, or narrow, and either high, medium, or low. This means that in the merely quantitative category of size, there are twenty-seven varieties of each of the two movements in each single beat,[1] and only one of these is perfectly in accordance with nature, in respect of length, breadth, and height, assuming of course that the movement of expansion, diastole, is equal to the movement of contraction or systole. Moreover, in the practical discernment of these twenty-seven sizes of pulse, no end of complications may arise, owing to the fact that the size of the movement in each of the three dimensions may be altered or concealed by the conditions of the tissues surrounding the artery, such as the fatness or thinness of the patient, or the wrinkled condition of the skin.

But this is only the beginning, for we have only been considering the beat's spacial dimensions. Variations in its many different qualities have now to be considered, as well as variations in the relations of systole to diastole in the single beat. The variations of the pulse may be considered under five different classes (γένη), four of which are concerned with the actual nature of the pulse itself: its size, which we have just described; its strength or force (σφοδρότης or τόνος); its speed, which is divided into two quite different categories, the speed of each single movement of diastole and/or systole, which makes it quick (ταχύς) or slow (βραδύς), and the speed or frequency of a series of pulses, in accordance with which it is frequent (πυκνός) or rare (ἀραιός). The fifth category of hardness or softness belongs, as we have already noted, not to the pulse itself, but to the condition of the coats of the arteries which makes the pulse either hard (σκληρός) or soft (μαλακός).

Pulsation consists of a double movement, dilation and contraction, which we will follow Galen in calling diastole and systole, and between each of these movements there is a pause which can be perceived by the touch of the expert, as well as being logically proved necessary.[2] Moreover,

ἀλλ' ἐν τῷ κατὰ φύσιν ἔχειν τὸ ζῷον συμμέτρως πάνυ διαστελλομένην εὑρήσεις τὴν ἀρτηρίαν· ἐν δὲ τῷ παρὰ φύσιν ἔχειν ἔστιν ὅπῃ τὸ μὲν ἐλλείπει, τὸ δ' ὑπερβάλλει καθ' ἡντιναοῦν διάστασιν. ἐν τούτῳ χρὴ μεμνημένον σε, οἷος ἦν ὁ κατὰ φύσιν σφυγμός, καὶ εἰ μὲν τῷ πλάτει μείζων ὁ παρὰ φύσιν εὑρίσκοιτο, πλατὴν καλεῖν, εἰ δὲ τῷ μήκει μακρόν, εἰ δὲ τῷ βάθει ὑψηλόν, καὶ τοὺς ἐναντίους αὐτοῖς, τοὺς ἐλάττους τοῦ κατὰ φύσιν ὀνομάζειν ἀνάλογον, στενὸν καὶ βραχὺν καὶ ταπεινόν. τῶν δὲ ἐν πάσαις ταῖς διαστάσεσιν ὁμοίως εἰς τὸ παρὰ φύσιν τρεπομένων, ὁ μὲν πάντῃ μειωθεὶς μικρός, ὁ δὲ πάντῃ αὐξηθεὶς μέγας ὀνομάζεται.

[1] Synopsis de pulsibus, 3, K. ix. 439: οὕτω δὴ τούτων ἑπτὰ καὶ εἴκοσι σφυγμῶν ὄντων κατὰ τὸ ποσὸν ἐν ταῖς τρισὶν ἅμα διαστάσεσιν.

[2] De diff. puls. i. 3, K. viii. 500: καὶ ταύτης τῆς διπλῆς κινήσεως ὀνομαζομένης σφυγμοῦ διττὰς ἀναγκαῖον αὐτῇ συμπίπτειν ἠρεμίας ἐφ' ἑκατέρᾳ· ἑτέραν μὲν ἐπὶ τῷ διασταλῆναι πρὸ τοῦ συστέλλεσθαι, δευτέραν δὲ ἐπὶ τῷ συσταλῆναι πρὸ τοῦ διαστέλλεσθαι, καὶ ταύτας τὰς δύο ἡσυχίας ἥ τε τῶν γεγυμνασμένων ἁφὴ γνωρίζει καὶ ὁ λόγος οὐδὲν ἧττον ἀποδείκνυσι. πρὶν γὰρ καταπαῦσαι τὴν προτέραν κίνησιν οὐκ ἂν ὑπάρξαιτο τῆς ἐναντίας ἡ ἀρτηρία. ἀλλὰ μὴν τὸ καταπαῦσαι στῆναί τε καὶ ἡσυχάσαι ἐστίν. ὥστε ἡσυχία μεταξύ ἐστι τῶν κινήσεων.

the two movements of diastole and systole may take place at different speeds, they may be quick, slow, or moderate, the moderate being the 'natural' rate.[1] And these classes are quite independent of the time relation of each beat to its predecessor or successors. And there are three kinds of motion the speed of which must be considered in accordance with the dimension in which it is taking place, each of which may be quick, moderate, or slow. This would make twenty-seven varieties with respect to the speed of each of the two movements of the single beat, only three of which would be perfectly in accordance with nature, and only three perfectly even, i.e. the same in each of the three dimensions.[2]

There is a third order of difference applicable to the single beat. It may be strong, weak, or faint, or again moderate, but the middle term has no technical name.[3] Finally there is still another category of differences, for which most physicians, particularly the younger ones, use the terms *full* and *empty*, the middle term again having no special name. Galen repudiates this terminology and prefers to use the words *hard* and *soft*, as describing more accurately the condition of the arteries perceived, since you cannot *feel* whether the artery is full or empty.[4]

The fourfold division of the interval between two beats of the pulse, which comprises the interval between the moment when the diastole of the artery can first be felt and that when diastole again becomes perceptible, was, as we have had reason to note, not accepted by many schools of contemporary medicine. Many of Galen's contemporaries denied the possibility that the movement of systole could be felt at all,[5] let alone the intervals of rest between the movements of diastole and systole. Though this somewhat simplified the fourfold Galenian system, it still left considerable scope for Herophilian complexities of rhythm,

---

[1] *De diff. puls.* i. 4, K. viii. 502: ἀνάγκη γὰρ ταύτην (κίνησιν) ἢ σύμμετρόν τε καὶ κατὰ φύσιν ὑπάρχειν, ἢ ὠκυτέραν πως ἢ βραδυτέραν γεγονέναι, ὡς εἶναι κατὰ τοῦτο τὸ γένος τρεῖς τὰς πάσας διαφορὰς σφυγμῶν, ταχὺν μὲν τὸν ἐν ὀλίγῳ χρόνῳ κινουμένης τῆς ἀρτηρίας γενόμενον, βραδὺν δὲ τὸν ἐν πολλῷ, σύμμετρον δὲ τὸν ἐν συμμέτρῳ.

[2] Ibid., 15, 532–3: οὕτω δὲ καὶ εἰ τρεῖς ὑποθέμενος διαφερούσας ἀλλήλων κινήσεις, καθ' ἑκάστην αὐτῶν τοὺς τρεῖς σφυγμοὺς ὑπαλλάττων συμπλέκοις ἑπτὰ μὲν καὶ εἴκοσι ἔσται τὰ πάντα σχήματα, τρία δ' ἐξ αὐτῶν εἰς ὁμαλότητα μεταπεσεῖν ἀναγκαῖον.

[3] Ibid., 5, 508: νυνὶ δὲ μεταβάντες ἐπὶ τὸ τρίτον γένος τῶν σφυγμῶν, τὸ κατὰ τὸν τόνον, εἴπωμεν καὶ τὰς τούτου διαφοράς. εἰσὶ δὲ τρεῖς, ὁ μέν τις εὔρωστος τῷ τόνῳ, καλεῖται δὲ σφοδρός, ὁ δέ τις ἄρρωστος, ὃν ἀμυδρὸν ὀνομάζουσι, τοῦ μέσου δ' αὐτῶν οὐκ ἔστιν ἴδιον ὄνομα.

[4] Ibid.: τὸ δὲ τέταρτον τῶν γενῶν τὸ κατὰ τὸ σῶμα τῆς ἀρτηρίας συνιστάμενον, εἰς τρεῖς τέμνεται καὶ αὐτὸ διαφοράς, καὶ καλεῖται παρὰ μὲν τοῖς πλείστοις τῶν ἰατρῶν, καὶ μάλιστα τοῖς νεωτέροις, τῷ τοῦ πλήρους ὀνόματι καὶ τῷ τοῦ κενοῦ. τὸ γὰρ μέσον ἀμφοῖν ἀνώνυμον κἀνταῦθα. παρ' ἡμῖν δ' οὐχ οὕτως, ἀλλ' ὁ μὲν ἕτερος αὐτῶν σκληρός, ὁ δ' ἕτερος μαλακὸς ὀνομάζεται, καὶ δηλοῦσιν ἀμφότεροι τῆς ἀρτηρίας τὴν σύστασιν. Cf. *Synopsis de pulsibus*, 4, K. ix. 441–2: τὸ γὰρ ἐγκεχυμένον αὐταῖς οὔθ' ὁπόσον ἐστίν, οὔθ' ὁποῖον αἰσθήσει διαγνῶναι δυνατόν.

[5] *De diff. puls.* i. 6, K. viii. 509–10: αἱ δ' ἄλλαι διαφοραὶ τῶν σφυγμῶν, τοῖς μὲν μηδ' ὅλως αἰσθάνεσθαι λέγουσι τῆς συστολῆς, ἔν τε τῷ χρόνῳ συνίστανται τῶν διαλειμμάτων, οὕτω γὰρ ὀνομάζουσι τὸν μεταξὺ χρόνον τῶν αἰσθητῶν κινήσεων, καὶ προσέτι τῷ λόγῳ τοῦ τε τῆς κινήσεως αὐτῆς χρόνου καὶ τοῦ τῆς ἡσυχίας.

since there could be varying time intervals between the beat (πληγή) which is what they called the diastole not the systole, and the subsequent 'interval', which had to be compared in their respective durations.[1] These complexities were, as we shall see, greatly increased by Galen's arrangement with its four time intervals, whose durations had to be measured and compared. Galen maintains that an accurate knowledge of the durations of these four intervals is useful to the physician, and insists that the time taken by diastole and that taken by systole, as well as the intervals between them, can actually be perceived by the touch, but that the interval of rest between the end of systole and the beginning of the next diastole cannot be measured quite so accurately. A knowledge of the proper natural sizes of these intervals and the proportions between them is essential, as well as a knowledge of the way in which they are altered by diseases. This is a matter which can only be acquired by long experience.[2]

Coming now to the time pattern, Galen carefully distinguishes between that of the single beat, which constitutes the rhythm, and that of the succession of beats. In each of these there is a possibility of regularity and several kinds of irregularity. To take first the single beat: the times taken by the movements of diastole and systole may or may not be equal. One may take many times as long as the other,[3] and each may therefore have a different relation to the two periods of rest. A perfectly even pulse would be one in which each of the four periods was equal, though the interval between the end of diastole and the beginning of systole cannot be measured accurately by touch. If we assume that each movement can be divided into three categories, fast, moderate, and slow, there are, as we have seen, another twenty-seven varieties of pulse, not taking into account the varying sizes of these four intervals, and of these only three

[1] Ibid., 510–11 : ὥστε εἶναι δύο χρόνων διάγνωσιν ἐν τῇ τοῦ σφυγμοῦ συμπληρώσει, προτέρου μὲν τοῦ τῆς κινήσεως, ἣν καὶ πληγὴν καὶ διαστολὴν ὀνομάζουσι, δευτέρου δὲ τῆς ἡσυχίας, ἣν καὶ διάλειμμα καὶ συστολὴν καλοῦσιν, γίγνεσθαι δὲ κατὰ μὲν τὸ τοῦ προτέρου χρόνου ποσόν, ἢ ταχὺν ἢ βραδύν, ἢ τὸν μέσον αὐτῶν σφυγμόν, κατὰ δὲ τοῦ δευτέρου πυκνόν, ἢ ἀραιόν, ἢ τὸν μέσον αὐτῶν, ὥστ' εἶναι ταχὺν μὲν σφυγμὸν τὸν ἐν ὀλίγῳ χρόνῳ τῆς ἀρτηρίας διαστελλομένης γιγνόμενον, πυκνὸν δὲ τὸν δι' ὀλίγου, καὶ βραδὺν μὲν τὸν ἐν πολλῷ χρόνῳ τῆς ἀρτηρίας διαστελλομένης γιγνόμενον, ἀραιὸν δὲ τὸν διὰ πολλοῦ.

[2] Ibid., 7, 514: ἔστι δὲ δηλονότι χρήσιμον ἰατρῷ τὸ ὑπὸ τὴν αἴσθησιν ἐρχόμενον· ὥστε καὶ χρόνον διαστολῆς ἢ συστολῆς τὸν αἰσθητὸν ἀναγκαῖον γνωρίζειν αὐτῷ. τὴν μὲν οὖν ἠρεμίαν, τὴν ἄνω καλουμένην, τὴν ἐπὶ τῇ διαστολῇ πρὸ τῆς συστολῆς, ἀκριβῶς δυνατὸν ἡλίκη τίς ἐστι γνῶναι διὰ τῆς ἁφῆς, τὴν κάτω δὲ οὐκ ἔτι ἀκριβῶς, διὰ τὸ προσλαμβάνειν ἑκατέρωθεν μόρια, κατὰ μὲν τὴν ἀρχὴν τὸ τῆς συστολῆς πέρας, κατὰ δὲ τὴν τελευτὴν τὰ πρῶτα τῆς διαστολῆς. μεμνῆσθαι δὲ χρὴ τῶν χρόνων τούτων τό τε κατὰ φύσιν ἑκάστου μέγεθος καὶ τὸν πρὸς ἀλλήλους λόγον, καὶ γνωρίζειν δύνασθαι πόσον ἐν τῷ νοσεῖν ἀλλοιοῦνται, καὶ τί δηλοῦν ἑκάστη τροπὴ πέφυκεν, ὃ τῇ τε τῆς αἰτίας εὑρέσει καὶ τῇ μακρᾷ πείρᾳ λαμβάνεται.

[3] Ibid., 8, 516: ἁπάντων δὲ τῶν ῥυθμῶν οἱ μὲν ἐν ἴσῳ λόγῳ συνίστανται, οἱ δ' ἐν ἀνίσῳ· ἐν ἴσῳ μέν, ὅταν ὁ τῆς διαστολῆς χρόνος ἴσος ὑπάρχῃ τῷ τῆς συστολῆς· ἐν ἀνίσῳ δέ, ὅταν θάτερος αὐτῶν ὑπερέχῃ. γίνεται δὲ τοῦτο ποτὲ μὲν ἐν ῥηταῖς, ποτὲ δὲ ἐν ἀρρήτοις ταῖς ὑπεροχαῖς· καὶ ἐν ῥηταῖς μὲν διχῶς, ἢ ὡς ἐν πολλαπλασίῳ λόγῳ, ἢ ὡς ἀριθμοῦ πρὸς ἀριθμόν, ὅσπερ καὶ ἐπιμόριος ὀνομάζεται.

are even, the rest displaying different kinds of unevenness.[1] We must distinguish evenness and unevenness from regularity and irregularity: the latter pair of terms can only be applied to a series of pulse beats, whereas the former can be applied, not only to temporal sequence, but also to differences in the qualitative characters of the pulse, such as size, speed, strength, etc.[2] Moreover the rhythm, the pattern of the single beat, changes naturally (κατὰ φύσιν) not only with age, but with seasons and with climate.

Passing now to regularity (ὁμαλότης) and irregularity (ἀνωμαλία) which apply to the series of beats, these terms can be used to describe not only the time-intervals between them, but also their qualities. To take the time-interval first: if this is maintained constant between a series of beats, then the succession is regular (τεταγμένος); if the intervals differ, then it is irregular (ἄτακτος). But there are different kinds of regularity. Every third or fourth beat might entail a longer interval between itself and its successor, and even in a series, though each interval was different, there might be a repetition of a pattern. Such a series would not be simply regular or simply irregular, but regular κατά τι.[3] This type of regularity is compared by Galen to the apparent motion of the planets in the sky with its annual repetition.[4] In the same way, there can be a regular pattern of the strength of the beats, e.g. each fourth beat might be stronger than the preceding three.[5]

With the details of the possible permutations and combinations of the differences of the pulse already described—and there are many more—we need not concern ourselves. The important thing is that Galen thought that he could perceive these differences by touch, or by what we may perhaps call immediate inference, and that a complete knowledge of

---

[1] See the passage quoted above, p. 401, n. 1.

[2] De diff. puls. i. 9, K. viii. 517–18: τὸ μὲν ἕτερον ἐν ᾧ τήν τε ὁμαλότητα καὶ τὴν ἀνωμαλίαν ἐπισκοπούμεθα, τὸ δ' ἕτερον ἐν ᾧ τάξιν τε καὶ ἀταξίαν. ὁμαλότης μὲν οὖν καὶ ἀνωμαλία καθ' ἕνα τε σφυγμὸν καὶ περὶ πλείονας γίνεται. τάξις δὲ καὶ ἀταξία περὶ πλείονας μόνον . . . ὁ μὲν γὰρ ἁπλῶς ὁμαλὸς οὔτε μέγεθος οὔτε τάχος οὔτ' ἄλλο οὐδὲν ἄνισον ἔχει. ὁ δὲ καθ' ἓν ὁτιοῦν ἅμα τῇ ἐκείνου προσηγορίᾳ λέγεσθαι βούλεται, κατὰ μέγεθος ὁμαλός, κατὰ τάχος, κατὰ σφοδρότητα, καθ' ἓν ὁτιοῦν ἄλλο.

[3] Ibid., 9, 521: ἔσθ' ὅτε γὰρ τρεῖς ἢ τέτταρες περίοδοι ἀλλήλαις ἄνισοι γενόμεναι τὰς ἑξῆς ἴσας ἀνάλογον ἴσχουσιν. ὥστ' εἰ τύχοι τὴν μὲν τετάρτην τῇ πρώτῃ, τὴν δὲ πέμπτην τῇ δευτέρᾳ, τὴν δ' ἕκτην τῇ τρίτῃ κατὰ πᾶν ἐξισοῦσθαι, τοιοῦτον τὸν σφυγμὸν εἰώθαμεν τεταγμένον κατὰ περίοδον καλεῖν, μέσον ὄντα τῶν ἁπλῶς λεγομένων τεταγμένων τε καὶ ἀτάκτων.

[4] Synopsis de pulsibus, 6, K. ix. 445: ἐπεὶ δ' ἐνίοτε διαφθείρεται μὲν ἡ ἐφεξῆς ἰσότης, καὶ διὰ τοῦτ' ἀνώμαλος ἡ κίνησις φαίνεται, καθάπερ ἐπὶ τῶν πλανήτων ἀστέρων, εὑρίσκεται μέντοι τις ἐν περιόδοις ἰσότης.

[5] De diff. puls. i. 9, K. viii. 520: ἔστωσαν γὰρ ὁ μὲν πρῶτος σφυγμὸς καὶ ὁ δεύτερος καὶ ὁ τρίτος ἴσοι κατὰ τὸ μέγεθος, ἄνισος δ' αὖ τοῖς ἐφεξῆς ἐπέσθω ὁ τέταρτος· δῆλον ὡς ἀνώμαλος κατὰ μέγεθος ὁ τοιοῦτός ἐστι σφυγμός, οὐ μὴν ἤδη πω δῆλον εἰ καὶ ἄτακτος· ἀλλὰ χρὴ περιμένειν ἄλλους τέτταρας, ἵν' εἰ μὲν οἱ τρεῖς, οἱ δεύτεροι καὶ ἀλλήλοις καὶ τοῖς ἐκ τῆς προτέρας περιόδου γεννηθεῖεν ἴσοι, καὶ μετ' αὐτοὺς ὁ τέταρτος τῷ τετάρτῳ, τεταγμένος ὁ τοιοῦτος λέγοιτο σφυγμὸς κατὰ μέγεθος.

them was clinically important for the purpose of diagnosis. To acquire
the habit of perceiving these differences, he tells us, requires very long
practice. It is not something that can be acquired immediately at will,[1]
and just as sculptors, painters, wine-tasters, cooks, scent-makers, or
musicians need many years to acquire their skills, in spite of the opportunity of unlimited practice on their materials in unlimited quantity, so
the physician needs even more time to acquire his.[2] What Galen meant
by accuracy of touch is not very easy to imagine, since he was firmly
convinced that he could 'feel' not only the diastole and systole of the
artery as two separate and different motions, but also variations in the
speed of the single motion. These refinements of sensibility of perception
were only acquired after years of practice. For a long time he could not
tell whether he could really distinguish clearly by touch the systole of
the arteries—a point on which, as we have already noted, there was
a difference of opinion among the leading authorities. Archigenes, who
followed Herophilus in this matter, believed that both diastole and
systole could be felt. Agathinus, on the other hand, and most of the
Empirics, denied that systole was perceptible to the touch. Galen decided
after some hesitation that he *could* feel the expansion of the artery, but the
systole or contraction evidently caused him a lot of difficulty. After years
of doubt and exploration, he finally came to the conclusion that he could
clearly perceive the movement of systole by touch, no less clearly than that
of diastole.[3] But the motion of systole was still not as easily felt as that
of diastole[4]—indeed it required, to be felt at all, a special sensitivity of
touch.[5]

A question discussed at length is whether we perceive the whole of the
diastole and the systole, or only part of each of them, and if a part of
them escapes our notice, which part is it, and how big?[6] Here Galen

---

[1] *De dignosc. puls.* i. 1, K. viii. 767: δεῖται δὲ λόγου μὲν ἥκιστα συχνοῦ τοῦτο, χρόνου δ' ὁμοῦ
τῶν ἄλλων ἁπάντων μακροτέρου. πρὸς γὰρ τὸ χρῆναι τὴν ἁφὴν ἀσκῆσαι, ὥστε τῆς παρὰ μικρὸν
ἀκριβῶς αἰσθάνεσθαι διαφορᾶς, οὐδ' ἐφ' ἡμῖν ἐστιν ἡ ἄσκησις αὐτῆς.

[2] Ibid., 768 f.: εἰ γὰρ οἱ πλαστικοὶ μὲν καὶ γραφικοὶ τὴν ὄψιν, οἰνοτροπικοὶ δὲ καὶ μαγειρικοὶ
τὴν γεῦσιν, τὴν ὄσφρησιν δὲ οἱ περὶ τὴν τῶν μύρων σκευασίαν, καὶ τὴν ἀκοὴν οἱ μουσικοί, καίτοι
τὴν ὕλην τῆς τέχνης ἄφθονον ἔχοντες, οὐχ ἡμεραῖς οὐδὲ μησίν, ἀλλ' ἔτεσι συχνοῖς εἰς ἀκρίβειαν
ἀσκοῦσιν, πόσου χρὴ δοκεῖν δεῖσθαι χρόνου τὸν ἰατρὸν εἰς τὴν τῆς ἁφῆς ἄσκησιν;

[3] *De dignosc. puls.* i. 1, 771–2: μόνον δὲ σχεδὸν τοῦθ' ἡμῖν ἐν πολλοῖς ἔτεσιν ἔγνωστο, κἀπὶ τῶν
ἐφεξῆς ἕν, ἢ τοῦ σφοδροῦ σφυγμοῦ διάγνωσις, τῶν δ' ἄλλων οὐδέπω γνώριμον ἦν, ἀλλ' ἐν
βαθείᾳ τινὶ κυλινδομένοις ἀπορίᾳ, συχνῶν ἐτῶν οὐ μὴν ἀφισταμένοις γε τῆς ζητήσεως ἀλλ' ἀεὶ καὶ
μᾶλλον λιπαρῶς ἐγκειμένοις ἐφαντάσθη ποτὲ συστολὴ σαφὴς τῇ ἁφῇ. τοὐντεῦθεν ἀσκοῦσιν ἐπὶ
πλέον, οὐ φάντασμα ἔτι ἀμυδρόν, ἀλλ' ἐναργὴς ἡ διάγνωσις αὐτῆς, οὐδὲν ἧττον τῆς διαστολῆς ἐγίνετο.

[4] *Synopsis de puls.* 9, K. ix. 461: τὸ μὲν οὖν τῆς διαστολῆς μέγεθος αἰσθήσει διαγνῶναι ῥᾷστόν
ἐστι, τὸ δὲ τῆς συστολῆς ἀδύνατον· ἐδείχθη γὰρ ἐν τοῖς περὶ διαγνώσεως σφυγμῶν ἐκφεῦγον
αὐτὴν τὸ πλεῖστον τῆς συστολῆς.

[5] Ibid., 7, 450: μαλακὴν δ' ἔχειν σε χρὴ τὴν ἁφὴν εὐαίσθητόν τε φύσει.

[6] *De dignosc. puls.* i. 8, K. viii. 806: ἑξῆς ἂν εἴη σκοπεῖσθαι πότερον ὅλης αἰσθανόμεθα τῆς τε
διαστολῆς καὶ τῆς συστολῆς, ἢ μόριον ἡμᾶς ἑκατέρας διαλανθάνει, καὶ εἰ διαλανθάνει τί τοῦτό ἐστι
καὶ πόσον.

indulges in a digression on his own clinical experience. In cases where the pulse is small and weak, like those of patients suffering from collapse and nearly all those who are about to die, some physicians say that they can at moments perceive the pulse, others that they cannot do so at all, and the same doctor will make contradictory statements after several applications of his hand to the same artery. Therefore it is plain that in these cases some part of the diastole escapes the touch.[1] Nor can we say that the physician of the finest natural constitution, who lays his hand on the artery with the most perfect technique, and has the most perfect and thorough practice, would perceive the whole of the diastole.[2] Even Galen himself is unable to make such a boast, not even in the case of an artery with no tissues at all lying above it, leave alone one with fat, membranes, or skin, which sometimes form a layer thicker than the artery itself.[3] In the last resort, even in the case of a very strong pulse, the actual beginning of the movement of diastole must escape detection, since the movement has to be communicated to the touch through layers of different tissues separating the artery of the patient from the doctor's finger— a process which must take some time.[4] Moreover the touch perceives the interval of quiescence after the artery has subsided and before the initiation of the new expansion or diastole, as much longer than it really is, so that on the same reasoning, the end-portion of the systole also escapes our perception.[5] The part of the motion of systole which is unperceived is somewhat greater than that of diastole, since we do not perceive quite so much of systole as we do of diastole.[6] The intervals of rest between the two motions are given the names outer and inner, the former being that after systole and before diastole, the latter the one between diastole and

---

[1] *De dignosc. puls.* I. 8, K. viii. 806–7: καὶ πρῶτον μὲν ἀναμνήσομεν ἡμᾶς αὐτούς, ὡς πολλάκις ἐπὶ πολλῶν ἀρρώστων μικροὺς καὶ ἀμυδροὺς ἐχόντων τοὺς σφυγμούς, οἷοι μάλιστα τοῖς τε συγκοπτομένοις γίνονται σχεδὸν ἅπασι τοῖς ἀποθνήσκουσι, τινὲς μὲν ἰατρῶν ἐπὶ βραχὺ τῆς κινήσεως αἰσθάνονται, τινὲς δ' οὐδ' ὅλως ... καὶ πολλάκις ὁ αὐτὸς ἰατρὸς ἐν ἑνὶ καιρῷ παρὰ τὰς διαφόρους ἐπιβολὰς τῆς χειρὸς ἐν μέρει τἀναντία φησί, δῆλον ὡς διαφεύγει μόριόν τι τῆς κινήσεως τὴν ἁφήν.

[2] Ibid., 807: ἴσως τις ἐρεῖ τὸν ἄριστα μὲν πεφυκότα κάλλιστα δ' ἐπιβάλλοντα τὴν χεῖρα τετριμμένον δ' ἀκριβῶς ἁπάσης αἰσθάνεσθαι τῆς διαστολῆς.

[3] Ibid.: ἐγὼ μὲν γὰρ οὐδ' ἐπὶ τῶν ἐκτὸς τούτων σωμάτων ὧν ἐστιν αὐτῶν ἅψασθαι μηδενὸς ἐπίπροσθεν ὄντος ἑτέρου, δυναίμην ἂν ἀλαζονεύσασθαι βεβαίαν διάγνωσιν, οὐχ ὅπως ἐπὶ σώματος οὗ πιμελὴ καὶ ὑμένες καὶ δέρμα πρόκειται παχύτερον αὐτοῦ πολλάκις τοῦ τῆς ἀρτηρίας σώματος.

[4] Ibid., 815–16: ἐμοὶ μὲν γὰρ δοκεῖ κἂν τούτοις διαφεύγειν ἔτι τὰ πρῶτα τῆς διαστολῆς ... μάθοις δ' ἄν, εἰ νοήσαις, ὡς ἀναγκαῖόν ἐστι τὴν ἐκ τῆς ἀρτηρίας ἀρχομένην κίνησιν διαδοθῆναι, πρώτοις μὲν τοῖς περικειμένοις σώμασιν, εἶτα τῷ δέρματι παντί, καὶ τότ' ἤδη τοῖς ἡμετέροις δακτύλοις. οὔκουν ἐνδέχεται παντάπασιν ἄχρονον εἶναι τὴν οὕτω γινομένην τῆς κινήσεως μετάληψιν.

[5] Ibid., 816: ἀλλὰ κἀκ τοῦ πολὺ μακροτέρας αἰσθάνεσθαι τὴν ἁφὴν τῆς μετὰ τὸ συνιζῆσαι τὴν ἀρτηρίαν πρὸ τοῦ διαστέλλεσθαι γιγνομένης ἡσυχίας, ἥπερ τῆς μετὰ τὸ διασταλῆναι πρὸ τοῦ συνιζάνειν, οὐκ ἀλόγως ἄν τις ὑπονοήσειεν ἐκφευγόντων ἡμᾶς μορίων τινῶν τῆς ἐντὸς κινήσεως τοῦτο γίνεσθαι. δῆλον γὰρ ὡς εἴπερ ἄληπτον τὸ πρῶτον τῆς διαστολῆς, εἴη ἂν καὶ τὸ τῆς συστολῆς ἔσχατον ἀδιάγνωστον.

[6] Ibid., 10, 818: ἐπειδή τοι ἴσον αἰσθανόμεθα τῆς συστολῆς ὅσον περ καὶ τῆς διαστολῆς, ἢ βραχεῖ τινι μεῖον, εἴη ἂν καὶ τὸ τῆς συστολῆς ἀναίσθητον, ἤτοι τοσοῦτον ὅσον καὶ τὸ τῆς διαστολῆς, ἢ βραχεῖ τινι πλέον.

systole. The outer rest can be perceived quite simply by laying your hand upon the artery, the inner one by the appropriate degree of pressure.[1]

But the perception of these infinitesimally small intervals is mere child's play in comparison with that of the speed of the motions of diastole and systole. For the speed of these motions depends not only on the time occupied by them, but also on the distance moved. It is, of course, greater when the pulse is 'larger', and depends also on the dimensions of the artery concerned. Speed is not a direct datum as such: it needs an inference (συλλογισμός) from the two components of time and distance. How can this inference be made instantaneously? To calculate these quantities needs time, but we do not in fact wait to perform these calculations when we are examining a patient: we immediately perceive the speed. In fact we perceive the swiftness or slowness in the first impulse we receive from the artery, which we should not do if we had to wait to make these calculations.[2]

The speed of the motion of diastole and systole seems therefore to be arrived at by what we might call unconscious inference. Galen appears to analyse our perception of a moving body into a succession of point-instants, percepts of a minimum duration covering a minimum area, a kind of spatio-temporal quanta. When we first cast our eyes upon it, we register it as being stationary in a minimum space for a minimum time, this forming as it were the point of reference from which we judge its change of place. Now when we look at a moving object in the far distance, it sometimes appears stationary for an appreciable length of time, even if it is moving very fast. From this fact it is clear that we judge it to be in motion not by direct perception, but by inference. For whenever the minimum perceptible area of a moving body remains in a minimum space for a duration less than the minimum perceptible time, then the body will appear to be in motion. These minimal quanta of space and time are in theory infinitely divisible, but in actual fact, and as measured by perception, they only exist as it were in quanta which are quasi-atomic. This proves that all motion is recognized by inference, not by direct perception as such. But as this inference is so close to perception,

---

[1] Ibid., 11, 818–19: ἤ τ' ἐντὸς καὶ ἡ ἐκτὸς ἡσυχία τῆς ἀρτηρίας· ἐπεὶ δὲ καὶ διὰ τούτων προγιγνώσκεταί τινα περὶ τῆς διαγνώσεως αὐτῶν ἀναγκαῖον εἰπεῖν. τὴν μὲν οὖν ἐκτὸς ἡσυχίαν ἁπλῶς ἐπιβάλλων τὴν χεῖρα μάλιστ' ἂν γνωρίσαις πηλίκη τίς ἐστιν . . . τὴν δὲ ἐντός, εἰ θλίβοις εἰς ὅσον ἡ παροῦσα σφοδρότης ἐγχωρεῖ, μάλιστ' ἂν οὕτως διαγνοίης. καὶ τὴν μὲν ἐκτὸς ἠρεμίαν ὅλην ἀκριβῶς διαγνώσῃ δεόντως, ἁπτόμενος. τὴν δ' ἐντός, ὡς καὶ πρόσθεν εἴρηται, σὺν τοῖς ἀναισθήτοις μορίοις ἑκατέρας τῶν κινήσεων, τοῦ τε τῆς συστολῆς πέρατος καὶ τῆς ἀρχῆς τοῦ διαστέλλεσθαι.

[2] Ibid., iii. 1, K. viii. 882: τὸ μὲν γὰρ τάχος τε καὶ τὴν βραδυτῆτα κατὰ τὴν πρώτην ὁρμὴν τῆς ἀρτηρίας γνωρίζομεν, τὸν δὲ λόγον τοῦ χρόνου πρὸς τὸν χρόνον, καὶ τῆς διαστάσεως πρὸς τὴν διάστασιν ἵν' ἐξεύροιμεν, παμπόλλου δεόμεθα χρόνον. ὥστ' οὐδ' ἀναμένομεν αὐτὰ λογίζεσθαι πρὸς τὴν ἐπὶ τῶν ἀρρώστων διάγνωσιν, ἀλλ' ὥσπερ εἰ καὶ παρόντα τινὰ θεασάμενοι τύχοιμεν, αὐτὸς ὁ ῥοῖζος τῆς ὁρμῆς ἱκανὸς τὸ τάχος ἐνδείξασθαι.

and the movement of the mind in making it so quick, we often think that motion is not inferred but directly perceived.[1] But this inference is not a conscious process of calculation. We are immediately aware of the quality of a motion, its quickness or its slowness: we do not have to stop to calculate it.[2] This perception of the quality of a motion also includes its evenness or unevenness.[3] Analogous considerations also apply to the size of the movement of diastole or systole, which cannot be perceived in their entirety, particularly in the dimension of length, since the whole body of the artery expands lengthwise, while our fingers are only in contact with a small part of it.[4] The best way of determining the length of a pulse is to apply no pressure, but to give the artery a superficial touch in many places.[5] In estimating the breadth and the height or depth of the arterial movements, both types of digital contact are required. First we must apply pressure, for though pressure may destroy not only the sensation of expansion, but also some of the actual movement itself, a superficial touch subsequently applied may enable us to perform the necessary, presumably unconscious, inference.[6] For our task is not to know all the

[1] *De dignosc. puls.* iii. 1, K. viii. 883–4: κατὰ γὰρ τὴν πρώτην ἐπιβολὴν τῆς ὄψεως ἀρρήτῳ τινὶ χρόνου βραχύτητι προσχρησάμενοι τὴν μονὴν τοῦ κινουμένου σώματος ἐγνωρίσαμεν. ἐφ᾿ ᾗ συνελογισάμεθα τὴν μετάβασιν. ὅσα γοῦν πόρρωθεν ὁρῶμεν, ἔστιν ὅτε ταῦτα μέχρι πλείονος ἡμῖν μένοντα φαντάζεται, κἂν ὅτι τάχιστα κινῆται, ᾧ καὶ δῆλον ὅτι συλλογισμῷ τὴν κίνησιν οὐκ αἰσθήσει γνωρίζομεν. ὅταν μὲν γὰρ ἕκαστον τῶν πρώτων αἰσθητῶν μορίων τοῦ κινουμένου σώματος ἐν τῷ πρώτῳ αἰσθητῷ τόπῳ τὸν πρῶτον αἰσθητὸν χρόνον ὑπομένῃ, τηνικαῦτα ἀκίνητον εἶναι δοκεῖ τὸ βλεπόμενον· ὅταν δὲ τὸ πρῶτον αἰσθητὸν μόριον ἐν τῷ πρώτῳ αἰσθητῷ τόπῳ τοῦ πρώτου αἰσθητοῦ χρόνου βραχύτερον ὑπομένῃ χρόνον, τηνικαῦτα κινεῖσθαι δοκεῖ. ἕκαστον μὲν γὰρ τῶν εἰρημένων εἰς ἄπειρον τέμνεσθαι δύναται, πρός γε τὴν φύσιν, αἰσθήσει δὲ μετρούμενα, πρῶτά τινα καὶ ἄτμητα κέκτηται μόρια, ᾧ καὶ δῆλον ὅτι συλλογισμῷ μὲν ἅπασα κίνησις, οὐκ αἰσθήσει διαγιγνώσκεται, τῷ δὲ παρακεῖσθαι μὲν αἰσθήσει τὸν συλλογισμόν, ταχίστην δ᾿ εἶναι τοῦ νοῦ τὴν μετάβασιν, οὐ συλλογισμῷ πολλάκις ἀλλ᾿ αἰσθήσει διαγινώσκεσθαι δοκεῖ.

[2] Ibid., 883: ὅπερ δὲ φαντάζεται μόνον ἡ αἴσθησις εἰς τὴν διάγνωσιν τῶν ταχέων τε καὶ βραδέων σφυγμῶν, τοῦτο ἀρκεῖ λεχθῆναι ... καὶ καλεῖσθαι τὴν μὲν ὠκεῖαν οὕτως, τὴν δὲ βραδεῖαν κατὰ τὰς τῶν τόπων ματαβάσεις τῆς αἰσθήσεως τὴν διάγνωσιν ποιουμένης οὐ κατὰ τὸν τῆς ὅλης κινήσεως χρόνον, οὔτ᾿ ἰδίᾳ καὶ μόνον οὔθ᾿ ὅσα τῷ ποσῷ παραβάλλεται· καὶ κατὰ τοῦθ᾿ ἡμῖν ἑτοίμη τοῦ τάχους τε καὶ τῆς βραδυτῆτος ἡ διάγνωσις γίγνεται, οὐκ ἂν γενομένη, εἴπερ ἀνεμένομεν ποσότητα χρόνων τε καὶ διαστάσεων λαβόντες τὰς ἐν αὐτοῖς ἀναλογίας σκοπεῖσθαι, ἀλλ᾿ οὐκ ἀναμένομεν δηλονότι.

[3] Ibid.: ἔτι δὲ μᾶλλον, εἰ τοὺς ἀνωμάλους κατὰ τάχος καὶ βραδυτῆτα σφυγμοὺς διαγινώσκειν μελετῴης, εὕροις ἂν ὡς ἐν τῷ ποιῷ κινήσεως ἡ γένεσις αὐτοῖς.

[4] Ibid., 2, 888–9: περὶ δὲ τοῦ κατὰ τὸ ποσὸν τῆς διαστολῆς ἐφεξῆς λέγωμεν· τριῶν δὴ διαστάσεων οὐσῶν τοῦ σώματος τῆς ἀρτηρίας, μήκους καὶ πλάτους καὶ βάθους, οὐδεμιᾶς οἷόν τε πάσης αἰσθέσθαι. τῆς μὲν κατὰ τὸ μῆκος ἄντικρυς δῆλον, μέχρι μὲν γὰρ ἐσχάτου πέρατος ἑκατέρωθεν ἡ ἀρτηρία σφύζει, βραχεῖ δ᾿ αὐτῆς μέρει τὴν ἀφὴν ὑποβάλλομεν.

[5] Ibid., 893: ἄθλιπτος μὲν οὖν πάντως ἔστω, πολλαχόθι δὲ καὶ ψαύων ἐπιβολῆς καὶ οἷον αἰωρῶν τὴν χεῖρα. χρηστὸς δ᾿ ὁ τοιοῦτος μάλιστα τρόπος ... καὶ διὰ ταῦτα ἀσφαλέστερόν ἐστιν εἰς τὴν τοῦ μήκους διάγνωσιν ἀθλίπτως ἐπιβάλλειν τὴν ἀφήν.

[6] Ibid., 896–7: ἀπόλλυται μὲν γάρ τι καὶ αὐτῆς τῆς κινήσεως ἐν ταῖς πλείσταις τῶν θλίψεων ... τὸ διάστημα δ᾿ οὐκέτι μικρόν, ἀλλ᾿ ὀλίγου δεῖν ὅλον διαφθείρεται· ψαύσας δ᾿ αὖ πάλιν ἐπιπολῆς οὐχ ἕξεις μαντεύσασθαι κατὰ πηλίκου διαστήματος ἡ κίνησις ἠνέχθη. ἡ μὲν οὖν ἀπορία τοιαύτη. λύσις δ᾿ αὐτῆς τὸ μὴ ζητεῖν πάντως αἰσθήσει διαγνῶναι τὸ ποσὸν τῆς διαστολῆς, ἀλλ᾿ εἰ καὶ συλλογισμῷ τινι δυνάμεθα, μηδὲν ἡγεῖσθαι βεβλάφθαι. πρόκειται γὰρ ἡμῖν οὐκ αἰσθήσει πάντως γνῶναι τὰ συμβεβηκότα τοῖς σφυγμοῖς, ἀλλ᾿ ἁπλῶς γνῶναι.

phenomena connected with the pulse *by direct perception*, but to *know* them.[1]

But enough of these sphygmological conundrums. The only interesting part of them today is to understand how Galen could have come to believe that he possessed such a subtle and so certain an intuition of so many shades of difference. To believe that he was merely a charlatan trying to display his own superiority under the cloak of an elaborate exhibition of false pretences would be quite unjustified. To dogmatize on problems of visual aesthetics, as any student of the history of art knows only too well, would be extremely risky. So I must leave these problems of tactile aesthetics raised by Galen's pulse-lore to be solved by others more competent than myself.

In comparing the descriptions given by Galen and his predecessors with tracings of the kymograph, there are one or two general features which are worth noticing. Galen was, of course, quite correct in assuming that his two movements of diastole and systole were separate and that each of them occupied a certain duration. The single beat occupies a perceptible time, and the ascent to the peak of the pressure wave (sometimes more than one peak), which corresponds to Galen's systole, is in most cases much quicker than the descent, which corresponds to his diastole. 'The rise or upstroke is much quicker than the fall. Its rapidity has often caused it to be overlooked', Ewart informs us. Indeed, 'Though aware of its occurrence, we may fail to notice it unless the whole attention is given to its perception.'[2] So too the doubt expressed, not so much by Galen as by some of his predecessors and colleagues, about the proportion of the movement of expansion that is actually perceptible to the touch, also finds an echo in Ewart: 'To follow the retraction of the artery requires great attention, a delicate touch, and a progressive pressure from the finger, usually only one half of the fall will be felt.'[3]

Fundamentally, it would appear, the study of the pulse inaugurated by Herophilus and continued by his successors, which culminated in the work of Galen, was on the right lines, notwithstanding their ignorance of hydrodynamics, and their failure, with the exception of Erasistratus, to grasp the significance of the propulsive power of the heart-muscles.

---

[1] In this connection it is interesting to compare this doctrine of Galen's with a paragraph taken from Ewart's little instructional monograph, *How to Feel the Pulse* (London, 1892), p. 29, in which one may be tempted to detect perhaps a far distant echo from our Greek sphygmologist: 'In addition to the form of manipulation (fingering) which addresses itself to the arterial wall, there is a *finer fingering* of the pulse itself, of which the systematic pressure applied to the artery is but a coarser mode. It can be more easily hinted at than described. It is a touch which tests the quality of the pulse *through and through*, sometimes playing at the surface, sometimes sounding, as it were, the depth of the arterial stream, sometimes bearing with full weight against the force of the pulse wave, sometimes pursuing its fall and floating up with its rise, a touch as soft and keen as that of the blind—in short a touch with a *mind* in it.'

[2] Ewart, *Heart Studies*, i, p. 80.   [3] Ibid., p. 84.

Their discrimination of the varying sensations and their analysis of their categories were quite surprisingly correct. Compare, for instance, the following paragraph from Broadbent's textbook:

The character of the beat is another matter for study, and brief as is the period occupied by it, each pulse-wave presents a rise, duration, and fall. It may strike the finger suddenly or lift it deliberately: the distension of the artery may be momentary only—or it may persist for some time: the full pressure finally may be abrupt or gradual. For the most part a sudden rise, brief duration, and abrupt fall go together and constitute the short pulse of large arteries and low blood-pressure; while a gradual rise, persistent fullness, and a slow decline are usually associated and give the long pulse of contracted arteries and high tension.[1]

Here the terminology differs somewhat from Galen's, but the fundamental notions are identical, 'big' and 'short' being Galen's 'quick' and 'slow'. Moreover the distinction between speed and frequency was still in use in Broadbent's time. But the purely geometrical distinctions of size no longer have any application. A large pulse is today measured by the strength of the cardiac systole and the tension of the arterial wall. A strong heartbeat and a yielding arterial wall constitute a large pulse, and a feeble systole and an inelastic undistendible arterial wall a small one. It may be noted that Galen's distinction of the hard and soft pulse as indicating the condition of the arterial wall has gained enormously in significance. But for his fundamental misunderstanding of the relation between the pulse and the heartbeat, his sphygmology would be almost modern.

Long before Galen, ever since the time of Herophilus, different kinds of pulse had been noted, some of which required no particular subtlety of tactile perception to distinguish. Various irregularities, such as 'dropped' beats, and what were interpreted as 'inserted' beats, to say nothing of palpitations and even the 'double-hammer' pulse had all been noted. The earliest of these unusual types had been discovered and named by Herophilus, one of them from the leaping of the gazelle, which we have called the 'gazelling' or 'capering' pulse. According to Galen it falls within the category of single-beat unevennesses and involves an interruption in the diastole of the artery, which starts dilating, stops, and then resumes the movement of expansion, the characteristic from which it acquired its name being that the second movement is much quicker and stronger than the first, so giving the impression of a leaping gazelle.[2] It is due to a condition in which the power of the artery to beat

---

[1] W. H. Broadbent, *The Pulse* (London, 1890), p. 32.

[2] *De diff. puls.* i. 28, K. viii. 556: καὶ ὁ δορκαδίζων δὲ κληθεὶς ὑπὸ Ἡροφίλου σφυγμὸς ἔστι μὲν ἐκ τῶν κατὰ μίαν διαστολὴν ἀνωμάλων . . . ὅταν καθ' ἓν μόριον ὁτιοῦν διακόπτηται τὴν κίνησιν ἡ ἀρτηρία, τηνικαῦτα μάλιστα γενόμενος, οὐχ ἁπλῶς, οὐ γὰρ ὅλον τοῦτο τὸ γένος δορκαδίζων ἐστὶ

keeps its normal tone, but is prevented from putting the motion into effect, either because of an excessive quantity of humours inside it, or because of obstruction or the pressure of surrounding organs. The expansion of the artery is therefore momentarily interrupted, and the second part of the movement must clearly be quicker and stronger, since the power of dilation or diastole has, as it were, collected itself and accumulated the extra force needed, and so it attacks its obstacle with greater strength and hastens to overcome the obstruction.[1] The 'gazelling',[2] as we have already noted,[3] has been identified with Corrigan's 'water-hammer' pulse, but considerable doubt still attaches to this identification; thus Broadbent noted that the name was applied differently by different writers, and that Rufus and Galen both insist that it is a pulse with a secondary beat, 'different from that of dicrotism, which is not easy to identify'.[4]

The observation of the 'double-hammer' pulse, to which Galen devoted a great deal of attention, is naturally of interest. As we have noted, this variety was given its picturesque name by Archigenes. Galen describes it in the following terms. It is quite different from the interrupted diastole just described. In this pulse there is quite a different kind of double beat. In the 'double-hammer' pulse the movement of expansion, the diastole, of the artery is completed, not interrupted. The artery starts receding from the finger and then returns to strike once more, so that there is an interval between the two beats.[5] The two beats are not of the same size, the second being much smaller than the first.[6] It is like the double blow of a hammer on an anvil, the first borne down on it

σφυγμός, ἀλλ' ὅταν ἡ μετὰ τὴν ἡσυχίαν δευτέρα κίνησις ὠκυτέρα καὶ σφοδροτέρα τῆς προτέρας ᾖ. τῷ γὰρ τοιούτῳ μόνῳ τοῦτο ἐπικεῖται τὸ ὄνομα, κατὰ τὴν πρὸς τὰ ζῷα τὰς δορκάδας ὁμοιότητα.

[1] De causis puls. ii. 7, K. ix. 80–1: ὁ μέντοι δορκαδίζων καλούμενος κοινὸν μὲν ἔχει πρὸς τὸν δίκροτον τὸ δὶς πλήττειν, οὐ κοινὴν δὲ τὴν αἰτίαν . . . ἀλλ' ὅταν ἡ δύναμις ὅσον μὲν ἐφ' ἑαυτῇ σώζῃ τὸν κατὰ φύσιν τόνον, ἴσχηται δὲ τῆς κινήσεως ἤτοι διὰ πλῆθος ἄμετρον, ἢ δι' ἔμφραξιν ἢ θλίψιν τῶν ὀργάνων, ἡσυχία τηνικαῦτα διακόπτει τὴν διαστολήν. δεόντως ἄρα τὸ δεύτερον μέρος αὐτῆς, τὸ μετὰ τὴν ἡσυχίαν, εὐρωστότερον φαίνεται τοῦ πρὸ τῆς ἡσυχίας. ἀθροίσασα γάρ, ὡς ἂν εἴποι τις, ἑαυτήν, καὶ συλλέξασα καὶ ῥώσασα καὶ ἀνακτησαμένη ἡ τέως νενικημένη δύναμις, ἐπιτίθεται σφοδρότερον, ἐκνικῆσαί τε καὶ διώσασθαι τὰ λυποῦντα σπεύδουσα.

[2] Ibid., 81: ἦν δέ ποτε καὶ κατὰ τὴν δευτέραν ὁρμὴν νικηθῇ, χείρων μὲν ἂν οὕτως εἴη τοῦ δορκαδίζοντος ὁ τοιοῦτος σφυγμός, ἀνώνυμος δέ ἐστιν.

[3] Broadbent, op. cit., p. 5.

[4] See above, p. 256. Cf. De diff. puls. i. 16, K. viii. 537: οἷός ἐστιν ὁ σφυγμὸς οὗτος ὁ πρὸς Ἀρχιγένους κεκλημένος.

[5] Ibid., 538: τὸ δὲ γένος τῶν δικρότων οὐχ οὕτως, ἀλλ' ἐπειδὰν πληρώσῃ τὴν διαστολὴν ἅπασαν εὐθὺς ἀποχωρεῖ πρὸς βραχὺ καὶ αὖθις παίει τὸ δεύτερον· ὥστε τῶν μὲν διαλειπόντων ἡσυχίαν μέσην εἶναι τῶν πληγῶν, τοῦ δὲ δικρότου συστολὴν ἢ σύνοδον ἢ ὑπονόστησιν, ἢ ὡς ἄν τις ἐθέλῃ καλεῖν, διὰ τοῦτό τινες δύο σφυγμοὺς εἶναί φασι, οὐχ ἕνα, τὸν δίκροτον· ἐροῦσι δὲ αὐτὸ μάλιστα οἱ μὴ παρακολουθοῦντες τῇ συστολῇ τῆς ἀρτηρίας, ἀλλ' ἐκ πληγῆς καὶ διαλείμματος τὸν σφυγμὸν συνεστάναι φάσκοντες.

[6] Ibid., 539: ἀλλὰ φανερῶς ἐκ βάθους πλέονος καὶ κατὰ μείζονος διαστάσεως ἡ προτέρα κίνησις ἐνηνέχθαι φαίνεται, αὐτόθεν δήπουθεν ἐγγύθεν ἡ δευτέρα.

violently from a great distance, and the second as if the hammer had just been lifted a little bit above the anvil and had fallen on it with much less force than the first, and from quite a short distance.[1] After the first blow, the artery does not contract, but it moves down in a confused motion or vibration as it were, and its descent from the limits of the first expansion is not divided by any clear interval of quiet when it contracts, but as soon as its upward motion has ceased, it begins to retreat, with a short confused oscillating motion, and then it strikes the finger once more.[2] In fact the whole movement of the dicrotic pulse is rather confused or shaky, so that even in the case of the first beat, it appears as if the artery were being lifted up and changing its whole position rather than expanding. The 'quivering' pulses are like that.[3] But if we wish to explain this pulse, we can only do so after we have examined the causes of the 'quivering' pulses. These occur when the pulsative power is strong, but its instrument, the artery, is hard, and the biological need is pressing. If any of these factors is absent, the 'quivering' pulse cannot arise, for it is essentially the product of the violent expansion of a hard artery.[4] The third of these factors, the pressing biological need, may arise from a variety of causes. Need is increased by an excess of heat or by expenditure of psychic spirit, and the refusal of the artery to function properly may be due to obstruction, compression, or induration; this latter being caused either by inflammation, the formation of lumps or hard patches, or by desiccation, tension, or refrigeration of the organs.[5] The 'double-hammer' pulse is produced as follows. When the parts of the artery on either side of that part to which we apply our fingers are harder and colder, the parts which are not in contact with our fingers become for that reason not easy to move; so when the middle part which

---

[1] De diff. puls. i. 16, K. viii. 540: ἔοικε γὰρ τὸ ἐπ' αὐτοῦ γιγνόμενον ταῖς τῆς σφυρᾶς διπλαῖς πρὸς τὸν ἄκμονα πληγαῖς, τῆς μὲν προτέρας ἐκ πολλοῦ μὲν διαστήματος καταφερομένης καὶ σφοδρῶς παιούσης, τῆς δευτέρας δὲ οἷον ἀναπαλλομένης τῆς σφυρᾶς ἀπὸ τοῦ ἄκμονος οὐκ ἐπὶ πολὺ καὶ αὖθις αὐτῷ προσπιπτούσης ἀρρωστότερόν τε ᾗ πρόσθεν καὶ ἐξ ὀλίγης διαστάσεως.

[2] Ibid.: οὐδὲ γὰρ συστέλλεται τότε ἡ ἀρτηρία, ἀλλά πως οἷον κλονουμένη καταφέρεται καὶ τὴν καταφορὰν αὐτῆς ἀπὸ τοῦ πέρατος τῆς πρώτης διαστολῆς οὐδεμία σαφὴς ἡσυχία διαιρεῖ, καθάπερ ἐπὶ τῆς συστολῆς φαίνεται, ἀλλ' εὐθὺς ἅμα τῷ παύσασθαι τῆς ἄνω φορᾶς ἡ ὑποχώρησις γίνεται, πρὸς ὀλίγον κλονουμένης αὐτῆς, εἶτ' αὖθις ἐμπιπτούσης.

[3] Ibid., 541: κλονώδη πάντως δεῖ τὴν κίνησιν εἶναι τοῦ δικρότου σφυγμοῦ, ὥστε καὶ κατ' αὐτὴν τὴν προτέραν πληγὴν οἷον ἐπαιρομένην καὶ τὸν τόπον ὅλον ἀλλάττουσαν τὴν ἀρτηρίαν ἄνω φέρεσθαι μᾶλλον ἢ διαστελλομένην· τοιοῦτοι γὰρ οἱ κλονώδεις.

[4] De causis puls. ii. 6, K. ix. 76: οὔκουν οἷόν τε τὰς αἰτίας αὐτῶν ἐξευρεῖν ἀκριβῶς, πρὶν τὰς τοῦ κλονώδους ἐπιμελῶς διασκέψασθαι. γίνεται τοίνυν οὗτος ὅταν ἡ μὲν δύναμις εὔρωστος ᾖ, τὸ δ' ὄργανον σκληρόν, ἐπειγῃ δ' ἡ χρεία. εἰ γὰρ ἕν τι τούτων ἐκλείπει, κλονώδης οὐκ ἂν γένοιτο. τὸ γάρ τοι συνέχον αὐτοῦ τὴν γένεσιν ἐστὶ βίαιος διαστολὴ σκληρᾶς ἀρτηρίας· οὐ γὰρ ἂν ἄλλως κραδαίνοιτό τε καὶ διασείοιτο παντῇ.

[5] Ibid., 77: λοιπὸν οὖν ἤτοι τῆς χρείας αὐξανομένης ἢ τῶν ὀργάνων ἀπειθούντων ... ἀλλ' ἡ μὲν χρεία τῇ πλεονεξίᾳ τῆς θερμότητος ἢ τῇ δαπάνῃ τοῦ ψυχικοῦ πνεύματος αὐξάνεται, δυσπαθῆ δὲ γίνεται ὄργανα δι' ἐμφράξεις ἢ θλίψεις ἢ σκληρότητας, αὗται δὲ αἱ σκληρότητες ἢ φλεγμαινόντων ἢ σκιρρωμένων ἢ σκληρυνομένων ἢ ξηραινομένων ἢ ψυχομένων ἢ τεινομένων γίνονται τῶν ὀργάνων.

is under our fingers starts moving, first in the movement of diastole, these surrounding parts pull it backwards, but when they start to expand in their turn, they carry up this middle portion again with them, so that of necessity the fingers feel a double beat.[1] The 'double-hammer' differs from the 'quivering' pulse in that the portions of the arteries involved in these different motions are much larger, whereas in the 'quivering' pulse each little portion of the artery is moving in a different direction.[2]

Galen seems to have changed his opinion about the 'double-hammer' pulse quite considerably. Here he seems to regard it as essentially an arterial phenomenon. In another passage, however, he looks upon it, as we shall see, as a single-beat version of the interrupted pulse, whose 'systematic' version is the intermittent, or 'beat-dropping' pulse, the principal cause of which lies in the defective functioning not only of the arteries, but also of the heart.[3]

To describe in any further detail all the different kinds of pulse distinguished by Galen would carry us far beyond the limits of this work. The principal work dealing with them as such is the treatise in four books named De differentiis pulsuum, which will be found in the eighth volume of Kühn's edition. Here Galen deals at length with all the traditional types of pulse which had been differentiated by Herophilus and his successors. To deal adequately with Galen's sphygmology would require a separate book. Here, therefore, we must confine ourselves to those elements in his teaching which throw some light on his ideas of the connections between the working of the heart and the arterial pulse. After dealing with the 'double-hammer' pulse and various other 'uneven' single-beat varieties such as the 'ant-crawling', and the one named by Democritus the 'worming', as well as various 'uneven' pulses due to conditions of the coats of the arteries or their contents, including that particularly obscure phenomenon the 'wave-like' pulse, Galen passes to the 'serially uneven' pulses, for which he uses the word 'systematic'. There are, he tells us, three kinds of irregularities, the 'mouse-tailed' or 'tapering' pulse, the intermittent or 'beat-dropping' pulse and its opposite the 'beat-inserting' pulse, and finally the 'nodding' pulse. The

---

[1] Ibid., 78: ὅταν τοῦ μέρους τῆς ἀρτηρίας, ᾧ τὴν ἀφὴν ἐπιβάλλομεν, σκληρότερα καὶ ψυχρότερα, καὶ διὰ τοῦτο δυσκινητότερα τὰ ἑκατέρωθεν, ὧν οὐκ ἁπτόμεθα γένηται, κἄπειτα προεξορμήσαν αὐτῶν εἰς τὴν διαστολὴν τὸ μέσον ἀντισπάσῃ πάλιν ἔσω καὶ αὖθις συνεξαίρῃ, δὶς ἀνάγκη πλήττεσθαι τὴν ἀφήν.

[2] Ibid., 78–80: ὁ μὲν οὖν τοιοῦτος σφυγμὸς δίκροτός ἐστι μόνον, οὐ μέντοι καὶ κλονώδης σαφῶς. ἕτερος δέ τις ἅμα καὶ κλονώδης ἱκανῶς ἐστι καὶ δίκροτος γίνεται κατὰ τοιόνδε τινὰ τρόπον . . . εὔδηλον οὖν ὅτι δίκροτος ὁ τοιοῦτος ἔσται, ταύτῃ πλεονεκτῶν τοῦ κλονώδους μόνον, ὅτι κατὰ μεγάλα μόρια τῆς ἀρτηρίας τὴν ἀνωμαλίαν τῆς κινήσεως ἐκτήσατο. τοῦ μὲν γὰρ ὑποπίπτοντος τοῖς δακτύλοις ἅπαντος ὁμοίως κινουμένου, πλὴν ὅσα κλονεῖται, τῶν δ' ἑκατέρωθεν αὐτοῦ διαφερόντων, ὁ δίκροτος γίνεται, τῷ κλονώδει δὲ μόνῳ οὐδὲν πλέον ὑπάρχει τοῦ κραδαίνεσθαι καὶ διασείεσθαι κατὰ μικρὸν ἅπαντα τὰ μόρια, τὴν δὲ ἐν οὕτω μεγάλοις μέρεσι διαφορὰν τῆς κινήσεως ὥσπερ ὁ δίκροτος οὐκ ἔχει.

[3] See below, p. 417.

phenomenon of tapering is to be observed in either of the two categories of size and strength, but it is the former which alone has generally been given the name by physicians.[1] A pulse is 'tapering' or 'mouse-tailed' when successive beats diminish gradually in size by equal amounts. Those which continue to taper finally end up in complete absence of motion, the pulse ceases altogether. These are called the intermittent or 'failing' taperers (διαλείπων μύουρος), but those which cease tapering are of two varieties. Some of them retain the size down to which they tapered, while others start increasing again in size, reversing the tapering process. These are called 'recurrent mouse-tailed'.[2] The cause of the 'tapering' or 'dying-away' pulse is a greatly enfeebled condition of the pulsative power or faculty. The 'recurrent taperers' indicate a smaller degree of weakness, since in their case the pulsative power is still fighting against its weakness, as it were, and recollecting itself returns repeatedly to its original size and tone, whereas the tapering pulses which remain weak indicate an extreme lack of strength.[3]

The intermittent or 'beat-dropping' pulse was regarded by Galen as deeply significant. The intermittent is different from the rare—or what we today would call the slow—pulse because it is necessarily uneven. It does not merely imply a long interval between beats, for that is consistent with regularity, but the 'beat-dropping' pulse must always be irregular, since it is found to drop a beat once every equivalent three, four, five, or even more beats.[4] The intermission of only one beat is

---

[1] De diff. puls. i. 11, K. viii. 525: ἐν μὲν δὴ τῇ κατὰ τὸ μέγεθος καὶ σμικρότητα ἀνωμαλίᾳ πάνυ σύνηθες τοῖς ἰατροῖς ὄνομα τὸ μύουρον. ἐν δὲ τῇ κατὰ σφοδρότητα καὶ ἀμυδρότητα καὶ τοῖς ἄλλοις γένεσιν οὐκ ἔθ' ὁμοίως ἐν ἔθει.

[2] Ibid., 10, 523-4: ἔστω τοίνυν ὁ μὲν δεύτερος σφυγμὸς τοῦ πρώτου βραχὺ μικρότερος, ὁ δὲ τρίτος τοῦ δευτέρου τοσούτῳ πάλιν, ἀλλὰ καὶ ὁ τέταρτος τοῦ τρίτου τῷ ἴσῳ, καὶ τοῦτ' ἄχρι πλείονος ἐφεξῆς γενέσθω, τοὺς τοιούτους σφυγμοὺς μειουρίζοντάς τε καὶ μειούρους καλοῦσιν ἀπὸ τῶν εἰς ὀξὺ τελευτώντων σχημάτων τοὔνομα μεταφέροντες. ὅσοι μὲν διὰ παντὸς αὐτῶν μειοῦνται καὶ οὐδέποτε παύονται τοῦδε τοῦ παθήματος, εἰς ἀκινησίαν παντελῆ τελευτῶσιν, καὶ καλοῦμεν αὐτοὺς ἐκλείποντας μυούρους. ὅσοι δὲ παύονται διττὴν ἔχουσι τὴν διαφοράν. τινὲς μὲν γὰρ αὐτῶν ἐν ᾗπερ πρώτῳ ἐπαύσαντο μειούμενοι σμικρότητι, ταύτην διὰ παντὸς φυλάττουσιν, τινὲς δ' αὐξάνονται πάλιν, οὓς μυούρους παλινδρομοῦντας καλοῦσι.

[3] De causis puls. ii. 2, K. ix. 64-5: εἰ δὲ τὰ μὲν τῶν ὀργάνων ἔχοι καλῶς, ἡ δύναμις δ' ἀσθενὴς εἴη μεγάλως, ἡ προειρημένη μὲν οὐκ ἂν εἴη, ἡ μέντοι μύουρος ὀνομαζομένη γένοιτ' ἂν ἀνωμαλία. And ibid., 3, 65: τὴν ἀσθένειαν τῆς τοὺς σφυγμοὺς ἐργαζομένης δυνάμεως οὐκ ἴσην ἐν πάσαις ταῖς διαθέσεσιν ὑπάρχειν ἀναγκαῖον . . . ἡ μὲν δὴ πρώτη καὶ βραχεῖα μικροτέρους μὲν καὶ ἀμυδροτέρους, οὐ μήν γε μυούρους ἐργάζεται τοὺς σφυγμούς. ἡ δὲ ἐπὶ ταύτῃ τοσούτῳ μείζων, ὡς ἤδη καὶ τοὺς ἐπιβαλλομένους δακτύλους ἄχθος εἶναι τῇ δυνάμει, τῶν μυούρων ἐστὶ σφυγμῶν ἀποτελεστική. διττῆς δ' οὔσης ἐν αὐτοῖς διαφορᾶς, οἱ μὲν γὰρ αὐτῶν εἰς τὴν ἐξ ἀρχῆς κίνησιν ἐπανέρχονται, καὶ καλοῦσιν αὐτοὺς μυούρους παλινδρομοῦντας, οἱ δ' αὐτόθι που καταστρέφουσιν, ἰστέον ὡς οἱ μὲν πρότεροι μικροτέραν δείκνυνται τὴν ἀσθένειαν. ἀναμάχεται γάρ πως ἡ δύναμις ἔτι, καὶ οἷον ἀθροίζουσα καὶ συστρέφουσα πολλάκις ἑαυτὴν αὔξει μὲν τὸ μέγεθος οὕτω τῶν σφυγμῶν, αὔξει δὲ καὶ τὸν τόνον. οἱ μέντοι καταμένοντες ἐν ἐσχάτῃ μικρότητι, καὶ μήκετ' ἐπανερχόμενοι μειζόνως ἢ κατὰ τούτους ἐμφαίνουσι λελύσθαι τὴν δύναμιν ὥσπερ εἰ καὶ τελέως ἐκλείποιεν ἐσχάτην τινὰ τὴν ἀρρωστίαν ἐνδείξονται.

[4] Synopsis de puls. 33, which has only come down in a Latin translation and is appended by Kühn to his text (K. ix. 544): 'Ac raritas quidem ab intermissione pulsuum distincta est

extremely moderate.¹ It is called a 'recurrent-intermittent' because after the interval caused by the 'drop', the artery begins again to move at its ordinary frequency.² The essential cause of these intermittent failures of the pulse to act is ultimately the weakness of the pulsative power, either in the heart or in the arteries themselves, relatively to the extra task imposed upon them by certain conditions, such as an excess of humours, or their thickness, which prevents the movement starting at the right moment, by blocking either the valves of the arteries connecting with the heart, through which it attracts and expels matter, or to some extent the narrowness of the lumen of these vessels themselves in the parts near to the valves. Often, too, the cause is external, in the form of a surfeit of thick humours in the tissues surrounding the arteries, which acts like a fetter, pressing heavily, like a packload on certain parts of the artery. Sometimes too the surrounding tissues occupy the space into which the artery should expand; at others, inflammation, induration, or swelling in these tissues prevents the arteries' diastole, and if such inflammation, etc., should occur in the coats of the arteries themselves, there is great danger. And if these morbid conditions should occur in the tissue of the heart itself, the danger is of the utmost gravity, for a patient with these morbid conditions collapses suddenly.³ A dyscrasia, that is to say a wrong mixture of the body's four elements, is not so deadly, as it is much less severe than an inflammation. But its consequence is a weakening of the pulsative power, and this also manifests itself in a feeble pulse. For when

prolixitate temporis; interdum vero etiam, quod raritas cum aequalitate aliquando consistat omnium percussionum. Intermittens vero pulsus necessario inaequalis fiat, interdum enim per tres, interdum per quatuor, aliquando per quinque percussiones, vel etiam plures intermittere invenitur.'

This passage is almost a word-for-word translation of one contained in the fourth chapter of the second book of the treatise *On prognostications from the pulse* (K. ix. 286 f.): ἀραιότης μὲν οὖν διαλείποντος σφυγμοῦ διώρισται τῷ μήκει τοῦ χρόνου· προσδιορισθήσεται δ' ἐνίοτε καὶ τῷ τὴν μὲν ἀραιότητα καὶ μεθ' ὁμαλότητός ποτε συνίστασθαι πάντων τῶν πληγῶν, τὸν διαλείποντα δὲ σφυγμὸν ἐξ ἀνάγκης ἀνώμαλον γίνεσθαι, ἐνίοτε μὲν γὰρ διὰ τριῶν, ἐνίοτε δὲ διὰ τεσσάρων, ἔστι δ' ὅτε διὰ πέντε πληγῶν ἢ καὶ πλειόνων εὑρίσκεται διαλείπων τε καὶ ἡσυχάζων ἕνα χρόνον ἢ καὶ πλέονα κινήσεως.

¹ Loc. cit.: 'Quies vero temporum unius pulsus intermissio est moderatissima.'
² *De diff. puls.* i. 11, K. viii. 526: παράκεινται δὲ τοῖς διαλείπουσι σφυγμοῖς οἱ καλούμενοι παλινδρομοῦντες ἐκλείποντες, ὅταν δύο ἢ καὶ τριῶν ἢ καὶ πλειόνων ἔτι σφυγμῶν χρόνον ἀκίνητος εἶναι δόξασα παντάπασιν ἡ ἀρτηρία, πάλιν ὑπάρξηται κινεῖσθαι.
³ *De praesag. ex puls.* ii. 4, K. ix. 280–1: τοὺς μὲν δὴ διαλείποντας σφυγμοὺς ἤτοι διὰ τὸ βαρύνεσθαι πρὸς τοῦ πλήθους ἡ δύναμις ἐργάζεται, κωλυομένη κατὰ τὸν προσήκοντα καιρὸν ἐπὶ τὴν κίνησιν ἐξορμᾶν διὰ πάχος ἢ πλῆθος χυμῶν ἐμφράττον ἤτοι τὰ στόματα τῶν πλησίων τῆς καρδίας ἀρτηριῶν, δι' ὧν ἕλκει τε καὶ αὖθις ἐκπέμπει τὰς ὕλας, ἢ καὶ μέχρι τινὸς ἀπὸ τῶν στομάτων ὅλην τῶν ἀγγείων τὴν εὐρύτητα, πολλάκις δ' ἔξωθεν αὐταῖς περιχυθὲν τὸ τοιοῦτον πλῆθος οἷον δεσμὸς γίνεται, τὸ μέν πού τι βαρῦνον αὐτὰς οἷον φόρτιον, ἔστι δ' ὅτε καὶ τὰς χώρας εἰς ἃς διαστέλλονται καταλαμβάνον, ἐνίοτε δὲ καὶ φλεγμονή τις ἢ σκίρρος ἤ τις ἕτερος ὄγκος τοιοῦτος ἐν τοῖς περιέχουσι τὰς ἀρτηρίας σώμασι συνιστάμενος, ἐμποδὼν ἵσταται ταῖς διαστολαῖς αὐτῶν· εἰ δὲ καὶ κατὰ τοὺς χιτῶνας αὐτῶν τῶν ἀρτηριῶν τοιοῦτόν τι συσταίη, μείζων ὁ κίνδυνος. εἰ δὲ καὶ κατὰ τὸ τῆς καρδίας αὐτῆς σῶμα, τοῦτο μὲν ἤδη κακὸν ἔσχατον, ἐξαιφνίδιον γὰρ οἱ τοιοῦτοι συγκόπτονται.

the condition of the heart is good, that is, when its mixture of elements is in the right proportions, it gives a strong pulse, when the mixture is bad, a faint one.¹ Here, it should be noted, a connection between the heart and the pulse is quite unequivocally laid down, but the connection is not one that has any meaning for us today, for it has nothing to do with what we call the heart's action. The wrong elemental mixture in the heart reduces its power of communicating to the arteries through their coats, *their* power of systole and diastole. It is the lack of this transmission which makes the pulse faint, not the feeble systole and diastole of the heart itself. The wrong mixture makes the pulse faint and small: its intermittence is due to the quantity of humours being too great relatively to this diminution in the pulsative power, both in the heart itself and in the arteries and veins which adjoin it (presumably the right auricle).²

Galen was evidently much impressed by the clinical significance of the 'dropped beat'. He regarded it as a very serious symptom indeed. As he put it, the fact that the artery does not move at all, which is called intermittence, whether in the case of the single beat, or in a series of beats, is a serious symptom, more serious than any other form of irregularity.³ The dropping of a single beat or a slightly longer interval of quiescence was quite commonly associated in his experience with recovery, particularly in the case of old patients.⁴ Indeed both in old people and in children dropped beats are less fatal than in persons in the prime of life.⁵ For old men and children can often recover completely from the suspension of a single beat, but men in the prime of life not even from this. The 'dropped beat' pulse must be carefully distinguished from the 'rare' or 'infrequent' pulse, since it is irregular. The drop may occur sometimes every three, sometimes every four, and sometimes every five or even more

---

¹ *De praesag. ex puls.* ii. 4, K. ix. 281: οὐ μὴν ἥ γε δυσκρασία τῆς καρδίας ὁμοίως ὀλέθριος, ἀλλ' ἐπιεικεστέρα μακρῷ φλεγμονῆς. ἕπεται δ' αὐτῇ δυνάμεως ἀρρωστία. καὶ ὅ γε ἀμυδρὸς σφυγμὸς οὐκ ἄλλου τινός ἐστιν ἢ τῆς τοιαύτης διαθέσεως γνώρισμα. συμμέτρως μὲν γὰρ ἔχουσα κράσεως ἡ καρδία τὸν σφοδρὸν σφυγμὸν ἀπεργάζεται, μοχθηρῶς δὲ τὸν ἀμυδρόν.

² Ibid., 281-2: ἀλλὰ μόνη μὲν ἡ δυσκρασία μικρὸν καὶ ἀμυδρὸν ἀποτελεῖ τὸν σφυγμόν, οὐ μὴν ἤδη γέ πω καὶ ἀνώμαλον, εἰ μὴ παραβαλλομένη τοῖς χυμοῖς ἡ δύναμις, ὅσοι τε κατ' αὐτὴν τὴν καρδίαν εἰσὶ καὶ ὅσοι κατὰ τὰς πλησίον αὐτῆς ἀρτηρίας τε καὶ φλέβας, ἐλάττων αὐτῶν φαίνοιτο κατὰ τὴν ἰσχύν, ὅπερ οὐδὲν ἄλλ' ἐστὶν ἢ τὸ πρὸς τὴν δύναμιν πλῆθος.

³ Ibid., 280: καὶ μὲν δὴ τὸ μηδόλως κινεῖσθαι τὴν ἀρτηρίαν, ὅπερ ὀνομάζεται διαλείπειν, ἄν τε καθ' ἕνα σφυγμὸν ἄν τε κατὰ σύστημα γένηται, χαλεπόν ἐστιν, ὡς οὐδὲν ἁπάντων τῶν εἰδῶν τῶν ἀνωμάλων γινομένων.

⁴ Ibid., 282-3: εἰ δὲ μὴ μόνον ἑνὸς σφυγμοῦ χρόνον ἡσυχάσειεν ἀλλὰ καὶ πλέονα, σαφέστερόν τ' ἂν ὁ τοιοῦτος διαλείπων φαίνοιτο καὶ κινδυνωδέστερος εἰς τοσοῦτον ἔσται τοῦ πρόσθεν εἰς ὅσον ἂν ἐπὶ πλέον ἡσυχάζῃ. ὥστε οὐκ οἶδα εἴ τινα σωθῆναι δυνατόν ἐστι δυοῖν σφυγμῶν χρόνον ἡσυχαζούσης τῆς ἀρτηρίας. ἑνὸς δὲ σφυγμοῦ χρόνον, ἢ καὶ βραχεῖ πλέον, πολλάκις ἐθεασάμεθα διαλειπούσης τῆς κινήσεως τῶν ἀρτηριῶν ἀναρρωθέντα τὸν ἄνθρωπον, καὶ μάλισθ' ὅταν ἄγῃ πρεσβυτικὴν ἡλικίαν, καίτοι τάχ' ἂν δόξειεν ἄλογον εἶναι τὸ τοιοῦτον.

⁵ Ibid., 283: γέροντες μὲν οὖν διὰ τοῦτο τοὺς διαλείποντας σφυγμοὺς ἧττον ὀλεθρίους ἔχουσι τῶν ἀκμαζόντων· οἱ δὲ δὴ παῖδες ἑξῆς.

beats, and the quiescence of the artery may be as long as one or more full beats.[1]

The 'dropped-beat' pulse was regarded by Galen as the 'systematic' variety of the intermittent or 'interrupted' pulse. Its single-beat varieties were of two kinds, the 'double-hammer' pulse which we have already described, in which the interruption appears to take place during systole, and another which involves an interruption of the diastole. It has several forms, of which all are dangerous and all involve a double motion. When the second motion is stronger than the first the case is less severe, but when the second movement is the fainter it is more serious. So too, slowness is a bad sign, speed is more favourable. For the 'interrupted' pulse is caused by nature fighting against morbid conditions. When she is able, as it were, to shake them off and loosen her bonds, the second beat or movement is quicker and stronger than the first.[2]

Another irregular pattern which also appears to have interested Galen was the so-called 'intercalating' pulse, which like the 'double-hammer' had also been dealt with by Archigenes. Here, instead of 'dropping' a beat, the heart and arteries at irregular intervals add an extra beat. The cause of this extra-beat phenomenon is almost always the exact opposite of that of the dropped beat, though the material conditions out of which it arises are the same as those just described, namely an excess of thick or heavy humours, and the obstruction of the arteries by the pressure of surrounding tissues, etc. In this case, however, the pulsative power is strong and makes an extra effort to overcome the obstacles to its proper functioning by making its pulsations larger, stronger, and quicker. In these circumstances the pulse is very high, and there are signs of an approaching crisis,[3] though not always a favourable one. The 'intercalated'

---

[1] Ibid., 286: ἡ δὲ περὶ τῶν ἑνὸς σφυγμοῦ χρόνων ἡσυχία μετριωτάτη τῶν διαλήψεών ἐστι καὶ πολλοὶ διεσώθησαν ἐκ ταύτης γέροντές τε καὶ παῖδες, ἀκμάζων δ' οὐδεὶς οὐδὲ ἐκ ταύτης.

[2] Ibid., 6, 294–6: ἔστι δὲ κἀνταυθοῖ χαλεπωτάτη πασῶν ἡ διαλείπουσα. γίνεται δ' αὕτη διακοπτούσης ἡσυχίας τὴν διαστολήν. ἰδέαι δὲ πλείους αὐτῆς, ἅπασαι μὲν χαλεπαί, διαφέρουσαι δ' ἀλλήλων τῷ μᾶλλόν τε καὶ ἧττον. ὅταν μὲν γὰρ ἡ δευτέρα κίνησις σφοδροτέρα γίνηται τῆς προτέρας, ἐπιεικέστερον, ὅταν δ' ἀμυδροτέρα χαλεπώτερον. οὕτω δὲ καὶ ἡ μὲν βραδυτέρα χαλεπώτερον σημεῖον, ἡ δὲ θάττων ἐπιεικέστερον. γίνονται γὰρ οἱ τοιοῦτοι σφυγμοὶ διαγωνιζομένης τε ἅμα καὶ ἐμποδιζομένης τῆς φύσεως ὑπὸ τῶν νοσωδῶν αἰτίων. ὅταν μὲν οὖν ἀποσείσασθαί πως αὐτὰ δυνηθεῖσα, καὶ οἷον ἐκ δεσμοῦ τινος ἀπολυθεῖσα, τὴν μετὰ τὴν ἡσυχίαν κίνησιν ἀμείνονα ποιήσεται τῆς ἔμπροσθεν, ἐπιεικέστερόν ἐστιν. ὁπόταν δὲ χείρονα χαλεπώτερον. βελτίων δὲ κίνησις ἡ σφοδρὰ καὶ ταχεῖα τῆς ἀμυδρᾶς καὶ βραδείας. ἡ μέντοι κατὰ μέγεθός τε καὶ σμικρότητα διαφορὰ τῆς προτέρας κινήσεως πρὸς τὴν δευτέραν οὐδεμίαν ἀξιόλογον ὑπεροχὴν ἔχει . . . κατὰ μέντοι σκληρότητά τε καὶ μαλακότητα διαφορὰ τῶν δύο προσβολῶν τῆς ἀρτηρίας οὐκ ἄν ποτε γένοιτο διὰ τὸ χρόνου πλέονος ἀεὶ δεῖσθαι τὴν τοιαύτην μεταβολήν . . . κλονωδεστέρα μέντοι πολλάκις ἡ δευτέρα προσβολὴ φαίνεται τῆς προτέρας.

[3] De causis puls. ii. 3, K. ix. 67 f.: ἡ δὲ τῶν παρεμπιπτόντων καλουμένων σφυγμῶν διάγνωσις ἐναντία τῇ τῶν διαλειπόντων ἐστίν . . . καὶ γίγνονται τῆς δυνάμεως ἐρρωμένης μέν, ἀλλ' ὑπὸ πλήθους χυμῶν ἢ ἐμφράξεως ὀργάνων ἐνοχλουμένης. ὡς οὖν ἵνα διώσηται τὰ λυποῦντα, μείζονας πολλάκις καὶ σφοδροτέρους καὶ ὠκυτέρους ἐργάζεται τοὺς σφυγμούς, οὕτω καὶ πλέονες ἐν ταῖς τοιαύταις διαθέσεσι μάλιστα καὶ ὑψηλοὶ γίνονται σφυγμοί, καὶ διὰ τοῦτο κριτικῆς ἐκκρίσεώς εἰσι σημεῖα.

pulse is much less dangerous than the 'intermittent',[1] though Archigenes wrongly thought otherwise.

In the last resort, the chief causes of these irregular pulses must be sought in the heart. For the principal function of both cardiac and arterial motion is a kind of respiration, the object of the heart's diastaltic power being to keep the innate heat in its proper condition and to evacuate the sooty superfluities.[2] The faulty action which these irregularities display is due to an uneven mixture of the elementary substances in its various parts.[3] This results in something like a battle of opposing forces in the organ itself, which tries to maintain its normal action but is sometimes defeated.

When the heart and its contents are evenly hot or cold, clear or turbid, all its parts react uniformly in performing their function; but when some parts are colder and others hotter, and some of its contents are completely pure while others are turbid with a surfeit of superfluous products, all of these parts do not have the same stimulus towards functioning. Some of them act earlier while others lag behind. Under these conditions the smaller and weaker parts follow the larger and stronger which have set themselves in motion to act . . . And just as the parts which are stimulating the heart to function strongly, when they are in a majority, bring the whole heart into action, so, on the other hand, when the parts stimulating action are in a minority and those making for stagnation and rest are in a majority, the whole heart is kept in a greater or longer state of quiescence. So too the actual quality of the motion is determined by the parts in it which prevail in the whole organ. For if the hotter parts take the lead in initiating the motion, the diastole starts sooner and is quicker and larger; but when the colder parts are in command, it is later, slower, and smaller.[4]

---

[1] *De praesag. ex puls.* ii. 5, K. ix. 290: εἰ δὲ ἐκ τῶν τοιούτων κρίσεων ἀπόλλυνταί τινες, οὐδὲν τοῦτο πρὸς τὸ χαλεπωτέραν εἶναι τὴν τῶν παρεμπιπτόντων διάθεσιν τῆς τῶν διαλειπόντων. πολὺ πλείους γὰρ ἐκ τῶν διαλειπόντων ἀπόλλυνται.

[2] Ibid., 7, 298: τὸ σῶμα τῆς καρδίας ἐν ἑαυτῷ τινα δύναμιν ἔχει διασταλτικήν τε καὶ συσταλτικήν. οὐ μάτην οὐδ᾽ ὡς ἔτυχεν οὔτε δοθεῖσαν ὑπὸ τῆς φύσεως, οὔτ᾽ ἐνεργοῦσαν . . . τοῦ φυλάττειν ἕνεκα τὴν ἔμφυτον θερμότητα. κατὰ μὲν οὖν τὰς συστολὰς ἀποχεῖ τὸ λιγνυῶδες περίττωμα, κατὰ δὲ τὰς διαστολὰς ἐπισπᾶται τὸ ἀναψῦχον αὐτήν.

[3] Ibid., 297–8: διὰ δὲ τὴν κοινωνίαν τοῦ λόγου καὶ τοὺς ἄλλους ἅπαντας ἀνωμάλους σφυγμούς, ὅσοι ταῖς τοῦ σώματος αὐτοῦ τῆς καρδίας ἀνωμάλοις ἀκολουθοῦσι δυσκρασίαις, ἐν τῷδε τῷ λόγῳ διέξιμεν ἀρξάμενοι κἀνταῦθα πάλιν ἀπὸ τῶν σαφεστέρων ἀνωμαλιῶν ἃς ὀνομάζουσι συστηματικάς.

[4] Ibid., 298–9: ὅταν μὲν οὖν ὁμαλῶς θερμὸν ἢ ψυχρόν, ἢ καθαρόν, ἢ τεθολωμένον ᾖ, πάντ᾽ αὐτοῦ τὰ μόρια πρὸς τὴν ἐνέργειαν ὡσαύτως ἐξορμᾷ. ὅταν δ᾽ ἤτοι τὰ μὲν θερμότερα, τὰ δὲ ψυχρότερα τύχοι τῶν μορίων αὐτοῦ, καὶ τὰ μὲν ἀκριβῶς καθαρά, τὰ δὲ τεθολωμένα τῷ πλήθει τῶν περιττωμάτων, οὐ τὴν αὐτὴν ὁρμὴν ἴσχει πρὸς τὴν ἐνέργειαν ἅπαντα, ἀλλὰ τὰ μὲν αὐτῶν φθάνει, τὰ δὲ μέλλει. κἂν τούτῳ τοῖς πλείοσί τε καὶ ἰσχυρότερον ἐξορμήσασι πρὸς τοὖργον ἕπεται τά τ᾽ ὀλιγώτερα καὶ ἀσθενέστερα . . . ὥσπερ δὲ τὰ πλείω τε καὶ σφοδρότερον ἐνεργεῖν ἐπειγόμενα σύμπασαν ἐξορμᾷ τὴν καρδίαν, οὕτω πάλιν, ὅταν ἐλάττω μὲν ᾖ τὰ πρὸς τὴν κίνησιν ἐπειγόμενα, πλείω δὲ τὰ μένοντα, σύμπασαν ἐν ἡσυχίᾳ κατέχει πλείονι. καὶ δὴ καὶ τὸ τῆς κινήσεως ποιὸν ἐκ τῶν κρατησάντων ἐν αὐτῇ μερῶν ὅλῳ τῷ σπλάγχνῳ γίνεται. εἰ μὲν γὰρ τὰ θερμότερα τῆς κινήσεως ἐξηγεῖται, πρωϊαίτερόν τε ἅμα καὶ θάττων καὶ μείζων ἡ διαστολὴ γίνεται, τῶν ψυχρῶν δ᾽ ἡγουμένων ὀψιαίτερόν τε καὶ βραδυτέρα καὶ μικροτέρα.

The determining factor may be of two kinds, either the relative sizes of the parts involved, or the magnitude of the biological need. Other things being equal, the greater need will provide a readier and stronger stimulus to action. In cases where one set of factors is much larger than the other, the whole organ functions accordingly, but when there is only a very small difference, or when the factors are exactly equal, each of them is unable thoroughly to master the other, and so prevailing in this part and mastered in that, they make the motions of the whole organ variable and uneven.[1] For example:

Suppose that the cold parts are greater in number, but not very much so, than the hot, then the first going-into-action of the heart is of necessity smaller and slower. Moreover, when the cold parts prevail, the period of rest is greater than it would have been were the hot parts more powerful. Now let the second going-into-action of the heart take place while the cold parts are still superior, this to be followed by a period of rest, and then a third and a fourth going-into-action followed by a period of rest, while the cold parts are still prevailing. Clearly the hotter parts, which require a larger, quicker, and more frequent motion, will not obtain sufficient satisfaction of their needs. So they will become hotter and communicate some of their heat to the parts surrounding them, with the result that the heart will not retain its original cold condition. More parts of it will become hot, and the parts which were hot will become hotter than before. So the time will come when the hot parts will prevail, and the heart will start into action earlier and make its movements quicker and larger than before, when the cold parts were in command, owing to the stimulation of their need. The reverse process will then happen. For the prevailing hot parts will receive a moderate refrigeration through the proper functioning of the systole, but the parts which are slightly cold will become colder, and so the original condition of the heart will be restored in the course of time. Furthermore, at this time the whole motion of the heart will inevitably be determined in accordance with its needs. Its diastole will again become small and slow and rare. And this alternating process will continue as long as the wrong elementary mixture of the heart continues to be present.[2]

---

[1] Ibid., 299: πολλάκις μὲν οὖν τῷ πλήθει τῶν μορίων ἡ τῆς κινήσεως ἡγεμονία συνέπεται, πολλάκις δὲ τῷ μεγέθει τῆς χρείας. ὅσα γὰρ ἱκανῶς δεῖταί τινος, ἑτοιμότερόν τε καὶ σφοδρότερον ἐπὶ τοὖργον ἐξορμᾷ μέν, κἂν ἴσα τῷ πλήθει ὑπάρχῃ τοῖς μὴ δεομένοις. ὅταν μὲν οὖν πολὺ πλείω τὰ ἕτερα τῶν ἑτέρων ᾖ, κατ᾽ ἐκεῖνα διὰ παντὸς κινεῖται καὶ ἐνεργεῖ τὸ σπλάγχνον. ὅταν δὲ ἤτοι βραχεῖ τινι τὰ ἕτερα τῶν ἑτέρων, ἢ πλείω, ἢ ἀκριβῶς ἴσα, διὰ παντὸς μὲν οὐκ ἐνδέχεται κρατεῖν τὰ ἕτερα, νικῶντα δὲ ἐν μέρει τε καὶ νικώμενα, ποικίλας τε καὶ ἀνωμάλους ἐργάζεται τὰς ὅλου τοῦ σπλάγχνου κινήσεις.

[2] Ibid., 299–301: ἔστω γάρ, εἰ τύχοι, πλείω μέν, οὐ μὴν πολλῷ γέ τινι τὰ ψυχρὰ μόρια τῶν θερμῶν, ἀνάγκη τὴν πρώτην ἐνέργειαν ἐλάττονά τε καὶ βραδυτέραν γίνεσθαι, καὶ μὲν δὴ καὶ τὴν ἡσυχίαν ἐν τούτοις κρατοῦσι μακροτέραν ἢ εἴπερ ἐκράτει τὰ θερμά. καὶ τοίνυν καὶ ἡ δευτέρα τῆς καρδίας ἐνέργεια τῶν ψυχρῶν κρατούντων γινέσθω, καὶ μετ᾽ αὐτὴν αὖθις ἡσυχία. καὶ τρίτη γε καὶ τετάρτη πρὸς ταύτας ἐνέργειά τε καὶ ἡσυχία κατὰ τὰ ψυχρὰ νικῶντα συντελείσθω. ἆρ᾽ οὐ πρόδηλον ὡς τὰ θερμότερα μόρια, τὰ μείζονός τε ἅμα καὶ θάττονος καὶ πυκνοτέρας δεόμενα τῆς κινήσεως, ἐνδεῶς ἀπολαύσει τῆς ἑαυτῶν χρείας; ὥστε ἐν τούτῳ θερμότερα γενήσεται καί τι καὶ τοῖς ὁμιλοῦσι μεταδώσει θερμότητος. οὐκοῦν ἔτι φυλαχθήσεται τῆς καρδίας ἡ ἐξ ἀρχῆς διάθεσις, εἴπερ καὶ πλείω γενήσεται τὰ θερμότερα μόρια καὶ μᾶλλον ἢ πρόσθεν θερμά. τούτου τοίνυν ἀεὶ συμβαίνοντος,

The need to which Galen is here referring is that provoked by the accumulation of sooty residues, which produce an uneven condition of faulty elemental mixture in the organ. This is passed on to the arteries in the form of a 'systematic' irregularity—though Galen never explains exactly how. He only tells us how the heart produces a 'single-beat' irregularity. It does this because the parts of the arteries directly connected with the hotter parts of the heart expand to a greater degree and move more quickly, while those in contact with the colder parts expand less and move more slowly.[1] Moreover, the arteries may have their own faulty elemental mixture, which may produce the same kind of irregularities as those of the heart, as regards size, quickness, frequency, etc., and in cases of very great departure from natural conditions even of strength.[2] The disordered functioning of these opposing forces resulting from this uneven faulty mixture of the elements, both in the heart and in the arteries, means that there are many different movements in a single beat, so that it seems sometimes to halt in the middle of its ascent, as often happens to the weary traveller. For these forces pulling in opposite directions not only make movements slower and make them come to a halt; they can make them fail to start altogether, and even sometimes actually reverse them.[3]

The 'double-hammer' pulse was evidently submitted by Galen to a prolonged study, and the subtleties of his descriptions of its varieties

ἔσται ποτὲ χρόνος ἐν ᾧ καὶ αὐτὰ κρατήσει τῶν ἐναντίων, ὥστε καὶ πρωϊαίτερον ἐπὶ τὴν ἐνέργειαν ἐξορμῆσαι, διὰ τὴν τῆς χρείας ἔπειξιν, αὐτήν τε τὴν κίνησιν ποιήσασθαι θάττονά τε καὶ μείζονα τῶν ἔμπροσθεν ἁπασῶν κινήσεων ὧν ἡγεῖτο τὰ ψυχρά. συμβήσεται τοιγαροῦν ἐν τούτῳ τὰ μὲν κρατοῦντα συμμέτρως ἀπολαύειν ἐμψύξεως, ὅσα δ' ἦν ψυχρότερα πλέον ἤδη καταψύχεσθαι, καὶ οὕτως μεταπεσεῖν αὖθις ἐν τῷ χρόνῳ τὴν διάθεσιν ὅλης τῆς καρδίας, ὡς κρατῆσαι τὰ ψυχρότερα . . . πάλιν δ' αὖ ἐν τούτῳ τῷ χρόνῳ τὴν κίνησιν ὅλης τῆς καρδίας ἀναγκαῖον ἔσται κατὰ τὴν τοιούτων χρείαν τυπωθῆναι καὶ γενέσθαι τὰς διαστολὰς αὐτῆς ἀραιὰς καὶ βραδείας καὶ μικράς, οἷαί περ ὑπέκειντο γίνεσθαι κατ' ἀρχάς. . . . οὕτω γὰρ οἶμαί σε πεισθήσεσθαι περὶ τῆς τῶν σφυγμῶν συνεχοῦς μεταπτώσεως ἄχρι περ ἂν ἡ εἰρημένη δυσκρασία κατὰ τὴν καρδίαν περιμένῃ.

[1] De praesag. ex puls. ii. 5, K. ix. 301 : κατὰ δὲ τὸν αὐτὸν λόγον ἐπειδὰν ἐν τῷ πλήθει τῶν λιγνυωδῶν περιττωμάτων ἀνώμαλός ἡ δυσκρασία κατὰ τὸ σπλάγχνον εἰς τὴν συστηματικὴν ἀνωμαλίαν καὶ ἡ τῶν σφυγμῶν κίνησις ἀχθήσεται. οὐδὲν δὲ δήπου θαυμαστὸν οὐδὲ τὴν καθ' ἕνα σφυγμὸν ἀνωμαλίαν ἐπὶ ταῖς τῆς καρδίας γίνεσθαι. τὰ μὲν γὰρ τοῖς θερμοτέροις αὐτῆς μέρεσι κατευθὺ τῶν ἀρτηριῶν μόρια θερμότερά τε γενήσεται τῶν ἄλλων καὶ διαστήσεται μεῖζον καὶ κινήσεται θᾶττον. τὰ δὲ τοῖς ψυχροτέροις αὐτὰ τ' ἔσται ψυχρότερα, καὶ βραδύτερον κινήσεται καὶ διαστήσεται μεῖον.

[2] Ibid., 302 : καὶ χωρὶς δὲ τῆς καρδίας οἰκεῖαί τινες γινόμεναι ταῖς ἀρτηρίαις δυσκρασίαι τάς τε εἰρημένας ἀνωμαλίας ἀποτελοῦσι, τὰς κατὰ μέγεθός καὶ μικρότητα καὶ τάχος καὶ βραδυτῆτα καὶ ἀραιότητα καὶ πυκνότητα, καὶ εἰ πολὺ τοῦ κατὰ τὴν φύσιν ἐκτρέποιντο, καὶ τὰς κατὰ σφοδρότητά τε καὶ ἀμυδρότητα.

[3] Ibid., 302–3 : καὶ μὲν δὴ κατὰ αὐτήν γε τὴν καρδίαν καὶ προσέτι τὰς ἀρτηρίας ἁπάσας, ἐκ τῆς κατὰ τὸ σπλάγχνον ἀνωμάλου δυσκρασίας, ἐν μιᾷ διαστολῇ πλείους γενήσονται διαφοραὶ τῶν κινήσεων, τῶν μὲν εἰς τάχος αὐτὴν ἐξορμώντων, ἐνίων δ' ἐπεχόντων τε καὶ βραδύνειν ἀναγκαζόντων. ὥστε ποτὲ καὶ στῆναι μεταξὺ κατὰ τὴν ἄνοδον, οἷόν τι συμβαίνει καὶ τοῖς ἐν ὁδοιπορίαις, ἢ καὶ ἄλλως ὁπωσοῦν ἕλκουσιν ἑτέρους βραδύνοντας. ἀντισπώμενοι γὰρ ὑπ' αὐτῶν ἀτάκτως, ἐκκόπτονταί τε καὶ διακόπτονται τὴν ὁρμήν, ὡς μήτε διαπαντὸς ὁμοίαν ποιεῖσθαι τὴν κίνησιν ἴσχεσθαί τε πολλάκις. εἰ δὲ καὶ ἀντιπράττοντάς τε καὶ ἀντισπῶντας ἕλκοιεν, οὐ μόνον ἴσχονται τῆς κινήσεως, ὡς ἤτοι βραδύτερον, ἢ μηδόλως ἐνίοτε βαδίζειν, ἀλλὰ καὶ ἀνθειλκύσθησάν ποτε εἰς τοὐπίσω.

and causes are not always easy to understand. The picturesque description of Archigenes loses its sharpness under a haze of logical distinctions and naïvely incorrect mechanics, which are perhaps worth quoting, to illustrate the *reductio ad absurdum* of Galen's sphygmology. Thus we are told that

if it so happens that at the same time some parts of the heart are very hot and others very choked with smoky fumes, the heart or artery will be stimulated to opposite movements. Some parts will attempt diastole and others systole. And so either, while the artery is in the process of dilation, the parts which are contracting begin to function, and contraction or systole will take the place of diastole without any period of rest between the two movements, or, while it is contracting, the expanding parts will start to work and the place of systole will be taken by diastole, again without any period of rest. And both of these movements will take place in various ways; for either the second motion will completely overcome the first, or it will pull against it for a short time and the first motion, having overcome it, will fulfil the measure allotted to itself. So there will be three differences in all in the pulsation of diastole and systole. The first, when in the process of diastole systole takes its place before it has fulfilled its allotted span, the second, when systole succeeds diastole at precisely the moment that diastole has been completed, the interval between the two movements being lost; the third, when, while the movement of diastole is still in being, the opposite movement pulls against it, and then becoming weaker permits the diastole to complete the remainder of its motion. In the same way also diastole can take the place of systole which is already in motion, sometimes not permitting the latter to maintain itself, sometimes breaking it off before it has completed its motion, overcoming it and taking its place, or at other times pulling counter to it for a while, but being finally overcome.[1]

And these morbid arterial motions can sometimes take place without the heart having any disease, either because the arteries themselves are affected with disease in the shape of an uneven wrong elemental mixture, or because their coats are hard, or merely on account of a weakness in their pulsative power.[2]

---

[1] Ibid., 8, 304–5: ἂν γὰρ ἅμα συμβῇ τὰ μὲν ἁπλῶς εἶναι πάνυ θερμά, τὰ δὲ καταπνίγεσθαι καπνώδει λιγύϊ, πρὸς τὰς ἐναντίας ἐξορμήσει κινήσεις, ὡς διαστέλλεσθαι μὲν ἐπιχειρεῖν τὰ ἕτερα, συστέλλεσθαι δὲ θάτερα. καὶ οὕτως ἤτοι διαστελλομένης τῆς ἀρτηρίας ἐνεργησάντων τῶν συστελλόντων διαδέξεταί ποτε τὴν διαστολὴν ἡ συστολὴ καὶ χωρὶς τῆς ἐκτὸς ἠρεμίας, ἢ συστελλομένης ἐνεργησάντων τῶν διαστελλόντων, ἢ διαδέξεται τὴν συστολὴν ἡ διαστολή, χωρὶς τῆς ἐντὸς ἡσυχίας. ἑκάτερον δὲ αὐτῶν ἔσται κατὰ πλείονας τρόπους, ἤτοι γὰρ ἐκνικήσει τελείως ἡ δευτέρα κίνησις τὴν προτέραν, ἢ ἐπ᾽ ὀλίγον μὲν ἀντισπάσει, νικήσασα δὲ ἡ προτέρα πληρώσει τὸ προκείμενον ἑαυτῇ μέτρον, ὥστε γίνεσθαι τρεῖς τὰς πάσας διαφορὰς σφυγμῶν ἔν τε τῷ διαστέλλεσθαι κἂν τῷ συστέλλεσθαι· πρώτην μέν, ἐπειδὰν ἐν τῷ διαστέλλεσθαι πρὶν πληρῶσαι τὸ μέτρον ἡ συστολὴ διαδέξηται, δευτέραν δ᾽ ὅταν ἀκριβῶς πληρωθεῖσαν ἐκδέξηται τῆς ἐκτὸς ἠρεμίας ἀπολλυμένης. τὴν τρίτην δ᾽ ὅταν ἔτι γιγνομένην τὴν διαστολὴν ἀντισπάσῃ μὲν ἡ ἐναντία κίνησις, ἀσθενεστέρα δὲ γενομένη συγχωρήσει τὸ λεῖπον ἐκπληρῶσαι. κατὰ ταὐτὰ δὲ καὶ τὴν συστολὴν ἡ διαστολὴ ποτὲ μὲν ἤδη γεγενημένην ἐνδέχεται, μὴ συγχωρήσασα στῆναι, ποτὲ δὲ καὶ πρὸ τοῦ πληρωθῆναι κολούσασά τε καὶ νικήσασα διεδέξατο, ποτὲ δ᾽ ἀντέσπασε μὲν ὀλίγον, ἐνικήθη δέ.

[2] Ibid., 305: τοιαῦται κινήσεις ἀρτηριῶν γίνονταί ποτε καὶ χωρὶς τοῦ τὴν καρδίαν πεπονθέναι, ἤτοι διὰ δυσκρασίαν ἀνώμαλον ἐν αὐταῖς συστᾶσαν, ἢ δι᾽ ἀρρωστίαν τῆς δυνάμεως, ἢ διὰ σκληρότητα

The faulty elemental mixture in the heart thus gives rise to various kinds of irregularity, namely the 'dicrotic' pulse and the pulse that has lost the period of rest between the two movements of diastole and systole, the one with the curtailed diastole, and also the interrupted pulse which drops a beat, to say nothing of irregularities of speed. All these are due to uneven faulty elemental mixture of the heart resulting in the battle between its hot and cold parts.[1]

We pass now to the changing conditions of the pulse in health and disease. The first of these to be considered here is what we moderns call the pulse rate. To Galen, as we have seen, this was rather a complicated affair, being composed of four distinct phases, diastole and systole and the two periods of rest interposed between them, like the pauses between breathing in and breathing out. Of these one was 'external', that following diastole and preceding systole, so called because the artery was at its fullest extension; the other 'internal', that following systole and preceding diastole. If they were shorter than their normal length, the pulse was 'frequent' and if less, 'rare'.[2] But here, as we have already noticed, endless complications began to arise, since the systole, though perceptible, was less so than the diastole, and it being uncertain how much of the systole was perceived, the boundary between a given systole and the diastole which followed it was also quite uncertain. Moreover, the quickness or slowness of diastole itself (and of course of systole) was not easily determined, because it depended on the size, *sensu Galenico*, of the pulse. If the pulse was 'small', the distance covered by the artery in expansion was small. Hence the time taken might be shorter than that taken by the diastole of a large pulse, though the movement would actually be slower. Ignorance of this distinction leads to many serious errors in prognosis.[3]

τοῦ χιτῶνος. This hardness of the arterial coat must not be confused with any modern notions of arteriosclerosis; it is regarded by Galen as a purely temporary phenomenon, not a permanent degenerative quality, though he did not think it was one which could be modified in an instant.

[1] *De praesag. ex puls.* ii. 8, K. ix. 309: ὡς ἐπὶ ταῖς ἀνωμάλοις δυσκρασίαις τῆς καρδίας . . . γίγνεται μὲν καὶ ὁ δὶς παίων σφυγμός, γίγνεται δὲ ὁ τὴν ἐκτὸς ἠρεμίαν ἀπολύς, ἔτι τε πρὸς τούτοις καὶ ὁ κολουόμενος τὴν διαστολήν. ἐδείχθη δ᾽ ὅτι καὶ οἱ διακοπτόμενοι τὴν κίνησιν ἡσυχίᾳ καὶ αὐτοὶ γίγνονται πάντες ἐπὶ ταῖς ἀνωμάλοις τῆς καρδίας δυσκρασίαις. οὐ μὴν ἀλλὰ καὶ ὅσοι χωρὶς τοῦ διακόπτεσθαι τὴν διαστολὴν ἀνώμαλοι φαίνονται κατὰ βραδυτῆτά τε καὶ τάχος . . . οὗτοι πρὸς ταῖς ἄλλαις αἰτίαις . . . ἔξουσιν . . . τὴν ἀνώμαλον τῆς καρδίας δυσκρασίαν, ὅταν ἐπὶ τοσοῦτον ἀλλήλοις διαμάχηται τὰ θερμὰ μόρια τοῖς ψυχροῖς.

[2] *Synopsis de puls.* 5, K. ix. 443 f.: ὅσοι μὲν οὖν ἀναισθήτην νομίζουσιν αὐτὴν (τὴν συστολὴν) ἐν τῷ μεταξὺ τοῦ πέρατος τῆς διαστολῆς καὶ τῆς ἀρχῆς τῆς συστολῆς, ἡσυχάζειν χρόνῳ φασὶ τὴν ἀρτηρίαν, ἀνάλογον τῇ μετὰ τὴν εἰσπνοὴν ἡσυχίᾳ τῶν ἀναπνευστικῶν ὀργάνων πρὸ τῆς ἐκπνοῆς. ὡσαύτως δὲ καὶ μετὰ τὴν συστολὴν πρὸ τῆς διαστολῆς ἡσυχάζειν αὖθις . . . εἰ μὲν οὖν μείζους εἶεν οἱ τῶν ἡσυχίων χρόνοι τοῦ κατὰ φύσιν, ἀραιὸν ὀνομάζουσι τὸν σφυγμόν, εἰ δ᾽ ἐλάττους πυκνόν, ὡς εἶναι δύο ἀραιότητας καὶ πυκνότητας, τὴν μὲν ἑτέραν ἐκτὸς ἐπὶ τῇ διαστολῇ πρὸ τῆς συστολῆς, τὴν δ᾽ ἑτέραν ἔνδον ἐπὶ τῇ συστολῇ πρὸ τῆς διαστολῆς.

[3] *De dignosc. puls.* ii. 1, K. viii. 824 f.: ἐμοὶ δ᾽ ἑτέρα μὲν ἡ τοῦ χρόνου φαίνεται διάγνωσις, ἄλλη δὲ ἡ κατὰ βραδυτῆτα καὶ τάχος. οὐ γὰρ εἰ βραχύτερος ὁ τῆς κινήσεως εἴη χρόνος, ἤδη καὶ τὸν

In all Galen's descriptions of the pulse we constantly meet with qualitative and quantitative terms involving different degrees, such as small, quick, slow, frequent, rare, strong, hard, etc., and each of these implies a middle term, which, being placed between the two extremes, represents the 'natural' or 'normal' or 'best' size, speed, force, etc.— a fundamental conception of Greek aesthetics, ethics, and metaphysics. In judging the pulse we need some standard. What then is the normal, natural, and best pulse-rate size, strength, etc., with respect to which we judge the pulse of a patient whom we have never seen? The essence of the answer is that the best pulse is determined by a large number of factors, each of which has to be taken into consideration, but the effects of which, owing to the complicated composition of causes, are very difficult to isolate. For the moderate pulse varies according to the age, sex, figure, 'temperament', or as we should call it, the constitution, of the patient, as well as his habits and mental condition, no less than the physical, as well as the climate and season of the year.[1] For the rhythm of the pulse depends on all these different factors. In searching therefore for a standard of comparison by which to judge the 'normal' pulse and the deviations from it, we must find a man of the best elemental mixture, and in the best of health, and make ourselves acquainted with the character of his pulse, by observing its behaviour under conditions when it is not disturbed by any external causes. For example, he must not have remained long in a condition of idleness, nor should his pulse be taken just after violent exercise or immediately after a meal, or after a long fast. He must, moreover, be free from emotional stress in a calm and clean state of soul.[2] The pulse of a man of this character is the measuring-rod of all the phenomena concerning the pulse, the golden mean in comparison with which we call other pulses slow, fat, large, small, or what not.[3]

σφυγμὸν ὠκύτερον εἶναί φημι . . . τὸ δ᾽ ἀληθὲς οὐχ οὕτως ἔχει. πολλάκις γὰρ ἡ τοῦ μακρότερον τὸν χρόνον ἔχοντος σφυγμοῦ κίνησις ὠκυτέρα τῆς τὸν βραχύτερον ἐχούσης ἐστίν. καὶ τοῦτ᾽ εἰ μή τις ἀκριβῶς διαγνοίη, πολλὰ καὶ μεγάλα τῶν ἐκ τῆς διὰ σφυγμῶν προγνώσεως εὑρισκομένων ἀγνοήσει.

[1] Ibid., 2, 844–5: καὶ πρῶτον μὲν τοῦτ᾽ ἴδωμεν, εἰ χρὴ καθ᾽ ἕκαστον γένος σφυγμῶν ἕνα ζητεῖν τὸν σύμμετρον ἢ πλείους, ἄλλον μὲν ὡς ἐν ἡλικίᾳ σύμμετρον, ἄλλον δ᾽ ὡς ἐν ἕξεσι σωμάτων, ἄλλον δ᾽ ἐν κράσεσιν, ἄλλον δ᾽ ὡς ἐν ὥραις ἢ χώραις, ἢ καταστάσεσιν, ἢ ἐπιτηδεύμασιν, ἢ ψυχικαῖς διαθέσεσιν. ἐν ἅπασι γὰρ τούτοις τοὺς μὲν μεγάλους, τοὺς δὲ μικρούς, τοὺς δὲ συμμέτρους λέγομεν εἶναι σφυγμοὺς καὶ τοὺς μὲν ταχεῖς, τοὺς δὲ βραδεῖς, τοὺς δὲ συμμέτρους, καὶ τὰς ἄλλας διαφορὰς ὡσαύτως.

[2] Ibid., 857: μάλιστα τὴν ἀρίστην τοῦ σώματος ἡμῶν ἐξευρόντας κατασκευὴν πρῶτα μὲν ἐπισκέψασθαι χρὴ ποῖοί τινες οἱ κατ᾽ αὐτὴν εἰσι σφυγμοί, καὶ τοῦθ᾽ οὐχ ἁπλῶς οὐδ᾽ ὡς ἔτυχε ποιητέον, ἀλλ᾽ ἐν τοιαύτῃ καταστάσει λαβόντας τὸν ἄνθρωπον, ἐν οἷα τὴν οἰκείαν κίνησιν οἱ σφυγμοὶ φυλάττουσιν ὑπὸ μηδενὸς τῶν ἔξωθεν αἰτίων τετραμμένοι, γίνοιτο δ᾽ ἂν τοῦτο μήτ᾽ ἀργίᾳ μακρᾷ κατεσχημένου μήθ᾽ ὑπόγυιον γεγυμνασμένου, ἀλλὰ μηδ᾽ ἐν ἀσιτίᾳ μακρᾷ γεγονότος ἢ καὶ ἀρτίως ἐδηδοκότος. εἶναι δὲ χρὴ καὶ τὸ περιέχον εὔκρατον δηλονότι καὶ τὸν ἄνθρωπον ἔξω τῶν ψυχικῶν παθημάτων ἐν γαλήνῃ καθαρᾷ τὴν ψυχὴν ἔχοντα.

[3] Ibid., 3, 860–1: μαθὼν οὖν τις πρότερον ὡς χρὴ τὴν ἀρίστην τοῦ σώματος ἡμῶν γνωρίζειν φύσιν . . . τὸν ἐν ταύτῃ σφυγμὸν μέσον ἁπασῶν τῶν ἄλλων ἴστω καὶ οἷόν τι μέτρον καὶ κανόνα τοῦτον ἐν ἁπάσαις ταῖς περὶ σφυγμῶν πραγματείαις, τὸν σύμμετρόν τε καὶ μέτριον ὑφ᾽ ἡμῶν

Interesting as they are, we must pass over Galen's rather elaborate explanations of Herophilus' conception of the characteristic pulses of the different ages and the different seasons and climates. Nor can we afford to linger over Galen's differentiation of the pulse-rates of the two sexes, except to point out that his idea that men have a rather slower pulse than women of the same age was confirmed in the nineteenth century by a French physician, Ozanan. The great French authority on the pulse at the end of the last century estimated the normal frequency of the adult male at seventy-two beats a minute, and that of the adult female at eighty.

Bodily shape and temperament, that is the particular type of elemental mixture, also have their effect on the pulse. The naturally hot have a much larger, quicker, and more frequent pulse, but not one which is much stronger.[1] Slender people, on the other hand, have a larger pulse but much rarer and only a little stronger.[2] For slenderness of itself means more room for the arteries to expand, since the tissues lying above them are lighter, which adds considerably to the size of their pulse, and as the physiological need is not greater, this means that their pulse will automatically be proportionally less frequent.[3] The pulse will appear stronger, not because it has acquired greater tone, but because it can exhibit the degree of tone it has more readily.[4]

We pass now to the effects on the pulse of certain bodily conditions, natural ones, like pregnancy, or sleep and wakening, as well as the acquired conditions resulting from certain forms of activity, such as bathing, taking exercise, or feeding. First take pregnancy. This makes the pulse larger, quicker, and more frequent, but does not change it in other

---

μεμνήσθω λεγόμενον, ᾧ παραβάλλοντες τοὺς ἄλλους ἅπαντας, ταχεῖς καὶ βραδεῖς καὶ μεγάλους καὶ μικροὺς εἶναί φαμεν . . . ἀλλ' ὥσπερ ἐν τῷ περὶ κράσεων λόγῳ τὴν ἀρίστην ἁπασῶν κρᾶσιν οὔτε θερμὴν ἔφαμεν οὔτε ψυχρὰν οὔτε ξηρὰν οὔθ' ὑγρὰν οὔτε μαλακὴν οὔτε σκληρὰν ὑπάρχειν . . . οὕτω καὶ νῦν οὔτε μέγαν οὔτε μικρὸν οὔτε ταχὺν οὔτε βραδύν, οὔτ' ἀλλ' οὐδὲν ὅσα τῆς μετριότητος ἐξίσταται, τὸν ἐν τῇ καλλίστῃ φύσει σφυγμὸν οὔτε προσαγορεύσομεν οὔτε νοήσομεν. οὐδὲ γὰρ αὐτὸν τὸν ἄνθρωπον ἐν ᾧ τοιοῦτον εὑρίσκομεν σφυγμόν . . . οὔτε γὰρ παχὺν οὔτ' ἰσχνὸν οὔτε θερμὸν οὔτε ψυχρόν . . . ἀλλ' εὔκρατόν τε καὶ σύμμετρον ἅπασι τοῖς μορίοις τοῦ σώματος ὀνομάζομεν. ἐν τούτῳ τοίνυν, ὅταν γε μάθῃς αὐτὸν διαγιγνώσκειν, ἁπάσας τὰς διαφορὰς τῶν σφυγμῶν ἐπισκεψάμενος, μέμνησό τε καὶ κρίνων πρὸς αὐτοὺς τοὺς ἄλλους ἅπαντας σφυγμούς, ἢ σκληροὺς οὕτως ἢ μαλακοὺς ἢ ἀραιοὺς ἢ πυκνοὺς ἤ τι τῶν ἄλλων ἀνάλογον κάλει. The parallel with the normative function of the 'reasonable man' in the English common law is certainly rather striking.

[1] De causis puls. iii. 3, K. ix. 115: οἱ δὲ φύσει θερμοὶ μείζονα μὲν καὶ ὠκύτερον καὶ πυκνότερον πολλῷ, σφοδρότερον δὲ οὐ πολλῷ.

[2] Ibid., 4, 117: οἱ δ' ἰσχνότεροι μείζονα μὲν καὶ ἀραιότερον πολλῷ, σφοδρότερον δ' ὀλίγῳ.

[3] Ibid.: ἰσχνότης οὖν αὐτὴ μόνη κατὰ ἑαυτῆς λόγον εὐρυτέρας μὲν τὰς χώρας τῶν ἀρτηριῶν ἐργαζομένη κουφότερα δὲ τὰ ἐπικείμενα σώματα, μέγεθος ἱκανὸν προσδίδωσι τοῖς σφυγμοῖς. ἔνθα δ' ἂν ἴσης τῆς χρείας μενούσης αὐξάνηται τὸ μέγεθος, ἀραιοτέρους ἐνταῦθα ἀναγκαῖον γίνεσθαι τοὺς σφυγμοὺς εἰς τοσοῦτον εἰς ὅσον καὶ μείζονας.

[4] Ibid., 118: οὐκ οὖν τῷ προσκτᾶσθαί τινα τόνον ἀλλὰ τῷ μᾶλλον ὃν ἔχουσιν ἐνδείκνυσθαι τοιοῦτοι φαίνονται.

respects, since the only factor changed by pregnancy is need. A pregnant woman has now to supply not only her own needs but those of the foetus. The strength of the pulse does not vary in pregnancy, neither does its hardness.[1] Sleep also alters the pulse. To begin with, it becomes smaller, fainter, and rarer, and later on its slowness and rareness gradually increase, most markedly after a meal. But if sleep be prolonged, it becomes bigger and stronger, it turns fainter, but it keeps its slowness and rareness.[2] In sleep the outward movement of the innate heat diminishes, and its movement inwards takes control: this means that systole gradually becomes quicker and diastole slower.[3] Moreover diastole becomes small, while systole becomes relatively large, since the artery does not expand to its full extent, though its contraction is at a maximum.[4] It expands only just so much as to counteract the movement of contraction. For during sleep there is a large production of 'superfluities', owing to the preparation of the humours, so that the artery wants to evacuate its smoky residues with greater force. Hence the movement inwards of the heat gains the upper hand. But when the working up of the humours from the products of digestion has finished, and the man continues asleep, both movements of the arteries become naturally smaller and slower and fainter and also rarer. For sleep, as the poets have told us, is the brother of death. Indeed it is a condition in which the only vital function which continues to be carried out is the digestion of food. All other functions are suspended, as if in death.[5] This is because during

[1] Ibid., 8, 131 : ἐν δὲ τῷ κύειν οἱ σφυγμοὶ μείζονες καὶ πυκνότεροι καὶ ὠκύτεροι γίνονται, τὰ δ' ἄλλα φυλάττουσιν. ἐπὶ τῶν κυουσῶν οὐδὲν παρήλλακται τῶν πρόσθεν ἢ τὰ τῆς χρείας. ἥ τις δ' ἂν ἥδε ᾖ, πάντως ἐπιτείνεταί τε καὶ προσαύξεται μηκέτι τῆς γυναικὸς ἑαυτῇ μόνον ἀναπνεῖν τε καὶ σφύζειν, ἀλλὰ καὶ τῷ κυουμένῳ δεομένης. ὥστ' εὐλόγως ὠκύτεροι μὲν καὶ μείζονες ἔσονται καὶ πυκνότεροι, οὐ μὴν σφοδρότεροί γε, ἢ ἀμυδρότεροι, ἢ σκληρότεροι, ἢ μαλακώτεροι, κατ' αὐτόν γε τὸν τοῦ κύειν λόγον.

[2] Ibid., 9, 131 : εἶεν δ' ἄν, εἴ πέρ τι ἄλλο, καὶ ὕπνοι κατὰ φύσιν. τρέπουσι δὲ καὶ οὗτοι τοὺς σφυγμούς, ἀρχόμενοι μὲν μικροτέρους καὶ ἀμυδροτέρους καὶ βραδυτέρους καὶ ἀραιοτέρους ἐργαζόμενοι, προϊόντες δὲ βραδυτῆτα ἐπιτείνουσι καὶ ἀραιότητα καὶ μάλιστα μετὰ τροφήν. μείζους δὲ γίνονται καὶ σφοδρότεροι, χρονίσαντες δὲ πάλιν τρέπονται εἰς ἀμυδρότητα, φυλάττουσι δὲ βραδυτῆτα καὶ ἀραιότητα.

[3] Ibid., 134 : ἐπειδὴ τοῖς κοιμωμένοις ἡ μὲν ἔξω κίνησις τοῦ θερμοῦ μεμείωται, κρατεῖ δ' ἡ ἔσω, τὴν μὲν συστολὴν εὔλογον γίνεσθαι θάττονα τὴν δὲ διαστολὴν βραδυτέραν.

[4] Ibid., 135 : καὶ μὲν δὴ καὶ μικρὸς κατὰ θάτερόν ἐστι τῶν ἑαυτοῦ μορίων τοῖς κοιμωμένοις ὁ σφυγμός. ἐπὶ πλεῖστον μὲν γὰρ συστέλλεται, διαστέλλεται δ' οὐκ ἐπὶ πλεῖστον, ἀλλ' ὅσον ἀνάγκη τὴν ἐναντίαν ἀποδοῦναι κίνησιν τῇ συστολῇ.

[5] Ibid., 137-8 : ἀλλὰ καὶ βραδὺς μὲν ἐν ταῖς διαστολαῖς, ταχὺς δὲ ἐν ταῖς συστολαῖς ἐστι, καὶ ὅλως εἴσω μᾶλλον κινεῖται. ὥστε καὶ σφοδρὸν αὐτὸν ἐν ταῖς συστολαῖς εἰπὼν οὐκ ἂν ἁμάρτοις. καὶ γὰρ οὖν καὶ τὸ περίττωμα τῆς τῶν χυμῶν ἐργασίας τὸ οἷον αἰθαλῶδες ἐκκρίνειν ἐφίεται σφοδρότερον ἡ ἀρτηρία κατὰ τοὺς ὕπνους, ὡς ἂν πλέον τότε γινόμενον, ὥστε καὶ διὰ τοῦτο τὰ τῆς ἔσω κινήσεως πλεονεκτεῖ. ὅταν μέντοι καταπαύσηται μὲν ἡ ἐργασία τῶν χυμῶν, μένῃ δ' ὑπνώττων ὁ ἄνθρωπος, ἄμετρος ἂν δήπουθεν ὁ τοιοῦτος ὕπνος εἴη, μικρότεραι δ' αἱ κινήσεις ἑκάτεραι καὶ βραδεῖαι καὶ ἄρρωστοι καὶ ἀραιαὶ γίνονται κατὰ λόγον. ὕπνος γάρ, ὡς καὶ τῶν ποιητῶν ἔστιν ἀκοῦσαι λεγόντων, ἀδελφός ἐστι θανάτου, καὶ ἐν αὐτῷ κοινὸν ὑπάρχει μόνον πρὸς τοὺς ζῶντας, ἡ περὶ τὴν τροφὴν ἐργασία, τὰ δ' ἄλλα πάντα τοῖς ἀποθνήσκουσιν ὅμοια, μὴ βλέπειν, μὴ ἀκούειν, μὴ φρονεῖν, μὴ νοεῖν, μὴ λαλεῖν, ἀναίσθητον, ἀκίνητον, ἀλόγιστον ἐρρίφθαι.

sleep a lot of steamy products from digestion have collected near the source of the innate heat itself, and in all the passages and tissues between the heart and the surface of the body.

The artificially acquired habits and conditions affecting the pulse, which Galen now proceeds to examine, are concerned almost entirely with those produced by exercise, hot and cold baths, and food and drink. Moderate exercise makes the pulse strong, large, quick, and frequent, but exercise taken greatly in excess of a man's strength makes it small, faint, and excessively quick and frequent.

Baths of a moderate heat make the pulse large, quick, frequent, and strong; but if they are too hot, the pulse becomes small and faint, as well as quick and frequent. If the patient is left in the baths a long time, the pulse becomes small, faint, slow, and rare.[1] Cold baths, on the other hand, momentarily make the pulse small, rather faint, slow, and rare but later, in accordance with the effect they ultimately happen to produce, which may be either numbness or strength. If the former, the pulse becomes small, faint, slow, and rare, if the latter, then it becomes large and strong, but only moderately quick and frequent.[2]

With regard to food and drink, Galen tells us that a large meal, sufficient to weigh down the digestive faculty, makes the pulse uneven and irregular and, according to Archigenes, quicker rather than more frequent. A moderate meal makes it large, quick, and frequent. Smaller meals, insufficient to provide adequate nutriment, produce a much smaller change in the pulse and one which lasts only a short time.[3] The effect of wine on the pulse is very much the same as that of food, but it is different in this respect: it takes place immediately and ceases more quickly than that of food. It increases the size and quickness of the pulse rather than its strength or frequency. Wine increases the size of the pulse by about the same amount as a moderate meal,[4] but its consumption at the wrong time produces, given sufficient vital force,

[1] De causis puls. iii. 14, K. ix. 145: λουτρὰ θερμὰ μὲν μεγάλους καὶ ταχεῖς καὶ πυκνοὺς καὶ σφοδρούς, ἔστ' ἂν ᾖ σύμμετρα. τὰ δ' ἄμετρα μικροὺς τε καὶ ἀμυδρούς, ὠκεῖς δ' ἔτι καὶ πυκνούς. εἰ δὲ ἐν τούτῳ παύσαιτο, μικροὺς καὶ ἀμυδροὺς καὶ βραδεῖς καὶ ἀραιούς.

[2] Ibid., 15, 147: ψυχρὰ δὲ λουτρὰ παραχρῆμα μὲν μικροὺς καὶ ἀμυδροτέρους καὶ βραδεῖς καὶ ἀραιούς, εἰς ὕστερον δὲ οἷον ἄν τι καὶ τύχῃ ἐργασάμενα. πάντως γὰρ ἢ ναρκώσει, ἢ ῥώσει. ναρκώσαντα μὲν οὖν καὶ καταψύξαντα μικροὺς καὶ ἀμυδροὺς καὶ βραδεῖς καὶ ἀραιούς, ἐκθερμήναντα δὲ καὶ ῥώσαντα μεγάλους μὲν καὶ σφοδρούς, ταχεῖ δὲ καὶ πυκνότητι συμμέτρους.

[3] Ibid., 16, 148–9: σιτία πολλὰ μὲν ὥστε βαρῦναι τὴν δύναμιν ἀνωμάλους τε καὶ ἀτάκτους τοὺς σφυγμοὺς ἐργάζεται. Ἀρχιγένης δέ φησιν ὠκυτέρους πλέον ἢ πυκνοτέρους. τὰ δὲ σύμμετρα μεγάλους καὶ ταχεῖς καὶ πυκνοὺς καὶ σφοδρούς. τὰ δ' ἐλάττω ἢ ὡς τρέφειν αὐτάρκως οὐχ ὁμοίως τοῖς συμμέτροις, ἀλλ' ἐλάττονά τε τὴν τροπὴν ἐργάζεται καὶ μέχρι χρόνου βραχέος.

[4] Ibid., 17, 152–3: οἶνος τὰ μὲν ἄλλα παραπλήσιος σιτίοις τρέπει τοὺς σφυγμούς, διαφέρει δὲ τῷ τε παραχρῆμα τὴν τροπὴν ἐργάζεσθαι ἀπ' οἴνου τῆς ἀπὸ σιτίων, καὶ τῷ τὸ τάχος πλέον αὔξειν καὶ τὸ μέγεθος ἤπερ τὴν σφοδρότητα καὶ πυκνότητα. σχεδὸν γὰρ ὅσῳ σφοδροτέραν τε καὶ διαρκεστέραν ἰσχὺν ἡ σύμμετρος τροφὴ παρέχει, τοσούτῳ καὶ τὸ μέγεθος ὁ οἶνος ἐξαίρει.

a rather rare pulse which, besides being strong, is both big and hard—
an almost contradictory condition—for hardness tends, as we have seen,
to diminish the size of the pulse. The pulse produced under the influence
of wine has the peculiarity that it makes the movement of systole most
easily perceptible.[1]

Galen now proceeds to examine the effects upon the pulse of various
kinds of emotion. Anger makes a high pulse, large, strong, quick, and
frequent.[2] Pleasure, on the other hand, makes the pulse large and rare
and slow, but makes no difference to its strength.[3] A strong attack of
fear, in the sense of swift present uncontrolled fright, makes the pulse
quick, quivery, irregular, and uneven, whereas the memory of a past
attack of fright has the same effect on the pulse as pain or sorrow.[4]
Pain also changes the pulse, particularly a fierce attack, or one in a vital
part, and so does inflammation.

Galen spends a lot of time describing, especially in the *De causis
pulsuum* and in the *De praesagitione ex pulsibus,* the different kinds of
pulse characteristically associated with various morbid conditions and
diseases. These include what we should still today call pleurisy and
pneumonia, though the latter under Galen's classification would also
have included bronchitis, *angina gutturis,* which probably besides croup
included diphtheria, dropsy, convulsions, epileptic fits, empyema, ele-
phantiasis (a very obscure disease not to be associated with that called by
the same name today), phrenitis, a disease characterized with delirium
(cf. 'brain fever'), lethargy, a condition of un- or semi-consciousness,
inflammation in general, the pulse characteristic of the terminal stages
of many diseases and, in one case, that caused by the administration of a drug, namely hellebore. Lack of space and also perhaps of
direct relevance to my main thesis unfortunately prevents me from reproducing these interesting observations, many of which must have been
based on clinical experience. It is, moreover, important to remember
that all these elaborate differentiations of the various pulses which to
us may appear absurd were to Galen of immense clinical significance,
since they were perhaps the chief instrument of one of the two principal

---

[1] *De dignosc. puls.* i. 6, K. viii. 801 : ἐλέχθη δ᾽ ὅτι καὶ ἡ σκληρότης συντελεῖ τι πρὸς τὴν τῆς
συστολῆς διάγνωσιν . . . τῷ γὰρ πληγῆς βιαίῳ μέγα συμβάλλεται καὶ ἡ τοῦ χιτῶνος τῆς ἀρτηρίας
σκληρότης . . . μέγας δὲ σφυγμὸς οὔτε ῥᾳδίως μίγνυται τῷ σκληρῷ . . . τοῖς ἰσχυροῖς μὲν τὴν ζωτικὴν δύναμιν, ἣν καὶ ζωτικὸν τόνον ἔνιοι τῶν ἰατρῶν καλοῦσι, πλημμελήσουσι δὲ κατὰ τὴν δίαιταν
ἄλλα τέ τινα, οὐχ ἥκιστα δὲ καὶ περὶ τὰς τῶν οἴνων οὐκ ἐν καιρῷ πόσεις οἱ τοιοῦτοι συμπί-
πτουσι σφυγμοί.

[2] *De causis puls.* iv. 2, K. ix. 157: θυμοῦ μὲν ὑψηλός ἐστιν ὁ σφυγμὸς καὶ μέγας καὶ σφοδρὸς
καὶ ταχὺς καὶ πυκνός.

[3] Ibid., 3, 159: ἡδονῆς δὲ μέγας καὶ ἀραιὸς καὶ βραδύς, οὐ μὴν σφοδρότητί γε διάφορος.

[4] Ibid., 4, 160: λύπης δὲ μικρὸς καὶ ἀμυδρὸς καὶ βραδὺς καὶ ἀραιός. Ibid., 5 : φόβου δὲ τοῦ μὲν
ὑπογυίου καὶ σφοδροῦ ταχὺς καὶ κλονώδης καὶ ἄτακτος καὶ ἀνώμαλος, τοῦ δὲ ἤδη κεχρονισμένου
οἷος ὁ τῆς λύπης.

tasks of the physician, laid down by medical tradition since the days of Hippocrates, namely prognosis, which by Galen's time was inseparably allied to what we now call diagnosis.

At the end of the fourth book of *On prognostications from the pulse*, Galen tries to sum up the practical purposes of his elaborate descriptions and explanations, namely prognosis. The diagnosis of any present illness is simply the discovery of the morbid condition; that of antecedents the discovery of the causes which created these conditions.[1] And prognosis is essentially the prediction of the future from the present. First and foremost, how the illness is going to terminate, in death or in recovery, and secondly, in what space of time. In all these cases, the prognosis is made from the morbid conditions, which will demonstrate the kind of illness that the patient is suffering and the degree of his strength or weakness. Now the nature of the illness is diagnosed from the location of the symptoms and from the condition of the part of the body in which they are found. And the strength of the patient is diagnosed from the nature of the elemental mixture of the solid or liquid constituents of the body.[2] Now the critical question is whether the strength of the patient is going to be able to tolerate the high point of the disease, that is to resist it when it reaches its maximum severity. If so, the patient will certainly recover, unless some external mishap intervenes. If not, the patient will certainly die.[3] Patients will recover at that point in time at which nature has completely overcome the morbid condition; they will die when the illness is so much stronger than their strength that one of the functions necessary to life is abolished.[4]

Now the loss or destruction of one of the functions necessary to life brings about suffocation or a collapse of the vital power, or something

---

[1] *De praesag. ex puls.* iv. 11, K. ix. 417: ἡ μὲν δὴ τῶν ἐνεστώτων διάγνωσις οὐδὲν ἄλλο ἐστὶν ἢ διαθέσεων εὕρεσις· ἡ δὲ τῶν προγεγονότων οὐδὲν αὖ πάλιν ἄλλο ⟨?ἢ⟩ τῶν τὰς διαθέσεις ἐργαζομένων αἰτίων.

[2] Ibid., 417–18: ὅτι δὲ καὶ ἡ τῶν μελλόντων πρόγνωσις ἐκ τῶν ἐνεστώτων γίνεται, πολλάκις μὲν ἤδη καὶ διὰ τῶν ἔμπροσθεν εἰρημένων ἐνεδειξάμεθα, καὶ νῦν δ' ἀναγκαῖον ἅπαντα διελθεῖν ἐπὶ κεφαλαίων τὸν λόγον ἀρχὴν αὐτῶν τήνδε ποιησαμένους τῆς περὶ τὸ μέλλον ἀποβήσεσθαι διαγνώσεως. ἐν μὲν πρῶτόν ἐστιν εἰς ὅ τι τελευτήσει τὸ νόσημα, πότερον εἰς ὄλεθρον, ἢ εἰς σωτηρίαν· ἕτερον δ' ἐπ' αὐτῷ δεύτερον, ἐν τίνι μάλιστα τοῦτ' ἔσται χρόνῳ. καὶ τρίτον δ' ἐπὶ τούτοις τίς ὁ τρόπος ἔσοιτο τοῦ τε θανάτου καὶ τῆς σωτηρίας. ἁπάντων δὲ τούτων ἡ πρόγνωσις ἐκ τῶν διαθέσεών ἐστιν. ἐξ αὐτῶν γάρ, ὡς ἐδείξαμεν, ἥ τε τοῦ νοσήματος ἰδέα καὶ τῆς δυνάμεως ἀρρωστία τε καὶ ῥώμη διαγιγνώσκεται. τούτων δ' ἀλλήλοις παραβαλλομένων τὰ μέλλοντα γενήσεσθαι προγινώσκεται. τοῦ μὲν γὰρ νοσήματος ἡ γνῶσις ἐκ τόπου τοῦ πεπονθότος ἐστὶ καὶ τῆς ἐν αὐτῷ διαθέσεως· τῆς δὲ δυνάμεως ἐκ τῆς εὐκρασίας τε καὶ δυσκρασίας τῶν στερεῶν σωμάτων.

[3] Ibid., 418: ἀλλήλοις δὲ τούτων παραβαλλομένων, εἰ μὲν οἷά τέ ἐστι τὴν ἀκμὴν τοῦ νοσήματος ἐνεγκεῖν ἡ δύναμις, ἀνάγκη σωθῆναι τὸν ἄνθρωπον, ἔξωθέν γε μηδενὸς ἁμαρτηθέντος· εἰ δ' οὐχ οἷά τε, πάντως τεθνήξεσθαι.

[4] Ibid., 418–19: τοῦ χρόνου δ' ἡ πρόγνωσις ἐν ᾧ τῶν εἰρημένων ἑκάτερον ἔσοιτο, διὰ τῶνδε γινώσκεται. σωθήσονται μὲν οἱ μέλλοντες σῴζεσθαι κατ' ἐκεῖνον τὸν χρόνον ἐν ᾧπερ ἂν ἡ φύσις ἐπικρατήσῃ τελεώτατα τῆς νοσώδους διαθέσεως· τεθνήξεται δὲ κατ' ἐκεῖνον τὸν χρόνον ἐν ᾧπερ τὸ νόσημα τῆς δυνάμεως εἰς τοσοῦτον ἔσται κρεῖττον ὡς ἐνέργειάν τινα τῶν πρὸς τὸ ζῆν ἀναγκαίων ἀπολέσθαι.

analogous to this collapse like suffocation. The big dyscrasies of the body of the heart, however they arise, whether directly from that organ itself or from morbid conditions transmitted by any other organ, bring on a collapse of the vital power, just as weaknesses of the psychic power follow the big dyscrasies of the brain, and suffocations as it were from congestion of the ventricles and the obstruction of the paths leading to them.[1]

Now the connecting link between these phenomena and the vital force is so to speak the pulse, for the pulse is essentially the activity of this force.[2] When the pulse is weak it is a sign that proportionately this vital force is failing in strength, a condition which affects the whole body, when it is the body of the heart which is in a state of dyscrasy, but only the particular part of the body when it is the arteries in that region which are suffering from this condition.[3]

From the historical point of view, the really interesting thing seems to me to be that in spite of their grotesquely faulty haemodynamics, the ancient Greeks did nevertheless succeed in observing and classifying so accurately so many different characteristics and variations of the pulse in an objective manner quite different from the fantastic descriptions of those other ancient champions of pulse-lore, the Chinese. Though the ancient Greeks had no intelligible concept of arterial elasticity, still less of blood-pressure, they were not so very far from the facts when they looked upon the pulse as a momentary change in the calibre of the artery expanding and contracting, both of which movements occupied a perceptible time. Nor was their distinction of speed from frequency wholly absurd, since it implied an inkling of the different kymographic patterns which modern medical techniques were to reveal. They had discovered, too, differences in the strength of the beat, though wholly unaware of the reasons for them, and they had stumbled upon a concept

---

[1] Ibid., 419–20: τῶν γὰρ ἀπολλυμένων ἐνεργειῶν ἀναγκαίων εἰς τὸ ζῆν ἔνιαι μὲν πνῖξιν ἐπιφέρουσιν, ἔνιαι δὲ τῆς ζωτικῆς δυνάμεως κατάπτωσιν, ἔνιαι δ' ἀνάλογον τῆς ζωτικῆς καταπτώσίν τε καὶ οἷον πνῖξιν. αἱ μὲν οὖν τῆς ζωτικῆς δυνάμεως ἐπιφέρουσαι πνῖξιν ἐκ τῶν τοῦ θώρακός τε καὶ πνεύμονος, ἔτι τε τραχείας ἀρτηρίας καὶ λάρυγγος καὶ φάρυγγος ὁρμῶνται διαθέσεων· ἔνιαι δὲ καὶ κατ' αὐτὴν εὐθέως συνίστανται τὴν καρδίαν. αἱ δὲ τὴν κατάπτωσιν ἔκ τε τῶν στομαχικῶν ὀνομαζομένων διαθέσεων, ἐφ' αἷς συγκόπτονται, καὶ προσέτι τῶν καθ' ἧπαρ χρονίων, ἐφ' αἷς ἀτροφοῦσι, καὶ ἀλγημάτων χρονίων ἢ σφοδρῶν, ἔτι τε τῶν ἑκτικῶν ἁπάντων πυρετῶν. συνελόντι δὲ φάναι, τοῦ τῆς καρδίας σώματος αἱ μεγάλαι δυσκρασίαι, καθ' ὃν ἄν τινα τρόπον ἢ αὐταὶ καθ' ἑαυτὰς εὐθὺς ἐξ ἀρχῆς, ἢ δι' ἕτερα σπλάγχνα πάθωσι, κατάπτωσιν ἐπάγουσι τῆς ζωτικῆς δυνάμεως. οὕτω δὲ καὶ τῆς ψυχικῆς δυνάμεως αἱ μὲν ἀρρωστίαι ταῖς ἐγκεφάλου μεγάλαις ἕπονται δυσκρασίαις, αἱ δ' οἷον πνίξεις ταῖς τε πληρώσεσι τῶν κοιλιῶν αὐτοῦ καὶ ταῖς ἐμφράξεσι τῶν εἰς αὐτὰς ἡκόντων πόρων.

[2] Ibid., 420: περὶ μὲν δὴ τῶν ἄλλων δυνάμεων ἐν ἑτέρῳ διώρισται, περὶ δὲ τῆς τοὺς σφυγμοὺς ἐργαζομένης, ἣν δὴ καὶ ζωτικὴν ὀνομάζομεν, εἴρηται μὲν καὶ ἐν τούτοις οὐκ ὀλίγα, λεχθήσεται δὲ καὶ νῦν.

[3] Ibid., 12, 421: ἐπειδὰν μὲν ἅπαντες ἀμυδροὶ τυγχάνωσιν ὄντες οἱ σφυγμοί, κατὰ τὸν ἑαυτῆς λόγον ἡ δύναμις ἀρρωστεῖ, καθ' ὅλον μὲν τὸ σῶμα τούτου γινομένου, τοῦ τῆς καρδίας σώματος ἔχοντος δυσκράτως, καθ' ἓν δὲ μόριον ἐκείνου μόνου τοῦ μορίου.

so important today, that of the hardness of the arterial coat, though what they thought they felt can only have been the increase in blood-pressure caused by the systole of the left ventricle. They also distinguished with considerable accuracy different patterns of pulse behaviour which are still recognized today—and all this in spite of the fact that they thought the chief (though not the only) content of the artery was not blood but *pneuma*. And if Galen carried to what must appear to us an absurd degree of complication the subdistinctions of his predecessors' already too elaborate categories, he certainly gives the impression of prolonged study and of a tactile sensibility which cannot just be dismissed as mere imagination. He was certainly the possessor of 'a touch with a mind in it'.

In conclusion we may once more sum up in a brief paragraph the reasons why none of the ancient Greeks, not even Galen, succeeded in arriving at any conception of the circulation. For this three principal theoretical errors, the implications of which have perhaps been developed in this study with unnecessary repetition, were chiefly responsible. Not one of them, curiously enough, is directly connected with the still inadequate knowledge of elementary physics possessed by the Greek scientist even after the great developments of Hellenistic times. The first arises out of their misconception of the nature and function of the pulse itself and the connection between the pulse and the movement of the heart. Erasistratus was nearly right but was misled by the pneumatic theory of Praxagoras, which, though modified, continued to mislead even those who realized that there was blood in the arteries. The second was the conception of the heart as the centre of the respiratory system. This mistaken notion of the functions of both the heart and the vascular system was an error in physiology rather than in physics. The third source of error was also physiological, a faulty, though by no means entirely false, conception of the function of the blood, which caused them all to make the logical deduction from their teleological premises, that the blood was entirely consumed in the replacement of wasted tissues. But for these misconceptions Galen might very well have got there, notwithstanding his rather curious physics. He knew that the right ventricle of the heart propelled blood into the lungs, and he also knew that the left ventricle propelled some blood into the aorta. He knew as well that the arterial and the venous systems were connected throughout the body by a system of capillaries. Had he discovered the valves in the veins, it is just possible that he might have realized that the traditional theory of blood-distribution by the veins was untenable. But even that can hardly be regarded as even probable. Galen's medical outlook was essentially conservative, and such a revolutionary discovery as that of the one-way traffic in the veins towards not away from the heart, which would have made nonsense of all previous physiological thinking, would, I cannot help feeling, have been almost impossible for him to accept. The built-in tradition of his too great physiological errors must have proved too strong. The whole history of the thought of the Renaissance leading up to Harvey seems to confirm this. It was thus that logical deductions drawn from incorrect teleological premises in the last resort prevented the ancient Greek physicians from arriving at the truth.

8 · HEART AND VASCULAR DISEASE

To conclude this study, I should like to add a few paragraphs on the interesting question of how much, or perhaps better how little, the ancient Greeks knew about heart disease. The difficulty of our investigation is greatly increased by one of the paradoxes of Greek medical terminology—the double meaning given to the word *kardia*, which means both the heart and the mouth of the oesophagus. Nor is our inquiry made any simpler by the different theories as to the seat of consciousness and the centre of the 'nervous' system. Thus the doctors who held that this was the heart would naturally attribute to the heart and/or the adjacent diaphragm (φρένες) all diseases resulting in disturbed mental conditions, delirium, and fainting or loss of consciousness. On the other hand, those who regarded the brain as the seat of consciousness would be more likely to associate the diseases of the heart with conditions of humoral imbalance in other parts of the body, such as the lungs and, as we shall see, the stomach. Representatives of both these schools of thought are included in the *Corpus*. Thus, for example, in the treatise *On girls' diseases*, we are told that when the flow of the *menses* is impeded in the growing girl owing to the blocking-up of the mouth of the womb, the menstrual blood, having no outlet, forces its way into the heart and the diaphragm. When this happens, the heart is made stupid. This stupefaction is followed by numbness, and numbness by derangement or madness.[1] So too in the appendix to *Regimen in acute diseases*, the author states that when internal pain arises owing to the influx of black bile and sharp or bitter humours, the veins are 'bitten' and become excessively dry; they are under extreme tension and become inflamed and are drawn tight. The blood is consequently corrupted (coagulated?) and the *pneumata* in it cannot find their natural channels. If the trouble reaches the heart or the liver, or the (great) vein, the patient is seized with fits and madness or paralysis as the result of the fluxions being discharged into the

[1] *On girls' diseases*, v. 1, L. viii. 466 : ὁκόταν οὖν τὸ στόμα τῆς ἐξόδου μὴ ᾖ ἀνεστομωμένον, τὸ δὲ αἷμα πλέον ἐπιρρέη διά τε τὰ σίτια καὶ τὴν αὔξησιν τοῦ σώματος, τηνικαῦτα οὐκ ἔχον τὸ αἷμα ἐκροῦν ἀναΐσσει ὑπὸ πλήθεος ἐς τὴν καρδίην καὶ ἐς τὴν διάφραξιν· ὁκόταν οὖν ταῦτα πληρηθέωσιν ἐμωρώθη ἡ καρδίη. εἶτα ἐκ τῆς μωρώσιος νάρκη· εἶτ' ἐκ τῆς νάρκης παράνοια ἔλαβεν.

surrounding parts, and (the blood-vessel?) drying up because the *pneumata* are not able to make their way through and out.[1]

In the *Coan prognoses* we seem to find a recognition of some connection between inflammation of the lung and heart failure, but it would be rash to build any hypothesis on so slender a foundation as the following of any real acquaintance with what we today call heart disease.[2]

In cases where the whole lung is inflamed, together with the heart, so that it is in contact with the ribs, the patient is wholly paralysed and lies cold and insensible. He dies on the second or third day. If this happens without involving the heart, and is not too severe, patients so affected may live longer and sometimes even recover.   [trs. Chadwick and Mann.]

In the treatise *On the sacred disease*, we also find the notion of the heart being affected by discharges of phlegm producing, *inter alia*, palpitations and air-hunger.[3]

If these discharges should make their way to the heart, the chest is attacked and palpitation or asthma supervenes: some patients even become humpbacked. For when cold phlegm reaches the lungs and the heart, the blood gets chilled, and the blood vessels, as the result of being violently chilled, beat against the lung and the heart, and the heart palpitates, so that under the compulsion of these conditions asthma and orthopnoea ensue. For the patient does not get as much *pneuma* as he wants, until the [cold] phlegm which has poured down has been overcome and after being warmed up has been dispersed into the blood vessels. When this has happened palpitations and asthma cease.[4]

---

[1] *Regimen in acute diseases*, L. ii. 404–6 : ὅταν ἀλγήματα προγένηται μελαίνης χολῆς καὶ δριμέων ῥευμάτων ἐπιρρύσιες γίγνονται· ἀλγέει δὲ τὰ ἐντὸς δακνούμενος· δηχθεῖσαι δὲ καὶ λίην ξηραὶ γενόμεναι αἱ φλέβες ἐντείνονταί τε καὶ φλεγμαίνουσαι ἐπισπῶνται τὰ ἐπιρρέοντα· ὅθεν διαφθαρέντος τοῦ αἵματος καὶ τῶν πνευμάτων οὐ δυναμένων ἐν αὐτῷ τὰς κατὰ φύσιν ὁδοὺς βαδίζειν, καταψύξιές τε γίνονται ὑπὸ τῆς στάσιος καὶ σκοτώσιες καὶ ἀφωνίη καὶ καρηβαρίη καὶ σπασμοί, ἣν ἤδη ἐπὶ τὴν καρδίην ἢ τὸ ἧπαρ ἢ ἐπὶ τὴν φλέβα ἔλθῃ, ἔνθεν ἐπίληπτοι γίγνονται ἢ παραπλῆγες, ἢν ἐς τοὺς περιέχοντας τόπους ἐμπέσῃ τὰ ῥεύματα καὶ ὑπὸ τῶν πνευμάτων οὐ δυναμένων διεξιέναι καταξηρανθῇ.

[2] *Coan prognoses*, ii. 20, L. v. 673 : οἷσι δ᾽ ἅπας ὁ πλεύμων φλεγμήνῃ μετὰ τῆς καρδίης ὥστε καὶ προσπεσέειν πρὸς τὴν πλευρήν, παραλύεται πᾶς ὁ νοσέων, καὶ κεῖται ψυχρὸς ὁ νοσέων ἀναίσθητος· θνήσκει δὲ δευτεραῖος ἢ τριταῖος. ἢν δὲ καὶ χωρὶς τῆς καρδίης συμβῇ καὶ ἧσσον πλέονα χρόνον ζώωσιν, ἔνιοι δὲ καὶ διασώζονται.

[3] *De morbo sacro*, L. vi. 368 : ἄρχεται δὲ φύεσθαι ἐπὶ τοῦ ἐμβρύου ἔτι ἐν τῇ μήτρῃ ἐόντος· καθαίρεται γὰρ καὶ ἀνθέει ὥσπερ τἄλλα μέρεα πρὶν γενέσθαι, καὶ ὁ ἐγκέφαλος ... ἢν δὲ κάθαρσις μὴ ἐπιγένηται, ἀλλὰ συστραφῇ τῷ ἐγκεφάλῳ, οὕτως ἀνάγκη φλεγματώδεα εἶναι. καὶ ὁκόσοισι μὲν παιδίοις ἐοῦσιν ἐξανθέει ἕλκεα καὶ ἐς τὴν κεφαλὴν καὶ ἐς τὰ οὔατα καὶ ἐς τὸν ἄλλον χρῶτα, καὶ σιαλώδεα γίνεται καὶ μυξόρροα, ταῦτα μὲν ῥήϊστα διάγει προϊούσης τῆς ἡλικίης. ἐνταῦθα γὰρ ἀφίει καὶ ἐκκαθαίρεται τὸ φλέγμα, ὃ ἐχρῆν ἐν τῇ μήτρῃ καθαρθῆναι· καὶ τὰ οὕτω καθαρθέντα οὐκ ἐπίληπτα γίνεται ταύτῃ τῇ νούσῳ ὡς ἐπὶ τὸ πουλύ.

[4] Ibid., 9 : ἢν δὲ ἐπὶ τὴν καρδίην ποιήσηται ὁ κατάρροος τὴν πορείην, παλμὸς ἐπιλαμβάνει καὶ ἆσθμα καὶ τὰ στήθεα διαφθείρεται, ἔνιοι δὲ καὶ κυφοὶ γίνονται· ὅταν γὰρ ἐπικατέλθῃ τὸ φλέγμα ψυχρὸν ἐπὶ τὸν πλεύμονα ἢ ἐπὶ τὴν καρδίην, ἀποψύχεται τὸ αἷμα· αἱ δὲ φλέβες πρὸς βίην ψυχόμεναι πρὸς τῷ πλεύμονι καὶ τῇ καρδίῃ πηδῶσι, καὶ ἡ καρδίη πάλλεται, ὥστε ὑπὸ τῆς ἀνάγκης ταύτης τό τε ἆσθμα ἐπιπίπτειν καὶ τὴν ὀρθοπνοίην. οὐ γὰρ δέχεται τὸ πνεῦμα ὅσον ἐθέλει, ἄχρι κρατηθῇ τοῦ φλέγματος τὸ ἐπιρρυὲν καὶ διαθερμανθὲν διαχυθῇ ἐς τὰς φλέβας· ἔπειτα παύεται τοῦ παλμοῦ καὶ τοῦ ἄσθματος.

Here, too, some connection between acute diseases of the chest like pneumonia and bronchitis and abnormal behaviour of the heart is plainly indicated, but of heart disease in its technical sense there is no sign of any intuition.

There was, however, one 'disease' which seems to have had a fairly long history, the so-called cardiac passion, which started as a violently painful disturbance of the mouth of the oesophagus and finished up as something not unlike heart-failure in the modern sense.[1] About this disease there would appear to have been marked differences of opinion as to its origin, at least since the time of Erasistratus. A full account of this *cardiaca passio* is found in the second book of the *De morbis acutis* of Caelius Aurelianus, which is presumably a translation of, or at any rate based on, the work of the Methodist Soranus.[2] Here the symptoms and treatment of the disease are gone into at some length. Two kinds are distinguished. Both would appear to be characterized by a biting pain in the mouth of the oesophagus, but one is distinguished from the other by two characteristic symptoms, profuse sweating and a particular type of weak pulse.

Our author next proceeds to discuss the seat of the disease. Some, of whom the first appears to have been Erasistratus, who was followed in this matter by Asclepiades, looked upon it as a tumour or swelling of the heart. Others, including, as we shall see, Galen, as well as the author of the *Definitiones medicae*, regarded the *passio cardiaca* as an affection of the oesophagus.[3] Others considered it a disease of the pericardium or of the diaphragm, others of the liver, or the lung.[4] It would appear that the disease was generally looked upon as seated in the first place in the oesophagus and the mouth of the stomach, resulting in a melting away of the innate 'tone', which must presumably be identified with the vital force, but some, we are told, believe that it is the result of an

---

[1] Caelius Aurelianus, *De morbis acutis*, II. xxx: 'Cardiacam passionem aiunt quidam duplici significatione nuncupari, communi et propria. Sed communem dicunt eam quae substantiam in stomacho atque ore ventris habuerit, ubi etiam mordicatio sequitur supradictarum partium, ut Hippocrates primo et secundo libro Epidemion commemorat, et Erasistratus libris quos De ventre scripsit. Propriam autem dicunt eam quae cum sudore fuerit atque pulsu imbecillo, de qua nunc dicere suscipimus.'

[2] Ibid., xxxi: 'Cognitio igitur sive intelligentia eius passionis ab Artemidoro Sidensi Erasistrati sectatore tradita est hoc modo: cardiaca, inquit, passio est tumor secundum cor. Item Asclepiadis sectatores aiunt tumorem secundum cor, corpusculorum coacervatione sive obtrusione effectum.'

[3] 'Galen', *Definitiones medicae*, def. cclxv, K. xix. 420 f.: καρδιακὴ διάθεσίς ἐστι τῆξις τοῦ ἐμφύτου τόνου καὶ πάρεσις. γίνεται δὲ τοὐπίπαν ἐπὶ στόματι γαστρὸς κακοπραγοῦντι καὶ στομάχῳ μεθ᾽ ἱδρώτων ἀκατασχέτων. τινὲς δὲ ᾠήθησαν ἐπὶ καρδίᾳ φλεγμαινούσῃ γίνεσθαι τὸ πάθημα καὶ διὰ ταύτην τοῦ τόνου τὴν ἔκλυσιν καρδιακὴν ἤτοι διάθεσιν ἢ συγκοπὴν ἐκάλεσαν τὸ συμβαῖνον.

[4] Caelius Aurelianus, op. cit., xxxiv: Praepati in cardiacis Erasistratus et Asclepiades cor dixerunt, alii membranam quae cor circumtegit, alii diaphragma, . . . alii stomachum, alii pulmonem, atque iecur.

inflammation of the heart which results in a dissolution of the vital tone of the heart and its syncope or collapse.

To the ear of the layman it might sound peculiar that the seat of an acute disease resulting in a sharp pain should remain so uncertain, but Siegel pointed out that

the Roman author was faced with the same difficulties which any contemporary physician encounters unless he is aided by modern diagnostic methods. On purely clinical evidence it is often absolutely impossible to make a definite diagnosis of an acute disease of stomach, gall-bladder, or heart.[1]

To what extent could the ancient physician distinguish the pain caused by gall-stones from that caused by angina pectoris? Asclepiades and his disciples thought that the heart-swelling was caused by the heaping up or obstruction of the pores of the heart wall, by atoms too large to pass through them.

Asclepiades differentiated the signs of the heart disease from those of a stomachic complaint by the fact that in the heart disease the pulse is always very small and weak, though the beating or leaping (*saltus*) of the heart itself is greater, indeed violent, and there is 'heaviness'—presumably a translation of the Greek πόνος, and perhaps best rendered into English in this context by the word *pain*—of the thorax and laboured breathing or suffocation, while in those suffering from a stomachic attack of pain, there is a strong pulse in the arteries, but the beating of the heart is found to be weak.[2] The symptom on which the cardiac, as opposed to the stomachic, theorists relied was that, once the attack had developed, palpitations of the heart supervened and pain, praecordial pain in the vicinity of the left nipple. They also laid stress on the great seriousness of these attacks, which proved that one of the most important organs of the body was involved, not merely the terminal portion of the oesophagus.

Soranus, as we have seen (p. 434, n. 1), seems to distinguish two forms of disease, each characterized by violent pain at the mouth of the stomach. The first, the 'common passion', would appear to be identical with καρδιωγμός to be described below, while the second, the 'cardiac passion' proper, is accompanied by profound sweating, and the collapse of the vital forces and terminal heart-failure. He maintained that there were no

---

[1] Siegel, 'Descriptions of circulatory collapse and coronary thrombosis in the fifth century A.D. by Caelius Aurelianus', *Am. J. Cardiol.* (1961), 427.

[2] Caelius Aurelianus, *De morb. ac.* II. xxxv: 'Asclepiades igitur haec discernens ait cardiacos atque eos qui stomachi supinitate decoquuntur ita internosci, quod in cardiacis omnis pulsus sit parvissimus atque imbecillus, cordis vero saltus maior et vehemens, cum gravedine thoracis atque spiratione praefocabili. In his vero qui stomacho patiente deficiunt atque coacervant caeteris arteriis pulsus cordis imbecillus invenitur exceptis caeteris accidentibus, quae symptomata Graeci vocaverunt. Nos vero magnitudinem pulsus in corde fieri cardiacis non invenimus.'

symptoms of swelling and that most authorities denied that the heart was involved at all. The whole body is involved and the dispute about the particular organ involved should be abandoned. The cardiac passion is an acute swift dissolution of the body through all its passages and pores. The antecedents of its onset are various, chronic indigestion and alcoholic indulgence, baths after a heavy meal, postprandial vomiting and even psychological disturbances like depression or fear. But its most frequent emergence is on the fifth or sixth day of non-intermittent fevers and those of a hot and burning nature.[1]

The various symptoms preceding and accompanying an attack are described at some length: acute, very rapid and inflammatory fever, pulse quick, frequent—no doubt the word πυκνός in the original was translated as *densus*—and low—i.e. the artery does not rise up to the finger—and, as it were, damp all through the time the attack is developing, sometimes even to the very end, and if the temperature drops at all, the pulse does not seem to get any stronger, indeed it appears even more submerged. Sometimes it becomes quite irregular, not that it drops beats, but compelled by their speed the jumps of the pulse are folded one upon the other, so that they merely lack order.[2] As the attack proceeds, the patient's limbs become cold and difficult to move, the pulse frequent, quick and small, empty and, as it were, liquid, and as the condition deteriorates, also submerged, difficult to distinguish, tremulous and ant-like and disordered and intermittent. Hallucinations occur, depression and continuous sleeplessness, and in some cases sudden, massive sweating throughout the whole body, sometimes watery and then thick, sticky, and evil-smelling. Respiration small, breathing difficult and painful, speech tremulous, face pale, sunken eyes, pains in the chest, fainting from weakness. . . . When the patient is sinking, the sight is darkened, the limbs be-

---

[1] Caelius Aurelianus, op. cit., xxxi: Soranus vero . . . tumoris inquit signum nullum subesse quod in cardiacis videatur. Item cor pati non valde plurimis probabile videtur. Sed ait cardiacam esse passionem solutionem celerem atque acutam qua disici corpora per omnes viarum particulas apprehendit. . . . Sed praecedentes causae quibus haec passio sufficitur multae atque variae sunt, magis autem iugis indigestio vel vinolentia aut post cibum lavacra, aut post coenam vomitus, aut maestitudo vel timor: in quae consentiens corpus solvitur in sudores. Emergit autem frequentius quinta vel sexta die in febribus continuis, vel ardentibus atque flammatis.

Cf. ibid., xxxiv: Nos vero cum Sorani iudicio totum videmus corpus in solutionem laxari, totum necessario pati accipimus. Et neque valde nobis de praepatienti loco certandum est.

[2] Ibid., xxxii: 'Intelligimus eos qui in cardiacam passionem declives atque proni videntur, et eos qui sunt iam in eadem constituti, ex his signis quae concurrunt. Sequitur enim in passionem pronos febris acuta atque celerrima et flammosa, pulsus celer densus humilis et quasi humectus toto accessionis tempore, aliquando etiam usque ad demissionem, ut etiam si fervoris relevatio fuerit quadam circumscriptione collecta, non tamen simili profectu pulsus quoque erigi videatur, quippe cum magis sui comparatione demersior esse noscatur. Aliquando etiam ut inordinatus occurrit, sed non ita ut deficiens intelligatur, sed celeritate coactus implicatis saltibus ordine careat modo.'

come livid and the nails clubbed, but most retain their mental clearness, palpitations of the heart become more frequent and then the heart-beat fails, the surface of the body becomes wrinkled, and symptoms common to the dying occur, such as bowel-movements. Involuntary weeping is also a dangerous sign and discharges from the eye, as well as disturbance of the digestion. An even more dangerous sign is delirium, since we are unable to restore strength by the administration of food to the patient who is melting away, and even worse, the recurrence of fever after a meal, and the subsequent invisible dissolution in sweat continuing for many days and terminating in a kind of rottenness. In certain cases the forces of the patient dissolve without any sweating, and their natural strength fades away and disperses in what the Greeks call invisible dissolution.[1] Siegel regards this account as containing an exact description of atrial fibrillation portending imminent vascular collapse. He remarks further:

Caelius Aurelianus gave an excellent description of circulatory collapse in connection with febrile diseases. He also seems to have observed cases of shock which accompany the acute onset of atrial fibrillation . . . The cardinal symptoms of acute coronary thrombosis also can be found in these chapters: precordial heaviness, pain (especially in the left side near the mamilla), the choking sensation, the collapse with clear mind, and poor prognosis.[2]

[1] Ibid.: At vero si iam fuerit praesens, sequitur aegros articulorum frigidus torpor, aliquando etiam omnium crurum vel manuum aut totius corporis. Pulsus densus, celer, parvus, imbecillis, inanis et quasi fluens, increscente passione etiam demersus, obscurus, tremulus et formicabilis, et inordinatus ac deserens, attestante hallucinatione, desponsione, cum vigiliis iugibus. Et quibusdam repentinus atque coacervatus per totum corpus sudor, quibusdam vero primum cervice tenus et vultus (-u?) parvus, tenuis, aquatus, dehinc per totum . . . corpus plurimus; tunc crassus et tractuosus atque viscosus, vel male redolens tamquam lotura carnis. Respiratio parva atque anhela et insustentabilis, et per profectum rara locutio ac tremula, ora pallida, oculi concavi, thoracis gravedo, debilitatis causa animi defectus imminentibus accessionibus. . . .

Deficiente aegro, visus obscuritas, articulorum livor, unguium uncatio, quam gryposin vocant, et plurimis mentis integer sensus, quibusdam vero falsitas intellectus, cordis saltus crebrior, dehinc deficiens, corporis superficies rugosa, et ea quae pereuntibus frequenter occurrunt ut solutio ventris. Perniciosum etiam signum est involuntaria lacrimatio, hoc est, sine ulla ratione, vel oculorum ex aliqua parte saniosa atque purulenta similitudo, vel ex oculi circulo qui nigro cum colore apparet albedo, que in unguis similitudinem vel nascentis vel crescentis lunae cornibus respondens, paulatim sumat augmentum: hunc Graeci onycha vocaverunt. Item coacervata atque non masticata cibi transvoratio, . . . Est etiam gravius diaphoreticum delirare, siquidem neque vini datione neque varietate ciborum ad sublevandas vires constantius uti possumus. Item gravius est post dationem ac resumptionem rursum in febres recurrere, tunc cum quadam maestitudine latenter disici per sudorem atque marcere. Etenim solubile ac dimissum sit aegrotantibus . . . multis diebus marcore quodam demersi moriuntur. . . . In quibusdam etiam sine sudore vires solvuntur, et naturalis vigor disiectione occulta, quam Graeci adelon diaphoresin vocant, extinguitur, cum omnis corporis habitudo laxior atque dimissa et friabilis fuerit facta . . .

[2] Siegel, op. cit., p. 428. 'Apparently he observed imminent vascular collapse resulting from atrial fibrillation. According to his exact description the pulse did not show any rhythm, but was not interrupted by pulseless periods. The pulse beats succeeded each other so fast and the little waves came so close together that he could hardly distinguish the single beats.'

Finally, a distinction is made of the *cardiaca passio* from another complaint called *cardimona*, which is a translation of the Greek καρδιωγμός. This is invariably accompanied by sharp pain of the mouth of the stomach generally called by laymen 'heart-pain'. But the 'cardiac passion' must not be confused with this; it is an acute and violent dissolutionary disease, though it may be accompanied by certain accidental tensions or swellings of the middle parts, which must not be regarded as of specific significance as peculiar symptoms or complications affecting cardiacs.[1] Siegel identifies καρδιωγμός with angina pectoris.[2]

Aretaeus, the famous Cappadocian physician—regarded until quite recently as a contemporary of Vespasian but now considered a contemporary of Galen—who wrote in the Ionic dialect of the *Hippocratic corpus*, definitely identified the 'cardiac passion' with syncope of the heart. He repudiates any idea that would attribute it to the oesophagus or the stomach. It is one of the great destroyers, an extremely acute and dangerous disease, which causes swift or sudden death. Once it has a tight hold it will not let go, but turns to dissolution, since it unties the bonds of life which are knotted in the heart.[3] He then goes on to describe the symptoms which accompany a death from heart failure which clearly indicate that it is the heart not the 'stomach' that is affected by them. These symptoms include a small and weak pulse, a noisy heart-beat, where the heart is leaping powerfully, fainting, blackouts, numbness and paralysis of the limbs, profuse ungovernable sweating, coldness of the whole body, loss of sensation and speech. He also appears to distinguish the symptoms of collapse due to poisons which affect the heart, from those forms of syncope derived from prolonged violent fevers.

---

[1] Caelius Aurelianus, op. cit., xxxv: 'Vocatur autem secundum aliquos quaedam passio etiam cardimona, quam Graeci cardiogmon vocaverunt, quam necessario sequitur dolor oris ventris, quem plurimi idiotae cordis dolorem vocaverunt. Generaliter autem cardiaca passio est solutionis atque una acutarum et vehementium passionum. Sed aliquando huic miscentur quaedam stricturae accidentia, ut tensio vel tumor partium mediarum, quae non speciali concursu ac significatione sint cardiacis adscribenda.'

In this connection, it must be remembered that καρδιωγμός already appears in the *Hippocratic corpus*, where it appears to be associated with the gall-bladder and not the heart. Thus in the *De morbis*, iv. 40, we are told: ἔχει δὲ καὶ τόδε ὅτι ἐς μὲν τὸ χωρίον τὸ ἐπὶ τῷ ἥπατι ἀπὸ τῶν βρωτῶν καὶ τῶν ποτῶν ἀποκρίνεται ἡ χολὴ μοῦνον· τὰ γὰρ φλέβια ἀσθενέα καὶ λεπτὰ ὑπάρχοντα οὐ δύναται ἕλκειν τὴν ἄλλην ἰκμάδα παχυτέρην καὶ βαρυτέρην ἐοῦσαν, καὶ ἅμα εὐρυχωρίη οὐκ ἔστι τῇ ἄλλῃ ἰκμάδι, ὥστε ἐν τούτῳ τῷ χωρίῳ εἶναι· σύνηθές τέ ἐστι τῇ χολῇ τοῦτο τὸ χωρίον κατὰ φύσιν μάλιστα, καὶ διὰ τοῦτο ἐν αὐτῷ οὐδεμία νοῦσος γίνεται ἄλλη ἢ ἥντινα καρδιωγμὸν οἱ ἄνθρωποι καλέουσιν.

[2] Siegel, op. cit., p. 430.

[3] Aretaeus, *On the causes and signs of acute diseases*, ii. 3 (*C.M.G.* vol. II, Berlin, 1958): τί μὲν γὰρ μέζον ἢ ὠκύτερον συγκοπῆς δυνάμιος; τί δὲ οὔνομα ἕτερον ἐς ἐπίκλησιν τοῦδε τοῦ πράγματος μᾶλλον εὔσημον; τί δὲ καρδίης ἄλλο καιριώτερον ἐς ζωὴν ἢ ἐς θάνατον; οὐδὲ τὴν συγκοπὴν ἄπιστον τῆς καρδίης νοῦσον ἔμμεναι, ἢ αὐτὴν σίνος τῆς ἐν αὐτέῃ τοῦ ζῆν δυνάμιος· τοσόνδε τάχος τοῦ ὀλέθρου, τοιήδε καὶ ἰδέη. ἔστι γὰρ τὸ πάθος λύσις τῶν δεσμῶν τῆς ἐς ζωὴν δυνάμιος, ἀντίξουν τῇ συστάσει τοῦ ἀνθρώπου ἐόν. τῆσδε γὰρ ἀπρὶξ λαβόμενον οὐ μεθίησι, ἀλλ᾽ εἰς διάλυσιν τρέπει.

The close neighbourhood of the mouth of the oesophagus (στόμαχος) to the heart is very important, since the heart draws from the stomachos its own proper nourishment as well as what is injurious to it, as indeed it draws *pneuma* through the lungs in respiration. But the lung is not the first mover (ἀρχή) of breathing in the same sense that the heart is. For the powers or functions do not exist in the organs themselves, but in the place where the principle of life and of force resides. But the stomachos is neither a first principle nor the seat of life. Now a patient can be injured also through the destruction of 'tone' (ἀτονία). Indeed the heart-hitting poisons (βρώματα) do not injure the stomachos, but through it the heart itself, since those who die from these poisons have the symptoms of an affection of the heart, namely small fast pulse, audible heart-beat and violent palpitation, blackout, loss of consciousness, numbness and paralysis of the limbs, profuse uncontrollable sweating, chilling, complete loss of sensation and loss of speech.[1]

Those who die of cardiac syncope (καρδιώσσοντες) have on the other hand rather different symptoms, particularly in the mental sphere. Their senses are abnormally sharp, of both sight and hearing, their judgement is more balanced and their soul is purer, and they are unerring seers of things present and to come. These powers do not arise from the stomachos, but from the heart, the seat of the soul and of the physis. Syncope is a disease of the heart, the dissolution of the 'tone' of the physis as the result of chilling and wetness. For the patients are without heat both within and without, they feel no thirst and their breath is cold, even if their condition arises out of burning fevers from which syncope results. For as long as the physis has force and remains in good elemental proportion, it can overcome all symptoms and keep the patient alive. But once the bond which holds the physis together, that is its 'tone', is loosened, then syncope occurs.[2] Aretaeus now goes on to describe the symptoms of the kind of fever which ends in syncope. Feeling of fire

---

[1] Ibid.: ἀλλὰ γὰρ τῆς καρδίης γειτόνημα καίριόν ἐστι ὁ στόμαχος, ἐξ οὗπερ ἕλκει ἡ καρδίη οἰκεῖον ἢ ἀξύμφορον. καὶ γὰρ καὶ διὰ πνεύμονος ἕλκει πνεῦμα εἰς ἀναπνοὴν ἡ καρδίη, ἀλλ' οὐχὶ πνεύμων ἐξ ἴσης ἀρχῆς ἀναπνεῖ. οὐ γὰρ ἐν τοῖσι ὀργάνοισι αἱ δυνάμιες, ἀλλ' ἔνθα ἡ ἀρχὴ ζωῆς ἦν καὶ ἰσχύος. στόμαχος δὲ οὔτε ἀρχὴ οὔτε χωρίον ζωῆς. βλαβήσεται δέ τις δι' ἀτονίην. καὶ γὰρ καὶ τὰ καρδιοβόλα βρώματα οὐ τὸν στόμαχον σίνεται, ἀλλὰ δι' αὐτέου τὴν καρδίην· ἐπεὶ καὶ οἱ ἐπὶ τοισίδε θνήσκοντες σημεῖα ἴσχουσι καρδίης πάθεος, σφυγμοὺς σμικρούς, ἀδρανέας, πάταγον τῆς καρδίης, ἐπὶ πηδήσει καρτερῇ, σκοτόδινος, λειποθυμίη, νάρκη καὶ παρέσιες μελέων, ἱδρὼς ἄσχετος πουλύς, ψῦξις ὅλου, ἀναισθησίη, ἀφωνίη.

[2] Ibid.: ἐπὶ δὲ τοῖσι καρδιώσσουσι καὶ αἴσθησις ὀξυτέρη, ὡς ἰδεῖν καὶ ἀκοῦσαι μᾶλλον ἢ πρόσθεν, καὶ γνώμη εὐσταθεστέρη καὶ ψυχὴ καθαρωτέρη· καὶ τάδε οὐκ ἐς τὰ παρεόντα μοῦνον ⟨ἀλλὰ⟩ καὶ ἐς τὰ μέλλοντα μάντιες ἀτρεκέες. μὴ ὦν καὶ αἵδε στομάχου [αἱ] δυνάμιες ἀλλὰ καρδίης, ἔνθα καὶ ἡ ψυχὴ καὶ ἡ φύσις αὐτέης ἦν, ἐς ἣν καὶ τὸ πάθος ᾖ τῶν τῆδε δυναμέων. ἔστι δὲ τῆσδε τῆς νόσου ἰδέη ἔκλυσις τοῦ τόνου τῆς φύσιος ἐπ' αἰτίῃ ψύξει καὶ ὑγρότητι· καὶ γὰρ ἄθερμοι, καὶ τὰ εἴσω καὶ τὰ ἔξω, καὶ ἄδιψοι καὶ ψυχρὸν ἀναπνέουσι, κἢν ἐκ μεγάλων καὶ καυσωδέων ἐστὶ πυρετῶν, ἐξ οὗπερ ἐξάπτεται ἡ ξυγκοπή. εὖτε μὲν γὰρ ἔρρωται ἡ φύσις καὶ ἐστὶν εὔκρατος, πάντων μὲν κρατέει, πᾶσι δὲ σημαίνει, καὶ ὑγρῷ, καὶ πνεύματι, καὶ στερεοῖσι, καὶ τῇ τούτων εὐταξίῃ καὶ ξυμμετρίῃ ἐς ζωὴν διέπει τὸν ἄνθρωπον. ἢν δὲ τῆς φύσιος ὁ δεσμός, τουτέστι ὁ τόνος, λυθῇ, τότε γίγνεται τὸ πάθος.

sharp and piercing, great air-hunger, dry tongue, lips, skin, sleeplessness, small, fast, disordered pulse, glittering bright eyes, high colour, cold extremities, etc. As the disease gets worse these symptoms are aggravated and delirium may result or even complete lack of knowledge of the environment, the fingers are cold but the palms of the hands very hot, the respiration very rapid, with beads of sweat on the forehead. If the extreme condition of heat and dryness is reached, then a sort of reversal takes place, what was hot becomes cold and what was dry wet. When syncope occurs, uncontrollable perspiration breaks out all over the body, the breath becomes cold, there is a lot of vapour in the nostrils, but no thirst, since all the thirst-producing organs like the mouth and the stomachos have been dried up. The belly mostly dry, but in some cases there is an abundance of fluid. The bones dissolve into liquid and from all the organs there is a movement outwards of liquid, like a river. Psychic condition, all the senses clean, the intelligence sharp, and the mind prophetic. The patient knows, first, that he is going to die, and then foretells to those who are present, things which will come to be in the future.[1]

With regard to the *cardiaca passio* with which we have been dealing, there is little that Galen adds to previous authorities. He is, of course, aware of the double meaning of the word καρδία, but he will not accept the heart as the primary seat of the disease. He uses, besides the term we have just been examining, *cardiac affection* (καρδιακὴ διάθεσις) and two others, namely, *cardalgia* and *cardiogmos*. The meaning of these latter two seems to be identical. Galen has no doubt that 'heart-burn' in all senses is clearly a stomach complaint, in spite of the fact that some physicians considered it to be an affection of the heart, and thought that καρδιωγμός was a leaping motion of that organ.[2] It is a biting pain accompanied

---

[1] Aretaeus, op. cit., ii. 4: πῦρ μὲν πάντῃ καὶ δριμὺ καὶ λεπτόν, μάλιστα δὲ τὰ εἴσω· ἀναπνοὴ θερμή, ὡς ἐκ πυρός· ἠέρος ὁλκὴ μεγάλη· ψυχροῦ ἐπιθυμίη· γλώσσης ξηρότης· αὐασμὸς χειλέων καὶ δέρματος· ἄκρεα ψυχρά· οὖρα χολόβαφα κατακορέως· ἀγρυπνίη· σφυγμοὶ πυκνοί, σμικροί, ἔκλυτοι· ὀφθαλμοὶ εὐαγέες, λαμπροί, ὑπέρυθροι· προσώπου εὐχροίη· ἢν δὲ ἐπὶ μᾶλλον αὔξῃ τὸ πάθος, μέζω τὰ πάντα καὶ κακίω· σφυγμοὶ σμικρότατοι καὶ πυκνότατοι· πῦρ ξηρότατον καὶ δριμύτατον· γνώμη παράφορος, πάντων ἀγνωσίη· διψώδεες· ψαῦσαι ψυχροῦ ἐπιθυμίη, τοίχου, ἐσθῆτος, ἐδάφεος, ὑγροῦ· χεῖρες ψυχραί, θέναρα θερμότατα· ὄνυχες πελιδνοί· ἀναπνοὴ πυκνή· νοτὶς περὶ μέτωπα καὶ κληῖδας. ἢν δὲ ἐς ἄκρον ξηρότητος καὶ θερμασίης ἥκῃ ἡ φύσις, τὸ μὲν θερμὸν ἐς ψυχρόν, ὁ δὲ αὐχμὸς ἐς ἐπομβρίην τρέπεται. αἱ γὰρ τῶν πρηγμάτων ἐς τὸ ἔσχατον ἐπιτάσιες ἐς τὴν ἐναντίην μεταβάλλουσι ἰδέην. ἐπὴν ὦν λυθῇ τῆς φύσιος τὰ δεσμά, τόδε ἐστὶ ἡ συγκοπή, τότε ἱδρὼς τοῦ σώματος πάντῃ ἄσχετος, ἀναπνοὴ ψυχρή· ἀτμὸς ἀνὰ ῥῖνας πουλύς· ἄδιψοι. ἐξήρανται γὰρ τἆλλα, ἀτὰρ καὶ τὰ ἄλλα διψαλέα ὄργανα, στόμα, στόμαχος· οὖρα λεπτά, ὑδατώδεα· κοιλίη τὰ πολλὰ μὲν ξηρή, ἔστι δὲ [καὶ] οἶσι ὑποφέρει βραχέα χολώδεα· πουλὺς πλάδος. διαρρέουσι δὲ καὶ τὰ ὀστέα λυόμενα, καὶ ἀπὸ πάντων ὡς ἐν ποταμῷ ἐς τὰ ἔξω ἡ φορή. ψυχῆς κατάστασις· αἴσθησις ξύμπασα καθαρή· διάνοια λεπτή· γνώμη μαντική. προγιγνώσκουσι μὲν ὦν πρώτιστα μὲν ωὑτέοισι τοῦ βίου τὴν μεταλλαγήν· ἔπειτα τοῖσι παρέουσι προλέγουσι τὰ αὖθις ἐσόμενα. . . .

[2] *Comment. in Hipp. Aphorism.* lxv, K. xviiʙ, 745–6: ὅτι μὲν οὖν . . . ἀλλὰ καὶ τὸ στόμα τῆς γαστρὸς οἱ παλαιοὶ καρδίαν ὠνόμαζον ἕν τι τῶν ὁμολογουμένων ἐστίν, ὥσπερ γε καὶ ὅτι καρδιαλγίαν τὰ τούτου τοῦ μέρους ἀλγήματα προσαγορεύουσι. τό γε μὴν καρδιώσσειν οἱ πλεῖστοι μὲν τῶν ἐξηγησαμένων τοὺς ἀφορισμοὺς ταυτὸν ἡγοῦνται σημαίνειν τῷ καρδιαλγεῖν. ἔνιοι δὲ τῆς καρδίας

by dizziness, vertigo, and blackouts. The large quantity of nerves connecting the brain with the stomach explains why, when the stomach is ill, the functions of the mind are also disturbed. The disease is due to an accumulation of bad humours in the mouth of the stomach.[1] The humour chiefly concerned is yellow bile, vomiting of yellow bile is accompanied by 'cardialgy'. An excess of yellow bile settling about the mouth of the stomach produces an extremely sharp biting pain as well as nausea and vomiting.[2] Galen is firmly convinced that the heart does not suffer pain,[3] at any rate of this nature. The disease is also characterized by 'syncope'. The exact nature of this gastric syncope is far from clear, nor is its relation to cardiac syncope easy to grasp, as explained by the rather vague notion of sympathy. Moreover, we shall see that cardiac syncope of an independent kind has quite a different explanation. We are told in the treatise *On the affected parts* that stomachic syncopes, by which word he no doubt means a sort of general collapse, produce a dissolution through the peculiar nature of the pain they involve, and perhaps also through the dyscrasia of the stomach penetrating—how is not explained—to the heart, with the result that when that organ is also involved in a great 'faulty humoral mixture', a complete collapse of all power takes place.[4]

Galen now goes on to enumerate the affections or diseases which arise in the heart itself. Most of these consist of various kinds of dyscrasies, even and uneven. Some of these occur at the beginning of attacks of cardiac inflammation or erysipelas. But the patient dies before these illnesses have reached their full development. These affections are also succeeded by cardiac syncopes, just like the stomachic ones, though these clearly imply a sympathetic, i.e. derivative, affection of the heart. Both

αὐτῆς, λέγω δὲ τοῦ σπλάγχνου, καρδιωγμὸν δηλοῦσθαί φασιν, ἐξηγούμενοί τε κίνησίν τινά φασι παλμώδη τὸν καρδιωγμὸν εἶναι.

[1] *Comment. in Hipp. Aphorism.* xvi, K. xviiB. 677 : ὁ δὲ καρδιωγμὸς δῆξίς ἐστι καρδίας, τουτέστι τοῦ στόματος τῆς γαστρός ... σκοτόδινος δ' ἐστίν, ἐπειδὰν ἅμα περιδινεῖσθαι δοκῇ τὰ βλεπόμενα, ἥ τε διὰ τῆς ὄψεως αἴσθησις ἐξαίφνης ἀπολεῖται, δοκούντων αὐτῶν σκότος περικεχύσθαι. γίγνεται δὲ τοῦτο τοῦ στόματος τῆς κοιλίας ὑπὸ μοχθηρῶν χυμῶν δακνομένου. διὰ γὰρ τὸ μέγεθος τῶν νεύρων τῶν ἐξ ἐγκεφάλου καθηκόντων εἰς αὐτὸ βλάπτεται τὰ τῆς ψυχῆς ἔργα κακοπραγοῦντος τοῦ μορίου.
[2] *De usu partium,* v. 4, K. iii. 356–7 : τίς γοῦν ἀγνοεῖ τῆς ξανθῆς χολῆς τὴν δύναμιν ἱκανῶς δριμεῖαν ὑπάρχουσαν δάκνουσάν τε καὶ ῥύπτουσαν ἅπαντα; ... τίς δ' οὐκ οἶδεν, ὡς ἐμέτου χολώδους ἄλλα τέ τινα παθήματα καὶ καρδιαλγία, δῆξις οὖσα τοῦ στόματος τῆς γαστρός, ἐξ ἀνάγκης προηγεῖται; ... εἰ μὲν οὖν ἐπιπολάσειεν ὁ χυμὸς οὗτος ἐπὶ τὸ στόμα τῆς γαστρός, ὡς ἂν αἰσθητικώτατον ὑπάρχον, ἀλγοῦσί τε σφοδρῶς δακνόμενοι πρὸς αὐτοῦ καὶ ναυτιῶσι καὶ ἐμοῦσιν.
[3] *De plac. Hipp. et Plat.* ii. 8, K. v. 275 : ἅπαντες οὗτοι δηλοῦσιν ἐναργῶς, τὸ στόμα τῆς γαστρὸς ὀνομάζεσθαι καρδίαν. ὥστε ταύτης μὲν τῆς καρδίας εἴη ἄν τι πάθος ἡ καρδιαλγία, τοῦ σπλάγχνου δ', ὑπὲρ οὗ πρόκειται σκοπεῖν, εἰ τὸ κυριεῦον τῆς ψυχῆς μόριον ἐν ἑαυτῷ περιέχει, τοιοῦτον πάθος οὐδέποτε γίγνεται.
[4] *De locis affectis,* v. 6, K. viii. 342 f. : αἱ στομαχικαὶ δὲ συγκοπαὶ διὰ τὴν ἰδιότητα τῶν κατ' αὐτὸν ἀλγημάτων ἔκλυσιν ἐπιφέρουσιν, ἴσως δὲ καὶ τῆς δυσκρασίας αὐτοῦ διϊκνουμένης εἰς τὴν καρδίαν, ὡς κἀκείνης ἐν δυσκρασίᾳ μεγάλῃ γινομένης ἀθρόαν κατάπτωσιν ἀκολουθῆσαι τῆς δυνάμεως.

the stomachic and the cardiac syncope are caused by the same circumstances, either merely a strong dyscrasia, or some poisonous liquidity, or even sometimes by erysipelas, inflammation, or some such tumour.[1]

In the fifth book of his treatise *On the affected parts* Galen tries to arrive at some notion of heart disease, distinguishing between heart disease proper, and what we might call functional disturbances due to 'sympathy' with other diseased organs. The heart being the fountain, as it were, of the innate heat, death must in the last resort be due to some kind of heart-failure, since unless the heart failed to function the person would not be dead. Death always follows on extreme 'dyscrasies' of the heart, since all parts of the body are also injured by defects of the heart. He has already demonstrated that the proper functioning of all the other parts of the body is due to the proper temperament, εὐκρασία, of the heart, so that it necessarily follows that when this is destroyed their functioning must also perish, including that of the two other principal organs, the brain and the liver. But not vice versa. For a creature that no longer preserves the power of perception or of voluntary action, or indeed of nutrition, like a hibernating animal, for example, can still be regarded as being able to live, so long as its heart has not suffered injury. But once the heart has been deprived of respiration the creature dies immediately. For this reason in cases of severe stroke, patients die immediately because of the injury to the brain, which paralyses the thoracic muscles and so prevents the heart respiring.[2]

---

[1] *De locis affectis*, v. 2, K. viii. 302: ἴδιον δὲ πάθος ἐν καρδίᾳ γίνεται κατὰ μὲν ἁπλῆν δυσκρασίαν πολλάκις, εἴτ' ἀνώμαλος εἴθ' ὁμαλὴς εἴη, κατά τε φλεγμονὴν ἢ ἐρυσίπελας ἀρχόμενον γίγνεσθαι· διαφθείρεται γὰρ παραυτίκα πρὶν αὐξηθῆναι τὰ πάθη τάδε τὸ ζῷον. ἕπονται δὲ πάλιν ταῖς τοιαύταις διαθέσεσιν αἱ καρδιακαὶ συγκοπαί, καθάπερ αἱ στομαχικαὶ ταῖς κατὰ τὸ τῆς κοιλίας στόμα, καλοῦσι δ' ἔνιοι καὶ τοῦτο στόμαχον. ἀλλὰ καὶ αὗται γίγνονται δηλονότι συμπασχούσης τῆς καρδίας. αἱ διαθέσεις δ' ἀμφοτέρων τῶν μορίων, τοῦ τε στόματος τῆς κοιλίας καὶ τῆς καρδίας, ἤτοι διὰ δυσκρασίαν μόνην ἰσχυράν, ἢ δι' ὑγρότητα φαρμακώδη καί ποτε καὶ δι' ἐρυσίπελας εἰώθασι γίγνεσθαι, καὶ διὰ φλεγμονὴν ἤ τινα παρὰ φύσιν ὄγκον ἕτερον τοιοῦτον.

[2] Ibid., v. 1, K. viii. 298 ff.: οὕτως καὶ ἐπὶ τῆς καρδίας διορίσασθαι χρή, τίνα μὲν ἰδιοπαθούσης ἢ πρωτοπαθούσης ... γίνεται συμπτώματα, τίνα δ' ἑτέροις μέρεσι συμπασχούσης.... ἐδείχθη, τῆς μὲν ἐμφύτου θερμασίας οἷον πηγή τις ὑπάρχειν ἡ καρδία, καὶ πάντως χρῆναι παθεῖν αὐτήν, εἰ μέλλοι τεθνήξεσθαι τὸ ζῷον. ἀρχῶν οὖν οὐσῶν τριῶν, αἷς διοικεῖται τὸ ζῷον ... ὁ μὲν θάνατος ἀεὶ ταῖς ἀμέτροις τῆς καρδίας ἕπεται δυσκρασίαις, ἅπαντα μὲν αὐτῇ συγκακοῦται τὰ μόρια· δεδειγμένου δ' ἡμῖν, ἐνεργεῖν αὐτὰ διὰ τὴν οἰκείαν καρδίας εὐκρασίαν, ἀναγκαῖόν ἐστιν, ἀπολομένης ταύτης συναπόλλυσθαι τὰς ἐνεργείας αὐτῶν, καὶ κατὰ τοῦτο καὶ τὰς ἐγκεφάλου τε καὶ ἥπατος, οὐ μὴν ταῖς ἐκείνων γε τὴν τῆς καρδίας. εἰ γὰρ μήτε τὰς αἰσθητικάς τε καὶ προαιρετικὰς ἐνεργείας ἔτι διασῴζοι τὸ ζῷον, ἀλλὰ μηδὲ τρέφοιτο, καθάπερ οὐδὲ τὰ φωλεύοντα, δυνατὸν ἄν τις εἶναι νομίσειεν ζῆν αὐτό, μέχρι περ ἂν ἡ καρδία μηδὲν ᾖ πεπονθυῖα ... εἰ δὲ τῆς ἀναπνοῆς στερήσειέ τις τὴν καρδίαν, αὐτίκα διαφθείρεται. ὅσοις οὖν ὁ θώραξ οὐδὲν ὅλως ἐδόκει συντελεῖν εἰς τὴν τῆς ἀναπνοῆς ἐνέργειαν, ἀποροῦσι τὴν αἰτίαν εὑρεῖν, δι' ἣν ἐν ταῖς ἰσχυραῖς ἀποπληξίαις ἀποθνήσκουσιν εὐθέως οἱ κάμνοντες, ἐπὶ μόνῃ τῇ βλάβῃ τῆς ἄνωθεν ἀρχῆς· ὑμεῖς δ' οὐκ ἀπορήσετε, πεπεισμένοι βεβαίως, ὑπὸ μυῶν διαστέλλεσθαι τὸν θώρακα, τὴν ἀρχὴν τῆς κινήσεως ἐχόντων ἐκ τῶν εἰς αὐτοὺς φερομένων νεύρων ἀπὸ τοῦ κατὰ τὸν αὐχένα νωτιαίου, στερουμένων τηνικαῦτα τῆς ἐπιρρεούσης ἐξ ἐγκεφάλου δυνάμεως αὐτοῖς κινητικῆς τῶν μυῶν.

This conception of the heart as the fountain of the innate heat and the centre or domicile of the vital powers, entails some interesting nosological implications which we must briefly examine, especially in regard to fever, the essence of which is an unnatural form of heat (παρὰ φύσιν θερμασία). This unnatural heat may be by origin of three kinds. It may arise primarily in the body of the heart itself, or in the humours, or in the pneuma.[1] But whatever its local origin, it does not become a fever until it communicates itself to the heart.[2] Now heat may be generated in a number of ways: (a) by motion, (b) by corruption, for Galen maintains that the rotting of what we would call organic matter always produces heat, (c) by contact with a hot body, what we should call conduction, (d) by the retention of a hot secretion, (e) by the admixture of a hot substance, for example from a boiling fountain. Fevers must be generated by one or more of these five sources.[3] The details of the origins of different kinds of fevers lie outside the scope of this study, except in so far as they affect the vascular system, but it is in this connection that some of Galen's notions need a brief explanation. Fevers are definitely conditions of the heart. They can arise from causes in the external environment, e.g. exposure to heat, from extra-cardiac conditions in the body, such as humoral imbalance and corruption of the humours, from blockage of the pores of the skin and the peripheral arterial system, and from overheating of the heart itself, the boiling of the blood described by Plato,[4] which is the result of anger, for the faculty of anger is located in the heart itself, and Galen tells us that this kind of fever has its beginning or principle (ἀρχή) in the motion and the boiling of the innate heat. Galen thus propounds a theory of direct psycho-physical interaction. Not only anger but pain and grief can also produce fever through their influence on the action of the heart.[5] The fevers arising out of the blockage of the pores and the blood vessels are the result of the failure of perspiration (διαπνοή) which prevents the innate heat being properly cooled by the air introduced

---

[1] De feb. diff. i. 3, K. vii. 281: αἱ διαφοραὶ δὲ κατὰ γένος τῆς θερμότητος, . . . ἀπὸ τῆς τῶν ὑλῶν διαφορᾶς ἐλαμβάνοντο τῶν δεχομένων τὴν πυρετώδη θερμασίαν, τριῶν οὐσῶν κατὰ γένος. ἤτοι γὰρ ἐν αὐτῷ τῷ σώματι τῆς καρδίας ἀνάπτεσθαι πρώτην αὐτὴν ἐλέγομεν, ἢ ἐν τοῖς χυμοῖς, ἢ ἐν τῷ πνεύματι.

[2] Ibid., 4, 283: ἔστι μὲν δήπου καὶ αὐτὸ τοῦτο παρὰ φύσιν θερμότης, οὐ μὴν ἤδη γέ πω πυρετός, εἰ μὴ καὶ συνεκθερμαίνῃ τὴν καρδίαν.

[3] Ibid., 282: ἐπεὶ τοίνυν ὁρῶμεν οὐχ ἕνα τρόπον οὔτε γενέσεως οὔτε αὐξήσεως τῆς θερμασίας, ὅτι μηδὲ αὐτοῦ τοῦ πυρός, ἀλλ' ἤτοι διὰ κίνησιν, ἢ διὰ σῆψιν, ἢ διὰ ὁμιλίαν ἑτέρας θερμότητος, ἢ δι' ἐπίσχεσιν ἀπορροῆς θερμῆς, ἢ δι' ἐπιμιξίαν οὐσίας θερμῆς, ὥσπερ γε ἐκ πηγῆς τινος ἀναζεούσης, . . . ἀνάγκη πάσας τὰς τῶν πυρετῶν αἰτίας εἰς τοὺς εἰρημένους ἀνάγεσθαι τρόπους.

[4] See above, p. 121.

[5] De feb. diff. i. 4, 283: ὁ δέ γε θυμὸς οἷον ζέσις τις καὶ κίνησις σφοδρὰ τῆς θυμοειδοῦς δυνάμεως ἐν τῷ σώματι τῆς καρδίας αὐτῷ καθιδρυμένης. συνεκθερμαίνεται δὲ αὐτῇ ποτὲ μὲν ἡ τοῦ πνεύματος, ἔστιν ὅτε δὲ ἡ τοῦ αἵματος οὐσία, καὶ ἢν ἐπιτηδείως ἔχοντα τύχῃ πρὸς τὸ τὰ δεξάμενα κατασχεῖν ἐπὶ πολὺ τὴν θερμότητα, κἂν τῆς καρδίας ἡ κίνησις καταστῇ, διαμένει ταῦτα παρὰ φύσιν θερμά, κἂν τῷδε πυρέττειν ἀνάγκη τὸν ἄνθρωπον. ὁ μὲν οὖν τοιοῦτος πυρετὸς ἀρχὴν ἔχει τὴν κίνησίν τε καὶ ζέσιν τῆς ἐμφύτου θερμασίας· ὁ δὲ ἐπὶ λύπαις οὐκέτι ζέσιν, ἀλλὰ κίνησιν μόνον.

into the arteries via the pores, and leads to a rotting of the humours.[1] The excess of yellow bile, a hot humour, in the blood is another cause of fever, particularly of tertian fever,[2] while inflammation, by producing heat, also causes fever.[3] In all these cases the fever is produced (by the conduction of the unnatural heat to the body of the heart. The effects of severe continuous fever on the body of the heart are of the greatest importance. They dry out the moisture of the heart's tissues, feeding upon it, as it were, like a flame through the wick. While this moisture still lasts out these fevers are called hectic, but when the natural moisture of the body of the heart is consumed the term marasmic is used.[4] The end of this marasmic process is of course death. But this drying up of the heart's tissues is not only produced by fevers, it is the essential characteristic of the irreversible process of old age, only here the drying of the heart's and other tissues is not the result of overheating, but the concomitant of the general cooling of the ageing body.[5]

Galen mentions two other heart conditions which may cause death. The first of these is a special kind of palpitation caused by the accumulation of a large amount of fluid in the sack of the pericardium which prevents the diastole of the ventricles. He tells us that in his animal dissections he has often found a lot of fluid like water in the pericardium, mentioning particularly the case of a monkey, which died before he was able to vivisect it. Here he found the pericardium swollen by a large volume of water like that of hydatid cysts. He concludes that similar conditions may also be found in human beings, as well as 'scirrous' tumours such as one he once found on the pericardium of a cock, which looked like thick membranes folded on top of each other. In this case there was no pericardial effusion.[6] The second is inflammation, which we have

---

[1] De. feb. diff. i. 5, 287: κατὰ μέντοι τὰς ἐμφράξεις τῶν πόρων καὶ σφηνώσεις τῶν χυμῶν . . . πυρέττει τὰ ζῷα τὸν ἐπὶ σηπεδόνι πυρετόν. ἑτοιμότατα γὰρ σήπεται πάνθ' ὅσα θερμὰ καὶ ὑγρὰ καὶ πολλὰ κατὰ θερμὸν χωρίον εἰ μὴ τύχῃ διαπνοῆς τε ἅμα καὶ ἀναψύξεως.

[2] Ibid., ii. 3, 339: ὁ μὲν γὰρ ἐπὶ τῇ ξανθῇ χολῇ διὰ τῶν αἰσθητικῶν σωμάτων φερομένη γιγνόμενος εἰσβάλλει τε μετὰ ῥίγους καὶ καυσώδης ἐστί, . . . τοῦ τοιούτου πυρετοῦ τὸ μῆκος τοῦ παροξυσμοῦ τὸ μέγιστον ὡρῶν ἐστιν ἰσημερινῶν δώδεκα. καὶ καλοῦμεν αὐτὸν ἀκριβῆ τριταῖον.

[3] Ibid., i. 5, 288: καὶ τὰ φλεγμαίνοντα δὲ μέρη τῆς σήψεως λόγῳ ἀνάπτει πυρετούς.

[4] Ibid., i. 10, 313: γίνονται τοίνυν οἱ ἑκτικοὶ καλούμενοι πυρετοὶ κατὰ διττὸν τρόπον, ὡς τὰ πολλὰ μὲν ἐπὶ τοῖς καυσώδεσιν, ἤτοι μηκυνθεῖσιν εἰς τοσοῦτον, ὡς ἐκδαπανῆσαι τῷ χρόνῳ τὴν ἰκμάδα τοῦ τῆς καρδίας σώματος ἢ καὶ μενούσης ἔτι συχνῆς. ἐνεῖνοι μὲν οὖν οὐχ ἑκτικοὶ μόνον εἰσίν, ἀλλὰ ἤδη καὶ μαρασμώδεις· οἱ δ' ἔτι μενούσης τῆς ὑγρότητος γιγνόμενοι, τὸ σῶμα τῆς καρδίας αὐτὸ καταλαβόντες, ἐντεῦθεν ἀνάπτονται μάλιστα, καθάπερ ἡ τῶν λύχνων φλὸξ ἐκ τῆς θρυαλλίδος.

[5] De marcore, 5, K. vii. 681: τὸν δὲ τοῦ γήρως μαρασμὸν ἀδύνατον δήπου καταλῦσαι, βοηθεῖσθαι δὲ ὡς ἐπιπλεῖστον ἐκταθῆναι δυνατόν, καὶ τό γε γηροκομικὸν ὀνομαζόμενον μέρος τῆς ἰατρικῆς αὐτὸ τοῦτ' ἐστι, σκοπὸν ἔχον . . . ἐνίστασθαι καὶ διακωλύειν ὡς οἷόν τε, μὴ ξηρανθῆναι τὸ σῶμα τῆς καρδίας εἰς τοσοῦτον, ὡς ἐνεργοῦν ποτε παύσασθαι. τοῦτο γὰρ δὴ τὸ πέρας ἐστὶ τῆς ζωῆς, παῦλα τοῦ τῆς καρδίας ἔργου, ὡς μέχρι ἂν ἥδε κινῆται κατὰ τὴν ἑαυτῆς ἐνέργειαν, ἀδύνατον ἀποθανεῖν τὸ ζῷον.

[6] De locis affectis, v. 2, K. viii. 303–4: ἕτερον δὲ παλμὸς τῆς καρδίας ἤτοι μόνος γιγνόμενος, ἢ μετά τινος ἐμφάσεως ἐν ὑγρῷ κινουμένης αὐτῆς (τῆς καρδίας)· καὶ θαυμαστὸν οὐδὲν ἀθροίζεσθαί

already mentioned. During his experience as a surgeon to gladiators he must have seen wounds which exposed the heart, and he notes that deaths very like those of patients who collapse from cardiac syncope taking place from obvious inflammation of the organ. If the wound penetrates the ventricles, particularly the left ventricle, death from haemorrhage takes place immediately, but if the weapon does not actually penetrate the ventricle but remains fixed in the body of the heart, the patients may survive for a short time, not only the remainder of the day in which the wound was inflicted, but even the following night. But they always die, clearly from inflammation. Their consciousness remains unimpaired, a fact which was adduced as a piece of evidence for the ancient doctrine that the heart is not the seat of the intelligence.[1]

It seems to be fairly clear that Galen thought that most, if not all, cases of cardiac syncope were the result of affections of other parts of the body, chiefly the stomach and the brain. He seems to have envisaged this 'sympathy' somewhat on the following lines. Both nerves and arteries served as conducting media. The centre of the trouble of 'cardialgy' is the stomach, and the more sensitive its nerves the greater the pain and the readier the transmission to the other two ἀρχαί, the brain and the heart. There are thus four conditions which combine to produce syncope: a strong and painful affection of the mouth of the stomach, a very delicate sensitivity of its nervous connections, and (what seems a little curious) a weakness in the nerves themselves or the arteries, as well as the brain and the heart.[2] Thus some patients through their lack of stomachic tone have epileptic fits, loss of consciousness, coma, seizures, spells of madness, and fits of melancholy, owing to the sympathetic reaction of the nervous system, the ruling centre (ἀρχή) of the

ποτε πλῆθος ὑγροῦ τοσοῦτον ἐν τῷ περιέχοντι χιτῶνι τὴν καρδίαν, ὡς ἐμποδίζειν αὐτῇ διαστελλομένῃ· καὶ γὰρ ἐπὶ τῶν ἀνατεμνομένων ζῴων ἐθεασάμεθα πολλάκις ὑγρὸν οὖρῳ παραπλήσιον ἐν τῷ περικαρδίῳ δαψιλές. εἰς δέ ποτε πίθηκος ἰσχνότερος ἑαυτοῦ γιγνόμενος οὐκ ἔφθασεν ἀνατμηθῆναι δι᾿ ἀσχολίας ἡμῶν ἀναγκαίας· ἀποθανόντος δ᾿ αὐτοῦ τὰ μὲν ἄλλα πάντα μόρια τοῦ σώματος ἦν ἀπαθῆ, ἐπέκειτο δὲ τῷ περικαρδίῳ χιτῶνι παρὰ φύσιν ὄγκος, ὑγρὸν ἐν ἑαυτῷ περιέχων ὅμοιον τῷ κατὰ τὰς ὑδατίδας· ἐπ᾿ ἀλεκτρυόνος δέ ποτε χωρὶς ὑγροῦ τοιοῦτος σκιρρώδης ὄγκος ἐπέκειτο τῷ περικαρδίῳ παραπλήσιος ὑμέσι παχέσι πολλοῖς κατ᾿ ἀλλήλων ἐπιβεβλημένοις. εἰκὸς οὖν ἐστι καὶ τοῖς ἀνθρώποις γίγνεσθαί τινα τοιαῦτα.

[1] De locis affectis, v. 2, K. viii. 304: φλεγμηνάσης δὲ φανερῶς καρδίας ἐπὶ μονομάχων ἐθεασάμεθα θάνατον ὁμοιότατον ἀκολουθήσαντα τοῖς συγκοπτομένοις καρδιακῶς. ἐὰν μὲν οὖν ἄχρι κοιλίας τινὸς τῶν ἐν αὐτῇ τὸ τρῶσαν ἀφίκηται, παραχρῆμα τελευτῶσιν αἱμορραγικῶς, καὶ μᾶλλον ὅταν ἡ ἀριστερὰ κοιλία τύχῃ τρωθεῖσα· μὴ διασχόντος δὲ τοῦ τρώσαντος εἰς κοιλίαν, ἀλλ᾿ ἐν τῷ σώματι τῆς καρδίας στηριχθέντος, οὐ μόνον αὐτὴν ἐκείνην τὴν ἡμέραν ἐν ᾗ τρωθέντες ἔτυχον, ἔνιοι διέζησαν ἀλλὰ καὶ τὴν ἐπιοῦσαν νύκτα, φλεγμονῆς δηλονότι λόγῳ τοῦ θανάτου γενομένου· φρονοῦσί γε μὴν ἅπαντες οὗτοι, μέχρι περ ἂν ζῶσιν, μαρτυροῦντος καὶ τούτου τοῦ φαινομένου τῷ παλαιῷ δόγματι περὶ τοῦ τὸ λογιζόμενον τῆς ψυχῆς οὐκ εἶναι κατὰ τὴν καρδίαν.

[2] De causis sympt. i. 7, K. vii. 136–7: καὶ ὅταν συνέλθῃ τὰ τέτταρα μέγιστον ἀνάγκη γενέσθαι τὸ πάθημα. τέσσαρα δὲ λέγω, τήν τε λυποῦσαν τὸν στόμαχον διάθεσιν ἰσχυρὰν γενομένην, καὶ τὴν αἴσθησιν αὐτῆς μάλιστα ἀκριβουμένην, καὶ τὸ τῶν νεύρων γένος, ἢ τὸ τῶν ἀρτηριῶν ἀσθενὲς ὑπάρχον, ἔτι δὲ πρὸς τούτοις ἤτοι τὸν ἐγκέφαλον, ἢ τὴν καρδίαν.

brain and the nerves; while the cardiac syncopes, as they are called, result from the sympathetic reaction of the heart and the arteries.[1] We have already noted that the final cardiac failure is due to the paralysis of the thoracic muscles, which deprives the heart of the refrigerating draught of *pneuma.*

In the third book of the treatise *On prognostication from the pulse*, Galen discusses the fundamental causes of disease, distinguishing them very carefully from the symptoms. These 'diatheses', which as we have seen the Latins translated as *passiones*, are the factors by which in the first place the functions of the body are impaired, while every condition which is not in accordance with nature Galen calls a 'pathos', or morbid state or happening. The 'affections' or 'diatheses' which give rise to disease are divided into two classes, those affecting the individual tissues (ὁμοιομερῆ), and those which affect the organs considered as wholes made up of different kinds of tissues or parts. They are either simple or compound, the simple ones implying excess of heat or of cold, of wetness or of dryness, while the compound consist of a combination of the two pairs, e.g. cold and dry, hot and wet, etc.[2] His interest in this thesis is to explain how the dyscrasies can affect the pulse. Those which do this may be dyscrasies, either of the heart itself or of the arteries, but the latter may exist without the former, while all dyscrasies of the heart must affect the arteries in greater or lesser degree.[3] He also tries to make a further distinction between those of the heart itself and those of its contents. Of the simple dyscrasies, the hot and cold pair are much the more important, both as affecting the heart itself and the arteries as such. At any given moment the dyscrasies in these two organs may be different, but they will react on one another. Thus the heart may be hot while the arteries are cold, and vice versa. Each of these conditions will affect the pulse, though the effect of one may counteract the effect of the other.

If the arteries are hotter than their natural condition while the heart

---

[1] *De causis sympt.* i. 7, 137: οὕτω γοῦν ἐπιληψίαι τε διὰ τὸν ἄτονον στόμαχον ἐνίοις ἐπιγίγνονται καὶ κάροι, καὶ κώματα, καὶ καταλήψεις, παραφροσύναι τε καὶ μελαγχολίαι, τῆς κατὰ τὸν ἐγκέφαλόν τε καὶ τὰ νεῦρα συμπαθούσης ἀρχῆς.

[2] *De praesag. ex puls.* iii. 1, K. ix. 330–1: πάθος μὲν οὖν ὀνομάζω νῦν ἅπαν τὸ παρὰ φύσιν . . . τὰ μέν εἰσι διαθέσεις τινές, ὑφ' ὧν πρώτως ἐνέργεια βλάπτεται, τὰ δὲ τούτων αἴτια, τὰ δὲ συμπτώματα, περὶ πρώτων τῶν διαθέσεων ῥητέον. ἐπεὶ δὲ καὶ τούτων ἐδείχθησαν αἱ μέν τινες ἴδιαι τῶν ὁμοιομερῶν σωμάτων, αἱ δὲ τῶν ὀργανικῶν, ἀπὸ τῶν ἐν τοῖς ὁμοιομερέσιν ὑπαρχουσῶν ἀρκτέον. εἰσὶ δὲ ὀκτὼ τὸν ἀριθμόν, ἅπασαι μὲν κατὰ δυσκρασίαν γιγνόμεναι, διαφέρουσαι δὲ τῷ τὰς μὲν ἁπλᾶς εἶναι τὰς δὲ συνθέτους. ἁπλαῖ μὲν οὖν εἰσι δυσκρασίαι θερμότης τε καὶ ξηρότης, ὑγρότης καὶ ψυχρότης· σύνθετοι δὲ ψυχρότης ἅμα ξηρότητι καὶ θερμότης ἅμα ὑγρότητι.

[3] *Ibid.*, 331: ἔτι δὲ πρὸς τούτοις ἀναμνηστέον ἐστὶν ὡς οὐκ ἄν ποτε σφυγμὸς ἀλλοιωθείη διὰ δυσκρασίαν χωρὶς τοῦ τὰς ἀρτηρίας τι παθεῖν ἢ τὴν καρδίαν, καὶ ὡς ἐνδέχεται ποτὲ τὰς μὲν ἀρτηρίας τι πεπονθέναι, τὴν καρδίαν δὲ ὑπάρχειν ἀπαθῆ. τῆς μέντοι καρδίας πασχούσης οὐκ ἐνδέχεται τὰς ἀρτηρίας ἀπαθεῖς διαμένειν, ἀλλ' ἀναγκαῖον ἀπολαύειν τι τῆς δυσκρασίας αὐτὰς ἔλαττον ἢ μεῖζον.

is colder, the result may be a pulse which is in the arteries equivalent to the natural as regards size and speed, though that of the heart is smaller and slower. This condition takes place without fever, when only the heart is cooled by cold, thick, sticky, humours. It is a rare condition, but it sometimes arises when these humours are in the lung, and the pulse becomes uneven, on account of the blocking of the mouths of the vessels growing out of the heart.[1] Presumably Galen is here referring only to those vessels which are connected with the lungs, and therefore the pulmonary and the bicuspid or mitral valves. Neither the aortal nor the tricuspid valve would appear to be involved.

So much for the 'affection' of the heart itself and those originating in it. We pass now to the secondary heart ailments, in which the heart participates through 'sympathy'. We have already examined a particular case, that of syncope communicated from the stomach. But all the organs can pass on their dyscrasies to the heart, and those most liable to do so are the lungs, on account of their contiguity and their vascular connections. Acute diseases of the chest only too often terminate in heart failures. In the fourth book of *On prognostication from the pulse*, Galen tabulates the effects on the arteries and the heart of disturbances in the various organs, varying from the brain to the testicles. Except in the case of those organs which lie close to it, like the lungs and the stomach, these effects are mediated mostly through the arteries and the nervous system. The lung is the organ which most quickly transfers any injury which it receives to the heart. The great blood vessels which connect the lung with both of its ventricles make the transfer of liquids from the lung to the heart through the valves inevitable while the physical proximity of the two organs makes the conduction of both heat and cold to the heart immediate. Dyscrasies of wetness and dryness are not so easily communicated as those of heat and cold, but they are more readily communicated by the lungs than by any other organ.[2]

---

[1] *De praesag. ex puls.* iii. 4, K. ix. 344–5: ἂν δὲ τῆς καρδίας ψυχροτέρας γεγενημένης αὗται θερμότεραι τοῦ κατὰ φύσιν ὦσιν, ἀλλοιώσουσι τὸν τῆς καρδίας σφυγμὸν εἰς τοσοῦτον εἰς ὅσον ἂν ἐκστῶσι τοῦ κατὰ φύσιν. ὥστε ποτὲ καὶ ἀκριβῶς ὅμοιος ἔσται τῷ κατὰ φύσιν ὁ κατὰ τὰς ἀρτηρίας, ὅσον γε ἐπὶ μεγέθει καὶ τάχει, τοῦ κατὰ τὴν καρδίαν ἐλάττονός τε καὶ βραδυτέρου γιγνομένου. εὔδηλον δ' ὡς αἱ τοιαῦται διαθέσεις ἄνευ πυρετῶν εἰσιν αὐτῆς τῆς καρδίας μόνης ψυχθείσης ὑπὸ χυμῶν ψυχρῶν τε ἅμα καὶ γλίσχρων καὶ παχέων. σπανίως μὲν οὖν ἐστιν ἡ τοιαύτη διάθεσις, ἀλλὰ γιγνομένη ποτέ, καὶ μάλισθ' ὅταν ἐν πνεύμονι τοιοῦτοι περιέχωνται χυμοί. συμβαίνει δ' ὡς τὰ πολλὰ τοῖς ἐπὶ τοιαύτῃ διαθέσει σφυγμοῖς εὐθὺς καὶ ἀνωμάλοις εἶναι διὰ τὰς ἐμφράξεις, ἃς οἱ προειρημένοι χυμοὶ κατὰ τὰ στόματα τῶν ἐκφυομένων τῆς καρδίας ἀγγείων ποιοῦσιν.

[2] Ibid., iv. 2, K. ix. 392–3: ταχίστην θ' ἅμα καὶ μεγίστην ἁπάντων ἐπιφέρει τῇ καρδίᾳ τὴν βλάβην ὁ πνεύμων. καὶ γὰρ τῇ θέσει πάντων ἔγγιστα καὶ τοῖς ἀγγείοις αὐτῇ συγγενέστατος ὑπάρχει, καὶ σύρρους μεγίστοις στόμασιν εἰς ἀμφοτέρας τὰς κοιλίας ἐστίν. εἰ γοῦν ἑαυτοῦ γένοιτό ποτε θερμότερος, αὐτίκα καὶ τὴν καρδίαν θερμαίνει, κἂν ᾖ ψυχρότερος, οὐδὲ τοῦτ' ἀναβάλλεται. τάς τε καθ' ὑγρότητά τε καὶ ξηρότητα δυσκρασίας οὐχ ὁμοίως μὲν ταῖς εἰρημέναις, θᾶττον δ' οὖν καὶ ταύτας ἁπάντων τῶν ἄλλων ὀργάνων ἐπιπέμπει τῇ καρδίᾳ.

Clearly in all these descriptions of the effects of the condition of the lungs on the heart, Galen is principally concerned with their influence on the pulse, the changes in which he regarded as being in many cases quite independent of the condition of the heart itself. There is little or nothing here which points to any knowledge of heart disease as we understand it today, a fact which is quite clearly recognized by Siegel.[1] This must not, however, be taken to imply that Galen did not observe accurately enough symptoms and syndromes which suggest heart diseases to the modern physician. Indeed one of his 'cases' has been identified by two of our contemporaries as describing mitral stenosis. The case in question is that of the physician Antipater, and Galen's description in the treatise *On the affected parts* is reproduced textually by Siegel in his book on Galen's system of physiology and medicine,[2] and also commented upon by Leibowich.[3] Both agree that the description of the irregularity of the pulse and Galen's diagnosis of blockage as the result of a narrowing of the passage of one of the big arteries in the lung point unequivocally to the atrial fibrillation associated with mitral stenosis.[4]

[1] Siegel, op. cit., p. 332.
[2] Siegel, op. cit., pp. 341 ff.
[3] J. O. Leibowich, 'On Galen's description of probable mitral stenosis, and on its translations', *Bull. Cleveland med. Libr.* 9 (Oct. 1962).
[4] *De locis affectis*, iv. 2, K. viii. 293 ff.: τὸ δ' Ἀντιπάτρῳ τῷ ἰατρῷ σύμβαν ἅπαντες ἔγνωσαν, ὡς οὐκ ἀφανῶς ἰατρεύοντι κατὰ τὴν Ῥωμαίων πόλιν. ἦν μὲν ὁ ἀνὴρ οὗτος ἡλικίαν ἄγων ἐτῶν ἐλαττόνων μὲν ἢ ἑξήκοντα πλεόνων δὲ ἢ πεντήκοντα, συνέβη δ' αὐτῷ ποτε πυρέξαντι τῶν ἐφημέρων τινὰ πυρετῶν ἐκ φανερᾶς προφάσεως, ἅψασθαι τῶν ἑαυτοῦ σφυγμῶν ἐν τῇ παρακμῇ τοῦ πυρετοῦ, χάριν τοῦ γνῶναι τί ποιητέον ἐστὶν αὐτῷ. πᾶσαν δ' εὑρὼν ἀνωμαλίαν ἐν τῇ τῶν ἀρτηριῶν κινήσει κατεπλάγη μὲν τὸ πρῶτον, ὡς δὲ σαφῶς ὕστερον ᾐσθάνετο μηκέτι πυρέττειν ἑαυτόν, ἐλούσατο μὲν εὐθέως· ἐπὶ κόποις τε γὰρ αὐτῷ καὶ ἀγρυπνίαις ἐκεκμήκει τὸ σῶμα· διῃτήθη δὲ πάνυ λεπτῶς ἄχρι τοῦ τὴν τρίτην ἀπὸ τῆς ἀρχῆς ἡμέραν διελθεῖν· ἐν ᾗ μηδενὸς ἔτι γενομένου πυρετοῦ, προῄει μὲν ἑκάστης ἡμέρας ὥσπερ καὶ πρόσθεν, ἁπτόμενος δὲ ἑαυτοῦ τῆς κατὰ τὸν καρπὸν ἀρτηρίας, ἐθαύμασε διαμενούσης ἐν τοῖς σφυγμοῖς τῆς ἀνωμαλίας. ἀπαντήσας οὖν μοί ποτε, προὔτεινε τὴν χεῖρα γελῶν, ἐκέλευσέ τε τῶν σφυγμῶν ἅψασθαι. κἀγὼ μειδιάσας, Τί τὸ αἴνιγμά ἐστιν, ὃ κελεύεις ἠρόμην· ὁ δ' αὖθις ὁμοίως γελῶν ἐδεῖτο πάντως ἅψασθαι. καὶ τοίνυν εὗρον ἁψάμενος ἀνωμαλίαν κατὰ τὸν σφυγμὸν ἅπασαν, οὐ μόνον ἐν ἀθροίσματι γινομένην, ἣν συστηματικὴν ὀνομάζουσιν ἀλλὰ καὶ κατὰ μίαν διαστολὴν τῆς ἀρτηρίας. ἐθαύμαζον οὖν ὅπως ἔτι ζῇ τοιοῦτον ἔχων σφυγμόν, ἐπυνθανόμην τε μή τις αὐτῷ δυσχέρεια κατὰ τὴν ἀναπνοὴν γίνεται· τοῦ δὲ οὐδεμίαν αἴσθητὴν ὁμολογοῦντος, ἐπετήρουν μὲν εἴ τινα μεταβολὴν ἕξοι ποτέ, συνεχῶς ἁπτόμενος τῆς κατὰ τὸν καρπὸν ἀρτηρίας ἐξ μηνῶν που χρόνῳ· πυνθανομένου δ' οὖν αὐτοῦ κατ' ἀρχάς, ἥ τις εἶναί μοι δοκεῖ διάθεσις ἐν τῷ σώματι, καὶ κατὰ τίνα τρόπον αὐτοῦ τοιοῦτον ἐργάζεσθαι δυναμένη τὸν σφυγμὸν ἄνευ πυρετοῦ, πρὸς τὴν ἐρώτησιν ἀπεκρινάμην, ἐν τῇ περὶ τῶν σφυγμῶν πραγματείᾳ δεδηλῶσθαί μοι περὶ τῆς τοιαύτης ἀνωμαλίας· ἡγοῦμαι γὰρ αὐτὴν ἐπὶ στενοχωρίᾳ τῶν ἐν τῷ πνεύμονι μεγάλων ἀρτηριῶν γίγνεσθαι· τὴν στενοχωρίαν δ' ἔφην, ἐπὶ μὲν φλεγμονῇ τοῦ σπλάγχνου, τό γε ἐπὶ σοῦ νῦν, ἀδύνατον ὑπάρχειν· ἐπύρεττες γὰρ ἄν. [I am wholly unable to follow or accept Siegel's translation of this passage, which makes Galen attribute the stenochoria to inflammation in the past.] ἀπολείπεται δ' ἤτοι δι' ἔμφραξιν ὑγρῶν καὶ γλίσχρων καὶ παχέων χυμῶν, ἢ διὰ φύματος ἀπέπτου γένεσιν, εἰς τὴν τοιαύτην ἀφῖχθαί σε διάθεσιν. ὁ δ' ὑπολαβών, Ἐχρῆν οὖν, ἔφη, ἀσθματικὴν ὀρθόπνοιαν εἶναί μοι. κἀγὼ πιθανῶς μὲν εἶπον λέγειν αὐτόν, οὐ μὴν ἀληθῶς· γίγνεσθαι μὲν γὰρ καὶ τὴν τοιαύτην ὀρθόπνοιαν διὰ τοιαύτην αἰτίαν, οὐ μὴν ἐν ταῖς λείαις ἀρτηρίαις, ἀλλ' ἐν ταῖς τραχείαις ἀθροιζομένου τοῦ γλίσχρου καὶ παχέος χυμοῦ. καὶ τοίνυν ἔδοξεν ἡμῖν, τήν τε δίαιταν πᾶσαν ὁμοίαν ποιεῖσθαι τοῖς τῶν ἀσθματικῶν. τά τε φάρμακα προσφέρεσθαι τὴν αὐτὴν ἐκείνοις ἔχοντα δύναμιν. ἐξ δὲ ἐν τῷ μεταξὺ γενομένων, ὡς ἔφην, μηνῶν, ᾔσθετό τινος οὐ μεγάλης δυσπνοίας ἅμα παλμῷ βραχεῖ τῆς καρδίας, τὸ

Galen, in his account of this case, tells how he met Antipater, who was worried about a prolonged irregularity in his pulse and insisted that he should feel his wrist and take it. He therefore complied, and found complete irregularity or unevenness, both in the single beat and in the succession of beats. He was surprised, he tells us, that anyone with such a pulse could continue to remain alive, and asked Antipater whether he was experiencing any difficulty in breathing. Antipater said that he was not. Galen kept him under observation, frequently taking his pulse over a period of six months to see whether any change in his condition was going to take place. Antipater had asked at an early stage what morbid condition Galen thought could be present, and how such a condition could produce a pulse like his without fever. Galen, after referring to his description of such an uneven pulse in his work on the pulse, expressed the opinion that it was due to a narrowing of the passage of one of the big arteries in the lung. This narrowing could not be due to an inflammation of the lung, as if it were, Antipater would be suffering from fever. The only alternative was that it was due to the blockage caused by moist, thick, and sticky discharges of humours, or to the growth of an undigested tubercle ($\phi\tilde{v}\mu a$). Antipater replied that he must have an asthmatic orthopnoea, but Galen, while admitting that this was a quite plausible explanation, said it was nevertheless not the true one. You can catch orthopnoea from asthma, but not in the smooth arteries (pulmonary veins) but only in the rough arteries (bronchial tubes), when thick sticky humours collect in them. During the six months he was under observation, Antipater had some, but not extreme, difficulties in breathing, together with some brief palpitations of the heart, but these symptoms gradually increased in severity, palpitations occurring at first only once, but then twice, three times, four times, and even more often a day, followed finally by a sudden collapse and death.

So much for the heart. There remains the question of vascular diseases. Two of these, aneurysm and varicose veins, were known to the ancient Greeks, and Galen deals with both of them. With regard to aneurysm, he describes it as follows:

When an artery undergoes a dilation, the morbid condition is called an aneurysm. It occurs as the result of a wound, when the skin surrounding it heals into a scar, but the wound in the artery itself remains, and does not close or cicatrize completely or become blocked with flesh. This condition is diagnosed from the beating of the arteries concerned. When these are compressed the swelling disappears entirely, the whole of the substance

μὲν πρῶτον ἅπαξ, εἶτα δίς που καὶ τρίς, εἶτα καὶ τετράκις τε καὶ πλεονάκις γιγνομένου, μετὰ τοῦ συναυξάνεσθαι τὴν δύσπνοιαν, ἐφ' ἡμέρας ὡς πέντε καὶ δέκα· μεθ' ἃς ἐξαίφνης δυσπνοιήσας σφοδρῶς, εἶτ' ἐκλυθείς, εὐθέως ἀπέθανεν, ὥσπερ ἄλλοι τινὲς ἐπὶ πάθεσι καρδίας, ὑπὲρ ὧν εἰρήσεται κατὰ τὸν ἐφεξῆς λόγον.

which caused it being withdrawn into the artery. This I showed in other works to be both light and bright blood mixed with a lot of light pneuma. This blood is definitely hotter than that in the veins, and if the aneurysm is pricked, it comes jumping out in a way which is difficult to stanch. Now in oedemata, the matter they contain is also made to retreat by pressure of the fingers and the swelling subsides, but here there is no arterial pulsation and the colour of the skin is paler.[1]

In another passage, in the treatise *On the method of medicine*, he tells us how an inexperienced young doctor, intending to perform a venesection in the arm of a patient, by mistake cut an artery, and how he, Galen, managed to heal this arterial wound without producing an aneurysm. In all other cases of wounds in an artery healing resulted in an aneurysm of greater or smaller size.[2] In the treatise *On treatment by phlebotomy*, he gives an account of his treatment of aneurysms. Having explained the difficulties of arresting haemorrhage from arterial wounds, he tells us that he knows several cases of death resulting from a wound in the artery lying under the vein on the inner side of the elbow, some in consequence of the tying of a ligature to arrest the haemorrhage which resulted in immediate necrosis (called by Galen gangrene), and some later, as the result of operations on the aneurysm itself, which had resulted from the healing of the arterial wound. For all operations on aneurysms entail interrupting the flow of blood in the vessel by ligature. That is why physicians fight shy of treating the greater arteries, while they neglect the smaller as being of no account. But he himself has seen great advantages to patients accruing from the healing of arteries without producing aneurysms. Even if the artery is one of the larger ones, it can be healed without forming an aneurysm—and this may often remove the danger of a haemorrhage—if the artery be cut right through, the ends on both sides of the cut being pulled, the one upwards and the

---

[1] *De tumoribus praeter naturam*, 11, K. vii. 725: ἀρτηρίας ἀναστομωθείσης τὸ πάθος ἀνεύρυσμα καλεῖται. γίνεται δὲ τρωθείσης αὐτῆς, ἐπειδὰν εἰς οὐλὴν μὲν ἀφίκηται τὸ προσκείμενον αὐτῇ δέρμα, μένῃ δὲ τῆς ἀρτηρίας ἕλκος μήτε συμφυθείσης μήτε συνουλωθείσης μήτε σαρκὶ φραχθείσης. διαγινώσκεται δὲ τὰ τοιαῦτα παθήματα τῶν σφυγμῶν τῶν ἐργασαμένων ἀρτηριῶν, ἀλλὰ καὶ θλιβομένων ἀφανίζεται πᾶς ὁ ὄγκος, παλινδρομούσης εἰς τὰς ἀρτηρίας τῆς ἐργαζομένης αὐτὸν οὐσίας, ἣν ἐδείξαμεν ἐν ἄλλοις ἅμα λεπτὸν καὶ ξανθὸν εἶναι αἷμά τι πνεύματι λεπτῷ καὶ πολλῷ συμμιγές. εὐθὺς δὲ καὶ θερμότερόν ἐστι τὸ αἷμα τοῦτο τοῦ κατὰ τὰς φλέβας καὶ τρωθέντος τοῦ ἀνευρύσματος ἐξακοντίζεται δυσεπισχέτως. ὑποχωρεῖ μὲν οὖν κἂν τοῖς οἰδήμασιν ἡ ὕλη θλιψάντων τῶν δακτύλων, καὶ βοθροῦται τὸ μέρος, ἀλλ' οὔτε σφυγμός ἐστιν ἐν τούτῳ τῷ πάθει καὶ ἡ χροιὰ λευκοτέρα.

[2] *De meth med.* v. 7, K. x. 334 f.: νεανίσκῳ δ' ἀγροικῷ ποτε... τμηθῆναι βουληθέντι... δήσαντος τὸν βραχίονα τοῦ μέλλοντος αὐτὸν φλεβοτομεῖν ἰατροῦ, συνέβη κυρτωθῆναι τὴν ἀρτηρίαν ... θεασάμενος δ' ἐγὼ τὸ γεγονός ... τῶν ἐναίμων τι φαρμάκων τῶν ἐμπλαστῶν παρασκευάσας ἐπιμελῶς τε πάνυ συναγαγὼν τὴν διαίρεσιν, ἐπέθηκά τε τὸ φάρμακον αὐτίκα καὶ σπόγγον μαλακώτατον ἔξωθεν ἐπέθησα. ... ἐπεὶ δὲ λύσαντες ἐν τῇ τετάρτῃ κεκολλημένην ἀκριβῶς εὕρομεν τὴν διαίρεσιν ... οὕτω μὲν ἐθεραπεύθη τὴν διαίρεσιν τῆς ἀρτηρίας ὁ ἄνθρωπος ἐκεῖνος μόνος· ὃν εἶδον ἐν ἀγκῶνι τμηθέντα ἀρτηρίαν· ἅπασι δὲ τοῖς ἄλλοις ἀνεύρυσμα τοῖς μὲν μεῖζον ἐπεγένετο, τοῖς δ' ἧττον.

other downwards. This procedure can also be applied to veins, but is more applicable to arteries.[1]

Galen also tells us how he came to practise this operation of arteriotomy. It was the result of two dreams, which induced him to perform it by severing an artery between the thumb and the index finger, and let the blood run until it stopped of itself. The total blood which escaped was under a litra—about half a pint. His patient was immediately relieved of a chronic pain near the place where the liver meets the diaphragm. The dreams mentioned came to him while he was a young man,[2] and he seems to have developed the practice of arteriotomy as a cure for a number of complaints, but he does not pretend that the operation was entirely his own invention. Thus it was customary for his contemporaries to divide the temporal arteries and those behind the ears, the former to relieve hot and 'pneumatic' fluxions in the eyes, the latter in cases of vertigo and chronic headaches. He does, however, claim the credit of being the first to apply this operation to other parts of the body.[3] To us it might appear rather curious that Galen never seems to have observed any cases of aneurysms, except in connection with wounded arteries, until we reflect that today by far the commonest cause of aneurysm is syphilis, a disease which almost certainly was unknown to the ancient world.

The existence of varicose veins was already known in the 'Hippocratic' age. Indeed we find them mentioned both in the *Aphorisms* and in the *Epidemics*. In the second book of the *Epidemics* there is an allusion

[1] *De curandi rat. per ven. sect.* 23, K. xi. 313–14: καὶ μέντοι καὶ ἀποθανόντας τινὰς ἴσμεν ἐκ τῆς ὑποκειμένης ἀρτηρίας τῇ κατ' ἀγκῶνα φλεβὶ τῇ ἔνδον. ἐνίους μὲν ἐν τῷ παραχρῆμα διὰ τὸν περιβληθέντα βρόχον, ἐθελησάντων τε τῶν ἰατρῶν ἐπέχειν, ὡς τὴν αἱμορραγίαν εἰς γάγγραιναν ἐλθεῖν, ἐνίους δ' ὕστερον ἐν τῇ τῶν ἀνευρυσμάτων χειρουργίᾳ διαφθαρέντας. ἀναγκαῖον γὰρ ἐν ταύτῃ βρόχῳ διαλαμβάνεσθαι τὸ ἀγγεῖον. τὰς μὲν οὖν ἀξιολόγους κατὰ τὸ μέγεθος ἀρτηρίας διὰ ταῦτα φεύγουσιν οἱ ἰατροί, τὰς δὲ μικρὰς ὡς οὐδὲν μέγα δυναμένας ἀνῦσαι. καίτοι καὶ αὗται πολλάκις ἡμῖν ὤφθησαν οὐ μικρὰν ὠφέλειαν ἐπιφέρουσαι μετὰ τοῦ συνουλοῦσθαι χωρὶς ἀνευρύσματος. καὶ μέντοι κἂν μείζων ἀρτηρία ᾖ, καὶ αὐτὴ χωρὶς ἀνευρύσματος συνουλοῦται διαιρεθεῖσα πᾶσα. καὶ πολλάκις τοῦτο αὐτὸ τὸν ἐκ τῆς αἱμορραγίας κίνδυνον ἰάσατο. φαίνεται γὰρ σαφῶς ὅθ' ὅλη δι' ὅλης ἑαυτῆς ἐγκαρσίως διακοπῇ, τῶν μερῶν ἑκατέρων ἀνασπωμένων ἑκατέρωσε, τὸ μὲν ἄνω τοῦ μορίου, τὸ δὲ κάτω. τοῦτο μέν γε καὶ ταῖς φλεψίν, ἀλλὰ μετρίου ὑπάρχει, ταῖς δ' ἀρτηρίαις ἀεὶ μᾶλλον τῶν φλεβῶν.

[2] Ibid., 314–15: ἔγωγ' οὖν ὅθεν ὁρμηθεὶς ἐπὶ τὸ διαιρεῖν ἀρτηρίας ἧκον ἤδη σοι φράσω. προτραπεὶς ὑπό τινων ὀνειράτων δυοῖν ἐναργῶς μοι γενομένων ἧκον ἐπὶ τὴν ἐν τῷ μεταξὺ λιχανοῦ τε καὶ μεγάλου δακτύλου τῆς δεξιᾶς χειρὸς ἀρτηρίαν, ἐπέτρεψά τε ῥεῖν ἄχρις ἂν αὐτομάτως παύσηται τὸ αἷμα, κελεύσαντος οὕτω τοῦ ὀνείρατος. ἐρρύη μὲν οὖν οὐδ' ὅλη λίτρα. παραχρῆμα δ' ἐπαύσατο χρόνιον ἄλγημα κατ' ἐκεῖνο μάλιστα τὸ μέρος ἐρεῖδον ἔνθα συμβάλλει τῷ διαφράγματι τὸ ἧπαρ. ἐμοὶ μὲν οὖν τοῦτο συνέβη νέῳ τὴν ἡλικίαν ὄντι.

[3] Ibid., 22, 312: οὕτω δὴ καὶ τὰς κατὰ τοὺς κροτάφους ἀρτηρίας καὶ τὰς τῶν ὤτων ὄπισθεν ἔθος ἐστὶ τοῖς ἰατροῖς διαιρεῖν, τὰς μὲν ἐν τοῖς κροτάφοις ἐπὶ τοῖς ἐν ὀφθαλμοῖς ῥεύμασιν, ὅσα θερμὰ καὶ πνευματώδη, τὰς δ' ὄπισθεν τῶν ὤτων ἐπὶ σκοτωματικοῖς μάλιστα καὶ ὅσοι χρονίοις ἀλγήμασι κεφαλῆς θερμοῖς καὶ πνευματώδεσι κάμνουσιν. ἤδη δὲ καὶ δι' ἄλλα πάθη περὶ τὴν κεφαλὴν συνιστάμενα χρόνια κέχρηνται τινὲς ἀρτηριοτομίᾳ τῶν ὤτων ὄπισθεν. οὐ μὴν ἐφ' ἑτέρου γέ τινος μορίου πάσχοντος ἐχρήσαντο τῷ βοηθήματι, καίτοι τῶν πολλῶν δεομένων αὐτοῦ μᾶλλον ἢ φλεβοτομίας.

to varicocele (varicose veins of the spermatic cord) where we are told that the emergence of these in both testicles is a cure for a thin voice.[1] In the *Aphorisms* we learn that varicose veins or haemorrhoids following on madness effect a cure; also that bald people do not get large varicose veins, but that if they do get any, they grow hair again.[2] These last statements cause Galen a good deal of difficulty, as he knows that they are not true. Baldness, he tells us, is incurable and has no connection at all with varicose veins. He does, however, find some excuse for Hippocrates' statements. There is a kind of baldness which is called by doctors μαδάρωσις due to bad humours, like ὀφιάσεις and ἀλωπεκίαι, complaints which do produce bald patches. These bad humours can be displaced to the legs, where they could produce varicose veins and so enable the hair to grow again, provided that this takes place before the roots of the hair have been destroyed.[3] 'Hippocrates' also regarded the formation of varices as a cure for spinal curvature affecting the lower vertebrae. Thus in the treatise *On joints* he tells us that when the spinal vertebrae are drawn into a hump, this is in most cases incurable when the hump is formed above the point where the spine is attached to the diaphragm, but curvatures formed below this point can be resolved by the formation of varicose veins in the legs, still more by varices in the veins of the groin.[4]

Galen also provides us with an explanation of the aetiology of varicose veins, and a description of surgical operation for their cure. Varicose veins, he tells us, were named by the ancients, the term being applied by them to all dilated veins. They are generally produced in the legs by the weakness of the veins, particularly when there is an excess of thick blood in the body, due to thick humours and black bile. Hence melancholy is sometimes

---

[1] The passage is quoted by Galen as follows in his commentary, K. xviiA. 468: ἰσχνοφωνίην κιρσὸς λύει, ἐς τὸν ἀριστερὸν καὶ τὸν δεξιὸν ὄρχιν. ἄνευ τουτέου τοῦ ἑτέρου οὐχ οἷόν τε λύεσθαι.

[2] Hippocrates, *Aphorisms* (ed. Loeb), 6. xxi and xxxiv: τοῖσι μαινομένοισι κιρσῶν ἢ αἱμορροΐδων ἐπιγινομένων, μανίης λύσις.

ὁκόσοι φαλακροί, τούτοισι κιρσοὶ μεγάλοι οὐ γίγνονται· ὁκόσοις ἂν φαλακροῖσι κιρσοὶ γένωνται, πάλιν γίγνονται δασέες.

[3] *Comment. in Aphorism.* xxiv, K. xviiiA. 55: ὁπόταν ἐν ἀνδρὸς φρονίμου συγγράμματι λόγος εὑρεθῇ προφάνως ψευδής, εἰκότως ἀπορεῖσθαι συμβαίνει τοὺς ἀναγιγνώσκοντας αὐτὸν καὶ πρῶτον μὲν ἑαυτοῖς ἀπιστεῖν, ὡς μηδὲ τὰ φανερὰ γιγνώσκουσι, εἶθ' ἑξῆς ὑποπτεύειν μή τι τῶν ὑποκειμένων ψευδὲς εἴη. τίς γὰρ οὐκ οἶδε ἀνίατόν τι πάθημα τὴν φαλάκρωσιν ὑπάρχουσαν; ἀλλὰ καὶ τὸ μηδέποτε ἐπιγίνεσθαι μεγάλους κιρσοὺς τοῖς φαλακροῖς οὐκ ἀληθές, ὥσπερ οὐδὲ τὸ γενομένων κιρσῶν παύεσθαι τὴν φαλάκρωσιν, εἰ μή τι ἄρα, καθάπερ ἔνιοί φασι, τὴν καλουμένην ὑπὸ τῶν ἰατρῶν μαδάρωσιν ὀνομάζει φαλάκρωσιν. ἐκείνη γὰρ ὑπὸ μοχθηρῶν χυμῶν γιγνομένη, καθάπερ αἵ τε ὀφιάσεις καὶ ἀλωπεκίαι ὀνομαζόμεναι, μεταστάντων εἰς τὰ σκέλη τῶν φαύλων χυμῶν ἐργάζεσθαι δύνανται κιρσοὺς ἀνακτήσασθαί τε τὰς τρίχας. εἰ γὰρ ἔμπροσθεν ὑπὸ μοχθηρῶν χυμῶν φθειρομένων αὐταῖς τῶν ῥιζῶν ἡ διαφθορὰ συνέβαινεν, εἰκότως νῦν ἐπὶ τῇ μεταστάσει τῶν χυμῶν, εἰς τὴν κατὰ φύσιν ἐπανήξουσι κατάστασιν.

[4] Hippocrates, *On joints*, 41: σπόνδυλοι δὲ οἱ κατὰ ῥάχιν, ὅσοισι μὲν ὑπὸ νοσημάτων ἕλκονται ἐς τὸ κυφόν. τὰ μὲν πλεῖστα ἀδύνατα λύεσθαι, ποτὶ καὶ ὅσα ἀνωτέρω τῶν φρενῶν τῆς προσφύσιος κυφοῦται. τῶν δὲ κατωτέρω μετεξέτερα λύουσι κιρσοὶ γενόμενοι ἐν τοῖς σκέλεσι, μᾶλλον δ' ἔτι ἐγγιγνόμενοι κιρσοὶ ἐν τῇ κατὰ ἰγνύην φλεβί.

cured by their appearance,[1] since the black bile, which is its cause, is thus concentrated in an unimportant organ like the veins of the legs.[2] In some cases, in the course of time, the skin above these varicose veins turns black, but if the varices contain only blood, this does not happen. If black bile, however, is present, there is a danger that if these veins are surgically removed the patient may be seized with melancholy, an occurrence which may also take place in the case of haemorrhoids caused by this humour.[3] Haemorrhoids were regarded by tradition not only as a disease, but also as a method employed by nature for ridding the body of superfluous blood.[4] Their suppression is cited by Galen as one of the causes of varicose veins. The retention of superfluities of black bile was regarded as the cause of most serious diseases, melancholia, phthisis, dropsy, cancer, and 'elephas'.[5]

With regard to surgical operation, Galen is convinced that this may sometimes be necessary, but he knows that it may sometimes lead to undesirable complications. Thus in the fourth book of *On the composition of drugs*, in a chapter dealing with the use of certain dry drugs in the treatment of wounds which refuse to heal, he tells us that if in the case of a leg-wound there should be higher up a large varicose vein, clearly visible, which by its colour shows that it contains not good but dark and black-bilious blood, this must be cut out. He knows of a case in which when the vein was excised, a wound below it, which had refused to heal for a whole year, healed immediately, but the place where the vein was divided in the excision developed a malignant wound which refused

---

[1] Galen, *De tumoribus praeter naturam*, 16, K. vii. 730: κιρσοὺς δὲ καὶ τὰς ἄλλας ἁπάσας (the exception being varicocele) φλέβας εὐρυνομένας ὀνομάζουσιν οἱ παλαιοί. . . . γίνονται δὲ καὶ κατὰ τὰ σκέλη κιρσοὶ δι' ἀρρωστίαν τῶν τῇδε φλεβῶν, καὶ μᾶλλον ὅταν αἷμα παχὺ πλεονάζῃ κατὰ τὸ σῶμα.

Comment. iii in Hipp. de alimento, K. xv. 331: ἔχουσι δὲ τὴν γένεσιν ἐκ τοῦ μελαγχολικοῦ περιττώματος, ὃ καὶ ἐργάζεται τὸν καλούμενον ἐλέφαντα, καὶ πολλάκις εἰς κιρσοὺς κατασκήπτει.

[2] *Comment. in Hipp. de humoribus*, iii. 26, K. xvi. 455: εἰσὶ γὰρ κιρσοὶ ἀνευρέσεις τῶν φλεβῶν τῶν ἐν τοῖς μηροῖς καὶ σκέλεσιν ἀπὸ παχέος καὶ μελαγχολικοῦ αἵματος γενόμενοι· οὗπερ εἰς τὰ ἀκυρώτερα μέρη ὠθουμένου ἡ μελαγχολία λύεται.

[3] *De atra bili*, 4, K. v. 118: καὶ μέντοι καὶ ἡ φύσις ἀποτίθεται τὸ τοιοῦτο αἷμα πολλάκις εἰς τὰς κατὰ τὰ σκέλη φλέβας, ὑφ' οὗ διατεινόμεναί τε καὶ διευρυνόμεναι, κιρσώδεις ἀποτελοῦνται, καὶ μελαίνεταί γε τῷ χρόνῳ τὸ δέρμα τὸ κατὰ τὰς τοιαύτας φλέβας. ἐφ' ὧν δ' αἵματος πλῆθος μόνον εἰσρέοι ἄνευ τοῦ μελαγχολικὸν ὑπάρχειν, ἀσθενεστέρας οὔσας φύσει τὰς τῇδε φλέβας ἀνευρύνει κατασκῆπτον, οὐδενὸς τοιούτου συμβαίνοντος, ὡς ἐφ' ὧν γε ἂν τὸ μελαγχολικὸν αἷμα τοὺς κιρσοὺς ἐργάσηται. κίνδυνος γὰρ ἐπὶ τούτων ἐστίν, ἐὰν ἐκτέμνῃ τις τὰς πεπονθυίας φλέβας, ἁλῶναι μελαγχολίᾳ· καὶ τοῦτο πολλάκις ἑωρᾶτο γιγνόμενον οὐ μόνον κατὰ τοὺς κιρσούς, ἀλλὰ καὶ κατὰ τὰς ὑπὸ τοιούτου χυμοῦ γιγνομένας αἱμορροΐδας.

[4] *De meth. med.* vii. 11, K. x. 512: ἑξῆς δ' ἐπ' ἀνδρῶν, εἰ ἡ συνήθης ἔκκρισις ἐπίσχηται (προσεπισκέπτου). πολλοῖς μὲν γὰρ αἱμορροῖς εἴθισται τὸ περιττὸν ἐκκενοῦν.

[5] *Comment. iii in Hipp. praedict. i*, 1. 333, K. xvi. 795: οἷς ἂν συνήθης κένωσις αἵματος ἐπίσχηται, τούτοις ἔσεσθαι νοσήματα πληθωρικά, ῥυέντος αὐτοῦ πρὸς ἐκεῖνα τὰ μόρια τοῦ σώματος, ὅσα πλησίον ἐστὶ τῶν ἐπεσχημένων ἐκρύσεων ἢ τῶν ἄλλων ἀσθενέστερα, κατὰ μέρος δὲ περὶ τῶν ἐξ αἱμορροΐδος, ὡς ἂν μελαγχολικὰ περιττώματα, τρεφόντων ἤτοι μελαγχολίαν ἢ φθίσιν ἢ ὕδερον ἢ κιρσοὺς ἢ καρκίνον ἢ ἐλέφαντα.

to heal.[1] Galen therefore recommends the following procedure, which appears to be an alternative to excision:

Having established the fact that your patient has sufficient strength, you should begin with phlebotomy, and immediately purge him with a drug which evacuates the melancholy humour, and with it also the phlegmatic, since this, too, often accumulates with the melancholic to form the varix. You then cut the vein above the wound along its length, and evacuate plenty of blood from it, and proceed to heal the division thus made in the vein first, and only when you see that it has properly healed up, do you then undertake the treatment of the originally malignant wound.[2]

In his great treatise *On the method of medicine*, Galen lays down the surgical treatment both of dilated arteries and of varicose veins, in connection with the operation of arteriotomy, just described, for the relief of certain eye-troubles. Sometimes these arise from the veins and arteries themselves, which have lost their tone, so that they become the receptacle of the surplus blood of the other vessels. In these cases we either cut out a piece of them, or cut them right through at a considerable depth. We thus interrupt their continuity through the formation of a solid hard scar, and so prevent any liquid passing from one part to the other. For varicose veins in the legs Galen appears to have practised the method of total excision in spite of the disadvantages he has detailed. When operating thus on veins it is not necessary as it is in arteriotomy, to use imperishable ligatures. For while in the case of arteries their constant pulsation keeps open the ends of the cut vessels, in the case of the veins once you have managed to close them, by whatever method, bandaging or astringent drugs, you will be able to let the flesh grown round them and so seal them by keeping the limb quiet and tilted up.[3] In the essay

---

[1] *De comp. med.* iv. 2, K. xiii. 667: εἴ τι πρόσθεν ἢ μοχθηρὸν . . . καὶ μάλισθ' ὅταν ἐν σκέλει τὸ ἕλκος ὑπάρχον ὑπερκειμένην ἔχοι φλέβα κιρσώδη· μεγάλης δ' οὔσης αὐτῆς καὶ κατὰ τὴν χρόαν ἐμφαινούσης οὔτε ἐρυθρὸν οὔτε χρηστὸν αἷμα περιέχειν, ἀλλὰ μελάντερον καὶ μελαγχολικώτερον, ἐκκόπτειν χρὴ τὴν φλέβα. συνέβη δέ ποτε φλεβὸς τοιαύτης ἐκκοπείσης, τὸ μὲν ἕλκος εὐθέως ἐπουλωθῆναι, καίτοι γ' ἐνιαυσιαῖον ὄν, ἀντ' αὐτοῦ δὲ κατὰ τὴν διαίρεσιν ὅθεν ἡ φλὲψ ἐξεκόπη γενέσθαι κακόηθες ἕλκος, ἐπουλωθῆναι μὴ δυνάμενον.

[2] Ibid., 668: ἄμεινον οὖν ἐπὶ τῶν τοιούτων τὴν ἰσχὺν τοῦ θεραπευομένου θεασάμενον ἀπὸ φλεβοτομίας μὲν ἄρξασθαι, καθῆραι δ' ἐφεξῆς φαρμάκῳ μελαγχολικὸν ἐκκενοῦντι χυμόν, καὶ σὺν τούτῳ καὶ φλεγματικόν, ἐπειδὴ καὶ οὗτος συνεπιρρεῖ ποτε τῷ μελαγχολικῷ κατὰ τὰς τῶν κιρσῶν γενέσεις. εἶθ' ἑξῆς αὐτὴν κατὰ τὸ μῆκος σχάσαι τὴν ὑπερκειμένην τοῦ ἕλκους φλέβα καὶ κενώσαντα δαψιλές, αὐτὴν ταύτην πρότερον ἰᾶσθαι τὴν γενομένην διαίρεσιν τῆς φλεβός, ὅταν δ' ἀκριβῶς ἤδη φαίνηται συνουλουμένη, τηνικαῦτα τῇ θεραπείᾳ τοῦ κακοήθους ἕλκους ἐπιχειρεῖν.

[3] *De meth. med.* xiii. 22, K. x. 940 ff.: ἐνίοτε δὲ τῶν ἀγγείων ἐστὶ τὸ πάθος ἤτοι τῶν φλεβῶν ἢ τῶν ἀρτηριῶν ἀτονωτέρων ὑπαρχουσῶν, ὡς δέχεσθαι τὴν τῶν ἄλλων ἀγγείων περιουσίαν. ἡνίκα ἐκτέμνοντές τι μέρος αὐτῶν ἢ καὶ διατέμνοντες ὅλα μέχρι πολλοῦ βάθους, διαλαμβάνομεν, οὐλῇ σκληρᾷ τὰ μεταξὺ διορίζοντες μόρια τοῦ τμηθέντος, ὡς μηκέτ' εἶναι συνεχῆ, μηδ' ἐπιρρεῖν ἐκ τοῦ ἑτέρου πρὸς τὸ ἕτερον. (943) τὰς μέντοι φλέβας, ὅτ' ἄν ποτε ἐκτέμνῃς τι μόριον αὐτῶν, οὐκ ἀναγκαῖον οὕτως ἀσήπτοις ὕλαις διαδεῖν, ἀλλ' ἀρκεῖ καὶ τῶν ἄλλων τις. ἐπὶ μὲν γὰρ τῶν ἀρτηριῶν ἡ διηνεκὴς κίνησις ἀνοίγνυσι τὰ στόματα τῶν τετμημένων ἀγγείων· ἐπὶ δὲ τῶν φλεβῶν, ὅταν ἅπαξ μύσῃ καθ' ὁντιναοῦν τρόπον ἤτοι πιληθέντα δι' ἐπιδέσεως ἢ στυφθέντα διὰ φαρμάκων, ἐπιτρέπει

called *Introduction or the doctor*, the genuineness of which has been doubted, though not by any means universally, the author gives a short account of an operation on varicose veins:

In operating on varicose veins in the legs, we first mark out their whole length on the surface, then bending the leg we take hold of the skin from the outside and cut it through, then we pull the varix with a hook towards us and bind it fast, and when we have done that after all the divisions, we either lift it up with an instrument specially designed for this purpose (κιρσουλκός), having cut through both the ends, or by means of a probe we pass a thread through the cavity of the varix and turn it over and pull it out.[1]

Finally we come to thrombosis, the formation of blood-clots in various organs which he discusses in *On affected places* more especially in connection with the bladder. When clots are formed in the bladder, and even more often, if they form in the intestines, the stomach, and the thorax, the patient grows pale and faints, and his pulse becomes small and faint and he becomes perplexed and dies. This often happens in the case of large wounds in the muscles. So that we wonder what is the cause of this phenomenon, namely that blood, which is of all substances the most proper to us, when it is poured outside its proper vessels, should be the cause of such great evils. For clots are followed by corruption and mortification of the parts.[2]

τῇ πέριξ σαρκὶ περιφύεσθαι, καὶ μάλισθ᾽ ὅταν ἀκίνητον ἔχῃ τὸ μέρος ὁ χειρουργηθεὶς ἄνθρωπος, ἔτι δὲ μᾶλλον, ἐὰν καὶ ἀνάρροπον ἔχῃ ἐπὶ κενῷ τῷ σύμπαντι σώματι.

[1] *Introductio sive medicus*, 19, K. xiv. 790: τοὺς δ᾽ ἐν σκέλεσι κιρσοὺς πρῶτον ἔξωθεν ἐπισημηνά-μενοι δι᾽ ὅλου ἐγχαράξεσιν εἶτα κλίναντες ἐξ ἐπιπολῆς λαβόμενοι τοῦ δέρματος, αὐτὸ πρῶτον διαιροῦμεν, εἶτα ἀγκίστρῳ ἐπισπώμενοι τὸν κιρσὸν διαδέομεν καὶ μετὰ πάσας τὰς διαιρέσεις τοῦτο ποιήσαντες, ἢ κιρσουλκῷ ἐξαιροῦμεν διακόπτοντες τὰ ἄκρα, ἢ διπυρήνῳ διαλαβόντες λίνῳ διὰ τῆς κοιλίας τοῦ κιρσοῦ κατ᾽ ἀναστροφὴν ἐξέλκομεν.

[2] *De locis affectis*, vi. 4, K. viii. 408 f.: ἐπὶ ταῖς καλουμέναις θρομβώσεσιν, οὐ μόνον ταῖς κατὰ κύστιν, ἀλλὰ καὶ τούτων ἔτι μᾶλλον εἰ κατ᾽ ἔντερά τε καὶ γαστέρα καὶ θώρακα γένοιτο, συμβαίνει λειποψυχεῖν τε καὶ ὠχριᾶν, καὶ μικροὺς καὶ ἀμυδροὺς καὶ πυκνοὺς ἴσχειν τοὺς σφυγμούς, ἀλύειν τε καὶ διαλύεσθαι. ταὐτὸ δὲ τοῦτο κἀπὶ τοῖς κατὰ τοὺς μῦς μεγάλοις τραύμασιν ἐπιγίγνεται πολλάκις· ὡς θαυμάσαι τὴν αἰτίαν τινὰ τοῦ συμβαίνοντος, εἰ τὸ πάντων οἰκειότατον ἡμῖν αἷμα τηλικούτων κακῶν ἐστι γεννητικὸν ἐκχυθὲν τῶν οἰκείων ἀγγείων· ἀκολουθοῦσι γὰρ αὐτῷ καὶ σηπεδόνες τῶν μορίων καὶ νεκρώσεις.

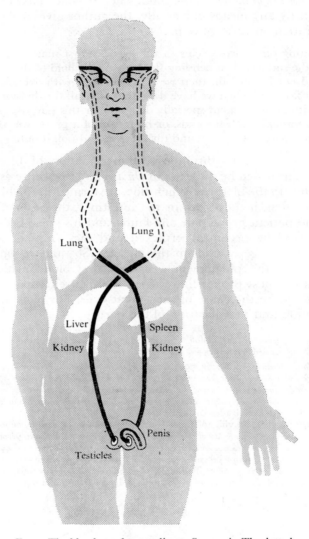

FIG. 1. The blood vessels according to Syennesis. The dotted lines represent blood vessels running dorsally, the solid lines, ventrally.

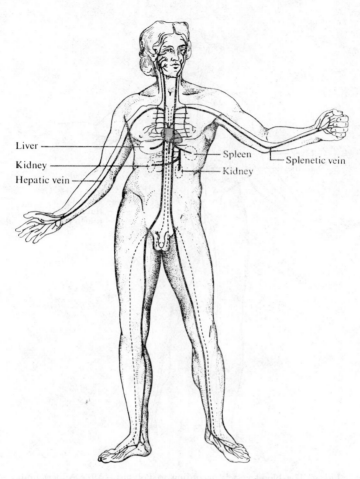

FIG. 2. The blood vessels according to Diogenes of Apollonia. (After Aubert und Wimmer's *Aristoteles Thierkunde*.)

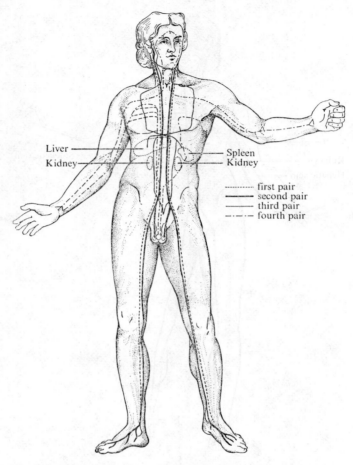

Liver

Kidney

Spleen

Kidney

.... first pair
———— second pair
———— third pair
—·—·— fourth pair

FIG. 3. The blood vessels according to Polybus. (After Aubert und
Wimmer's *Aristoteles Thierkunde*.)

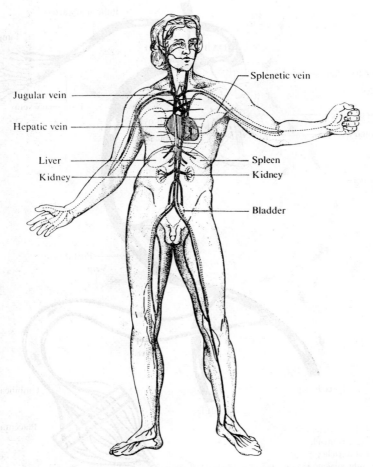

Jugular vein

Hepatic vein

Liver

Kidney

Splenetic vein

Spleen

Kidney

Bladder

Fig. 4. The blood vessels according to Aristotle. (After Aubert und
Wimmer's *Aristoteles Thierkunde*.)

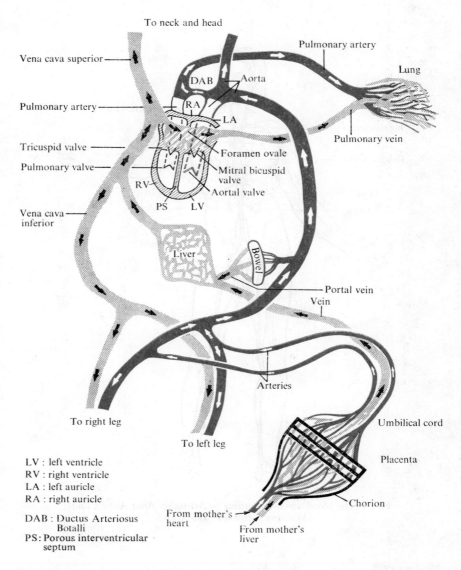

To neck and head

Vena cava superior

Pulmonary artery

DAB

Aorta

RA

Pulmonary artery

LA

Tricuspid valve

Pulmonary valve

Foramen ovale

Mitral bicuspid valve

Aortal valve

RV

PS   LV

Vena cava inferior

Pulmonary artery

Lung

Pulmonary vein

Liver

Bowel

Portal vein

Vein

Arteries

To right leg

To left leg

Umbilical cord

Placenta

LV : left ventricle
RV : right ventricle
LA : left auricle
RA : right auricle

DAB : Ductus Arteriosus
        Botalli
PS : Porous interventricular
        septum

From mother's heart

From mother's liver

Chorion

FIG. 5. The author's diagram of Galen's conception of vascular arrangements in the embryo.

INDEX

Abel, K.-H., 2, 50 n., 81, 84–5, 92 n., 121
Abscess, Aristotle's views on, 163
Ackerknecht, E., 73 n.
Aegimius of Elis, 182
Aesthetics, 133
Aetius, 5, 8, 25 n., 26, 104 n., 107, 177, 236 n.
Agathinus, 191, 237, 251, 254, 405
Air
  all-powerful, 43–4
  as cause of disease, 31, 44
  identified with soil, 28, 38
  source of consciousness, 42
  transformed into 'spirits', 225
  universe composed of, 20
  vital principle, 41
Air-hunger, 433
Alcmaeon of Croton
  arteries bloodless, 8
  date, 4–6
  discovery of optic nerve, 6, 7, 8, 99, 150
  distinction of types of blood vessels, 8, 58, 59
  doctrine of primacy of brain, 5–7, 11, 27, 42, 103
  immortality of the soul, 11
  operation on human eye, 6
  originated theory of direct respiration of pneuma to brain, 7, 26
  possible dissection of human body, 6, 7, 89
  relation to Pythagoras, 4, 9–10
  theory of disease, 5, 7, 9, 14
  theory of 'psychic' spirit, 8
  theory of sleep, 8, 15
Alexander of Tralles, 236 n.
Alexandria
  dissection of human body in, 177, 178, 234
  Erasistratus practised in, 178
  human skeletons available in, 234
  library, 30, 177
  School of, 7, 33, 36, 89, 98, 106, 136, 177–233, 235, 380
  De corde attributed to, 85
  discovery of nervous system, 99, 162, 236
  founded by Praxagoras of Cos, 108
Allbutt, Sir C., 187, 235

Amacher, M. P., 382 n., 387, 388
Anatomy
  contributions of Herophilus, 178–81
  established in Rome, 235
  state of knowledge before fourth century
    B.C., 35–7, 102–3
  state of knowledge in fourth century B.C.,
    98–103
Anaxagoras
  soul equated with hot air, 28, 395
  theory of respiration of fishes, 28 n.
Anaximenes
  influence on Diogenes, 20
  influence on Hippocratic corpus, 43
  theory of monistic air-substance, 8, 9, 28, 34, 75, 236 n.
Aneurysm, 449–51
Anonymous Londoner, 13, 19, 32, 98, 116, 162, 180, 209, 212, 214, 218, 224, 394
Anonymous Parisian, 33, 98, 104, 106, 107, 109 n., 110 n., 111, 114, 223
Antioch, 178
Antipater, case of, 448–9
Antyllus, 236 n., 239, 243
Apollonius of Pergamum, 241
Archidamus, 106
Archigenes of Apamea, 81, 185, 190–1, 235–6, 238, 242, 248, 251–60, 262, 265, 411, 417, 426
Aretaeus, 81, 235, 438
Aristogenes, 81
Ariston, 114
Aristotelian School (Lyceum), 200
Aristotle
  blood
    clotting, 141–2
    diseases connected with, 141
    fibrous content of, 142–3, 162
    formation of, 136–7, 141
    none in brain, 148
    variations in kind and quantity, 135–6, 140–3, 160, 334
  brain
    bloodless, 148
    functions of, 99, 135–6

Aristotle (*cont.*):
    digestion, 136–9, 158–9, 168
    heart
        air-cooled, 170, 172
        beating of, 136, 163–5
        bone in, 134
        centre of vascular system, 25, 39, 122,
            125, 158, 196
        contains own blood supply, 134
        description of, 122–4
        endowed with nerves, 162
        first organ formed, 173
        no knowledge of valves, 136, 160
        passage of *pneuma* to, 155–7
        primacy of, 104, 121, 160, 173
        properties related to character, 166–
            7
        seat of consciousness, 121, 160, 168
        'sinews' in ventricles, 123
        teleological philosophy of, 133–4
        third ventricle, 37, 121–33
            explained by Aubert and Wimmer,
            132; D'Arcy Thompson, 129–31;
            Huxley, 127–9; Mühsam, 132
    heat, innate
        extinction causes death, 171–2
        function of, 167–8
        not fuelled by respiration, 170, 346
        relation to scale of nature, 168
    liver, 328
    lungs, 154–7
    pneuma
        description of, 165–6
        equated with nourishment, 81
        function of, 165–7
        relation to sperm, 166
    quoted in *Hippocratic corpus*, 39, 51
    reproduction, 139
    residues, useful and useless, 138
    respiration
        function of, 165, 168–71, 320, 346
        of fishes, 28
    scale of nature, 168
    soul
        immortality of, 166
        not localized, 237
    tissue-formation, 138
    vascular system
        anatomy of blood vessels, 122, 148, 150–
            4
        cites Diogenes, 21–2
        cites Syennesis, 20–1
        connections between lungs and heart,
            154–7
        great vein (aorta and vena cava), 123–4,
            131–2, 149, 155–6, 159
        intestinal vein, 137, 158, 159

        no distinction between arteries and
            veins, 122, 139, 144
        pulsation of veins, 163
Aristoxenus, 187
Arteries, *see* Blood vessels
Asclepiades, 12, 111 n., 112, 179, 208, 228,
    244 n., 252, 434–5
Athenaeus, 81, 235, 237–8
Athens, 117
Atomism, 12, 34
    Asclepides' postulates, 219, 221
    Erasistratus' theories, 218–22
    Strato's theories, 202–3
Atrial fibrillation, 437
Atrio-ventricular bundle, 110
Attraction (ὁλκή), physiological power of,
    74, 218–19, 309, 326–31
    competition between organs, 369–72
    differs in different organs, 309
    operation of, 369
    'qualitative', 372
Aubert, H. (editor of Aristotle), 23, 132, 145,
    156
Augustine, Saint, 104
Aulus Gellius, 80 n.

Baccheius, 258, 263
Baldness, 452
Bañuelos, M., 2–3, 310–11
Bardong, K., 108 n.
Beltrani, J. R., 5 n.
Bernard, C., 133, 150
Bidez, J., 84 n., 86, 89
Bile
    black, 13, 74, 222, 327, 332–3, 366–7, 432
    yellow, 13, 36, 74, 91, 149, 222–3, 300,
        325–7, 332–3, 441, 444
Bladder, urinary, 36, 53, 56, 67, 82, 151,
    158, 271, 292, 330
Blood
    Aristotle's views on, 135–8, 141–54, 159–60
    as humour, 13, 74, 83
    circulation of
        guessed by Chinese?, 1–2
        known to Egyptians?, 115
        known to Greeks?, 2–3, 37, 46–50, 263,
            310–15, 366
        not known to Aristotle, 124–35
        not known to Erasistratus, 197–8, 263,
            366
        pulmonary (Galen), 304–5, 312–14,
            319–21, 323, 332–3
    constituents of, 141–3
    corruption of, 432
    formed in liver, 197, 325–30
    Galen's views on, 285, 303, 332–3, 363
    Hippocrates' views on, 43, 74, 81, 83

instrument of thought, 14
menstrual, 138–9, 291, 432
movement of, 15, 18
seat of intelligence, 18, 19, 28, 44
source of, 74, 83, 136–7
vehicle of innate heat, 14, 43
Blood vessels
  arteries
    ambiguity of term, 10, 24, 39, 54, 57,
      63–6, 72, 82, 108, 109 147, 156, 176,
      249
    beneath lung, 199
    bloodless, 8
    connections between, 46, 48, 52
    empty in dead bodies, 92
    expansion of (Erasistratus), 198–9
    function in nutrition, 363–5, 374
    function in respiration, 374
    function of systole and diastole in, 282,
      364
    originate in head, 9, 20, 45, 49, 80
    pulsation of, 49
    rough and smooth (Galen), 340
  arteries (by name)
    aorta, 23, 25, 36, 37, 46, 54, 57, 59–61,
      66, 73, 76–7, 85–6, 91–3, 106, 109–10,
      122–3, 131, 144–6, 159, 162, 199,
      210, 292–4, 308, 323, 336, 339, 368
    carotid, 25, 40, 357
    condyloid, 377–8
    iliac, 152
    innominate, 21
    intercostal, 57
    meningeal, 357
    occipital, 357
    pulmonary, 38, 64–5, 72–3, 86, 90–1, 94,
      98, 123–4, 126, 128–32, 146–7, 155,
      157, 179, 199, 200, 210, 213, 265, 281,
      284–7, 312–13, 333–4, 367
  capillaries, 282–3, 322, 334, 364, 366–7,
    374
  connecting heart and lung, 38
  contain *pneuma*, 45, 84, 91
  descriptions of
    by Aristotle, 33, 143–54, 163
    by Diogenes of Apollonia, 21–2
    by Empedocles, 37
    by 'Hippocrates', 40–3, 45, 47–9, 50–73
    by Syennesis, 20–1
  distinction between arteries and veins, 36,
    52, 59
    attributed to Euryphon, 84
    blood moves more slowly in veins, 332,
      363–4
    both absorb food (Herophilus), 181
    described by Herophilus, 24, 179, 265,
      281

difference in texture (Aristotle), 144
foreshadowed by Alcmaeon?, 8, 59, 93
in *Hippocratic corpus*, 36, 57–61
intercommunications of, 62
recognized by Praxagoras?, 24, 25, 43,
  57, 72, 79–80, 83–6
distinction between great vein and aorta,
  36, 40–3, 108, 146, 323
double system of, 25, 40, 48, 83
portal system, 36, 137, 210, 236, 330–1
rete, 62
start from head, 20, 33
veins
  originate in liver, 25, 80
veins (by name)
  azygos, 146–7, 210
  cerebral, 359
  great, hollow, or thick, 20–2, 36, 40,
    47–8, 58, 61–4, 66, 76–7, 98, 106,
    127–31, 137, 144, 146–9, 152, 154,
    158–9, 273, 432
  hemi-azygos, 147
  hepatic vein, 21–2, 40, 45, 48, 60–1, 71,
    149, 213, 288
  iliac, 152
  innominate, 21, 59, 130
  intercostal, 147
  jugular, 25, 40, 74, 130, 147–8
  pulmonary vein, 25, 38, 46, 59–60,
    64–6, 68, 73, 90, 98, 124–5, 131–2,
    154–5, 179, 210–11, 265, 274, 281,
    284–7, 308, 312–14, 336, 367
  spermatic vein, 22
  splenetic vein, 21–2, 40, 45, 48, 61, 71
  subclarian vein, 130
  vena cava, 23, 25, 36, 63–4, 73, 79, 86,
    90, 122, 127–30, 132, 143–6, 148, 180,
    197, 210, 275, 288–9, 293, 323–5,
    328, 333–4, 368
venous sinuses, 359, 361
Booth, W. B., 17
Borelli, 214
Brain
  Aristotle's views on, 135–6, 148, 159
  blood vessels leading to, 148
  dissection of, 357–8
  mind installed in, 33
  parts of
    choroid plexus, 354–5, 357–61, 366
    corpus callosum, 361
    diploon, 362
    dura mater, 355, 357, 358, 362
    foramen ovale, 295–6, 357
    foramen orbito-rotundum, 357
    hypophysis, 357
    infundibulum, 357
    pia mater, 362

Brain, parts of (*cont.*):
    pineal gland, 355
    pituitary gland, 357
    retiform plexus, 230 n., 311, 354–62
    ventricles, 355, 359, 360, 361
    primacy of, 5, 6, 9, 37, 42
    psychic spirit elaborated in, 351, 355–62
    seat of intelligence, 6–7, 27–8, 41–2, 95, 115–17, 236, 432
    vascular arrangements of (Galen), 360
Breathing (respiration), 40–2
Broadbent, Sir W., 410–11
Brock, A. J., 221
Bronchi, 36
Bronchioles, 124, 156–7, 309
Burnet, J., 5 n.
Bylebyl, J. J., 321 n.
βρόγχος, meaning of word, 63

Caelius Aurelianus, 108 n., 177, 181, 434, 437
Cagliostro, A., 11
Cartilage, 62, 330
Celsus, 178
Censorinus, 18
Chadwick, J., 433
Chalcidius, 6
Chicoyneau, F., 383
Chinese medicine, 1–2, 99, 429
Chirac, Dr. P., 383
Chorion, 290–1
Chrysermus, 187
Chrysippus, 38, 89, 195, 203, 206, 228
Cicero, 18, 235
Clement of Alexandria, 5 n., 23
Cnidos, School of, 19, 33, 37, 48, 84, 89, 98, 105, 109, 114, 136, 177, 195, 197, 223, 228, 236, 332
Cohen, M. R., 352
Colombo, Realdo, 321–2
Concoction, Aristotle's conception of, 136–41
Cornelio de Cosenza, Thomaso, 383
Cornford, F., 170
Corrigan, D. J., 266, 411
Cos, School of, 24, 31, 33, 37–8, 84, 98, 104–5, 109, 177, 195
Cosmic process (Hippocrates), 75–6
Critias, 18 n.
Croton, 4, 5
Ctesibius, 203
Cysts, hydatid, 101, 444

Da Vinci, Leonardo, 124, 302
Daremberg, C., 3, 173–4, 175, 263, 268–70, 294

De la Granda, 3, 311
De Waal, J., 53, 382–3
Death, 35, 43, 170–2, 181, 444
Deichgräber, K., 4, 32 n., 97, 98, 108
Democritus, 11, 34, 201–2, 218–19, 221, 230, 413
Diaphragm, 36, 40, 47, 53, 54, 60, 62, 70–1, 106, 149, 325, 329
    early connection with mind, 114, 432
    inflammation causes phrenitis, 106, 114 n.
    primacy of, 114
Diels, H., 104 n., 201 n., 202, 221, 237
Diels–Kranz (D–K), 15, 22, 80
Diepgen, P., 2, 52, 85
Dietetics, 31
Digestion, 78, 136–8, 326–33
Diller, H., 2, 80, 81, 85, 206
Diocles, 36, 84, 92
    acquainted with two ventricles, 105, 135
    doctrine of vital spirit as vaporization of blood, 107–8
    fever as symptom, 205
    heart as source of blood, 105
    ignorant of distinction between arteries and veins, 104–5
    influenced by Philistion, 38
    pneuma, 105, 108
    primacy of heart, 94–5, 103–4, 115, 162
    relation between brain and heart, 105 n., 115
    relation to Empedocles and Diogenes of Apollonia, 104
    respiration, 106, 112
    theory of headache, 105
    theory of phrenetic passion, 105, 106, 111, 114
    wrote on dissection, 36
Diogenes of Apollonia
    description of vascular system, 21–2, 41, 48, 53 n., 57, 59–61, 68, 72, 120–1, 154
    doctrine of air-soul, 8, 38, 75, 79, 104 n.
    founder of Pneumatist theory, 26–8
    located intelligence in brain, 27–8
Diogenes Laertius, 4, 5, 9, 116
Dionysius of Syracuse, 19, 117
Dioxippus, 170 n.
Diseases
    angina pectoris, 435–6
    apoplexy, 109
    asthma, 64, 433
    bronchitis, 434
    causes of, 19, 20, 31, 43, 49, 116–17, 421, 428–9, 432
    consumption, 64
    coronary thrombosis, 435, 437
    croup, 427
    delirium, 109

diphtheria, 427
dropsy, 427
empyema, 64
epilepsy, 42, 44, 427, 445
heart-burn, 440
lethargy, 427
mania, 110–11
mitral stenosis, 448
paralysis, 110
phrenetic passion, 105
pleurisy, 427, 434
pneumonia, 427, 434
religious frenzy, 111
stroke, 442
Diseases, see Heart-disease
Dissection
  animal, 21, 35–6, 62
    described by Galen, 272, 333, 357, 444
    difficulties described by Aristotle, 143
    practised at Alexandria, 234–5
  human, 85, 89
    banned before Erasistratus and Hero-
      philus?, 24–5
    brain dissected by Herophilus, 357
    practice discussed by commentators,
      101–3
    practised at Alexandria, 234–5
Dittinger, 23
Dobson, J. F., 178 n., 198
Dodds, E. R., 10
Dogmatists, 235, 236, 257
Drabkin, E., 352
Ductus arteriosus Botallo, 145, 294, 300,
  302
Ductus venosus Arantii, 292, 300
Dyscrasia, 7, 429, 441, 446

Eclectic School, 235, 238, 251, 257
Edelstein, L., 4, 5, 9, 29, 30, 31 n., 32, 97,
  101, 234
Egyptian medicine, 114–15, 177
Eleatics, 34
Embryo, 173
Empedocles, 4–5, 10–19, 28, 35, 37
  blood as soul, 18–20, 28, 350
  blood vessels, 37, 78, 104, 106
  date, 4–5
  founder of Sicilian School?, 19
  relation to Orphism and Pythagoreanism,
    10–11
  a Shaman?, 10
  theory of blood movement, 18–19
  theory of four elements, 13
  theory of respiration, 15–18, 116, 119, 212,
    241, 243
Empiric School, 193, 235, 238, 225, 405
Entralgo, Lain, 3, 311

Epicureanism, 222
Epicurus, 201, 218, 219, 221
Epidemics, 43, 44
Epiglottis, 54, 86, 158, 170, 342, 393–6
Epiphanius, 201 n.
Erasistratans, 226, 255
Erasistratus, 30, 37, 86
  arteries bloodless, 8, 132, 180, 200–10,
    298, 343
  blood production, 149, 197, 200
  blood vessels start from heart, 196, 323
  described valves of heart, 84, 95, 196–8,
    200, 276, 393
  failed to discover circulation, 197–9, 267
  heart as pump, 181, 211–13, 229
  horror vacui, 203–10, 215–16
  innate heat, 222
  knowledge of vascular system, 196, 210–11,
    323, 331, 333
  leaky epiglottis, 395
  mechanistic physiology, 214, 222–5, 227
  nervous system, 219–22, 229–33
  pioneer of human dissection, 177
  pneuma, 66, 225, 338–9
  postulated capillary system, 196, 215, 282
  quasi-atomic theory, 12, 203
  theory of disease, 206, 223, 434
  theory of fear, 205
  theory of humours, 222
  theory of muscle contraction, 214, 364
  theory of nutrition, 213–15, 342
  theory of pulse, 122, 184, 227–9, 378, 380,
    397, 430
  theory of respiration, 211–12, 225–7
  theory of threefold skin, 176, 217–20, 232
  tissues as blood deposits, 217–18, 327–8
Erhard, H., 4, 7 n., 20, 21, 23, 26, 27, 28 n.
Ethics, 133
Eucrasia, 14
Eudoxus, 38, 89
Euryphon of Cnidos, 24, 84, 108
Ewart, W., 194, 229, 409
Experiments, physiological
  by Erasistratus, 224, 378
  by Galen, 282, 297, 315–17, 342, 345–6,
    353–4, 378–80, 389

Fabricius of Aquapendente, 216, 312
Fåhraeus, Dr., 93
Fat, 330
Fernel, J., 321
Fever, 43, 443–4
Fleming, D., 3, 306, 314, 331, 370
Foetal respiration (Hippocrates), 77
Form, 34
Forrester, J. M., 381, 386–7
Foster, Sir M., 351–2, 370–1

Four elements, theory of, 11–14, 34, 35, 38, 78, 238
Four humours, theory of, 12, 332
Fracastorius, 392
Franklin, D. M., 292
Franklin, K. J., 216
Fraser, P. M., 177–8
Fredrich, C., 2, 8, 9 n., 24, 84
Fuchs, R., 33, 102, 107
Furley, D. J., 17 n.

Galen
    anastomoses of capillary system, 282–3
    arteries, contain blood and *pneuma*, 275, 294, 336–9, 363, 378
        function of, 363
        motion of, 374, 378–88, 390–2, 397–8
    blood, description of, 332–4, 363, 367
        motion of, 364, 367, 371–2
        production of, 325–30, 333, 367
        purification of, 336–7, 343, 348, 366–7
        waste products of, 287, 303, 305–6, 335, 337, 340–1, 343, 346, 348, 398–9
    brain, 359–60
    capillary system, 364
    comments on *Hippocratic corpus*, 41 n., 46, 50–1, 62, 80, 83, 95
    conception of double vascular system, 323
    criticism of Empedocles, 12
    criticism of Erasistratus, 204–9, 214–19, 222–9
    criticism of Praxagoras, 110
    did not dissect human heart, 268
    did not know of valves in veins, 322, 333
    distinction between veins and arteries, 281–2, 304
    doctrine of nerves and tendons, 37
    embryology, 287–303
    epiglottis, leaky, 393–5
    fever, 443
    heart, description of, 89, 95, 268–87, 303, 314, 363–4, 392–3
        not centre of vascular system, 25
        source of arteries, 80
        valves of, 95, 226, 284–7, 298–9, 302, 305, 308, 310, 312–16, 318, 368, 371, 393–6
    heart-disease, 434–9, 445–9
    innate heat, 371, 374–8, 418, 443
    interventricular septum, porous, 280, 305, 314–15, 322, 333–6
    knew about circulation?, 2–3, 8, 268, 322
    liver, 36, 80, 324–32, 366
    lungs, 285, 303–4, 307–10, 327, 335, 363, 365–7
    muscles, 364
    nutrition, 363–4, 366, 374, 418

pericardial fluid, 86, 393–5
physiological attraction, 326–31, 369–73
pneuma, theory of, 275, 294, 320, 326, 336–46, 349–51, 353–4, 358, 363–6, 374
psychic spirit, 358–62
pulse theory, 337, 397–431
respiration, 283–7, 339–49, 363, 374, 418
retiform plexus, 230 n., 351, 354–62
spleen, 366–7
surgical experience, 388, 390–2
three principal animal functions, 326, 352
varicose veins, 452
vascular system as irrigation, 373
vital spirit, 94, 107, 398, 429
vivisection, 390
Gall-bladder, 36, 54, 70, 300, 330, 332
Gall-stones, 435
Glaucias, 80 n.
Gods, 34, 118, 119
Goss, G. M., 357–8, 361
Gossen, J. C. G., 2
Gottschalk, H. B., 201 n., 203
Granjel, Professor, 3, 310, 311
Grapow, H., 115
Gray's *Anatomy*, 49, 85, 147 n.
Grensemann, H., 114 n.
Grossmann, J. D., 357 n.
Guthrie, D.,

Haemorrhoids, 453
Haeser, H., 305
Hall, R., 3, 338, 339, 351
Harvey, 48, 49 n., 73, 96, 97, 196, 211, 317, 321, 334, 381–3, 392, 431
Head, 74
    blood vessels start from, 38, 40–2, 45, 47, 50
    primacy of (Hippocrates), 39
    seat of intelligence, 33
Heart
    Aristotle's description of, 37, 122–34, 160–2, 170, 173, 269
    auricles, 25, 63, 87, 91, 93, 105, 126–30, 132, 180, 264–5, 273
    auricular septum, 132, 294, 315
    bone of, 134, 287
    centre of consciousness, 34, 71, 73, 95
    centre of vascular system, 25, 39, 49, 71–3, 79, 83–4
    chordae tendineae, 89, 161, 179
    connection with blood vessels, 21, 40, 47–50, 53, 55, 57–60, 63–4
    connection with lung, 66
    early knowledge of, 36
    first organ formed, 18
    foetal anatomy of, 293–5
    functions of, 118–19
    Galen's views on, 85, 268–86, 333

Hippocrates' description of, 76, 82, 86–9, 105

infundibulum, 179

interventricular septum, 305, 314, 322, 333–4

liquid in pericardial sack, 54, 85–6, 158, 170, 444

movements of, 18, 66

musculi papillares, 161, 179

pericardial membrane, 54, 85

Plato's description of, 21

Pneumatics' description of, 240

primacy of, 6, 7, 18–19, 37–9, 104–5, 108, 116, 121–2, 432

propulsive power, 211

seat of innate heat, 79

seat of intelligence, 7, 18–19, 28, 33, 38, 94

source of blood, 54, 74, 105, 122, 125, 128

valves of, 37, 83–95, 136, 179, 200, 215, 226, 241, 275–9, 308–9, 333, 390–6, 447

ventricles, 25, 37, 59, 86–7, 91–4, 104–5, 122–32, 144–5, 157–8, 179, 197, 213–14, 274, 288, 303, 333–6, 339–41, 445

Heart-beat

  Aristotles's views on, 136, 163–5

  cause of (Hippocrates), 42

  Erasistratus' views on, 226

  Galen's views on, 317

  pathological, 42–3

Heart-disease, 432–55

  Aristotle's views on, 173–5

  cardiac passion, 434–41, 446

  cardiac syncope, 432–4

  Galen's theory of, 422, 442, 445

  heart-failure, 181, 432–55

  Hippocrates' views on, 74–5, 433

Heat as supreme principle, 75, 79–80

Heat, innate, see Innate heat

Heidel, W. A., 4, 10

Heinemann, F., 103 n.

Heliodorus, 63

Heracleitus, 34, 75, 107

Hero of Alexandria, 201, 202, 203

Herophilus

  anatomical knowledge, 179–81, 230 n., 354, 357

  description of heart, 178–80

  description of vascular system, 179, 265

  discovered nervous system?, 178, 186, 232

  distinguished between arteries and veins, 24, 30, 34, 108, 179, 181, 210, 281

  heart failure, 181

  location of soul, 330

  pulse theory, 181–95, 229, 244, 256, 266 n., 378, 405, 409

    criticized by Galen, 192–9

Hett, W. S., 121 n., 172, 176

Hippocrates

  acquainted with circulation of blood?, 2, 46, 50, 80

  acquainted with valves in veins?, 312

  authorship of *Hippocratic corpus*, 28–34, 38, 97–9

  date, 31

  description of pulse, 185–6

  description of vascular system, 39–96, 184, 323

  doctrine of organic sympathy, 80, 376, 396

  impurity of body constituents, 310, 394

  innate heat, 375–7

  leaky epiglottis, 393

  theory of baldness and varicose veins, 452

  theory of dyscrasia, 7

  theory of four elements and humours, 12–14, 216–17, 238, 332

  theory of nutrition, 369

Hippocratic corpus

  anatomical knowledge in, 36

  authorship of, 29–33, 80, 85, 117

  date of, 3, 29–33, 72, 79, 80–1, 84, 97

  doctrine of elements and humours, 12, 14

  Erotion's canon, 80

  Galen's system based on, 267

  Kapferer's re-arrangement, 51–3, 72

  on the heart and vascular system, 81–3, 90–6, 108, 157, 320

  pathology in, 99–101

  primacy of the head, 33, 39

  primacy of the heart, 33, 50

  treatises dealing with vascular system, 39

  views on respiration, 27

Hippocratic medicine, 30, 103, 116

Hippocratic School, 12, 48, 110

Hofman, L., 321

Homer, 3, 31 n., 143, 185

Horror vacui, 200, 201–5, 209–10, 225–7, 229, 243, 318, 329, 333, 340, 371–3

Humours

  Erasistratus recognized two, 222

  Galen recognized, four, 332

  implicated in fever, 443

  in Hippocratic doctrine, 74, 216–17

  phlegm, 42–3, 74, 333, 433

  water, 74

  see also Bile, Four humours

Hunain ibn Ishaq, 352, 357 n.

Hunter, John and William, 291

Hurlbutt, F. R., 19, 84, 86

Huxley, T. H., 127–31, 133, 145–6, 156–7

Hwang-Ti, 1

Iatro-chemists, 224

Iatro-physicists, 244

Ibn-an Nafis, 198, 322
Ilberg, J., 34 n.
Indian medicine, 99
Innate heat, 14, 43, 79, 87, 90–1, 443
    Aristotle's theory of, 137–9, 159, 167–8
    contained in left ventricle, 304
    externally caused, 111, 222
    functions not exclusively physical, 374
    generated by pneumatic friction, 239
    identified with innate *pneuma*, 138, 376
    maintained or cooled by respiration?, 79,
        94, 243–4, 344–9, 374
    nourished by arteries, 363, 366
    refines blood, 287, 303–5
    source of physiological activity, 374–5
Intestines, 36, 54, 150
Issel, E., 216 n.
Italo-Sicilian School, 33

Jablonski, W., 92 n.
Jaeger, W., 103–4
Jaundice, 223
Johannitus, 352
Joly, R., 30
Jones, W. H. S., 29 n., 30 n., 31–2, 114 n.,
    221
Jowett, B., 121 n.
Junker, H., 115

Kapferer, Dr. R., 2, 38–9, 50–73, 85, 88–90,
    121
kardia, double meaning of, 432
Keele, K. D., 124 n., 303 n.
Kidneys, 40, 45, 54, 56, 147, 150
    described by Hippocrates, 56
    function of, 56, 330–2
    vascular system of, 50, 60, 67, 70, 82, 151
Killian, H. F., 294 n.
Körner, O., 3–4
Krause, E., 23, 25, 27
Kudlien, F., 4 n., 32, 97, 98, 103, 235 n.
Kühn, C. G., 293

Laodicea, 235
Laurentianus, 341
Lavoisier, 320, 338
Lebouc, G., 84 n., 86, 89
Leibowich, J. O., 448
Leucippus, 11, 34
Liddell and Scott's *Greek Lexicon*, 154, 156,
    221, 338
Ligaments, 271, 330
Ligamentum arteriosum, 146
Lister, Lord, 82
Littré, E., 2, 25, 32, 41, 45 n., 46, 48–9, 51,
    53 n., 56, 62, 73, 80, 83–4, 90, 97, 103,
    122, 183

Liver, 36, 40, 54, 60, 62, 432
    bile separated in, 325–7
    blood produced in, 325–30
    blood vessels of, 70, 80, 149, 288, 324–5,
        366
    contains innate heat, 374
    contains 'natural' *pneuma*, 351
    described by Hippocrates, 82
    distributes blood to organs, 333
    distributive function of, 328
    embryonic development of, 288
    five-lobed, 53
    formation of, 78
    function of, 149
    inflammation of, 223
    seat of faculty of nutrition, 328
    source of veins, 25, 80, 323
Lonie, I. M., 34 n., 197, 200
Louis, P., 23
Lungs, 36, 50, 81–2, 93, 432–3
    Aristotle's conception of, 123–5, 131, 155,
        168–9
    blood vessels of, 40, 45, 63, 130–1, 146–7
    compared to bellows, 169
    connection with heart, 39, 63–6, 165
    described by Hippocrates, 82
    Erasistratus' conception of, 198–9, 210–11
        criticized by Galen, 199, 211
    formation of, 78
    Galen's description of, 283–5
    nutrition of, 94, 285–7, 309–13, 335, 363,
        366
    Plato's conception of, 118–19
    respiratory motion described, 169–70, 226,
        340–2
    tubercles discovered in, 100

Macrobius, 18
Madrid, 93
Magnus, 254
Malato, M. T., 380–1, 383 n. 387–8
Mann, W. N., 433
Markellinos, 190–1, 228, 357–61
Marullus, 389
Marx, K. F. H., 186
May, Mrs. T., 270 n., 293 n., 297
Mediastinum, 329
Mehwaldt, 80
Menétrier, H., 263
Meninx, 148, 230
Meno, 30, 31, 98
Menoneia, *see* Anonymous Londoner
Menstruation, 432
Mesentery, 150–1
Methodists, School of, 235, 238, 434
Michler, M., 4, 19, 73
Milesians, 34

Milk, 81, 138–9, 359
Milne, J. S., 386
Mitchell, G. A. G., 4 n.
Mitral stenosis, 448
Monistic theories, 8, 13, 20, 34
Montpellier, 383
Moschion, 244 n., 258, 262–3
Mühsam, E., 126, 146, 157, 200
Mummification, 177–8
Muscle, 270–1, 363–4

Needham, J., 292 n., 302
Nei Ching, 1
Nero, 80
Nerves
    ambiguity of early descriptions, 37, 62,
      160–2, 220–1
    nervous system discovered by Herophilus?,
      178
    origin in heart, 110, 160–2
    relation to vascular system, 162
Nestle, W., 27, 32 n.
Neuburger, M., 103 n.
Neuenar, Count, 94
Newton, Sir Isaac, 11
Nicarchos, 108, 267
Nourishment, 74, 81–2, 91, 94–5
Nous, see Soul
Nutrition, 168, 329

O'Brien, D., 17 n.
Octavius Horatianus, 94
Oesophagus, 36, 47, 158, 434
Ogle, W., 16–17, 127, 129, 174–5
Omentum, 149
Operations, surgical, 389–90
Oribasius, 63, 111 n., 177, 236 n., 239,
    243 n.
Ostium venosum, 64, 65 n.
Ozanan, Dr., 424

Padua, 274
Pagel, J., 102, 306
Pagel, W., 24, 100, 101, 321 n., 334 n.
Palpitation (παλμός), 182–4, 433
    cardiac, 42
Pancreas, 150
Papyrus Ebers, 114–15
Parenchyma, 217–18, 322
Parmenides, 34
Patterson, E. L., 4 n.
Paul of Aegina, 236 n.
Pauly, A. F. von, 2, 29 n., 80 n.
Pauly–Wissowa, 2, 29 n., 80 n.
Peck, A., 23, 123–4, 136–7, 144–7, 152,
    156, 159, 165, 174
Peller, S., 3

Pelops, 46
Penis, 45, 67–8, 151
Pergamum, 235, 241, 388
Pericardium, 329
Pericles, 34
Pericranium, 362
Peritoneum, 36
Petron of Aegina, 114
Pezopoulos, S. N., 2, 215
Pharynx, 158
Pherecydes, 80 n.
Philistion
    adopted some Empedoclean ideas, 37–8,
      116, 118
    author of some Hippocratic works?, 80,
      117
    founder of Sicilian School, 13, 17, 19, 84,
      103
    source of Plato's medical doctrines, 86,
      117–19
    theory of leaky epiglottis, 86, 169–70
    theory of mental disease, 42
    theory of respiration, 17, 106, 116, 203
Philolaus of Tarentum, 5, 116–17
Philonides, 251–2
Philoponus, 18 n.
Phlegm, 13, 42–3, 74, 433
Phylotimus, 80, 111
Placenta, 290–1, 300
Plato, 6, 19
    conception of world-soul, 236
    debt to Hippocratic corpus, 30–1
    description of vascular system, 21, 120–1
    doctrine of four elements, 118
    doctrine of tripartite soul, 116–18, 237,
      328
    function of innate heat, 79, 311, 374–5
    function of respiration, 119–20, 203
    functioning of the heart, 118–19, 121
    influenced by Philistion, 117
    knowledge of tracheal and vascular con-
      nections, 119
    liquid in windpipe, 54, 86, 158, 170
Platt, A., 125–7
Pliny, 190 n., 191 n.
Plutarch, 83, 239
Pneuma
    Aristotle's theory of, 155–7, 164–6
    as air, 107, 164–6, 337–8, 349
    as instrument of sensation and thought,
      7–8, 27, 37
    as nourishment, 81
    as vital spirit, 38, 107–8
    as world-soul, 26
    breathed direct to brain, 7, 38, 40, 336
    Diocles' theory of, 108
    Erasistratus' theory of, 211–14, 353

Pneuma (*cont.*):
　Galen's theory of, 320, 326, 351, 363–6
　Hippocrates' theory of, 40–3, 106–7
　innate
　　Aristotle's theory of, 138, 165–7
　　Diocles' theory of, 104
　　Stoic doctrine of, 238
　inner, 26
　natural, 326, 349–52, 365
　obstruction of, 20, 41, 44
　path to heart, 66
　Philiston's theory of, 38
　present in blood vessels, 26, 40–1, 43, 320,
　　363–6
　psychic, 38, 94, 326, 329, 349–51, 355–63
　School of Cos, theory of, 38
　source of, 349–51
　Stoic doctrine of, 243–4
　vital, 326, 329, 349–50, 358–62, 364,
　　398
Pneumatist School, 7, 38, 81, 95, 235–51
　definition of blood, 240
　description of heart, 240
　doctrine of *pneuma*, 238, 240–1
　doctrine of pulse, 244–51, 333
　double function of respiration, 239–41
　founded by Athenaeus of Attalia, 235
　relation between vascular and respiratory
　　systems, 240
　theory of nutrition, 243
Pohlenz, M., 29 n., 32 n.
Polybus, 12, 23, 33, 60, 332
Pores, 282, 443–4
Porphyrius, 4
Poschenrieder, F., 131
Poseidonius, 235, 237
Praxagoras, 53, 57
　arteries bloodless, 8, 91, 108–9, 113, 132,
　　180, 195, 197, 204, 216, 267–8, 283,
　　367, 430
　bubble theory, 111–13
　date, 24, 103
　distinguished between arteries and veins,
　　24, 81, 83–4, 136
　innate heat, 111
　nature of *pneuma*, 112
　nerves originating in heart, 110, 160–1
　primacy of heart, 108, 113–14
　pulse theory, 109, 111–12, 181–2, 184, 194,
　　367
　theory of diseases, 109–10
　theory of humours, 111
　vascular system as motor, 162, 184
Prendergast, J. S., 3, 312–14, 391
Prognosis, 428
Prostate, 67
Psyche, *see* Soul

Psychic spirit
　theory developed by Erasistratus and
　　Galen, 38, 94, 165, 225
　theory founded by Alcmaeon?, 8
Ptolemy Philadelphus, 200
Ptolemy Physkon, 234
Pulse
　Archigenes' theory of, 252–6
　Aristotle's theory of, 163, 176
　clinical importance of, 228
　definition of, 182–4
　Erasistratus' theory of, 227–9, 378, 396
　Galen's experiment on, 378–80
　Galen's theory of, 282, 337–8, 397–431
　Herophilus' theory of, 181–95
　Hippocrates' theory of, 50
　Markellinos' theory of, 257–61
　normal frequency of, 194
　Pneumatist doctrine of, 237, 244–51, 264
　Praxagoras' theory of, 111–13
　Rufus of Ephesus' theory of, 262–6, 392,
　　397, 411
　sign of health or disease, 81
　Soranus' theory of, 261–6
Pus, 81–2, 163
Pythagoras, 4–6, 9–10, 116
Pythagoreanism, 6, 9, 11–12

Regis, Dr., 383
Renan, E., 11
Repulsion, physiological, 371, 373
Respiration, 66, 79, 94
　Aristotle's theory of, 163–5, 168–9
　arterial, 37
　Erasistratus' theory of, 211–13
　foetal, 177
　function of, 37–8, 106, 168–9, 172, 181, 239
　Hippocrates' theory of, 40–1
　necessary to life, 37
　Plato's description of, 119–21
　Pneumatic doctrine of, 239–41
　poral theory of, 15–18, 37, 116, 181, 242
　varies with age, 81
Rhode, E., 236 n.
Richter, G., 334 n.
Riolanus, 341
Rose, V., 237, 261
Ross, Sir D., 4
Rouve, Dr., 383
Ruelle, C. E., 263
Rufus of Ephesus, 66, 82, 177, 181, 184–5,
　187–8, 189 n., 195, 238, 264, 265
Rüsche, Fr., 14, 18 n., 28 n., 43, 79, 104, 107,
　164, 238

Sacred disease, *see* Diseases (epilepsy)
Sambursky, S., 238, 244 n.

Santorio Capo d'Istria, 224
Saunders, J. B., 115 n.
Scaliger, J. C., 17
Scarano, G. B., 380-1, 383 n., 387-8
Schoene, H., 216 n., 257
Schöner, E., 13
School of Alexandria, 33
Schumacher, J., 12
Semen, 68, 94, 138-9, 359
Sensation, 168
Servetus, 198, 322
Sextus Empiricus, 201 n.
Sicilian School, 17, 19, 84-5, 89, 103, 105,
     115, 169, 228, 236
Siegel, E., 279 n., 291, 299-304, 314-21,
     338, 344-7, 357 n., 358, 435-8, 448
Sigerist, H. E., 4, 6, 7, 11, 29 n., 32, 33 n.,
     36, 75, 103
Simplicius, 27 n., 201 n.
Singer, C., 125 n., 180, 222, 371
Sisson, S., 357 n.
Skull, 361-2
Sleep, 8, 44, 159-60
Sloane, Sir H., 224
Soranus, 228, 235, 236 n., 261, 434
Soul
     Aristotle's concept of, 166, 168, 328
     as hot air, 80
     choroid plexus first instrument of, 358
     innate heat of, 168
     nature and location of, 9, 17, 27-8, 38, 91
     not identified with pneuma, 357
     Platonic doctrine of, 117-18, 236
     Pythagorean doctrine of, 9, 116
     theory of Philolaus, 6
Spalteholz, W., 358
Spasm (σπασμός), 182-3
Spermatic cord, 359
Spigelius, 341
Spinal curvature, 452
Spinal marrow, 68
Spine, 45, 151
Spirit, psychic, 225
Spleen, 36, 40, 45, 54, 70, 74, 330, 332, 366-7
Steckerl, F., 104, 108 n., 111 n., 112-13
Stella, L. A., 4 n., 8
Sternum, 60, 389-91
Stever, R. O., 115 n.
Sticker, G., 2, 32 n.
Stoics, 7, 14, 26, 38, 92 n., 104, 201, 228,
     236-9, 243-4
Stomach, 36, 40, 330
Strato of Lampsacus, 200-4, 210-11, 216,
     219-20, 222, 230
Stroppiana, L., 47
Susemihl, F., 177
Swammerdam, J., 233

Sweat, 153
Sydenham, T., 224
Syennesis of Cyprus, 20-1, 24, 46
Synanastomoses between arteries and veins,
     196, 215, 282-4, 306, 308-9, 322, 339-41,
     373
Syncope, cardiac, 434-5, 438, 446
Syphilis, 451

Temkin, O., 98, 103, 118 n., 351, 352 n., 365
Tendon, 271
Tertullian, 18
Testicles, 20, 22, 45-8, 67-9
Thales, 34, 172
Thebesius, 334
Theodore Priscian, 94 n., 104
Theodoret, 18 n.
Theodoretus, 201 n.
Theophrastus, 7, 11, 14, 26, 27 n., 156, 200-1
Thessalus, 80
Thompson, D'Arcy W., 129-31, 145, 156-7,
     199 n.
Thorax, 71, 143-4, 210, 285-7, 367
Töply, Ritter von, 102, 126
Torcular Herophili, 359, 361
Trajan, 235, 262
Tremor (τρόμος), 182-4
Tubercles, 24, 99-100, 449
Tuberculosis, 24
τρῆμα (Aristotle), 155-7

Umbilical cord, 288-91, 293
Ureters, 151
Urine, 56, 331
Uterus, 151, 271, 290-1, 330

Vacuum, 202-4
Vaporization (ἀναθυμίασις), 80, 94, 107-8,
     136, 350, 353-5, 358-9, 360-1
Variciform plexus, 359
Varicose veins, 449, 451-5
Vascular system
     compared to framework, 154
     compared to irrigation system, 152, 373
     confusion with tracheal system, 41, 65-6,
          90
     described by Diogenes, 20
     described by Hippocrates, 39, 44
     described by Syennesis, 20
     heart as centre, see Heart
     instrument of movement, 162
     see also Blood vessels, Heart
Verbecke, G., 231, 236 n., 243
Vertebrae, 60
Vesalius, A., 126-7, 334, 381 n., 382
Vieussens, R., 334, 383-5, 387
Villi, 290

Vindicianus, 23 n., 92, 95 n., 104–7
Viscera as blood-deposits, 125
Vitalism, 222–3, 227
Vivisection, 178, 390
Vlastos, G., 9
Voluntary movement, 168

Waste products
  digestive, 336
  evacuation of, 303, 305–6, 331–2, 337,
    340, 398–9
  of veins in brain, 362
  produced in heart, 287, 305
  sooty, 335, 341, 346, 398
  urine, 331
Wehrle, F. R., 201 n.
Wellmann, M., 4, 7, 8 n., 17–19, 23–5, 33 n.,
  37–8, 42, 79, 83–4, 89, 92, 103–5, 111,

114 n., 117, 162, 177–8, 188 n., 195, 203,
  210, 220, 228, 231, 236, 239, 251, 253–4
Weygoldt, G. P., 23, 25
Whitam, M., 383
Wiberg, J., 2
Wilamowitz-Moellendorff, U. von, 29, 31
Willis, circle of, 357–8, 361
Wilson, L., 322
Wimmer, Fr. (editor of Aristotle), 23, 132,
  145, 156
Windpipe, 158, 170
Wissowa, G., 2, 29 n., 80 n.
Wong, K. C., 1
World soul, 236, 243
Wu Lien-Teh, 1

Zeler, E., 25, 27
Zeno, 236, 238

LIST OF WORKS CITED

Aetius, *On the doctrines of the philosophers*, 5, 8 n., 14, 15, 25 n., 26, 197

Anaxagoras, *Fragments*, 395

Aretaeus, *On the causes and signs of acute diseases*, 438

Aristotle
  On dissections (lost), 155
  The generation of animals, 138–40, 151, 154, 161, 165–6, 172–3
  The history of animals, 20, 22, 33, 60, 122–3, 126, 128–9, 134–5, 141–4, 146–50, 152, 154–6, 158, 161–2
  On length of life, 168
  Metaphysics, 4, 12, 14
  The motion of animals, 165
  The parts of animals, 122, 125, 133–4, 136–8, 142–4, 149, 152–4, 158, 160, 167, 169, 173–4
  Politics, 30 n.
  On respiration, 15, 17, 28 n., 121, 162–4, 168–70, 172
  On the sky, 164, 166
  On sleep and wakefulness, 125, 135–6, 158–9
  On the soul, 11
  On youth and old age, 167–8, 171

Aristotle (?), *On breath*, 81, 160, 164, 175 n.

Aristoxenus, *Fragments*, 187

Caelius Aurelianus
  On acute diseases, 434–8
  On chronic diseases, 108, 181

Celsus, *On medicine*, 178

Censorinus, *On the day of birth*, 18

Chalcidius, *On the Timaeus*, 6

Cicero, *Tusculan disputations*, 18

Clement of Alexandria
  Pedagogus, 23
  Protrepticus, 5

Diogenes Laertius, *The lives of the philosophers*, 4, 9, 10

Epiphanius, *Against heresies*, 201 n.

Galen
  On the affected parts, 199, 211, 226, 232, 333, 441–2, 444–5, 448–9, 455
  On anatomical procedures, 133, 180, 196, 234, 269–74, 276, 281–2, 316, 361, 379–80, 389–92
  For beginners, 256, 400
  On the best sect, 180
  On black bile, 222–3, 327, 453
  On blood in the arteries, 112, 180, 201, 268, 282, 342–3, 380
  On the causes of diseases, 363
  On the causes of the pulses, 256, 282, 398–400, 411–12, 414, 417, 424–7
  On the causes of symptoms, 183, 442–3
  Commentary on the aphorisms of Hippocrates, 290, 376, 440–1
  Commentary on Hippocrates on humours, 183, 363, 453
  Commentary I on Hippocrates on the nature of man, 12, 205
  Commentary II on Hippocrates on the nature of man, 377
  Commentary III on Hippocrates on nourishment, 326, 352, 363, 376, 453
  Commentary III on Hippocrates' prognosis, 453
  Commentary IV on Hippocrates on nourishment, 286, 303
  Commentary V on Hippocrates' epidemics VI, 337, 350, 375
  Commentary on Hippocrates' regimen in acute diseases, 117
  On diagnosing the pulses, 108, 189–92, 245 n., 254–5, 282, 400, 405–8, 427
  On the differences of fevers, 253, 440–1
  On the differences of the pulses, 109, 182–6, 188, 192, 195, 226–9, 244, 251–5, 258, 401–4, 410, 412, 415
  On dissection of the uterus, 290
  On dissection of veins and arteries, 126, 284, 294, 325
  On errors of the mind, 184
  On the formation of the foetus, 288–9
  On fullness, 108, 263
  Glossary, 50
  The great art (= *The method of medicine*), 218, 351–3, 388–9, 450, 454
  On Hippocrates' elements, 333
  Introduction or the doctor, 205–6, 217, 238, 352, 455

Galen (cont.):
Is blood naturally contained in the arteries?, 206, 208
Medical definitions, 213, 235–8, 240–1, 244–9, 352, 411, 434
On the mixing of medicines, 454
On the mixing of simple drugs, 344, 376
Natural faculties, 195, 208, 214–16, 219–20, 222–3, 231, 281, 283, 305 n., 329, 331–4, 337, 340, 364, 368–74
On the opinions of Hippocrates and Plato, 46, 110, 112, 179–80, 182, 200, 228, 230–1, 237, 271, 273, 275, 283–4, 292, 303, 323–4, 328, 330, 332–3, 336–7, 339, 350–1, 353, 355, 358–9, 362–4, 367, 377, 393, 441
On philosophical history, 201, 205, 230
On phlebotomy, 195–6, 374, 378
On prognosis, 229
On prognostics from the pulse, 188, 191–2, 256–7, 415–23, 428–9, 446–7
On the pulse to Antonius, 182, 249–51
On the pulse theory of Archigenes (lost), 252
On the pulse theory of Herophilus (lost), 191
On sperm, 288, 363–4
Synopsis of the books on the pulse, 188, 190, 193, 227
Synopsis on the pulses, 187, 256, 352, 401, 404–5, 414
On treatment by phlebotomy, 451
On trembling, palpitation, convulsions, and cramps, 109, 111, 183–5, 222
On unnatural tumours, 450, 453
On the use of breathing, 112, 179, 211, 225–6, 342–3, 345, 347–8, 353, 376–7
On the use of the parts, 179, 195, 204–5, 209, 212, 218, 225, 230–1, 269, 271, 273–81, 283–7, 289, 291–3, 295, 297–8, 300, 303–10, 313, 325–8, 331–2, 335–6, 339–42, 346, 349, 356–62, 364–6, 391, 393–4, 441
On the use of the pulses, 196, 213, 218, 226–7, 242, 282, 354, 364, 396–8
On wasting away, 5, 253, 375–6, 444

Hero of Alexandria Pneumatics, 201–3
Hippocrates
Airs, waters, and places, 98
On anatomy, 82
Aphorisms, 98
The art, 98
On breaths, 43–4, 108
On diseases, 34, 38–9, 73–5, 83, 98, 100, 438 n.
On the eight-month child, 156
Epidemics, 60, 97–8
On fleshes, 36, 75–98, 108, 131

On fractures, 88
On girls' diseases, 432
On healthy diet, 117
On the heart, 34, 50, 83, 85–91, 97, 131, 157, 241, 274
On internal affections, 101
On joints, 52, 98, 100–1
On the nature of the bones, 37–8, 50–73, 157
On the nature of the child, 73, 79
The nature of man, 33, 45, 60, 98
On nourishment, 31, 50, 81–2, 97
On places in man, 34, 47–8, 50
Prognostics, 97
Regimen, 35, 80, 98
Regimen in acute diseases, 98, 432–3
The sacred disease, 23, 33, 38, 40–3, 98, 106–7, 433
Homer, Iliad, 40, 49, 185

Londoner, Anonymous, 98, 116, 162, 180, 209, 212, 214, 218, 224, 394

Macrobius, Scipio's dream, 18
Markellinos, On the pulses, 190, 228, 257–61

Oribasius, Collected works, 63, 239, 243

Papyrus Ebers, 115
Parisian, Anonymous
AMG (1894), 33, 104 n., 105–7, 109 n., 110 n., 111, 114, 223
AMG (1895), 98
Philoponus, Commentary on Aristotle on the soul, 18 n.
Plato
Epistles, 117
Phaedrus, 30
Protagoras, 30
Timaeus, 18, 21, 42, 54, 71, 117, 119–21, 158
Pliny, Natural history, 190 n., 191 n.
Plutarch, Table-talk, 83

Rufus of Ephesus
On the anatomy of human parts, 264–5
On the names of human parts, 37 n., 82, 179, 264–5
Synopsis on the pulses, 184, 188–9, 266

Sextus Empiricus, Hypotyposes, 201 n.
Simplicius
Commentary on Aristotle's physics, 27
Commentary on Aristotle on the sky, 201
Soranus (?), Medical questions, 228, 261

Tertullian, On the soul, 18
Theodoretus, The cure of Greek diseases, 201 n.
Theophrastus
The history of plants, 156
On sense, 7, 26–7